2nd Edition

HARRISON'S™

HEMATOLOGY AND ONCOLOGY

Derived from Harrison's Principles of Internal Medicine, 18th Edition

Editors

DAN L. LONGO, MD
Professor of Medicine, Harvard Medical School; Senior Physician, Brigham and Women's Hospital; Deputy Editor, New England Journal of Medicine, Boston, Massachusetts

ANTHONY S. FAUCI, MD
Chief, Laboratory of Immunoregulation; Director, National Institute of Allergy and Infectious Diseases, National Institutes of Health, Bethesda, Maryland

DENNIS L. KASPER, MD
William Ellery Channing Professor of Medicine, Professor of Microbiology and Molecular Genetics, Harvard Medical School; Director, Channing Laboratory, Department of Medicine, Brigham and Women's Hospital, Boston, Massachusetts

STEPHEN L. HAUSER, MD
Robert A. Fishman Distinguished Professor and Chairman, Department of Neurology, University of California, San Francisco, San Francisco, California

J. LARRY JAMESON, MD, PhD
Robert G. Dunlop Professor of Medicine; Dean, University of Pennsylvania School of Medicine; Executive Vice-President of the University of Pennsylvania for the Health System, Philadelphia, Pennsylvania

JOSEPH LOSCALZO, MD, PhD
Hersey Professor of the Theory and Practice of Medicine, Harvard Medical School; Chairman, Department of Medicine; Physician-in-Chief, Brigham and Women's Hospital, Boston, Massachusetts

2nd Edition

HARRISON'S™

HEMATOLOGY AND ONCOLOGY

Dan L. Longo, MD

Professor of Medicine, Harvard Medical School; Senior Physician, Brigham and Women's Hospital; Deputy Editor, New England Journal of Medicine, Boston, Massachusetts

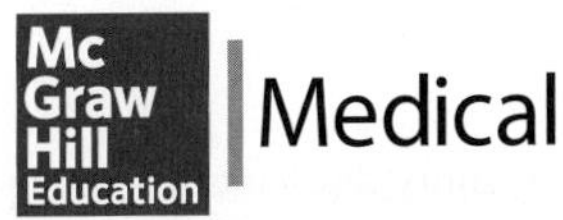

New York Chicago San Francisco Lisbon London Madrid Mexico City
Milan New Delhi San Juan Seoul Singapore Sydney Toronto

Harrison's Hematology and Oncology, Second Edition

Dr. Fauci's work as an editor and author was performed outside the scope of his employment as a U.S. government employee. This work represents his personal and professional views and not necessarily those of the U.S. government.

1 2 3 4 5 6 7 8 9 0 CTP/CTP 18 17 16 15 14 13

ISBN 978-0-07-181490-4
MHID 0-07-181490-6

This book was set in Bembo by Cenveo Publisher Services. The editors were James F. Shanahan and Kim J. Davis. The production supervisor was Catherine H. Saggese. Project management was provided by Sandhya Gola of Cenveo® Publisher Services. The cover design was by Thomas DePierro. Cover illustration, oxygen-starved cancer cells, microscopic view, from Nancy Kedersha.

China Translation & Printing Services, Ltd. was the printer and binder.

Library of Congress Cataloging-in Publication Data

Harrison's hematology and oncology/editor, Dan L. Longo. — 2nd ed.
p. ; cm.
Hematology and oncology
Based on 18th edition of Harrison's principles of internal medicine.
Includes bibliographical references and index.
ISBN 978-0-07-181490-4 (pbk. : alk. paper)—ISBN 0-07-181490-6 (pbk. : alk. paper)
I. Longo, Dan L. (Dan Louis), 1949- II. Harrison, Tinsley Randolph, 1900-1978. III. Harrison's principles of internal medicine. IV. Title: Hematology and oncology.
[DNLM: 1. Hematologic Diseases. 2. Neoplasms. WH 120]
616.99'418—dc23

2012040189

CONTENTS

SECTION VII
BIOLOGY OF CANCER

SECTION VIII
PRINCIPLES OF CANCER PREVENTION AND TREATMENT

SECTION IX
NEOPLASTIC DISORDERS

SECTION X
ENDOCRINE NEOPLASIA

SECTION XI
REMOTE EFFECTS OF CANCER

SECTION XII

ONCOLOGIC EMERGENCIES AND LATE EFFECTS COMPLICATIONS

CONTRIBUTORS

Numbers in brackets refer to the chapter(s) written or co-written by the contributor.

James L. Abbruzzese, MD
Professor and Chair, Department of GI Medical Oncology; M.G. and Lillie Johnson Chair for Cancer Treatment and Research, University of Texas, MD Anderson Cancer Center, Houston, Texas [47]

John W. Adamson, MD
Clinical Professor of Medicine, Department of Hematology/Oncology, University of California, San Diego, San Diego, California [2, 7]

Kenneth C. Anderson, MD
Kraft Family Professor of Medicine, Harvard Medical School; Chief, Jerome Lipper Multiple Myeloma Center, Dana-Farber Cancer Institute, Boston, Massachusetts [12, 17]

Frederick R. Appelbaum, MD
Director, Division of Clinical Research, Fred Hutchinson Cancer Research Center, Seattle, Washington [30]

Wiebke Arlt, MD, DSc, FRCP, FMedSci
Professor of Medicine, Centre for Endocrinology, Diabetes and Metabolism, School of Clinical and Experimental Medicine, University of Birmingham; Consultant Endocrinologist, University Hospital Birmingham, Birmingham, United Kingdom [51]

Valder R. Arruda, MD, PhD
Associate Professor of Pediatrics, University of Pennsylvania School of Medicine; Division of Hematology, The Children's Hospital of Philadelphia, Philadelphia, Pennsylvania [20]

Robert C. Basner, MD
Professor of Clinical Medicine, Division of Pulmonary, Allergy, and Critical Care Medicine, Columbia University College of Physicians and Surgeons, New York, New York [Appendix]

Robert S. Benjamin, MD
P.H. and Fay E. Robinson Distinguished Professor and Chair, Department of Sarcoma Medical Oncology, University of Texas MD Anderson Cancer Center, Houston, Texas [45]

Edward J. Benz, Jr., MD
Richard and Susan Smith Professor of Medicine, Professor of Pediatrics, Professor of Genetics, Harvard Medical School; President and CEO, Dana-Farber Cancer Institute; Director, Dana-Farber/Harvard Cancer Center (DF/HCC), Boston, Massachusetts [8]

Clara D. Bloomfield, MD
Distinguished University Professor; William G. Pace, III Professor of Cancer Research; Cancer Scholar and Senior Advisor, The Ohio State University Comprehensive Cancer Center; Arthur G. James Cancer Hospital and Richard J. Solove Research Institute, Columbus, Ohio [14]

George J. Bosl, MD
Professor of Medicine, Weill Cornell Medical College; Chair, Department of Medicine; Patrick M. Byrne Chair in Clinical Oncology, Memorial Sloan-Kettering Cancer Center, New York, New York [43]

Otis W. Brawley, MD
Chief Medical Officer, American Cancer Society Professor of Hematology, Oncology, Medicine, and Epidemiology, Emory University, Atlanta, Georgia [27]

Cynthia D. Brown, MD
Assistant Professor of Medicine, Division of Pulmonary and Critical Care Medicine, University of Virginia, Charlottesville, Virginia [Review and Self-Assessment]

Brian I. Carr, MD, PhD, FRCP
Professor of Oncology and Hepatology, IRCCS De Bellis Medical Research Institute, Castellana Grotte, Italy [39]

Irene Chong, MRCP, FRCR
Clinical Research Fellow, Royal Marsden NHS Foundation Trust, London and Sutton, United Kingdom [40]

Francis S. Collins, MD, PhD
Director, National Institutes of Health, Bethesda, Maryland [24]

Jennifer M. Croswell, MD, MPH
Acting Director, Office of Medical Applications of Research, National Institutes of Health, Bethesda, Maryland [27]

David Cunningham, MD, FRCP
Professor of Cancer Medicine, Royal Marsden NHS Foundation Trust, London and Sutton, United Kingdom [40]

Josep Dalmau, MD, PhD
ICREA Research Professor, Institute for Biomedical Investigations, August Pi i Sunyer (IDIBAPS)/Hospital Clinic, Department of Neurology, University of Barcelona, Barcelona, Spain; Adjunct Professor of Neurology University of Pennsylvania, Philadelphia, Pennsylvania [53]

Lisa M. DeAngelis, MD
Professor of Neurology, Weill Cornell Medical College; Chair, Department of Neurology, Memorial Sloan-Kettering Cancer Center, New York, New York [46]

Janice Dutcher, MD
Department of Oncology, New York Medical College, Montefiore, Bronx, New York [54]

Jeffery S. Dzieczkowski, MD
Physician, St. Alphonsus Regional Medical Center; Medical Director, Coagulation Clinic, Saint Alphonsus Medical Group, International Medicine and Travel Medicine, Boise, Idaho [12]

Andrew J. Einstein, MD, PhD
Assistant Professor of Clinical Medicine, Columbia University College of Physicians and Surgeons; Department of Medicine, Division of Cardiology, Department of Radiology, Columbia University Medical Center and New York-Presbyterian Hospital, New York, New York [Appendix]

Ezekiel J. Emanuel, MD, PhD
Vice Provost for Global Initiatives and Chair, Department of Medical Ethics and Health Policy, University of Pennsylvania, Philadelphia, Pennsylvania [32]

Robert Finberg, MD
Chair, Department of Medicine, University of Massachusetts Medical School, Worcester, Massachusetts [29]

Jane E. Freedman, MD
Professor, Department of Medicine, University of Massachusetts Medical School, Worcester, Massachusetts [21]

Carl E. Freter, MD, PhD
Professor, Department of Internal Medicine, Division of Hematology/Medical Oncology, University of Missouri; Ellis Fischel Cancer Center, Columbia, Missouri [55]

Robert F. Gagel, MD
Professor of Medicine and Head, Division of Internal Medicine, University of Texas MD Anderson Cancer Center, Houston, Texas [50]

John I. Gallin, MD
Director, Clinical Center, National Institutes of Health, Bethesda, Maryland [5]

Samuel Z. Goldhaber, MD
Professor of Medicine, Harvard Medical School; Director, Venous Thromboembolism Research Group, Cardiovascular Division, Brigham and Women's Hospital, Boston, Massachusetts [22]

Rasim Gucalp, MD
Professor of Clinical Medicine, Albert Einstein College of Medicine; Associate Chairman for Educational Programs, Department of Oncology; Director, Hematology/Oncology Fellowship, Montefiore Medical Center, Bronx, New York [54]

Anna R. Hemnes, MD
Assistant Professor, Division of Allergy, Pulmonary, and Critical Care Medicine, Vanderbilt University Medical Center, Nashville, Tennessee [Review and Self-Assessment]

Patrick H. Henry, MD
Clinical Adjunct Professor of Medicine, University of Iowa, Iowa City, Iowa [4]

Katherine A. High, MD
Investigator, Howard Hughes Medical Institute; William H. Bennett Professor of Pediatrics, University of Pennsylvania School of Medicine; Director, Center for Cellular and Molecular Therapeutics, Children's Hospital of Philadelphia, Philadelphia, Pennsylvania [20]

A. Victor Hoffbrand, DM
Professor Emeritus of Haematology, University College, London; Honorary Consultant Haematologist, Royal Free Hospital, London, United Kingdom [9]

Steven M. Holland, MD
Chief, Laboratory of Clinical Infectious Diseases, National Institute of Allergy and Infectious Diseases, National Institutes of Health, Bethesda, Maryland [5]

Leora Horn, MD, MSc
Division of Hematology and Medical Oncology, Vanderbilt University School of Medicine, Nashville, Tennessee [35]

J. Larry Jameson, MD, PhD
Robert G. Dunlop Professor of Medicine; Dean, University of Pennsylvania School of Medicine; Executive Vice President of the University of Pennsylvania for the Health System, Philadelphia, Pennsylvania [48, 52]

Robert T. Jensen, MD
Digestive Diseases Branch, National Institute of Diabetes; Digestive and Kidney Diseases, National Institutes of Health, Bethesda, Maryland [49]

David H. Johnson, MD, FACP
Donald W. Seldin Distinguished Chair in Internal Medicine; Professor and Chairman, Department of Internal Medicine, University of Texas Southwestern Medical School, Dallas, Texas [35]

Barbara Konkle, MD
Professor of Medicine, Hematology, University of Washington; Director, Translational Research, Puget Sound Blood Center, Seattle, Washington [3, 19]

Barnett S. Kramer, MD, MPH
Director, Division of Cancer Prevention, National Cancer Institute, Bethesda, Maryland [27]

Alexander Kratz, MD, PhD, MPH
Associate Professor of Pathology and Cell Biology, Columbia University College of Physicians and Surgeons; Director, Core Laboratory, Columbia University Medical Center, New York, New York [Appendix]

Marc E. Lippman, MD, MACP
Kathleen and Stanley Glaser Professor; Chairman, Department of Medicine, Deputy Director, Sylvester Comprehensive Cancer Center, University of Miami Miller School of Medicine, Miami, Florida [37]

Dan L. Longo, MD
Professor of Medicine, Harvard Medical School; Senior Physician, Brigham and Women's Hospital; Deputy Editor, New England Journal of Medicine, Boston, Massachusetts [1, 2, 4, 6, 15, 16, 17, 25, 26, 28, 31, 36, 51, 52, 55]

Joseph Loscalzo, MD, PhD
Hersey Professor of the Theory and Practice of Medicine, Harvard Medical School; Chairman, Department of Medicine; Physician-in-Chief, Brigham and Women's Hospital, Boston, Massachusetts [21]

Lucio Luzzatto, MD, FRCP, FRCPath
Professor of Haematology, University of Genova, Scientific Director Istituto Toscano Tumori, Italy [10]

Guido Marcucci, MD
Professor of Medicine; John B. and Jane T. McCoy Chair in Cancer Research; Associate Director of Translational Research, Comprehensive Cancer Center, The Ohio State University College of Medicine, Columbus, Ohio [14]

Robert J. Mayer, MD
Stephen B. Kay Family Professor of Medicine, Harvard Medical School, Boston, Massachusetts [38]

Pat J. Morin, PhD
Senior Investigator, Laboratory of Molecular Biology and Immunology, National Institute on Aging, National Institutes of Health, Baltimore, Maryland [24]

Robert J. Motzer, MD
Professor of Medicine, Weill Cornell Medical College; Attending Physician, Genitourinary Oncology Service, Memorial Sloan-Kettering Cancer Center, New York, New York [41, 43]

Nikhil C. Munshi, MD
Associate Professor of Medicine, Harvard Medical School; Associate Director, Jerome Lipper Multiple Myeloma Center, Dana Farber Cancer Institute, Boston, Massachusetts [17]

Hari Nadiminti, MD
Clinical Instructor, Department of Dermatology, Emory University School of Medicine, Atlanta, Georgia [33]

Hartmut P. H. Neumann, MD
Head, Section Preventative Medicine, Department of Nephrology and General Medicine, Albert-Ludwigs-University of Freiburg, Germany [51]

William Pao, MD, PhD
Associate Professor of Medicine, Cancer Biology, and Pathology, Division of Hematology and Medical Oncology, Vanderbilt University School of Medicine, Nashville, Tennessee [35]

Shreyaskumar R. Patel, MD
Center Medical Director, Sarcoma Center; Professor of Medicine; Deputy Chairman, Department of Sarcoma Medical Oncology, MD Anderson Cancer Center, Houston, Texas [45]

Michael A. Pesce, PhD
Professor Emeritus of Pathology and Cell Biology, Columbia University College of Physicians and Surgeons; Columbia University Medical Center, New York, New York [Appendix]

Myrna R. Rosenfeld, MD, PhD
Professor of Neurology and Chief, Division of Neuro-oncology, University of Pennsylvania, Philadelphia, Pennsylvania [53]

Edward A. Sausville, MD, PhD
Professor, Department of Medicine, University of Maryland School of Medicine; Deputy Director and Associate Director for Clinical Research, University of Maryland Marlene and Stewart Greenebaum Cancer Center, Baltimore, Maryland [28]

David T. Scadden, MD
Gerald and Darlene Jordan Professor of Medicine, Harvard Stem Cell Institute, Harvard Medical School; Department of Stem Cell and Regenerative Biology, Massachusetts General Hospital, Boston, Massachusetts [1]

Howard I. Scher, MD
Professor of Medicine, Weill Cornell Medical College; D. Wayne Calloway Chair in Urologic Oncology; Chief, Genitourinary Oncology Service, Department of Medicine, Memorial Sloan-Kettering Cancer Center, New York, New York [41, 42]

Michael V. Seiden, MD, PhD
Professor of Medicine; President and CEO, Fox Chase Cancer Center, Philadelphia, Pennsylvania [44]

David C. Seldin, MD, PhD
Chief, Section of Hematology-Oncology, Department of Medicine; Director, Amyloid Treatment and Research Program, Boston University School of Medicine; Boston Medical Center, Boston, Massachusetts [18]

Martha Skinner, MD
Professor, Department of Medicine, Boston University School of Medicine, Boston, Massachusetts [18]

Jerry L. Spivak, MD
Professor of Medicine and Oncology, Hematology Division, Johns Hopkins University School of Medicine, Baltimore, Maryland [13]

Jeffrey M. Trent, PhD, FACMG
President and Research Director, Translational Genomics Research Institute, Phoenix, Arizona; Van Andel Research Institute, Grand Rapids, Michigan [24]

Walter J. Urba, MD, PhD
Director of Cancer Research, Robert W. Franz Cancer Research Center, Providence Portland Medical Center, Portland, Oregon [33]

Gauri R. Varadhachary, MD
Associate Professor, Department of Gastrointestinal Medical Oncology, University of Texas MD Anderson Cancer Center, Houston, Texas [47]

Camilo Jimenez Vasquez, MD
Assistant Professor, Department of Endocrine Neoplasia and Hormonal Disorders, Division of Internal Medicine, University of Texas MD Anderson Cancer Center, Houston, Texas [50]

Bert Vogelstein, MD
Professor of Oncology and Pathology; Investigator, Howard Hughes Medical Institute; Sidney Kimmel Comprehensive Cancer Center; Johns Hopkins University School of Medicine, Baltimore, Maryland [24]

Everett E. Vokes, MD
John E. Ultmann Professor and Chairman, Department of Medicine; Physician-in-Chief, University of Chicago Medical Center, Chicago, Illinois [34]

Carl V. Washington, MD
Associate Professor of Dermatology, Winship Cancer Center, Emory University School of Medicine, Atlanta, Georgia [33]

Anthony P. Weetman, MD
University of Sheffield School of Medicine, Sheffield, United Kingdom [48]

Jeffrey I. Weitz, MD, FRCP(C), FACP
Professor of Medicine and Biochemistry; Executive Director, Thrombosis and Atherosclerosis Research Institute; HSFO/J. F. Mustard Chair in Cardiovascular Research, Canada Research Chair (Tier 1) in Thrombosis, McMaster University, Hamilton, Ontario, Canada [23]

Patrick Y. Wen, MD
Professor of Neurology, Harvard Medical School; Dana-Farber Cancer Institute, Boston, Massachusetts [46]

Meir Wetzler, MD, FACP
Professor of Medicine, Roswell Park Cancer Institute, Buffalo, New York [14]

Charles M. Wiener, MD
Dean/CEO Perdana University Graduate School of Medicine, Selangor, Malaysia; Professor of Medicine and Physiology, Johns Hopkins University School of Medicine, Baltimore, Maryland [Review and Self-Assessment]

Neal S. Young, MD
Chief, Hematology Branch, National Heart, Lung and Blood Institute, National Institutes of Health, Bethesda, Maryland [11]

PREFACE

Harrison's Principles of Internal Medicine has a long and distinguished tradition in the field of hematology. Maxwell Wintrobe, whose work actually established hematology as a distinct subspecialty of medicine, was a founding editor of the book and participated in the first seven editions, taking over for Tinsley Harrison as editor-in-chief on the sixth and seventh editions. Wintrobe, born in 1901, began his study of blood in earnest in 1927 as an assistant in medicine at Tulane University in New Orleans. He continued his studies at Johns Hopkins from 1930 to 1943 and moved to the University of Utah in 1943, where he remained until his death in 1986. He invented a variety of the measures that are routinely used to characterize red blood cell abnormalities, including the hematocrit, the red cell indices, and erythrocyte sedimentation rate, and defined the normal and abnormal values for these parameters, among many other important contributions in a 50-year career.

Oncology began as a subspecialty much later. It came to life as a specific subdivision within hematology. A subset of hematologists with a special interest in hematologic malignancies began working with chemotherapeutic agents to treat leukemia and lymphoma in the mid-1950s and early 1960s. As new agents were developed and the principles of clinical trial research were developed, the body of knowledge of oncology began to become larger and mainly independent from hematology. Informed by the laboratory study of cancer biology and an expansion in focus beyond hematologic neoplasms to tumors of all organ systems, oncology developed as a separable discipline from hematology. This separation was also fueled by the expansion of the body of knowledge about clotting and its disorders, which became a larger part of hematology.

In most academic medical centers, hematology and oncology remain connected. However, conceptual distinctions between hematology and oncology have been made. Differences are reinforced by separate fellowship training programs (although many joint training programs remain), separate board certification examinations, separate professional organizations, and separate textbooks describing separate bodies of knowledge. In some academic medical centers, oncology is not merely a separate subspecialty division in a Department of Medicine but is an entirely distinct department in the medical school with the same standing as the Department of Medicine. Economic forces are also at work to separate hematology and oncology.

Perhaps I am only reflecting the biases of an old dog, but I am unenthusiastic about the increasing fractionation of medicine subspecialties. There are now invasive and noninvasive cardiologists, gastroenterologists who do and others who do not use endoscopes, and organ-focused subspecialists (diabetologists, thyroidologists) instead of organ system–focused subspecialists (endocrinologists). At a time when the body of knowledge that must be mastered is increasing dramatically, the duration of training has not been increased to accommodate the additional learning that is necessary to become highly skilled. Extraordinary attention has been focused on the hours that trainees work. Apparently, the administrators are more concerned about undocumented adverse effects of every third night call on trainees than they are about the well-documented adverse effects on patients of frequent handoffs of patient responsibility to multiple caregivers.

Despite the sub-sub-subspecialization that is pervasive in modern medicine, students, trainees, general internists, family medicine physicians, physicians' assistants, nurse practitioners, and specialists in nonmedicine specialties still require access to information in hematology and oncology that can assist them in meeting the needs of their patients. Given the paucity of single sources of integrated information on hematology and oncology, the editors of *Harrison's Principles of Internal Medicine* decided to pull together the chapters in the "mother book" related to hematology and oncology and bind them together in a subspecialty themed book called *Harrison's Hematology and Oncology*. The first edition of this book appeared in 2010 and was based on the 17th edition of *Harrison's Principles of Internal Medicine*. Encouraged by the response to that book, we have embarked upon a second edition based on 18th edition of *Harrison's Principles of Internal Medicine*.

The book contains 55 chapters organized into 12 sections: (I) The Cellular Basis of Hematopoiesis, (II) Cardinal Manifestations of Hematologic Diseases, (III) Anemias, (IV) Myeloproliferative Disorders, (V) Hematologic Malignancies, (VI) Disorders of Hemostasis, (VII) Biology of Cancer, (VIII) Principles of Cancer Prevention and Treatment, (IX) Neoplastic Disorders, (X) Endocrine Neoplasia, (XI) Remote Effects of Cancer, and (XII) Oncologic Emergencies and Late Effects Complications.

The chapters have been written by physicians who have made seminal contributions to the body of knowledge in their areas of expertise. The information is authoritative and as current as we can make it, given the time requirements of producing books. Each chapter contains the relevant information on the genetics, cell biology, pathophysiology, and treatment of specific disease entities. In addition, separate chapters on hematopoiesis, cancer cell biology, and cancer prevention reflect the rapidly growing body of knowledge in these areas that are the underpinning of our current concepts of diseases in hematology and oncology. In addition to the factual information presented in the chapters, a section of test questions and answers is provided to reinforce important principles. A narrative explanation of what is wrong with the wrong answers should be of further value in the preparation of the reader for board examinations.

The bringing together of hematology and oncology in a single text is unusual and we hope it is useful. Like many areas of medicine, the body of knowledge relevant to the practice of hematology and oncology is expanding rapidly. New discoveries with clinical impact are being made at an astounding rate; nearly constant effort is required to try to keep pace. It is our hope that this book is helpful to you in the struggle to master the daunting volume of new findings relevant to the care of your patients.

We are extremely grateful to Kim Davis and James Shanahan at McGraw-Hill for their invaluable assistance in the preparation of this book.

Dan L. Longo, MD

NOTICE

Review and self-assessment questions and answers were taken from Wiener CM, Brown CD, Hemnes AR (eds). *Harrison's Self-Assessment and Board Review*, 18th ed. New York, McGraw-Hill, 2012, ISBN 978-0-07-177195-5.

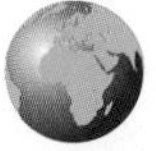
The global icons call greater attention to key epidemiologic and clinical differences in the practice of medicine throughout the world.

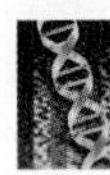
The genetic icons identify a clinical issue with an explicit genetic relationship.

SECTION I

THE CELLULAR BASIS OF HEMATOPOIESIS

CHAPTER 1

HEMATOPOIETIC STEM CELLS

David T. Scadden ■ Dan L. Longo

All of the cell types in the peripheral blood and some cells in every tissue of the body are derived from hematopoietic (*hemo*: blood; *poiesis*: creation) stem cells. If the hematopoietic stem cell is damaged and can no longer function (e.g., due to a nuclear accident), a person would survive 2–4 weeks in the absence of extraordinary support measures. With the clinical use of hematopoietic stem cells, tens of thousands of lives are saved each year (Chap. 30). Stem cells produce tens of billions of blood cells daily from a stem cell pool that is estimated to be only in the hundreds of thousands. How stem cells do this, how they persist for many decades despite the production demands, and how they may be better used in clinical care are important issues in medicine.

The study of blood cell production has become a paradigm for how other tissues may be organized and regulated. Basic research in hematopoiesis that includes defining stepwise molecular changes accompanying functional changes in maturing cells, aggregating cells into functional subgroups, and demonstrating hematopoietic stem cell regulation by a specialized microenvironment are concepts worked out in hematology, but they offer models for other tissues. Moreover, these concepts may not be restricted to normal tissue function but extend to malignancy. Stem cells are rare cells among a heterogeneous population of cell types, and their behavior is assessed mainly in experimental animal models involving reconstitution of hematopoiesis. Thus, much of what we know about stem cells is imprecise and based on inferences from genetically manipulated animals.

CARDINAL FUNCTIONS OF HEMATOPOIETIC STEM CELLS

All stem cell types have two cardinal functions: self-renewal and differentiation (Fig. 1-1). Stem cells exist to generate, maintain, and repair tissues. They function successfully if they can replace a wide variety of shorter-lived mature cells over prolonged periods. The process of self-renewal (discussed later) assures that a stem cell population can be sustained over time. Without self-renewal, the stem cell pool would become exhausted, and tissue maintenance would not be possible. The process of differentiation leads to production of the effectors of tissue function: mature cells. Without proper differentiation, the integrity of tissue function would be compromised, and organ failure would ensue.

In the blood, mature cells have variable average life spans, ranging from 7 h for mature neutrophils to a few months for red blood cells to many years for memory lymphocytes. However, the stem cell pool is the central, durable source of all blood and immune cells, maintaining a capacity to produce a broad range of cells from a single cell source yet keeping itself vigorous over decades of life. As an individual stem cell divides, it has the capacity to accomplish one of three division outcomes: two stem cells, two cells destined for differentiation, or one stem cell and one differentiating cell. The former two outcomes are the result of symmetric cell division, whereas the latter indicates a different outcome for the two daughter cells—an event termed *asymmetric cell division*. The relative balance for these types of outcomes may change during development and under particular kinds of demands on the stem cell pool.

DEVELOPMENTAL BIOLOGY OF HEMATOPOIETIC STEM CELLS

During development, blood cells are produced at different sites. Initially, the yolk sac provides oxygen-carrying red blood cells, and then the placenta and several sites of intraembryonic blood cell production become involved. These intraembryonic sites engage in sequential order, moving from the genital ridge at a site where the aorta,

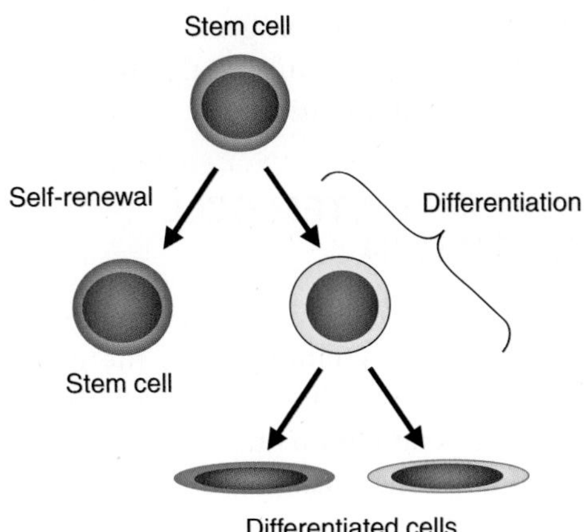

FIGURE 1-1
Signature characteristics of the stem cell. Stem cells have two essential features: the capacity to differentiate into a variety of mature cell types and the capacity for self-renewal. Intrinsic factors associated with self-renewal include expression of Bmi-1, Gfi-1, PTEN, STAT5, Tel/Atv6, p21, p18, MCL-1, Mel-18, RAE28, and HoxB4. Extrinsic signals for self-renewal include Notch, Wnt, SHH, and Tie2/Ang-1. Based mainly on murine studies, hematopoietic stem cells express the following cell surface molecules: CD34, Thy-1 (CD90), c-Kit receptor (CD117), CD133, CD164, and c-Mpl (CD110, also known as the thrombopoietin receptor).

gonadal tissue, and mesonephros are emerging to the fetal liver and then, in the second trimester, to the bone marrow and spleen. As the location of stem cells changes, the cells they produce also change. The yolk sac provides red cells expressing embryonic hemoglobins while intraembryonic sites of hematopoiesis generate red cells, platelets, and the cells of innate immunity. The production of the cells of adaptive immunity occurs when the bone marrow is colonized and the thymus forms. Stem cell proliferation remains high, even in the bone marrow, until shortly after birth, when it appears to dramatically decline. The cells in the bone marrow are thought to arrive by the bloodborne transit of cells from the fetal liver after calcification of the long bones has begun. The presence of stem cells in the circulation is not unique to a time window in development. Rather, hematopoietic stem cells appear to circulate throughout life. The time that cells spend freely circulating appears to be brief (measured in minutes in the mouse), but the cells that do circulate are functional and can be used for transplantation. The number of stem cells that circulate can be increased in a number of ways to facilitate harvest and transfer to the same or a different host.

MOBILITY OF HEMATOPOIETIC STEM CELLS

Cells entering and exiting the bone marrow do so through a series of molecular interactions. Circulating stem cells (through CD162 and CD44) engage the lectins P- and E-selectin on the endothelial surface to slow the movement of the cells to a rolling phenotype. Stem cell integrins are then activated and accomplish firm adhesion between the stem cell and vessel wall, with a particularly important role for stem cell VCAM-1 engaging endothelial VLA-4. The chemokine CXCL12 (SDF1) interacting with stem cell CXCR4 receptors also appears to be important in the process of stem cells getting from the circulation to where they engraft in the bone marrow. This is particularly true in the developmental move from fetal liver to bone marrow; however, the role for this molecule in adults appears to be more related to retention of stem cells in the bone marrow rather the process of getting them there. Interrupting that retention process through specific molecular blockers of the CXCR4/CXCL12 interaction, cleavage of CXCL12, or downregulation of the receptor can all result in the release of stem cells into the circulation. This process is an increasingly important aspect of recovering stem cells for therapeutic use as it has permitted the harvesting process to be done by leukapheresis rather than bone marrow punctures in the operating room. Refining our knowledge of how stem cells get into and out of the bone marrow may improve our ability to obtain stem cells and make them more efficient at finding their way to the specific sites for blood cell production, the so-called stem cell niche.

HEMATOPOIETIC STEM CELL MICROENVIRONMENT

The concept of a specialized microenvironment, or stem cell niche, was first proposed to explain why cells derived from the bone marrow of one animal could be used in transplantation and again be found in the bone marrow of the recipient. This niche is more than just a housing site for stem cells, however. It is an anatomic location where regulatory signals are provided that allow the stem cells to thrive, to expand if needed, and to provide varying amounts of descendant daughter cells. In addition, unregulated growth of stem cells may be problematic based on their undifferentiated state and self-renewal capacity. Thus, the niche must also regulate the number of stem cells produced. In this manner, the niche has the dual function of serving as a site of nurture but imposing limits for stem cells: in effect, acting as both a nutritive and constraining home.

The niche for blood stem cells changes with each of the sites of blood production during development, but for most of human life, it is located in the bone marrow. Within the bone marrow, at least two niche sites have been proposed: on trabecular bone surfaces and in the perivascular space. Stem cells may be found in both places by histologic analysis, and functional regulation has been shown at the highly vascular bone surface. Specifically, bone-forming mesenchymal cells, osteoblastic cells, participate in hematopoietic stem cell function, affecting their location, proliferation, and number. The basis for this interaction is through a number of molecules mediating location, such as the chemokine CXCL12 (SDF1), through proliferation signals mediated by angiopoietin 1, and signaling to modulate self-renewal or survival by factors such as Notch ligands, kit ligand, and Wnts. Other bone components, such as the extracellular matrix glycoprotein, osteopontin, and the high ionic calcium found at trabecular surfaces, contribute to the unique microenvironment, or stem cell niche, on trabecular bone. This physiology has practical applications. First, medications altering niche components may have an effect on stem cell function. This has now been shown for a number of compounds, and some are being clinically tested. Second, it is now possible to assess whether the niche participates in disease states and to examine whether targeting the niche with medications may alter the outcome of certain diseases.

EXCESS CAPACITY OF HEMATOPOIETIC STEM CELLS

In the absence of disease, one never runs out of hematopoietic stem cells. Indeed, serial transplantation studies in mice suggest that sufficient stem cells are present to reconstitute several animals in succession, with each animal having normal blood cell production. The fact that allogeneic stem cell transplant recipients also never run out of blood cells in their life span, which can extend for decades, argues that even the limiting numbers of stem cells provided to them are sufficient. How stem cells respond to different conditions to increase or decrease their mature cell production remains poorly understood. Clearly, negative feedback mechanisms affect the level of production of most of the cells, leading to the normal tightly regulated blood cell counts. However, many of the regulatory mechanisms that govern production of more mature progenitor cells do not apply or apply differently to stem cells. Similarly, most of the molecules shown to be able to change the size of the stem cell pool have little effect on more mature blood cells. For example, the growth factor erythropoietin, which stimulates red blood cell production from more mature precursor cells, has no effect on stem cells. Similarly, granulocyte colony-stimulating factor drives the rapid proliferation of granulocyte precursors but has little or no effect on the cell cycling of stem cells. Rather, it changes the location of stem cells by indirect means, altering molecules such as CXCL12 that tether stem cells to their niche. Molecules shown to be important for altering the proliferation, self renewal or survival of stem cells, such as cyclin-dependent kinase inhibitors, transcription factors such as Bmi-1, or microRNAs such as miR125a, have little or different effects on progenitor cells. Hematopoietic stem cells have governing mechanisms that are distinct from the cells they generate.

HEMATOPOIETIC STEM CELL DIFFERENTIATION

Hematopoietic stem cells sit at the base of a branching hierarchy of cells, culminating in the many mature cell types that comprise the blood and immune system (Fig. 1-2). The maturation steps leading to terminally differentiated and functional blood cells take place both as a consequence of intrinsic changes in gene expression and niche- and cytokine-directed changes in the cells. Our knowledge of the details remains incomplete. As stem cells mature to progenitors, precursors, and, finally, mature effector cells, they undergo a series of functional changes. These include the obvious acquisition of functions defining mature blood cells, such as phagocytic capacity or hemoglobin synthesis. They also include the progressive loss of plasticity (i.e., the ability to become other cell types). For example, the myeloid progenitor can make all cells in the myeloid series but none in the lymphoid series. As common myeloid progenitors mature, they become precursors for either monocytes and granulocytes or erythrocytes and megakaryocytes, but not both. Some amount of reversibility of this process may exist early in the differentiation cascade, but that is lost beyond a distinct stage. As cells differentiate, they may also lose proliferative capacity (Fig. 1-3). Mature granulocytes are incapable of proliferation and only increase in number by increased production from precursors. Lymphoid cells retain the capacity to proliferate but have linked their proliferation to the recognition of particular proteins or peptides by specific antigen receptors on their surface. In most tissues, the proliferative cell population is a more immature progenitor population. In general, cells within the highly proliferative progenitor cell compartment are also relatively short-lived, making their way through the differentiation process in a defined molecular program involving the sequential activation of particular sets of genes. For any particular cell type, the differentiation program is difficult to speed up. The time it takes for hematopoietic progenitors to become mature cells is ~10–14 days in humans, evident clinically by the interval between cytotoxic chemotherapy and blood count recovery in patients.

SELF-RENEWAL

The hematopoietic stem cell must balance its three potential fates: apoptosis, self-renewal, and differentiation. The proliferation of cells is generally not associated with the ability to undergo a self-renewing division except among memory T and B cells and among stem

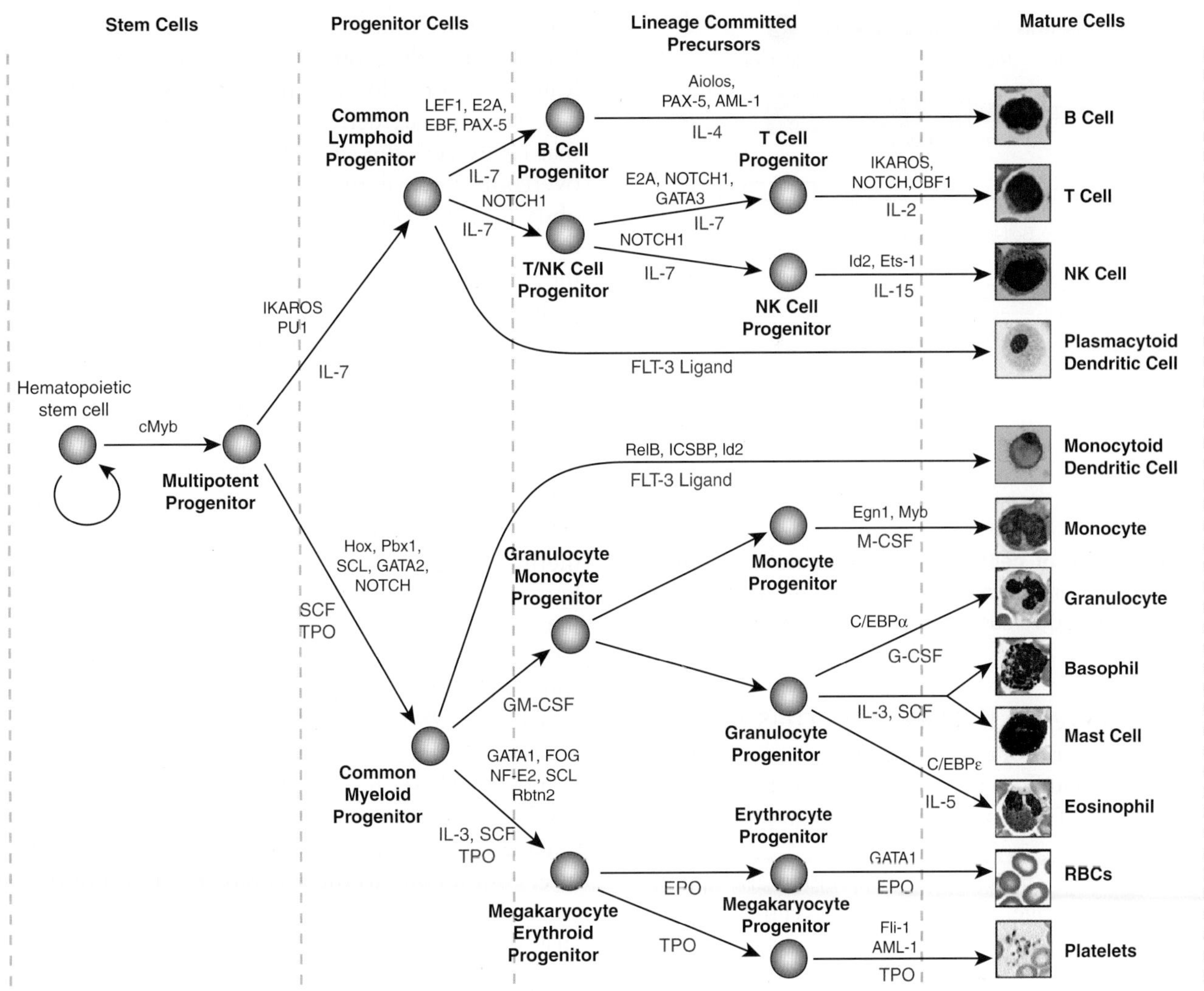

FIGURE 1-2

Hierarchy of hematopoietic differentiation. *Stem cells* are multipotent cells that are the source of all descendant cells and have the capacity to provide either long-term (measured in years) or short-term (measured in months) cell production. *Progenitor cells* have a more limited spectrum of cells they can produce and are generally a short-lived, highly proliferative population also known as transient amplifying cells. *Precursor cells* are cells committed to a single blood cell lineage but with a continued ability to proliferate; they do not have all the features of a fully mature cell. *Mature cells* are the terminally differentiated product of the differentiation process and are the effector cells of specific activities of the blood and immune system. Progress through the pathways is mediated by alterations in gene expression. The regulation of the differentiation by soluble factors and cell–cell communications within the bone marrow niche are still being defined. The transcription factors that characterize particular cell transitions are illustrated on the arrows; the soluble factors that contribute to the differentiation process are in blue. EPO, erythropoietin; SCF, stem cell factor; TPO, thrombopoietin. M-CSF is macrophage-colony-stimulating factor; GM-CSF is granulocyte-macrophage-colony stimulating factor; G-CSF is granulocyte-colony-stimulating factor.

cells. Self-renewal capacity gives way to differentiation as the only option after cell division when cells leave the stem cell compartment until they have the opportunity to become memory lymphocytes. In addition to this self-renewing capacity, stem cells have an additional feature characterizing their proliferation machinery. Stem cells in many mature adult tissues may be heterogeneous with some being deeply quiescent, serving as a deep reserve, while others are more proliferative and replenish the short-lived progenitor population. In the hematopoietic system, stem cells are generally cytokine-resistant, remaining dormant even when cytokines drive bone marrow progenitors to proliferation rates measured in hours. Stem cells, in contrast, are thought to divide at far longer intervals measured in months to years, for the most quiescent cells. This quiescence is difficult to overcome in vitro, limiting the ability to effectively expand human hematopoietic stem cells. The process may be controlled by particularly high levels of cyclin-dependent kinase inhibitors that restrict entry of

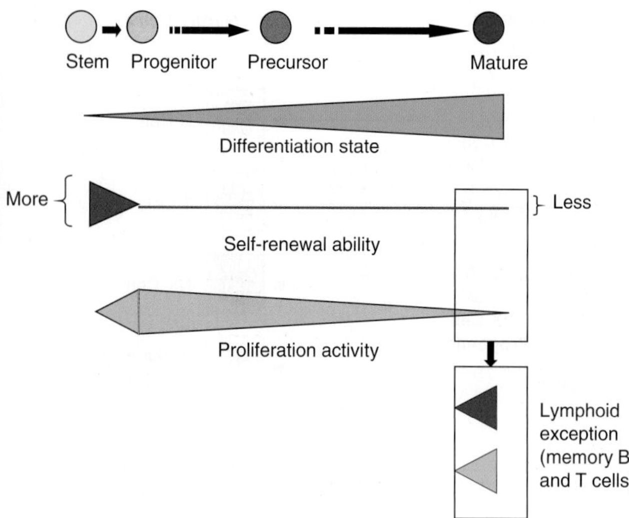

FIGURE 1-3

Relative function of cells in the hematopoietic hierarchy. The boxes represent distinct functional features of cells in the myeloid (*upper box*) versus lymphoid (*lower box*) lineages.

stem cells into cell cycle, blocking the G1–S transition. Exogenous signals from the niche also appear to enforce quiescence, including the activation of the tyrosine kinase receptor Tie2 on stem cells by angiopoietin 1 on osteoblasts.

The regulation of stem cell proliferation also appears to change with age. In mice, the cyclin-dependent kinase inhibitor p16INK4a accumulates in stem cells in older animals and is associated with a change in five different stem cell functions, including cell cycling. Lowering expression of p16INK4a in older animals improves stem cell cycling and the capacity to reconstitute hematopoiesis in adoptive hosts, making them similar to younger animals. Mature cell numbers are unaffected. Therefore, molecular events governing the specific functions of stem cells are being gradually made clear and offer the potential of new approaches to changing stem cell function for therapy. One critical stem cell function that remains poorly defined is the molecular regulation of self-renewal.

For medicine, self-renewal is perhaps the most important function of stem cells because it is critical in regulating the number of stem cells. Stem cell number is a key limiting parameter for both autologous and allogeneic stem cell transplantation. Were we to have the ability to use fewer stem cells or expand limited numbers of stem cells ex vivo, it might be possible to reduce the morbidity and expense of stem cell harvests and enable use of other stem cell sources. Specifically, umbilical cord blood is a rich source of stem cells. However, the volume of cord blood units is extremely small and, therefore, the total number of hematopoietic stem cells that can be obtained is generally only sufficient to transplant an individual weighing <40 kg. This limitation restricts what would otherwise be an extremely promising source of stem cells. Two features of cord blood stem cells are particularly important. (1) They are derived from a diversity of individuals that far exceeds the adult donor pool and therefore can overcome the majority of immunologic cross-matching obstacles. (2) Cord blood stem cells have a large number of T cells associated with them, but (paradoxically) they appear to be associated with a lower incidence of graft-versus-host disease when compared with similarly mismatched stem cells from other sources. If stem cell expansion by self-renewal could be achieved, the number of cells available might be sufficient for use in larger adults. An alternative approach to this problem is to improve the efficiency of engraftment of donor stem cells. Graft engineering is exploring methods of adding cell components that may enhance engraftment. Furthermore, at least some data suggest that depletion of host natural killer (NK) cells may lower the number of stem cells necessary to reconstitute hematopoiesis.

Some limited understanding of self-renewal exists and, intriguingly, implicates gene products that are associated with the chromatin state, a high-order organization of chromosomal DNA that influences transcription. These include members of the polycomb family, a group of zinc finger–containing transcriptional regulators that interact with the chromatin structure, contributing to the accessibility of groups of genes for transcription. One member, *Bmi-1*, is important in enabling hematopoietic stem cell self-renewal through modification of cell cycle regulators such as the cyclin-dependent kinase inhibitors. In the absence of *Bmi-1* or of the transcriptional regulator, Gfi-1, hematopoietic stem cells decline in number and function. In contrast, dysregulation of *Bmi-1* has been associated with leukemia; it may promote leukemic stem cell self-renewal when it is overexpressed. Other transcription regulators have also been associated with self-renewal, particularly homeobox, or "hox," genes. These transcription factors are named for their ability to govern large numbers of genes, including those determining body patterning in invertebrates. HoxB4 is capable of inducing extensive self-renewal of stem cells through its DNA-binding motif. Other members of the hox family of genes have been noted to affect normal stem cells, but they are also associated with leukemia. External signals that may influence the relative self-renewal versus differentiation outcomes of stem cell cycling include the Notch ligands and specific Wnt ligands. Intracellular signal transducing intermediates are also implicated in regulating self-renewal but, interestingly, are not usually associated with the pathways activated by Notch or Wnt receptors. They include PTEN, an inhibitor of the AKT pathway, and STAT5, both of which are usually downstream of activated growth factor receptors and necessary for normal stem cell functions including, self-renewal, at least in mouse models. The connections between these molecules remain to be defined, and their role in physiologic regulation of stem cell self-renewal is still poorly understood.

CANCER IS SIMILAR TO AN ORGAN WITH SELF-RENEWING CAPACITY

The relationship of stem cells to cancer is an important evolving dimension of adult stem cell biology. Cancer may share principles of organization with normal tissues. Cancer might have the same hierarchical organization of cells with a base of stem-like cells capable of the signature stem-cell features, self-renewal, and differentiation. These stem-like cells might be the basis for perpetuation of the tumor and represent a slowly dividing, rare population with distinct regulatory mechanisms, including a relationship with a specialized microenvironment. A subpopulation of self-renewing cells has been defined for some, but not all, cancers. A more sophisticated understanding of the stem-cell organization of cancers may lead to improved strategies for developing new therapies for the many common and difficult-to-treat types of malignancies that have been relatively refractory to interventions aimed at dividing cells.

Does the concept of cancer stem cells provide insight into the cellular origin of cancer? The fact that some cells within a cancer have stem cell–like properties does not necessarily mean that the cancer arose in the stem cell itself. Rather, more mature cells could have acquired the self-renewal characteristics of stem cells. Any single genetic event is unlikely to be sufficient to enable full transformation of a normal cell to a frankly malignant one. Rather, cancer is a multistep process, and for the multiple steps to accumulate, the cell of origin must be able to persist for prolonged periods. It must also be able to generate large numbers of daughter cells. The normal stem cell has these properties and, by virtue of its having intrinsic self-renewal capability, may be more readily converted to a malignant phenotype. This hypothesis has been tested experimentally in the hematopoietic system. Taking advantage of the cell-surface markers that distinguish hematopoietic cells of varying maturity, stem cells, progenitors, precursors, and mature cells can be isolated. Powerful transforming gene constructs were placed in these cells, and it was found that the cell with the greatest potential to produce a malignancy was dependent on the transforming gene. In some cases it was the stem cell, but in others, the progenitor cell functioned to initiate and per-petuate the cancer. This shows that cells can acquire stem cell-like properties in malignancy.

WHAT ELSE CAN HEMATOPOIETIC STEM CELLS DO?

Some experimental data have suggested that hematopoietic stem cells or other cells mobilized into the circulation by the same factors that mobilize hematopoietic stem cells are capable of playing a role in healing the vascular and tissue damage associated with stroke and myocardial infarction. These data are controversial, and the applicability of a stem-cell approach to nonhematopoietic conditions remains experimental. However, the application of the evolving knowledge of hematopoietic stem cell biology may lead to wide-ranging clinical uses.

The stem cell, therefore, represents a true dual-edged sword. It has tremendous healing capacity and is essential for life. Uncontrolled, it can threaten the life it maintains. Understanding how stem cells function, the signals that modify their behavior, and the tissue niches that modulate stem cell responses to injury and disease are critical for more effectively developing stem cell–based medicine. That aspect of medicine will include the use of the stem cells and the use of drugs to target stem cells to enhance repair of damaged tissues. It will also include the careful balance of interventions to control stem cells where they may be dysfunctional or malignant.

SECTION II

CARDINAL MANIFESTATIONS OF HEMATOLOGIC DISEASE

CHAPTER 2

ANEMIA AND POLYCYTHEMIA

John W. Adamson ■ Dan L. Longo

HEMATOPOIESIS AND THE PHYSIOLOGIC BASIS OF RED CELL PRODUCTION

Hematopoiesis is the process by which the formed elements of blood are produced. The process is regulated through a series of steps beginning with the hematopoietic stem cell. Stem cells are capable of producing red cells, all classes of granulocytes, monocytes, platelets, and the cells of the immune system. The precise molecular mechanism—either intrinsic to the stem cell itself or through the action of extrinsic factors—by which the stem cell becomes committed to a given lineage is not fully defined. However, experiments in mice suggest that erythroid cells come from a common erythroid/megakaryocyte progenitor that does not develop in the absence of expression of the GATA-1 and FOG-1 (friend of GATA-1) transcription factors (Chap. 1). Following lineage commitment, hematopoietic progenitor and precursor cells come increasingly under the regulatory influence of growth factors and hormones. For red cell production, erythropoietin (EPO) is the regulatory hormone. EPO is required for the maintenance of committed erythroid progenitor cells that, in the absence of the hormone, undergo programmed cell death (*apoptosis*). The regulated process of red cell production is *erythropoiesis*, and its key elements are illustrated in Fig. 2-1.

In the bone marrow, the first morphologically recognizable erythroid precursor is the pronormoblast. This cell can undergo four to five cell divisions, which result in the production of 16–32 mature red cells. With increased EPO production, or the administration of EPO as a drug, early progenitor cell numbers are amplified and, in turn, give rise to increased numbers of erythrocytes. The regulation of EPO production itself is linked to tissue oxygenation.

In mammals, O_2 is transported to tissues bound to the hemoglobin contained within circulating red cells. The mature red cell is 8 μm in diameter, anucleate, discoid in shape, and extremely pliable in order to traverse the microcirculation successfully; its membrane integrity is maintained by the intracellular generation of ATP. Normal red cell production results in the daily replacement of 0.8–1% of all circulating red cells in the body, since the average red cell lives 100–120 days. The organ responsible for red cell production is called the *erythron*. The erythron is a dynamic organ made up of a rapidly proliferating pool of marrow erythroid precursor cells and a large mass of mature circulating red blood cells. The size of the red cell mass reflects the balance of red cell production and destruction. The physiologic basis of red cell production and destruction provides an understanding of the mechanisms that can lead to anemia.

The physiologic regulator of red cell production, the glycoprotein hormone EPO, is produced and released by peritubular capillary lining cells within the kidney. These cells are highly specialized epithelial-like cells. A small amount of EPO is produced by hepatocytes. The fundamental stimulus for EPO production is the availability of O_2 for tissue metabolic needs. Key to EPO gene regulation is hypoxia-inducible factor (HIF)-1α. In the presence of O_2, HIF-1α is hydroxylated at a key proline, allowing HIF-1α to be ubiquitinylated and degraded via the proteasome pathway. If O_2 becomes limiting, this critical hydroxylation step does not occur, allowing HIF-1α to partner with other proteins, translocate to the nucleus, and upregulate the EPO gene, among others.

Impaired O_2 delivery to the kidney can result from a decreased red cell mass (*anemia*), impaired O_2 loading of the hemoglobin molecule or a high O_2 affinity mutant hemoglobin (*hypoxemia*), or, rarely, impaired blood flow to the kidney (renal artery stenosis). EPO governs the day-to-day production of red cells, and ambient levels of the hormone can be measured in the plasma by sensitive immunoassays—the normal

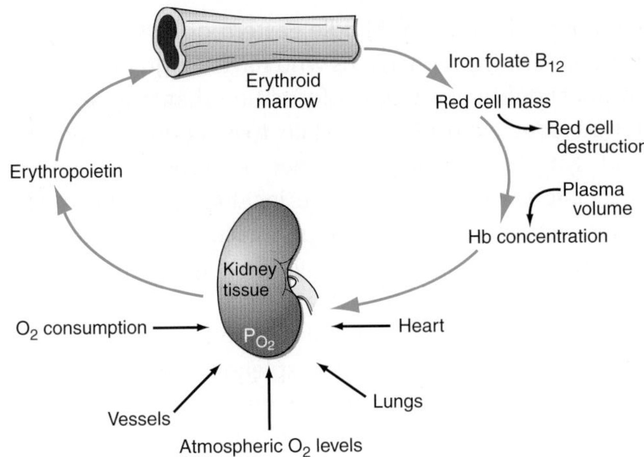

FIGURE 2-1
The physiologic regulation of red cell production by tissue oxygen tension. Hb, hemoglobin.

level being 10–25 U/L. When the hemoglobin concentration falls below 100–120 g/L (10–12 g/dL), plasma EPO levels increase in proportion to the severity of the anemia (Fig. 2-2). In circulation, EPO has a half-clearance time of 6–9 h. EPO acts by binding to specific receptors on the surface of marrow erythroid precursors, inducing them to proliferate and to mature. With EPO stimulation, red cell production can increase four- to fivefold within a 1- to 2-week period, but only in the presence of adequate nutrients, especially iron. The functional capacity of the erythron, therefore, requires normal renal production of EPO, a functioning erythroid marrow, and an adequate supply of substrates for hemoglobin synthesis. A defect in any of these key components can lead to anemia. Generally, anemia is recognized in the laboratory when a patient's hemoglobin level or hematocrit is reduced below an expected value (the normal range). The likelihood and severity of anemia are defined based on the deviation of the patient's hemoglobin/hematocrit from values expected for age- and sex-matched normal subjects. The hemoglobin concentration in adults has a Gaussian distribution. The mean hematocrit value for adult males is 47% (± SD 7) and that for adult females is 42% (± 5). Any single hematocrit or hemoglobin value carries with it a likelihood of associated anemia. Thus, a hematocrit of ≤39% in an adult male or <35% in an adult female has only about a 25% chance of being normal. Suspected low hemoglobin or hematocrit values are more easily interpreted if previous values for the same patient are known for comparison. The World Health Organization (WHO) defines anemia as a hemoglobin level <130 g/L (13 g/dL) in men and <120 g/L (12 g/dL) in women.

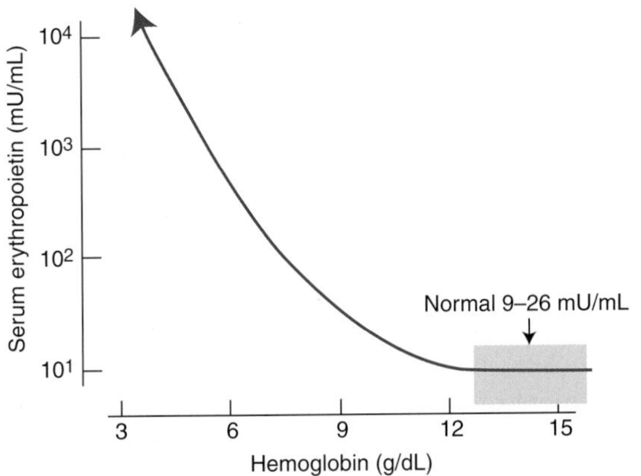

FIGURE 2-2
Erythropoietin (EPO) levels in response to anemia. When the hemoglobin level falls to 120 g/L (12 g/dL), plasma EPO levels increase logarithmically. In the presence of chronic kidney disease or chronic inflammation, EPO levels are typically lower than expected for the degree of anemia. As individuals age, the level of EPO needed to sustain normal hemoglobin levels appears to increase. *(From RS Hillman et al: Hematology in Clinical Practice, 5th ed. New York, McGraw-Hill, 2010.)*

The critical elements of erythropoiesis—EPO production, iron availability, the proliferative capacity of the bone marrow, and effective maturation of red cell precursors—are used for the initial classification of anemia (discussed later).

ANEMIA

CLINICAL PRESENTATION OF ANEMIA

Signs and symptoms

Anemia is most often recognized by abnormal screening laboratory tests. Patients less commonly present with advanced anemia and its attendant signs and symptoms. Acute anemia is due to blood loss or hemolysis. If blood loss is mild, enhanced O_2 delivery is achieved through changes in the O_2–hemoglobin dissociation curve mediated by a decreased pH or increased CO_2 (*Bohr effect*). With acute blood loss, hypovolemia dominates the clinical picture, and the hematocrit and hemoglobin levels do not reflect the volume of blood lost. Signs of vascular instability appear with acute losses of 10–15% of the total blood volume. In such patients, the issue is not anemia but hypotension and decreased organ perfusion. When >30% of the blood volume is lost suddenly, patients are unable to compensate with the usual mechanisms of vascular contraction and changes in regional blood flow. The patient prefers to remain supine and will show postural hypotension and tachycardia. If the volume of blood lost is >40% (i.e., >2 L in the average-sized adult), signs of hypovolemic shock including confusion, dyspnea, diaphoresis, hypotension, and tachycardia appear (Chap. 10). Such patients have significant deficits in vital organ perfusion and require immediate volume replacement.

With acute hemolysis, the signs and symptoms depend on the mechanism that leads to red cell destruction. Intravascular hemolysis with release of free hemoglobin may be associated with acute back pain, free hemoglobin in the plasma and urine, and renal failure. Symptoms associated with more chronic or progressive anemia depend on the age of the patient and the adequacy of blood supply to critical organs. Symptoms associated with moderate anemia include fatigue, loss of stamina, breathlessness, and tachycardia (particularly with physical exertion). However, because of the intrinsic compensatory mechanisms that govern the O_2–hemoglobin dissociation curve, the gradual onset of anemia—particularly in young patients—may not be associated with signs or symptoms until the anemia is severe (hemoglobin <70–80 g/L [7–8 g/dL]). When anemia develops over a period of days or weeks, the total blood volume is normal to slightly increased, and changes in cardiac output and regional blood flow help compensate for the overall loss in O_2-carrying capacity. Changes in the position of the O_2–hemoglobin dissociation curve account for some of the compensatory response to anemia. With chronic anemia, intracellular levels of 2,3-bisphosphoglycerate rise, shifting the dissociation curve to the right and facilitating O_2 unloading. This compensatory mechanism can only maintain normal tissue O_2 delivery in the face of a 20–30 g/L (2–3 g/dL) deficit in hemoglobin concentration. Finally, further protection of O_2 delivery to vital organs is achieved by the shunting of blood away from organs that are relatively rich in blood supply, particularly the kidney, gut, and skin.

Certain disorders are commonly associated with anemia. Chronic inflammatory states (e.g., infection, rheumatoid arthritis, cancer) are associated with mild to moderate anemia, whereas lymphoproliferative disorders, such as chronic lymphocytic leukemia and certain other B-cell neoplasms, may be associated with autoimmune hemolysis.

APPROACH TO THE PATIENT Anemia

The evaluation of the patient with anemia requires a careful history and physical examination. Nutritional history related to drugs or alcohol intake and family history of anemia should always be assessed. Certain geographic backgrounds and ethnic origins are associated with an increased likelihood of an inherited disorder of the hemoglobin molecule or intermediary metabolism. Glucose-6-phosphate dehydrogenase (G6PD) deficiency and certain hemoglobinopathies are seen more commonly in those of Middle Eastern or African origin, including African Americans who have a high frequency of G6PD deficiency. Other information that may be useful includes exposure to certain toxic agents or drugs and symptoms related to other disorders commonly associated with anemia. These include symptoms and signs such as bleeding, fatigue, malaise, fever, weight loss, night sweats, and other systemic symptoms. Clues to the mechanisms of anemia may be provided on physical examination by findings of infection, blood in the stool, lymphadenopathy, splenomegaly, or petechiae. Splenomegaly and lymphadenopathy suggest an underlying lymphoproliferative disease, and petechiae suggest platelet dysfunction. Past laboratory measurements are helpful to determine a time of onset.

In the anemic patient, physical examination may demonstrate a forceful heartbeat, strong peripheral pulses, and a systolic "flow" murmur. The skin and mucous membranes may be pale if the hemoglobin is <80–100 g/L (8–10 g/dL). This part of the physical examination should focus on areas where vessels are close to the surface such as the mucous membranes, nail beds, and palmar creases. If the palmar creases are lighter in color than the surrounding skin when the hand is hyperextended, the hemoglobin level is usually <80 g/L (8 g/dL).

LABORATORY EVALUATION Table 2-1 lists the tests used in the initial workup of anemia. A routine complete blood count (CBC) is required as part of the evaluation and includes the hemoglobin, hematocrit, and red cell indices: the mean cell volume (MCV) in femtoliters, mean cell hemoglobin (MCH) in picograms per cell, and mean concentration of hemoglobin per volume of red cells (MCHC) in grams per liter (non-SI: grams per deciliter). The red cell indices are calculated as shown in Table 2-2, and the normal variations in the hemoglobin and hematocrit with age are shown in Table 2-3. A number of physiologic factors affect the CBC, including age, sex, pregnancy, smoking, and altitude. High-normal hemoglobin values may be seen in men and women who live at high altitude or smoke heavily. Hemoglobin elevations from smoking reflect normal compensation due to the displacement of O_2 by CO in hemoglobin binding. Other important information is provided by the reticulocyte count and measurements of iron supply, including *serum iron, total iron-binding capacity* (TIBC; an indirect measure of the transferrin level), and *serum ferritin.* Marked alterations in the red cell indices usually reflect disorders of maturation or iron deficiency. A careful evaluation of the peripheral blood smear is important, and clinical laboratories often provide a description of both the red and white cells, a white cell differential count, and the platelet count. In patients with severe anemia and abnormalities in red blood cell morphology and/or low reticulocyte counts, a

TABLE 2-1

LABORATORY TESTS IN ANEMIA DIAGNOSIS

I. Complete blood count (CBC)
   A. Red blood cell count
      1. Hemoglobin
      2. Hematocrit
      3. Reticulocyte count
   B. Red blood cell indices
      1. Mean cell volume (MCV)
      2. Mean cell hemoglobin (MCH)
      3. Mean cell hemoglobin concentration (MCHC)
      4. Red cell distribution width (RDW)
   C. White blood cell count
      1. Cell differential
      2. Nuclear segmentation of neutrophils
   D. Platelet count
   E. Cell morphology
      1. Cell size
      2. Hemoglobin content
      3. Anisocytosis
      4. Poikilocytosis
      5. Polychromasia

II. Iron supply studies
   A. Serum iron
   B. Total iron-binding capacity
   C. Serum ferritin

III. Marrow examination
   A. Aspirate
      1. M/E ratio[a]
      2. Cell morphology
      3. Iron stain
   B. Biopsy
      1. Cellularity
      2. Morphology

[a]M/E ratio, ratio of myeloid to erythroid precursors.

bone marrow aspirate or biopsy can assist in the diagnosis. Other tests of value in the diagnosis of specific anemias are discussed in chapters on specific disease states.

The components of the CBC also help in the classification of anemia. *Microcytosis* is reflected by a lower than normal MCV (<80), whereas high values (>100) reflect *macrocytosis*. The MCH and MCHC reflect defects in hemoglobin synthesis (*hypochromia*). Automated cell counters describe the red cell volume distribution width (RDW). The MCV (representing the peak of the distribution curve) is insensitive to the appearance of small populations of macrocytes or microcytes. An

TABLE 2-2

RED BLOOD CELL INDICES

INDEX	NORMAL VALUE
Mean cell volume (MCV) = (hematocrit × 10)/(red cell count × 10^6)	90 ± 8 fL
Mean cell hemoglobin (MCH) = (hemoglobin × 10)/(red cell count × 10^6)	30 ± 3 pg
Mean cell hemoglobin concentration = (hemoglobin × 10)/hematocrit, or MCH/MCV	33 ± 2%

TABLE 2-3

CHANGES IN NORMAL HEMOGLOBIN/HEMATOCRIT VALUES WITH AGE AND PREGNANCY

AGE/SEX	HEMOGLOBIN g/dL	HEMATOCRIT %
At birth	17	52
Childhood	12	36
Adolescence	13	40
Adult man	16 (±2)	47 (±6)
Adult woman (menstruating)	13 (±2)	40 (±6)
Adult woman (postmenopausal)	14 (±2)	42 (±6)
During pregnancy	12 (±2)	37 (±6)

Source: From RS Hillman et al: Hematology in Clinical Practice, 5th ed. New York, McGraw-Hill, 2010.

experienced laboratory technician will be able to identify minor populations of large or small cells or hypochromic cells before the red cell indices change.

Peripheral Blood Smear The peripheral blood smear provides important information about defects in red cell production (Chap. 6). As a complement to the red cell indices, the blood smear also reveals variations in cell size (*anisocytosis*) and shape (*poikilocytosis*). The degree of anisocytosis usually correlates with increases in the RDW or the range of cell sizes. Poikilocytosis suggests a defect in the maturation of red cell precursors in the bone marrow or fragmentation of circulating red cells. The blood smear may also reveal *polychromasia*—red cells that are slightly larger than normal and grayish blue in color on the Wright-Giemsa stain. These cells are reticulocytes that have been prematurely released from the bone marrow, and their color represents residual amounts of ribosomal RNA. These cells appear in circulation in response to EPO stimulation or to architectural damage of the bone marrow (fibrosis, infiltration of the marrow by malignant cells, etc.) that results in their disordered release from the marrow. The appearance of nucleated red cells, Howell-Jolly bodies, target cells, sickle cells, and others may provide clues to specific disorders (Figs. 2-3 to 2-11).

Reticulocyte Count An accurate reticulocyte count is key to the initial classification of anemia. Normally, reticulocytes are red cells that have been recently released from the bone marrow. They are identified by staining with a supravital dye that precipitates the ribosomal RNA (Fig. 2-12). These precipitates appear as blue or black punctate spots. This residual RNA is metabolized over the first 24–36 h of the reticulocyte's life span in circulation. Normally, the reticulocyte count ranges from 1 to 2% and reflects the daily replacement of 0.8–1.0% of the

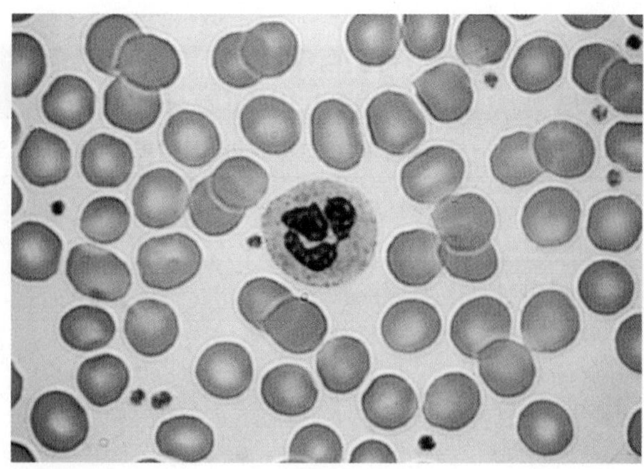

FIGURE 2-3
Normal blood smear (Wright stain). High-power field showing normal red cells, a neutrophil, and a few platelets. (*From RS Hillman et al: Hematology in Clinical Practice, 5th ed. New York, McGraw-Hill, 2010.*)

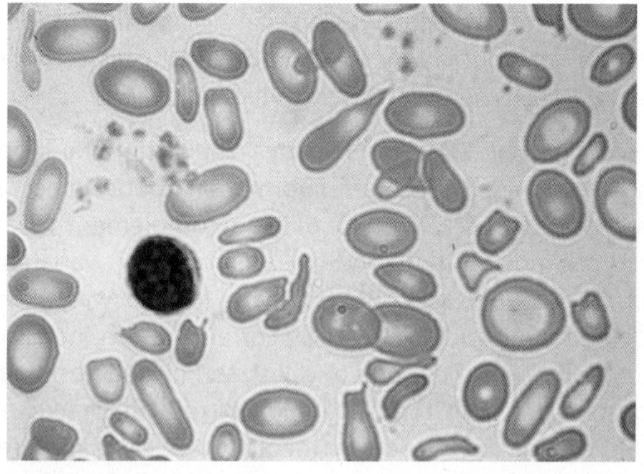

FIGURE 2-4
Severe iron-deficiency anemia. Microcytic and hypochromic red cells smaller than the nucleus of a lymphocyte associated with marked variation in size (anisocytosis) and shape (poikilocytosis). (*From RS Hillman et al: Hematology in Clinical Practice, 5th ed. New York, McGraw-Hill, 2010.*)

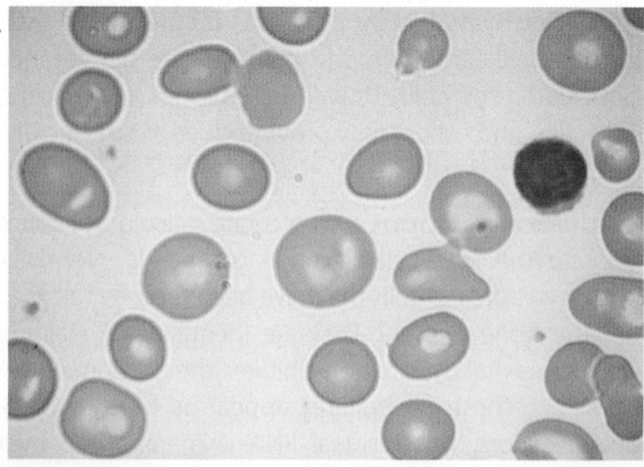

FIGURE 2-5
Macrocytosis. Red cells are larger than a small lymphocyte and well hemoglobinized. Often macrocytes are oval shaped (macro-ovalocytes).

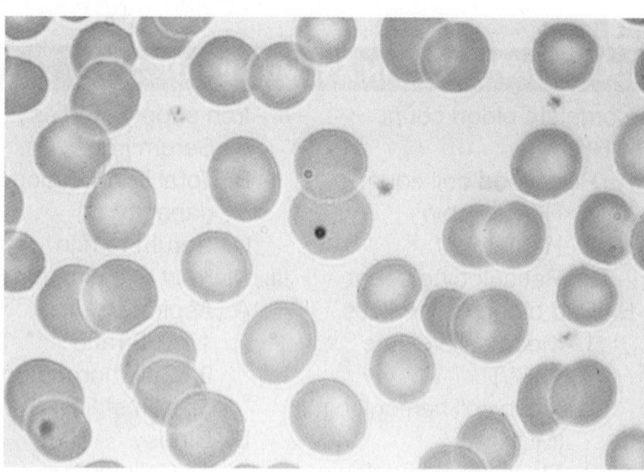

FIGURE 2-6
Howell-Jolly bodies. In the absence of a functional spleen, nuclear remnants are not culled from the red cells and remain as small homogeneously staining blue inclusions on Wright stain. (*From RS Hillman et al: Hematology in Clinical Practice, 5th ed. New York, McGraw-Hill, 2010.*)

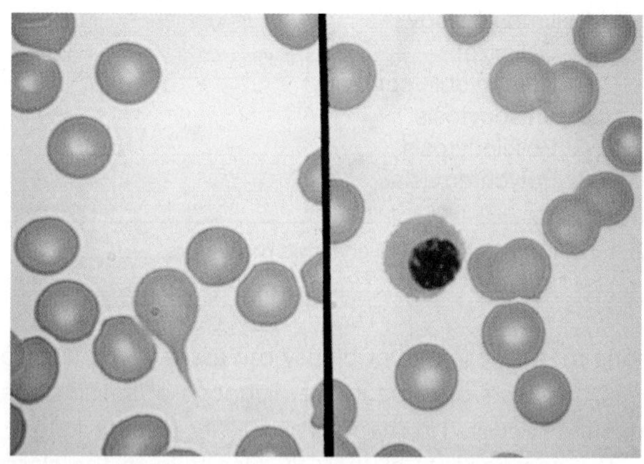

FIGURE 2-7
Red cell changes in myelofibrosis. The left panel shows a teardrop-shaped cell. The right panel shows a nucleated red cell. These forms are seen in myelofibrosis.

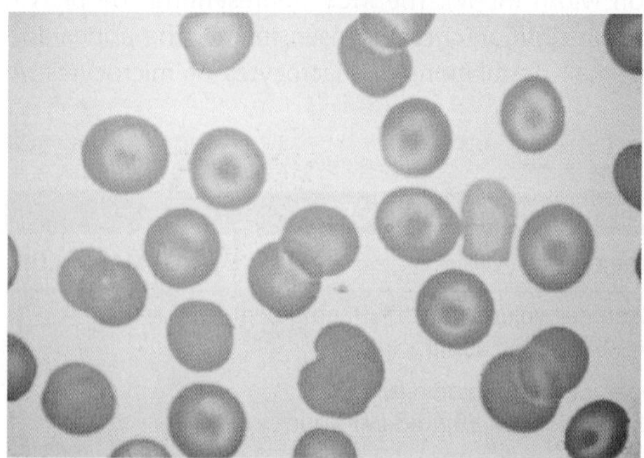

FIGURE 2-8
Target cells. Target cells have a bull's-eye appearance and are seen in thalassemia and in liver disease. (*From RS Hillman et al: Hematology in Clinical Practice, 5th ed. New York, McGraw-Hill, 2010.*)

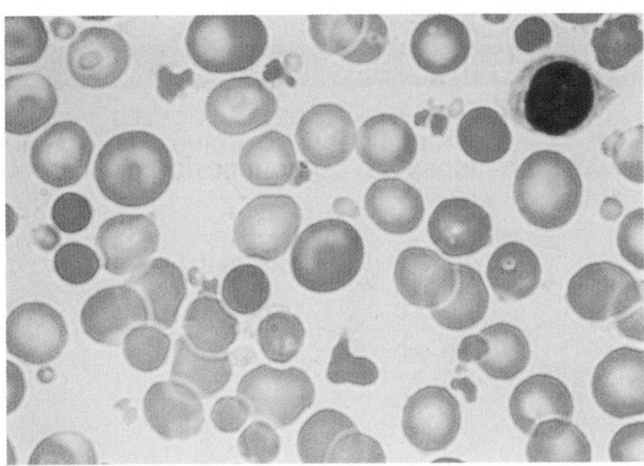

FIGURE 2-9
Red cell fragmentation. Red cells may become fragmented in the presence of foreign bodies in the circulation, such as mechanical heart valves, or in the setting of thermal injury. *(From RS Hillman et al: Hematology in Clinical Practice, 5th ed. New York, McGraw-Hill, 2010.)*

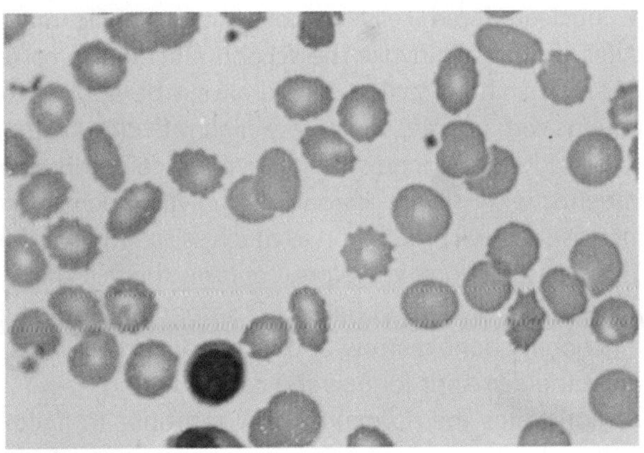

FIGURE 2-10
Uremia. The red cells in uremia may acquire numerous regularly spaced, small, spiny projections. Such cells, called burr cells or echinocytes, are readily distinguishable from irregularly spiculated acanthocytes shown in Fig. 2-11.

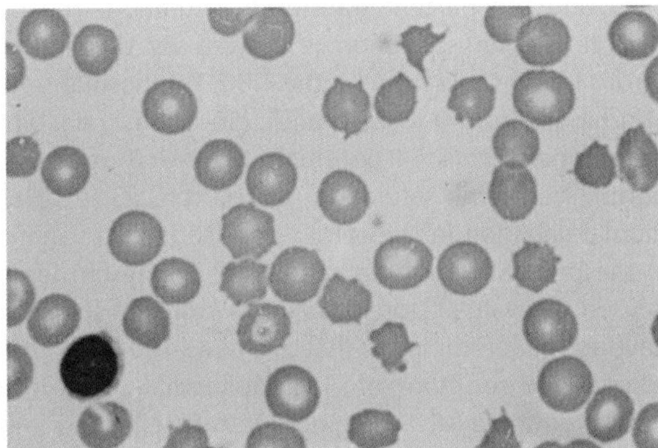

FIGURE 2-11
Spur cells. Spur cells are recognized as distorted red cells containing several irregularly distributed thornlike projections. Cells with this morphologic abnormality are also called acanthocytes. *(From RS Hillman et al: Hematology in Clinical Practice, 5th ed. New York, McGraw-Hill, 2010.)*

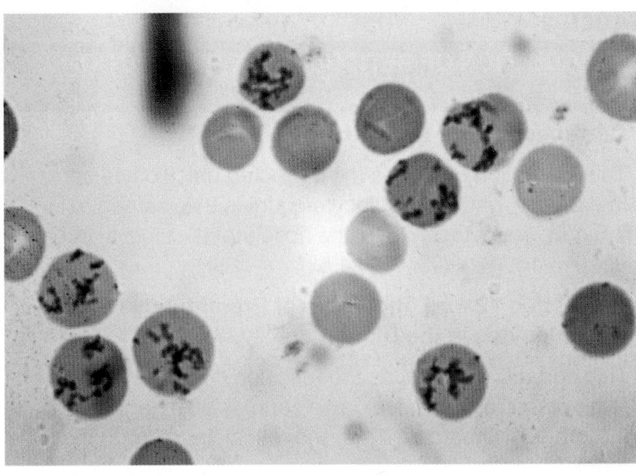

FIGURE 2-12
Reticulocytes. Methylene blue stain demonstrates residual RNA in newly made red cells. *(From RS Hillman et al: Hematology in Clinical Practice, 5th ed. New York, McGraw-Hill, 2010.)*

circulating red cell population. A corrected reticulocyte count provides a reliable measure of red cell production.

In the initial classification of anemia, the patient's reticulocyte count is compared with the expected reticulocyte response. In general, if the EPO and erythroid marrow responses to moderate anemia (hemoglobin <100 g/L [10 g/dL]) are intact, the red cell production rate increases to two to three times normal within 10 days following the onset of anemia. In the face of established anemia, a reticulocyte response less than two to three times normal indicates an inadequate marrow response.

In order to use the reticulocyte count to estimate marrow response, two corrections are necessary. The first correction adjusts the reticulocyte count based on the reduced number of circulating red cells. With anemia, the percentage of reticulocytes may be increased while the absolute number is unchanged. To correct for this effect, the reticulocyte percentage is multiplied by the ratio of the patient's hemoglobin or hematocrit to the expected hemoglobin or hematocrit for the age and gender of the patient (Table 2-4). This provides an estimate of the reticulocyte count corrected for anemia. In order to convert the corrected reticulocyte count to an index of marrow production, a further correction is required, depending on whether some of the reticulocytes in circulation have been released from the marrow prematurely. For this second correction, the peripheral blood smear is examined to see if there are polychromatophilic macrocytes present.

These cells, representing prematurely released reticulocytes, are referred to as "shift" cells, and the relationship between the degree of shift and the necessary shift correction factor is shown in Fig. 2-13. The correction is necessary because these prematurely released cells survive as reticulocytes in circulation for >1 day, thereby providing a falsely high estimate of daily red cell production. If polychromasia is increased, the reticulocyte

TABLE 2-4

CALCULATION OF RETICULOCYTE PRODUCTION INDEX

Correction #1 for Anemia:

This correction produces the corrected reticulocyte count
In a person whose reticulocyte count is 9%, hemoglobin 7.5 g/dL, hematocrit 23%, the absolute reticulocyte count = 9 × (7.5/15) [or × (23/45)]= 4.5%

Correction #2 for Longer Life of Prematurely Released Reticulocytes in the Blood:

This correction produces the reticulocyte production index
In a person whose reticulocyte count is 9%, hemoglobin 7.5 gm/dL, hematocrit 23%, the reticulocyte production index

$$= 9 \times \frac{(7.5/15)(\text{hemoglobin correction})}{2(\text{maturation timecorrection})} = 2.25$$

TABLE 2-5

NORMAL MARROW RESPONSE TO ANEMIA

HEMATOCRIT	PRODUCTION INDEX	RETICULOCYTES (INCLUDING CORRECTIONS)	MARROW M/E RATIO
45	1	1	3:1
35	2.0–3.0	4.8%/3.8/2.5	2:1–1:1
25	3.0–5.0	14%/8/4.0	1:1–1:2
15	3.0–5.0	30%/10/4.0	1:1–1:2

count, already corrected for anemia, should be divided again by 2 to account for the prolonged reticulocyte maturation time. The second correction factor varies from 1 to 3 depending on the severity of anemia. In general, a correction of 2 is commonly used. An appropriate correction is shown in Table 2-4. If polychromatophilic cells are not seen on the blood smear, the second correction is not required. The now doubly corrected reticulocyte count is the *reticulocyte production index*, and it provides an estimate of marrow production relative to normal.

Premature release of reticulocytes is normally due to increased EPO stimulation. However, if the integrity of the bone marrow release process is lost through tumor infiltration, fibrosis, or other disorders, the appearance of nucleated red cells or polychromatophilic macrocytes should still invoke the second reticulocyte correction. The shift correction should always be applied to a patient with anemia and a very high reticulocyte count to provide a true index of effective red cell production. Patients with severe chronic hemolytic anemia may increase red cell production as much as six- to sevenfold. This measure alone, therefore, confirms the fact that the patient has an appropriate EPO response, a normally functioning bone marrow, and sufficient iron available to meet the demands for new red cell formation. Table 2-5 demonstrates the normal marrow response to anemia. If the reticulocyte production index is <2 in the face of established anemia, a defect in erythroid marrow proliferation or maturation must be present.

Tests of Iron Supply and Storage The laboratory measurements that reflect the availability of iron for hemoglobin synthesis include the serum iron, the TIBC, and the percent transferrin saturation. The percent transferrin saturation is derived by dividing the serum iron level (× 100) by the TIBC. The normal serum iron ranges from 9 to 27 μmol/L (50–150 μg/dL), while the normal TIBC is 54–64 μmol/L (300–360 μg/dL); the normal transferrin saturation ranges from 25 to 50%. A diurnal variation in the serum iron leads to a variation in the percent transferrin saturation. The serum ferritin is used to evaluate total body iron stores. Adult males have serum ferritin levels that average ~100 μg/L, corresponding to iron stores of ~1 g. Adult females have lower serum ferritin levels averaging 30 μg/L, reflecting lower iron stores (~300 mg). A serum ferritin level of 10–15 μg/L represents depletion of body iron stores. However, ferritin is also an acute-phase reactant and, in the presence of acute or chronic inflammation, may rise severalfold above baseline levels. As a rule, a serum ferritin >200 μg/L means there is at least some iron in tissue stores.

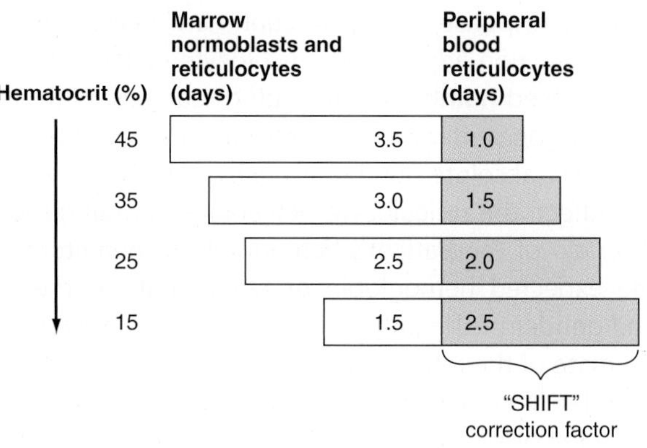

FIGURE 2-13

Correction of the reticulocyte count. In order to use the reticulocyte count as an indicator of effective red cell production, the reticulocyte percentage must be corrected based on the level of anemia and the circulating life span of the reticulocytes. Erythroid cells take ~4.5 days to mature. At a normal hemoglobin, reticulocytes are released to the circulation with ~1 day left as reticulocytes. However, with different levels of anemia, reticulocytes (and even earlier erythroid cells) may be released from the marrow prematurely. Most patients come to clinical attention with hematocrits in the mid-20s, and thus a correction factor of 2 is commonly used because the observed reticulocytes will live for 2 days in the circulation before losing their RNA.

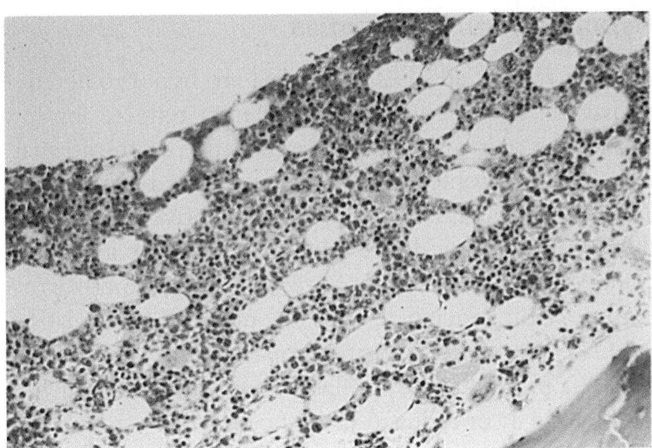

FIGURE 2-14
Normal bone marrow. This is a low-power view of a section of a normal bone marrow biopsy stained with hematoxylin and eosin (H&E). Note that the nucleated cellular elements account for ~40–50% and the fat (clear areas) accounts for ~50–60% of the area. (*From RS Hillman et al: Hematology in Clinical Practice, 5th ed. New York, McGraw-Hill, 2010.*)

Bone Marrow Examination A bone marrow aspirate and smear or a needle biopsy can be useful in the evaluation of some patients with anemia. In patients with hypoproliferative anemia and normal iron status, a bone marrow biopsy is indicated. Marrow examination can diagnose primary marrow disorders such as myelofibrosis, a red cell maturation defect, or an infiltrative disease (Figs. 2-14 to 2-16). The increase or decrease of one cell lineage (myeloid vs. erythroid) compared with another is obtained by a differential count of nucleated cells in a bone marrow smear (the myeloid/erythroid [M/E] ratio). A patient with a hypoproliferative anemia (see below) and a reticulocyte production index <2 will demonstrate an M/E ratio of 2 or 3:1. In contrast, patients with hemolytic disease and a production index >3 will have an M/E ratio of at least 1:1. Maturation disorders are identified from the discrepancy between the M/E ratio and the reticulocyte production index discussed later). Either the marrow smear or biopsy can be stained for the presence of iron stores or iron in developing red cells. The storage iron is in the form of ferritin or *hemosiderin*. On carefully prepared bone marrow smears, small ferritin granules can normally be seen under oil immersion in 20–40% of developing erythroblasts. Such cells are called *sideroblasts*.

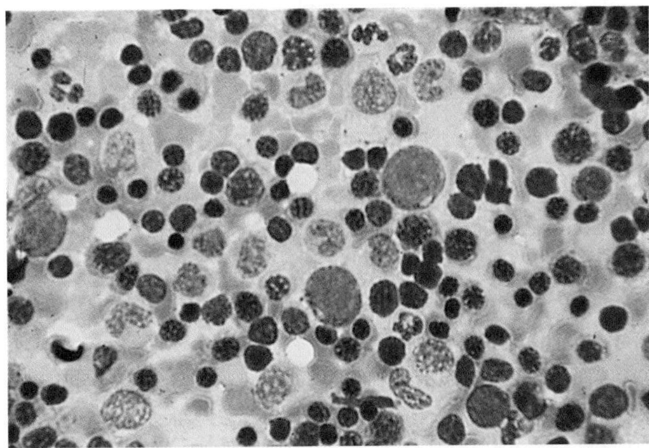

FIGURE 2-15
Erythroid hyperplasia. This marrow shows an increase in the fraction of cells in the erythroid lineage as might be seen when a normal marrow compensates for acute blood loss or hemolysis. The myeloid/erythroid ratio is about 1:1. (*From RS Hillman et al: Hematology in Clinical Practice, 5th ed. New York, McGraw-Hill, 2010.*)

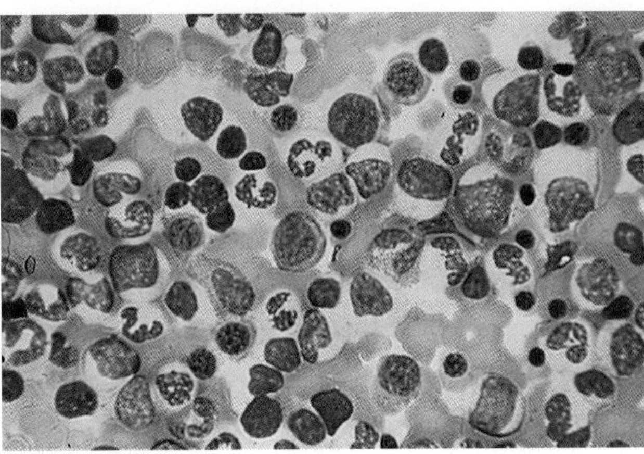

FIGURE 2-16
Myeloid hyperplasia. This marrow shows an increase in the fraction of cells in the myeloid or granulocytic lineage as might be seen in a normal marrow responding to infection. The myeloid/erythroid ratio is >3:1. (*From RS Hillman et al: Hematology in Clinical Practice, 5th ed. New York, McGraw-Hill, 2010.*)

OTHER LABORATORY MEASUREMENTS Additional laboratory tests may be of value in confirming specific diagnoses. For details of these tests and how they are applied in individual disorders, see Chaps. 7 to 11.

DEFINITION AND CLASSIFICATION OF ANEMIA

Initial classification of anemia

The functional classification of anemia has three major categories. These are (1) marrow production defects (*hypoproliferation*), (2) red cell maturation defects (*ineffective erythropoiesis*), and (3) decreased red cell survival (*blood loss or hemolysis*). The classification is shown in Fig. 2-17. A hypoproliferative anemia is typically seen with a low reticulocyte production index together with little or no change in red cell morphology (a normocytic, normochromic anemia) (Chap. 7). Maturation disorders typically have a slight to moderately elevated reticulocyte production index that is accompanied by

Algorithm of the Physiologic Classification of Anemia

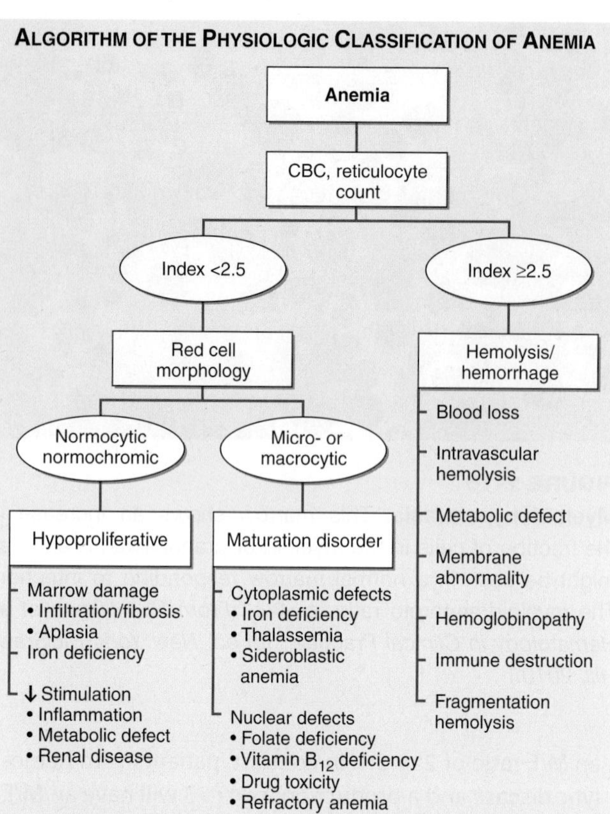

FIGURE 2-17

The physiologic classification of anemia. CBC, complete blood count.

either macrocytic (Chap. 9) or microcytic (Chaps. 7 and 8) red cell indices. Increased red blood cell destruction secondary to hemolysis results in an increase in the reticulocyte production index to at least three times normal (Chap. 10), provided sufficient iron is available. Hemorrhagic anemia does not typically result in production indices of more than 2.0–2.5 times normal because of the limitations placed on expansion of the erythroid marrow by iron availability.

In the first branch point of the classification of anemia, a reticulocyte production index >2.5 indicates that hemolysis is most likely. A reticulocyte production index <2 indicates either a hypoproliferative anemia or maturation disorder. The latter two possibilities can often be distinguished by the red cell indices, by examination of the peripheral blood smear, or by a marrow examination. If the red cell indices are normal, the anemia is almost certainly hypoproliferative in nature. Maturation disorders are characterized by ineffective red cell production and a low reticulocyte production index. Bizarre red cell shapes—macrocytes or hypochromic microcytes—are seen on the peripheral blood smear. With a hypoproliferative anemia, no erythroid hyperplasia is noted in the marrow, whereas patients with ineffective red cell production have erythroid hyperplasia and an M/E ratio <1:1.

Hypoproliferative anemias

At least 75% of all cases of anemia are hypoproliferative in nature. A hypoproliferative anemia reflects absolute or relative marrow failure in which the erythroid marrow has not proliferated appropriately for the degree of anemia. The majority of hypoproliferative anemias are due to mild to moderate iron deficiency or inflammation. A hypoproliferative anemia can result from marrow damage, iron deficiency, or inadequate EPO stimulation. The last may reflect impaired renal function, suppression of EPO production by inflammatory cytokines such as interleukin 1, or reduced tissue needs for O_2 from metabolic disease such as hypothyroidism. Only occasionally is the marrow unable to produce red cells at a normal rate, and this is most prevalent in patients with renal failure. With diabetes mellitus or myeloma, the EPO deficiency may be more marked than would be predicted by the degree of renal insufficiency. In general, hypoproliferative anemias are characterized by normocytic, normochromic red cells, although microcytic, hypochromic cells may be observed with mild iron deficiency or long-standing chronic inflammatory disease. The key laboratory tests in distinguishing between the various forms of hypoproliferative anemia include the serum iron and iron-binding capacity, evaluation of renal and thyroid function, a marrow biopsy or aspirate to detect marrow damage or infiltrative disease, and serum ferritin to assess iron stores. An iron stain of the marrow will determine the pattern of iron distribution. Patients with the anemia of acute or chronic inflammation show a distinctive pattern of serum iron (low), TIBC (normal or low), percent transferrin saturation (low), and serum ferritin (normal or high). These changes in iron values are brought about by hepcidin, the iron regulatory hormone that is increased in inflammation (Chap. 7). A distinct pattern of results is noted in mild to moderate iron deficiency (low serum iron, high TIBC, low percent transferrin saturation, low serum ferritin) (Chap. 7). Marrow damage by drugs, infiltrative disease such as leukemia and lymphoma, and marrow aplasia are diagnosed from the peripheral blood and bone marrow morphology. With infiltrative disease or fibrosis, a marrow biopsy is required.

Maturation disorders

The presence of anemia with an inappropriately low reticulocyte production index, macro- or microcytosis on smear, and abnormal red cell indices suggests a maturation disorder. Maturation disorders are divided into two categories: nuclear maturation defects, associated with macrocytosis, and cytoplasmic maturation defects, associated with microcytosis and hypochromia usually from defects in hemoglobin synthesis. The inappropriately low reticulocyte production index is a reflection of the ineffective erythropoiesis that results from the destruction within the marrow of developing erythroblasts. Bone marrow examination shows erythroid hyperplasia.

Nuclear maturation defects result from vitamin B_{12} or folic acid deficiency, drug damage, or myelodysplasia. Drugs that interfere with cellular DNA synthesis, such as methotrexate or alkylating agents, can produce a nuclear maturation defect. Alcohol, alone, is also capable of producing macrocytosis and a variable degree of anemia, but this is usually associated with folic acid deficiency. Measurements of folic acid and vitamin B_{12} are critical not only in identifying the specific vitamin deficiency but also because they reflect different pathogenetic mechanisms (Chap. 9).

Cytoplasmic maturation defects result from severe iron deficiency or abnormalities in globin or heme synthesis. Iron deficiency occupies an unusual position in the classification of anemia. If the iron-deficiency anemia is mild to moderate, erythroid marrow proliferation is blunted, and the anemia is classified as hypoproliferative. However, if the anemia is severe and prolonged, the erythroid marrow will become hyperplastic despite the inadequate iron supply, and the anemia will be classified as ineffective erythropoiesis with a cytoplasmic maturation defect. In either case, an inappropriately low reticulocyte production index, microcytosis, and a classic pattern of iron values make the diagnosis clear and easily distinguish iron deficiency from other cytoplasmic maturation defects such as the thalassemias. Defects in heme synthesis, in contrast to globin synthesis, are less common and may be acquired or inherited. Acquired abnormalities are usually associated with myelodysplasia, may lead to either a macro- or microcytic anemia, and are frequently associated with mitochondrial iron loading. In these cases, iron is taken up by the mitochondria of the developing erythroid cell but not incorporated into heme. The iron-encrusted mitochondria surround the nucleus of the erythroid cell, forming a ring. Based on the distinctive finding of so-called ringed sideroblasts on the marrow iron stain, patients are diagnosed as having a sideroblastic anemia—almost always reflecting myelodysplasia. Again, studies of iron parameters are helpful in the differential diagnosis of these patients.

Blood loss/hemolytic anemia

In contrast to anemias associated with an inappropriately low reticulocyte production index, hemolysis is associated with red cell production indices ≥2.5 times normal. The stimulated erythropoiesis is reflected in the blood smear by the appearance of increased numbers of polychromatophilic macrocytes. A marrow examination is rarely indicated if the reticulocyte production index is increased appropriately. The red cell indices are typically normocytic or slightly macrocytic, reflecting the increased number of reticulocytes. Acute blood loss is not associated with an increased reticulocyte production index because of the time required to increase EPO production and, subsequently, marrow proliferation. Subacute blood loss may be associated with modest reticulocytosis. Anemia from chronic blood loss presents more often as iron deficiency than with the picture of increased red cell production.

The evaluation of blood loss anemia is usually not difficult. Most problems arise when a patient presents with an increased red cell production index from an episode of acute blood loss that went unrecognized. The cause of the anemia and increased red cell production may not be obvious. The confirmation of a recovering state may require observations over a period of 2–3 weeks, during which the hemoglobin concentration will be seen to rise and the reticulocyte production index fall (Chap. 10).

Hemolytic disease, while dramatic, is among the least common forms of anemia. The ability to sustain a high reticulocyte production index reflects the ability of the erythroid marrow to compensate for hemolysis and, in the case of extravascular hemolysis, the efficient recycling of iron from the destroyed red cells to support red cell production. With intravascular hemolysis, such as paroxysmal nocturnal hemoglobinuria, the loss of iron may limit the marrow response. The level of response depends on the severity of the anemia and the nature of the underlying disease process.

Hemoglobinopathies, such as sickle cell disease and the thalassemias, present a mixed picture. The reticulocyte index may be high but is inappropriately low for the degree of marrow erythroid hyperplasia (Chap. 8).

Hemolytic anemias present in different ways. Some appear suddenly as an acute, self-limited episode of intravascular or extravascular hemolysis, a presentation pattern often seen in patients with autoimmune hemolysis or with inherited defects of the Embden-Meyerhof pathway or the glutathione reductase pathway. Patients with inherited disorders of the hemoglobin molecule or red cell membrane generally have a lifelong clinical history typical of the disease process. Those with chronic hemolytic disease, such as hereditary spherocytosis, may actually present not with anemia but with a complication stemming from the prolonged increase in red cell destruction such as symptomatic bilirubin gallstones or splenomegaly. Patients with chronic hemolysis are also susceptible to aplastic crises if an infectious process interrupts red cell production.

The differential diagnosis of an acute or chronic hemolytic event requires the careful integration of family history, the pattern of clinical presentation, and—whether the disease is congenital or acquired—a careful examination of the peripheral blood smear.

Precise diagnosis may require more specialized laboratory tests, such as hemoglobin electrophoresis or a screen for red cell enzymes. Acquired defects in red cell survival are often immunologically mediated and require a direct or indirect antiglobulin test or a cold agglutinin titer to detect the presence of hemolytic antibodies or complement-mediated red cell destruction (Chap. 10).

TREATMENT Anemia

An overriding principle is to initiate treatment of mild to moderate anemia only when a specific diagnosis is made. Rarely, in the acute setting, anemia may be so severe that red cell transfusions are required before a specific diagnosis is made. Whether the anemia is of acute or gradual onset, the selection of the appropriate treatment is determined by the documented cause(s) of the anemia. Often, the cause of the anemia is multifactorial. For example, a patient with severe rheumatoid arthritis who has been taking anti-inflammatory drugs may have a hypoproliferative anemia associated with chronic inflammation as well as chronic blood loss associated with intermittent gastrointestinal bleeding. In every circumstance, it is important to evaluate the patient's iron status fully before and during the treatment of any anemia. Transfusion is discussed in Chap. 12; iron therapy is discussed in Chap. 7; treatment of megaloblastic anemia is discussed in Chap. 9; treatment of other entities is discussed in their respective chapters (sickle cell anemia, Chap. 8; hemolytic anemias, Chap. 10; aplastic anemia and myelodysplasia, Chap. 11).

Therapeutic options for the treatment of anemias have expanded dramatically during the past 25 years. Blood component therapy is available and safe. Recombinant EPO as an adjunct to anemia management has transformed the lives of patients with chronic renal failure on dialysis and reduced transfusion needs of anemic cancer patients receiving chemotherapy. Eventually, patients with inherited disorders of globin synthesis or mutations in the globin gene, such as sickle cell disease, may benefit from the successful introduction of targeted genetic therapy.

POLYCYTHEMIA

Polycythemia is defined as an increase in the hemoglobin above normal. This increase may be real or only apparent because of a decrease in plasma volume (spurious or relative polycythemia). The term *erythrocytosis* may be used interchangeably with *polycythemia*, but some draw a distinction between them: erythrocytosis implies documentation of increased red cell mass, whereas polycythemia refers to any increase in red cells. Often patients with polycythemia are detected through an incidental finding of elevated hemoglobin or hematocrit levels. Concern that the hemoglobin level may be abnormally high is usually triggered at 170 g/L (17 g/dL) for men and 150 g/L (15 g/dL) for women. Hematocrit levels >50% in men or >45% in women may be abnormal. Hematocrits >60% in men and >55% in women are almost invariably associated with an increased red cell mass. Given that the machine that quantitates red cell parameters actually measures hemoglobin concentrations and calculates hematocrits, hemoglobin levels may be a better index.

Features of the clinical history that are useful in the differential diagnosis include smoking history; current living at high altitude; or a history of congenital heart disease, sleep apnea, or chronic lung disease.

Patients with polycythemia may be asymptomatic or experience symptoms related to the increased red cell mass or the underlying disease process that leads to the increased red cell mass. The dominant symptoms from an increased red cell mass are related to hyperviscosity and thrombosis (both venous and arterial) because the blood viscosity increases logarithmically at hematocrits >55%. Manifestations range from digital ischemia to Budd-Chiari syndrome with hepatic vein thrombosis. Abdominal vessel thromboses are particularly common. Neurologic symptoms such as vertigo, tinnitus, headache, and visual disturbances may occur. Hypertension is often present. Patients with *polycythemia vera* may have aquagenic pruritus and symptoms related to hepatosplenomegaly. Patients may have easy bruising, epistaxis, or bleeding from the gastrointestinal tract. Peptic ulcer disease is common. Patients with hypoxemia may develop cyanosis on minimal exertion or have headache, impaired mental acuity, and fatigue.

The physical examination usually reveals a ruddy complexion. Splenomegaly favors polycythemia vera as the diagnosis (Chap. 13). The presence of cyanosis or evidence of a right-to-left shunt suggests congenital heart disease presenting in the adult, particularly tetralogy of Fallot or Eisenmenger's syndrome. Increased blood viscosity raises pulmonary artery pressure; hypoxemia can lead to increased pulmonary vascular resistance. Together, these factors can produce cor pulmonale.

Polycythemia can be spurious (related to a decrease in plasma volume; Gaisbock's syndrome), primary, or secondary in origin. The secondary causes are all associated with increases in EPO levels: either a physiologically adapted appropriate elevation based on tissue hypoxia (lung disease, high altitude, CO poisoning, high-affinity hemoglobinopathy) or an abnormal overproduction (renal cysts, renal artery stenosis, tumors with ectopic EPO production). A rare familial form of polycythemia is associated with normal EPO levels but hyperresponsive EPO receptors due to mutations.

APPROACH TO THE PATIENT Polycythemia

As shown in Fig. 2-18, the first step is to document the presence of an increased red cell mass using the principle of isotope dilution by administering ^{51}Cr-labeled autologous red blood cells to the patient and sampling blood radioactivity over a 2-h period. If the red cell mass is normal (<36 mL/kg in men, <32 mL/kg in women), the patient has spurious or relative polycythemia. If the red cell mass is increased (>36 mL/kg in men, >32 mL/kg in women), serum EPO levels should be measured. If EPO levels are low or unmeasurable, the patient most likely has polycythemia vera. Tests that support this diagnosis include an elevated white blood cell count, increased absolute basophil count, and thrombocytosis. A mutation in *JAK-2* (Val617Phe), a key member of the cytokine intracellular signaling pathway, can be found in 70–95% of patients with polycythemia vera.

If serum EPO levels are elevated, one needs to distinguish whether the elevation is a physiologic response to hypoxia or is related to autonomous EPO production. Patients with low arterial O_2 saturation (<92%) should be further evaluated for the presence of heart or lung disease if they are not living at high altitude. Patients with normal O_2 saturation who are smokers may have elevated EPO levels because of CO displacement of O_2. If carboxyhemoglobin (COHb) levels are high, the diagnosis is "smoker's polycythemia." Such patients should be urged to stop smoking. Those who cannot stop smoking require phlebotomy to control their polycythemia. Patients with normal O_2 saturation who do not smoke either have an abnormal hemoglobin that does not deliver O_2 to the tissues (evaluated by finding elevated O_2–hemoglobin affinity) or have a source of EPO production that is not responding to the normal feedback inhibition. Further workup is dictated by the differential diagnosis of EPO-producing neoplasms. Hepatoma, uterine leiomyoma, and renal cancer or cysts are all detectable with abdominopelvic CT scans. Cerebellar hemangiomas may produce EPO, but they present with localizing neurologic signs and symptoms rather than polycythemia-related symptoms.

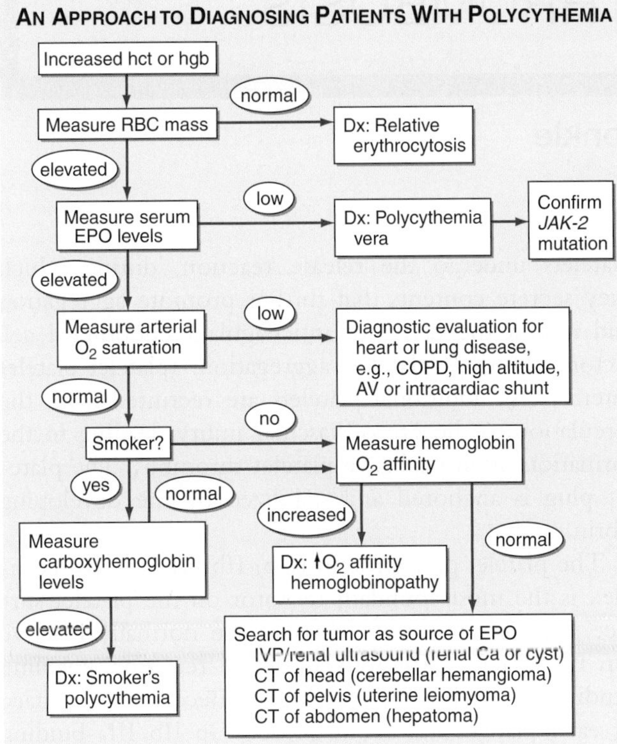

FIGURE 2-18

An approach to the differential diagnosis of patients with an elevated hemoglobin (possible polycythemia). AV, atrioventricular; COPD, chronic obstructive pulmonary disease; CT, computed tomography; Dx, diagnosis; EPO, erythropoietin; hct, hematocrit; IVP, intravenous pyelogram; RBC, red blood cell.

CHAPTER 3

BLEEDING AND THROMBOSIS

Barbara Konkle

The human hemostatic system provides a natural balance between procoagulant and anticoagulant forces. The procoagulant forces include platelet adhesion and aggregation and fibrin clot formation; anticoagulant forces include the natural inhibitors of coagulation and fibrinolysis. Under normal circumstances, hemostasis is regulated to promote blood flow; however, it is also prepared to clot blood rapidly to arrest blood flow and prevent exsanguination. After bleeding is successfully halted, the system remodels the damaged vessel to restore normal blood flow. The major components of the hemostatic system, which function in concert, are (1) platelets and other formed elements of blood, such as monocytes and red cells; (2) plasma proteins (the coagulation and fibrinolytic factors and inhibitors); and (3) the vessel wall.

STEPS OF NORMAL HEMOSTASIS

PLATELET PLUG FORMATION

On vascular injury, platelets adhere to the site of injury, usually the denuded vascular intimal surface. Platelet adhesion is mediated primarily by von Willebrand factor (VWF), a large multimeric protein present in both plasma and the extracellular matrix of the subendothelial vessel wall, which serves as the primary "molecular glue," providing sufficient strength to withstand the high levels of shear stress that would tend to detach them with the flow of blood. Platelet adhesion is also facilitated by direct binding to subendothelial collagen through specific platelet membrane collagen receptors.

Platelet adhesion results in subsequent platelet activation and aggregation. This process is enhanced and amplified by humoral mediators in plasma (e.g., epinephrine, thrombin); mediators released from activated platelets (e.g., adenosine diphosphate, serotonin); and vessel wall extracellular matrix constituents that come in contact with adherent platelets (e.g., collagen, VWF). Activated platelets undergo the release reaction, during which they secrete contents that further promote aggregation and inhibit the naturally anticoagulant endothelial cell factors. During platelet aggregation (platelet-platelet interaction), additional platelets are recruited from the circulation to the site of vascular injury, leading to the formation of an occlusive platelet thrombus. The platelet plug is anchored and stabilized by the developing fibrin mesh.

The platelet glycoprotein (Gp) IIb/IIIa ($\alpha_{IIb}\beta_3$) complex is the most abundant receptor on the platelet surface. Platelet activation converts the normally inactive Gp IIb/IIIa receptor into an active receptor, enabling binding to fibrinogen and VWF. Because the surface of each platelet has about 50,000 Gp IIb/IIIa-binding sites, numerous activated platelets recruited to the site of vascular injury can rapidly form an occlusive aggregate by means of a dense network of intercellular fibrinogen bridges. Since this receptor is the key mediator of platelet aggregation, it has become an effective target for antiplatelet therapy.

FIBRIN CLOT FORMATION

Plasma coagulation proteins (*clotting factors*) normally circulate in plasma in their inactive forms. The sequence of coagulation protein reactions that culminate in the formation of fibrin was originally described as a *waterfall* or a *cascade*. Two pathways of blood coagulation have been described in the past: the so-called extrinsic, or tissue factor, pathway and the so-called intrinsic, or contact activation, pathway. We now know that coagulation is normally initiated through tissue factor (TF) exposure and activation through the classic *extrinsic pathway* but with critically important amplification through elements of the classic *intrinsic pathway*, as illustrated in Fig. 3-1. These reactions take place on phospholipid surfaces, usually the activated platelet surface. Coagulation testing in the laboratory can reflect other influences

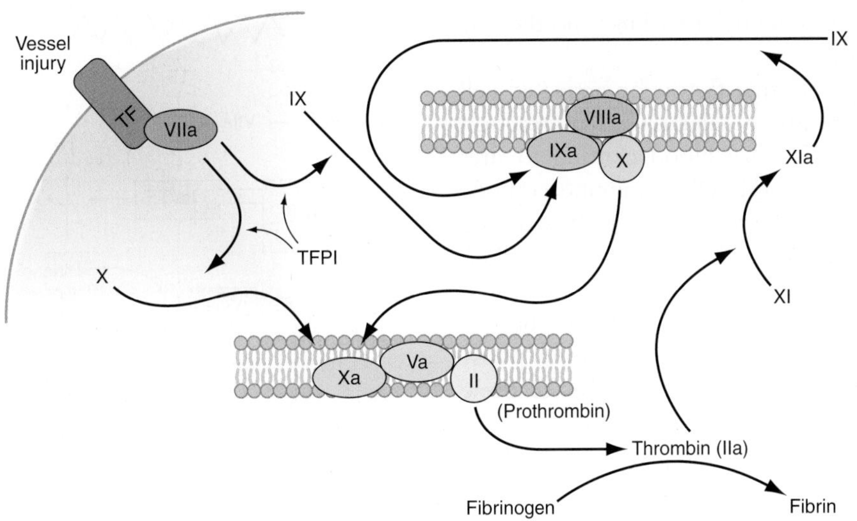

FIGURE 3-1

Coagulation is initiated by tissue factor (TF) exposure, which, with factor (F)VIIa, activates FIX and FX, which in turn, with FVIII and FV as cofactors, respectively, results in thrombin formation and subsequent conversion of fibrinogen to fibrin. Thrombin activates FXI, FVIII, and FV, amplifying the coagulation signal. Once the TF/FVIIa/FXa complex is formed, tissue factor pathway inhibitor (TFPI) inhibits the TF/FVIIa pathway, making coagulation dependent on the amplification loop through FIX/FVIII. Coagulation requires calcium (not shown) and takes place on phospholipid surfaces, usually the activated platelet membrane.

due to the artificial nature of the in vitro systems used (discussed later).

The immediate trigger for coagulation is vascular damage that exposes blood to TF that is constitutively expressed on the surfaces of subendothelial cellular components of the vessel wall, such as smooth muscle cells and fibroblasts. TF is also present in circulating microparticles, presumably shed from cells including monocytes and platelets. TF binds the serine protease factor VIIa; the complex activates factor X to factor Xa. Alternatively, the complex can indirectly activate factor X by initially converting factor IX to factor IXa, which then activates factor X. The participation of factor XI in hemostasis is not dependent on its activation by factor XIIa but rather on its positive feedback activation by thrombin. Thus, factor XIa functions in the propagation and amplification, rather than in the initiation, of the coagulation cascade.

Factor Xa can be formed through the actions of either the tissue factor/factor VIIa complex or factor IXa (with factor VIIIa as a cofactor) and converts prothrombin to thrombin, the pivotal protease of the coagulation system. The essential cofactor for this reaction is factor Va. Like the homologous factor VIIIa, factor Va is produced by thrombin-induced limited proteolysis of factor V. Thrombin is a multifunctional enzyme that converts soluble plasma fibrinogen to an insoluble fibrin matrix. Fibrin polymerization involves an orderly process of intermolecular associations (Fig. 3-2). Thrombin also activates factor XIII (fibrin-stabilizing factor)

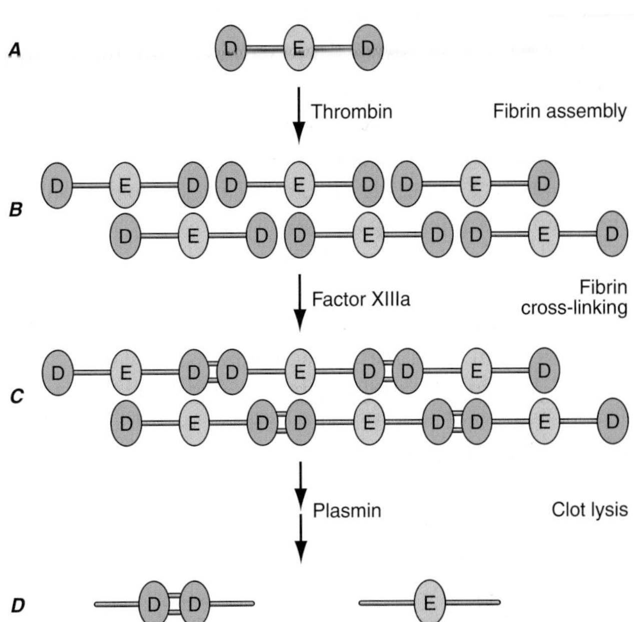

FIGURE 3-2

Fibrin formation and dissolution. (***A***). Fibrinogen is a trinodular structure consisting of 2 D domains and 1 E domain. Thrombin activation results in an ordered lateral assembly of protofibrils (***B***) with noncovalent associations. FXIIIa cross-links the D domains on adjacent molecules (***C***). Fibrin and fibrinogen (not shown) lysis by plasmin occurs at discrete sites and results in intermediary fibrin(ogen) degradation products (not shown). D-Dimers are the product of complete lysis of fibrin (***D***), maintaining the cross-linked D domains.

to factor XIIIa, which covalently cross-links and thereby stabilizes the fibrin clot.

The assembly of the clotting factors on activated cell membrane surfaces greatly accelerates their reaction rates and also serves to localize blood clotting to sites of vascular injury. The critical cell membrane components, acidic phospholipids, are not normally exposed on resting cell membrane surfaces. However, when platelets, monocytes, and endothelial cells are activated by vascular injury or inflammatory stimuli, the procoagulant head groups of the membrane anionic phospholipids become translocated to the surfaces of these cells or released as part of microparticles, making them available to support and promote the plasma coagulation reactions.

ANTITHROMBOTIC MECHANISMS

Several physiologic antithrombotic mechanisms act in concert to prevent clotting under normal circumstances. These mechanisms operate to preserve blood fluidity and to limit blood clotting to specific focal sites of vascular injury. Endothelial cells have many antithrombotic effects. They produce prostacyclin, nitric oxide, and ectoADPase/CD39, which act to inhibit platelet binding, secretion, and aggregation. Endothelial cells produce anticoagulant factors including heparan proteoglycans, antithrombin, TF pathway inhibitor, and thrombomodulin. They also activate fibrinolytic mechanisms through the production of tissue plasminogen activator 1, urokinase, plasminogen activator inhibitor, and annexin-2. The sites of action of the major physiologic antithrombotic pathways are shown in Fig. 3-3.

Antithrombin (or antithrombin III) is the major plasma protease inhibitor of thrombin and the other clotting factors in coagulation. Antithrombin neutralizes thrombin and other activated coagulation factors by forming a complex between the active site of the enzyme and the reactive center of antithrombin. The rate of formation of these inactivating complexes increases by a factor of several thousand in the presence of heparin. Antithrombin inactivation of thrombin and other activated clotting factors occurs physiologically on vascular surfaces, where glycosoaminoglycans, including heparan sulfates, are present to catalyze these reactions. Inherited quantitative or qualitative deficiencies of antithrombin lead to a lifelong predisposition to venous thromboembolism.

Protein C is a plasma glycoprotein that becomes an anticoagulant when it is activated by thrombin. The thrombin-induced activation of protein C occurs physiologically on thrombomodulin, a transmembrane proteoglycan-binding site for thrombin on endothelial cell surfaces. The binding of protein C to its receptor on endothelial cells places it in proximity to the

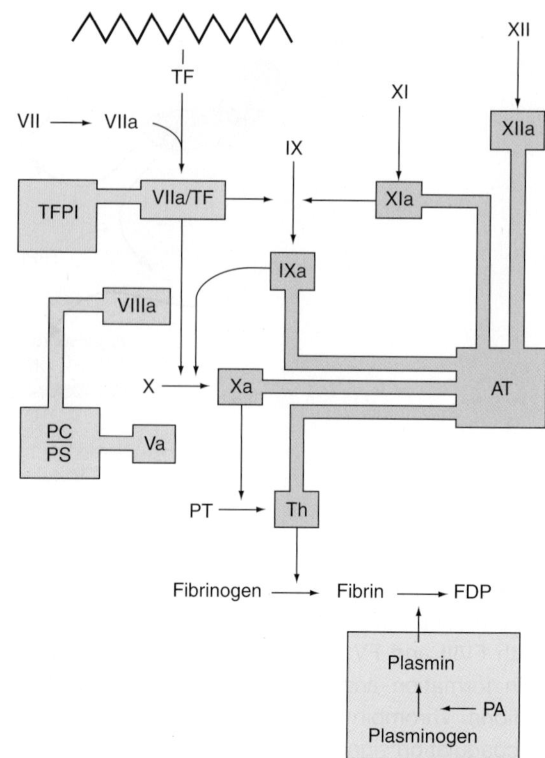

FIGURE 3-3
Sites of action of the four major physiologic antithrombotic pathways: antithrombin (AT); protein C/S (PC/PS); tissue factor pathway inhibitor (TFPI); and the fibrinolytic system, consisting of plasminogen, plasminogen activator (PA), and plasmin. FDP, fibrin(ogen) degradation products. PT, prothrombin; Th, thrombin; (*Modified from BA Konkle, AI Schafer, in DP Zipes et al [eds]: Braunwald's Heart Disease, 7th ed. Philadelphia, Saunders, 2005.*)

thrombin–thrombomodulin complex, thereby enhancing its activation efficiency. Activated protein C acts as an anticoagulant by cleaving and inactivating activated factors V and VIII. This reaction is accelerated by a cofactor, protein S, which, like protein C, is a glycoprotein that undergoes vitamin K–dependent posttranslational modification. Quantitative or qualitative deficiencies of protein C or protein S, or resistance to the action of activated protein C by a specific mutation at its target cleavage site in factor Va (factor V Leiden), lead to hypercoagulable states.

Tissue factor pathway inhibitor (TFPI) is a plasma protease inhibitor that regulates the TF-induced extrinsic pathway of coagulation. TFPI inhibits the TF/FVIIa/FXa complex, essentially turning off the TF/FVIIa initiation of coagulation, which then becomes dependent on the "amplification loop" via FXI and FVIII activation by thrombin. TFPI is bound to lipoprotein and can also be released by heparin from endothelial cells, where it is bound to glycosoaminoglycans, and from platelets. The heparin-mediated release of TFPI may play a role in the anticoagulant effects of unfractionated and low-molecular-weight heparins.

THE FIBRINOLYTIC SYSTEM

Any thrombin that escapes the inhibitory effects of the physiologic anticoagulant systems is available to convert fibrinogen to fibrin. In response, the endogenous fibrinolytic system is then activated to dispose of intravascular fibrin and thereby maintain or reestablish the patency of the circulation. Just as thrombin is the key protease enzyme of the coagulation system, plasmin is the major protease enzyme of the fibrinolytic system, acting to digest fibrin to fibrin degradation products. The general scheme of fibrinolysis and its control is shown in Fig. 3-4.

The plasminogen activators, tissue type plasminogen activator (tPA) and the urokinase type plasminogen activator cleave (uPA), cleave the Arg560-Val561 bond of plasminogen to generate the active enzyme plasmin. The lysine-binding sites of plasmin (and plasminogen) permit it to bind to fibrin, so that physiologic fibrinolysis is "fibrin specific." Both plasminogen (through its lysine-binding sites) and tPA possess specific affinity for fibrin and thereby bind selectively to clots. The assembly of a ternary complex, consisting of fibrin, plasminogen, and tPA, promotes the localized interaction between plasminogen and tPA and greatly accelerates the rate of plasminogen activation to plasmin. Moreover, partial degradation of fibrin by plasmin exposes new plasminogen and tPA-binding sites in carboxy-terminus lysine residues of fibrin fragments to enhance these reactions further. This creates a highly efficient mechanism to generate plasmin focally on the fibrin clot, which then becomes plasmin's substrate for digestion to fibrin degradation products. Plasmin cleaves fibrin at distinct sites of the fibrin molecule, leading to the generation of characteristic fibrin fragments during the process of fibrinolysis (Fig. 3-2). The sites of plasmin cleavage of fibrin are the same as those in fibrinogen. However, when plasmin acts on covalently cross-linked fibrin, D-dimers are released; hence, D-dimers can be measured in plasma as a relatively specific test of fibrin (rather than fibrinogen) degradation. D-dimer assays can be used as sensitive markers of blood clot formation, and some have been validated for clinical use to exclude the diagnosis of deep-venous thrombosis (DVT) and pulmonary embolism in selected populations.

Physiologic regulation of fibrinolysis occurs primarily at three levels: (1) plasminogen activator inhibitors (PAIs), specifically PAI-1 and PAI-2, inhibit the physiologic plasminogen activators; (2) the thrombin-activatable fibrinolysis inhibitor (TAFI) limits fibrinolysis; and (3) α_2-antiplasmin inhibits plasmin. PAI1 is the primary inhibitor of tPA and uPA in plasma. TAFI cleaves the N-terminal lysine residues of fibrin, which aid in localization of plasmin activity. α_2-Antiplasmin is the main inhibitor of plasmin in human plasma, inactivating any non–fibrin clot–associated plasmin.

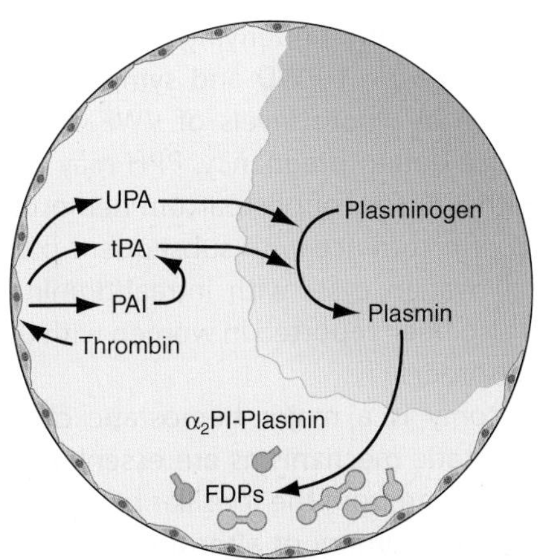

FIGURE 3-4

A schematic diagram of the fibrinolytic system. Tissue plasminogen activator (tPA) is released from endothelial cells, binds the fibrin clot, and activates plasminogen to plasmin. Excess fibrin is degraded by plasmin to distinct degradation products (FDPs). Any free plasmin is complexed with α_2-antiplasmin (α_2PI). PAI, plasminogen activator inhibitor; UPA, urokinase type plasminogen activator.

APPROACH TO THE PATIENT: Bleeding and Thrombosis

CLINICAL PRESENTATION Disorders of hemostasis may be either inherited or acquired. A detailed personal and family history is key in determining the chronicity of symptoms and the likelihood of the disorder being inherited, and it provides clues to underlying conditions that have contributed to the bleeding or thrombotic state. In addition, the history can give clues as to the etiology by determining (1) the bleeding (mucosal and/or joint) or thrombosis (arterial and/or venous) site and (2) whether an underlying bleeding or clotting tendency was enhanced by another medical condition or the introduction of medications or dietary supplements.

History of Bleeding A history of bleeding is the most important predictor of bleeding risk. In evaluating a patient for a bleeding disorder, a history of at-risk situations, including the response to past surgeries, should be assessed. Does the patient have a history of spontaneous or trauma- or surgery-induced bleeding? Spontaneous hemarthroses are a hallmark of moderate and severe factor VIII and IX deficiency and, in rare circumstances, of other clotting factor deficiencies. Mucosal bleeding symptoms are more suggestive of underlying platelet disorders or von Willebrand disease (VWD), termed *disorders of primary hemostasis or platelet plug formation.* Disorders affecting primary hemostasis are shown in Table 3-1.

A bleeding score has been validated as a tool to predict patients more likely to have Type 1 VWD. Studies are under way to validate additional formats, including ones that are easier to administer and improving performance in pediatric populations. Bleeding symptoms that appear to be more common in patients with bleeding disorders include prolonged bleeding with surgery, dental procedures and extractions, and/or trauma; menorrhagia or postpartum hemorrhage; and large bruises (often described with lumps).

Easy bruising and menorrhagia are common complaints in patients with and without bleeding disorders. Easy bruising can also be a sign of medical conditions in which there is no identifiable coagulopathy; instead, the conditions are caused by an abnormality of blood vessels or their supporting tissues. In Ehlers-Danlos syndrome, there may be posttraumatic bleeding and a history of joint hyperextensibility. Cushing's syndrome, chronic steroid use, and aging result in changes in skin and subcutaneous tissue, and subcutaneous bleeding occurs in response to minor trauma. The latter has been termed *senile purpura.*

TABLE 3-1

PRIMARY HEMOSTATIC (PLATELET PLUG) DISORDERS
Defects of Platelet Adhesion
Von Willebrand disease
Bernard-Soulier syndrome (absence of dysfunction of GpIb-IX-V)
Defects of Platelet Aggregation
Glanzmann's thrombasthenia (absence or dysfunction of GpIIbIIIa)
Afibrinogenemia
Defects of Platelet Secretion
Decreased cyclooxygenase activity
Drug-induced (aspirin, nonsteroidal anti-inflammatory agents, thienopyridines)
Inherited
Granule storage pool defects
Inherited
Acquired
Nonspecific inherited secretory defects
Nonspecific drug effects
Uremia
Platelet coating (e.g., paraprotein, penicillin)
Defect of Platelet Coagulant Activity
Scott's syndrome

Epistaxis is a common symptom, particularly in children and in dry climates, and may not reflect an underlying bleeding disorder. However, it is the most common symptom in hereditary hemorrhagic telangiectasia and in boys with VWD. Clues that epistaxis is a symptom of an underlying bleeding disorder include lack of seasonal variation and bleeding that requires medical evaluation or treatment, including cauterization. Bleeding with eruption of primary teeth is seen in children with more severe bleeding disorders, such as moderate and severe hemophilia. It is uncommon in children with mild bleeding disorders. Patients with disorders of primary hemostasis (platelet adhesion) may have increased bleeding after dental cleanings and other procedures that involve gum manipulation.

Menorrhagia is defined quantitatively as a loss of >80 mL of blood per cycle, based on blood loss required to produce iron-deficiency anemia. A complaint of heavy menses is subjective and has a poor correlation with excessive blood loss. Predictors of menorrhagia include bleeding resulting in iron-deficiency anemia or a need for blood transfusion, passage of clots >1 inch in diameter, and changing a pad or tampon more than hourly. Menorrhagia is a common symptom in women with underlying bleeding disorders and is reported in the majority of women with VWD and factor XI deficiency and in symptomatic carriers of hemophilia A. Women with underlying bleeding disorders are more likely to have other bleeding symptoms, including bleeding after dental extractions, postoperative bleeding, and postpartum bleeding, and are much more likely to have menorrhagia beginning at menarche than women with menorrhagia due to other causes.

Postpartum hemorrhage (PPH) is a common symptom in women with underlying bleeding disorders. In women with type 1 VWD and symptomatic carriers of hemophilia in whom levels of VWF and FVIII usually normalize during pregnancy, PPH may be delayed. Women with a history of postpartum hemorrhage have a high risk of recurrence with subsequent pregnancies. Rupture of ovarian cysts with intraabdominal hemorrhage has also been reported in women with underlying bleeding disorders.

Tonsillectomy is a major hemostatic challenge, as intact hemostatic mechanisms are essential to prevent excessive bleeding from the tonsillar bed. Bleeding may occur early after surgery or after approximately 7 days postoperatively, with loss of the eschar at the operative site. Similar delayed bleeding is seen after colonic polyp resection. Gastrointestinal (GI) bleeding and hematuria are usually due to underlying pathology, and procedures to identify and treat the bleeding site should be undertaken, even in patients with known bleeding disorders. VWD, particularly types 2 and 3, has been associated with angiodysplasia of the bowel and GI bleeding.

Hemarthroses and spontaneous muscle hematomas are characteristic of moderate or severe congenital factor VIII or IX deficiency. They can also be seen in moderate and severe deficiencies of fibrinogen; prothrombin; and of factors V, VII, and X. Spontaneous hemarthroses occur rarely in other bleeding disorders except for severe VWD, with associated FVIII levels <5%. Muscle and soft tissue bleeds are also common in acquired FVIII deficiency. Bleeding into a joint results in severe pain and swelling, as well as loss of function, but is rarely associated with discoloration from bruising around the joint. Life-threatening sites of bleeding include bleeding into the oropharynx, where bleeding can obstruct the airway, into the central nervous system, and into the retroperitoneum. Central nervous system bleeding is the major cause of bleeding-related deaths in patients with severe congenital factor deficiencies.

Prohemorrhagic Effects of Medications and Dietary Supplements Aspirin and other nonsteroidal anti-inflammatory drugs (NSAIDs) that inhibit cyclooxygenase 1 impair primary hemostasis and may exacerbate bleeding from another cause or even unmask a previously occult mild bleeding disorder such as VWD. All NSAIDs, however, can precipitate GI bleeding, which may be more severe in patients with underlying bleeding disorders. The aspirin effect on platelet function as assessed by aggregometry can persist for up to 7 days, although it has frequently returned to normal by 3 days after the last dose. The effect of other NSAIDs is shorter, as the inhibitor effect is reversed when the drug is removed. Thienopyridines (clopidogrel and prasugrel) inhibit ADP-mediated platelet aggregation and like NSAIDs can precipitate or exacerbate bleeding symptoms.

Many herbal supplements can impair hemostatic function (Table 3-2). Some are more convincingly associated with a bleeding risk than others. Fish oil or concentrated omega 3 fatty acid supplements impair platelet function. They alter platelet biochemistry to produce more PGI3, a more potent platelet inhibitor than prostacyclin (PGI2), and more thromboxane A3, a less potent platelet activator than thromboxane A2. In fact, diets naturally rich in omega 3 fatty acids can result in a prolonged bleeding time and abnormal platelet aggregation studies, but the actual associated bleeding risk is unclear. Vitamin E appears to inhibit protein kinase C–mediated platelet aggregation and nitric oxide production. In patients with unexplained bruising or bleeding, it is prudent to review any new medications or supplements and discontinue those that may be associated with bleeding.

Underlying Systemic Diseases That Cause or Exacerbate a Bleeding Tendency Acquired bleeding disorders are commonly secondary to, or associated with, systemic disease. The clinical evaluation of a patient with a bleeding tendency must therefore include a thorough assessment for evidence of underlying disease. Bruising or mucosal bleeding may be the presenting complaint in liver disease, severe renal impairment, hypothyroidism, paraproteinemias or amyloidosis, and conditions causing bone marrow failure. All coagulation factors are synthesized in the liver, and hepatic failure results in combined factor deficiencies. This is often compounded by thrombocytopenia from splenomegaly due to portal hypertension. Coagulation factors II, VII, IX, X and proteins C, S, and Z are dependent on vitamin K for posttranslational modification. Although vitamin K is required in both procoagulant and anticoagulant processes, the phenotype of vitamin K deficiency or the warfarin effect on coagulation is bleeding.

The normal blood platelet count is 150,000–450,000/μL. Thrombocytopenia results from decreased production, increased destruction, and/or sequestration. Although the bleeding risk varies somewhat by the reason for the thrombocytopenia, bleeding rarely occurs in isolated thrombocytopenia at counts <50,000/μL and usually not until <10,000–20,000/μL. Coexisting coagulopathies, as is seen in liver failure or disseminated coagulation, infection, platelet-inhibitory drugs, and underlying medical conditions, can all increase the risk of bleeding in the thrombocytopenic patient. Most procedures can be performed in patients with a platelet count of 50,000/μL. The level needed for major surgery will depend on the type of surgery and the patient's

TABLE 3-2

HERBAL SUPPLEMENTS ASSOCIATED WITH INCREASED BLEEDING

Herbs With Potential Antiplatelet Activity
Ginkgo (*Ginkgo biloba L.*)
Garlic (*Allium sativum*)
Bilberry (*Vaccinium myrtillus*)
Ginger (*Gingiber officinale*)
Dong quai (*Angelica sinensis*)
Feverfew (*Tanacetum parthenium*)
Asian ginseng (*Panax ginseng*)
American ginseng (*Panax quinquefolius*)
Siberian ginseng/eleuthero (*Eleutherococcus senticosus*)
Turmeric (*Circuma longa*)
Meadowsweet (*Filipendula ulmaria*)
Willow (*Salix spp.*)
Coumarin-Containing Herbs
Motherworth (*Leonurus cardiaca*)
Chamomile (*Matricaria recutita, Chamaemelum mobile*)
Horse chestnut (*Aesculus hippocastanum*)
Red clover (*Trifolium pratense*)
Fenugreek (*Trigonella foenum-graecum*)

underlying medical state, although a count of approximately 80,000/µL is likely sufficient.

HISTORY OF THROMBOSIS The risk of thrombosis, like that of bleeding, is influenced by both genetic and environmental influences. The major risk factor for arterial thrombosis is atherosclerosis, while for venous thrombosis, the risk factors are immobility, surgery, underlying medical conditions such as malignancy, medications such as hormonal therapy, obesity, and genetic predispositions. Factors that increase risks for venous and for both venous and arterial thromboses are shown in Table 3-3.

The most important point in a history related to venous thrombosis is determining whether the thrombotic event was idiopathic (meaning there was no clear precipitating factor) or was a precipitated event. In patients without underlying malignancy, having an idiopathic event is the strongest predictor of recurrence of venous thromboembolism. In patients who have a vague history of thrombosis, a history of being treated with warfarin suggests a past DVT. Age is an important risk factor for venous thrombosis—the risk of DVT increasing per decade, with an approximate incidence of 1/100,000 per year in early childhood to 200 per year among octogenarians. Family history is helpful in determining if there is a genetic predisposition and how strong that predisposition appears to be. A genetic thrombophilia that confers a relatively small increased risk, such as being a heterozygote for the prothrombin G20210A or factor V Leiden mutation, may be a minor determinant of risk in an elderly individual undergoing a high-risk surgical procedure. As illustrated in Fig. 3-5, a thrombotic event usually has more than one contributing factor. Predisposing factors must be carefully assessed to determine the risk of recurrent thrombosis and, with consideration of the patient's bleeding risk, determine the length of anticoagulation. Similar consideration should be given in determining the need to test the patient and family members for thrombophilias.

LABORATORY EVALUATION Careful history taking and clinical examination are essential components in the assessment of bleeding and thrombotic risk. The use of laboratory tests of coagulation complement, but

TABLE 3-3

RISK FACTORS FOR THROMBOSIS

VENOUS	VENOUS AND ARTERIAL
Inherited	**Inherited**
Factor V Leiden	Homocystinuria
Prothrombin G20210A	Dysfibrinogenemia
Antithrombin deficiency	**Mixed (inherited and acquired)**
Protein C deficiency	Hyperhomocysteinemia
Protein S deficiency	**Acquired**
Elevated FVIII	Malignancy
Acquired	Antiphospholipid antibody syndrome
Age	Hormonal therapy
Previous thrombosis	Polycythemia vera
Immobilization	Essential thrombocythemia
Major surgery	Paroxysmal nocturnal hemoglobinuria
Pregnancy and puerperium	Thrombotic thrombocytopenic purpura
Hospitalization	Heparin-induced thrombocytopenia
Obesity	Disseminated intravascular coagulation
Infection APC resistance, nongenetic	
Smoking	
Unknown[a]	
Elevated factor II, IX, XI	
Elevated TAFI levels	
Low levels of TFPI	

[a]Unknown whether risk is inherited or acquired.

Abbreviations: APC, activated protein C; TAFI, thrombin-activatable fibrinolysis inhibitor; TFPI, tissue factor pathway inhibitor.

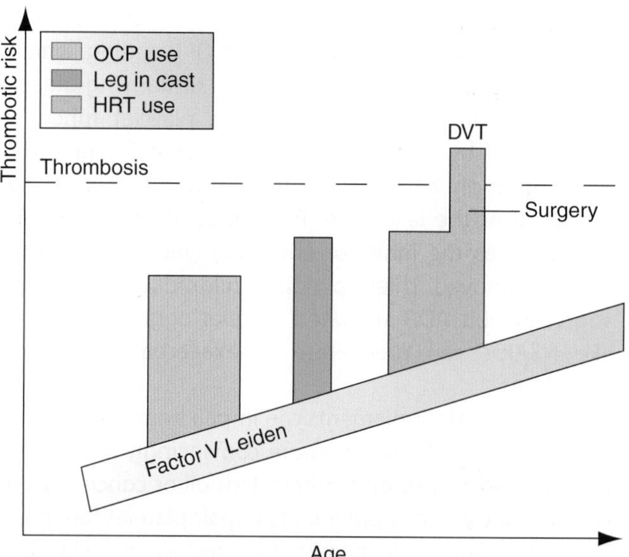

FIGURE 3-5

Thrombotic risk over time. Shown schematically is an individual's thrombotic risk over time. An underlying factor V Leiden mutation provides a "theoretically" constant increased risk. The thrombotic risk increases with age and, intermittently, with oral contraceptive (OCP) or hormone replacement (HRT) use; other events may increase the risk further. At some point the cumulative risk may increase to the threshold for thrombosis and result in deep-venous thrombosis (DVT). Note: The magnitude and duration of risk portrayed in the figure is meant for example only and may not precisely reflect the relative risk determined by clinical study. *(From BA Konkle, A Schafer, in DP Zipes et al [eds]: Braunwald's Heart Disease, 7th ed. Philadelphia, Saunders, 2005; modified with permission from FR Rosendaal: Venous thrombosis: A multicausal disease. Lancet 353:1167, 1999.)*

cannot substitute for, clinical assessment. No test exists that provides a global assessment of hemostasis. The bleeding time has been used to assess bleeding risk; however, it does not predict bleeding risk with surgery and it is not recommended for this indication. The PFA-100, an instrument that measures platelet-dependent coagulation under flow conditions, is more sensitive and specific for platelet disorders and VWD than the bleeding time; however it is not sensitive enough to rule out underlying mild bleeding disorders. Also, its utility in predicting bleeding risk has not been determined.

For routine preoperative and preprocedure testing, an abnormal prothrombin time (PT) may detect liver disease or vitamin K deficiency that had not been previously appreciated. Studies have not confirmed the usefulness of an activated partial thromboplastin time (aPTT) in preoperative evaluations in patients with a negative bleeding history. The primary use of coagulation testing should be to confirm the presence and type of bleeding disorder in a patient with a suspicious clinical history.

Because of the nature of coagulation assays, proper sample acquisition and handling is critical to obtaining valid results. In patients with abnormal coagulation assays who have no bleeding history, repeat studies with attention to these factors frequently results in normal values. Most coagulation assays are performed in sodium citrate anticoagulated plasma that is recalcified for the assay. Because the anticoagulant is in liquid solution and needs to be added to blood in proportion to the plasma volume, incorrectly filled or inadequately mixed blood collection tubes will give erroneous results. Vacutainer tubes should be filled to >90% of the recommended fill, which is usually denoted by a line on the tube. An elevated hematocrit (>55%) can result in a false value due to a decreased plasma to anticoagulant ratio.

Screening Assays The most commonly used screening tests are the PT, aPTT, and platelet count. The PT assesses the factors I (fibrinogen), II (prothrombin), V, VII, and X (Fig. 3-6). The PT measures the time for clot formation of the citrated plasma after recalcification and addition of thromboplastin, a mixture of TF and phospholipids. The sensitivity of the assay varies by the source of thromboplastin. The relationship between defects in secondary hemostasis (fibrin formation) and coagulation test abnormalities is shown in Table 3-4. To adjust for this variability, the overall sensitivity of different thromboplastins to reduction of the vitamin K–dependent clotting factors II, VII, IX, and X in anticoagulation patients is now expressed as the International Sensitivity Index (ISI). An inverse relationship exists between ISI and thromboplastin sensitivity. The international normalized ratio (INR) is then determined based on the formula: $INR = (PT_{patient}/PT_{normal\ mean})^{ISI}$.

The INR was developed to assess anticoagulation due to reduction of vitamin K–dependent coagulation factors; it is commonly used in the evaluation of patients with liver disease. While it does allow comparison among laboratories, reagent sensitivity as used to determine the ISI is not the same in liver disease as with warfarin anticoagulation. In addition, progressive liver failure is associated with variable changes in coagulation factors; the degree of prolongation of either the PT or the INR only roughly predicts the bleeding risk. Thrombin generation has been shown to be normal in many patients with mild to moderate liver dysfunction. As the PT only measures one aspect of hemostasis affected by liver dysfunction, we likely overestimate the bleeding risk of a mildly elevated INR in this setting.

The aPTT assesses the intrinsic and common coagulation pathways, factors XI, IX, VIII, X, V, II; fibrinogen; and also prekallikrein, high-molecular-weight kininogen, and factor XII (Fig. 3-6). The aPTT reagent contains phospholipids derived from either animal or vegetable sources that function as a platelet substitute in the coagulation pathways and includes an activator of the intrinsic coagulation system, such as nonparticulate ellagic acid or the particulate activators kaolin, celite, or micronized silica.

The phospholipid composition of aPTT reagents varies, which influences the sensitivity of individual reagents to clotting factor deficiencies and to inhibitors such as heparin and lupus anticoagulants. Thus, aPTT

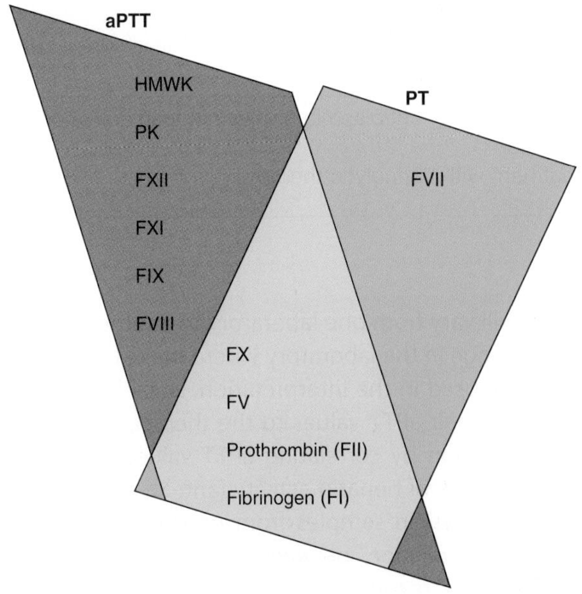

FIGURE 3-6
Coagulation factor activity tested in the activated partial thromboplastin time (aPTT) in red and prothrombin time (PT) in green, or both. F, factor; HMWK, high-molecular-weight kininogen; PK, prekallikrein.

TABLE 3-4

HEMOSTATIC DISORDERS AND COAGULATION TEST ABNORMALITIES

Prolonged Activated Partial Thromboplastin Time (aPTT)
No clinical bleeding—↓ factors XII, high-molecular-weight kininogen, prekallikrein
Variable, but usually mild, bleeding—↓ factor XI, mild↓ FVIII and FIX
Frequent, severe bleeding—severe deficiencies of FVIII and FIX
Heparin
Prolonged Prothrombin Time (PT)
Factor VII deficiency
Vitamin K deficiency—early
Warfarin anticoagulation
Prolonged aPTT and PT
Factor II, V, X, or fibrinogen deficiency
Vitamin K deficiency—late
Direct thrombin inhibitors
Prolonged Thrombin Time
Heparin or heparin-like inhibitors
Mild or no bleeding—dysfibrinogenemia
Frequent, severe bleeding—afibrinogenemia
Prolonged PT and/or aPTT Not Correct with Mixing with Normal Plasma
Bleeding—specific factor inhibitor
No symptoms, or clotting and/or pregnancy loss—lupus anticoagulant
Disseminated intravascular coagulation
Heparin or direct thrombin inhibitor
Abnormal Clot Solubility
Factor XIII deficiency
Inhibitors or defective cross-linking
Rapid Clot Lysis
Deficiency of α_2-antiplasmin or plasminogen activator inhibitor 1
Treatment with fibrinolytic therapy

results will vary from one laboratory to another, and the normal range in the laboratory where the testing occurs should be used in the interpretation. Local laboratories can relate their aPTT values to the therapeutic heparin anticoagulation by correlating aPTT values with direct measurements of heparin activity (anti-Xa or protamine titration assays) in samples from heparinized patients, although correlation between these assays is often poor. The aPTT reagent will vary in sensitivity to individual factor deficiencies and usually becomes prolonged with individual factor deficiencies of 30–50%.

Mixing Studies Mixing studies are used to evaluate a prolonged aPTT or, less commonly PT, to distinguish between a factor deficiency and an inhibitor. In this assay, normal plasma and patient plasma are mixed in a 1:1 ratio, and the aPTT or PT is determined immediately and after incubation at 37°C for varying times, typically 30, 60, and/or 120 min. With isolated factor deficiencies, the aPTT will correct with mixing and stay corrected with incubation. With aPTT prolongation due to a lupus anticoagulant, the mixing and incubation will show no correction. In acquired neutralizing factor antibodies, such as an acquired factor VIII inhibitor, the initial assay may or may not correct immediately after mixing but will prolong or remain prolonged with incubation at 37°C. Failure to correct with mixing can also be due to the presence of other inhibitors or interfering substances such as heparin, fibrin split products, and paraproteins.

Specific Factor Assays Decisions to proceed with specific clotting factor assays will be influenced by the clinical situation and the results of coagulation screening tests. Precise diagnosis and effective management of inherited and acquired coagulation deficiencies necessitate quantitation of the relevant factors. When bleeding is severe, specific assays are often urgently required to guide appropriate therapy. Individual factor assays are usually performed as modifications of the mixing study, where the patient's plasma is mixed with plasma deficient in the factor being studied. This will correct all factor deficiencies to >50%, thus making prolongation of clot formation due to a factor deficiency dependent on the factor missing from the added plasma.

Testing for Antiphospholipid Antibodies Antibodies to phospholipids (cardiolipin) or phospholipid-binding proteins (β_2-microglobulin and others) are detected by enzyme-linked immunosorbent assay (ELISA). When these antibodies interfere with phospholipid-dependent coagulation tests, they are termed *lupus anticoagulants*. The aPTT has variability sensitivity to lupus anticoagulants, depending in part on the aPTT reagents used. An assay using a sensitive reagent has been termed an *LA-PTT*. The dilute Russell viper venom test (dRVVT) and the tissue thromboplastin inhibition (TTI) test are modifications of standard tests with the phospholipid reagent decreased, thus increasing the sensitivity to antibodies that interfere with the phospholipid component. The tests, however, are not specific for lupus anticoagulants, as factor deficiencies or other inhibitors will also result in prolongation. Documentation of a lupus anticoagulant requires not only prolongation of a phospholipid-dependent coagulation test but also lack of correction when mixed with normal plasma and correction with the addition of activated platelet membranes or certain phospholipids, e.g. hexagonal phase.

Other Coagulation Tests The thrombin time and the reptilase time measure fibrinogen conversion to fibrin and are prolonged when the fibrinogen level is low (usually <80–100 mg/dL) or qualitatively abnormal, as seen in inherited or acquired dysfibrinogenemias, or when fibrin/fibrinogen degradation products interfere. The thrombin time, but not the reptilase time, is prolonged in the presence of heparin. Measurement of anti–factor Xa plasma inhibitory activity is a test frequently used to assess low-molecular-weight heparin (LMWH) levels or as a direct measurement of unfractionated heparin (UFH) activity. Heparin in the patient sample inhibits the enzymatic conversion of a Xa-specific chromogenic substrate to colored product by factor Xa. Standard curves are created using multiple concentrations of UFH and LMWH and are used to calculate the concentration of anti-Xa activity in the patient plasma.

Laboratory Testing for Thrombophilia Laboratory assays to detect thrombophilic states include molecular diagnostics and immunologic and functional assays. These assays vary in their sensitivity and specificity for the condition being tested. Furthermore, acute thrombosis, acute illnesses, inflammatory conditions, pregnancy, and medications affect levels of many coagulation factors and their inhibitors. Antithrombin is decreased by heparin and in the setting of acute thrombosis. Protein C and S levels may be increased in the setting of acute thrombosis and are decreased by warfarin. Antiphospholipid antibodies are frequently transiently positive in acute illness. Testing for genetic thrombophilias should, in general, only be performed when there is a strong family history of thrombosis and results would affect clinical decision making.

Because thrombophilia evaluations are usually performed to assess the need to extend anticoagulation, testing should be performed in a steady state, remote from the acute event. In most instances, warfarin anticoagulation can be stopped after the initial 3–6 months of treatment, and testing performed at least 3 weeks later. Sensitive markers of coagulation activation, notably the D-dimer assay and the thrombin generation test, hold promise as predictors, when elevated, of recurrent thrombosis when measured at least 1 month from discontinuation of warfarin.

Measures of Platelet Function The bleeding time has been used to assess bleeding risk; however, it has not been found to predict bleeding risk with surgery, and it is not recommended for use for this indication. The PFA-100 and similar instruments that measure platelet-dependent coagulation under flow conditions are generally more sensitive and specific for platelet disorders and VWD than the bleeding time; however, data are insufficient to support their use to predict bleeding risk or monitor response to therapy. When they are used in the evaluation of a patient with bleeding symptoms, abnormal results, as with the bleeding time, require specific testing, such as VWF assays and/or platelet aggregation studies. Since all of these "screening" assays may miss patients with mild bleeding disorders, further studies are needed to define their role in hemostasis testing.

For classic platelet aggregometry, various agonists are added to the patient's platelet-rich plasma, and platelet aggregation is observed. Tests of platelet secretion in response to agonists can also be measured. These tests are affected by many factors, including numerous medications, and the association between minor defects in aggregation or secretion in these assays and bleeding risk is not clearly established.

ACKNOWLEDGMENT

Robert I. Handin, MD, contributed this chapter in the 16th edition of Harrison's Principles of Internal Medicine and some material from that chapter has been retained here.

CHAPTER 4

ENLARGEMENT OF LYMPH NODES AND SPLEEN

Patrick H. Henry ■ Dan L. Longo

This chapter is intended to serve as a guide to the evaluation of patients who present with enlargement of the lymph nodes (*lymphadenopathy*) or the spleen (*splenomegaly*). Lymphadenopathy is a rather common clinical finding in primary care settings, whereas palpable splenomegaly is less so.

LYMPHADENOPATHY

Lymphadenopathy may be an incidental finding in patients being examined for various reasons, or it may be a presenting sign or symptom of the patient's illness. The physician must eventually decide whether the lymphadenopathy is a normal finding or one that requires further study, up to and including biopsy. Soft, flat, submandibular nodes (<1 cm) are often palpable in healthy children and young adults; healthy adults may have palpable inguinal nodes of up to 2 cm, which are considered normal. Further evaluation of these normal nodes is not warranted. In contrast, if the physician believes the node(s) to be abnormal, then pursuit of a more precise diagnosis is needed.

APPROACH TO THE PATIENT Lymphadenopathy

Lymphadenopathy may be a primary or secondary manifestation of numerous disorders, as shown in Table 4-1. Many of these disorders are infrequent causes of lymphadenopathy. In primary care practice, more than two-thirds of patients with lymphadenopathy have nonspecific causes or upper respiratory illnesses (viral or bacterial) and <1% have a malignancy. In one study, 84% of patients referred for evaluation of lymphadenopathy had a "benign" diagnosis. The remaining 16% had a malignancy (lymphoma or metastatic adenocarcinoma). Of the patients with benign lymphadenopathy, 63% had a nonspecific or reactive etiology (no causative agent found), and the remainder had a specific cause demonstrated, most commonly infectious mononucleosis, toxoplasmosis, or tuberculosis. Thus, the vast majority of patients with lymphadenopathy will have a nonspecific etiology requiring few diagnostic tests.

CLINICAL ASSESSMENT The physician will be aided in the pursuit of an explanation for the lymphadenopathy by a careful medical history, physical examination, selected laboratory tests, and perhaps an excisional lymph node biopsy.

The *medical history* should reveal the setting in which lymphadenopathy is occurring. Symptoms such as sore throat, cough, fever, night sweats, fatigue, weight loss, or pain in the nodes should be sought. The patient's age, sex, occupation, exposure to pets, sexual behavior, and use of drugs such as diphenylhydantoin are other important historic points. For example, children and young adults usually have benign (i.e., nonmalignant) disorders that account for the observed lymphadenopathy such as viral or bacterial upper respiratory infections; infectious mononucleosis; toxoplasmosis; and, in some countries, tuberculosis. In contrast, after age 50 years, the incidence of malignant disorders increases and that of benign disorders decreases.

The *physical examination* can provide useful clues such as the extent of lymphadenopathy (localized or generalized), size of nodes, texture, presence or absence of nodal tenderness, signs of inflammation over the node, skin lesions, and splenomegaly. A thorough ear, nose, and throat (ENT) examination is indicated in adult patients with cervical adenopathy and a history of tobacco use. Localized or regional adenopathy implies involvement of a single anatomic area. Generalized

TABLE 4-1

DISEASES ASSOCIATED WITH LYMPHADENOPATHY

1. Infectious diseases
   a. Viral—infectious mononucleosis syndromes (EBV, CMV), infectious hepatitis, herpes simplex, herpesvirus-6, varicella-zoster virus, rubella, measles, adenovirus, HIV, epidemic keratoconjunctivitis, vaccinia, herpesvirus-8
   b. Bacterial—streptococci, staphylococci, cat-scratch disease, brucellosis, tularemia, plague, chancroid, melioidosis, glanders, tuberculosis, atypical mycobacterial infection, primary and secondary syphilis, diphtheria, leprosy
   c. Fungal—histoplasmosis, coccidioidomycosis, paracoccidioidomycosis
   d. Chlamydial—lymphogranuloma venereum, trachoma
   e. Parasitic—toxoplasmosis, leishmaniasis, trypanosomiasis, filariasis
   f. Rickettsial—scrub typhus, rickettsialpox, Q fever
2. Immunologic diseases
   a. Rheumatoid arthritis
   b. Juvenile rheumatoid arthritis
   c. Mixed connective tissue disease
   d. Systemic lupus erythematosus
   e. Dermatomyositis
   f. Sjögren's syndrome
   g. Serum sickness
   h. Drug hypersensitivity—diphenylhydantoin, hydralazine, allopurinol, primidone, gold, carbamazepine, etc.
   i. Angioimmunoblastic lymphadenopathy
   j. Primary biliary cirrhosis
   k. Graft-vs.-host disease
   l. Silicone-associated
   m. Autoimmune lymphoproliferative syndrome
3. Malignant diseases
   a. Hematologic—Hodgkin's disease, non-Hodgkin's lymphomas, acute or chronic lymphocytic leukemia, hairy cell leukemia, malignant histiocytosis, amyloidosis
   b. Metastatic—from numerous primary sites
4. Lipid storage diseases—Gaucher's, Niemann-Pick, Fabry, Tangier
5. Endocrine diseases—hyperthyroidism
6. Other disorders
   a. Castleman's disease (giant lymph node hyperplasia)
   b. Sarcoidosis
   c. Dermatopathic lymphadenitis
   d. Lymphomatoid granulomatosis
   e. Histiocytic necrotizing lymphadenitis (Kikuchi's disease)
   f. Sinus histiocytosis with massive lymphadenopathy (Rosai-Dorfman disease)
   g. Mucocutaneous lymph node syndrome (Kawasaki's disease)
   h. Histiocytosis X
   i. Familial Mediterranean fever
   j. Severe hypertriglyceridemia
   k. Vascular transformation of sinuses
   l. Inflammatory pseudotumor of lymph node
   m. Congestive heart failure

Abbreviations: CMV, cytomegalovirus; EBV, Epstein-Barr virus.

adenopathy has been defined as involvement of three or more noncontiguous lymph node areas. Many of the causes of lymphadenopathy (Table 4-1) can produce localized *or* generalized adenopathy, so this distinction is of limited utility in the differential diagnosis. Nevertheless, generalized lymphadenopathy is frequently associated with nonmalignant disorders such as infectious mononucleosis (Epstein-Barr virus [EBV] or cytomegalovirus [CMV]), toxoplasmosis, AIDS, other viral infections, systemic lupus erythematosus (SLE), and mixed connective tissue disease. Acute and chronic lymphocytic leukemias and malignant lymphomas also produce generalized adenopathy in adults.

The site of localized or regional adenopathy may provide a useful clue about the cause. Occipital adenopathy often reflects an infection of the scalp, and preauricular adenopathy accompanies conjunctival infections and cat-scratch disease. The most frequent site of regional adenopathy is the neck, and most of the causes are benign—upper respiratory infections, oral and dental lesions, infectious mononucleosis, or other viral illnesses. The chief malignant causes include metastatic cancer from head and neck, breast, lung, and thyroid primaries. Enlargement of supraclavicular and scalene nodes is always abnormal. Because these nodes drain regions of the lung and retroperitoneal space, they can reflect lymphomas, other cancers, or infectious processes arising in these areas. Virchow's node is an enlarged left supraclavicular node infiltrated with metastatic cancer from a gastrointestinal primary. Metastases to supraclavicular nodes also occur from lung, breast, testis, or ovarian cancers. Tuberculosis, sarcoidosis, and toxoplasmosis are nonneoplastic causes of supraclavicular adenopathy. Axillary adenopathy is usually due to injuries or localized infections of the ipsilateral upper extremity. Malignant causes include melanoma or lymphoma and, in women, breast cancer. Inguinal lymphadenopathy is usually secondary to infections or trauma of the lower extremities and may accompany sexually transmitted diseases such as lymphogranuloma venereum, primary syphilis, genital herpes, or chancroid. These nodes may also be involved by lymphomas and metastatic cancer from primary lesions of the rectum, genitalia, or lower extremities (melanoma).

The size and texture of the lymph node(s) and the presence of pain are useful parameters in evaluating a patient with lymphadenopathy. Nodes <1.0 cm^2 in area (1.0 cm × 1.0 cm or less) are almost always secondary to benign, nonspecific reactive causes. In one retrospective analysis of younger patients (9–25 years) who had a lymph node biopsy, a maximum diameter of >2 cm served as one discriminant for predicting that the biopsy would reveal malignant or granulomatous disease. Another study showed that a lymph node size of 2.25 cm^2 (1.5 cm × 1.5 cm) was the best size limit for distinguishing malignant or granulomatous lymphadenopathy from other causes of lymphadenopathy. Patients with node(s) ≤1.0 cm^2 should be observed after excluding infectious mononucleosis and/or toxoplasmosis unless there are symptoms and signs of an underlying systemic illness.

The texture of lymph nodes may be described as soft, firm, rubbery, hard, discrete, matted, tender, movable, or fixed. Tenderness is found when the capsule is stretched during rapid enlargement, usually secondary to an inflammatory process. Some malignant diseases such as acute leukemia may produce rapid enlargement and pain in the nodes. Nodes involved by lymphoma tend to be large, discrete, symmetric, rubbery, firm, mobile, and nontender. Nodes containing metastatic cancer are often hard, nontender, and nonmovable because of fixation to surrounding tissues. The coexistence of splenomegaly in the patient with lymphadenopathy implies a systemic illness such as infectious mononucleosis, lymphoma, acute or chronic leukemia, SLE, sarcoidosis, toxoplasmosis, cat-scratch disease, or other less common hematologic disorders. The patient's story should provide helpful clues about the underlying systemic illness.

Nonsuperficial presentations (thoracic or abdominal) of adenopathy are usually detected as the result of a symptom-directed diagnostic workup. Thoracic adenopathy may be detected by routine chest radiography or during the workup for superficial adenopathy. It may also be found because the patient complains of a cough or wheezing from airway compression; hoarseness from recurrent laryngeal nerve involvement; dysphagia from esophageal compression; or swelling of the neck, face, or arms secondary to compression of the superior vena cava or subclavian vein. The differential diagnosis of mediastinal and hilar adenopathy includes primary lung disorders and systemic illnesses that characteristically involve mediastinal or hilar nodes. In the young, mediastinal adenopathy is associated with infectious mononucleosis and sarcoidosis. In endemic regions, histoplasmosis can cause unilateral paratracheal lymph node involvement that mimics lymphoma. Tuberculosis can also cause unilateral adenopathy. In older patients, the differential diagnosis includes primary lung cancer (especially among smokers), lymphomas, metastatic carcinoma (usually lung), tuberculosis, fungal infection, and sarcoidosis.

Enlarged intraabdominal or retroperitoneal nodes are usually malignant. Although tuberculosis may present as mesenteric lymphadenitis, these masses usually contain lymphomas or, in young men, germ cell tumors.

LABORATORY INVESTIGATION The laboratory investigation of patients with lymphadenopathy must be tailored to elucidate the etiology suspected from the patient's history and physical findings. One study from a family practice clinic evaluated 249 younger patients with "enlarged lymph nodes, not infected" or "lymphadenitis." No laboratory studies were obtained in 51%. When studies were performed, the most common were a complete blood count (CBC) (33%), throat culture (16%), chest x-ray (12%), or monospot test (10%). Only eight patients (3%) had a node biopsy, and half of those were normal or reactive. The CBC can provide useful data for the diagnosis of acute or chronic leukemias, EBV or CMV mononucleosis, lymphoma with a leukemic component, pyogenic infections, or immune cytopenias in illnesses such as SLE. Serologic studies may demonstrate antibodies specific to components of EBV, CMV, HIV, and other viruses; *Toxoplasma gondii*; *Brucella*; etc. If SLE is suspected, antinuclear and anti-DNA antibody studies are warranted.

The chest x-ray findings are usually negative, but the presence of a pulmonary infiltrate or mediastinal lymphadenopathy would suggest tuberculosis, histoplasmosis, sarcoidosis, lymphoma, primary lung cancer, or metastatic cancer and demands further investigation.

A variety of imaging techniques (computed tomography [CT], magnetic resonance imaging [MRI], ultrasonography color Doppler ultrasonography) have been employed to differentiate benign from malignant lymph nodes, especially in patients with head and neck cancer. CT and MRI are comparably accurate (65–90%) in the diagnosis of metastases to cervical lymph nodes. Ultrasonography has been used to determine the long (L) axis, short (S) axis, and a ratio of long to short axis in cervical nodes. An L/S ratio of <2.0 has a sensitivity and a specificity of 95% for distinguishing benign and malignant nodes in patients with head and neck cancer. This ratio has greater specificity and sensitivity than palpation or measurement of either the long or the short axis alone.

The indications for lymph node biopsy are imprecise, yet it is a valuable diagnostic tool. The decision to biopsy may be made early in a patient's evaluation or delayed for up to 2 weeks. Prompt biopsy should occur if the patient's history and physical findings suggest a malignancy; examples include a solitary, hard, nontender cervical node in an older patient who is a chronic user of tobacco; supraclavicular adenopathy; and solitary or generalized adenopathy that is firm, movable, and suggestive of lymphoma. If a primary head and neck cancer is suspected as the basis of a solitary, hard cervical node, then a careful ENT examination should be performed. Any mucosal lesion that is suspicious for a primary neoplastic process should be biopsied first. If no mucosal lesion is detected, an excisional biopsy of the largest node should be performed. Fine-needle aspiration should not be performed as the first diagnostic procedure. Most diagnoses require more tissue than such aspiration can provide, and it often delays a definitive diagnosis. Fine-needle aspiration should be reserved for thyroid nodules and for confirmation of relapse in patients whose primary diagnosis is known. If the primary physician is uncertain about whether to proceed to biopsy, consultation with a hematologist or medical oncologist should be helpful. In primary care practices, <5% of lymphadenopathy patients will require a biopsy. That percentage will be considerably larger in referral practices, i.e., hematology, oncology, or ENT.

Two groups have reported algorithms that they claim will identify more precisely those lymphadenopathy patients who should have a biopsy. Both reports were retrospective analyses in referral practices. The first study involved patients 9–25 years of age who had a node biopsy performed. Three variables were identified that predicted those young patients with peripheral lymphadenopathy who should undergo biopsy; lymph node size >2 cm in diameter and abnormal chest x-ray had positive predictive values, whereas recent ENT symptoms had negative predictive values. The second study evaluated 220 lymphadenopathy patients in a hematology unit and identified five variables (lymph node size, location [supraclavicular or nonsupraclavicular], age [>40 years or <40 years], texture [nonhard or hard], and tenderness) that were used in a mathematical model to identify patients requiring a biopsy. Positive predictive value was found for age >40 years, supraclavicular location, node size >2.25 cm^2, hard texture, and lack of pain or tenderness. Negative predictive value was evident for age <40 years, node size <1.0 cm^2, nonhard texture, and tender or painful nodes. Ninety-one percent of those who required biopsy were correctly classified by this model. Because both of these studies were retrospective analyses and one was limited to young patients, it is not known how useful these models would be if applied prospectively in a primary care setting.

Most lymphadenopathy patients do not require a biopsy, and at least half require no laboratory studies. If the patient's history and physical findings point to a benign cause for lymphadenopathy, careful follow-up at a 2- to 4-week interval can be employed. The patient should be instructed to return for reevaluation if there is an increase in the size of the nodules. Antibiotics are not indicated for lymphadenopathy unless strong evidence of a bacterial infection is present. Glucocorticoids should not be used to treat lymphadenopathy because their lympholytic effect obscures some diagnoses (lymphoma, leukemia, Castleman's disease), and they contribute to delayed healing or activation of underlying infections. An exception to this statement is the life-threatening pharyngeal obstruction by enlarged lymphoid tissue in Waldeyer's ring that is occasionally seen in infectious mononucleosis.

SPLENOMEGALY

STRUCTURE AND FUNCTION OF THE SPLEEN

The spleen is a reticuloendothelial organ that has its embryologic origin in the dorsal mesogastrium at about 5 weeks' gestation. It arises in a series of hillocks, migrates to its normal adult location in the left upper quadrant (LUQ), and is attached to the stomach via the gastrolienal ligament and to the kidney via the lienorenal ligament. When the hillocks fail to unify into a single tissue mass, accessory spleens may develop in around 20% of persons. The function of the spleen has been elusive. Galen believed it was the source of "black bile" or melancholia, and the word *hypochondria* (literally, beneath the ribs) and the idiom "to vent one's spleen" attest to the beliefs that the spleen had an important influence on the psyche and emotions. In humans, its normal physiologic roles seem to be the following:

1. Maintenance of quality control over erythrocytes in the red pulp by removal of senescent and defective red blood cells. The spleen accomplishes this function through a unique organization of its parenchyma and vasculature (Fig. 4-1).
2. Synthesis of antibodies in the white pulp.
3. Removal of antibody-coated bacteria and antibody-coated blood cells from the circulation.

An increase in these normal functions may result in splenomegaly.

The spleen is composed of *red pulp* and *white pulp*, which are Malpighi's terms for the red blood–filled sinuses and reticuloendothelial cell–lined cords and the white lymphoid follicles arrayed within the red pulp matrix. The spleen is in the portal circulation. The reason for this is unknown but may relate to the fact that lower blood pressure allows less rapid flow and minimizes damage to normal erythrocytes. Blood flows into the spleen at a rate of about 150 mL/min through the splenic artery, which ultimately ramifies into central arterioles. Some blood goes from the arterioles to capillaries and then to splenic veins and out of the spleen, but the majority of blood from central arterioles flows into the macrophage-lined sinuses and cords. The blood entering the sinuses reenters the circulation through the splenic venules, but the blood entering the cords is subjected to an inspection of sorts. To return to the circulation, the blood cells in the cords must squeeze through slits in the cord lining to enter the sinuses that lead to the venules. Old and damaged erythrocytes are less deformable and are retained in the cords, where they are destroyed and their components recycled. Red cell–inclusion bodies such as parasites, nuclear residua (Howell-Jolly bodies, or denatured hemoglobin (Heinz bodies) are pinched off in the process of passing through

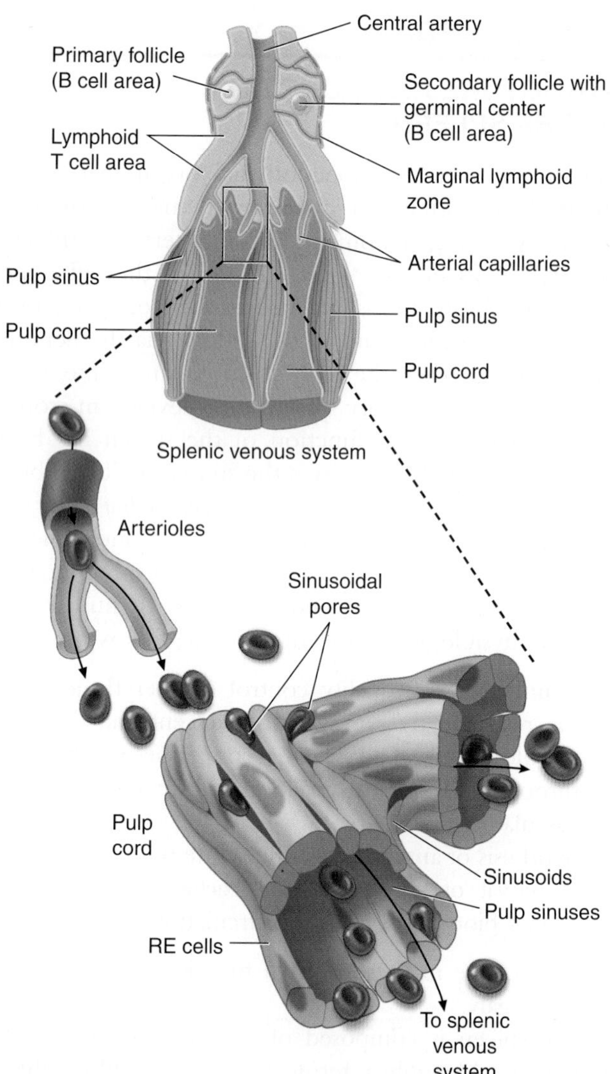

FIGURE 4-1

Schematic spleen structure. The spleen comprises many units of red and white pulp centered around small branches of the splenic artery, called *central arteries*. White pulp is lymphoid in nature and contains B cell follicles, a marginal zone around the follicles, and T cell–rich areas sheathing arterioles. The red pulp areas include pulp sinuses and pulp cords. The cords are dead ends. In order to regain access to the circulation, red blood cells must traverse tiny openings in the sinusoidal lining. Stiff, damaged, or old red cells cannot enter the sinuses. RE, reticuloendthelial. (*Bottom portion of figure from RS Hillman, KA Ault: Hematology in Clinical Practice, 4th ed. New York, McGraw-Hill, 2005.*)

the slits, a process called *pitting*. The culling of dead and damaged cells and the pitting of cells with inclusions appear to occur without significant delay because the blood transit time through the spleen is only slightly slower than in other organs.

The spleen is also capable of assisting the host in adapting to its hostile environment. It has at least three adaptive functions: (1) clearance of bacteria and particulates from the blood, (2) the generation of immune responses to certain pathogens, and (3) the generation of cellular components of the blood under circumstances in which the marrow is unable to meet the needs (i.e., extramedullary hematopoiesis). The latter adaptation is a recapitulation of the blood-forming function the spleen plays during gestation. In some animals, the spleen also serves a role in the vascular adaptation to stress because it stores red blood cells (often hemoconcentrated to higher hematocrits than normal) under normal circumstances and contracts under the influence of β-adrenergic stimulation to provide the animal with an autotransfusion and improved oxygen-carrying capacity. However, the normal human spleen does not sequester or store red blood cells and does not contract in response to sympathetic stimuli. The normal human spleen contains approximately one-third of the total body platelets and a significant number of marginated neutrophils. These sequestered cells are available when needed to respond to bleeding or infection.

APPROACH TO THE PATIENT Splenomegaly

CLINICAL ASSESSMENT The most common *symptoms* produced by diseases involving the spleen are pain and a heavy sensation in the LUQ. Massive splenomegaly may cause early satiety. Pain may result from acute swelling of the spleen with stretching of the capsule, infarction, or inflammation of the capsule. For many years, it was believed that splenic infarction was clinically silent, which, at times, is true. However, Soma Weiss, in his classic 1942 report of the self-observations by a Harvard medical student on the clinical course of subacute bacterial endocarditis, documented that severe LUQ and pleuritic chest pain may accompany thromboembolic occlusion of splenic blood flow. Vascular occlusion, with infarction and pain, is commonly seen in children with sickle cell crises. Rupture of the spleen, from either trauma or infiltrative disease that breaks the capsule, may result in intraperitoneal bleeding, shock, and death. The rupture itself may be painless.

A palpable spleen is the major *physical sign* produced by diseases affecting the spleen and suggests enlargement of the organ. The normal spleen weighs <250 g, decreases in size with age, normally lies entirely within the rib cage, has a maximum cephalocaudad diameter of 13 cm by ultrasonography or maximum length of 12 cm and/or width of 7 cm by radionuclide scan, and is usually not palpable. However, a palpable spleen was found in 3% of 2200 asymptomatic, male, freshman college students. Follow-up at 3 years revealed that 30% of those students still had a palpable spleen without any increase in disease prevalence. Ten-year follow-up found no evidence for lymphoid malignancies. Furthermore, in some tropical countries (e.g., New Guinea), the incidence of splenomegaly may reach 60%. Thus, the presence of a palpable spleen does not always equate with presence of disease. Even when disease is present, splenomegaly may not reflect the primary disease but rather a reaction to it. For example, in patients with Hodgkin's disease, only two-thirds of the palpable spleens show involvement by the cancer.

Physical examination of the spleen uses primarily the techniques of palpation and percussion. Inspection may reveal fullness in the LUQ that descends on inspiration, a finding associated with a massively enlarged spleen. Auscultation may reveal a venous hum or friction rub.

Palpation can be accomplished by bimanual palpation, ballotment, and palpation from above (Middleton maneuver). For bimanual palpation, which is at least as reliable as the other techniques, the patient is supine with flexed knees. The examiner's left hand is placed on the lower rib cage and pulls the skin toward the costal margin, allowing the fingertips of the right hand to feel the tip of the spleen as it descends while the patient inspires slowly, smoothly, and deeply. Palpation is begun with the right hand in the left lower quadrant with gradual movement toward the left costal margin, thereby identifying the lower edge of a massively enlarged spleen. When the spleen tip is felt, the finding is recorded as centimeters below the left costal margin at some arbitrary point, e.g. 10–15 cm, from the midpoint of the umbilicus or the xiphisternal junction. This allows other examiners to compare findings or the initial examiner to determine changes in size over time. Bimanual palpation in the right lateral decubitus position adds nothing to the supine examination.

Percussion for splenic dullness is accomplished with any of three techniques described by Nixon, Castell, or Barkun:

1. *Nixon's method*: The patient is placed on the right side so that the spleen lies above the colon and stomach. Percussion begins at the lower level of pulmonary resonance in the posterior axillary line and proceeds diagonally along a perpendicular line toward the lower midanterior costal margin. The upper border of dullness is normally 6–8 cm above the costal margin. Dullness >8 cm in an adult is presumed to indicate splenic enlargement.
2. *Castell's method*: With the patient supine, percussion in the lowest intercostal space in the anterior axillary line (8th or 9th) produces a resonant note if the spleen is normal in size. This is true during expiration or full inspiration. A dull percussion note on full inspiration suggests splenomegaly.
3. *Percussion of Traube's semilunar space*: The borders of Traube's space are the sixth rib superiorly, the left midaxillary line laterally, and the left costal margin inferiorly. The patient is supine with the left arm slightly abducted. During normal breathing, this space is percussed from medial to lateral margins, yielding a normal resonant sound. A dull percussion note suggests splenomegaly.

Studies comparing methods of percussion and palpation with a standard of ultrasonography or scintigraphy have revealed sensitivity of 56–71% for palpation and 59–82% for percussion. Reproducibility among examiners is better for palpation than percussion. Both techniques are less reliable in obese patients and patients who have just eaten. Thus, the physical examination techniques of palpation and percussion are imprecise at best. It has been suggested that the examiner perform percussion first and, if results are positive, proceed to palpation; if the spleen is palpable, then one can be reasonably confident that splenomegaly exists. However, not all LUQ masses are enlarged spleens; gastric or colon tumors and pancreatic or renal cysts or tumors can mimic splenomegaly.

The presence of an enlarged spleen can be more precisely determined, if necessary, by liver–spleen radionuclide scan, CT, MRI, or ultrasonography. The latter technique is the current procedure of choice for routine assessment of spleen size (normal = a maximum cephalocaudad diameter of 13 cm) because it has high sensitivity and specificity and is safe, noninvasive, quick, mobile, and less costly. Nuclear medicine scans are accurate, sensitive, and reliable but are costly, require greater time to generate data, and use immobile equipment. They have the advantage of demonstrating accessory splenic tissue. CT and MRI provide accurate determination of spleen size, but the equipment is immobile and the procedures are expensive. MRI appears to offer no advantage over CT. Changes in spleen structure such as mass lesions, infarcts, inhomogeneous infiltrates, and cysts are more readily assessed by CT, MRI, or ultrasonography. None of these techniques is very reliable in the detection of patchy infiltration (e.g., Hodgkin's disease).

DIFFERENTIAL DIAGNOSIS Many of the diseases associated with splenomegaly are listed in Table 4-2. They are grouped according to the presumed basic mechanisms responsible for organ enlargement:

1. Hyperplasia or hypertrophy related to a particular splenic function such as reticuloendothelial hyperplasia (work hypertrophy) in diseases such as hereditary spherocytosis or thalassemia syndromes that require removal of large numbers of defective red blood cells, immune hyperplasia in response to systemic infection (infectious mononucleosis, subacute bacterial endocarditis) and or immunologic diseases (immune thrombocytopenia, SLE, Felty's syndrome).

TABLE 4-2

DISEASES ASSOCIATED WITH SPLENOMEGALY GROUPED BY PATHOGENIC MECHANISM

Enlargement Due to Increased Demand for Splenic Function	
Reticuloendothelial system hyperplasia (for removal of defective erythrocytes)	Malaria
Spherocytosis	Leishmaniasis
Early sickle cell anemia	Trypanosomiasis
Ovalocytosis	Ehrlichiosis
Thalassemia major	**Disordered immunoregulation**
Hemoglobinopathies	Rheumatoid arthritis (Felty's syndrome)
Paroxysmal nocturnal hemoglobinuria	Systemic lupus erythematosus
Pernicious anemia	Collagen vascular diseases
Immune hyperplasia	Serum sickness
Response to infection (viral, bacterial, fungal, parasitic)	Immune hemolytic anemias
Infectious mononucleosis	Immune thrombocytopenias
AIDS	Immune neutropenias
Viral hepatitis	Drug reactions
Cytomegalovirus	Angioimmunoblastic lymphadenopathy
Subacute bacterial endocarditis	Sarcoidosis
Bacterial septicemia	Thyrotoxicosis (benign lymphoid hypertrophy)
Congenital syphilis	Interleukin-2 therapy
Splenic abscess	**Extramedullary hematopoiesis**
Tuberculosis	Myelofibrosis
Histoplasmosis	Marrow damage by toxins, radiation, strontium
	Marrow infiltration by tumors, leukemias, Gaucher's disease
Enlargement Due to Abnormal Splenic or Portal Blood Flow	
Cirrhosis	Splenic artery aneurysm
Hepatic vein obstruction	Hepatic schistosomiasis
Portal vein obstruction, intrahepatic or extrahepatic	Congestive heart failure
Cavernous transformation of the portal vein	Hepatic echinococcosis
Splenic vein obstruction	Portal hypertension (any cause including the above): "Banti's disease"
Infiltration of the Spleen	
Intracellular or extracellular depositions	Hodgkin's disease
Amyloidosis	Myeloproliferative syndromes (e.g., polycythemia vera, essential thrombocytosis)
Gaucher's disease	Angiosarcomas
Niemann-Pick disease	Metastatic tumors (melanoma is most common)
Tangier disease	Eosinophilic granuloma
Hurler's syndrome and other mucopolysaccharidoses	Histiocytosis X
Hyperlipidemias	Hamartomas
Benign and malignant cellular infiltrations	Hemangiomas, fibromas, lymphangiomas
Leukemias (acute, chronic, lymphoid, myeloid, monocytic)	Splenic cysts
Lymphomas	
Unknown Etiology	
Idiopathic splenomegaly	Iron-deficiency anemia
Berylliosis	

2. Passive congestion due to decreased blood flow from the spleen in conditions that produce portal hypertension (cirrhosis, Budd-Chiari syndrome, congestive heart failure).
3. Infiltrative diseases of the spleen (lymphomas, metastatic cancer, amyloidosis, Gaucher's disease, myeloproliferative disorders with extramedullary hematopoiesis).

The differential diagnostic possibilities are much fewer when the spleen is "massively enlarged" or palpable more than 8 cm below the left costal margin or when its drained weight is ≥1000 g (Table 4-3). The vast majority of such patients will have non-Hodgkin's lymphoma, chronic lymphocytic leukemia, hairy cell leukemia, chronic myeloid leukemia, myelofibrosis with myeloid metaplasia, or polycythemia vera.

TABLE 4-3

DISEASES ASSOCIATED WITH MASSIVE SPLENOMEGALY*

Chronic myeloid leukemia	Gaucher's disease
Lymphomas	Chronic lymphocytic leukemia
Hairy cell leukemia	Sarcoidosis
Myelofibrosis with myeloid metaplasia	Autoimmune hemolytic anemia
Polycythemia vera	Diffuse splenic hemangiomatosis

*The spleen extends >8 cm below left costal margin and/or weighs >1000 g.

LABORATORY ASSESSMENT The major laboratory abnormalities accompanying splenomegaly are determined by the underlying systemic illness. Erythrocyte counts may be normal, decreased (thalassemia major syndromes, SLE, cirrhosis with portal hypertension), or increased (polycythemia vera). Granulocyte counts may be normal, decreased (Felty's syndrome, congestive splenomegaly, leukemias), or increased (infections or inflammatory disease, myeloproliferative disorders). Similarly, the platelet count may be normal, decreased when there is enhanced sequestration or destruction of platelets in an enlarged spleen (congestive splenomegaly, Gaucher's disease, immune thrombocytopenia), or increased in the myeloproliferative disorders such as polycythemia vera.

The CBC may reveal cytopenia of one or more blood cell types, which should suggest *hypersplenism*. This condition is characterized by splenomegaly, cytopenia(s), normal or hyperplastic bone marrow, and a response to splenectomy. The latter characteristic is less precise because reversal of cytopenia, particularly granulocytopenia, is sometimes not sustained after splenectomy. The cytopenias result from increased destruction of the cellular elements secondary to reduced flow of blood through enlarged and congested cords (congestive splenomegaly) or to immune-mediated mechanisms. In hypersplenism, various cell types usually have normal morphology on the peripheral blood smear, although the red cells may be spherocytic due to loss of surface area during their longer transit through the enlarged spleen. The increased marrow production of red cells should be reflected as an increased reticulocyte production index, although the value may be less than expected due to increased sequestration of reticulocytes in the spleen.

The need for additional laboratory studies is dictated by the differential diagnosis of the underlying illness of which splenomegaly is a manifestation.

SPLENECTOMY

Splenectomy is infrequently performed for diagnostic purposes, especially in the absence of clinical illness or other diagnostic tests that suggest underlying disease. More often, splenectomy is performed for symptom control in patients with massive splenomegaly, for disease control in patients with traumatic splenic rupture, or for correction of cytopenias in patients with hypersplenism or immune-mediated destruction of one or more cellular blood elements. Splenectomy is necessary for staging of patients with Hodgkin's disease only in those with clinical stage I or II disease in whom radiation therapy alone is contemplated as the treatment. Noninvasive staging of the spleen in Hodgkin's disease is not a sufficiently reliable basis for treatment decisions because one-third of normal-sized spleens will be involved with Hodgkin's disease and one-third of enlarged spleens will be tumor-free. The widespread use of systemic therapy to test all stages of Hodgkin's disease has made staging laparotomy with splenectomy unnecessary. Although splenectomy in chronic myeloid leukemia (CML) does not affect the natural history of disease, removal of the massive spleen usually makes patients significantly more comfortable and simplifies their management by significantly reducing transfusion requirements. The improvements in therapy of CML have reduced the need for splenectomy for symptom control. Splenectomy is an effective secondary or tertiary treatment for two chronic B cell leukemias, hairy cell leukemia and prolymphocytic leukemia, and for the very rare splenic mantle cell or marginal zone lymphoma. Splenectomy in these diseases may be associated with significant tumor regression in bone marrow and other sites of disease. Similar regressions of systemic disease have been noted after splenic irradiation in some types of lymphoid tumors, especially chronic lymphocytic leukemia and prolymphocytic leukemia. This has been termed the *abscopal effect*. Such systemic tumor responses to local therapy directed at the spleen suggest that some hormone or growth factor produced by the spleen may affect tumor cell proliferation, but this conjecture is not yet substantiated. A common therapeutic indication for splenectomy is traumatic or iatrogenic splenic rupture. In a fraction of patients with splenic rupture, peritoneal seeding of splenic fragments can lead to *splenosis*—the presence of multiple rests of spleen tissue not connected to the portal circulation. This ectopic spleen tissue may cause pain or gastrointestinal obstruction, as in endometriosis. A large number of hematologic, immunologic, and congestive causes of splenomegaly can lead to destruction of one or more cellular blood elements. In the majority of such cases, splenectomy can correct the cytopenias, particularly anemia and thrombocytopenia. In a large series of patients seen in two tertiary care centers, the indication for splenectomy was diagnostic in 10% of patients, therapeutic in 44%, staging for Hodgkin's disease in 20%, and incidental to another procedure in 26%. Perhaps the only contraindication to splenectomy is the presence of marrow failure, in which the enlarged spleen is the only source of hematopoietic tissue.

The absence of the spleen has minimal long-term effects on the hematologic profile. In the immediate postsplenectomy period, leukocytosis (≤25,000/μL) and thrombocytosis (≤1 × 10^6/μL) may develop, but within 2–3 weeks, blood cell counts and survival of each cell lineage are usually normal. The chronic manifestations of splenectomy are marked variation in size and shape of erythrocytes (anisocytosis, poikilocytosis) and the presence of Howell-Jolly bodies (nuclear remnants), Heinz bodies (denatured hemoglobin), basophilic stippling, and an occasional nucleated erythrocyte in the peripheral blood. When such erythrocyte abnormalities appear in a patient whose spleen has not been removed, one should suspect splenic infiltration by tumor that has interfered with its normal culling and pitting function.

The most serious consequence of splenectomy is increased susceptibility to bacterial infections, particularly those with capsules such as *Streptococcus pneumoniae*, *Haemophilus influenzae*, and some gram-negative enteric organisms. Patients younger than age 20 years are particularly susceptible to overwhelming sepsis with *S. pneumoniae*, and the overall actuarial risk of sepsis in patients who have had their spleens removed is about 7% in 10 years. The case-fatality rate for pneumococcal sepsis in splenectomized patients is 50–80%. About 25% of patients without spleens will develop a serious infection at some time in their; oves. The frequency is highest within the first 3 years after splenectomy. About 15% of the infections are polymicrobial, and lung, skin, and blood are the most common sites. No increased risk of viral infection has been noted in patients who have no spleen. The susceptibility to bacterial infections relates to the inability to remove opsonized bacteria from the bloodstream and a defect in making antibodies to T cell–independent antigens such as the polysaccharide components of bacterial capsules. Pneumococcal vaccine should be administered to all patients 2 weeks before elective splenectomy. The Advisory Committee on Immunization Practices recommends that these patients receive repeat vaccination 5 years postsplenectomy. Efficacy has not been proven for this group, and the recommendation discounts the possibility that administration of the vaccine may actually lower the titer of specific pneumococcal antibodies. A more effective pneumococcal conjugate vaccine that involves T cells in the response is now available (Prevenar, 7-valent). The vaccine to *Neisseria meningitidis* should also be given to patients in whom elective splenectomy is planned. Although efficacy data for *H. influenzae* type b vaccine are not available for older children or adults, it may be given to patients who have had a splenectomy.

Splenectomized patients should be educated to consider any unexplained fever as a medical emergency. Prompt medical attention with evaluation and treatment of suspected bacteremia may be life-saving. Routine chemoprophylaxis with oral penicillin can result in the emergence of drug-resistant strains and is not recommended.

In addition to an increased susceptibility to bacterial infections, splenectomized patients are also more susceptible to the parasitic disease babesiosis. Splenectomized patient should avoid areas where the parasite *Babesia* is endemic (e.g., Cape Cod, MA).

Surgical removal of the spleen is an obvious cause of hyposplenism. Patients with sickle cell disease often suffer from autosplenectomy as a result of splenic destruction by the numerous infarcts associated with sickle cell crises during childhood. Indeed, the presence of a palpable spleen in a patient with sickle cell disease after age 5 years suggests a coexisting hemoglobinopathy, e.g., thalassemia or hemoglobin C. In addition, patients who receive splenic irradiation for a neoplastic or autoimmune disease are also functionally hyposplenic. The term *hyposplenism* is preferred to *asplenism* in referring to the physiologic consequences of splenectomy because asplenia is a rare, specific, and fatal congenital abnormality in which there is a failure of the left side of the coelomic cavity (which includes the splenic anlagen) to develop normally. Infants with asplenia have no spleens, but that is the least of their problems. The right side of the developing embryo is duplicated on the left so there is liver where the spleen should be, there are two right lungs, and the heart comprises two right atria and two right ventricles.

CHAPTER 5

DISORDERS OF GRANULOCYTES AND MONOCYTES

Steven M. Holland ■ John I. Gallin

Leukocytes, the major cells comprising inflammatory and immune responses, include neutrophils, T and B lymphocytes, natural killer (NK) cells, monocytes, eosinophils, and basophils. These cells have specific functions, such as antibody production by B lymphocytes or destruction of bacteria by neutrophils, but in no single infectious disease is the exact role of the cell types completely established. Thus, whereas neutrophils are classically thought to be critical to host defense against bacteria, they may also play important roles in defense against viral infections.

The blood delivers leukocytes to the various tissues from the bone marrow, where they are produced. Normal blood leukocyte counts are 4.3–10.8 × 10^9/L, with neutrophils representing 45–74% of the cells, bands 0–4%, lymphocytes 16–45%, monocytes 4–10%, eosinophils 0–7%, and basophils 0–2%. Variation among individuals and among different ethnic groups can be substantial, with lower leukocyte numbers for certain African-American ethnic groups. The various leukocytes are derived from a common stem cell in the bone marrow. Three-fourths of the nucleated cells of bone marrow are committed to the production of leukocytes. Leukocyte maturation in the marrow is under the regulatory control of a number of different factors, known as colony-stimulating factors (CSFs) and interleukins (ILs). Because an alteration in the number and type of leukocytes is often associated with disease processes, total white blood cell (WBC) count (cells per μL) and differential counts are informative. This chapter focuses on neutrophils, monocytes, and eosinophils.

NEUTROPHILS

MATURATION

Important events in neutrophil life are summarized in Fig. 5-1. In normal humans, neutrophils are produced only in the bone marrow. The minimum number of stem cells necessary to support hematopoiesis is estimated to be 400–500 at any one time. Human blood monocytes, tissue macrophages, and stromal cells produce CSFs, hormones required for the growth of monocytes and neutrophils in the bone marrow. The hematopoietic system not only produces enough neutrophils (~1.3 × 10^{11} cells per 80-kg person per day) to carry out physiologic functions but also has a large reserve stored in the marrow, which can be mobilized in response to inflammation or infection. An increase in the number of blood neutrophils is called *neutrophilia*, and the presence of immature cells is termed a *shift to the left*. A decrease in the number of blood neutrophils is called *neutropenia*.

Neutrophils and monocytes evolve from pluripotent stem cells under the influence of cytokines and CSFs (Fig. 5-2). The proliferation phase through the metamyelocyte takes about 1 week, while the maturation phase from metamyelocyte to mature neutrophil takes another week. The myeloblast is the first recognizable precursor cell and is followed by the *promyelocyte*. The promyelocyte evolves when the classic lysosomal granules, called the *primary*, or *azurophil, granules* are produced. The primary granules contain hydrolases, elastase, myeloperoxidase, cathepsin G, cationic proteins, and bactericidal/permeability-increasing protein, which is important for killing gram-negative bacteria. Azurophil granules also contain *defensins*, a family of cysteine-rich polypeptides with broad antimicrobial activity against bacteria, fungi, and certain enveloped viruses. The promyelocyte divides to produce the *myelocyte*, a cell responsible for the synthesis of the *specific*, or *secondary, granules*, which contain unique (specific) constituents such as lactoferrin, vitamin B_{12}–binding protein, membrane components of the reduced nicotinamide-adenine dinucleotide phosphate (NADPH)

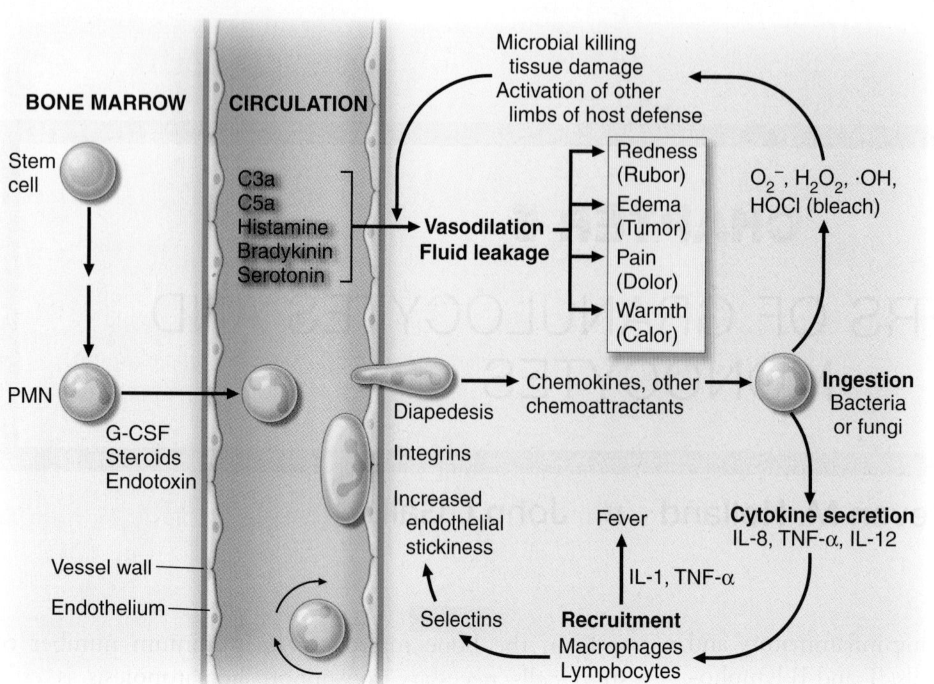

FIGURE 5-1

Schematic events in neutrophil production, recruitment, and inflammation. The four cardinal signs of inflammation (rubor, tumor, calor, dolor) are indicated, as are the interactions of neutrophils with other cells and cytokines. G-CSF, granulocyte colony-stimulating factor; IL, interleukin; PMN, polymorphonuclear leukocyte; TNF-α, tumor necrosis factor α.

Cell	Stage	Surface Markers[a]	Characteristics
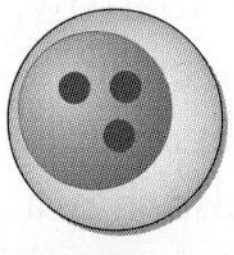	MYELOBLAST	CD33, CD13, CD15	Prominent nucleoli
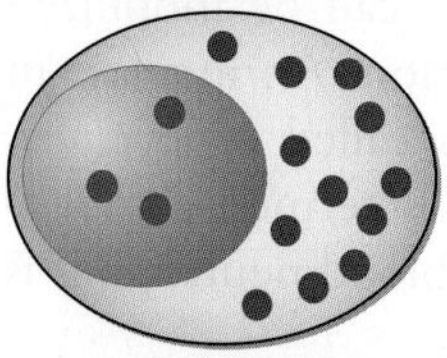	PROMYELOCYTE	CD33, CD13, CD15	Large cell Primary granules appear
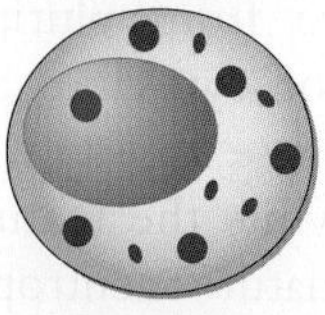	MYELOCYTE	CD33, CD13, CD15, CD14, CD11b	Secondary granules appear
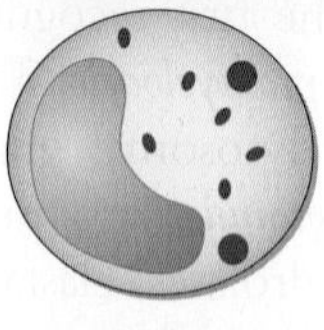	METAMYELOCYTE	CD33, CD13, CD15, CD14, CD11b	Kidney bean-shaped nucleus
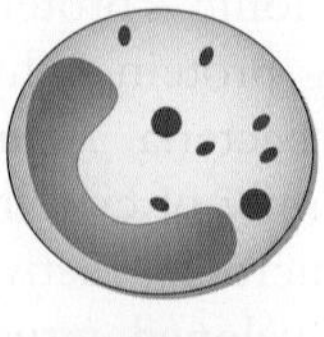	BAND FORM	CD33, CD13, CD15, CD14, CD11b CD10, CD16	Condensed, band-shaped nucleus
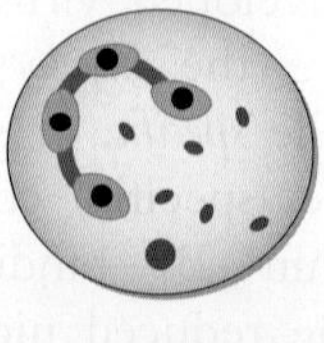	NEUTROPHIL	CD33, CD13, CD15, CD14, CD11b CD10, CD16	Condensed, multilobed nucleus

[a]CD= Cluster determinant; ● Nucleolus; ● Primary granule; • Secondary granule.

FIGURE 5-2

Stages of neutrophil development shown schematically. G-CSF (granulocyte colony-stimulating factor) and GM-CSF (granulocyte-macrophage colony-stimulating factor) are critical to this process. Identifying cellular characteristics and specific cell-surface markers are listed for each maturational stage.

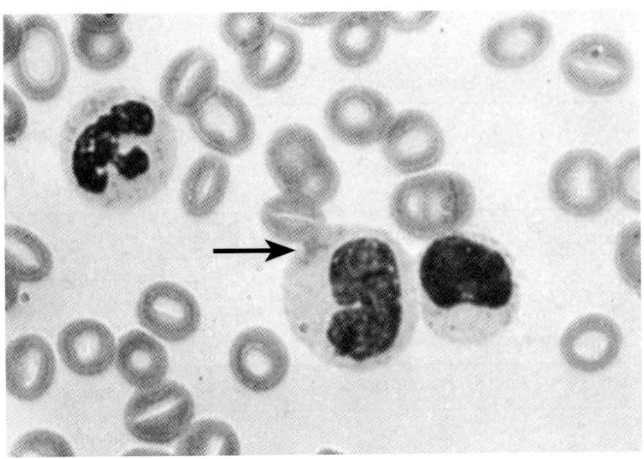

FIGURE 5-3
Neutrophil band with Döhle body. The neutrophil with a sausage-shaped nucleus in the center of the field is a band form. Döhle bodies are discrete, blue-staining nongranular areas found in the periphery of the cytoplasm of the neutrophil in infections and other toxic states. They represent aggregates of rough endoplasmic reticulum.

oxidase required for hydrogen peroxide production, histaminase, and receptors for certain chemoattractants and adherence-promoting factors (CR3) as well as receptors for the basement membrane component, laminin. The secondary granules do not contain acid hydrolases and therefore are not classic lysosomes. Packaging of secondary granule contents during myelopoiesis is controlled by CCAAT/enhancer binding protein-ε. Secondary granule contents are readily released extracellularly, and their mobilization is important in modulating inflammation. During the final stages of maturation, no cell division occurs, and the cell passes through the metamyelocyte stage and then to the band neutrophil with a sausage-shaped nucleus (Fig. 5-3). As the band cell matures, the nucleus assumes a lobulated configuration. The nucleus of neutrophils normally contains up to four segments (Fig. 5-4). Excessive segmentation (more than five nuclear lobes) may be a manifestation of folate or vitamin B_{12} deficiency or the congenital neutropenia syndrome of warts, hypogammaglobulinemia, infections, and myelokathexis (WHIM) described later. The Pelger-Hüet anomaly (Fig. 5-5), an infrequent dominant benign inherited trait, results in neutrophils with distinctive bilobed nuclei that must be distinguished from band forms. Acquired bilobed nuclei, pseudo Pelger-Hüet anomaly, can occur with acute infections or in myelodysplastic syndromes. The physiologic role of the normal multilobed nucleus of neutrophils is unknown, but it may allow great deformation of neutrophils during migration into tissues at sites of inflammation.

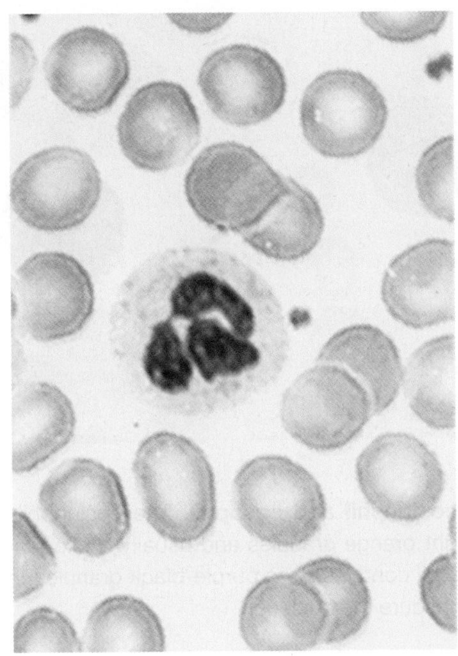

FIGURE 5-4
Normal granulocyte. The normal granulocyte has a segmented nucleus with heavy, clumped chromatin; fine neutrophilic granules are dispersed throughout the cytoplasm.

In severe acute bacterial infection, prominent neutrophil cytoplasmic granules, called *toxic granulations*, are occasionally seen. Toxic granulations are immature or abnormally staining azurophil granules. Cytoplasmic inclusions, also called *Döhle bodies* (Fig. 5-3), can be seen during infection and are fragments of ribosome-rich endoplasmic reticulum. Large neutrophil vacuoles are often present in acute bacterial infection and probably represent pinocytosed (internalized) membrane.

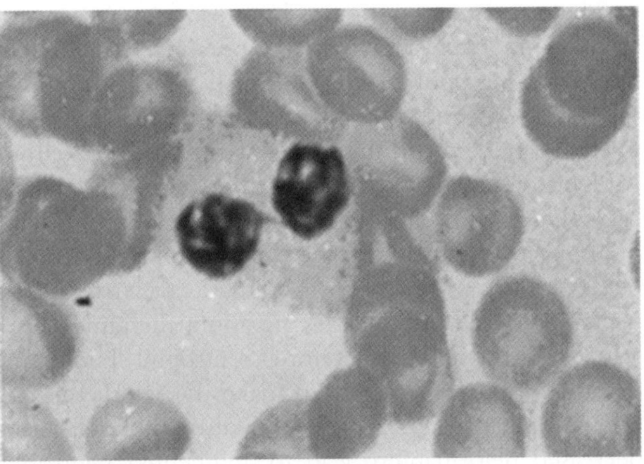

FIGURE 5-5
Pelger-Hüet anomaly. In this benign disorder, the majority of granulocytes are bilobed. The nucleus frequently has a spectacle-like, or "pince-nez," configuration.

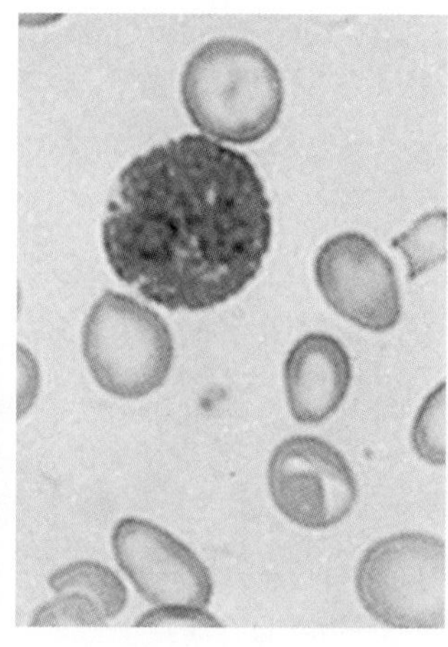
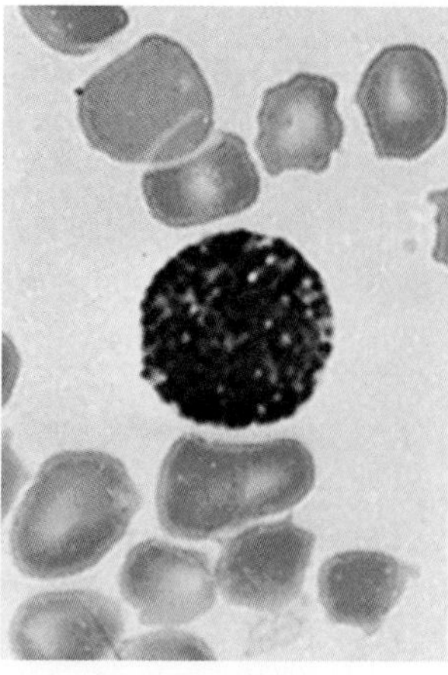

FIGURE 5-6
Normal eosinophil and basophil. The eosinophil contains large, bright orange granules and usually a bilobed nucleus. The basophil contains large purple-black granules that fill the cell and obscure the nucleus.

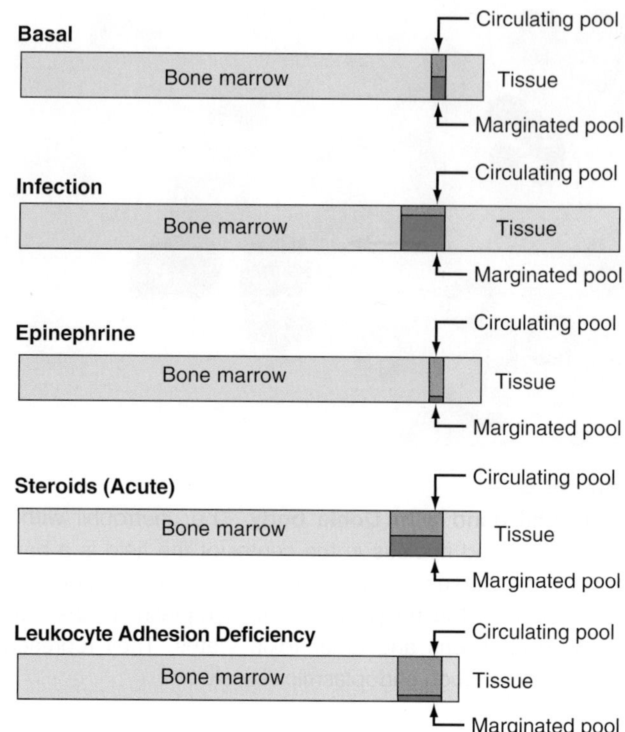

FIGURE 5-7
Schematic neutrophil distribution and kinetics between the different anatomic and functional pools.

Neutrophils are heterogeneous in function. Monoclonal antibodies have been developed that recognize only a subset of mature neutrophils. The meaning of neutrophil heterogeneity is not known.

The morphology of eosinophils and basophils is shown in Fig. 5-6.

MARROW RELEASE AND CIRCULATING COMPARTMENTS

Specific signals, including IL-1, tumor necrosis factor α (TNF-α), the CSFs, complement fragments, and chemokines, mobilize leukocytes from the bone marrow and deliver them to the blood in an unstimulated state. Under normal conditions, ~90% of the neutrophil pool is in the bone marrow, 2–3% in the circulation, and the remainder in the tissues (Fig. 5-7).

The circulating pool exists in two dynamic compartments: one freely flowing and one marginated. The freely flowing pool is about one-half the neutrophils in the basal state and is composed of those cells that are in the blood and not in contact with the endothelium. Marginated leukocytes are those that are in close physical contact with the endothelium (Fig. 5-8). In the pulmonary circulation, where an extensive capillary bed (~1000 capillaries per alveolus) exists, margination occurs because the capillaries are about the same size as a mature neutrophil. Therefore, neutrophil fluidity and deformability are necessary to make the transit through the pulmonary bed. Increased neutrophil rigidity and decreased deformability lead to augmented neutrophil trapping and margination in the lung. In contrast, in the systemic postcapillary venules, margination is mediated by the interaction of specific cell-surface molecules called *selectins*. Selectins are glycoproteins expressed on neutrophils and endothelial cells, among others, that cause a low-affinity interaction, resulting in "rolling" of the neutrophil along the endothelial surface. On neutrophils, the molecule L-selectin (cluster determinant [CD] 62L) binds to glycosylated proteins on endothelial cells (e.g., glycosylation-dependent cell adhesion molecule [GlyCAM1] and CD34). Glycoproteins on neutrophils, most importantly sialyl-Lewis^x (SLe^x, CD15s), are targets for binding of selectins expressed on endothelial cells (E-selectin [CD62E] and P-selectin [CD62P]) and other leukocytes. In response to chemotactic stimuli from injured tissues (e.g., complement product C5a, leukotriene B_4, IL-8) or bacterial products (e.g., *N*-formylmethionylleucylphenylalanine [f-metleuphe]), neutrophil adhesiveness increases, and the cells "stick" to the endothelium through *integrins*. The integrins are leukocyte glycoproteins that exist as complexes of a common CD18 β chain with CD11a (LFA-1), CD11b (called Mac-1, CR3, or the C3bi receptor), and CD11c (called p150,95 or CR4). CD11a/CD18 and CD11b/CD18 bind to specific endothelial receptors (intercellular adhesion molecules [CAM] 1 and 2).

On cell stimulation, L-selectin is shed from neutrophils, and E-selectin increases in the blood, presumably because it is shed from endothelial cells; receptors for chemoattractants and opsonins are mobilized; and the phagocytes orient toward the chemoattractant source in the extravascular space, increase their motile activity

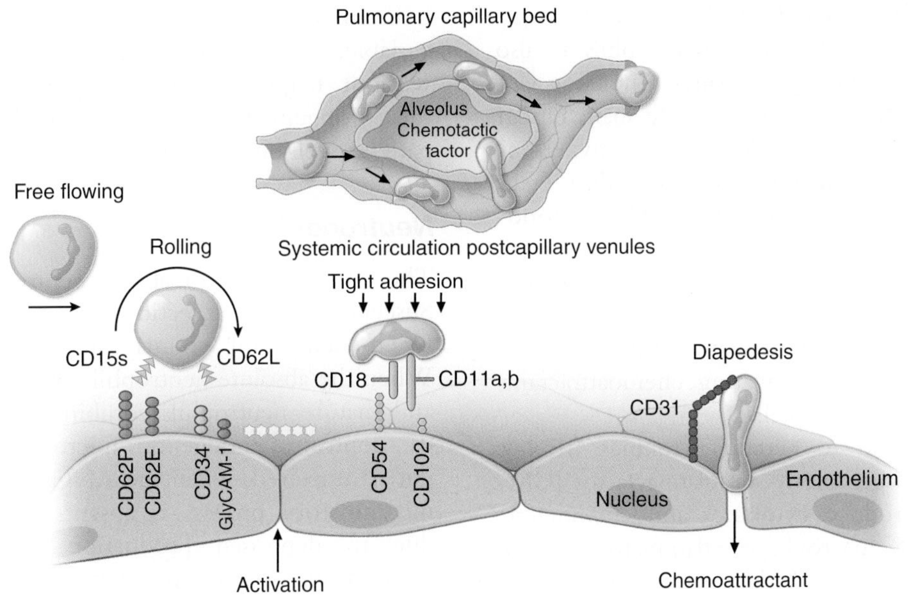

FIGURE 5-8

Neutrophil travel through the pulmonary capillaries is dependent on neutrophil deformability. Neutrophil rigidity (e.g., caused by C5a) enhances pulmonary trapping and response to pulmonary pathogens in a way that is not so dependent on cell-surface receptors. Intraalveolar chemotactic factors, such as those caused by certain bacteria (e.g., *Streptococcus pneumoniae*), lead to diapedesis of neutrophils from the pulmonary capillaries into the alveolar space. Neutrophil interaction with the endothelium of the systemic postcapillary venules is dependent on molecules of attachment. The neutrophil "rolls" along the endothelium using selectins: neutrophil CD15s (sialyl-Lewis^x) binds to CD62E (E-selectin) and CD62P (P-selectin) on endothelial cells; CD62L (l-selectin) on neutrophils binds to CD34 and other molecules (e.g., GlyCAM-1) expressed on endothelium. Chemokines or other activation factors stimulate integrin-mediated "tight adhesion": CD11a/CD18 (LFA-1) and CD11b/CD18 (Mac-1, CR3) bind to CD54 (ICAM-1) and CD102 (ICAM-2) on the endothelium. Diapedesis occurs between endothelial cells: CD31 (PECAM-1) expressed by the emigrating neutrophil interacts with CD31 expressed at the endothelial cell–cell junction. CD, cluster determinant; GlyCAM, glycosylation-dependent cell adhesion molecule; ICAM, intercellular adhesion molecule; PECAM, platelet/endothelial cell adhesion molecule.

(chemokinesis), and migrate directionally (chemotaxis) into tissues. The process of migration into tissues is called *diapedesis* and involves the crawling of neutrophils between postcapillary endothelial cells that open junctions between adjacent cells to permit leukocyte passage. Diapedesis involves platelet/endothelial cell adhesion molecule (PECAM) 1 (CD31), which is expressed on both the emigrating leukocyte and the endothelial cells. The endothelial responses (increased blood flow from increased vasodilation and permeability) are mediated by anaphylatoxins (e.g., C3a and C5a) as well as vasodilators such as histamine, bradykinin, serotonin, nitric oxide, vascular endothelial growth factor (VEGF), and prostaglandins E and I. Cytokines regulate some of these processes (e.g., TNF-α induction of VEGF, interferon [IFN] γ inhibition of prostaglandin E).

In a healthy adult, most neutrophils leave the body by migration through the mucous membrane of the gastrointestinal tract. Normally, neutrophils spend a short time in the circulation (half-life, 6–7 h). Senescent neutrophils are cleared from the circulation by macrophages in the lung and spleen. Once in the tissues, neutrophils release enzymes, such as collagenase and elastase, which may help establish abscess cavities. Neutrophils ingest pathogenic materials that have been opsonized by IgG and C3b. Fibronectin and the tetrapeptide tuftsin also facilitate phagocytosis.

With phagocytosis comes a burst of oxygen consumption and activation of the hexose-monophosphate shunt. A membrane-associated NADPH oxidase, consisting of membrane and cytosolic components, is assembled and catalyzes the reduction of oxygen to superoxide anion, which is then converted to hydrogen peroxide and other toxic oxygen products (e.g., hydroxyl radical). Hydrogen peroxide + chloride + neutrophil myeloperoxidase generate hypochlorous acid (bleach), hypochlorite, and chlorine. These products oxidize and halogenate microorganisms and tumor cells and, when uncontrolled, can damage host tissue. Strongly cationic proteins, defensins, elastase, cathepsins, and probably nitric oxide also participate in microbial killing. Lactoferrin chelates iron, an important growth factor for microorganisms, especially fungi. Other enzymes, such as lysozyme and acid proteases, help digest microbial debris. After 1–4 days in tissues, neutrophils die. The apoptosis of neutrophils is also cytokine-regulated; granulocyte colony-stimulating factor (G-CSF) and IFN-γ prolong their life span. Under certain conditions, such as in delayed-type hypersensitivity, monocyte accumulation occurs within 6–12 h of initiation of inflammation. Neutrophils, monocytes, microorganisms in various states of digestion, and altered local tissue cells make up the inflammatory exudate, pus. Myeloperoxidase confers the characteristic green color to pus and may participate in turning off the inflammatory process by inactivating chemoattractants and immobilizing phagocytic cells.

Neutrophils respond to certain cytokines (IFN-γ, granulocyte-macrophage colony-stimulating factor [GM-CSF], IL-8) and produce cytokines and chemotactic signals (TNF-α, IL-8, macrophage inflammatory protein [MIP] 1) that modulate the inflammatory response. In the presence of fibrinogen, f-metleuphe or leukotriene B_4 induces IL-8 production by neutrophils, providing autocrine amplification of inflammation. *Chemokines* (*chemo*attractant cyto*kines*) are small proteins produced by many different cell types, including endothelial cells, fibroblasts, epithelial cells, neutrophils, and monocytes, that regulate neutrophil, monocyte, eosinophil, and lymphocyte recruitment and activation. Chemokines transduce their signals through heterotrimeric G protein–linked receptors that have seven cell membrane–spanning domains, the same type of cell-surface receptor that mediates the response to the classic chemoattractants f-metleuphe and C5a. Four major groups of chemokines are recognized based on the cysteine structure near the N terminus: C, CC, CXC, and CXXXC. The CXC cytokines such as IL-8 mainly attract neutrophils; CC chemokines such as MIP-1 attract lymphocytes, monocytes, eosinophils, and basophils; the C chemokine lymphotactin is T cell tropic; the CXXXC chemokine fractalkine attracts neutrophils, monocytes, and T cells. These molecules and their receptors not only regulate the trafficking and activation of inflammatory cells, but specific chemokine receptors serve as co-receptors for HIV infection and have a role in other viral infections such as West Nile infection and atherogenesis.

NEUTROPHIL ABNORMALITIES

Defects in the neutrophil life cycle can lead to dysfunction and compromised host defenses. Inflammation is often depressed, and the clinical result is often recurrent, with severe bacterial and fungal infections. Aphthous ulcers of mucous membranes (gray ulcers without pus) and gingivitis and periodontal disease suggest a phagocytic cell disorder. Patients with congenital phagocyte defects can have infections within the first few days of life. Skin, ear, upper and lower respiratory tract, and bone infections are common. Sepsis and meningitis are rare. In some disorders, the frequency of infection is variable, and patients can go for months or even years without major infection. Aggressive management of these congenital diseases has extended the life span of patients well beyond 30 years.

Neutropenia

The consequences of absent neutrophils are dramatic. Susceptibility to infectious diseases increases sharply when neutrophil counts fall below 1000 cells/μL. When the absolute neutrophil count (ANC; band forms and mature neutrophils combined) falls to <500 cells/μL, control of endogenous microbial flora (e.g., mouth, gut) is impaired; when the ANC is <200/μL, the local inflammatory process is absent. Neutropenia can be due to depressed production, increased peripheral destruction, or excessive peripheral pooling. A falling neutrophil count or a significant decrease in the number of neutrophils below steady-state levels, together with a failure to increase neutrophil counts in the setting of infection or other challenge, requires investigation. Acute neutropenia, such as that caused by cancer chemotherapy, is more likely to be associated with increased risk of infection than neutropenia of long duration (months to years) that reverses in response to infection or carefully controlled administration of endotoxin (see "Laboratory Diagnosis and Management," later in the chapter).

Some causes of inherited and acquired neutropenia are listed in **Table 5-1**. The most common neutropenias are iatrogenic, resulting from the use of cytotoxic or immunosuppressive therapies for malignancy or control of autoimmune disorders. These drugs cause neutropenia because they result in decreased production of rapidly growing progenitor (stem) cells of the marrow. Certain antibiotics such as chloramphenicol, trimethoprim–sulfamethoxazole, flucytosine, vidarabine, and the antiretroviral drug zidovudine may cause neutropenia by inhibiting proliferation of myeloid precursors. Azathioprine and 6-mercaptopurine are metabolized by the enzyme thiopurine methyltransferase (TMPT), hypofunctional polymorphisms in which can lead to accumulation of 6-thioguanine and profound marrow toxicity. The marrow suppression is generally dose-related and dependent on continued administration of the drug. Cessation of the offending agent and recombinant human G-CSF usually reverse these forms of neutropenia.

Another important mechanism for iatrogenic neutropenia is the effect of drugs that serve as immune haptens and sensitize neutrophils or neutrophil precursors to immune-mediated peripheral destruction. This form of drug-induced neutropenia can be seen within 7 days of exposure to the drug; with previous drug exposure, resulting in preexisting antibodies, neutropenia may

TABLE 5-1

CAUSES OF NEUTROPENIA

Decreased Production
Drug-induced—alkylating agents (nitrogen mustard, busulfan, chlorambucil, cyclophosphamide); antimetabolites (methotrexate, 6-mercaptopurine, 5-flucytosine); noncytotoxic agents (antibiotics [chloramphenicol, penicillins, sulfonamides], phenothiazines, tranquilizers [meprobamate], anticonvulsants [carbamazepine], antipsychotics [clozapine], certain diuretics, anti-inflammatory agents, antithyroid drugs, many others)
Hematologic diseases—idiopathic, cyclic neutropenia, Chédiak-Higashi syndrome, aplastic anemia, infantile genetic disorders (see text)
Tumor invasion, myelofibrosis
Nutritional deficiency—vitamin B_{12}, folate (especially with alcoholism)
Infection—tuberculosis, typhoid fever, brucellosis, tularemia, measles, infectious mononucleosis, malaria, viral hepatitis, leishmaniasis, AIDS
Peripheral Destruction
Antineutrophil antibodies and/or splenic or lung trapping
Autoimmune disorders—Felty's syndrome, rheumatoid arthritis, lupus erythematosus
Drugs as haptens—aminopyrine, α-methyldopa, phenylbutazone, mercurial diuretics, some phenothiazines
Granulomatosis with polyangiitis (Wegener's)
Peripheral Pooling (Transient Neutropenia)
Overwhelming bacterial infection (acute endotoxemia)
Hemodialysis
Cardiopulmonary bypass

occur a few hours after administration of the drug. Although any drug can cause this form of neutropenia, the most frequent causes are commonly used antibiotics, such as sulfa-containing compounds, penicillins, and cephalosporins. Fever and eosinophilia may also be associated with drug reactions, but often these signs are not present. Drug-induced neutropenia can be severe, but discontinuation of the sensitizing drug is sufficient for recovery, which is usually seen within 5–7 days and is complete by 10 days. Readministration of the sensitizing drug should be avoided, since abrupt neutropenia will often result. For this reason, diagnostic challenge should be avoided.

Autoimmune neutropenias caused by circulating antineutrophil antibodies are another form of acquired neutropenia that results in increased destruction of neutrophils. Acquired neutropenia may also be seen with viral infections, including infection with HIV. Acquired neutropenia may be cyclic in nature, occurring at intervals of several weeks. Acquired cyclic or stable neutropenia may be associated with an expansion of large granular lymphocytes (LGLs), which may be T cells, NK cells, or NK-like cells. Patients with large granular lymphocytosis may have moderate blood and bone marrow lymphocytosis, neutropenia, polyclonal hypergammaglobulinemia, splenomegaly, rheumatoid arthritis, and absence of lymphadenopathy. Such patients may have a chronic and relatively stable course. Recurrent bacterial infections are frequent. Benign and malignant forms of this syndrome occur. In some patients, a spontaneous regression has occurred even after 11 years, suggesting an immunoregulatory defect as the basis for at least one form of the disorder. Glucocorticoids, cyclosporine, and methotrexate are commonly used to manage these cytopenias.

Hereditary neutropenias

Hereditary neutropenias are rare and may manifest in early childhood as a profound constant neutropenia or agranulocytosis. Congenital forms of neutropenia include Kostmann's syndrome (neutrophil count <100/μL), which is often fatal and due to mutations in the anti-apoptosis gene HAX-1; severe chronic neutropenia (neutrophil count of 300–1500/μL) due to mutations in neutrophil elastase (ELA-2); hereditary cyclic neutropenia, or, more appropriately, cyclic hematopoiesis, also due to mutations in neutrophil elastase (ELA-2); the cartilage-hair hypoplasia syndrome due to mutations in the mitochondrial RNA-processing endoribonuclease RMRP; Shwachman-Diamond syndrome associated with pancreatic insufficiency due to mutations in the Shwachman-Bodian-Diamond syndrome gene *SBDS*; the WHIM (*w*arts, *h*ypogammaglobulinemia, *i*nfections, *m*yelokathexis [retention of WBCs in the marrow]) syndrome, characterized by neutrophil hypersegmentation and bone marrow myeloid arrest due to mutations in the chemokine receptor CXCR4; and neutropenias associated with other immune defects, such as X-linked agammaglobulinemia, Wiskott-Aldrich syndrome, and CD40 ligand deficiency. Mutations in the G-CSF receptor can develop in severe congenital neutropenia and are linked to leukemia. Absence of both myeloid and lymphoid cells is seen in reticular dysgenesis, due to mutations in the nuclear genome-encoded mitochondrial enzyme adenylate kinase-2 (AK2).

Maternal factors can be associated with neutropenia in the newborn. Transplacental transfer of IgG directed against antigens on fetal neutrophils can result in peripheral destruction. Drugs (e.g., thiazides) ingested during pregnancy can cause neutropenia in the newborn by either depressed production or peripheral destruction.

In Felty's syndrome—the triad of rheumatoid arthritis, splenomegaly, and neutropenia spleen-produced antibodies can shorten neutrophil life span, while LGLs can attack marrow neutrophil precursors. Splenectomy may increase the neutrophil count in Felty's syndrome and lower serum neutrophil-binding IgG. Some Felty's syndrome patients also have neutropenia associated with an increased number of LGLs. Splenomegaly with peripheral trapping and destruction of neutrophils is also seen in lysosomal storage diseases and in portal hypertension.

Neutrophilia

Neutrophilia results from increased neutrophil production, increased marrow release, or defective margination (Table 5-2). The most important acute cause of neutrophilia is infection. Neutrophilia from acute infection represents both increased production and increased marrow release. Increased production is also associated with chronic inflammation and certain myeloproliferative diseases. Increased marrow release and mobilization of the marginated leukocyte pool are induced by glucocorticoids. Release of epinephrine, as with vigorous exercise, excitement, or stress, will demarginate neutrophils in the spleen and lungs and double the neutrophil count in minutes. Cigarette smoking can elevate neutrophil counts above the normal range. Leukocytosis with cell counts of 10,000–25,000/μL occurs in response to infection and other forms of acute inflammation and results from both release of the marginated pool and mobilization of marrow reserves. Persistent neutrophilia with cell counts of ≥30,000–50,000/μL is called a *leukemoid reaction*, a term often used to distinguish this degree of neutrophilia from leukemia. In a leukemoid reaction, the circulating neutrophils are usually mature and not clonally derived.

TABLE 5-2

CAUSES OF NEUTROPHILIA
Increased Production
Idiopathic
Drug-induced—glucocorticoids, G-CSF
Infection—bacterial, fungal, sometimes viral
Inflammation—thermal injury, tissue necrosis, myocardial and pulmonary infarction, hypersensitivity states, collagen vascular diseases
Myeloproliferative diseases—myelocytic leukemia, myeloid metaplasia, polycythemia vera
Increased Marrow Release
Glucocorticoids
Acute infection (endotoxin)
Inflammation—thermal injury
Decreased or Defective Margination
Drugs—epinephrine, glucocorticoids, nonsteroidal anti-inflammatory agents
Stress, excitement, vigorous exercise
Leukocyte adhesion deficiency type 1 (CD18); leukocyte adhesion deficiency type 2 (selectin ligand, CD15s); leukocyte adhesion deficiency type 3 (Kindlin-3)
Miscellaneous
Metabolic disorders—ketoacidosis, acute renal failure, eclampsia, acute poisoning
Drugs—lithium
Other—metastatic carcinoma, acute hemorrhage or hemolysis

Abbreviation: G-CSF, granulocyte colony-stimulating factor.

Abnormal neutrophil function

Inherited and acquired abnormalities of phagocyte function are listed in Table 5-3. The resulting diseases are best considered in terms of the functional defects of adherence, chemotaxis, and microbicidal activity. The distinguishing features of the important inherited disorders of phagocyte function are shown in Table 5-4.

Disorders of adhesion

Three main types of leukocyte adhesion deficiency (LAD) have been described. All are autosomal recessive and result in the inability of neutrophils to exit the circulation to sites of infection, leading to leukocytosis and increased susceptibility to infection (Fig. 5-8). Patients with LAD 1 have mutations in CD18, the common component of the integrins LFA-1, Mac-1, and p150,95, leading to a defect in tight adhesion between neutrophils and the endothelium. The heterodimer formed by CD18/CD11b (Mac-1) is also the receptor for the complement-derived opsonin C3bi (CR3). The *CD18* gene is located on distal chromosome 21q. The severity of the defect determines the severity of clinical disease. Complete lack of expression of the leukocyte integrins results in a severe phenotype in which inflammatory stimuli do not increase the expression of leukocyte integrins on neutrophils or activated T and B cells. Neutrophils (and monocytes) from patients with LAD 1 adhere poorly to endothelial cells and protein-coated surfaces and exhibit defective spreading, aggregation, and chemotaxis. Patients with LAD 1 have recurrent bacterial infections involving the skin, oral and genital mucosa, and respiratory and intestinal tracts; persistent leukocytosis (resting neutrophil counts of 15,000–20,000/μL) because cells do not marginate; and, in severe cases, a history of delayed separation of the umbilical stump. Infections, especially of the skin, may become necrotic with progressively enlarging borders, slow healing, and development of dysplastic scars. The most common bacteria are *Staphylococcus aureus* and enteric gram-negative bacteria. LAD 2 is caused by an abnormality of fucosylation of SLe^x (CD15s), the ligand on neutrophils that interacts with selectins on endothelial cells and is responsible for neutrophil rolling along the endothelium. Infection susceptibility in LAD 2 appears to be less severe than in LAD 1. LAD 2 is also known as *congenital disorder of glycosylation IIc* (CDGIIc) due to mutation in a GDP-fucose transporter (SLC35C1). LAD 3 is characterized by infection susceptibility, leukocytosis, and petechial hemorrhage due to

TABLE 5-3

TYPES OF GRANULOCYTE AND MONOCYTE DISORDERS

	CAUSE OF INDICATED DYSFUNCTION		
FUNCTION	**DRUG-INDUCED**	**ACQUIRED**	**INHERITED**
Adherence-aggregation	Aspirin, colchicine, alcohol, glucocorticoids, ibuprofen, piroxicam	Neonatal state, hemodialysis	Leukocyte adhesion deficiency types 1, 2, and 3
Deformability		Leukemia, neonatal state, diabetes mellitus, immature neutrophils	
Chemokinesis-chemotaxis	Glucocorticoids (high dose), auranofin, colchicine (weak effect), phenylbutazone, naproxen, indomethacin, IL-2	Thermal injury, malignancy, malnutrition, periodontal disease, neonatal state, systemic lupus erythematosus, rheumatoid arthritis, diabetes mellitus, sepsis, influenza virus infection, herpes simplex virus infection, acrodermatitis enteropathica, AIDS	Chédiak-Higashi syndrome, neutrophil-specific granule deficiency, hyper IgE–recurrent infection (Job's) syndrome (in some patients), Down syndrome, α-mannosidase deficiency, leukocyte adhesion deficiencies, Wiskott-Aldrich syndrome
Microbicidal activity	Colchicine, cyclophosphamide, glucocorticoids (high dose), TNF-α blocking antibodies	Leukemia, aplastic anemia, certain neutropenias, tuftsin deficiency, thermal injury, sepsis, neonatal state, diabetes mellitus, malnutrition, AIDS	Chédiak-Higashi syndrome, neutrophil-specific granule deficiency, chronic granulomatous disease, defects in IFN- /IL-12 axis

Abbreviations: IFN, interferon; IL, interleukin; TNF-α, tumor necrosis factor alpha.

TABLE 5-4

INHERITED DISORDERS OF PHAGOCYTE FUNCTION: DIFFERENTIAL FEATURES

CLINICAL MANIFESTATIONS	CELLULAR OR MOLECULAR DEFECTS	DIAGNOSIS
Chronic Granulomatous Diseases (70% X-linked, 30% Autosomal Recessive)		
Severe infections of skin, ears, lungs, liver, and bone with catalase-positive microorganisms such as *Staphylococcus aureus, Burkholderia cepacia, Aspergillus* spp., *Chromobacterium violaceum*; often hard to culture organism; excessive inflammation with granulomas, frequent lymph node suppuration; granulomas can obstruct GI or GU tracts; gingivitis, aphthous ulcers, seborrheic dermatitis	No respiratory burst due to the lack of one of five NADPH oxidase subunits in neutrophils, monocytes, and eosinophils	DHR or NBT test; no superoxide and H_2O_2 production by neutrophils; immunoblot for NADPH oxidase components; genetic detection
Chédiak-Higashi Syndrome (Autosomal Recessive)		
Recurrent pyogenic infections, especially with *S. aureus;* many patients get lymphoma-like illness during adolescence; periodontal disease; partial oculocutaneous albinism, nystagmus, progressive peripheral neuropathy, mental retardation in some patients	Reduced chemotaxis and phagolysosome fusion, increased respiratory burst activity, defective egress from marrow, abnormal skin window; defect in *CHS1*	Giant primary granules in neutrophils and other granule-bearing cells (Wright's stain); genetic detection
Specific Granule Deficiency (Autosomal Recessive)		
Recurrent infections of skin, ears, and sinopulmonary tract; delayed wound healing; decreased inflammation; bleeding diathesis	Abnormal chemotaxis, impaired respiratory burst and bacterial killing, failure to upregulate chemotactic and adhesion receptors with stimulation, defect in transcription of granule proteins; defect in C/EBPε	Lack of secondary (specific) granules in neutrophils (Wright's stain), no neutrophil-specific granule contents (i.e., lactoferrin), no defensins, platelet α granule abnormality; genetic detection

(*continued*)

TABLE 5-4

INHERITED DISORDERS OF PHAGOCYTE FUNCTION: DIFFERENTIAL FEATURES (*CONTINUED*)

CLINICAL MANIFESTATIONS	CELLULAR OR MOLECULAR DEFECTS	DIAGNOSIS
Myeloperoxidase Deficiency (Autosomal Recessive)		
Clinically normal except in patients with underlying disease such as diabetes mellitus; then candidiasis or other fungal infections	No myeloperoxidase due to pre- and posttranslational defects in myeloperoxidase deficiency	No peroxidase in neutrophils; genetic detection
Leukocyte Adhesion Deficiency		
Type 1: Delayed separation of umbilical cord, sustained neutrophilia, recurrent infections of skin and mucosa, gingivitis, periodontal disease Type 2: Mental retardation, short stature, Bombay (hh) blood phenotype, recurrent infections, neutrophilia Type 3: Petechial hemorrhage, recurrent infections	Impaired phagocyte adherence, aggregation, spreading, chemotaxis, phagocytosis of C3bi-coated particles; defective production of CD18 subunit common to leukocyte integrins Impaired phagocyte rolling along endothelium due to defects in fucose transporter Impaired signaling for integrin activation resulting in impaired adhesion due to mutation in *FERMT3*	Reduced phagocyte surface expression of the CD18-containing integrins with monoclonal antibodies against LFA-1 (CD18/CD11a), Mac-1 or CR3 (CD18/CD11b), p150,95 (CD18/CD11c); genetic detection Reduced phagocyte surface expression of Sialyl-Lewis^x, with monoclonal antibodies against CD15s; genetic detection Reduced signaling for adhesion through integrins; genetic detection
Phagocyte Activation Defects (X-linked and Autosomal Recessive)		
NEMO deficiency: mild hypohidrotic ectodermal dysplasia; broad-based immune defect: pyogenic and encapsulated bacteria, viruses, *Pneumocystis*, mycobacteria; X-linked IRAK4 and MyD88 deficiency: susceptibility to pyogenic bacteria such as staphylococci, streptococci, clostridia; resistant to candida; autosomal recessive	Impaired phagocyte activation by IL-1, IL-18, TLR, CD40L, TNF-α leading to problems with inflammation and antibody production Impaired phagocyte activation by endotoxin through TLR and other pathways; TNF-α signaling preserved	Poor in vitro response to endotoxin; lack of NF-κB activation; genetic detection Poor in vitro response to endotoxin; lack of NF-κB activation by endotoxin; genetic detection
Hyper IgE–Recurrent Infection Syndrome (Autosomal Dominant) (Job's Syndrome)		
Eczematoid or pruritic dermatitis, "cold" skin abscesses, recurrent pneumonias with *S. aureus* with bronchopleural fistulas and cyst formation, mild eosinophilia, mucocutaneous candidiasis, characteristic facies, restrictive lung disease, scoliosis, delayed primary dental deciduation DOCK8 deficiency (autosomal recessive), severe eczema, atopic dermatitis, cutaneous abscesses, HSV, HPV, and molluscum infections, severe allergies, cancer	Reduced chemotaxis in some patients, reduced suppressor T cell activity. Mutation in *STAT3* Impaired T cell proliferation to mitogens	Somatic and immune features involving lungs, skeleton, and immune system; serum IgE >2000 IU/mL; genetic testing Severe allergies, viral infections, high IgE, eosinophilia, low IgM, progressive lymphopenia, genetic detection
Mycobacteria Susceptibility (Autosomal Dominant and Recessive Forms)		
Severe extrapulmonary or disseminated infections with bacille Calmette-Guérin nontuberculous mycobacteria, salmonella, histoplasmosis, coccidioidomycosis, poor granuloma formation	Inability to kill intracellular organisms due to low IFN-γ production or response; mutations in IFN-γ receptors, IL-12 receptor, IL-12 p40, STAT1, NEMO	Low or very high levels of IFN-γ receptor 1; functional assays of cytokine production and response; genetic detection

Abbreviations: C/EBPε, CCAAT/enhancer binding protein-ε; DHR, dihydrorhodamine (oxidation test); DOCK8, dedicator of cytokinesis 8; GI, gastrointestinal; GU, genitourinary; HPV, human papilloma virus; HSV, herpes simplex virus; IFN, interferon; IL, interleukin; IRAK4, IL-1 receptor–associated kinase 4; LFA-1, leukocyte function–associated antigen 1; MyD88, myeloid differentiation primary response gene 88; NADPH, nicotinamide-adenine dinueleotide phosphate; NBT, nitroblue tetrazolium (dye test); NEMO, NF-κB essential modulator; NF-κB, nuclear factor κB; STAT1, -3, signal transducer and activator of transcription 1, –3; TLR, Toll-like receptor; TNF, tumor necrosis factor.

impaired integrin activation caused by mutations in the gene *FERMT3*.

Disorders of neutrophil granules

The most common neutrophil defect is myeloperoxidase deficiency, a primary granule defect inherited as an autosomal recessive trait; the incidence is ~1 in 2000 persons. Isolated myeloperoxidase deficiency is not associated with clinically compromised defenses, presumably because other defense systems such as hydrogen peroxide generation are amplified. Microbicidal activity of neutrophils is delayed but not absent. Myeloperoxidase deficiency may make other acquired host defense defects more serious. An acquired form of myeloperoxidase deficiency occurs in myelomonocytic leukemia and acute myeloid leukemia.

Chédiak-Higashi syndrome (CHS) is a rare disease with autosomal recessive inheritance due to defects in the lysosomal transport protein LYST, encoded by the gene *CHS1* at 1q42. This protein is required for normal packaging and disbursement of granules. Neutrophils (and all cells containing lysosomes) from patients with CHS characteristically have large granules (Fig. 5-9), making it a systemic disease. Patients with CHS have nystagmus, partial oculocutaneous albinism, and an increased number of infections resulting from many bacterial agents. Some CHS patients develop an "accelerated phase" in childhood with a hemophagocytic syndrome and an aggressive lymphoma requiring bone marrow transplantation. CHS neutrophils and monocytes have impaired chemotaxis and abnormal rates of microbial killing due to slow rates of fusion of the lysosomal granules with phagosomes. NK cell function is also impaired. CHS patients may develop a severe disabling peripheral neuropathy in adulthood that can lead to bed confinement.

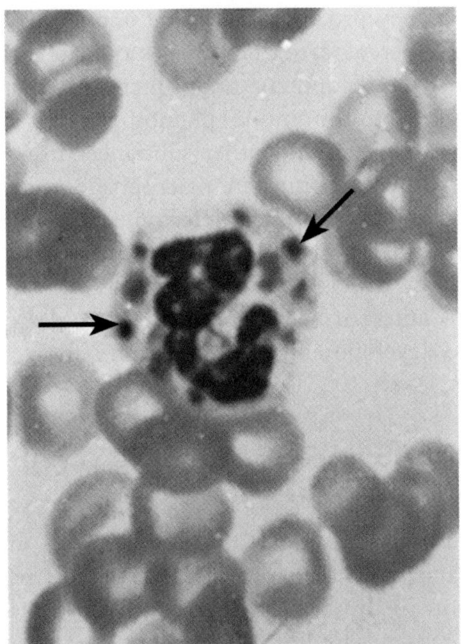

FIGURE 5-9
Chédiak-Higashi syndrome. The granulocytes contain huge cytoplasmic granules formed from aggregation and fusion of azurophilic and specific granules (*arrows*). Large abnormal granules are found in other granule-containing cells throughout the body.

Specific granule deficiency is a rare autosomal recessive disease in which the production of secondary granules and their contents, as well as the primary granule component defensins, is defective. The defect in bacterial killing leads to severe bacterial infections. One type of specific granule deficiency is due to a mutation in the CCAAT/enhancer binding protein-ε, a regulator of expression of granule components.

Chronic granulomatous disease

Chronic granulomatous disease (CGD) is a group of disorders of granulocyte and monocyte oxidative metabolism. Although CGD is rare, with an incidence of 1 in 200,000 individuals, it is an important model of defective neutrophil oxidative metabolism. Most often CGD is inherited as an X-linked recessive trait; 30% of patients inherit the disease in an autosomal recessive pattern. Mutations in the genes for the five proteins that assemble at the plasma membrane account for all patients with CGD. Two proteins (a 91-kDa protein, abnormal in X-linked CGD, and a 22-kDa protein, absent in one form of autosomal recessive CGD) form the heterodimer cytochrome b-558 in the plasma membrane. Three other proteins (40-, 47-, and 67-kDa, abnormal in the other autosomal recessive forms of CGD) are cytoplasmic in origin and interact with the cytochrome after cell activation to form NADPH oxidase, required for hydrogen peroxide production. Leukocytes from patients with CGD have severely diminished hydrogen peroxide production. The genes involved in each of the defects have been cloned and sequenced and the chromosome locations identified. Patients with CGD characteristically have increased numbers of infections due to catalase-positive microorganisms (organisms that destroy their own hydrogen peroxide). When patients with CGD become infected, they often have extensive inflammatory reactions, and lymph node suppuration is common despite the administration of appropriate antibiotics. Aphthous ulcers and chronic inflammation of the nares are often present. Granulomas are frequent and can obstruct the gastrointestinal or genitourinary tracts. The excessive inflammation reflects failure to downregulate inflammation, reflecting failure to inhibit the synthesis, degradation of, or response to chemoattractants or residual antigens, leading to persistent neutrophil accumulation. Impaired killing of intracellular microorganisms by macrophages may lead to persistent cell-mediated immune activation and granuloma formation. Autoimmune complications such as immune thrombocytopenic purpura and juvenile rheumatoid arthritis are also increased in CGD. In addition, discoid lupus is more common in X-linked carriers. Late complications, including nodular regenerative hyperplasia and portal hypertension, are increasingly recognized in long-term survivors of severe CGD.

Disorders of phagocyte activation

Phagocytes depend on cell-surface stimulation to induce signals that evoke multiple levels of the inflammatory response, including cytokine synthesis, chemotaxis, and antigen presentation. Mutations affecting the major pathway that signals through NF-κB have been noted in patients with a variety of infection susceptibility syndromes. If the defects are at a very late stage of signal transduction, in the protein critical for NF-κB activation known as the NF-κB essential modulator (NEMO), then affected males develop ectodermal dysplasia and severe immune deficiency with susceptibility to bacteria, fungi, mycobacteria, and viruses. If the defects in NF-κB activation are closer to the cell-surface receptors, in the proteins transducing Toll-like receptor signals, IL-1 receptor–associated kinase 4 (IRAK4), and myeloid differentiation primary response gene 88 (MyD88), then children have a marked susceptibility to pyogenic infections early in life but develop resistance to infection later.

MONONUCLEAR PHAGOCYTES

The mononuclear phagocyte system is composed of monoblasts, promonocytes, and monocytes in addition to the structurally diverse tissue macrophages that make up what was previously referred to as the reticuloendothelial system. Macrophages are long-lived phagocytic cells capable of many of the functions of neutrophils. They are also secretory cells that participate in many immunologic and inflammatory processes distinct from neutrophils. Monocytes leave the circulation by diapedesis more slowly than neutrophils and have a half-life in the blood of 12–24 h.

After blood monocytes arrive in the tissues, they differentiate into macrophages ("big eaters") with specialized functions suited for specific anatomic locations. Macrophages are particularly abundant in capillary walls of the lung, spleen, liver, and bone marrow, where they function to remove microorganisms and other noxious elements from the blood. Alveolar macrophages, liver Kupffer cells, splenic macrophages, peritoneal macrophages, bone marrow macrophages, lymphatic macrophages, brain microglial cells, and dendritic macrophages all have specialized functions. Macrophage-secreted products include lysozyme, neutral proteases, acid hydrolases, arginase, complement components, enzyme inhibitors (plasmin, α_2-macroglobulin), binding proteins (transferrin, fibronectin, transcobalamin II), nucleosides, and cytokines (TNF-α; IL-1, -8, -12, -18). IL-1 has many functions, including initiating fever in the hypothalamus, mobilizing leukocytes from the bone marrow, and activating lymphocytes and neutrophils. TNF-α is a pyrogen that duplicates many of the actions of IL-1 and plays an important role in the pathogenesis of gram-negative shock. TNF-α stimulates production of hydrogen peroxide and related toxic oxygen species by macrophages and neutrophils. In addition, TNF-α induces catabolic changes that contribute to the profound wasting (cachexia) associated with many chronic diseases.

Other macrophage-secreted products include reactive oxygen and nitrogen metabolites, bioactive lipids (arachidonic acid metabolites and platelet-activating factors), chemokines, CSFs, and factors stimulating fibroblast and vessel proliferation. Macrophages help regulate the replication of lymphocytes and participate in the killing of tumors, viruses, and certain bacteria (*Mycobacterium tuberculosis* and *Listeria monocytogenes*). Macrophages are key effector cells in the elimination of intracellular microorganisms. Their ability to fuse to form giant cells that coalesce into granulomas in response to some inflammatory stimuli is important in the elimination of intracellular microbes and is under the control of IFN-γ. Nitric oxide induced by IFN-γ is an important effector against intracellular parasites, including tuberculosis and *Leishmania*.

Macrophages play an important role in the immune response. They process and present antigen to lymphocytes and secrete cytokines that modulate and direct lymphocyte development and function. Macrophages participate in autoimmune phenomena by removing immune complexes and other substances from the circulation. Polymorphisms in macrophage receptors for immunoglobulin (FcγRII) determine susceptibility to some infections and autoimmune diseases. In wound healing, they dispose of senescent cells, and they contribute to atheroma development. Macrophage elastase mediates development of emphysema from cigarette smoking.

DISORDERS OF THE MONONUCLEAR PHAGOCYTE SYSTEM

Many disorders of neutrophils extend to mononuclear phagocytes. Thus, drugs that suppress neutrophil production in the bone marrow can cause monocytopenia. Transient monocytopenia occurs after stress or glucocorticoid administration. Monocytosis is associated with tuberculosis, brucellosis, subacute bacterial endocarditis, Rocky Mountain spotted fever, malaria, and visceral leishmaniasis (kala azar). Monocytosis also occurs with malignancies, leukemias, myeloproliferative syndromes, hemolytic anemias, chronic idiopathic neutropenias, and granulomatous diseases such as sarcoidosis, regional enteritis, and some collagen vascular diseases. Patients with LAD, hyperimmunoglobulin E–recurrent infection (Job's) syndrome, CHS, and CGD all have defects in the mononuclear phagocyte system.

Monocyte cytokine production or response is impaired in some patients with disseminated nontuberculous mycobacterial infection who are not infected with HIV. Genetic defects in the pathways regulated by IFN-γ and IL-12 lead to impaired killing of intracellular bacteria, mycobacteria, salmonellae, and certain viruses (Fig. 5-10).

Certain viral infections impair mononuclear phagocyte function. For example, influenza virus infection causes abnormal monocyte chemotaxis. Mononuclear phagocytes can be infected by HIV using CCR5, the chemokine receptor that acts as a co-receptor with CD4 for HIV. T lymphocytes produce IFN-γ, which induces FcR expression and phagocytosis and stimulates hydrogen peroxide production by mononuclear phagocytes

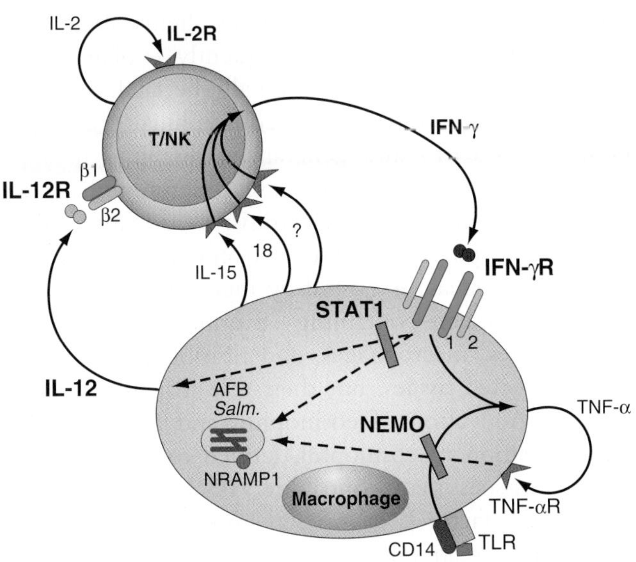

FIGURE 5-10

Lymphocyte–macrophage interactions underlying resistance to mycobacteria and other intracellular parasites such as *Salmonella*. Mycobacteria infect macrophages, leading to the production of IL-12, which activates T or NK cells through its receptor, leading to production of IL-2 and IFN-γ. IFN-γ acts through its receptor on macrophages to upregulate TNF-γ and IL-12 and kill intracellular parasites. Mutant forms of the cytokines and receptors shown in large type have been found in severe cases of nontuberculous mycobacterial infection and salmonellosis. AFB, acid-fast bacilli; IFN, interferon; IL, interleukin; NEMO, NF-κB essential modulator; NK, natural killer; STAT1, signal transducer and activator of transcription 1; TLR, Toll-like receptor; TNF, tumor necrosis factor.

and neutrophils. In certain diseases, such as AIDS, IFN-γ production may be deficient, whereas in other diseases, such as T cell lymphomas, excessive release of IFN-γ may be associated with erythrophagocytosis by splenic macrophages.

Autoinflammatory diseases are characterized by abnormal cytokine regulation, leading to excess inflammation in the absence of infection. These diseases can mimic infectious or immunodeficient syndromes. Gain-of-function mutations in the TNF-α receptor cause TNF-α receptor–associated periodic syndrome (TRAPS), which is characterized by recurrent fever in the absence of infection, due to persistent stimulation of the TNF-α receptor. Diseases with abnormal IL-1 regulation leading to fever include familial Mediterranean fever due to mutations in *PYRIN*. Mutations in *cold-induced autoinflammatory syndrome 1* (*CIAS1*) lead to neonatal-onset multisystem autoinflammatory disease, familial cold urticaria, and Muckle-Wells syndrome. The syndrome of pyoderma gangrenosum, acne, and sterile pyogenic arthritis (PAPA syndrome) is caused by mutations in *CD2BP1*. In contrast to these syndromes of overexpression of proinflammatory cytokines, blockade of TNF-α by the antagonists infliximab, adalimumab, certolizumab, or etanercept has been associated with severe infections due to tuberculosis, nontuberculous mycobacteria, and fungi.

Monocytopenia occurs with acute infections, with stress, and after treatment with glucocorticoids. Monocytopenia also occurs in aplastic anemia, hairy cell leukemia, and acute myeloid leukemia and as a direct result of myelotoxic drugs.

EOSINOPHILS

Eosinophils and neutrophils share similar morphology, many lysosomal constituents, phagocytic capacity, and oxidative metabolism. Eosinophils express a specific chemoattractant receptor and respond to a specific chemokine, eotaxin, but little is known about their required role. Eosinophils are much longer lived than neutrophils, and unlike neutrophils, tissue eosinophils can recirculate. During most infections, eosinophils appear unimportant. However, in invasive helminthic infections, such as hookworm, schistosomiasis, strongyloidiasis, toxocariasis, trichinosis, filariasis, echinococcosis, and cysticercosis, the eosinophil plays a central role in host defense. Eosinophils are associated with bronchial asthma, cutaneous allergic reactions, and other hypersensitivity states.

The distinctive feature of the red-staining (Wright's stain) eosinophil granule is its crystalline core consisting of an arginine-rich protein (major basic protein) with histaminase activity, important in host defense against parasites. Eosinophil granules also contain a unique eosinophil peroxidase that catalyzes the oxidation of many substances by hydrogen peroxide and may facilitate killing of microorganisms.

Eosinophil peroxidase, in the presence of hydrogen peroxide and halide, initiates mast cell secretion in vitro and thereby promotes inflammation. Eosinophils contain cationic proteins, some of which bind to heparin and reduce its anticoagulant activity. Eosinophil-derived neurotoxin and eosinophil cationic protein are ribonucleases that can kill respiratory syncytial virus. Eosinophil cytoplasm contains Charcot-Leyden crystal protein, a hexagonal bipyramidal crystal first observed in a patient with leukemia and then in sputum of patients with asthma; this protein is lysophospholipase and may function to detoxify certain lysophospholipids.

Several factors enhance the eosinophil's function in host defense. T cell–derived factors enhance the ability of eosinophils to kill parasites. Mast cell–derived eosinophil chemotactic factor of anaphylaxis (ECFa) increases the number of eosinophil complement receptors and enhances eosinophil killing of parasites. Eosinophil CSFs (e.g., IL-5) produced by macrophages increase eosinophil production in the bone marrow and activate eosinophils to kill parasites.

EOSINOPHILIA

Eosinophilia is the presence of >500 eosinophils per μL of blood and is common in many settings besides parasite infection. Significant tissue eosinophilia can occur without an elevated blood count. A common cause of eosinophilia is allergic reaction to drugs (iodides, aspirin, sulfonamides, nitrofurantoin, penicillins, and cephalosporins). Allergies such as hay fever, asthma, eczema, serum sickness, allergic vasculitis, and pemphigus are associated with eosinophilia. Eosinophilia also occurs in collagen vascular diseases (e.g., rheumatoid arthritis, eosinophilic fasciitis, allergic angiitis, and periarteritis nodosa) and malignancies (e.g., Hodgkin's disease; mycosis fungoides; chronic myeloid leukemia; and cancer of the lung, stomach, pancreas, ovary, or uterus), as well as in Job's syndrome, DOCK8 deficiency (discussed later), and CGD. Eosinophilia is commonly present in helminthic infections. IL-5 is the dominant eosinophil growth factor. Therapeutic administration of the cytokines IL-2 and GM-CSF frequently leads to transient eosinophilia. The most dramatic hypereosinophilic syndromes are Loeffler's syndrome, tropical pulmonary eosinophilia, Loeffler's endocarditis, eosinophilic leukemia, and idiopathic hypereosinophilic syndrome (50,000–100,000/μL). IL-5 is the dominant eosinophil growth factor and can be specifically inhibited with the monoclonal antibody mepolizumab.

The idiopathic hypereosinophilic syndrome represents a heterogeneous group of disorders with the common feature of prolonged eosinophilia of unknown cause and organ system dysfunction, including the heart, central nervous system, kidneys, lungs, gastrointestinal tract, and skin. The bone marrow is involved in all affected individuals, but the most severe complications involve the heart and central nervous system. Clinical manifestations and organ dysfunction are highly variable. Eosinophils are found in the involved tissues and likely cause tissue damage by local deposition of toxic eosinophil proteins such as eosinophil cationic protein and major basic protein. In the heart, the pathologic changes lead to thrombosis, endocardial fibrosis, and restrictive endomyocardiopathy. The damage to tissues in other organ systems is similar. Some cases are due to mutations involving the platelet-derived growth factor receptor, and these are extremely sensitive to the tyrosine kinase inhibitor imatinib. Glucocorticoids, hydroxyurea, and IFN-α each have been used successfully, as have therapeutic antibodies against IL-5. Cardiovascular complications are managed aggressively.

The *eosinophilia–myalgia syndrome* is a multisystem disease, with prominent cutaneous, hematologic, and visceral manifestations, that frequently evolves into a chronic course and can occasionally be fatal. The syndrome is characterized by eosinophilia (eosinophil count >1000/μL) and generalized disabling myalgias without other recognized causes. Eosinophilic fasciitis, pneumonitis, and myocarditis; neuropathy culminating in respiratory failure; and encephalopathy may occur. The disease is caused by ingesting contaminants in L-tryptophan–containing products. Eosinophils, lymphocytes, macrophages, and fibroblasts accumulate in the affected tissues, but their role in pathogenesis is unclear. Activation of eosinophils and fibroblasts and the deposition of eosinophil-derived toxic proteins in affected tissues may contribute. IL-5 and transforming growth factor β have been implicated as potential mediators. Treatment is withdrawal of products containing L-tryptophan and the administration of glucocorticoids. Most patients recover fully, remain stable, or show slow recovery, but the disease can be fatal in up to 5% of patients.

EOSINOPENIA

Eosinopenia occurs with stress, such as acute bacterial infection, and after treatment with glucocorticoids. The mechanism of eosinopenia of acute bacterial infection is unknown but is independent of endogenous glucocorticoids, since it occurs in animals after total adrenalectomy. There is no known adverse effect of eosinopenia.

HYPERIMMUNOGLOBULIN E–RECURRENT INFECTION SYNDROME

The hyperimmunoglobulin E–recurrent infection syndrome, or Job's syndrome, is a rare multisystem disease in which the immune and somatic systems are affected, including neutrophils, monocytes, T cells, B cells, and osteoclasts. Autosomal dominant mutations in signal transducer and activator of transcription 3 (STAT3) lead to inhibition of normal STAT signaling with broad and profound effects. Patients have characteristic facies with broad noses, kyphoscoliosis and osteoporosis, and eczema. The primary teeth erupt normally but do not deciduate, often requiring extraction. Patients develop recurrent sinopulmonary and cutaneous infections that tend to be much less inflamed than appropriate for the degree of infection and have been referred to as "cold abscesses." Characteristically, pneumonias cavitate, leading to pneumatoceles. Coronary artery aneurysms are common, as are cerebral demyelinated plaques that accumulate with age. Importantly, IL-17–producing cells, which are thought responsible for protection against extracellular and mucosal infections, are profoundly reduced in Job's syndrome. Despite very high IgE levels, these patients do not have elevated levels of allergy. An important syndrome with clinical overlap with STAT3 deficiency is due to autosomal recessive defects in dedicator of cytokinesis 8 (DOCK8). In DOCK8 deficiency, IgE elevation is joined to severe allergy, viral susceptibility, and increased rates of cancer.

LABORATORY DIAGNOSIS AND MANAGEMENT

Initial studies of WBC and differential and often a bone marrow examination may be followed by assessment of bone marrow reserves (steroid challenge test), marginated circulating pool of cells (epinephrine challenge test), and marginating ability (endotoxin challenge test) (Fig. 5-7). In vivo assessment of inflammation is possible with a Rebuck skin window test or an in vivo skin blister assay, which measures the ability of leukocytes and inflammatory mediators to accumulate locally in the skin. In vitro tests of phagocyte aggregation, adherence, chemotaxis, phagocytosis, degranulation, and microbicidal activity (for *S. aureus*) may help pinpoint cellular or humoral lesions. Deficiencies of oxidative metabolism are detected with either the nitroblue tetrazolium (NBT) dye test or the dihydrorhodamine (DHR) oxidation test. These tests are based on the ability of products of oxidative metabolism to alter the oxidation states of reporter molecules so that they can be detected microscopically (NBT) or by flow cytometry (DHR). Qualitative studies of superoxide and hydrogen peroxide production may further define neutrophil oxidative function.

Patients with leukopenias or leukocyte dysfunction often have delayed inflammatory responses. Therefore, clinical manifestations may be minimal despite overwhelming infection, and unusual infections must always be suspected. Early signs of infection demand prompt, aggressive culturing for microorganisms, use of antibiotics, and surgical drainage of abscesses. Prolonged courses of antibiotics are often required. In patients with CGD, prophylactic antibiotics (trimethoprim–sulfamethoxazole) and antifungals (itraconazole) markedly diminish the frequency of life-threatening infections. Glucocorticoids may relieve gastrointestinal or genitourinary tract obstruction by granulomas in patients with CGD. Although TNF-α blocking agents may markedly relieve inflammatory bowel symptoms, extreme caution must be exercised in their use in CGD inflammatory bowel disease, as it profoundly increases these patients' already heightened susceptibility to infection. Recombinant human IFN-γ, which nonspecifically stimulates phagocytic cell function, reduces the frequency of infections in patients with CGD by 70% and reduces the severity of infection. This effect of IFN-γ in CGD is additive to the effect of prophylactic antibiotics. The recommended dose is 50 μg/m^2 subcutaneously three times weekly. IFN-γ has also been used successfully in the treatment of leprosy, nontuberculous mycobacteria, and visceral leishmaniasis.

Rigorous oral hygiene reduces but does not eliminate the discomfort of gingivitis, periodontal disease, and aphthous ulcers; chlorhexidine mouthwash and tooth brushing with a hydrogen peroxide–sodium bicarbonate paste helps many patients. Oral antifungal agents (fluconazole, itraconazole, voriconazole, posaconazole) have reduced mucocutaneous candidiasis in patients with Job's syndrome. Androgens, glucocorticoids, lithium, and immunosuppressive therapy have been used to restore myelopoiesis in patients with neutropenia due to impaired production. Recombinant G-CSF is useful in the management of certain forms of neutropenia due to depressed neutrophil production, especially those related to cancer chemotherapy. Patients with chronic neutropenia with evidence of a good bone marrow reserve need not receive prophylactic antibiotics. Patients with chronic or cyclic neutrophil counts <500/μL may benefit from prophylactic antibiotics and G-CSF during periods of neutropenia. Oral trimethoprim–sulfamethoxazole (160/800 mg) twice daily can prevent infection. Increased numbers of fungal infections are not seen in patients with CGD on this regimen. Oral quinolones such as levofloxacin and ciprofloxacin are alternatives.

In the setting of cytotoxic chemotherapy with severe, persistent neutropenia, trimethoprim–sulfamethoxazole prevents *Pneumocystis jirovecii* pneumonia. These patients and patients with phagocytic cell dysfunction should avoid heavy exposure to airborne soil, dust, or decaying matter (mulch, manure), which are often rich in *Nocardia* spp. and the spores of *Aspergillus* spp. and other fungi. Restriction of activities or social contact has no proven role in reducing risk of infection.

Although aggressive medical care for many patients with phagocytic disorders can allow them to go for years without a life-threatening infection, there may still be delayed effects of prolonged antimicrobials and other inflammatory complications. Cure of most congenital phagocyte defects is possible by bone marrow transplantation, and rates of success are improving (Chap. 30). The identification of specific gene defects in patients with LAD 1, CGD, and other immunodeficiencies has led to gene therapy trials in a number of genetic WBC disorders.

CHAPTER 6

ATLAS OF HEMATOLOGY AND ANALYSIS OF PERIPHERAL BLOOD SMEARS

Dan L. Longo

Some of the relevant findings in peripheral blood, enlarged lymph nodes, and bone marrow are illustrated in this chapter. Systematic histologic examination of the bone marrow and lymph nodes is beyond the scope of a general medicine textbook. However, every internist should know how to examine a peripheral blood smear.

The examination of a peripheral blood smear is one of the most informative exercises a physician can perform. Although advances in automated technology have made the examination of a peripheral blood smear by a physician seem less important, the technology is not a completely satisfactory replacement for a blood smear interpretation by a trained medical professional who also knows the patient's clinical history, family history, social history, and physical findings. It is useful to ask the laboratory to generate a Wright's-stained peripheral blood smear and examine it.

The best place to examine blood cell morphology is the feathered edge of the blood smear where red cells lie in a single layer, side by side, just barely touching one another but not overlapping. The author's approach is to look at the smallest cellular elements, the platelets, first and work his way up in size to red cells and then white cells.

Using an oil immersion lens that magnifies the cells 100-fold, one counts the platelets in five to six fields, averages the number per field, and multiplies by 20,000 to get a rough estimate of the platelet count. The platelets are usually 1–2 μm in diameter and have a blue granulated appearance. There is usually 1 platelet for every 20 or so red cells. Of course, the automated counter is much more accurate, but gross disparities between the automated and manual counts should be assessed. Large platelets may be a sign of rapid platelet turnover, as young platelets are often larger than old ones; alternatively, certain rare inherited syndromes can produce large platelets. Platelet clumping visible on the smear can be associated with falsely low automated platelet counts. Similarly, neutrophil fragmentation can be a source of falsely elevated automated platelet counts.

Next one examines the red blood cells. One can gauge their size by comparing the red cell with the nucleus of a small lymphocyte. Both are normally about 8 μm wide. Red cells that are smaller than the small lymphocyte nucleus may be microcytic; those larger than the small lymphocyte nucleus may be macrocytic. Macrocytic cells also tend to be more oval than spherical in shape and are sometimes called macroovalocytes. The automated mean corpuscular volume (MCV) can assist in making a classification. However, some patients may have both iron and vitamin B_{12} deficiency, which will produce an MCV in the normal range but wide variation in red cell size. When the red cells vary greatly in size, *anisocytosis* is said to be present. When the red cells vary greatly in shape, *poikilocytosis* is said to be present. The electronic cell counter provides an independent assessment of variability in red cell size. It measures the range of red cell volumes and reports the results as "red cell distribution width" (RDW). This value is calculated from the MCV; thus, cell width is not being measured but cell volume is. The term is derived from the curve displaying the frequency of cells at each volume, also called the distribution. The width of red cell volume distribution curve is what determines the RDW. The RDW is calculated as follows: RDW = (standard deviation of MCV ÷ mean MCV) × 100. In the presence of morphologic anisocytosis, RDW (normally 11–14%) increases to 15–18%. The RDW is useful in at least two clinical settings. In patients with microcytic anemia, the differential diagnosis is generally between iron deficiency and thalassemia. In thalassemia, the small red cells are generally of uniform size with a normal small RDW. In iron deficiency, the size variability and the RDW are large. In addition, a large

RDW can suggest a dimorphic anemia when a chronic atrophic gastritis can produce both vitamin B_{12} malabsorption to produce macrocytic anemia and blood loss to produce iron deficiency. In such settings, RDW is also large. An elevated RDW also has been reported as a risk factor for all-cause mortality in population-based studies (Patel KV, Ferrucci L, Ershler WB, et al: Red blood cell distribution width and the risk of death in middle-aged and older adults. *Arch Intern Med* 169:515, 2009), a finding that is unexplained currently.

After red cell size is assessed, one examines the hemoglobin content of the cells. They are either normal in color (*normochromic*) or pale in color (*hypochromic*). They are never "hyperchromic." If more than the normal amount of hemoglobin is made, the cells get larger—they do not become darker. In addition to hemoglobin content, the red cells are examined for inclusions. Red cell inclusions are the following:

1. *Basophilic stippling*—diffuse fine or coarse blue dots in the red cell usually representing RNA residue—especially common in lead poisoning
2. *Howell-Jolly bodies*—dense blue circular inclusions that represent nuclear remnants—their presence implies defective splenic function
3. *Nuclei*—red cells may be released or pushed out of the marrow prematurely before nuclear extrusion—often implies a myelophthisic process or a vigorous narrow response to anemia, usually hemolytic anemia
4. *Parasites*—red cell parasites include malaria and babesia
5. *Polychromatophilia*—the red cell cytoplasm has a bluish hue, reflecting the persistence of ribosomes still actively making hemoglobin in a young red cell

Vital stains are necessary to see precipitated hemoglobin called *Heinz bodies*.

Red cells can take on a variety of different shapes. All abnormally shaped red cells are *poikilocytes*. Small red cells without the central pallor are *spherocytes*; they can be seen in hereditary spherocytosis, hemolytic anemias of other causes, and clostridial sepsis. *Dacrocytes* are teardrop-shaped cells that can be seen in hemolytic anemias, severe iron deficiency, thalassemias, myelofibrosis, and myelodysplastic syndromes. *Schistocytes* are helmet-shaped cells that reflect microangiopathic hemolytic anemia or fragmentation on an artificial heart valve. *Echinocytes* are spiculated red cells with the spikes evenly spaced; they can represent an artifact of abnormal drying of the blood smear or reflect changes in stored blood. They also can be seen in renal failure and malnutrition and are often reversible. *Acanthocytes* are spiculated red cells with the spikes irregularly distributed. This process tends to be irreversible and reflects underlying renal disease, abetalipoproteinemia, or splenectomy. *Elliptocytes* are elliptical-shaped red cells that can reflect an inherited defect in the red cell membrane, but they also are seen in iron deficiency, myelodysplastic syndromes, megaloblastic anemia, and thalassemias. *Stomatocytes* are red cells in which the area of central pallor takes on the morphology of a slit instead of the usual round shape. Stomatocytes can indicate an inherited red cell membrane defect and also can be seen in alcoholism. *Target cells* have an area of central pallor that contains a dense center, or bull's eye. These cells are seen classically in thalassemia, but they are also present in iron deficiency, cholestatic liver disease, and some hemoglobinopathies. They also can be generated artifactually by improper slide making.

One last feature of the red cells to assess before moving to the white blood cells is the distribution of the red cells on the smear. In most individuals, the cells lie side by side in a single layer. Some patients have red cell clumping (called *agglutination*) in which the red cells pile upon one another; it is seen in certain paraproteinemias and autoimmune hemolytic anemias. Another abnormal distribution involves red cells lying in single cell rows on top of one another like stacks of coins. This is called *rouleaux formation* and reflects abnormal serum protein levels.

Finally, one examines the white blood cells. Three types of granulocytes are usually present: neutrophils, eosinophils, and basophils, in decreasing frequency. Neutrophils are generally the most abundant white cell. They are round, are 10–14 μm wide, and contain a lobulated nucleus with two to five lobes connected by a thin chromatin thread. Bands are immature neutrophils that have not completed nuclear condensation and have a U-shaped nucleus. Bands reflect a left shift in neutrophil maturation in an effort to make more cells more rapidly. Neutrophils can provide clues to a variety of conditions. Vacuolated neutrophils may be a sign of bacterial sepsis. The presence of 1- to 2-μm blue cytoplasmic inclusions, called *Döhle bodies*, can reflect infections, burns, or other inflammatory states. If the neutrophil granules are larger than normal and stain a darker blue, "toxic granulations" are said to be present, and they also suggest a systemic inflammation. The presence of neutrophils with more than five nuclear lobes suggests megaloblastic anemia. Large misshapen granules may reflect the inherited Chédiak-Higashi syndrome.

Eosinophils are slightly larger than neutrophils, have bilobed nuclei, and contain large red granules. Diseases of eosinophils are associated with too many of them rather than any morphologic or qualitative change. They normally total less than one-thirtieth the number of neutrophils. Basophils are even more rare than eosinophils in the blood. They have large dark blue granules and may be increased as part of chronic myeloid leukemia.

Lymphocytes can be present in several morphologic forms. Most common in healthy individuals are small lymphocytes with a small dark nucleus and scarce cytoplasm. In the presence of viral infections, more of the lymphocytes are larger, about the size of neutrophils, with abundant cytoplasms and a less condensed nuclear chromatin. These cells are called *reactive lymphocytes*. About 1% of lymphocytes are larger and contain blue granules in a light blue cytoplasm; they are called *large granular lymphocytes*. In chronic lymphoid leukemia, the small lymphocytes are increased in number, and many of them are ruptured in making the blood smear, leaving a smudge of nuclear material without a surrounding cytoplasm or cell membrane; they are called *smudge cells* and are rare in the absence of chronic lymphoid leukemia.

Monocytes are the largest white blood cells, ranging from 15 to 22 μm in diameter. The nucleus can take on a variety of shapes but usually appears to be folded; the cytoplasm is gray.

Abnormal cells may appear in the blood. Most often the abnormal cells originate from neoplasms of bone marrow–derived cells, including lymphoid cells, myeloid cells, and occasionally red cells. More rarely, other types of tumors can get access to the bloodstream, and rare epithelial malignant cells may be identified. The chances of seeing such abnormal cells is increased by examining blood smears made from buffy coats, the layer of cells that is visible on top of sedimenting red cells when blood is left in the test tube for an hour. Smears made from finger sticks may include rare endothelial cells.

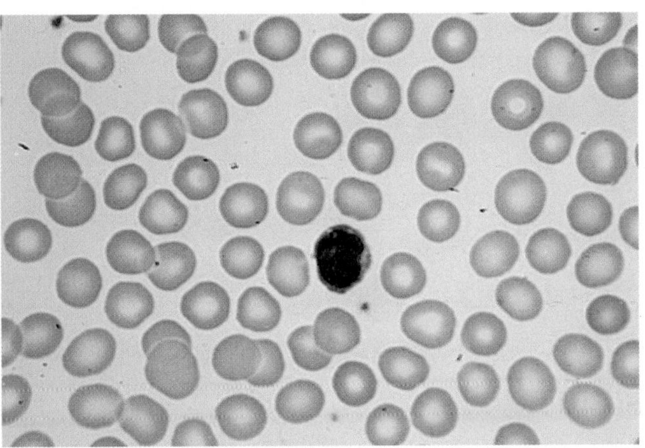

FIGURE 6-1
Normal peripheral blood smear. Small lymphocyte in center of field. Note that the diameter of the red blood cell is similar to the diameter of the small lymphocyte nucleus.

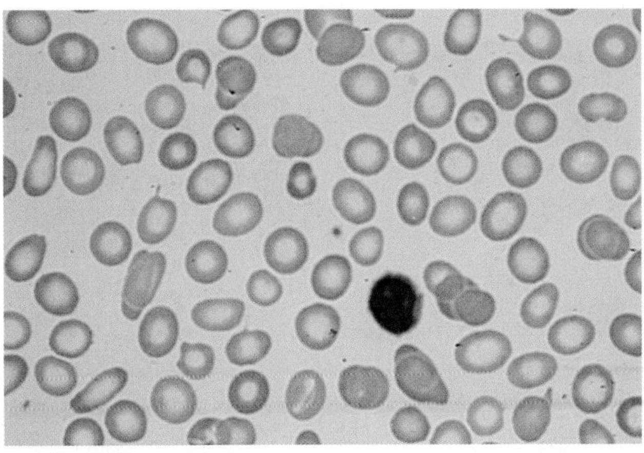

FIGURE 6-3
Hypochromic microcytic anemia of iron deficiency. Small lymphocyte in field helps assess the red blood cell size.

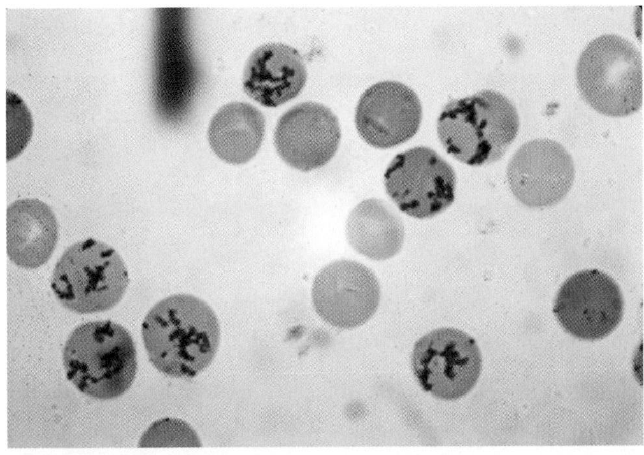

FIGURE 6-2
Reticulocyte count preparation. This new methylene blue–stained blood smear shows large numbers of heavily stained reticulocytes (the cells containing the dark blue–staining RNA precipitates).

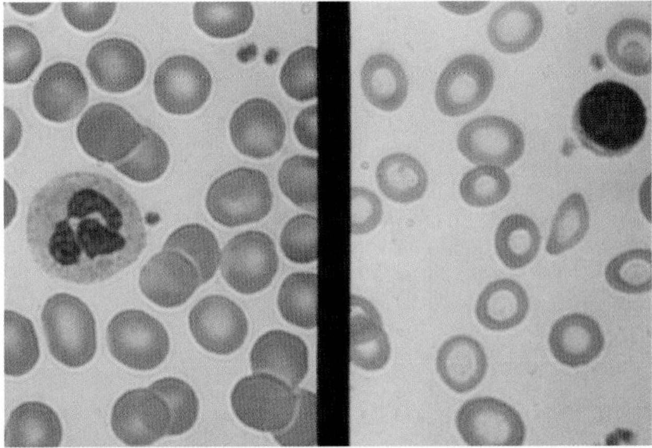

FIGURE 6-4
Iron deficiency anemia next to normal red blood cells. Microcytes (*right panel*) are smaller than normal red blood cells (cell diameter <7 μm) (*left panel*) and may or may not be poorly hemoglobinized (hypochromic).

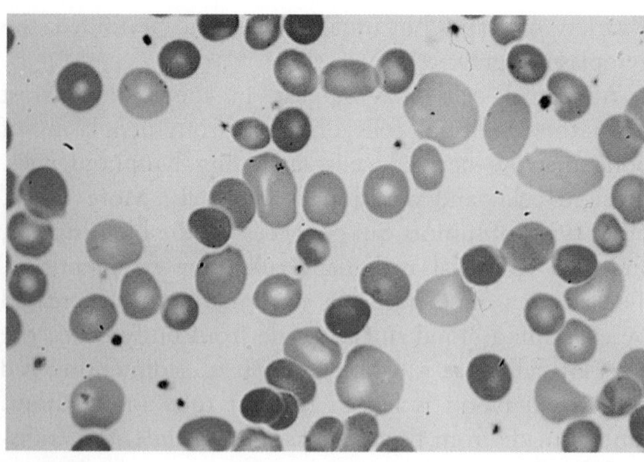

FIGURE 6-5
Polychromatophilia. Note large red cells with light purple coloring.

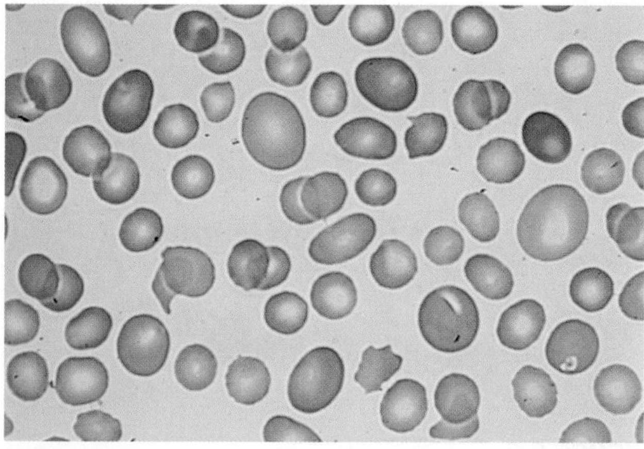

FIGURE 6-6
Macrocytosis. These cells are both larger than normal (mean corpuscular volume >100) and somewhat oval in shape. Some morphologists call these cells macroovalocytes.

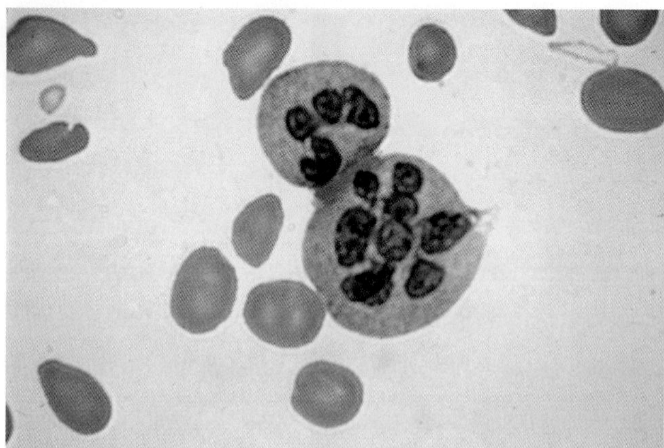

FIGURE 6-7
Hypersegmented neutrophils. Hypersegmented neutrophils (multilobed polymorphonuclear leukocytes) are larger than normal neutrophils with five or more segmented nuclear lobes. They are commonly seen with folic acid or vitamin B_{12} deficiency.

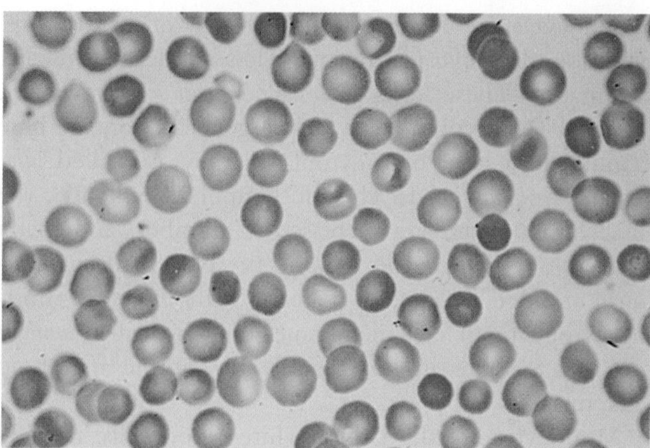

FIGURE 6-8
Spherocytosis. Note small hyperchromatic cells without the usual clear area in the center.

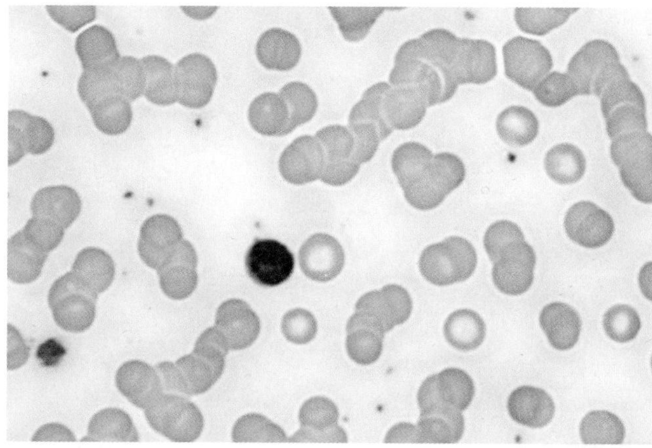

FIGURE 6-9
Rouleaux formation. Small lymphocyte in center of field. These red cells align themselves in stacks and are related to increased serum protein levels.

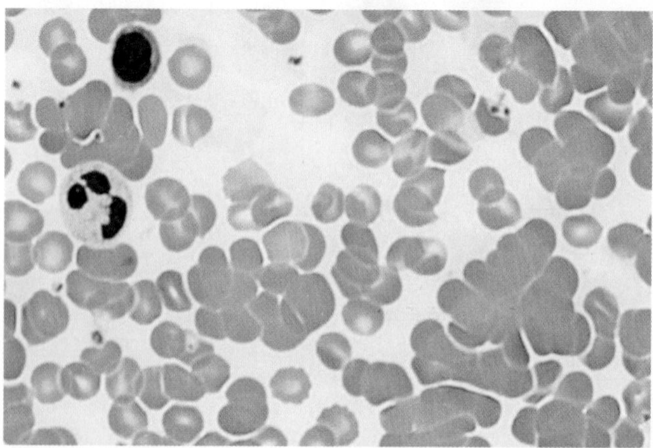

FIGURE 6-10
Red cell agglutination. Small lymphocyte and segmented neutrophil in the upper left center. Note the irregular collections of aggregated red cells.

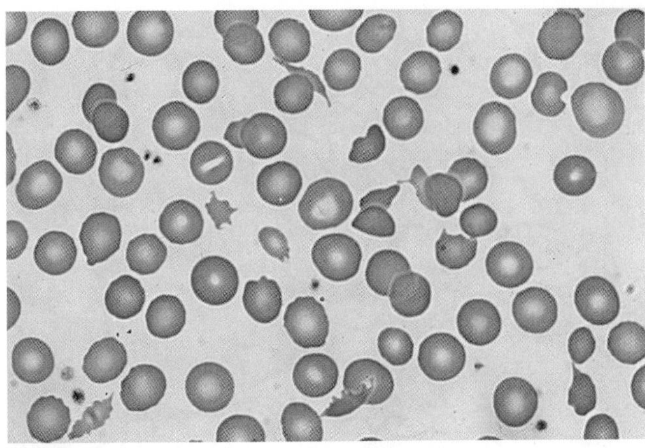

FIGURE 6-11
Fragmented red cells. Heart valve hemolysis.

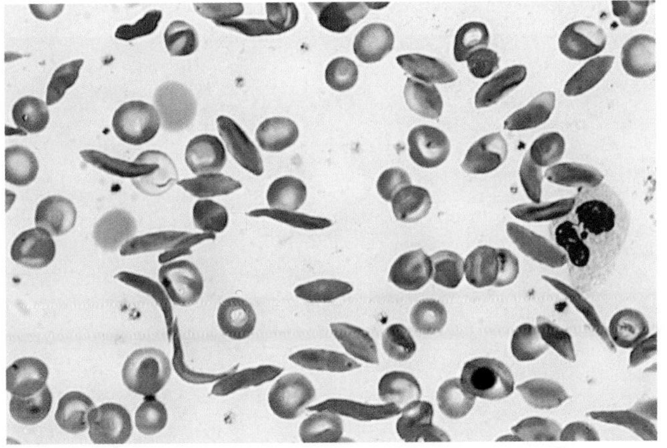

FIGURE 6-12
Sickle cells. Homozygous sickle cell disease. A nucleated red cell and neutrophil are also in the field.

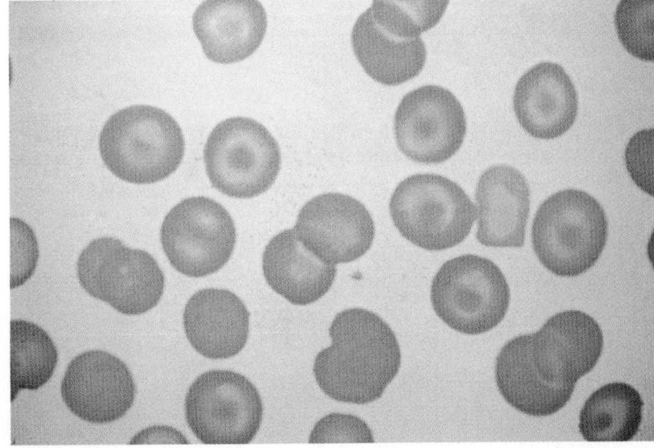

FIGURE 6-13
Target cells. Target cells are recognized by the bull's-eye appearance of the cell. Small numbers of target cells are seen with liver disease and thalassemia. Larger numbers are typical of hemoglobin C disease.

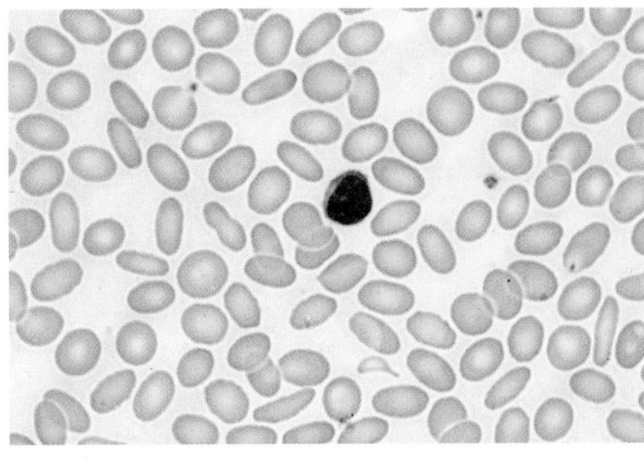

FIGURE 6-14
Elliptocytosis. Small lymphocyte in center of field. Elliptical shape of red cells related to weakened membrane structure, usually due to mutations in spectrin.

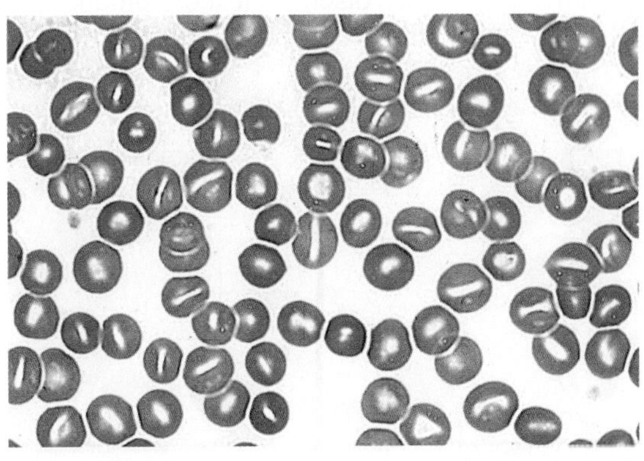

FIGURE 6-15
Stomatocytosis. Red cells characterized by a wide transverse slit or stoma. This often is seen as an artifact in a dehydrated blood smear. These cells can be seen in hemolytic anemias and in conditions in which the red cells are overhydrated or dehydrated.

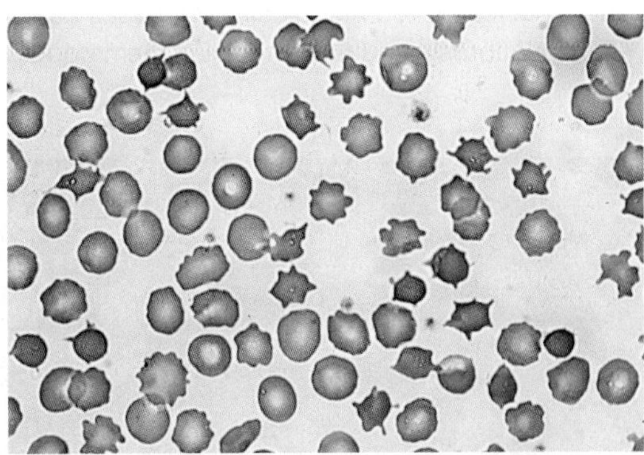

FIGURE 6-16
Acanthocytosis. Spiculated red cells are of two types: *acanthocytes* are contracted dense cells with irregular membrane projections that vary in length and width; *echinocytes* have small, uniform, and evenly spaced membrane projections. Acanthocytes are present in severe liver disease, in patients with abetalipoproteinemia, and in rare patients with McLeod blood group. Echinocytes are found in patients with severe uremia, in glycolytic red cell enzyme defects, and in microangiopathic hemolytic anemia.

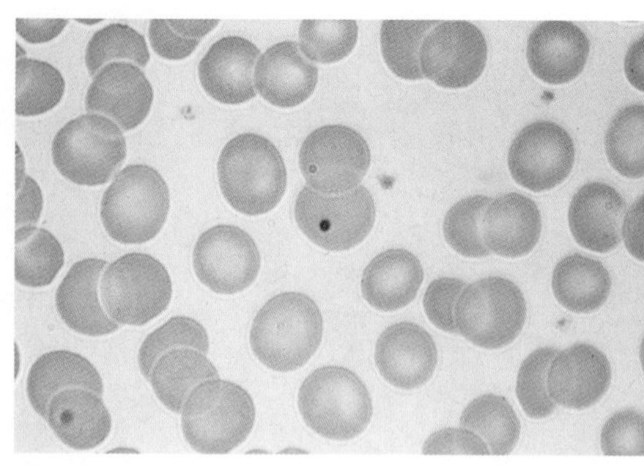

FIGURE 6-17
Howell-Jolly bodies. Howell-Jolly bodies are tiny nuclear remnants that normally are removed by the spleen. They appear in the blood after splenectomy (defect in removal) and with maturation/dysplastic disorders (excess production).

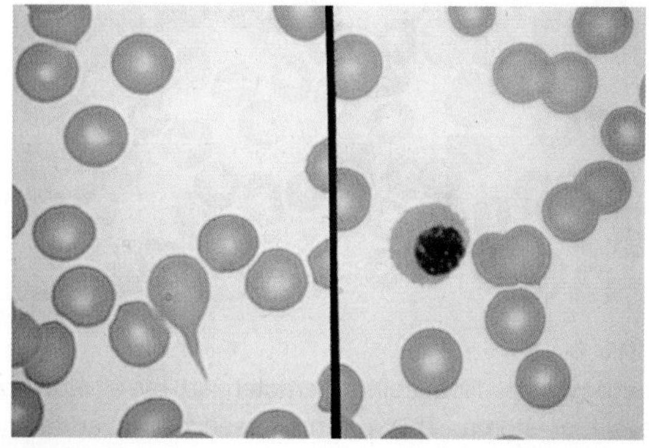

FIGURE 6-18
Teardrop cells and nucleated red blood cells characteristic of myelofibrosis. A teardrop-shaped red blood cell (*left panel*) and a nucleated red blood cell (*right panel*) as typically seen with myelofibrosis and extramedullary hematopoiesis.

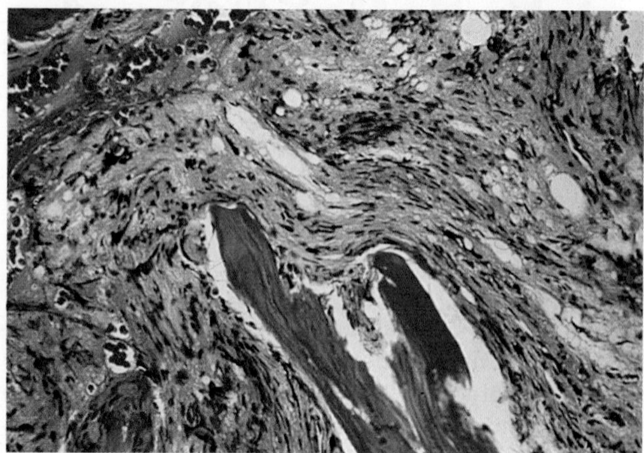

FIGURE 6-19
Myelofibrosis of the bone marrow. Total replacement of marrow precursors and fat cells by a dense infiltrate of reticulin fibers and collagen (H&E stain).

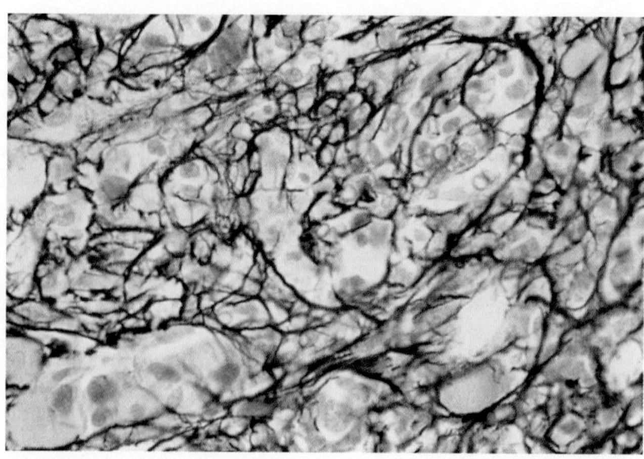

FIGURE 6-20
Reticulin stain of marrow myelofibrosis. Silver stain of a myelofibrotic marrow showing an increase in reticulin fibers (black-staining threads).

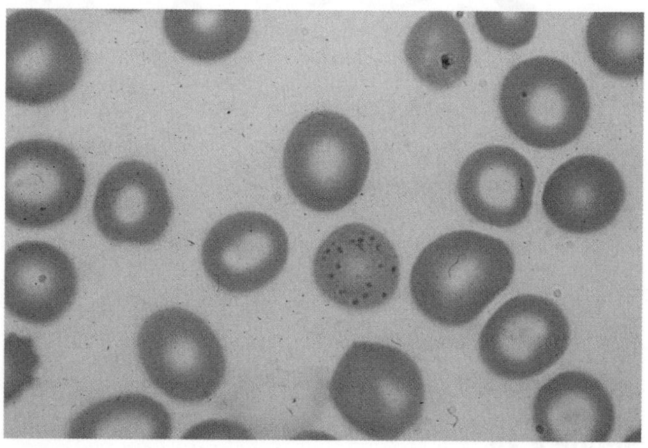

FIGURE 6-21
Stippled red cell in lead poisoning. Mild hypochromia. Coarsely stippled red cell.

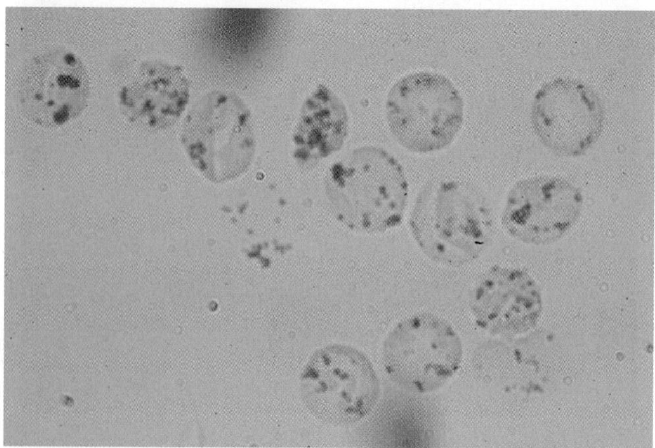

FIGURE 6-22
Heinz bodies. Blood mixed with hypotonic solution of crystal violet. The stained material is precipitates of denatured hemoglobin within cells.

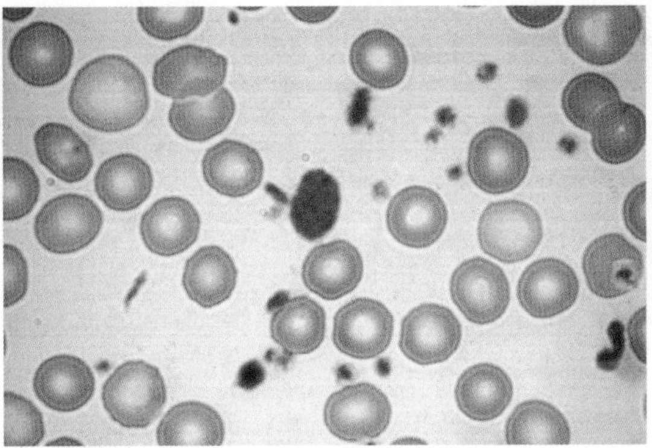

FIGURE 6-23

Giant platelets. Giant platelets, together with a marked increase in the platelet count, are seen in myeloproliferative disorders, especially primary thrombocythemia.

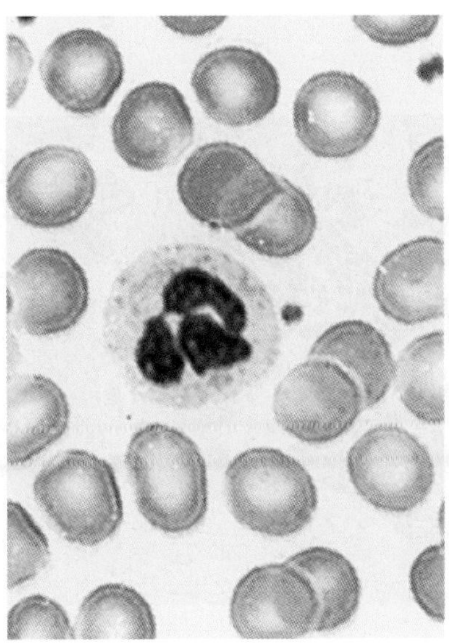

FIGURE 6-24

Normal granulocytes. The normal granulocyte has a segmented nucleus with heavy, clumped chromatin; fine neutrophilic granules are dispersed throughout the cytoplasm.

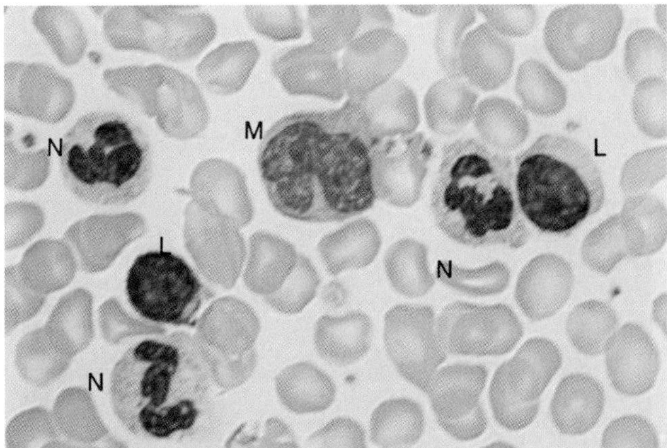

FIGURE 6-25

Normal monocytes. The film was prepared from the buffy coat of the blood from a normal donor. L, lymphocyte; M monocyte; N, neutrophil.

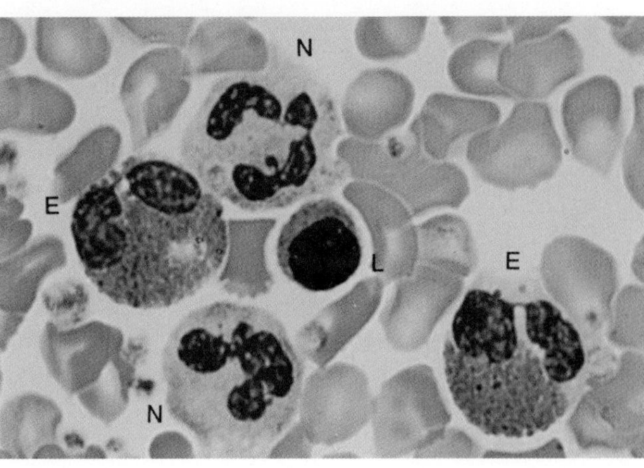

FIGURE 6-26

Normal eosinophils. The film was prepared from the buffy coat of the blood from a normal donor. E, eosinophil; L, lymphocyte. N, neutrophil;

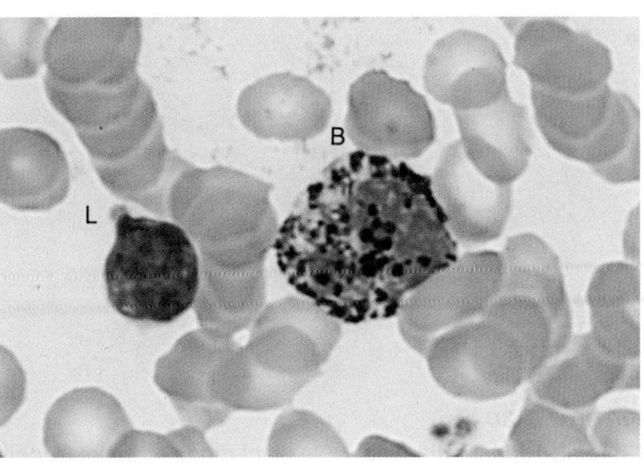

FIGURE 6-27

Normal basophil. The film was prepared from the buffy coat of the blood from a normal donor. B, basophil; L, lymphocyte.

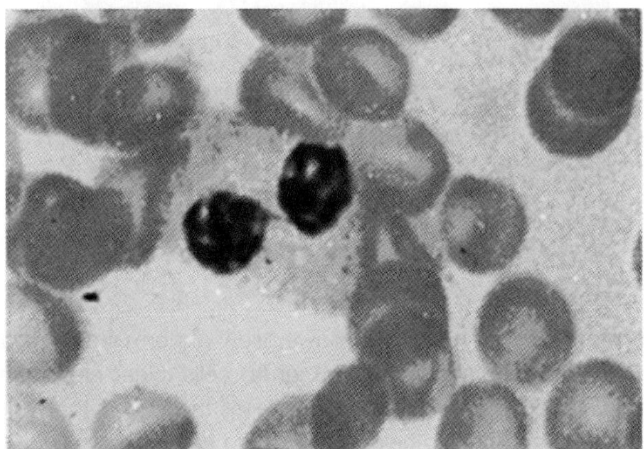

FIGURE 6-28

Pelger-Hüet anomaly. In this benign disorder, the majority of granulocytes are bilobed. The nucleus frequently has a spectacle-like, or "pince-nez," configuration.

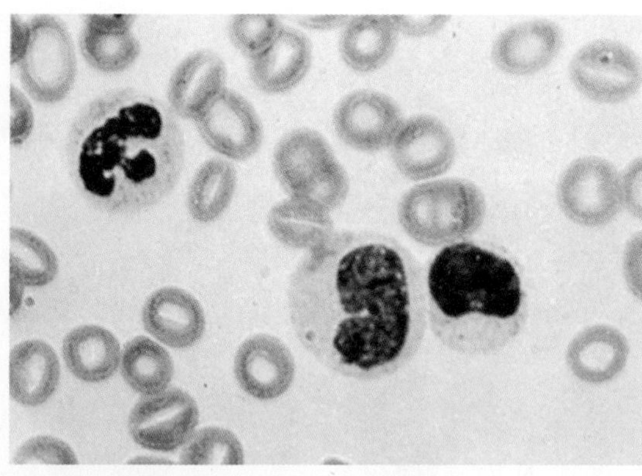

FIGURE 6-29
Döhle body. Neutrophil band with Döhle body. The neutrophil with a sausage-shaped nucleus in the center of the field is a band form. Döhle bodies are discrete, blue-staining nongranular areas found in the periphery of the cytoplasm of the neutrophil in infections and other toxic states. They represent aggregates of rough endoplasmic reticulum.

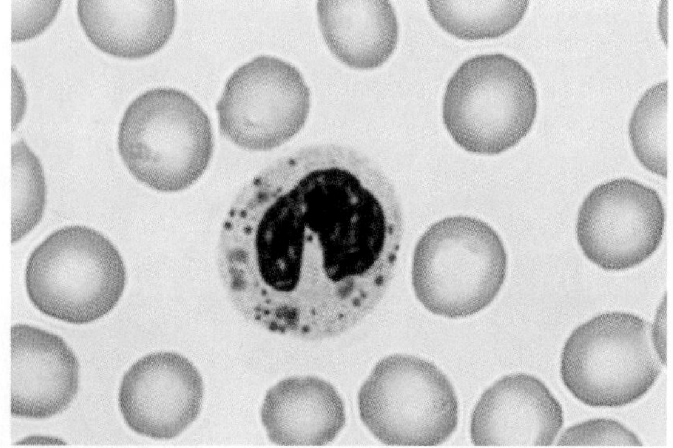

FIGURE 6-30
Chédiak-Higashi disease. Note giant granules in neutrophil.

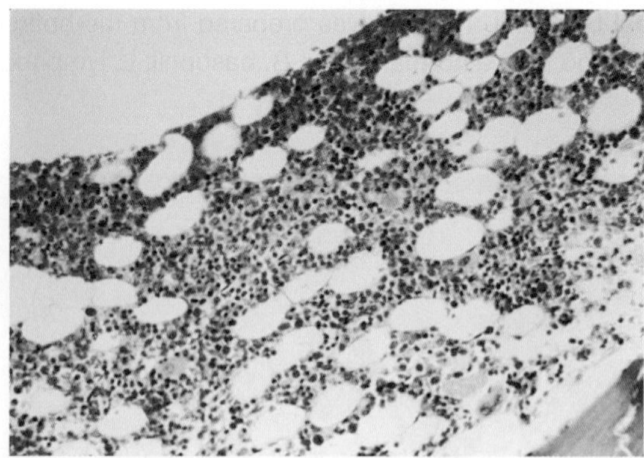

FIGURE 6-31
Normal bone marrow. Low-power view of normal adult marrow (H&E stain), showing a mix of fat cells (clear areas) and hematopoietic cells. The percentage of the space that consists of hematopoietic cells is referred to as *marrow cellularity*. In adults, normal marrow cellularity is 35–40%. If demands for increased marrow production occur, cellularity may increase to meet the demand. As people age, the marrow cellularity decreases and the marrow fat increases. Patients >70 years old may have a 20–30% marrow cellularity.

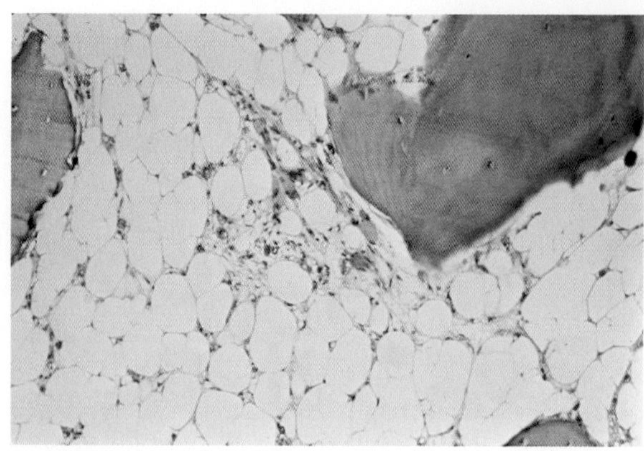

FIGURE 6-32
Aplastic anemia bone marrow. Normal hematopoietic precursor cells are virtually absent, leaving behind fat cells, reticuloendothelial cells, and the underlying sinusoidal structure.

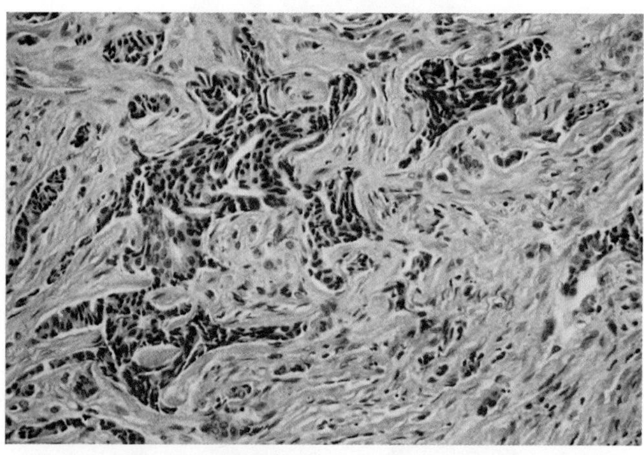

FIGURE 6-33
Metastatic cancer in the bone marrow. Marrow biopsy specimen infiltrated with metastatic breast cancer and reactive fibrosis (H&E stain).

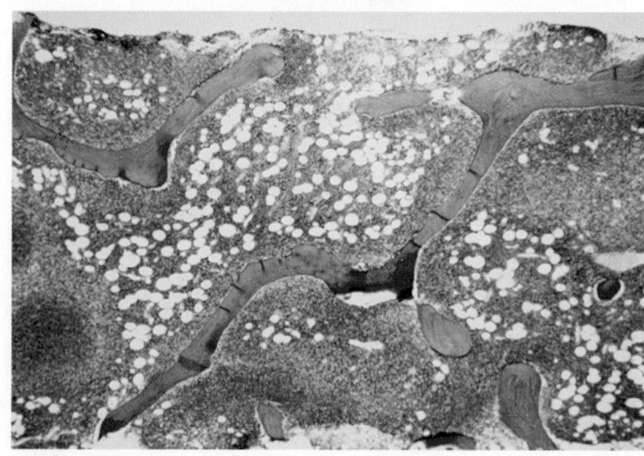

FIGURE 6-34
Lymphoma in the bone marrow. Nodular (follicular) lymphoma infiltrate in a marrow biopsy specimen. Note the characteristic paratrabecular location of the lymphoma cells.

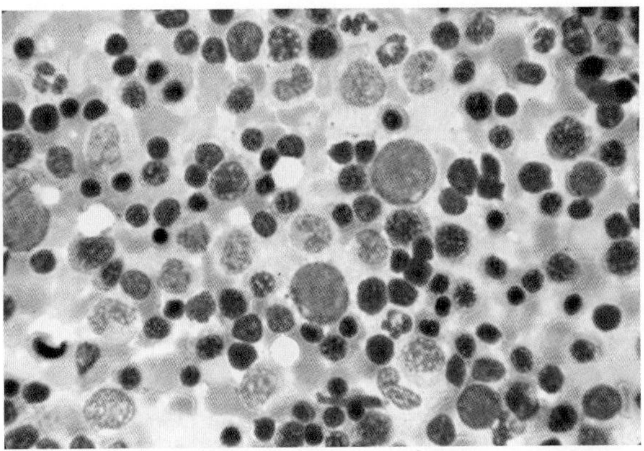

FIGURE 6-35
Erythroid hyperplasia of the marrow. Marrow aspirate specimen with a myeloid/erythroid ratio (M/E ratio) of 1:1–2, typical for a patient with a hemolytic anemia or one recovering from blood loss.

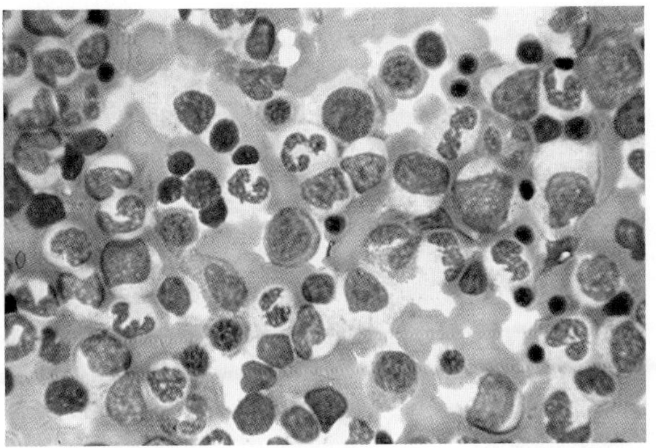

FIGURE 6-36
Myeloid hyperplasia of the marrow. Marrow aspirate specimen showing a myeloid/erythroid ratio of ≥ 3:1, suggesting either a loss of red blood cell precursors or an expansion of myeloid elements.

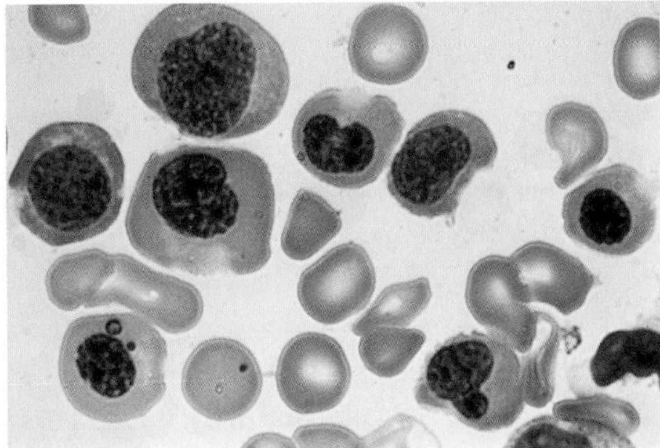

FIGURE 6-37
Megaloblastic erythropoiesis. High-power view of megaloblastic red blood cell precursors from a patient with a macrocytic anemia. Maturation is delayed, with late normoblasts showing a more immature-appearing nucleus with a lattice-like pattern with normal cytoplasmic maturation.

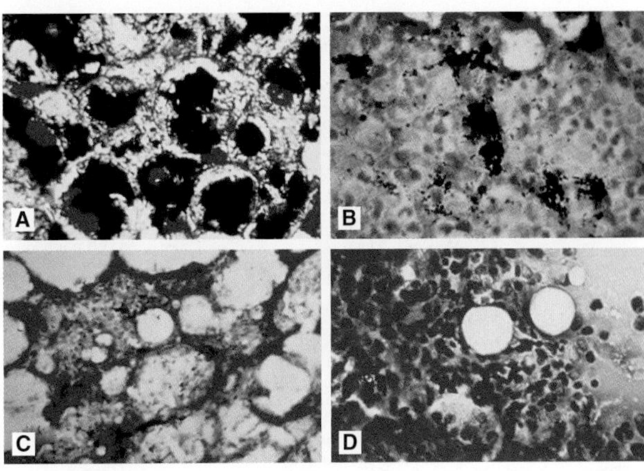

FIGURE 6-38
Prussian blue staining of marrow iron stores. Iron stores can be graded on a scale of 0 to 4+. ***A:*** a marrow with excess iron stores (>4+); ***B:*** normal stores (2–3+); ***C:*** minimal stores (1+); and ***D:*** absent iron stores (0).

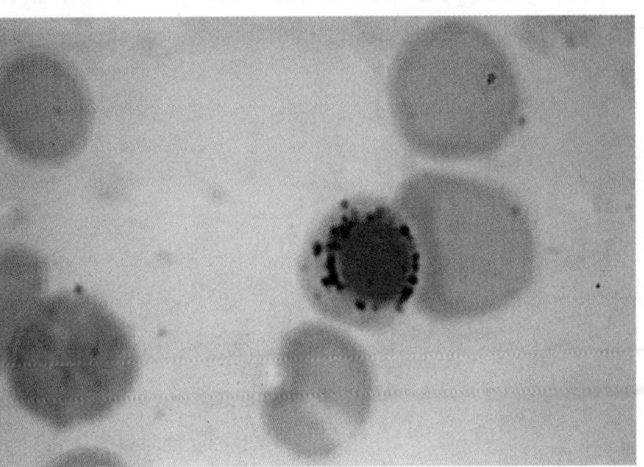

FIGURE 6-39
Ringed sideroblast. An orthochromatic normoblast with a collar of blue granules (mitochondria encrusted with iron) surrounding the nucleus.

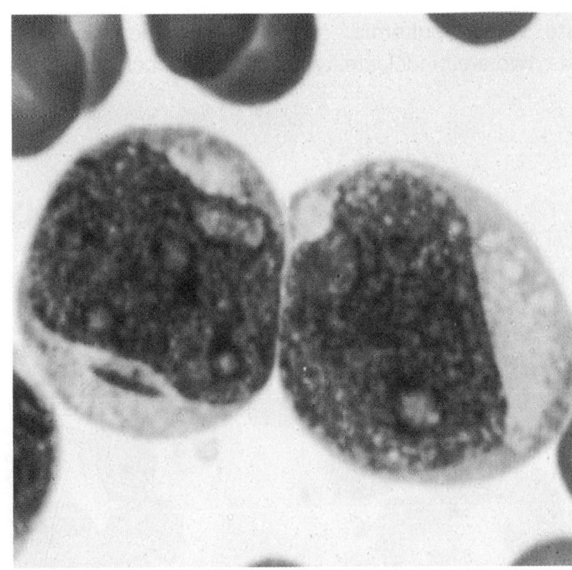

FIGURE 6-40
Acute myeloid leukemia. Leukemic myeloblast with an Auer rod. Note two to four large, prominent nucleoli in each cell.

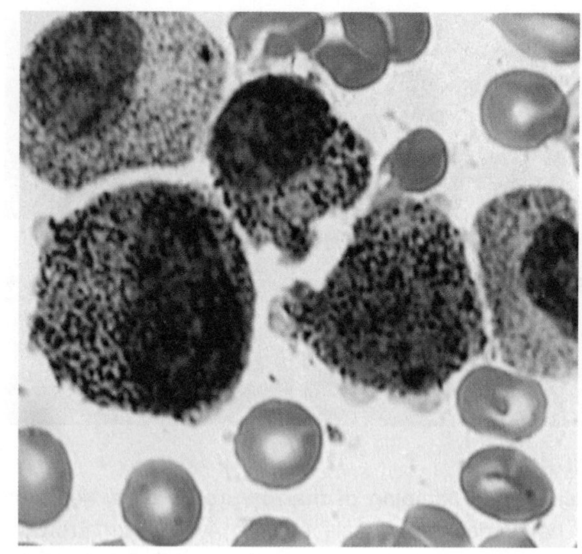

FIGURE 6-41
Acute promyelocytic leukemia. Note prominent cytoplasmic granules in the leukemia cells.

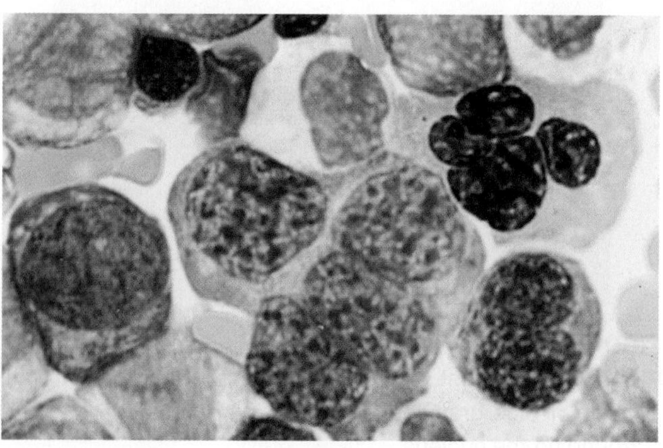

FIGURE 6-42
Acute erythroleukemia. Note giant dysmorphic erythroblasts; two are binucleate, and one is multinucleate.

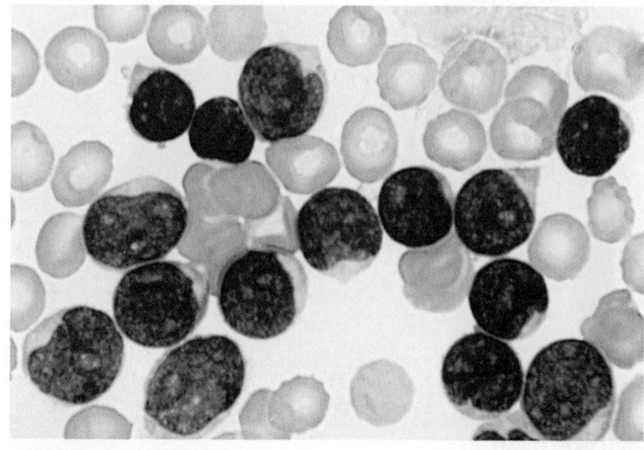

FIGURE 6-43
Acute lymphoblastic leukemia.

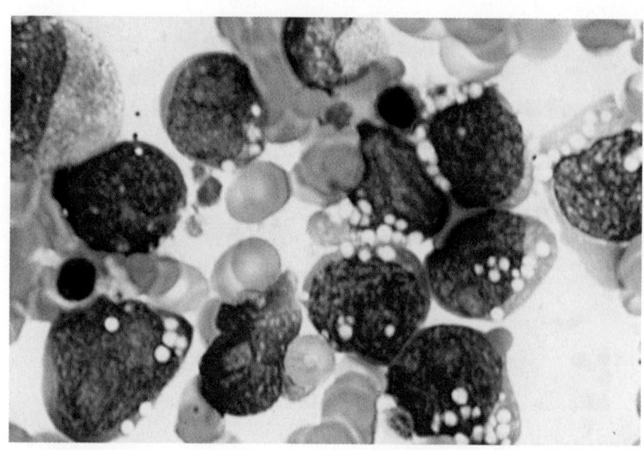

FIGURE 6-44
Burkitt's leukemia, acute lymphoblastic leukemia.

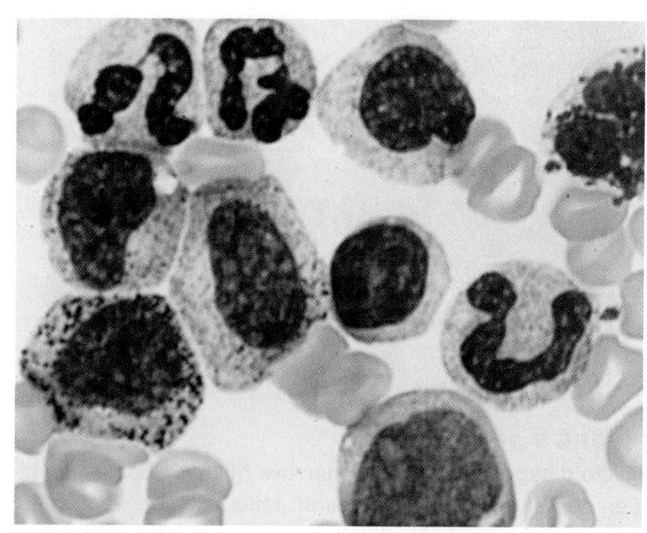

FIGURE 6-45
Chronic myeloid leukemia in the peripheral blood.

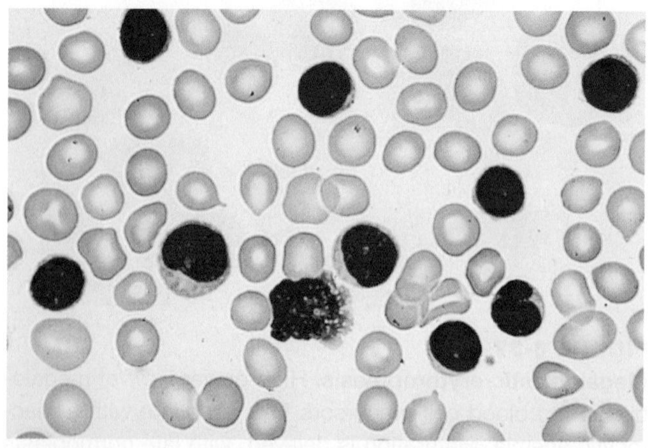

FIGURE 6-46
Chronic lymphoid leukemia in the peripheral blood.

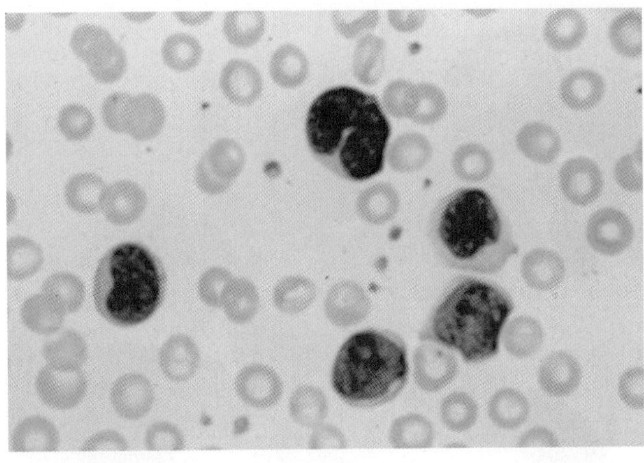

FIGURE 6-47
Sézary's syndrome. Lymphocytes with frequently convoluted nuclei (Sézary cells) in a patient with advanced mycosis fungoides.

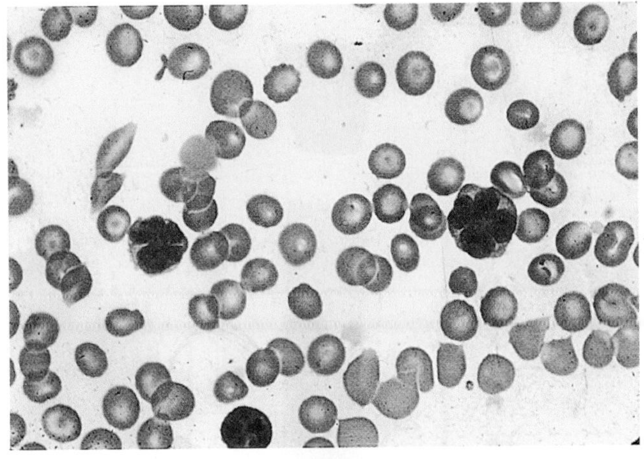

FIGURE 6-48
Adult T cell leukemia. Peripheral blood smear showing leukemia cells with typical "flower-shaped" nucleus.

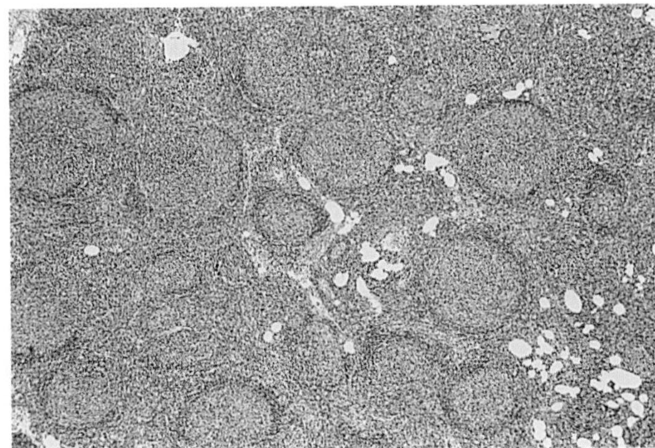

FIGURE 6-49
Follicular lymphoma in a lymph node. The normal nodal architecture is effaced by nodular expansions of tumor cells. Nodules vary in size and contain predominantly small lymphocytes with cleaved nuclei along with variable numbers of larger cells with vesicular chromatin and prominent nucleoli.

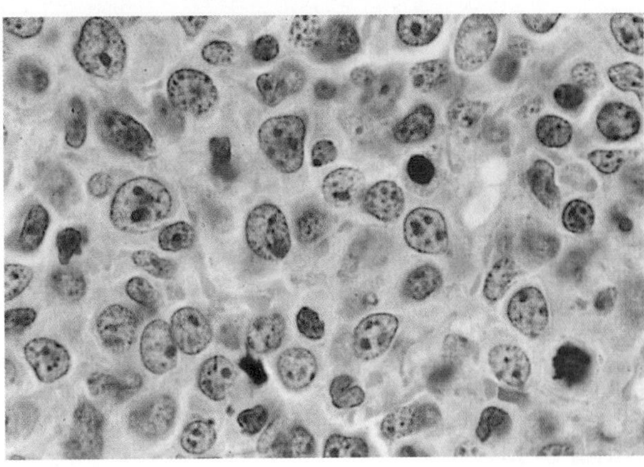

FIGURE 6-50
Diffuse large B cell lymphoma in a lymph node. The neoplastic cells are heterogeneous but predominantly large cells with vesicular chromatin and prominent nucleoli.

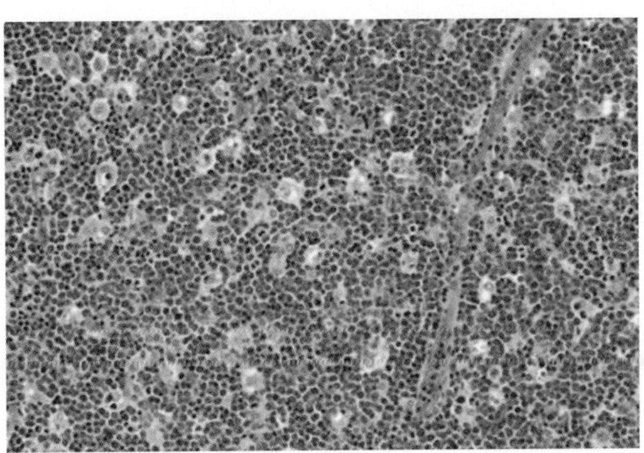

FIGURE 6-51
Burkitt's lymphoma in a lymph node. Burkitt's lymphoma with starry-sky appearance. The lighter areas are macrophages attempting to clear dead cells.

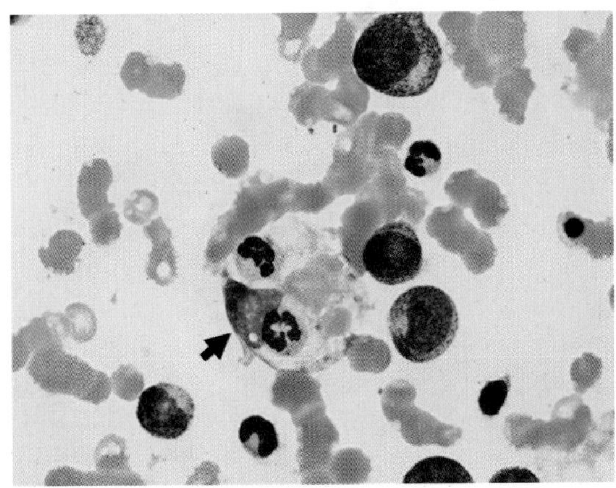

FIGURE 6-52
Erythrophagocytosis accompanying aggressive lymphoma. The central macrophage is ingesting red cells, neutrophils, and platelets. (*Courtesy of Dr. Kiyomi Tsukimori, Kyushu University, Fukuoka, Japan.*)

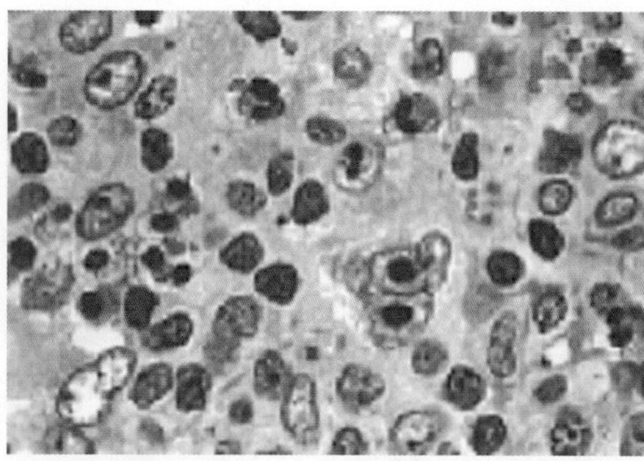

FIGURE 6-53
Hodgkin's disease. A Reed-Sternberg cell is present near the center of the field; a large cell with a bilobed nucleus and prominent nucleoli giving an "owl's eyes" appearance. The majority of the cells are normal lymphocytes, neutrophils, and eosinophils that form a pleiomorphic cellular infiltrate.

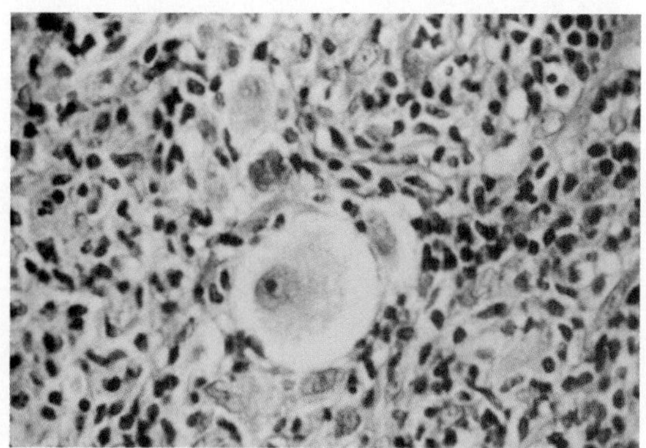

FIGURE 6-54
Lacunar cell; Reed-Sternberg cell variant in nodular sclerosing Hodgkin's disease. High-power view of single mononuclear lacunar cell with retracted cytoplasm in a patient with nodular sclerosing Hodgkin's disease.

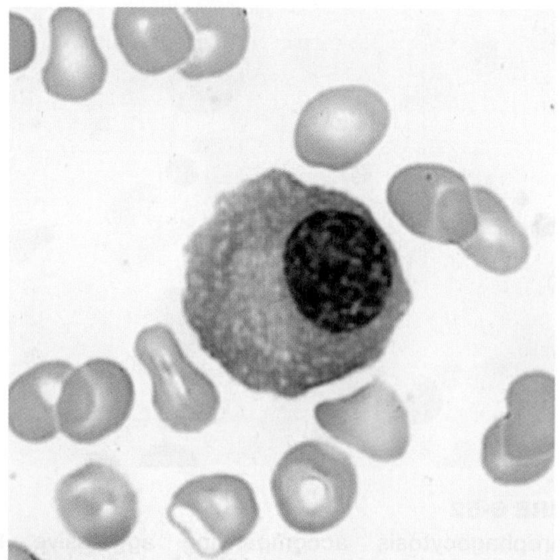

FIGURE 6-55
Normal plasma cell.

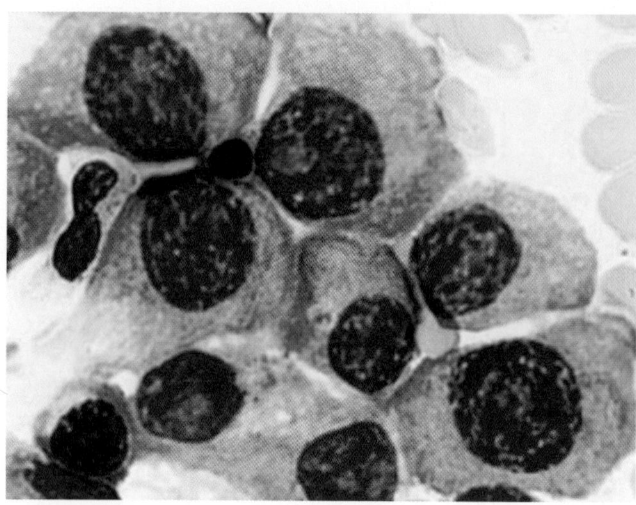

FIGURE 6-56
Multiple myeloma.

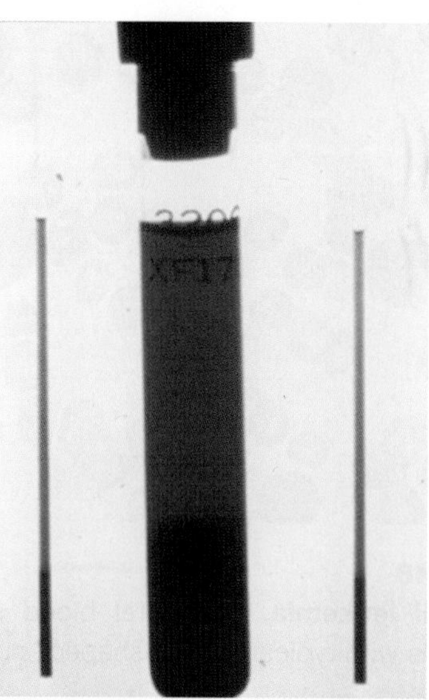

FIGURE 6-57
Color serum in hemoglobinemia. The distinctive red coloration of plasma (hemoglobinemia) in a spun blood sample in a patient with intravascular hemolysis.

ACKNOWLEDGMENT

Figures in this chapter were borrowed from Lichtman M, et al (eds): *Williams Hematology,* 7th edition. New York, McGraw-Hill, 2005; Hillman RS, Ault KA: *Hematology in General Practice,* 4th edition. New York, McGraw-Hill, 2005.

SECTION III

ANEMIAS

CHAPTER 7

IRON DEFICIENCY AND OTHER HYPOPROLIFERATIVE ANEMIAS

John W. Adamson

Anemias associated with normocytic and normochromic red cells and an inappropriately low reticulocyte response (reticulocyte index <2–2.5) are *hypoproliferative anemias*. This category includes early iron deficiency (before hypochromic microcytic red cells develop), acute and chronic inflammation (including many malignancies), renal disease, hypometabolic states such as protein malnutrition and endocrine deficiencies, and anemias from marrow damage. Marrow damage states are discussed in Chap. 11.

Hypoproliferative anemias are the most common anemias, and anemia associated with chronic inflammation is the most common of these. The anemia of inflammation, similar to iron deficiency, is related in part to abnormal iron metabolism. The anemias associated with renal disease, inflammation, cancer, and hypometabolic states are characterized by an abnormal erythropoietin response to the anemia.

IRON METABOLISM

Iron is a critical element in the function of all cells, although the amount of iron required by individual tissues varies during development. At the same time, the body must protect itself from free iron, which is highly toxic in that it participates in chemical reactions that generate free radicals such as singlet O_2 or OH^-. Consequently, elaborate mechanisms have evolved that allow iron to be made available for physiologic functions while at the same time conserving this element and handling it in such a way that toxicity is avoided.

The major role of iron in mammals is to carry O_2 as part of hemoglobin. O_2 is also bound by myoglobin in muscle. Iron is a critical element in iron-containing enzymes, including the cytochrome system in mitochondria. Iron distribution in the body is shown in Table 7-1. Without iron, cells lose their capacity for electron transport and energy metabolism. In erythroid cells, hemoglobin synthesis is impaired, resulting in anemia and reduced O_2 delivery to tissue.

THE IRON CYCLE IN HUMANS

Figure 7-1 outlines the major pathways of internal iron exchange in humans. Iron absorbed from the diet or released from stores circulates in the plasma bound to *transferrin*, the iron transport protein. Transferrin is a bilobed glycoprotein with two iron binding sites. Transferrin that carries iron exists in two forms—*monoferric* (one iron atom) or *diferric* (two iron atoms). The turnover (half-clearance time) of transferrin-bound iron is very rapid—typically 60–90 min. Because almost all of the iron transported by transferrin is delivered to the erythroid marrow, the clearance time of transferrin-bound iron from the circulation is affected most by the plasma iron level and the erythroid marrow activity. When erythropoiesis is markedly stimulated, the pool of erythroid cells requiring iron increases, and the clearance time of iron from the circulation decreases. The half-clearance time of iron in the presence of iron deficiency is as short as 10–15 min. With suppression of erythropoiesis, the plasma iron level typically increases, and the

TABLE 7-1

BODY IRON DISTRIBUTION

	IRON CONTENT, mg	
	ADULT MALE, 80 kg	**ADULT FEMALE, 60 kg**
Hemoglobin	2500	1700
Myoglobin/enzymes	500	300
Transferrin iron	3	3
Iron stores	600–1000	0–300

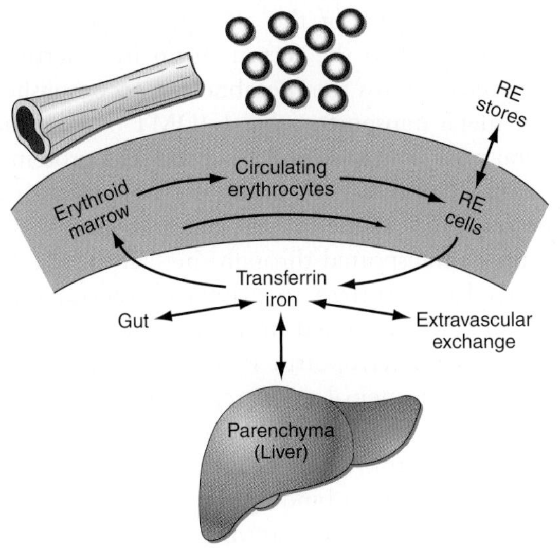

FIGURE 7-1

Internal iron exchange. Normally approximately 80% of iron passing through the plasma transferrin pool is recycled from broken-down red cells. Absorption of approximately 1 mg/d is required from the diet in men and 1.4 mg/d in women to maintain homeostasis. As long as transferrin saturation is maintained between 20–60% and erythropoiesis is not increased, use of iron stores is not required. However, in the event of blood loss, dietary iron deficiency, or inadequate iron absorption, up to 40 mg/d of iron can be mobilized from stores. RE, reticuloendothelial.

half-clearance time may be prolonged to several hours. Normally, the iron bound to transferrin turns over 6–8 times per day. Assuming a normal plasma iron level of 80–100 μg/dL, the amount of iron passing through the transferrin pool is 20–24 mg/d.

The iron–transferrin complex circulates in the plasma until it interacts with specific *transferrin receptors* on the surface of marrow erythroid cells. Diferric transferrin has the highest affinity for transferrin receptors; apotransferrin (not carrying iron) has very little affinity. Although transferrin receptors are found on cells in many tissues within the body—and all cells at some time during development will display transferrin receptors—the cell having the greatest number of receptors (300,000 to 400,000/cell) is the developing erythroblast.

Once the iron-bearing transferrin interacts with its receptor, the complex is internalized via clathrin-coated pits and transported to an acidic endosome, where the iron is released at the low pH. The iron is then made available for heme synthesis while the transferrin–receptor complex is recycled to the surface of the cell, where the bulk of the transferrin is released back into circulation and the transferrin receptor reanchors into the cell membrane. At this point, a certain amount of the transferrin receptor protein may be released into circulation and can be measured as soluble transferrin receptor protein. Within the erythroid cell, iron in excess of the amount needed for hemoglobin synthesis binds to a storage protein, *apoferritin*, forming *ferritin*. This mechanism of iron exchange also takes place in other cells of the body expressing transferrin receptors, especially liver parenchymal cells, where the iron can be incorporated into heme-containing enzymes or stored. The iron incorporated into hemoglobin subsequently enters the circulation as new red cells are released from the bone marrow. The iron is then part of the red cell mass and will not become available for reutilization until the red cell dies.

In a normal individual, the average red cell life span is 120 days. Thus, 0.8–1% of red cells turn over each day. At the end of its life span, a red cell is recognized as senescent by the cells of the *reticuloendothelial (RE) system*, and the cell undergoes phagocytosis. Once within the RE cell, the hemoglobin from the ingested red cell is broken down, the globin and other proteins are returned to the amino acid pool, and the iron is shuttled back to the surface of the RE cell, where it is presented to circulating transferrin. It is the efficient and highly conserved recycling of iron from senescent red cells that supports steady state (and even mildly accelerated) erythropoiesis.

Because each milliliter of red cells contains 1 mg of elemental iron, the amount of iron needed to replace red cells lost through senescence amounts to 20 mg/d (assuming an adult with a red cell mass of 2 L). Any additional iron required for daily red cell production comes from the diet. Normally, an adult male will need to absorb at least 1 mg of elemental iron daily to meet needs, while females in the childbearing years will need to absorb an average of 1.4 mg/d. However, to achieve a maximum proliferative erythroid marrow response to anemia, additional iron must be available. With markedly stimulated erythropoiesis, demands for iron are increased by as much as six- to eightfold. With extravascular hemolytic anemia, the rate of red cell destruction is increased, but the iron recovered from the red cells is efficiently reutilized for hemoglobin synthesis. In contrast, with intravascular hemolysis or blood loss anemia, the rate of red cell production is limited by the amount of iron that can be mobilized from stores. Typically, the rate of mobilization under these circumstances will not support red cell production more than 2.5 times normal. If the delivery of iron to the stimulated marrow is suboptimal, the marrow's proliferative response is blunted, and hemoglobin synthesis is impaired. The result is a hypoproliferative marrow accompanied by microcytic, hypochromic anemia.

Whereas blood loss or hemolysis places a demand on the iron supply, inflammatory conditions interfere with iron release from stores and can result in a rapid decrease in the serum iron (discussed later).

NUTRITIONAL IRON BALANCE

The balance of iron in humans is tightly controlled and designed to conserve iron for reutilization. There is no regulated excretory pathway for iron, and the only mechanisms by which iron is lost are blood loss (via gastrointestinal [GI] bleeding, menses, or other forms of bleeding) and the loss of epithelial cells from the skin, gut, and genitourinary tract. Normally, the only route by which iron comes into the body is via absorption from food or from medicinal iron taken orally. Iron may also enter the body through red-cell transfusions or injection of iron complexes. The margin between the amount of iron available for absorption and the requirement for iron in growing infants and adult females is narrow; this accounts for the great prevalence of iron deficiency worldwide—currently estimated at one-half billion people.

The amount of iron required from the diet to replace losses averages approximately 10% of body iron content a year in men and 15% in women of childbearing age. Dietary iron content is closely related to total caloric intake (~6 mg of elemental iron per 1000 calories). Iron bioavailability is affected by the nature of the foodstuff, with heme iron (e.g., red meat) being most readily absorbed. In the United States, the average iron intake in an adult male is 15 mg/d with 6% absorption; for the average female, the daily intake is 11 mg/d with 12% absorption. An individual with iron deficiency can increase iron absorption to approximately 20% of the iron present in a meat-containing diet but only 5–10% of the iron in a vegetarian diet. As a result, one-third of the female population in the United States has virtually no iron stores. Vegetarians are at an additional disadvantage because certain foodstuffs that include phytates and phosphates reduce iron absorption by approximately 50%. When ionizable iron salts are given together with food, the amount of iron absorbed is reduced. When the percentage of iron absorbed from individual food items is compared with the percentage for an equivalent amount of ferrous salt, iron in vegetables is only about one-twentieth as available, egg iron one-eighth, liver iron one-half, and heme iron one-half to two-thirds.

Infants, children, and adolescents may be unable to maintain normal iron balance because of the demands of body growth and lower dietary intake of iron. During the last two trimesters of pregnancy, daily iron requirements increase to 5–6 mg. That is the reason why iron supplements are strongly recommended for pregnant women in developed countries.

Iron absorption takes place largely in the proximal small intestine and is a carefully regulated process. For absorption, iron must be taken up by the luminal cell. That process is facilitated by the acidic contents of the stomach, which maintains the iron in solution. At the brush border of the absorptive cell, the ferric iron is converted to the ferrous form by a ferrireductase. Transport across the membrane is accomplished by divalent metal transporter type 1 (DMT-1, also known as natural resistance macrophage-associated protein type 2 [Nramp 2] or DCT-1). DMT-1 is a general cation transporter. Once inside the gut cell, iron may be stored as ferritin or transported through the cell to be released at the basolateral surface to plasma transferrin through the membrane-embedded iron exporter, ferroportin. The function of ferroportin is negatively regulated by hepcidin, the principal iron regulatory hormone. In the process of release, iron interacts with another ferroxidase, hephaestin, which oxidizes the iron to the ferric form for transferrin binding. Hephaestin is similar to ceruloplasmin, the copper-carrying protein.

Iron absorption is influenced by a number of physiologic states. Erythroid hyperplasia stimulates iron absorption even in the face of normal or increased iron stores, and hepcidin levels are inappropriately low. The molecular mechanism underlying this relationship is not known. Thus, patients with anemias associated with high levels of ineffective erythropoiesis absorb excess amounts of dietary iron. Over time, this may lead to iron overload and tissue damage. In iron deficiency, hepcidin levels are low, and iron is much more efficiently absorbed; the contrary is true in states of secondary iron overload. A normal individual can reduce iron absorption in situations of excessive intake or medicinal iron intake; however, while the percentage of iron absorbed goes down, the absolute amount goes up. This accounts for the acute iron toxicity occasionally seen when children ingest large numbers of iron tablets. Under these circumstances, the amount of iron absorbed exceeds the transferrin binding capacity of the plasma, resulting in free iron that affects critical organs such as cardiac muscle cells.

IRON-DEFICIENCY ANEMIA

Iron deficiency is one of the most prevalent forms of malnutrition. Globally, 50% of anemia is attributable to iron deficiency and accounts for approximately 841,000 deaths annually worldwide. Africa and parts of Asia bear 71% of the global mortality burden; North America represents only 1.4% of the total morbidity and mortality associated with iron deficiency.

STAGES OF IRON DEFICIENCY

The progression to iron deficiency can be divided into three stages (Fig. 7-2). The first stage is *negative iron balance*, in which the demands for (or losses of) iron

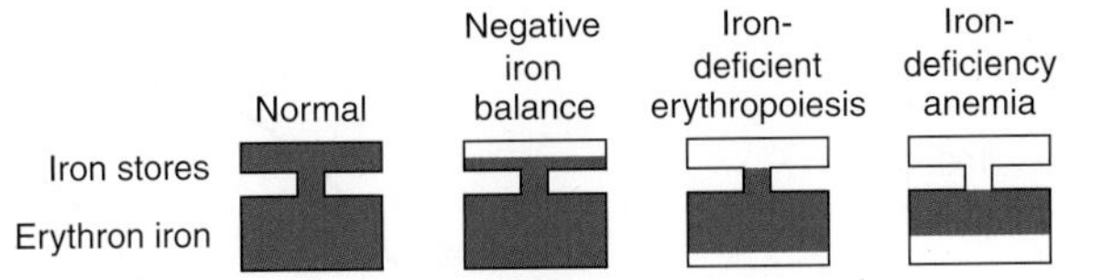

	Normal	Negative iron balance	Iron-deficient erythropoiesis	Iron-deficiency anemia
Iron stores				
Erythron iron				
Marrow iron stores	1–3+	0-1+	0	0
Serum ferritin (μg/L)	50–200	<20	<15	<15
TIBC (μg/dL)	300–360	>360	>380	>400
SI (μg/dL)	50–150	NL	<50	<30
Saturation (%)	30–50	NL	<20	<10
Marrow sideroblasts (%)	40–60	NL	<10	<10
RBC protoporphyrin (μg/dL)	30–50	NL	>100	>200
RBC morphology	NL	NL	NL	Microcytic/ hypochromic

FIGURE 7-2

Laboratory studies in the evolution of iron deficiency. Measurements of marrow iron stores, serum ferritin, and total iron-binding capacity (TIBC) are sensitive to early iron-store depletion. Iron-deficient erythropoiesis is recognized from additional abnormalities in the serum iron (SI), percent transferrin saturation, the pattern of marrow sideroblasts, and the red cell protoporphyrin level. Patients with iron-deficiency anemia demonstrate all the same abnormalities plus hypochromic microcytic anemia. NL, normal; RBC, red blood cell. (*From RS Hillman, CA Finch: Red Cell Manual, 7th ed. Philadelphia, Davis, 1996, with permission.*)

exceed the body's ability to absorb iron from the diet. This stage results from a number of physiologic mechanisms, including blood loss, pregnancy (in which the demands for red cell production by the fetus outstrip the mother's ability to provide iron), rapid growth spurts in an adolescent, or inadequate dietary iron intake. Blood loss in excess of 10–20 mL of red cells per day is greater than the amount of iron that the gut can absorb from a normal diet. Under these circumstances, the iron deficit must be made up by mobilization of iron from RE storage sites. During this period, iron stores—reflected by the serum ferritin level or the appearance of stainable iron on bone marrow aspirations—decrease. As long as iron stores are present and can be mobilized, the serum iron, total iron-binding capacity (TIBC), and red cell protoporphyrin levels remain within normal limits. At this stage, red cell morphology and indices are normal.

When iron stores become depleted, the serum iron begins to fall. Gradually, the TIBC increases, as do red cell protoporphyrin levels. By definition, marrow iron stores are absent when the serum ferritin level is <15 μg/L. As long as the serum iron remains within the normal range, hemoglobin synthesis is unaffected despite the dwindling iron stores. Once the transferrin saturation falls to 15–20%, hemoglobin synthesis becomes impaired. This is a period of *iron-deficient erythropoiesis*. Careful evaluation of the peripheral blood smear reveals the first appearance of microcytic cells, and if the laboratory technology is available, one finds hypochromic reticulocytes in circulation. Gradually, the hemoglobin and hematocrit begin to fall, reflecting *iron-deficiency anemia*. The transferrin saturation at this point is 10–15%.

When moderate anemia is present (hemoglobin 10–13 g/dL), the bone marrow remains hypoproliferative. With more severe anemia (hemoglobin 7–8 g/dL), hypochromia and microcytosis become more prominent, target cells and misshapen red cells (poikilocytes) appear on the blood smear as cigar- or pencil-shaped forms, and the erythroid marrow becomes increasingly ineffective. Consequently, with severe prolonged iron-deficiency anemia, erythroid hyperplasia of the marrow develops rather than hypoproliferation.

CAUSES OF IRON DEFICIENCY

Conditions that increase demand for iron, increase iron loss, or decrease iron intake or absorption can produce iron deficiency (Table 7-2).

CLINICAL PRESENTATION OF IRON DEFICIENCY

Certain clinical conditions carry an increased likelihood of iron deficiency. Pregnancy, adolescence, periods of rapid growth, and an intermittent history of blood loss of any kind should alert the clinician to possible iron deficiency. A cardinal rule is that the appearance of iron deficiency in an adult male means GI blood loss

TABLE 7-2

CAUSES OF IRON DEFICIENCY
Increased Demand for Iron
Rapid growth in infancy or adolescence
Pregnancy
Erythropoietin therapy
Increased Iron Loss
Chronic blood loss
Menses
Acute blood loss
Blood donation
Phlebotomy as treatment for polycythemia vera
Decreased Iron Intake or Absorption
Inadequate diet
Malabsorption from disease (sprue, Crohn's disease)
Malabsorption from surgery (postgastrectomy)
Acute or chronic inflammation

until proven otherwise. Signs related to iron deficiency depend on the severity and chronicity of the anemia in addition to the usual signs of anemia—fatigue, pallor, and reduced exercise capacity. *Cheilosis* (fissures at the corners of the mouth) and *koilonychia* (spooning of the fingernails) are signs of advanced tissue iron deficiency. The diagnosis of iron deficiency is typically based on laboratory results.

LABORATORY IRON STUDIES

Serum iron and total iron-binding capacity

The serum iron level represents the amount of circulating iron bound to transferrin. The TIBC is an indirect measure of the circulating transferrin. The normal range for the serum iron is 50–150 μg/dL; the normal range for TIBC is 300–360 μg/dL. Transferrin saturation, which is normally 25–50%, is obtained by the following formula: serum iron × 100 ÷ TIBC. Iron-deficiency states are associated with saturation levels below 20%. There is a diurnal variation in the serum iron. A transferrin saturation >50% indicates that a disproportionate amount of the iron bound to transferrin is being delivered to non-erythroid tissues. If this persists for an extended time, tissue iron overload may occur.

Serum ferritin

Free iron is toxic to cells, and the body has established an elaborate set of protective mechanisms to bind iron in various tissue compartments. Within cells, iron is stored complexed to protein as ferritin or hemosiderin. Apoferritin binds to free ferrous iron and stores it in the ferric state. As ferritin accumulates within cells of the RE system, protein aggregates are formed as hemosiderin. Iron in ferritin or hemosiderin can be extracted for release by the RE cells, although hemosiderin is less readily available. Under steady-state conditions, the serum ferritin level correlates with total body iron stores; thus, the serum ferritin level is the most convenient laboratory test to estimate iron stores. The normal value for ferritin varies according to the age and gender of the individual (Fig. 7-3). Adult males have serum ferritin values averaging 100 μg/L, while adult females have levels averaging 30 μg/L. As iron stores are depleted, the serum ferritin falls to <15 μg/L. Such levels are diagnostic of absent body iron stores.

Evaluation of bone marrow iron stores

Although RE cell iron stores can be estimated from the iron stain of a bone marrow aspirate or biopsy, the measurement of serum ferritin has largely supplanted bone marrow aspirates for determination of storage iron (Table 7-3). The serum ferritin level is a better

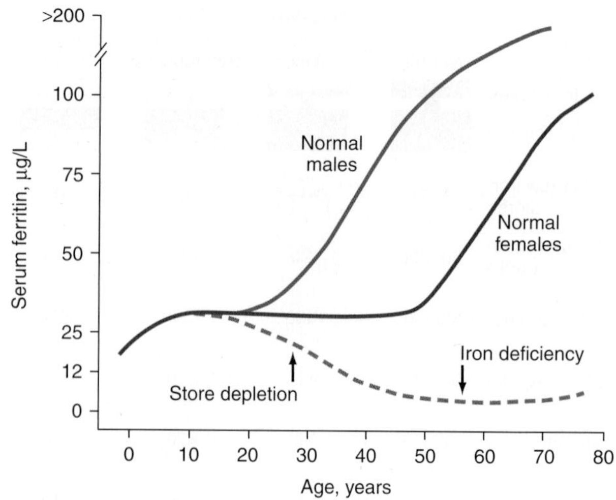

FIGURE 7-3

Serum ferritin levels as a function of sex and age. Iron store depletion and iron deficiency are accompanied by a decrease in serum ferritin level below 20 μg/L. (*From RS Hillman et al: Hematology in Clinical Practice, 5th ed. New York, McGraw-Hill, 2010, with permission.*)

indicator of iron overload than the marrow iron stain. However, in addition to storage iron, the marrow iron stain provides information about the effective delivery of iron to developing erythroblasts. Normally, when the marrow smear is stained for iron, 20–40% of developing erythroblasts—called *sideroblasts*—will have visible ferritin granules in their cytoplasms. This represents iron in excess of that needed for hemoglobin synthesis. In states in which release of iron from storage sites is blocked, RE iron will be detectable, and there will be few or no sideroblasts. In the myelodysplastic syndromes, mitochondrial dysfunction can occur, and accumulation of iron in mitochondria appears in a necklace fashion around the nucleus of the erythroblast. Such cells are referred to as *ringed sideroblasts*.

Red cell protoporphyrin levels

Protoporphyrin is an intermediate in the pathway to heme synthesis. Under conditions in which heme synthesis is impaired, protoporphyrin accumulates within

TABLE 7-3

IRON STORE MEASUREMENTS

IRON STORES	MARROW IRON STAIN, 0-4+	SERUM FERRITIN, μg/L
0	0	<15
1–300 mg	Trace to 1+	15–30
300–800 mg	2+	30–60
800–1000 mg	3+	60–150
1–2 g	4+	>150
Iron overload	—	>500–1000

the red cell. This reflects an inadequate iron supply to erythroid precursors to support hemoglobin synthesis. Normal values are <30 μg/dL of red cells. In iron deficiency, values in excess of 100 μg/dL are seen. The most common causes of increased red cell protoporphyrin levels are absolute or relative iron deficiency and lead poisoning.

Serum levels of transferrin receptor protein

Because erythroid cells have the highest numbers of transferrin receptors of any cell in the body and because transferrin receptor protein (TRP) is released by cells into the circulation, serum levels of TRP reflect the total erythroid marrow mass. Another condition in which TRP levels are elevated is absolute iron deficiency. Normal values are 4–9 μg/L determined by immunoassay. This laboratory test is becoming increasingly available and, along with the serum ferritin, has been proposed to distinguish between iron deficiency and the anemia of chronic inflammation (discussed later).

DIFFERENTIAL DIAGNOSIS

Other than iron deficiency, only three conditions need to be considered in the differential diagnosis of a hypochromic microcytic anemia (Table 7-4). The first is an inherited defect in globin chain synthesis: the thalassemias. These are differentiated from iron deficiency most readily by serum iron values; normal or increased serum iron levels and transferrin saturation are characteristic of the thalassemias. In addition, the red blood cell distribution width (RDW) index is generally small in thalassemia and elevated in iron deficiency.

The second condition is the anemia of chronic inflammation with inadequate iron supply to the erythroid marrow. The distinction between true iron-deficiency anemia and the anemia associated with chronic inflammation is among the most common diagnostic problem encountered by clinicians (see below). Usually the anemia of chronic inflammation is normocytic and normochromic. The iron values usually make the differential diagnosis clear, as the ferritin level is normal or increased and the percent transferrin saturation and TIBC are typically below normal.

Finally, the myelodysplastic syndromes represent the third and least common condition. Occasionally, patients with myelodysplasia have impaired hemoglobin synthesis with mitochondrial dysfunction, resulting in impaired iron incorporation into heme. The iron values again reveal normal stores and more than an adequate supply to the marrow, despite the microcytosis and hypochromia.

TREATMENT Iron-Deficiency Anemia

The severity and cause of iron-deficiency anemia will determine the appropriate approach to treatment. As an example, symptomatic elderly patients with severe iron-deficiency anemia and cardiovascular instability may require red cell transfusions. Younger individuals who have compensated for their anemia can be treated more conservatively with iron replacement. The foremost issue for the latter patient is the precise identification of the cause of the iron deficiency.

For the majority of cases of iron deficiency (pregnant women, growing children and adolescents, patients with infrequent episodes of bleeding, and those with inadequate dietary intake of iron), oral iron therapy will suffice. For patients with unusual blood loss or malabsorption, specific diagnostic tests and appropriate therapy take priority. Once the diagnosis of iron-deficiency anemia and its cause is made, there are three major therapeutic approaches.

RED CELL TRANSFUSION Transfusion therapy is reserved for individuals who have symptoms of anemia, cardiovascular instability, continued and excessive blood loss from whatever source, and require immediate intervention. The management of these patients is less

TABLE 7-4

DIAGNOSIS OF MICROCYTIC ANEMIA

TEST	IRON DEFICIENCY	INFLAMMATION	THALASSEMIA	SIDEROBLASTIC ANEMIA
Smear	Micro/hypo	Normal micro/hypo	Micro/hypo with targeting	Variable
SI	<30	<50	Normal to high	Normal to high
TIBC	>360	<300	Normal	Normal
Percent saturation	<10	10–20	30–80	30–80
Ferritin (μg/L)	<15	30–200	50–300	50–300
Hemoglobin pattern on electrophoresis	Normal	Normal	Abnormal with β thalassemia; can be normal with α thalassemia	Normal

Abbreviations: SI, serum iron; TIBC, total iron-binding capacity.

related to the iron deficiency than it is to the consequences of the severe anemia. Not only do transfusions correct the anemia acutely, but the transfused red cells also provide a source of iron for reutilization, assuming they are not lost through continued bleeding. Transfusion therapy will stabilize the patient while other options are reviewed.

ORAL IRON THERAPY In an asymptomatic patient with established iron-deficiency anemia, treatment with oral iron is usually adequate. Multiple preparations are available, ranging from simple iron salts to complex iron compounds designed for sustained release throughout the small intestine (Table 7-5). Although the various preparations contain different amounts of iron, they are generally all absorbed well and are effective in treatment. Some come with other compounds designed to enhance iron absorption, such as ascorbic acid. It is not clear whether the benefits of such compounds justify their costs. Typically, for iron replacement therapy, up to 300 mg of elemental iron per day is given, usually as three or four iron tablets (each containing 50–65 mg elemental iron) given over the course of the day. Ideally, oral iron preparations should be taken on an empty stomach, since food may inhibit iron absorption. Some patients with gastric disease or prior gastric surgery require special treatment with iron solutions, as the retention capacity of the stomach may be reduced. The retention capacity is necessary for dissolving the shell of the iron tablet before the release of iron. A dose of 200–300 mg of elemental iron per day should result in the absorption of iron up to 50 mg/d. This supports a red cell production level of two to three times normal in an individual with a normally functioning marrow and appropriate erythropoietin stimulus. However, as the hemoglobin level rises, erythropoietin stimulation decreases, and the amount of iron absorbed is reduced. The goal of therapy in individuals with iron-deficiency anemia is not only to repair the anemia but also to provide stores of at least 0.5–1 g of iron. Sustained treatment for a period of 6–12 months after correction of the anemia will be necessary to achieve this.

TABLE 7-5

ORAL IRON PREPARATIONS

GENERIC NAME	TABLET (IRON CONTENT), mg	ELIXIR (IRON CONTENT), mg IN 5 mL
Ferrous sulfate	325 (65)	300 (60)
	195 (39)	90 (18)
Extended release	525 (105)	
Ferrous fumarate	325 (107)	
	195 (64)	100 (33)
Ferrous gluconate	325 (39)	300 (35)
Polysaccharide iron	150 (150)	100 (100)
	50 (50)	

Of the complications of oral iron therapy, GI distress is the most prominent and is seen in 15–20% of patients. Abdominal pain, nausea, vomiting, or constipation may lead to noncompliance. Although small doses of iron or iron preparations with delayed release may help somewhat, the GI side effects are a major impediment to the effective treatment of a number of patients.

The response to iron therapy varies, depending on the erythropoietin stimulus and the rate of absorption. Typically, the reticulocyte count should begin to increase within 4–7 days after initiation of therapy and peak at 1–1½ weeks. The absence of a response may be due to poor absorption, noncompliance (which is common), or a confounding diagnosis. A useful test in the clinic to determine the patient's ability to absorb iron is the *iron tolerance test*. Two iron tablets are given to the patient on an empty stomach, and the serum iron is measured serially over the subsequent 2 hours. Normal absorption will result in an increase in the serum iron of at least 100 μg/dL. If iron deficiency persists despite adequate treatment, it may be necessary to switch to parenteral iron therapy.

PARENTERAL IRON THERAPY Intravenous iron can be given to patients who are unable to tolerate oral iron; whose needs are relatively acute; or who need iron on an ongoing basis, usually due to persistent GI blood loss. Parenteral iron use has been increasing rapidly in the last several years with the recognition that recombinant erythropoietin (EPO) therapy induces a large demand for iron—a demand that frequently cannot be met through the physiologic release of iron from RE sources or oral iron absorption. The safety of parenteral iron—particularly iron dextran—has been a concern. The serious adverse reaction rate to intravenous high-molecular weight iron dextran is 0.7%. Fortunately, newer iron complexes are available in the United States, such as sodium ferric gluconate (Ferrlecit) and iron sucrose (Venofer) that have much lower rates of adverse effects.

Parenteral iron is used in two ways: one is to administer the total dose of iron required to correct the hemoglobin deficit and provide the patient with at least 500 mg of iron stores; the second is to give repeated small doses of parenteral iron over a protracted period. The latter approach is common in dialysis centers, where it is not unusual for 100 mg of elemental iron to be given weekly for 10 weeks to augment the response to recombinant EPO therapy. The amount of iron needed by an individual patient is calculated by the following formula:

Body weight (kg) × 2.3 × (15–patient's hemoglobin, g/dL) + 500 or 1000 mg (for stores).

In administering intravenous iron dextran, anaphylaxis is a concern. Anaphylaxis is much rarer with the newer preparations. The factors that have correlated with an anaphylactic-like reaction include a history of multiple allergies or a prior allergic reaction to dextran (in the case of iron dextran). Generalized symptoms appearing several days after the infusion of a large dose of iron can include arthralgias, skin rash, and low-grade fever. These may be dose-related, but they do not preclude the further use of parenteral iron in the patient. To date, patients with sensitivity to iron dextran have been safely treated with iron gluconate. If a large dose of iron dextran is to be given (>100 mg), the iron preparation should be diluted in 5% dextrose in water or 0.9% NaCl solution. The iron solution can then be infused over a 60- to 90-minute period (for larger doses) or at a rate convenient for the attending nurse or physician. Although a test dose (25 mg) of parenteral iron dextran is recommended, in reality, a slow infusion of a larger dose of parenteral iron solution will afford the same kind of early warning as a separately injected test dose. Early in the infusion of iron, if chest pain, wheezing, a fall in blood pressure, or other systemic symptoms occur, the infusion of iron should be stopped immediately.

OTHER HYPOPROLIFERATIVE ANEMIAS

In addition to mild to moderate iron-deficiency anemia, the hypoproliferative anemias can be divided into four categories: (1) chronic inflammation, (2) renal disease, (3) endocrine and nutritional deficiencies (hypometabolic states), and (4) marrow damage (Chap. 11). With chronic inflammation, renal disease, or hypometabolism, endogenous EPO production is inadequate for the degree of anemia observed. For the anemia of chronic inflammation, the erythroid marrow also responds inadequately to stimulation, due in part to defective *iron reutilization*. As a result of the lack of adequate EPO stimulation, an examination of the peripheral blood smear will disclose only an occasional polychromatophilic ("shift") reticulocyte. In cases of iron deficiency or marrow damage, appropriate elevations in endogenous EPO levels are typically found, and shift reticulocytes will be present on the blood smear.

ANEMIA OF ACUTE AND CHRONIC INFLAMMATION/INFECTION (THE ANEMIA OF INFLAMMATION)

The anemia of inflammation—which encompasses inflammation, infection, tissue injury, and conditions (e.g., cancer) associated with the release of proinflammatory cytokines—is one of the most common forms of anemia seen clinically. It is the most important anemia in the differential diagnosis of iron deficiency because many of the features of the anemia are brought about by inadequate iron delivery to the marrow, despite the presence of normal or increased iron stores. This is reflected by a low serum iron, increased red cell protoporphyrin, a hypoproliferative marrow, transferrin saturation in the range of 15–20%, and a normal or increased serum ferritin. The serum ferritin values are often the most distinguishing features between true iron-deficiency anemia and the iron-restricted erythropoiesis associated with inflammation. Typically, serum ferritin values increase threefold over basal levels in the face of inflammation. These changes are due to the effects of inflammatory cytokines and hepcidin, the key iron regulatory hormone, acting at several levels of erythropoiesis (Fig. 7-4).

Interleukin 1 (IL-1) directly decreases EPO production in response to anemia. IL-1, acting through accessory cell release of interferon γ (IFN-γ), suppresses the response of the erythroid marrow to EPO—an effect that can be overcome by EPO administration in vitro and in vivo. In addition, tumor necrosis factor (TNF), acting through the release of IFN-γ by marrow stromal cells, also suppresses the response to EPO. Hepcidin, made by the liver, is increased in inflammation and acts to suppress iron absorption and iron release from storage sites. The overall result is a chronic hypoproliferative anemia with classic changes in iron metabolism. The anemia is further compounded by a mild to moderate shortening in red cell survival.

With chronic inflammation, the primary disease will determine the severity and characteristics of the anemia. For example, many patients with cancer also have anemia that is typically normocytic and normochromic. In

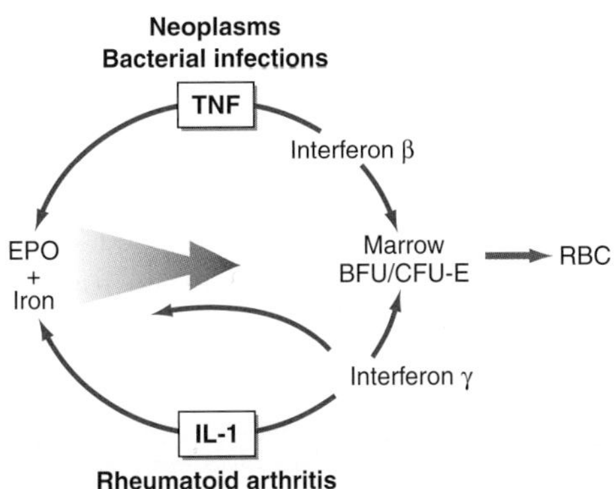

FIGURE 7-4
Suppression of erythropoiesis by inflammatory cytokines. Through the release of tumor necrosis factor (TNF) and interferon γ (IFN-γ), neoplasms and bacterial infections suppress erythropoietin (EPO) production and the proliferation of erythroid progenitors (erythroid burst-forming units and erythroid colony-forming units [BFU/CFU-E]). The mediators in patients with vasculitis and rheumatoid arthritis include interleukin 1 (IL-1) and IFN-γ The *red arrows* indicate sites of inflammatory cytokine inhibitory effects.

contrast, patients with long-standing active rheumatoid arthritis or chronic infections such as tuberculosis will have a microcytic, hypochromic anemia. In both cases, the bone marrow is hypoproliferative, but the differences in red cell indices reflect differences in the availability of iron for hemoglobin synthesis. Occasionally, conditions associated with chronic inflammation are also associated with chronic blood loss. Under these circumstances, a bone marrow aspirate stained for iron may be necessary to rule out absolute iron deficiency. However, the administration of iron in this case will correct the iron deficiency component of the anemia and leave the inflammatory component unaffected.

The anemia associated with acute infection or inflammation is typically mild but becomes more pronounced over time. Acute infection can produce a decrease in hemoglobin levels of 2–3 g/dL within 1 or 2 days; this is largely related to the hemolysis of red cells near the end of their natural life span. The fever and cytokines released exert a selective pressure against cells with more limited capacity to maintain the red cell membrane. In most individuals, the mild anemia is reasonably well tolerated, and symptoms, if present, are associated with the underlying disease. Occasionally, in patients with preexisting cardiac disease, moderate anemia (hemoglobin 10–11 g/dL) may be associated with angina, exercise intolerance, and shortness of breath. The erythropoietic profile that distinguishes the anemia of inflammation from the other causes of hypoproliferative anemias is shown in Table 7-6.

ANEMIA OF CHRONIC KIDNEY DISEASE (CKD)

Progressive CKD is usually associated with a moderate to severe hypoproliferative anemia; the level of the anemia correlates with the stage of CKD. Red cells are typically normocytic and normochromic, and reticulocytes are decreased. The anemia is primarily due to a failure of EPO production by the diseased kidney and a reduction in red cell survival. In certain forms of acute renal failure, the correlation between the anemia and renal function is weaker. Patients with the hemolytic-uremic syndrome increase erythropoiesis in response to the hemolysis, despite renal failure requiring dialysis. Polycystic kidney disease also shows a smaller degree of EPO deficiency for a given level of renal failure. By contrast, patients with diabetes or myeloma have more severe EPO deficiency for a given level of renal failure.

Assessment of iron status provides information to distinguish the anemia of CKD from the other forms of hypoproliferative anemia (Table 7-6) and to guide management. Patients with the anemia of CKD usually present with normal serum iron, TIBC, and ferritin levels. However, those maintained on chronic hemodialysis may develop iron deficiency from blood loss through the dialysis procedure. Iron must be replenished in these patients to ensure an adequate response to EPO therapy (discussed later).

ANEMIA IN HYPOMETABOLIC STATES

Patients who are starving, particularly for protein, and those with a variety of endocrine disorders that produce lower metabolic rates may develop a mild to moderate hypoproliferative anemia. The release of EPO from the kidney is sensitive to the need for O_2, not just O_2 levels. Thus, EPO production is triggered at lower levels of blood O_2 content in disease states (e.g., hypothyroidism and starvation) where metabolic activity, and thus O_2 demand, is decreased.

Endocrine deficiency states

The difference in the levels of hemoglobin between men and women is related to the effects of androgen and estrogen on erythropoiesis. Testosterone and anabolic steroids augment erythropoiesis; castration and estrogen administration to males decrease erythropoiesis. Patients who are hypothyroid or have deficits in pituitary hormones also may develop a mild anemia. Pathogenesis may be complicated by other nutritional deficiencies because iron and folic acid absorption can

TABLE 7-6

DIAGNOSIS OF HYPOPROLIFERATIVE ANEMIAS

TESTS	IRON DEFICIENCY	INFLAMMATION	RENAL DISEASE	HYPOMETABOLIC STATES
Anemia	Mild to severe	Mild	Mild to severe	Mild
MCV (fL)	60–90	80–90	90	90
Morphology	Normo-microcytic	Normocytic	Normocytic	Normocytic
SI	<30	<50	Normal	Normal
TIBC	>360	<300	Normal	Normal
Saturation (%)	<10	10–20	Normal	Normal
Serum ferritin (μg/L)	<15	30–200	115–150	Normal
Iron stores	0	2–4+	1–4+	Normal

Abbreviations: MCV, mean corpuscular volume; SI, serum iron; TIBC, total iron-binding capacity.

be affected by these disorders. Usually, correction of the hormone deficiency reverses the anemia.

Anemia may be more severe in Addison's disease, depending on the level of thyroid and androgen hormone dysfunction; however, anemia may be masked by decreases in plasma volume. Once such patients are given cortisol and volume replacement, the hemoglobin level may fall rapidly. Mild anemia complicating hyperparathyroidism may be due to decreased EPO production as a consequence of the renal effects of hypercalcemia or to impaired proliferation of erythroid progenitors.

Protein starvation

Decreased dietary intake of protein may lead to mild to moderate hypoproliferative anemia; this form of anemia may be prevalent in the elderly. The anemia can be more severe in patients with a greater degree of starvation. In marasmus, where patients are both protein and calorie deficient, the release of EPO is impaired in proportion to the reduction in metabolic rate; however, the degree of anemia may be masked by volume depletion and becomes apparent after refeeding. Deficiencies in other nutrients (iron, folate) may also complicate the clinical picture but may not be apparent at diagnosis. Changes in the erythrocyte indices on refeeding should prompt evaluation of iron, folate, and B_{12} status.

Anemia in liver disease

A mild hypoproliferative anemia may develop in patients with chronic liver disease from nearly any cause. The peripheral blood smear may show spur cells and stomatocytes from the accumulation of excess cholesterol in the membrane from a deficiency of lecithin-cholesterol acyltransferase. Red cell survival is shortened, and the production of EPO is inadequate to compensate. In alcoholic liver disease, nutritional deficiencies are common and complicate the management. Folate deficiency from inadequate intake, as well as iron deficiency from blood loss and inadequate intake, can alter the red cell indices.

TREATMENT Hypoproliferative Anemias

Many patients with hypoproliferative anemias experience recovery of normal hemoglobin levels when the underlying disease is appropriately treated. For those in whom such reversals are not possible—such as patients with end-stage kidney disease, cancer, and chronic inflammatory diseases—symptomatic anemia requires treatment. The two major forms of treatment are transfusions and EPO.

TRANSFUSIONS Thresholds for transfusion should be altered based on the patient's symptoms. In general, patients without serious underlying cardiovascular or pulmonary disease can tolerate hemoglobin levels above 8 g/dL and do not require intervention until the hemoglobin falls below that level. Patients with more physiologic compromise may need to have their hemoglobin levels kept above 11 g/dL. A typical unit of packed red cells increases the hemoglobin level by 1 g/dL. Transfusions are associated with certain infectious risks (Chap. 12), and chronic transfusions can produce iron overload. Importantly, the liberal use of blood has been associated with increased morbidity and mortality, particularly in the intensive care setting. Therefore, in the absence of documented tissue hypoxia, a conservative approach to the use of red cell transfusions is preferable.

ERYTHROPOIETIN (EPO) EPO is particularly useful in anemias in which endogenous EPO levels are inappropriately low, such as CKD or the anemia of chronic inflammation. Iron status must be evaluated and iron repleted to obtain optimal effects from EPO. In patients with CKD, the usual dose of EPO is 50–150 U/kg three times a week intravenously. Hemoglobin levels of 10–12 g/dL are usually reached within 4–6 weeks if iron levels are adequate; 90% of these patients respond. Once a target hemoglobin level is achieved, the EPO dose can be decreased. A decrease in hemoglobin level occurring in the face of EPO therapy usually signifies the development of an infection or iron depletion. Aluminum toxicity and hyperparathyroidism can also compromise the EPO response. When an infection intervenes, it is best to interrupt the EPO therapy and rely on transfusion to correct the anemia until the infection is adequately treated. The dose needed to correct the anemia in patients with cancer is higher, up to 300 U/kg three times a week, and only approximately 60% of patients respond. Because of evidence that tumor progression may result from EPO administration, the risks and benefits of using EPO in patients with chemotherapy-induced anemia must be weighed carefully, and the target hemoglobin should be that necessary to avoid transfusions.

Longer-acting preparations of EPO can reduce the frequency of injections. Darbepoetin alfa, a molecularly modified EPO with additional carbohydrate, has a half-life in the circulation that is three to four times longer than recombinant human EPO, permitting weekly or every other week dosing.

CHAPTER 8
DISORDERS OF HEMOGLOBIN

Edward J. Benz, Jr.

Hemoglobin is critical for normal oxygen delivery to tissues; it is also present in erythrocytes in such high concentrations that it can alter red cell shape, deformability, and viscosity. Hemoglobinopathies are disorders affecting the structure, function, or production of hemoglobin. These conditions are usually inherited and range in severity from asymptomatic laboratory abnormalities to death in utero. Different forms may present as hemolytic anemia, erythrocytosis, cyanosis, or vaso-occlusive stigmata.

PROPERTIES OF THE HUMAN HEMOGLOBINS

HEMOGLOBIN STRUCTURE

Different hemoglobins are produced during embryonic, fetal, and adult life (Fig. 8-1). Each consists of a tetramer of globin polypeptide chains: a pair of α-like chains 141 amino acids long and a pair of β-like chains 146 amino acids long. The major adult hemoglobin, HbA, has the structure $\alpha_2\beta_2$. HbF ($\alpha_2\gamma_2$) predominates during most of gestation, and HbA_2 ($\alpha_2\delta_2$) is minor adult hemoglobin. Embryonic hemoglobins need not be considered here.

Each globin chain enfolds a single heme moiety, consisting of a protoporphyrin IX ring complexed with a single iron atom in the ferrous state (Fe^{2+}). Each heme moiety can bind a single oxygen molecule; a molecule of hemoglobin can transport up to four oxygen molecules.

The amino acid sequences of the various globins are highly homologous to one another. Each has a highly helical *secondary structure*. Their globular *tertiary structures* cause the exterior surfaces to be rich in polar (hydrophilic) amino acids that enhance solubility and the interior to be lined with nonpolar groups, forming a hydrophobic pocket into which heme is inserted. The tetrameric *quaternary structure* of HbA contains two $\alpha\beta$ dimers. Numerous tight interactions (i.e., $\alpha_1\beta_1$ contacts) hold the α and β chains together. The complete tetramer is held together by interfaces (i.e., $\alpha_1\beta_2$ contacts) between the α-like chain of one dimer and the non-α chain of the other dimer.

The hemoglobin tetramer is highly soluble, but individual globin chains are insoluble. Unpaired globin precipitates, forming inclusions that damage the cell. Normal globin chain synthesis is balanced so that each newly synthesized α or non-α globin chain will have an available partner with which to pair.

Solubility and reversible oxygen binding are the key properties deranged in hemoglobinopathies. Both depend most on the hydrophilic surface amino acids, the hydrophobic amino acids lining the heme pocket, a key histidine in the F helix, and the amino acids forming the $\alpha_1\beta_1$ and $\alpha_1\beta_2$ contact points. Mutations in these strategic regions tend to be the ones that alter oxygen affinity or solubility.

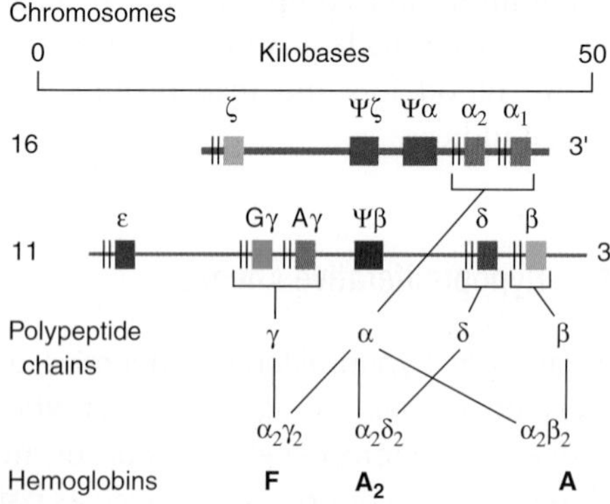

FIGURE 8-1

The globin genes. The α-like genes (α,ζ) are encoded on chromosome 16; the β-like genes (β,γ,δ,ε) are encoded on chromosome 11. The ζ and ε genes encode embryonic globins.

FUNCTION OF HEMOGLOBIN

To support oxygen transport, hemoglobin must bind O_2 efficiently at the partial pressure of oxygen (PO_2) of the alveolus, retain it, and release it to tissues at the PO_2 of tissue capillary beds. Oxygen acquisition and delivery over a relatively narrow range of oxygen tensions depend on a property inherent in the tetrameric arrangement of heme and globin subunits within the hemoglobin molecule called *cooperativity* or *heme–heme interaction.*

At low oxygen tensions, the hemoglobin tetramer is fully deoxygenated (Fig. 8-2). Oxygen binding begins slowly as O_2 tension rises. However, as soon as some oxygen has been bound by the tetramer, an abrupt increase occurs in the slope of the curve. Thus, hemoglobin molecules that have bound some oxygen develop a higher oxygen affinity, greatly accelerating their ability to combine with more oxygen. This S-shaped oxygen equilibrium curve (Fig. 8-2), along which substantial amounts of oxygen loading *and unloading* can occur over a narrow range of oxygen tensions, is physiologically more useful than the high-affinity hyperbolic curve of individual monomers.

Oxygen affinity is modulated by several factors. The Bohr effect is the ability of hemoglobin to deliver more oxygen to tissues at low pH. It arises from the stabilizing action of protons on deoxyhemoglobin, which binds protons more readily than oxyhemoglobin because the latter is a weaker acid (Fig. 8-2). Thus, hemoglobin has a lower oxygen affinity at low pH. The major small molecule that alters oxygen affinity in humans is 2,3-bisphosphoglycerate (2,3-BPG, formerly 2,3-DPG), which lowers oxygen affinity when bound to hemoglobin. HbA has a reasonably high affinity for 2,3-BPG. HbF does not bind 2,3-BPG, so it tends to have a higher oxygen affinity in vivo. Hemoglobin also binds nitric oxide reversibly; this interaction influences vascular tone, but its clinical relevance remains controversial.

Proper oxygen transport depends on the tetrameric structure of the proteins, the proper arrangement of the charged amino acids, and interaction with protons or 2,3-BPG.

DEVELOPMENTAL BIOLOGY OF HUMAN HEMOGLOBINS

Red cells first appearing at about 6 weeks after conception contain the embryonic hemoglobins Hb Portland ($\zeta_2\gamma_2$), Hb Gower I ($\zeta_2\varepsilon_2$), and Hb Gower II ($\alpha_2\varepsilon_2$). At 10–11 weeks, fetal hemoglobin (HbF; $\alpha_2\gamma_2$) becomes predominant. The switch to nearly exclusive synthesis of adult hemoglobin (HbA; $\alpha_2\beta_2$) occurs at about 38 weeks (Fig. 8-1). Fetuses and newborns therefore require α-globin but not β-globin for normal gestation. A major advance in understanding the HbF-to-HbA

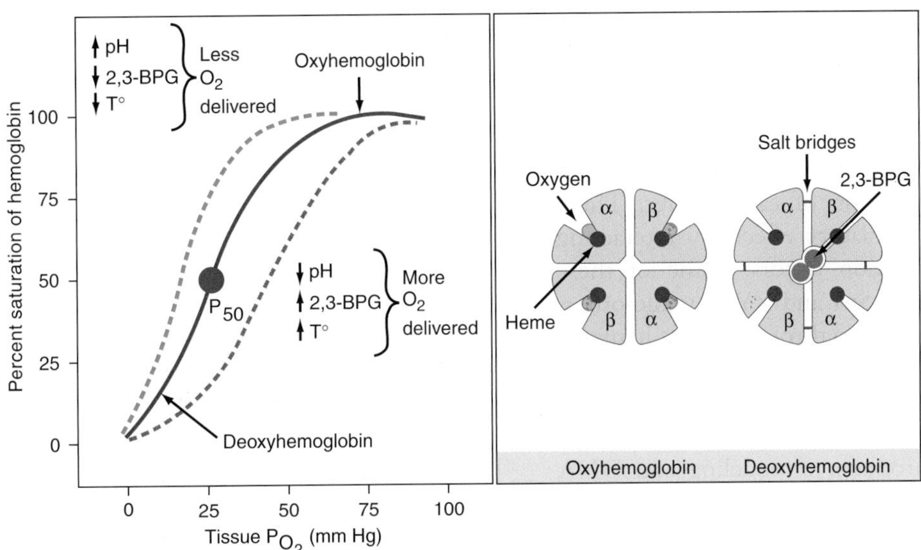

FIGURE 8-2

Hemoglobin–oxygen dissociation curve. The hemoglobin tetramer can bind up to four molecules of oxygen in the iron-containing sites of the heme molecules. As oxygen is bound, 2,3-BPG and CO_2 are expelled. Salt bridges are broken, and each of the globin molecules changes its conformation to facilitate oxygen binding. Oxygen release to the tissues is the reverse process, salt bridges being formed and 2,3-BPG and CO_2 bound. Deoxyhemoglobin does not bind oxygen efficiently until the cell returns to conditions of higher pH, the most important modulator of O_2 affinity (Bohr effect). When acid is produced in the tissues, the dissociation curve shifts to the right, facilitating oxygen release and CO_2 binding. Alkalosis has the opposite effect, reducing oxygen delivery.

transition has been the demonstration that the transcription factor Bcl11a plays a pivotal role in its regulation. Small amounts of HbF are produced during postnatal life. A few red cell clones called *F cells* are progeny of a small pool of immature committed erythroid precursors (BFU-e) that retain the ability to produce HbF. Profound erythroid stresses, such as severe hemolytic anemias, bone marrow transplantation, or cancer chemotherapy, cause more of the F-potent BFU-e to be recruited. HbF levels thus tend to rise in some patients with sickle cell anemia or thalassemia. This phenomenon probably explains the ability of hydroxyurea to increase levels of HbF in adults. Agents such as butyrate and histone deacetylase inhibitors can also activate fetal globin genes partially after birth.

GENETICS AND BIOSYNTHESIS OF HUMAN HEMOGLOBIN

The human hemoglobins are encoded in two tightly linked gene clusters; the α-like globin genes are clustered on chromosome 16, and the β-like genes on chromosome 11 (Fig. 8-1). The α-like cluster consists of two α-globin genes and a single copy of the ζ gene. The non-α gene cluster consists of a single ε gene, the Gγ and Aγ fetal globin genes, and the adult δ and β genes.

Important regulatory sequences flank each gene. Immediately upstream are typical promoter elements needed for the assembly of the transcription initiation complex. Sequences in the 5′ flanking region of the γ and the β genes appear to be crucial for the correct developmental regulation of these genes, while elements that function like classic enhancers and silencers are in the 3′ flanking regions. The locus control region (LCR) elements located far upstream appear to control the overall level of expression of each cluster. These elements achieve their regulatory effects by interacting with *trans*-acting transcription factors. Some of these factors are ubiquitous (e.g., Sp1 and YY1), while others are more or less limited to erythroid cells or hematopoietic cells (e.g., GATA-1, NFE-2, and EKLF). The LCR controlling the α-globin gene cluster is modulated by a SWI/SNF-like protein called *ATRX*; this protein appears to influence chromatin remodeling and DNA methylation. The association of α thalassemia with mental retardation and myelodysplasia in some families appears to be related to mutations in the ATRX pathway. This pathway also modulates genes specifically expressed during erythropoiesis, such as those that encode the enzymes for heme biosynthesis. Normal red blood cell (RBC) differentiation requires the coordinated expression of the globin genes with the genes responsible for heme and iron metabolism. RBC precursors contain a protein, α-hemoglobin-stabilizing protein (AHSP), that enhances the folding and solubility of α globin, which is otherwise easily denatured, leading to insoluble precipitates. These precipitates play an important role in the thalassemia syndromes and certain unstable hemoglobin disorders. Polymorphic variation in the amounts and/or functional capacity of AHSP might explain some of the clinical variability seen in patients inheriting identical thalassemia mutations.

CLASSIFICATION OF HEMOGLOBINOPATHIES

There are five major classes of hemoglobinopathies (Table 8-1). *Structural hemoglobinopathies* occur when mutations alter the amino acid sequence of a globin chain, altering the physiologic properties of the variant hemoglobins and producing the characteristic clinical abnormalities. The most clinically relevant variant hemoglobins polymerize abnormally, as in sickle cell anemia, or exhibit altered solubility or oxygen-binding affinity. *Thalassemia syndromes* arise from mutations

TABLE 8-1

CLASSIFICATION OF HEMOGLOBINOPATHIES

I. Structural hemoglobinopathies—hemoglobins with altered amino acid sequences that result in deranged function or altered physical or chemical properties
   A. Abnormal hemoglobin polymerization—HbS, hemoglobin sickling
   B. Altered O_2 affinity
      1. High affinity—polycythemia
      2. Low affinity—cyanosis, pseudoanemia
   C. Hemoglobins that oxidize readily
      1. Unstable hemoglobins—hemolytic anemia, jaundice
      2. M hemoglobins—methemoglobinemia, cyanosis
II Thalassemias—defective biosynthesis of globin chains
   A. α Thalassemias
   B. β Thalassemias
   C. δβ, γδβ, αβ Thalassemias
III. Thalassemic hemoglobin variants—structurally abnormal Hb associated with co-inherited thalassemic phenotype
   A. HbE
   B. Hb Constant Spring
   C. Hb Lepore
IV. Hereditary persistence of fetal hemoglobin—persistence of high levels of HbF into adult life
V. Acquired hemoglobinopathies
   A. Methemoglobin due to toxic exposures
   B. Sulfhemoglobin due to toxic exposures
   C. Carboxyhemoglobin
   D. HbH in erythroleukemia
   E. Elevated HbF in states of erythroid stress and bone marrow dysplasia

that impair production or translation of globin mRNA, leading to deficient globin chain biosynthesis. Clinical abnormalities are attributable to the inadequate supply of hemoglobin and the imbalances in the production of individual globin chains, leading to premature destruction of erythroblasts and RBC. *Thalassemic hemoglobin variants* combine features of thalassemia (e.g., abnormal globin biosynthesis) and of structural hemoglobinopathies (e.g., an abnormal amino acid sequence). *Hereditary persistence of fetal hemoglobin* (HPFH) is characterized by synthesis of high levels of fetal hemoglobin in adult life. *Acquired hemoglobinopathies* include modifications of the hemoglobin molecule by toxins (e.g., acquired methemoglobinemia) and clonal abnormalities of hemoglobin synthesis (e.g., high levels of HbF production in preleukemia and α thalassemia in myeloproliferative disorders).

EPIDEMIOLOGY

Hemoglobinopathies are especially common in areas in which malaria is endemic. This clustering of hemoglobinopathies is assumed to reflect a selective survival advantage for the abnormal RBC, which presumably provide a less hospitable environment during the obligate RBC stages of the parasitic life cycle. Very young children with α thalassemia are *more* susceptible to infection with the nonlethal *Plasmodium vivax*. Thalassemia might then favor a natural protection against infection with the more lethal *P. falciparum*.

Thalassemias are the most common genetic disorders in the world, affecting nearly 200 million people worldwide. About 15% of American blacks are silent carriers for α thalassemia; α-thalassemia trait (minor) occurs in 3% of American blacks and in 1–15% of persons of Mediterranean origin. β-Thalassemia has a 10–15% incidence in individuals from the Mediterranean and Southeast Asia and 0.8% in American blacks. The number of severe cases of thalassemia in the United States is about 1000. Sickle cell disease is the most common structural hemoglobinopathy, occurring in heterozygous form in ~8% of American blacks and in homozygous form in 1 in 400. Between 2 and 3% of American blacks carry a hemoglobin C allele.

INHERITANCE AND ONTOGENY

Hemoglobinopathies are autosomal codominant traits—compound heterozygotes who inherit a different abnormal mutant allele from each parent exhibit composite features of each. For example, patients inheriting sickle β thalassemia exhibit features of β thalassemia and sickle cell anemia. The α chain is present in HbA, HbA_2, and HbF; α-chain mutations thus cause abnormalities in all three. The α-globin hemoglobinopathies are symptomatic in utero and after birth because normal function of the α-globin gene is required throughout gestation and adult life. In contrast, infants with β-globin hemoglobinopathies tend to be asymptomatic until 3–9 months of age, when HbA has largely replaced HbF. Prevention or partial reversion of the switch should thus be an effective therapeutic strategy for β-chain hemoglobinopathies.

DETECTION AND CHARACTERIZATION OF HEMOGLOBINOPATHIES—GENERAL METHODS

Electrophoretic techniques are widely used for hemoglobin analysis. Electrophoresis at pH 8.6 on cellulose acetate membranes is especially simple, inexpensive, and reliable for initial screening. Agar gel electrophoresis at pH 6.1 in citrate buffer is often used as a complementary method because each method detects different variants. Some important variants are electrophoretically silent. These mutant hemoglobins can usually be characterized by more specialized techniques such as isoelectric focusing and/or high-pressure liquid chromatography (HPLC), which is rapidly replacing electrophoresis for initial analysis.

Quantitation of the hemoglobin profile is often desirable. HbA_2 is frequently elevated in β thalassemia trait and depressed in iron deficiency. HbF is elevated in HPFH, some β-thalassemia syndromes, and occasional periods of erythroid stress or marrow dysplasia. For characterization of sickle cell trait, sickle thalassemia syndromes, or HbSC disease, and for monitoring the progress of exchange transfusion therapy to lower the percentage of circulating HbS, quantitation of individual hemoglobins is also required. In most laboratories, quantitation is performed only if the test is specifically ordered. Complete characterization, including amino acid sequencing or gene cloning and sequencing, is readily available from several reference laboratories.

Because some variants can comigrate with HbA or HbS (sickle hemoglobin), electrophoretic assessment should always be regarded as incomplete unless functional assays for hemoglobin sickling, solubility, or oxygen affinity are also performed, as dictated by the clinical presentation. The best sickling assays involve measurement of the degree to which the hemoglobin sample becomes insoluble, or gelated, as it is deoxygenated (i.e., sickle solubility test). Unstable hemoglobins are detected by their precipitation in isopropanol or after heating to 50°C. High-O_2 affinity and low-O_2 affinity variants are detected by quantitating the P_{50}, the partial pressure of oxygen at which the hemoglobin sample becomes 50% saturated with oxygen. Direct tests for the percentage carboxyhemoglobin and methemoglobin, employing spectrophotometric techniques, can readily be obtained from most clinical laboratories on an urgent basis.

Laboratory evaluation remains an adjunct rather than the primary diagnostic aid. Diagnosis is best established by recognition of a characteristic history, physical findings, peripheral blood smear morphology, and abnormalities of the complete blood cell count (e.g., profound microcytosis with minimal anemia in thalassemia trait).

STRUCTURALLY ABNORMAL HEMOGLOBINS

SICKLE CELL SYNDROMES

The sickle cell syndromes are caused by a mutation in the β-globin gene that changes the sixth amino acid from glutamic acid to valine. HbS ($\alpha_2\beta_2^{6\ Glu\rightarrow Val}$) polymerizes reversibly when deoxygenated to form a gelatinous network of fibrous polymers that stiffen the RBC membrane, increase viscosity, and cause dehydration due to potassium leakage and calcium influx (Fig. 8-3). These changes also produce the sickle shape. Sickled cells lose the pliability needed to traverse small capillaries. They possess altered "sticky" membranes that are abnormally adherent to the endothelium of small venules. These abnormalities provoke unpredictable episodes of microvascular vasoocclusion and premature RBC destruction (hemolytic anemia). Hemolysis occurs because the spleen destroys the abnormal RBC. The rigid adherent cells clog small capillaries and venules, causing tissue ischemia, acute pain, and gradual end-organ damage. This venoocclusive component usually dominates the clinical course. Prominent manifestations include episodes of ischemic pain (i.e., painful crises) and ischemic malfunction or frank infarction in the spleen, central nervous system, bones, liver, kidneys, and lungs (Fig. 8-3).

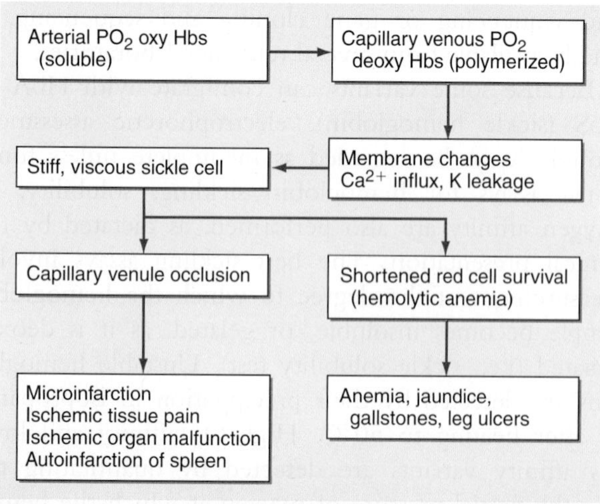

FIGURE 8-3
Pathophysiology of sickle cell crisis.

Several sickle syndromes occur as the result of inheritance of HbS from one parent and another hemoglobinopathy, such as β thalassemia or HbC ($\alpha_2\beta_2^{6\ Glu\rightarrow Lys}$), from the other parent. The prototype disease, sickle cell anemia, is the homozygous state for HbS (Table 8-2).

Clinical manifestations of sickle cell anemia

Most patients with sickling syndromes have hemolytic anemia, with hematocrits from 15 to 30%, and significant reticulocytosis. Anemia was once thought to exert protective effects against vasoocclusion by reducing blood viscosity. However, natural history and drug therapy trials suggest that an *increase* in the hematocrit and feedback inhibition of reticulocytosis might be beneficial, even at the expense of increased blood viscosity. The role of adhesive reticulocytes in vasoocclusion might account for these paradoxical effects.

Granulocytosis is common. The white count can fluctuate substantially and unpredictably during and between painful crises, infectious episodes, and other intercurrent illnesses.

Vasoocclusion causes protean manifestations. Intermittent episodes of vasoocclusion in connective and musculoskeletal structures produce ischemia manifested by acute pain and tenderness, fever, tachycardia, and anxiety. These recurrent episodes, called *painful crises*, are the most common clinical manifestation. Their frequency and severity vary greatly. Pain can develop almost anywhere in the body and may last from a few hours to 2 weeks. Repeated crises requiring hospitalization (>3 per year) correlate with reduced survival in adult life, suggesting that these episodes are associated with accumulation of chronic end-organ damage. Provocative factors include infection, fever, excessive exercise, anxiety, abrupt changes in temperature, hypoxia, and hypertonic dyes.

Repeated micro-infarction can destroy tissues having microvascular beds prone to sickling. Thus, the spleen is frequently lost within the first 18–36 months of life, causing susceptibility to infection, particularly by pneumococci. Acute venous obstruction of the spleen (*splenic sequestration crisis*), a rare occurrence in early childhood, may require emergency transfusion and/or splenectomy to prevent trapping of the entire arterial output in the obstructed spleen. Occlusion of retinal vessels can produce hemorrhage, neovascularization, and eventual detachments. Renal papillary necrosis invariably produces isosthenuria. More widespread renal necrosis leads to renal failure in adults, a common late cause of death. Bone and joint ischemia can lead to aseptic necrosis, especially of the femoral or humeral heads; chronic arthropathy; and unusual susceptibility to osteomyelitis,

TABLE 8-2

CLINICAL FEATURES OF SICKLE HEMOGLOBINOPATHIES

CONDITION	CLINICAL ABNORMALITIES	HEMOGLOBIN LEVEL g/L (g/dL)	MCV, fL	HEMOGLOBIN ELECTROPHORESIS
Sickle cell trait	None; rare painless hematuria	Normal	Normal	Hb S/A:40/60
Sickle cell anemia	Vasoocclusive crises with infarction of spleen, brain, marrow, kidney, lung; aseptic necrosis of bone; gallstones; priapism; ankle ulcers	70–100 (7–10)	80–100	Hb S/A:100/0 Hb F:2–25%
S/β° thalassemia	Vasoocclusive crises; aseptic necrosis of bone	70–100 (7–10)	60–80	Hb S/A:100/0 Hb F:1–10%
S/β$^+$ thalassemia	Rare crises and aseptic necrosis	100–140 (10–14)	70–80	Hb S/A:60/40
Hemoglobin SC	Rare crises and aseptic necrosis; painless hematuria	100–140 (10–14)	80–100	Hb S/A:50/0 Hb C:50%

which may be caused by organisms, such as *Salmonella*, rarely encountered in other settings. The *hand–foot syndrome* is caused by painful infarcts of the digits and dactylitis. Stroke is especially common in children; a small subset tend to experience repeated episodes. Stroke is less common in adults and is often hemorrhagic. A particularly painful complication in males is priapism, due to infarction of the penile venous outflow tracts; permanent impotence is a frequent consequence. Chronic lower leg ulcers probably arise from ischemia and superinfection in the distal circulation.

Acute chest syndrome is a distinctive manifestation characterized by chest pain, tachypnea, fever, cough, and arterial oxygen desaturation. It can mimic pneumonia, pulmonary emboli, bone marrow infarction and embolism, myocardial ischemia, or in situ lung infarction. Acute chest syndrome is thought to reflect in situ sickling within the lung, producing pain and temporary pulmonary dysfunction. Often it is difficult or impossible to distinguish among other possibilities. Pulmonary infarction and pneumonia are the most frequent underlying or concomitant conditions in patients with this syndrome. Repeated episodes of acute chest pain correlate with reduced survival. Acutely, reduction in arterial oxygen saturation is especially ominous because it promotes sickling on a massive scale. Chronic acute or subacute pulmonary crises lead to pulmonary hypertension and cor pulmonale, an increasingly common cause of death as patients survive longer. Considerable controversy exists about the possible role played by free plasma HbS in scavenging NO_2, thus raising pulmonary vascular tone. Trials of sildenafil to restore NO_2 levels were terminated because of adverse effects.

Sickle cell syndromes are remarkable for their clinical heterogeneity. Some patients remain virtually asymptomatic into or even through adult life, while others have repeated crises requiring hospitalization from early childhood. Patients with sickle thalassemia and sickle-HbE tend to have similar, slightly milder, symptoms, perhaps because of the ameliorating effects of production of other hemoglobins within the RBC. Hemoglobin SC disease, one of the more common variants of sickle cell anemia, is frequently marked by lesser degrees of hemolytic anemia and a greater propensity for the development of retinopathy and aseptic necrosis of bones. In most respects, however, the clinical manifestations resemble sickle cell anemia. Some rare hemoglobin variants actually aggravate the sickling phenomenon.

The clinical variability in different patients inheriting the same disease-causing mutation (sickle hemoglobin) has made sickle cell disease the focus of efforts to identify modifying genetic polymorphisms in other genes that might account for the heterogeneity. The complexity of the data obtained thus far has dampened the expectation that genomewide analysis will yield individualized profiles that predict a patient's clinical course. Nevertheless, a number of interesting patterns have emerged from these modifying gene analyses. For example, genes affecting the inflammatory response or cytokine expression appear to be modifying candidates. Genes that affect transcriptional regulation of lymphocytes may be involved. Thus, it appears likely that key polymorphic changes in the patient's inflammatory response to the damages provoked by sickle red cells or in the response to chronic or recurrent infections may prove to be important for prognosticating the clinical severity of disease.

Clinical manifestations of sickle cell trait

Sickle cell trait is usually asymptomatic. Anemia and painful crises are rare. An uncommon but highly distinctive symptom is painless hematuria often occurring in adolescent males, probably due to papillary necrosis. Isosthenuria is a more common manifestation of the same process. Sloughing of papillae with urethral obstruction has been reported, as have isolated cases of massive sickling or sudden death due to exposure to high altitudes or extremes of exercise and dehydration. Avoidance of dehydration and extreme physical stress should be advised.

Diagnosis

Sickle cell syndromes are suspected on the basis of hemolytic anemia, RBC morphology (Fig. 8-4), and intermittent episodes of ischemic pain. Diagnosis is confirmed by hemoglobin electrophoresis and the sickling tests already discussed. Thorough characterization of the exact hemoglobin profile of the patient is important because sickle thalassemia and hemoglobin SC disease have distinct prognoses and clinical features. Diagnosis is usually established in childhood, but occasional patients, often with compound heterozygous states, do not develop symptoms until the onset of puberty, pregnancy, or early adult life. Genotyping of family members and potential parental partners is critical for genetic counseling. Details of the childhood history establish prognosis and need for aggressive or experimental therapies. Factors associated with increased morbidity and reduced survival are more than three crises requiring hospitalization per year, chronic neutrophilia, a history of splenic sequestration or hand–foot syndrome, and second episodes of acute chest syndrome. Patients with a history of cerebrovascular accidents are at higher risk for repeated episodes and require partial exchange transfusion and especially close monitoring using Doppler carotid flow measurements. Patients with severe or repeated episodes of acute chest syndrome may need lifelong transfusion support, utilizing partial exchange transfusion, if possible.

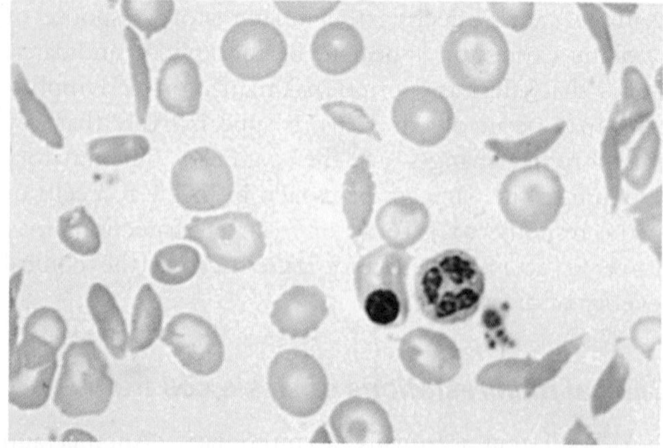

FIGURE 8-4
Sickle cell anemia. The elongated and crescent-shaped red blood cells seen on this smear represent circulating irreversibly sickled cells. Target cells and a nucleated red blood cell are also seen.

TREATMENT Sickle Cell Syndromes

Patients with sickle cell syndromes require ongoing continuity of care. Familiarity with the pattern of symptoms provides the best safeguard against excessive use of the emergency department, hospitalization, and habituation to addictive narcotics. Additional preventive measures include regular slit-lamp examinations to monitor development of retinopathy; antibiotic prophylaxis appropriate for splenectomized patients during dental or other invasive procedures; and vigorous oral hydration during or in anticipation of periods of extreme exercise, exposure to heat or cold, emotional stress, or infection. Pneumococcal and *Haemophilus influenzae* vaccines are less effective in splenectomized individuals. Thus, patients with sickle cell anemia should be vaccinated early in life.

The management of acute painful crisis includes vigorous hydration, thorough evaluation for underlying causes (e.g., infection), and aggressive analgesia administered by a standing order and/or patient-controlled analgesia (PCA) pump. Morphine (0.1–0.15 mg/kg every 3–4 h) should be used to control severe pain. Bone pain may respond as well to ketorolac (30–60 mg initial dose, then 15–30 mg every 6–8 h). Inhalation of nitrous oxide can provide short-term pain relief, but great care must be exercised to avoid hypoxia and respiratory depression. Nitrous oxide also elevates O_2 affinity, reducing O_2 delivery to tissues. Its use should be restricted to experts. Many crises can be managed at home with oral hydration and oral analgesia. Use of the emergency department should be reserved for especially severe symptoms or circumstances in which other processes, e.g., infection, are strongly suspected. Nasal oxygen should be employed as appropriate to protect arterial saturation. Most crises resolve in 1–7 days. Use of blood transfusion should be reserved for extreme cases: transfusions do not shorten the duration of the crisis.

No tests are definitive to diagnose acute painful crises. Critical to good management is an approach that recognizes that most patients reporting crisis symptoms do indeed have crisis or another significant medical problem. Diligent diagnostic evaluation for underlying causes is imperative, even though these are found infrequently. In adults, the possibility of aseptic necrosis or sickle arthropathy must be considered, especially if pain and immobility become repeated or chronic at a single site. Nonsteroidal anti-inflammatory agents are often effective for sickle cell arthropathy.

Acute chest syndrome is a medical emergency that may require management in an intensive care unit. Hydration should be monitored carefully to avoid the development of pulmonary edema, and oxygen therapy should be especially vigorous for protection of arterial saturation. Diagnostic evaluation for pneumonia and pulmonary embolism should be especially thorough, since these may occur with atypical symptoms. Critical interventions are transfusion to maintain a hematocrit >30, and emergency exchange transfusion if arterial saturation drops to <90%. As patients with sickle cell syndrome increasingly survive into their fifth and sixth decades, end-stage renal failure and pulmonary hypertension are becoming increasingly prominent causes of end-stage morbidity. A sickle cell cardiomyopathy and/or premature coronary artery disease may compromise cardiac function in later years. Sickle cell patients have received kidney transplants, but they often experience an increase in the frequency and severity of crises, possibly due to increased infection as a consequence of immunosuppression.

The most significant advance in the therapy of sickle cell anemia has been the introduction of hydroxyurea as a mainstay of therapy for patients with severe symptoms. Hydroxyurea (10–30 mg/kg per day) increases fetal hemoglobin and may also exert beneficial affects on RBC hydration, vascular wall adherence, and suppression of the granulocyte and reticulocyte counts; dosage is titrated to maintain a white cell count between 5000 and 8000 per μL. White cells and reticulocytes may play a major role in the pathogenesis of sickle cell crisis, and their suppression may be an important benefit of hydroxyurea therapy.

Hydroxyurea should be considered in patients experiencing repeated episodes of acute chest syndrome or with more than three crises per year requiring hospitalization. The utility of this agent for reducing the incidence of other complications (priapism, retinopathy) is under evaluation, as are the long-term side effects. Hydroxyurea offers broad benefits to most patients whose disease is severe enough to impair their functional status, and it may improve survival. HbF levels increase in most patients within a few months.

The antitumor drug 5-azacytidine was the first agent found to elevate HbF. It never achieved widespread use because of concerns about acute toxicity and carcinogenesis. However, low doses of the related agent 5-deoxyazacytidine (decitabine) can elevate HbF with more acceptable toxicity.

Bone marrow transplantation can provide definitive cures but is known to be effective and safe only in children. Partially myeloablative conditioning regimens ("mini" transplants) may allow more widespread use of this modality. Prognostic features justifying bone marrow transplant are the presence of repeated crises early in life, a high neutrophil count, or the development of hand–foot syndrome. Children at risk for stroke can now be identified through the use of Doppler ultrasound techniques. Prophylactic exchange transfusion appears to substantially reduce the risk of stroke in this population. Children who do suffer a cerebrovascular accident should be maintained for at least 3–5 years on a program of vigorous exchange transfusion, as the risk of second strokes is extremely high.

Gene therapy for sickle cell anemia is being intensively pursued, but no safe measures are currently available. Agents blocking RBC dehydration or vascular adhesion, such as clotrimazole or magnesium, may have value as an adjunct to hydroxyurea therapy, pending the completion of ongoing trials. Combinations of clotrimazole and magnesium are being evaluated.

UNSTABLE HEMOGLOBINS

Amino acid substitutions that reduce solubility or increase susceptibility to oxidation produce unstable hemoglobins that precipitate, forming inclusion bodies injurious to the RBC membrane. Representative mutations are those that interfere with contact points between the α and β subunits (e.g., Hb Philly [$\beta^{35Tyr\rightarrow Phe}$]), alter the helical segments (e.g., Hb Genova [$\beta^{28Leu\rightarrow Pro}$]), or disrupt interactions of the hydrophobic pockets of the globin subunits with heme (e.g., Hb Koln [$\beta^{98Val\rightarrow Met}$]) (Table 8-3). The inclusions, called *Heinz bodies*, are clinically detectable by staining with supravital dyes such as crystal violet. Removal of these inclusions by the spleen generates pitted, rigid cells that have shortened life spans, producing hemolytic anemia of variable severity, sometimes requiring chronic transfusion

TABLE 8-3

REPRESENTATIVE ABNORMAL HEMOGLOBINS WITH ALTERED SYNTHESIS OR FUNCTION

DESIGNATION	MUTATION	POPULATION	MAIN CLINICAL EFFECTS[a]
Sickle or S	$\beta^{6Glu\rightarrow Val}$	African	Anemia, ischemic infarcts
C	$\beta^{6Glu\rightarrow Lys}$	African	Mild anemia; interacts with HbS
E	$\beta^{26Glu\rightarrow Lys}$	Southeast Asian	Microcytic anemia, splenomegaly, thalassemic phenotype
Köln	$\beta^{98Val\rightarrow Met}$	Sporadic	Hemolytic anemia, Heinz bodies when splenectomized
Yakima	$\beta^{99Asp\rightarrow His}$	Sporadic	Polycythemia
Kansas	$\beta^{102Asn\rightarrow Lys}$	Sporadic	Mild anemia
M. Iwata	$\alpha^{87His\rightarrow Tyr}$	Sporadic	Methemoglobinemia

[a]See text for details.

support. Splenectomy may be needed to correct the anemia. Leg ulcers and premature gallbladder disease due to bilirubin loading are frequent stigmata.

Unstable hemoglobins occur sporadically, often by spontaneous new mutations. Heterozygotes are often symptomatic because a significant Heinz body burden can develop even when the unstable variant accounts for only a portion of the total hemoglobin. Symptomatic unstable hemoglobins tend to be β-globin variants because sporadic mutations affecting only one of the four α globins would generate only 20–30% abnormal hemoglobin.

HEMOGLOBINS WITH ALTERED OXYGEN AFFINITY

High-affinity hemoglobins (e.g., Hb Yakima [$\beta^{99Asp \rightarrow His}$]) bind oxygen more readily but deliver less O_2 to tissues at normal capillary PO_2 levels (Fig. 8-2). Mild tissue hypoxia ensues, stimulating RBC production and erythrocytosis (Table 8-3). In extreme cases, the hematocrits can rise to 60–65%, increasing blood viscosity and producing typical symptoms (headache, somnolence, or dizziness). Phlebotomy may be required. Typical mutations alter interactions within the heme pocket or disrupt the Bohr effect or salt-bond site. Mutations that impair the interaction of HbA with 2,3-BPG can increase O_2 affinity because 2,3-BPG binding lowers O_2 affinity.

Low-affinity hemoglobins (e.g., Hb Kansas [$\beta^{102Asn \rightarrow Lys}$]) bind sufficient oxygen in the lungs, despite their lower oxygen affinity, to achieve nearly full saturation. At capillary oxygen tensions, they lose sufficient amounts of oxygen to maintain homeostasis at a low hematocrit (Fig. 8-2) (*pseudoanemia*). Capillary hemoglobin desaturation can also be sufficient to produce clinically apparent cyanosis. Despite these findings, patients usually require no specific treatment.

METHEMOGLOBINEMIAS

Methemoglobin is generated by oxidation of the heme iron moieties to the ferric state, causing a characteristic bluish-brown muddy color resembling cyanosis. Methemoglobin has such high oxygen affinity that virtually no oxygen is delivered. Levels >50–60% are often fatal.

Congenital methemoglobinemia arises from globin mutations that stabilize iron in the ferric state (e.g., HbM Iwata [$\alpha^{87His \rightarrow Tyr}$], Table 8-3) or from mutations that impair the enzymes that reduce methemoglobin to hemoglobin (e.g., methemoglobin reductase, NADP diaphorase). Acquired methemoglobinemia is caused by toxins that oxidize heme iron, notably nitrate and nitrite-containing compounds, including drugs commonly used in cardiology and anesthesiology.

DIAGNOSIS AND MANAGEMENT OF PATIENTS WITH UNSTABLE HEMOGLOBINS, HIGH-AFFINITY HEMOGLOBINS, AND METHEMOGLOBINEMIA

Unstable hemoglobin variants should be suspected in patients with nonimmune hemolytic anemia, jaundice, splenomegaly, or premature biliary tract disease. Severe hemolysis usually presents during infancy as neonatal jaundice or anemia. Milder cases may present in adult life with anemia or only as unexplained reticulocytosis, hepatosplenomegaly, premature biliary tract disease, or leg ulcers. Because spontaneous mutation is common, family history of anemia may be absent. The peripheral blood smear often shows anisocytosis, abundant cells with punctate inclusions, and irregular shapes (i.e., poikilocytosis).

The two best tests for diagnosing unstable hemoglobins are the Heinz body preparation and the isopropanol or heat stability test. Many unstable Hb variants are electrophoretically silent. A normal electrophoresis does not rule out the diagnosis.

Severely affected patients may require transfusion support for the first 3 years of life because splenectomy before age 3 years is associated with a significantly higher immune deficit. Splenectomy is usually effective thereafter, but occasional patients may require lifelong transfusion support. After splenectomy, patients can develop cholelithiasis and leg ulcers, hypercoagulable states, and susceptibility to overwhelming sepsis. Splenectomy should be avoided or delayed unless it is the only alternative. Precipitation of unstable hemoglobins is aggravated by oxidative stress, e.g., infection and antimalarial drugs, which should be avoided when possible.

High-O_2 affinity hemoglobin variants should be suspected in patients with erythrocytosis. The best test for confirmation is measurement of the P_{50}. A high-O_2 affinity Hb causes a significant left shift (i.e., lower numeric value of the P_{50}); confounding conditions, e.g., tobacco smoking or carbon monoxide exposure, can also lower the P_{50}.

High-affinity hemoglobins are often asymptomatic; rubor or plethora may be telltale signs. When the hematocrit reaches to 55–60%, symptoms of high blood viscosity and sluggish flow (e.g., headache, lethargy, dizziness) may be present. These persons may benefit from judicious phlebotomy. Erythrocytosis represents an appropriate attempt to compensate for the impaired oxygen delivery by the abnormal variant. Overzealous phlebotomy may stimulate increased erythropoiesis or aggravate symptoms by thwarting this compensatory mechanism. The guiding principle of phlebotomy should be to improve oxygen delivery by reducing blood viscosity and increasing blood flow rather than restoration of a normal hematocrit. Modest iron deficiency may aid in control.

Low-affinity hemoglobins should be considered in patients with cyanosis or a low hematocrit with no other reason apparent after thorough evaluation. The P_{50} test confirms the diagnosis. Counseling and reassurance are the interventions of choice.

Methemoglobin should be suspected in patients with hypoxic symptoms who appear cyanotic but have a PaO_2 sufficiently high that hemoglobin should be fully saturated with oxygen. A history of nitrite or other oxidant ingestions may not always be available; some exposures may be inapparent to the patient, and others may result from suicide attempts. The characteristic muddy appearance of freshly drawn blood can be a critical clue. The best diagnostic test is methemoglobin assay, which is usually available on an emergency basis.

Methemoglobinemia often causes symptoms of cerebral ischemia at levels >15%; levels >60% are usually lethal. Intravenous injection of 1 mg/kg of methylene blue is effective emergency therapy. Milder cases and follow-up of severe cases can be treated orally with methylene blue (60 mg three to four times each day) or ascorbic acid (300–600 mg/d).

THALASSEMIA SYNDROMES

The thalassemia syndromes are inherited disorders of α- or β-globin biosynthesis. The reduced supply of globin diminishes production of hemoglobin tetramers, causing hypochromia and microcytosis. Unbalanced accumulation of α and β subunits occurs because the synthesis of the unaffected globins proceeds at a normal rate. Unbalanced chain accumulation dominates the clinical phenotype. Clinical severity varies widely, depending on the degree to which the synthesis of the affected globin is impaired, altered synthesis of other globin chains, and coinheritance of other abnormal globin alleles.

CLINICAL MANIFESTATIONS OF β-THALASSEMIA SYNDROMES

Mutations causing thalassemia can affect any step in the pathway of globin gene expression: transcription, processing of the mRNA precursor, translation, and post-translational metabolism of the β-globin polypeptide chain. The most common forms arise from mutations that derange splicing of the mRNA precursor or prematurely terminate translation of the mRNA.

Hypochromia and microcytosis characterize all forms of β thalassemia because of the reduced amounts of hemoglobin tetramers (Fig. 8-5). In heterozygotes (β-thalassemia trait), this is the only abnormality seen. Anemia is minimal. In more severe homozygous states, unbalanced α- and β-globin accumulation causes accumulation of highly insoluble unpaired α chains. They

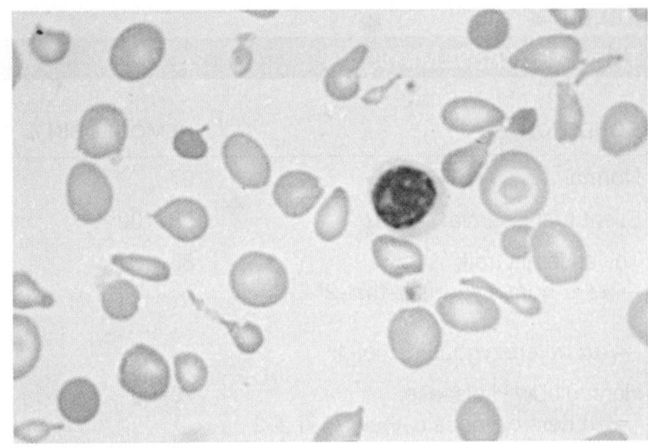

FIGURE 8-5
β-Thalassemia intermedia. Microcytic and hypochromic red blood cells are seen that resemble the red blood cells of severe iron deficiency anemia. Many elliptical and teardrop-shaped red blood cells are noted.

form toxic inclusion bodies that kill developing erythroblasts in the marrow. Few of the proerythroblasts beginning erythroid maturation survive. The surviving RBCs bear a burden of inclusion bodies that are detected in the spleen, shortening the RBC life span and producing severe hemolytic anemia. The resulting profound anemia stimulates erythropoietin release and compensatory erythroid hyperplasia, but the marrow response is sabotaged by the ineffective erythropoiesis. Anemia persists. Erythroid hyperplasia can become exuberant and produce masses of extramedullary erythropoietic tissue in the liver and spleen.

Massive bone marrow expansion deranges growth and development. Children develop characteristic "chipmunk" facies due to maxillary marrow hyperplasia and frontal bossing. Thinning and pathologic fracture of long bones and vertebrae may occur due to cortical invasion by erythroid elements and profound growth retardation. Hemolytic anemia causes hepatosplenomegaly, leg ulcers, gallstones, and high-output congestive heart failure. The conscription of caloric resources to support erythropoiesis leads to inanition; susceptibility to infection; endocrine dysfunction; and in the most severe cases, death during the first decade of life. Chronic transfusions with RBCs improve oxygen delivery, suppress the excessive ineffective erythropoiesis, and prolong life, but the inevitable side effects, notably iron overload, usually prove fatal by age 30 years.

Severity is highly variable. Known modulating factors are those that ameliorate the burden of unpaired α-globin inclusions. Alleles associated with milder synthetic defects and coinheritance of α-thalassemia trait reduce clinical severity by reducing accumulation of excess α globin. HbF persists to various degrees in β thalassemias. γ-Globin gene chains can substitute for

TABLE 8-4

THE α THALASSEMIAS

CONDITION	HEMOGLOBIN A, %	HEMOGLOBIN H (β^4), %	HEMOGLOBIN LEVEL, g/L (g/dL)	MCV, fL
Normal	97	0	150 (15)	90
Silent thalassemia: –α/αα	98–100	0	150 (15)	90
Thalassemia trait: —α/–α homozygous α-thal-2[a] or —/αα heterozygous α-thal-1[a]	85–95	Rare red blood cell inclusions	120–130 (12–13)	70–80
Hemoglobin H disease: —/–α heterozygous α-thal-1/α-thal-2	70–95	5–30	60–100 (6–10)	60–70
Hydrops fetalis: —/– homozygous α-thal-1	0	5–10[b]	Fatal in utero or at birth	

[a]When both α alleles on one chromosome are deleted, the locus is called α-thal-1; when only a single α allele on one chromosome is deleted, the locus is called α-thal-2.
[b]90–95% of the hemoglobin is hemoglobin Barts (tetramers of γ chains).

β chains, generating more hemoglobin and reducing the burden of α-globin inclusions. The terms *β-thalassemia major* and *β-thalassemia intermedia* are used to reflect the clinical heterogeneity. Patients with β-thalassemia major require intensive transfusion support to survive. Patients with β-thalassemia intermedia have a somewhat milder phenotype and can survive without transfusion. The terms *β-thalassemia minor* and *β-thalassemia trait* describe asymptomatic heterozygotes for β thalassemia.

THALASSEMIA SYNDROMES

The four classic α thalassemias, most common in Asians, are α-thalassemia-2 trait, in which one of the four α-globin loci is deleted; α-thalassemia-1 trait, with two deleted loci; HbH disease, with three loci deleted; and hydrops fetalis with Hb Barts, with all four loci deleted (Table 8-4). Nondeletion forms of α thalassemia also exist.

α-Thalassemia-2 trait is an asymptomatic, silent carrier state. *α-Thalassemia-1 trait* resembles β-thalassemia minor. Offspring doubly heterozygous for α-thalassemia-2 and α-thalassemia-1 exhibit a more severe phenotype called *HbH disease*. Heterozygosity for a deletion that removes both genes from the same chromosome (*cis* deletion) is common in Asians and in those from the Mediterranean region, as is homozygosity for α-thalassemia-2 (*trans* deletion). Both produce asymptomatic hypochromia and microcytosis.

In *HbH disease*, HbA production is only 25–30% normal. Fetuses accumulate some unpaired γ chains (Hb Barts; γ-chain tetramers). In adults, unpaired β chains accumulate and are soluble enough to form β_4 tetramers called HbH. HbH forms few inclusions in erythroblasts and precipitates in circulating RBC. Patients with HbH disease have thalassemia intermedia characterized by moderately severe hemolytic anemia but milder ineffective erythropoiesis. Survival into midadult life without transfusions is common.

The homozygous state for the α-thalassemia-1 *cis* deletion (hydrops fetalis) causes total absence of α-globin synthesis. No physiologically useful hemoglobin is produced beyond the embryonic stage. Excess γ globin forms tetramers called *Hb Barts* (γ_4), which has a very high oxygen affinity. It delivers almost no O_2 to fetal tissues, causing tissue asphyxia, edema (hydrops fetalis), congestive heart failure, and death in utero. α-Thalassemia-2 trait is common (15–20%) among people of African descent. The *cis* α-thalassemia-1 deletion is almost never seen, however. Thus, α-thalassemia-2 and the *trans* form of α-thalassemia-1 are very common, but HbH disease and hydrops fetalis are rare.

It has been known for some time that some patients with myelodysplasia or erythroleukemia produce RBC clones containing HbH. This phenomenon is due to mutations in the ATRX pathway that affect the LCR of the α-globin gene cluster.

DIAGNOSIS AND MANAGEMENT OF THALASSEMIAS

The diagnosis of β-thalassemia major is readily made during childhood on the basis of severe anemia accompanied by the characteristic signs of massive ineffective erythropoiesis: hepatosplenomegaly; profound microcytosis; a characteristic blood smear (Fig. 8-5); and elevated levels of HbF, HbA_2, or both. Many patients require chronic hypertransfusion therapy designed to maintain a hematocrit of at least 27–30% so that erythropoiesis is suppressed. Splenectomy is required if the annual transfusion requirement (volume of RBCs per kilogram of body weight per year) increases by >50%.

Folic acid supplements may be useful. Vaccination with Pneumovax in anticipation of eventual splenectomy is advised, as is close monitoring for infection, leg ulcers, and biliary tract disease. Many patients develop endocrine deficiencies as a result of iron overload. Early endocrine evaluation is required for glucose intolerance, thyroid dysfunction, and delayed onset of puberty or secondary sexual characteristics.

Patients with β-thalassemia intermedia exhibit similar stigmata but can survive without chronic hypertransfusion. Management is particularly challenging because a number of factors can aggravate the anemia, including infection, onset of puberty, and development of splenomegaly and hypersplenism. Some patients may eventually benefit from splenectomy. The expanded erythron can cause absorption of excessive dietary iron and hemosiderosis, even without transfusion.

β-Thalassemia minor (i.e., thalassemia trait) usually presents as profound microcytosis and hypochromia with target cells but only minimal or mild anemia. The mean corpuscular volume is rarely >75 fL; the hematocrit is rarely <30–33%. Hemoglobin analysis classically reveals an elevated HbA_2 (3.5–7.5%), but some forms are associated with normal HbA_2 and/or elevated HbF. Genetic counseling and patient education are essential. Patients with β-thalassemia trait should be warned that their blood picture resembles iron deficiency and can be misdiagnosed. They should eschew empirical use of iron, yet iron deficiency can develop during pregnancy or from chronic bleeding.

Persons with α-thalassemia trait may exhibit mild hypochromia and microcytosis usually without anemia. HbA_2 and HbF levels are normal. Affected individuals usually require only genetic counseling. HbH disease resembles β-thalassemia intermedia, with the added complication that the HbH molecule behaves like moderately unstable hemoglobin. Patients with HbH disease should undergo splenectomy if excessive anemia or a transfusion requirement develops. Oxidative drugs should be avoided. Iron overload leading to death can occur in more severely affected patients.

PREVENTION

Antenatal diagnosis of thalassemia syndromes is now widely available. DNA diagnosis is based on polymerase chain reaction amplification of fetal DNA, obtained by amniocentesis or chorionic villus biopsy followed by hybridization to allele-specific oligonucleotides probes or direct DNA sequencing.

THALASSEMIC STRUCTURAL VARIANTS

Thalassemic structural variants are characterized by both defective synthesis and abnormal structure.

HEMOGLOBIN LEPORE

Hb Lepore ($\alpha_2[\delta\beta]_2$) arises by an unequal crossover and recombination event that fuses the proximal end of the δ-gene with the distal end of the closely linked β-gene. It is common in the Mediterranean basin. The resulting chromosome contains only the fused δβ gene. The Lepore (δβ) globin is synthesized poorly because the fused gene is under the control of the weak δ-globin promoter. Hb Lepore alleles have a phenotype like β thalassemia, except for the added presence of 2–20% Hb Lepore. Compound heterozygotes for Hb Lepore and a classic β-thalassemia allele may also have severe thalassemia.

HEMOGLOBIN E

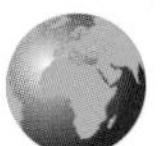

HbE (i.e., $\alpha_2\beta_2^{26Glu\rightarrow Lys}$) is extremely common in Cambodia, Thailand, and Vietnam. The gene has become far more prevalent in the United States as a result of immigration of Asian persons, especially in California, where HbE is the most common variant detected. HbE is mildly unstable but not enough to affect RBC life span significantly. Heterozygotes resemble individuals with a mild β-thalassemia trait. Homozygotes have somewhat more marked abnormalities but are asymptomatic. Compound heterozygotes for HbE and a β-thalassemia gene can have β-thalassemia intermedia or β-thalassemia major, depending on the severity of the coinherited thalassemic gene.

The β^E allele contains a single base change in codon 26 that causes the amino acid substitution. However, this mutation activates a cryptic RNA splice site, generating a structurally abnormal globin mRNA that cannot be translated from about 50% of the initial pre-mRNA molecules. The remaining 40–50% are normally spliced and generate functional mRNA that is translated into β^E-globin because the mature mRNA carries the base change that alters codon 26.

Genetic counseling of the persons at risk for HbE should focus on the interaction of HbE with β thalassemia rather than HbE homozygosity, a condition associated with asymptomatic microcytosis, hypochromia, and hemoglobin levels rarely <100 g/L (<10 g/dL).

HEREDITARY PERSISTENCE OF FETAL HEMOGLOBIN

HPFH is characterized by continued synthesis of high levels of HbF in adult life. No deleterious effects are apparent, even when all of the hemoglobin produced is HbF. These rare patients demonstrate convincingly that prevention or reversal of the fetal to adult hemoglobin switch would provide effective therapy for sickle cell anemia and β thalassemia.

ACQUIRED HEMOGLOBINOPATHIES

The two most important acquired hemoglobinopathies are carbon monoxide poisoning and methemoglobinemia (discussed earlier). Carbon monoxide has a higher affinity for hemoglobin than does oxygen; it can replace oxygen and diminish O_2 delivery. Chronic elevation of carboxyhemoglobin levels to 10 or 15%, as occurs in smokers, can lead to secondary polycythemia. Carboxyhemoglobin is cherry red in color and masks the development of cyanosis usually associated with poor O_2 delivery to tissues.

Abnormalities of hemoglobin biosynthesis have also been described in blood dyscrasias. In some patients with myelodysplasia, erythroleukemia, or myeloproliferative disorders, elevated HbF or a mild form of HbH disease may also be seen. The abnormalities are not severe enough to alter the course of the underlying disease.

TREATMENT Transfusional Hemosiderosis

Chronic blood transfusion can lead to bloodborne infection, alloimmunization, febrile reactions, and lethal iron overload (Chap. 12). A unit of packed RBCs contains 250–300 mg iron (1 mg/mL). The iron assimilated by a single transfusion of two units of packed RBCs is thus equal to a 1- to 2-year intake of iron. Iron accumulates in chronically transfused patients because no mechanisms exist for increasing iron excretion: an expanded erythron causes especially rapid development of iron overload because accelerated erythropoiesis promotes excessive absorption of dietary iron. Vitamin C should not be supplemented because it generates free radicals in iron excess states.

Patients who receive >100 units of packed RBCs usually develop hemosiderosis. The ferritin level rises, followed by early endocrine dysfunction (glucose intolerance and delayed puberty), cirrhosis, and cardiomyopathy. Liver biopsy shows both parenchymal and reticuloendothelial iron. The superconducting quantum-interference device (SQUID) is accurate at measuring hepatic iron but is not widely available. Cardiac toxicity is often insidious. Early development of pericarditis is followed by dysrhythmia and pump failure. The onset of heart failure is ominous, often presaging death within a year.

The decision to start long-term transfusion support should also prompt one to institute therapy with iron-chelating agents. Desferoxamine (Desferal) is for parenteral use. Its iron-binding kinetics require chronic slow infusion via a metering pump. The constant presence of the drug improves the efficiency of chelation and protects tissues from occasional releases of the most toxic fraction of iron—low-molecular-weight iron—which may not be sequestered by protective proteins.

Desferoxamine is relatively nontoxic. Occasional cataracts; deafness; and local skin reactions, including urticaria, occur. Skin reactions can usually be managed with antihistamines. Negative iron balance can be achieved, even in the face of a high transfusion requirement, but this alone does not prevent long-term morbidity and mortality in chronically transfused patients. Irreversible end-organ deterioration develops at relatively modest levels of iron overload, even if symptoms do not appear for many years thereafter. To enjoy a significant survival advantage, chelation must begin before 5–8 years of age in β-thalassemia major.

Deferasirox is an oral iron-chelating agent. Single daily doses of 20 to 30 mg/kg deferasirox produced reductions in liver iron concentration comparable to desferoxamine in long-term transfused adult and pediatric patients. Deferasirox produces some elevations in liver enzymes and slight but persistent increases in serum creatinine without apparent clinical consequence. Other toxicities are similar to those of desferoxamine. Its toxicity profile is acceptable, although long-term effects are still being evaluated.

EXPERIMENTAL THERAPIES

BONE MARROW TRANSPLANTATION, GENE THERAPY, AND MANIPULATION OF HBF

Bone marrow transplantation provides stem cells able to express normal hemoglobin; it has been used in a large number of patients with β thalassemia and a smaller number of patients with sickle cell anemia. Early in the course of disease, before end-organ damage occurs, transplantation is curative in 80–90% of patients. In highly experienced centers, the treatment-related mortality rate is <10%. Since survival into adult life is possible with conventional therapy, the decision to transplant is best made in consultation with specialized centers.

Gene therapy of thalassemia and sickle cell disease has proved to be an elusive goal. Uptake of gene vectors into the nondividing hematopoietic stem cells has been inefficient. Lentiviral-type vectors that can transduce nondividing cells may solve this problem.

Reestablishing high levels of fetal hemoglobin synthesis should ameliorate the symptoms of β chain hemoglobinopathies. Cytotoxic agents such as hydroxyurea and cytarabine promote high levels of HbF synthesis, probably by stimulating proliferation of the primitive HbF-producing progenitor cell population (i.e., F cell progenitors). Unfortunately, this regimen has not yet been effective in β thalassemia. Butyrates stimulate HbF production but only transiently. Pulsed or intermittent administration has been found to sustain HbF induction in the majority of patients with sickle cell disease. It is unclear whether butyrates will have similar activity in patients with β thalassemia.

APLASTIC AND HYPOPLASTIC CRISIS IN PATIENTS WITH HEMOGLOBINOPATHIES

Patients with hemolytic anemias sometimes exhibit an alarming decline in hematocrit during and immediately after acute illnesses. Bone marrow suppression occurs in almost everyone during acute inflammatory illnesses. In patients with short RBC life spans, suppression can affect RBC counts more dramatically. These hypoplastic crises are usually transient and self-correcting before intervention is required.

Aplastic crisis refers to a profound cessation of erythroid activity in patients with chronic hemolytic anemias. It is associated with a rapidly falling hematocrit. Episodes are usually self-limited. Aplastic crises are caused by infection with a particular strain of parvovirus, B19A. Children infected with this virus usually develop permanent immunity. Aplastic crises do not often recur and are rarely seen in adults. Management requires close monitoring of the hematocrit and reticulocyte count. If anemia becomes symptomatic, transfusion support is indicated. Most crises resolve spontaneously within 1–2 weeks.

CHAPTER 9

MEGALOBLASTIC ANEMIAS

A. Victor Hoffbrand

The megaloblastic anemias are a group of disorders characterized by the presence of distinctive morphologic appearances of the developing red cells in the bone marrow. The marrow is usually cellular, and the anemia is based on ineffective erythropoiesis. The cause is usually a deficiency of either cobalamin (vitamin B_{12}) or folate, but megaloblastic anemia may occur because of genetic or acquired abnormalities that affect the metabolism of these vitamins or because of defects in DNA synthesis not related to cobalamin or folate (Table 9-1). Cobalamin and folate absorption and metabolism are described next, followed by the biochemical basis, clinical and laboratory features, causes, and treatment of megaloblastic anemia.

COBALAMIN

Cobalamin (vitamin B_{12}) exists in a number of different chemical forms. All have a cobalt atom at the center of a corrin ring. In nature, the vitamin is mainly in the 2-deoxyadenosyl (ado) form, which is located in mitochondria. It is the cofactor for the enzyme methylmalonyl coenzyme A (CoA) mutase. The other major natural cobalamin is methylcobalamin, the form in human plasma and in cell cytoplasm. It is the cofactor for methionine synthase. There are also minor amounts of hydroxocobalamin to which methyl- and adocobalamin are converted rapidly by exposure to light.

Dietary sources and requirements

Cobalamin is synthesized solely by microorganisms. Ruminants obtain cobalamin from the foregut, but the only source for humans is food of animal origin, e.g., meat, fish, and dairy products. Vegetables, fruits, and other foods of nonanimal origin are free from cobalamin unless they are contaminated by bacteria. A normal Western diet contains 5–30 μg of cobalamin daily. Adult daily losses (mainly in the urine and feces) are 1–3 μg (~0.1% of body stores), and as the body does not have the ability to degrade cobalamin, daily requirements are also about 1–3 μg. Body stores are of the order of 2–3 mg, sufficient for 3–4 years if supplies are completely cut off.

Absorption

Two mechanisms exist for cobalamin absorption. One is passive, occurring equally through buccal, duodenal, and ileal mucosa; it is rapid but extremely inefficient, with <1% of an oral dose being absorbed by this process. The normal physiologic mechanism is active; it occurs through the ileum and is efficient for small (a few micrograms) oral doses of cobalamin, and it is mediated by gastric intrinsic factor (IF). Dietary cobalamin is released from protein complexes by enzymes in the stomach, duodenum, and jejunum; it combines rapidly with a salivary glycoprotein that belongs to the family of cobalamin-binding proteins known as HC (HCs). In the

TABLE 9-1

CAUSES OF MEGALOBLASTIC ANEMIA
Cobalamin deficiency or abnormalities of cobalamin metabolism (see Tables 9-3 and 9-4)
Folate deficiency or abnormalities of folate metabolism (see Table 9-5)
Therapy with antifolate drugs (e.g., methotrexate)
Independent of either cobalamin or folate deficiency and refractory to cobalamin and folate therapy:
Some cases of acute myeloid leukemia, myelodysplasia
Therapy with drugs interfering with synthesis of DNA (e.g., cytosine arabinoside, hydroxyurea, 6-mercaptopurine, azidothymidine [AZT])
Orotic aciduria (responds to uridine)
Thiamine-responsive

intestine, the HC is digested by pancreatic trypsin and the cobalamin is transferred to IF.

IF (gene at chromosome 11q13 coding for 9 exons) is produced in the gastric parietal cells of the fundus and body of the stomach, and its secretion parallels that of hydrochloric acid. Normally, there is a vast excess of IF. The IF–cobalamin complex passes to the ileum, where IF attaches to a specific receptor (cubilin) on the microvillus membrane of the enterocytes. Cubilin also is present in yolk sac and renal proximal tubular epithelium. Cubulin appears to traffic by means of amnionless (AMN), an endocytic receptor protein that directs sub-localization and endocytosis of cubulin with its ligand IF–cobalamin complex. The cobalamin–IF complex enters the ileal cell, where IF is destroyed. After a delay of about 6 h, the cobalamin appears in portal blood attached to transcobalamin (TC) II.

Between 0.5 and 5 μg of cobalamin enters the bile each day. This binds to IF, and a major portion of biliary cobalamin normally is reabsorbed together with cobalamin derived from sloughed intestinal cells. Because of the appreciable amount of cobalamin undergoing enterohepatic circulation, cobalamin deficiency develops more rapidly in individuals who malabsorb cobalamin than it does in vegans, in whom reabsorption of biliary cobalamin is intact.

Transport

Two main cobalamin transport proteins exist in human plasma; they both bind cobalamin—one molecule for one molecule. One HC, known as TC I, is closely related to other cobalamin-binding HCs in milk, gastric juice, bile, saliva, and other fluids. The gene *TCNL* is at chromosome 11q11-q12.3 and has 9 exons. These HCs differ from each other only in the carbohydrate moiety of the molecule. TC I is derived primarily from the specific granules in neutrophils. Normally, it is about two-thirds saturated with cobalamin, which it binds tightly. TC I does not enhance cobalamin entry into tissues. Glycoprotein receptors on liver cells are involved in the removal of TC I from plasma, and TC I may play a role in the transport of cobalamin analogues (which it binds more effectively than IF) to the liver for excretion in bile.

The other major cobalamin transport protein in plasma is TC II. The gene is on chromosome 22q11-q13.1. As for IF and HC, there are 9 exons. The three proteins are likely to have a common ancestral origin. TC II is synthesized by liver and by other tissues, including macrophages, ileum, and vascular endothelium. It normally carries only 20–60 ng of cobalamin per liter of plasma and readily gives up cobalamin to marrow, placenta, and other tissues, which it enters by receptor-mediated endocytosis involving the TC II receptor and megalin (encoded by the *LRP-2* gene). The TC II cobalamin is internalized by endocytosis via clathrin-coated pits; the complex is degraded, but the receptor probably is recycled to the cell membrane as is the case for transferrin. Export of "free" cobalamin is via the ATP-binding cassette drug transporter alias multidrug resistance protein 1.

FOLATE

Dietary folate

Folic (pteroylglutamic) acid is a yellow, crystalline, water-soluble substance. It is the parent compound of a large family of natural folate compounds, which differ from it in three respects: (1) they are partly or completely reduced to di- or tetrahydrofolate (THF) derivatives, (2) they usually contain a single carbon unit (Table 9-2), and (3) 70–90% of natural folates are folate-polyglutamates.

Most foods contain some folate. The highest concentrations are found in liver, yeast, spinach, other greens, and nuts (>100 μg/100 g). The total folate content of an average Western diet is ~250 μg daily, but the amount varies widely according to the type of food eaten and the method of cooking. Folate is easily destroyed by heating, particularly in large volumes of water. Total-body folate in an adult is ~10 mg, with the liver containing the largest store. Daily adult requirements are ~100 μg, so stores are sufficient for only 3–4 months in normal adults, and severe folate deficiency may develop rapidly.

Absorption

Folates are absorbed rapidly from the upper small intestine. The absorption of folate polyglutamates is less efficient than that of monoglutamates; on average, ~50% of food folate is absorbed. Polyglutamate forms are hydrolyzed to the monoglutamate derivatives either in the lumen of the intestine or within the mucosa. All dietary folates are converted to 5-methyl-THF (5-MTHF) within the small-intestinal mucosa before entering portal plasma. The monoglutamates are actively transported across the enterocyte by a carrier-mediated mechanism. Pteroylglutamic acid at doses >400 μg is absorbed largely unchanged and converted to natural folates in the liver. Lower doses are converted to 5-MTHF during absorption through the intestine.

About 60–90 μg of folate enters the bile each day and is excreted into the small intestine. Loss of this folate, together with the folate of sloughed intestinal cells, accelerates the speed with which folate deficiency develops in malabsorption conditions.

TABLE 9-2

BIOCHEMICAL REACTIONS OF FOLATE COENZYMES

REACTION	COENZYME FORM OF FOLATE INVOLVED	SINGLE CARBON UNIT TRANSFERRED	IMPORTANCE
Formate activation	THF	–CHO	Generation of 10-formyl-THF
Purine synthesis			
Formation of glycinamide ribonucleotide	5,10-MethyleneTHF	–CHO	Formation of purines needed for DNA, RNA synthesis, but reactions probably not rate-limiting
Formylation of amino-imidazole carboxamide ribonucleotide (AICAR)	10-Formyl (CHO)THF		
Pyrimidine synthesis			
Methylation of deoxyuridine monophosphate (dUMP) to thymidine monophosphate (dTMP)	5,10-MethyleneTHF	$-CH_3$	Rate limiting in DNA synthesis Oxidizes THF to DHF Some breakdown of folate at the C-9–N-10 bond
Amino acid interconversion			
Serine–glycine interconversion	THF	$=CH_2$	Entry of single carbon units into active pool
Homocysteine to methionine	5-Methyl(M)THF	$-CH_3$	Demethylation of 5-MTHF to THF; also requires cobalamin, flavine adenine dinucleotide, ATP, and adenosylmethionine
Forminoglutamic acid to glutamic acid in histidine catabolism	THF	-HN–CH=	

Abbreviations: ATP, adenosine triphosphate; DHF, dihydrofolate; THF, tetrahydrofolate.

Transport

Folate is transported in plasma; about one-third is loosely bound to albumin, and two-thirds is unbound. In all body fluids (plasma, cerebrospinal fluid, milk, bile) folate is largely, if not entirely, 5-MTHF in the monoglutamate form. Two types of folate-binding protein are involved in the entry of MTHF into cells. A high-affinity proton-coupled folate receptor (PCFT/HCPI) takes folate into cells by endocytosis and is internalized by clathrin-coated pits or in a vesicle (caveola), which is then acidified, releasing folate. It accounts for the bulk of folate absorption. Folate then is carried by the membrane folate transporter into the cytoplasm. The high-affinity receptor is attached to the outer surface of the cell membrane by glycosyl phosphatidylinositol linkages. It may be involved in transport of oxidized folates and folate breakdown products to the liver for excretion in bile. An independent low-affinity reduced-folate carrier also mediates uptake of physiologic folates into cells but also regulates the uptake of methotrexate.

Biochemical functions

Folates (as the intracellular polyglutamate derivatives) act as coenzymes in the transfer of single-carbon units (Fig. 9-1 and Table 9-2). Two of these reactions are involved in purine synthesis and one in pyrimidine synthesis necessary for DNA and RNA replication. Folate is also a coenzyme for methionine synthesis, in which methylcobalamin is also involved and in which THF is regenerated. THF is the acceptor of single carbon units newly entering the active pool via conversion of serine to glycine. Methionine, the other product of the methionine synthase reaction, is the precursor for *S*-adenosylmethionine (SAM), the universal methyl donor involved in >100 methyltransferase reactions (**Fig. 9-1**).

During thymidylate synthesis, 5,10-methylene-THF is oxidized to DHF (dihydrofolate). The enzyme DHF reductase converts this to THF. The drugs methotrexate, pyrimethamine, and (mainly in bacteria) trimethoprim inhibit DHF reductase and so prevent formation of active THF coenzymes from DHF. A small fraction of the folate coenzyme is not recycled during thymidylate synthesis but is degraded.

BIOCHEMICAL BASIS OF MEGALOBLASTIC ANEMIA

The common feature of all megaloblastic anemias is a defect in DNA synthesis that affects rapidly dividing cells in the bone marrow. All conditions that give rise

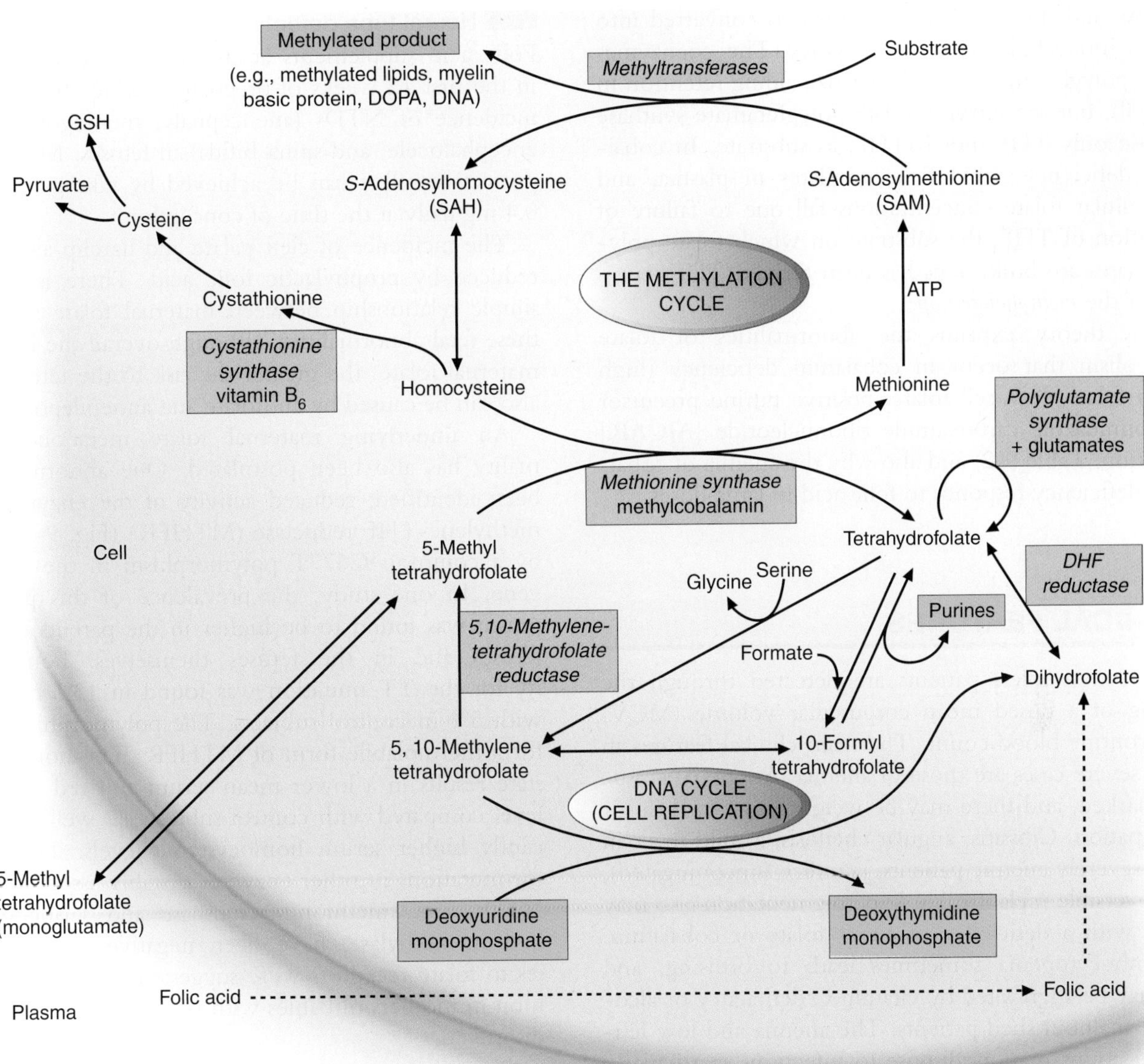

FIGURE 9-1
The role of folates in DNA synthesis and in formation of S-adenosylmethionine (SAM), which is involved in numerous methylation reactions. ATP, adenosine triphosphate; (*Reprinted from Hoffbrand AV, et al [eds]: Postgraduate Haematology, 5th ed, Oxford, UK, Blackwell Publishing, 2005; with permission.*)

to megaloblastic changes have in common a disparity in the rate of synthesis or availability of the four immediate precursors of DNA: the deoxyribonucleoside triphosphates (dNTPs)—dA(adenine)TP and dG(guanine)TP (purines), dT(thymine)TP and dC(cytosine)TP (pyrimidines). In deficiencies of either folate or cobalamin, there is failure to convert deoxyuridine monophosphate (dUMP) to deoxythymidine monophosphate (dTMP), the precursor of dTTP (Fig. 9-1). This is the case because folate is needed as the coenzyme 5,10-methylene-THF polyglutamate for conversion of dUMP to dTMP; the availability of 5,10-methylene-THF is reduced in either cobalamin or folate deficiency. An alternative theory for megaloblastic anemia in cobalamin or folate deficiency is misincorporation of uracil into DNA because of a buildup of deoxyuridine triphosphate (dUTP) at the DNA replication fork as a consequence of the block in conversion of dUMP to dTMP.

Cobalamin–folate relations

Folate is required for many reactions in mammalian tissues. Only two reactions in the body are known to require cobalamin. Methylmalonyl CoA isomerization requires adocobalamin, and the methylation of homocysteine to methionine requires both methylcobalamin and 5-MTHF (Fig. 9-1). This reaction is the first step in the pathway by which 5-MTHF, which enters bone marrow and other cells from plasma, is converted into all the intracellular folate coenzymes. The coenzymes are all polyglutamated (the larger size aiding retention in the cell), but the enzyme folate polyglutamate synthase can use only THF, not MTHF, as substrate. In cobalamin deficiency, MTHF accumulates in plasma, and intracellular folate concentrations fall due to failure of formation of THF, the substrate on which folate polyglutamates are built. This has been termed *THF starvation*, or the *methylfolate trap*.

This theory explains the abnormalities of folate metabolism that occur in cobalamin deficiency (high serum folate, low cell folate, positive purine precursor aminoimidazole carboxamide ribonucleotide [AICAR] excretion; Table 9-2) and also why the anemia of cobalamin deficiency responds to folic acid in large doses.

CLINICAL FEATURES

Many symptomless patients are detected through the finding of a raised mean corpuscular volume (MCV) on a routine blood count. The main clinical features in more severe cases are those of anemia. Anorexia is usually marked, and there may be weight loss, diarrhea, or constipation. Glossitis, angular cheilosis, a mild fever in more severely anemic patients, jaundice (unconjugated), and reversible melanin skin hyperpigmentation also may occur with a deficiency of either folate or cobalamin. Thrombocytopenia sometimes leads to bruising, and this may be aggravated by vitamin C deficiency or alcohol in malnourished patients. The anemia and low leukocyte count may predispose to infections, particularly of the respiratory and urinary tracts. Cobalamin deficiency has also been associated with impaired bactericidal function of phagocytes.

General tissue effects of cobalamin and folate deficiencies

Epithelial surfaces

After the marrow, the next most frequently affected tissues are the epithelial cell surfaces of the mouth, stomach, and small intestine and the respiratory, urinary, and female genital tracts. The cells show macrocytosis, with increased numbers of multinucleate and dying cells. The deficiencies may cause cervical smear abnormalities.

Complications of pregnancy

The gonads are also affected, and infertility is common in both men and women with either deficiency. Maternal folate deficiency has been implicated as a cause of prematurity, and both folate deficiency and cobalamin deficiency have been implicated in recurrent fetal loss and neural tube defects (NTDs), as discussed later.

Neural tube defects

Folic acid supplements at the time of conception and in the first 12 weeks of pregnancy reduce by ~70% the incidence of NTDs (anencephaly, meningomyelocele, encephalocele, and spina bifida) in fetuses. Most of this protective effect can be achieved by taking folic acid, 0.4 mg daily at the time of conception.

The incidence of cleft palate and harelip also can be reduced by prophylactic folic acid. There is no clear simple relationship between maternal folate status and these fetal abnormalities, although overall the lower the maternal folate, the greater the risk to the fetus. NTDs also can be caused by antifolate and antiepileptic drugs.

An underlying maternal folate metabolic abnormality has also been postulated. One abnormality has been identified: reduced activity of the enzyme 5,10-methylene-THF reductase (MTHFR) (Fig. 9-1) caused by a common C677T polymorphism in the *MTHFR* gene. In one study, the prevalence of this polymorphism was found to be higher in the parents of NTD fetuses and in the fetuses themselves: homozygosity for the TT mutation was found in 13% compared with 5% in control subjects. The polymorphism codes for a thermolabile form of MTHFR. The homozygous state results in a lower mean serum and red cell folate level compared with control subjects, as well as significantly higher serum homocysteine levels. Test results for mutations in other enzymes possibly associated with NTDs, e.g., methionine synthase and serine–glycine hydroxymethylase, have been negative. Autoantibodies to folate receptors were suggested to be more common in mothers of babies with NTDs, but this has been disproved.

Cardiovascular disease

Children with severe homocystinuria (blood levels ≥100 μmol/L) due to deficiency of one of three enzymes, methionine synthase, MTHFR, or cystathionine synthase (Fig. 9-1), have vascular disease, e.g., ischemic heart disease, cerebrovascular disease, or pulmonary embolus, as teenagers or in young adulthood. Lesser degrees of raised serum homocysteine and low levels of serum folate and homozygous inherited mutations of MTHFR have been found to be associated with cerebrovascular, peripheral vascular, and coronary heart disease and with deep vein thrombosis. Prospective randomized trials of lowering homocysteine levels with supplements of folic acid, vitamin B_{12}, and vitamin B_6 against placebo over a 5-year period in patients with vascular disease or diabetes have not, however, shown a reduction of major cardiovascular events, nor have these supplements reduced the risk of recurrent cardiovascular disease after an acute myocardial infarct. It is possible that these trials were not sufficiently powered to detect a small (e.g., 10%) benefit or that another underlying factor is responsible for both the vascular damage and the raised homocysteine. Alternatively, the beneficial effects of lowering homocysteine were offset in these trials by the vitamins stimulating endothelial cell proliferation. Meta-analysis has suggested that folic acid supplementation reduces the risk of stroke by 18%. The results of longer and larger trials are needed to resolve these uncertainties.

Malignancy

Prophylactic folic acid in pregnancy has been found in some but not all studies to reduce the subsequent incidence of acute lymphoblastic leukemia (ALL) in childhood. A significant negative association has also been found with the *MTHFR* C677T polymorphism and leukemias with mixed lineage leukemia (MLL) translocations but a positive association with hyperdiploidy in infants with ALL or acute myeloid leukemia or with childhood ALL. A second polymorphism in the *MTHFR* gene, A1298C, is also strongly associated with hyperdiploid leukemia. There are various positive and negative associations between polymorphisms in folate-dependent enzymes and the incidence of adult ALL. The C677T polymorphism is thought to lead to increased thymidine pools and "better quality" of DNA synthesis by shunting 1-carbon groups toward thymidine and purine synthesis. This may explain its reported association with a lower risk for colorectal cancer. Most but not all studies suggest that prophylactic folic acid also protects against colon adenomas. Other tumors that have been associated with folate polymorphisms or status include follicular lymphoma, breast cancer, and gastric cancer. Because folic acid may "feed" tumors, it probably should be avoided in those with established tumors unless there is severe megaloblastic anemia due to folate deficiency.

Neurologic manifestations

Cobalamin deficiency may cause a bilateral peripheral neuropathy or degeneration (demyelination) of the posterior and pyramidal tracts of the spinal cord and, less frequently, optic atrophy or cerebral symptoms.

The patient, more frequently male, presents with paresthesias, muscle weakness, or difficulty in walking and sometimes dementia, psychotic disturbances, or visual impairment. Long-term nutritional cobalamin deficiency in infancy leads to poor brain development and impaired intellectual development. Folate deficiency has been suggested to cause organic nervous disease, but this is uncertain, although methotrexate injected into the cerebrospinal fluid may cause brain or spinal cord damage.

An important clinical problem is the nonanemic patient with neurologic or psychiatric abnormalities and a low or borderline serum cobalamin level. In such patients, it is necessary to try to establish whether there is significant cobalamin deficiency, e.g., by careful examination of the blood film, tests for serum gastrin level and for antibodies to IF or parietal cells, along with serum methylmalonic acid (MMA) measurement if available. A trial of cobalamin therapy for at least 3 months will usually also be needed to determine whether the symptoms improve.

The biochemical basis for cobalamin neuropathy remains obscure. Its occurrence in the absence of methylmalonic aciduria in TC II deficiency suggests that the neuropathy is related to the defect in homocysteine–methionine conversion. Accumulation of *S*-adenosylhomocysteine in the brain, resulting in inhibition of transmethylation reactions, has been suggested.

Psychiatric disturbance is common in both folate and cobalamin deficiencies. This, like the neuropathy, has been attributed to a failure of the synthesis of SAM, which is needed in methylation of biogenic amines (e.g., dopamine) as well as that of proteins, phospholipids, and neurotransmitters in the brain (Fig. 9-1). Associations between lower serum folate or cobalamin levels and higher homocysteine levels and the development of decreased cognitive function and dementia in Alzheimer's disease have been reported. A 2-year double-blind placebo-controlled randomized clinical trial involving healthy subjects >65 years old given folate, cobalamin, and vitamin B_6 supplements showed no benefit for cognitive performance, whereas a 3-year (FACIT) study did show benefit.

HEMATOLOGIC FINDINGS

Peripheral blood

Oval macrocytes, usually with considerable anisocytosis and poikilocytosis, are the main feature (Fig. 9-2*A*). The MCV is usually >100 fL unless a cause of microcytosis (e.g., iron deficiency or thalassemia trait) is present. Some of the neutrophils are hypersegmented (more than five nuclear lobes). There may be leukopenia due to a reduction in granulocytes and lymphocytes, but this is usually $>1.5 \times 10^9$/L; the platelet count may be moderately reduced, rarely to $<40 \times 10^9$/L. The severity of all these changes parallels the degree of anemia. In a nonanemic patient, the presence of a few macrocytes and hypersegmented neutrophils in the peripheral blood may be the only indication of the underlying disorder.

Bone marrow

In a severely anemic patient, the marrow is hypercellular with an accumulation of primitive cells due to selective death by apoptosis of more mature forms. The erythroblast nucleus maintains a primitive appearance despite maturation and hemoglobinization of the cytoplasm. The cells are larger than normoblasts, and an increased

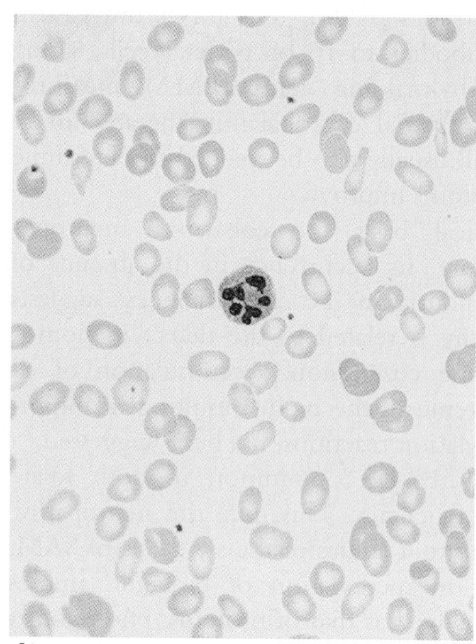

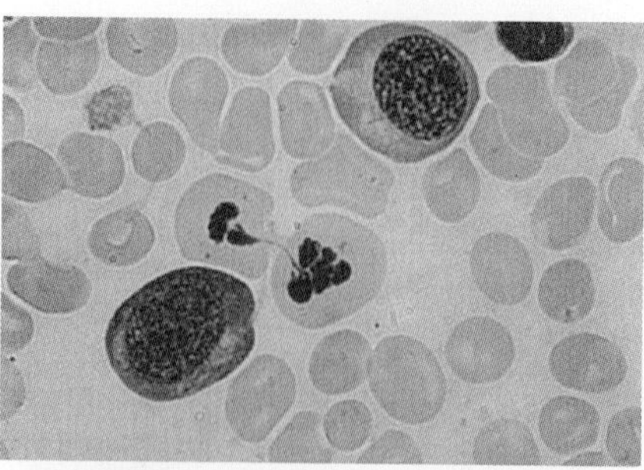

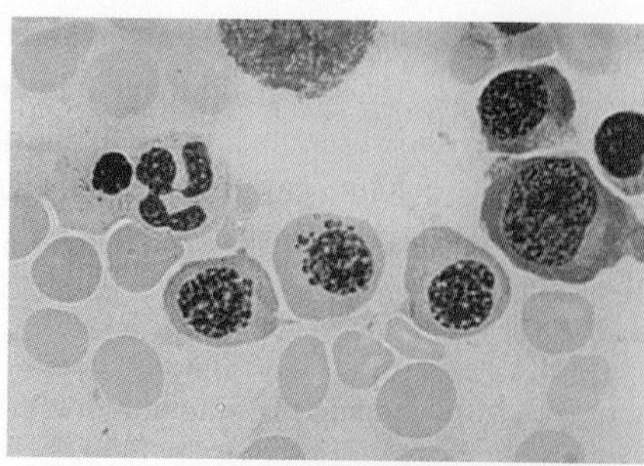

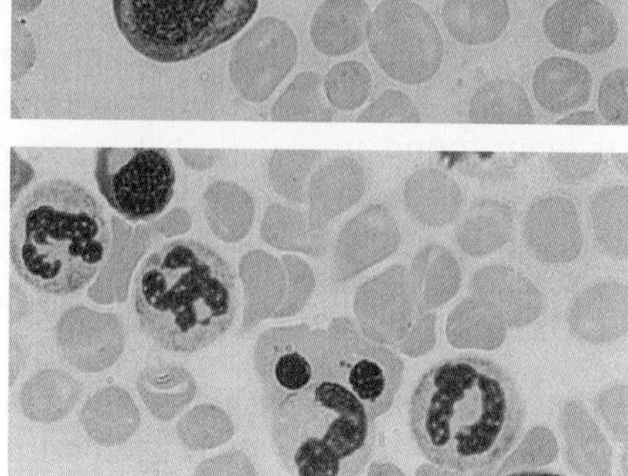

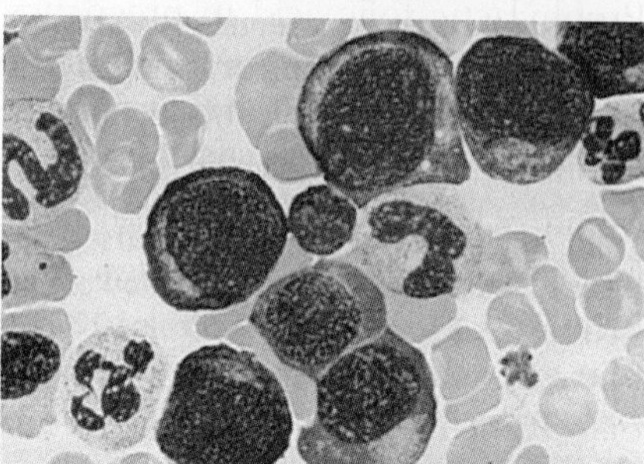

A B

FIGURE 9-2

A. The peripheral blood in severe megaloblastic anemia. ***B.*** The bone marrow in severe megaloblastic anemia. (*Reprinted from AV Hoffbrand et al [eds], Postgraduate Haematology, 5th ed, Oxford, UK, Blackwell Publishing, 2005; with permission.*)

number of cells with eccentric lobulated nuclei or nuclear fragments may be present (Fig. 9-2*B*). Giant and abnormally shaped metamyelocytes and enlarged hyperpolyploid megakaryocytes are characteristic. In less anemic patients, the changes in the marrow may be difficult to recognize. The terms *intermediate*, *mild*, and *early* have been used. The term *megaloblastoid* does not mean mildly megaloblastic. Rather, it is used to describe cells with both immature-appearing nuclei and defective hemoglobinization and is usually seen in myelodysplasia.

Chromosomes

Bone marrow cells, transformed lymphocytes, and other proliferating cells in the body show a variety of changes, including random breaks, reduced contraction, spreading of the centromere, and exaggeration of secondary chromosomal constrictions and overprominent satellites. Similar abnormalities may be produced by antimetabolite drugs (e.g., cytosine arabinoside, hydroxyurea, and methotrexate) that interfere with either DNA replication or folate metabolism and that also cause megaloblastic appearances.

Ineffective hematopoiesis

There is an accumulation of unconjugated bilirubin in plasma due to the death of nucleated red cells in the marrow (ineffective erythropoiesis). Other evidence for this includes raised urine urobilinogen, reduced haptoglobins and positive urine hemosiderin, and a raised serum lactate dehydrogenase. A weakly positive direct antiglobulin test due to complement can lead to a false diagnosis of autoimmune hemolytic anemia.

CAUSES OF COBALAMIN DEFICIENCY

Cobalamin deficiency is usually due to malabsorption. The only other cause is inadequate dietary intake.

Inadequate dietary intake

Adults

Dietary cobalamin deficiency arises in vegans who omit meat, fish, eggs, cheese, and other animal products from their diet. The largest group in the world consists of Hindus, and it is likely that many millions of Indians are at risk of deficiency of cobalamin on a nutritional basis. Subnormal serum cobalamin levels are found in up to 50% of randomly selected, young, adult Indian vegans, but the deficiency usually does not progress to megaloblastic anemia since the diet of most vegans is not totally lacking in cobalamin, and the enterohepatic circulation of cobalamin is intact. Dietary cobalamin deficiency may also arise rarely in nonvegetarian individuals who exist on grossly inadequate diets because of poverty or psychiatric disturbance.

Infants

Cobalamin deficiency has been described in infants born to severely cobalamin-deficient mothers. These infants develop megaloblastic anemia at about 3–6 months of age, presumably because they are born with low stores of cobalamin and because they are fed breast milk with low cobalamin content. The babies have also shown growth retardation, impaired psychomotor development, and other neurologic sequelae.

Gastric causes of cobalamin malabsorption

See Tables 9-3 and 9-4.

Pernicious anemia

Pernicious anemia (PA) may be defined as a severe lack of IF due to gastric atrophy. It is a common disease in north Europeans but occurs in all countries and ethnic groups. The overall incidence is about 120 per 100,000 population in the United Kingdom (UK). The ratio of incidence in men and women among whites is ~1:1.6, and the peak age of onset is 60 years, with only 10% of patients being <40 years of age. However, in some ethnic groups, notably black individuals and Latin Americans, the age at onset of PA is generally lower. The disease occurs more commonly than by chance in close relatives and in persons with other organ-specific autoimmune diseases, e.g., thyroid diseases, vitiligo, hypoparathyroidism, and Addison's disease. It is also associated with hypogammaglobulinemia, with premature graying or blue eyes, and persons of blood group A. An association with human leukocyte antigen (HLA) 3 has been reported in some but not all series and, in those with endocrine disease, with HLA-B8, -B12, and -BW15. Life expectancy is normal in women once regular treatment has begun. Men have a slightly subnormal life expectancy as a result of a higher incidence of carcinoma of the stomach than in control subjects. Gastric output of hydrochloric acid, pepsin, and IF is severely reduced. The serum gastrin level is raised, and serum pepsinogen I levels are low.

TABLE 9-3

CAUSES OF COBALAMIN DEFICIENCY SUFFICIENTLY SEVERE TO CAUSE MEGALOBLASTIC ANEMIA

Nutritional	Vegans
Malabsorption	Pernicious anemia
Gastric causes	Congenital absence of intrinsic factor or functional abnormality Total or partial gastrectomy
Intestinal causes	Intestinal stagnant loop syndrome: jejunal diverticulosis, ileocolic fistula, anatomic blind loop, intestinal stricture, etc. Ileal resection and Crohn's disease Selective malabsorption with proteinuria Tropical sprue Transcobalamin II deficiency Fish tapeworm

TABLE 9-4

MALABSORPTION OF COBALAMIN MAY OCCUR IN THE FOLLOWING CONDITIONS BUT IS NOT USUALLY SUFFICIENTLY SEVERE AND PROLONGED TO CAUSE MEGALOBLASTIC ANEMIA

Gastric causes
- Simple atrophic gastritis (food cobalamin malabsorption)
- Zollinger–Ellison syndrome
- Gastric bypass surgery
- Use of proton pump inhibitors

Intestinal causes
- Gluten-induced enteropathy
- Severe pancreatitis
- HIV infection
- Radiotherapy
- Graft-vs.-host disease

Deficiencies of cobalamin, folate, protein, ?riboflavin, ?nicotinic acid

Therapy with colchicine, para-aminosalicylate, neomycin, slow-release potassium chloride, anticonvulsant drugs, metformin, phenformin, cytotoxic drugs

Alcohol

Gastric biopsy

This usually shows atrophy of all layers of the body and fundus, with loss of glandular elements, an absence of parietal and chief cells and replacement by mucous cells, a mixed inflammatory cell infiltrate, and perhaps intestinal metaplasia. The infiltrate of plasma cells and lymphocytes contains an excess of CD4 cells. The antral mucosa is usually well preserved. *Helicobacter pylori* infection occurs infrequently in PA, but it has been suggested that *H. pylori* gastritis occurs at an early phase of atrophic gastritis and presents in younger patients as iron-deficiency anemia but in older patients as PA. *H. pylori* is suggested to stimulate an autoimmune process directed against parietal cells, with the *H. pylori* infection then being gradually replaced, in some individuals, by an autoimmune process.

Serum antibodies

Two types of IF immunoglobulin G antibody may be found in the sera of patients with PA. One, the "blocking," or type I, antibody, prevents the combination of IF and cobalamin, whereas the "binding," or type II, antibody prevents attachment of IF to ileal mucosa. Type I occurs in the sera of ~55% of patients and type II in 35%. IF antibodies cross the placenta and may cause temporary IF deficiency in a newborn infant. Patients with PA also show cell-mediated immunity to IF. Type I antibody has been detected rarely in the sera of patients without PA but with thyrotoxicosis, myxedema, Hashimoto's disease, or diabetes mellitus and in relatives of PA patients. IF antibodies also have been detected in gastric juice in ~80% of PA patients. These gastric antibodies may reduce absorption of dietary cobalamin by combining with small amounts of remaining IF.

Parietal cell antibody is present in the sera of almost 90% of adult patients with PA but is frequently present in other subjects. Thus, it occurs in as many as 16% of randomly selected female subjects age >60 years. The parietal cell antibody is directed against the α and β subunits of the gastric proton pump (H^+,K^+-ATPase).

Juvenile pernicious anemia

This usually occurs in older children and resembles PA of adults. Gastric atrophy, achlorhydria, and serum IF antibodies are all present, although parietal cell antibodies are usually absent. About one-half of these patients show an associated endocrinopathy such as autoimmune thyroiditis, Addison's disease, or hypoparathyroidism; in some, mucocutaneous candidiasis occurs.

Congenital intrinsic factor deficiency or functional abnormality

An affected child usually presents with megaloblastic anemia in the first to third year of life; a few have presented as late as the second decade. The child usually has no demonstrable IF but has a normal gastric mucosa and normal secretion of acid. The inheritance is autosomal recessive. Parietal cell and IF antibodies are absent. Variants have been described in which the child is born with IF that can be detected immunologically but is unstable or functionally inactive, unable to bind cobalmin or to facilitate its uptake by ileal receptors.

Gastrectomy

After total gastrectomy, cobalamin deficiency is inevitable, and prophylactic cobalamin therapy should be commenced immediately after the operation. After partial gastrectomy, 10–15% of patients also develop this deficiency. The exact incidence and time of onset are most influenced by the size of the resection and the preexisting size of cobalamin body stores.

Food cobalamin malabsorption

Failure of release of cobalamin from binding proteins in food is believed to be responsible for this condition, which is more common in the elderly. It is associated with low serum cobalamin levels, with or without raised serum levels of MMA and homocysteine. Typically, these patients have normal cobalamin absorption, as measured with crystalline cobalamin, but show malabsorption when a modified test using food-bound cobalamin is used. The frequency of progression to severe cobalamin deficiency and the reasons for this progression are not clear.

Intestinal causes of cobalamin malabsorption

Intestinal stagnant loop syndrome

Malabsorption of cobalamin occurs in a variety of intestinal lesions in which there is colonization of the upper small intestine by fecal organisms. This may occur in patients with jejunal diverticulosis, enteroanastomosis, or an intestinal stricture or fistula or with an anatomic blind loop due to Crohn's disease, tuberculosis, or an operative procedure.

Ileal resection

Removal of ≥1.2 m of terminal ileum causes malabsorption of cobalamin. In some patients after ileal resection, particularly if the ileocecal valve is incompetent, colonic bacteria may contribute further to the onset of cobalamin deficiency.

Selective malabsorption of cobalamin with proteinuria (Imerslund syndrome: Imerslund-Gräsbeck syndrome; congenital cobalamin malabsorption; autosomal recessive megaloblastic anemia, MGA1)

This autosomally recessive disease is the most common cause of megaloblastic anemia due to cobalamin deficiency in infancy in Western countries. More than 200 cases have been reported, with familial clusters in Finland, Norway, the Middle East, and North Africa. The patients secrete normal amounts of IF and gastric acid but are unable to absorb cobalamin. In Finland, impaired synthesis, processing, or ligand binding of cubilin due to inherited mutations is found. In Norway, mutation of the gene for AMN has been reported. Other tests of intestinal absorption are normal. Over 90% of these patients show nonspecific proteinuria, but renal function is otherwise normal, and renal biopsy has not shown any consistent renal defect. A few have shown aminoaciduria and congenital renal abnormalities, such as duplication of the renal pelvis.

Tropical sprue

Nearly all patients with acute and subacute tropical sprue show malabsorption of cobalamin; this may persist as the principal abnormality in the chronic form of the disease, when the patient may present with megaloblastic anemia or neuropathy due to cobalamin deficiency. Absorption of cobalamin usually improves after antibiotic therapy and, in the early stages, folic acid therapy.

Fish tapeworm infestation

The fish tapeworm (*Diphyllobothrium latum*) lives in the small intestine of humans and accumulates cobalamin from food, rendering the cobalamin unavailable for absorption. Individuals acquire the worm by eating raw or partly cooked fish. Infestation is common around the lakes of Scandinavia, Germany, Japan, North America, and Russia. Megaloblastic anemia or cobalamin neuropathy occurs only in those with a heavy infestation.

Gluten-induced enteropathy

Malabsorption of cobalamin occurs in ~30% of untreated patients (presumably those in whom the disease extends to the ileum). Cobalamin deficiency is not severe in these patients and is corrected with a gluten-free diet.

Severe chronic pancreatitis

In this condition, lack of trypsin is thought to cause dietary cobalamin attached to gastric non-IF (R) binder to be unavailable for absorption. It also has been proposed that in pancreatitis, the concentration of calcium ions in the ileum falls below the level needed to maintain normal cobalamin absorption.

HIV infection

Serum cobalamin levels tend to fall in patients with HIV infection and are subnormal in 10–35% of those with AIDS. Malabsorption of cobalamin not corrected by IF has been shown in some, but not all, patients with subnormal serum cobalamin levels. Cobalamin deficiency sufficiently severe to cause megaloblastic anemia or neuropathy is rare.

Zollinger–Ellison syndrome

Malabsorption of cobalamin has been reported in the Zollinger–Ellison syndrome. It is thought that there is a failure to release cobalamin from R-binding protein due to inactivation of pancreatic trypsin by high acidity, as well as interference with IF binding of cobalamin.

Radiotherapy

Both total-body irradiation and local radiotherapy to the ileum (e.g., as a complication of radiotherapy for carcinoma of the cervix) may cause malabsorption of cobalamin.

Graft-versus-host disease

This commonly affects the small intestine. Malabsorption of cobalamin due to abnormal gut flora, as well as damage to ileal mucosa, is common.

Drugs

The drugs that have been reported to cause malabsorption of cobalamin are listed in Table 9-4. Megaloblastic anemia due to these drugs is, however, rare.

Abnormalities of cobalamin metabolism

Congenital transcobalamin II deficiency or abnormality

Infants with TC II deficiency usually present with megaloblastic anemia within a few weeks of birth. Serum cobalamin and folate levels are normal, but the anemia responds to massive (e.g., 1 mg three times weekly) injections of cobalamin. Some cases show neurologic complications. The protein may be present but functionally inert. Genetic abnormalities found include mutations of an intra-exonic cryptic splice site, extensive deletion, single nucleotide deletion, nonsense mutation, and an RNA editing defect. Malabsorption of cobalamin occurs in all cases, and serum immunoglobulins are usually reduced. Failure to institute adequate cobalamin therapy or treatment with folic acid may lead to neurologic damage.

Congenital methylmalonic acidemia and aciduria

Infants with this abnormality are ill from birth with vomiting, failure to thrive, severe metabolic acidosis, ketosis, and mental retardation. Anemia, if present, is normocytic and normoblastic. The condition may be due to a functional defect in either mitochondrial methylmalonyl CoA mutase or its cofactor adocobalamin. Mutations in the methylmalonyl CoA mutase are not responsive, or only poorly responsive, to treatment with cobalamin. A proportion of infants with failure of adocobalamin synthesis respond to cobalamin in large doses. Some children have combined methylmalonic aciduria and homocystinuria due to defective formation of both cobalamin coenzymes. This usually presents in the first year of life with feeding difficulties, developmental delay, microcephaly, seizures, hypotonia, and megaloblastic anemia.

Acquired abnormality of cobalamin metabolism: nitrous oxide inhalation

Nitrous oxide irreversibly oxidizes methylcobalamin to an inactive precursor; this inactivates methionine synthase. Megaloblastic anemia has occurred in patients undergoing prolonged N_2O anesthesia (e.g., in intensive care units). A neuropathy resembling cobalamin neuropathy has been described in dentists and anesthetists who are exposed repeatedly to N_2O. Methylmalonic aciduria does not occur as adocobalamin is not inactivated by N_2O.

CAUSES OF FOLATE DEFICIENCY

(Table 9-5)

Nutritional

Dietary folate deficiency is common. Indeed, in most patients with folate deficiency, a nutritional element is present. Certain individuals are particularly prone to have diets containing inadequate amounts of folate (Table 9-5). In the United States and other countries where fortification of the diet with folic acid has been

TABLE 9-5

CAUSES OF FOLATE DEFICIENCY

Dietary[a]
Particularly in: old age, infancy, poverty, alcoholism, chronic disabilities, and the people with mental illnesses; may be associated with scurvy or kwashiorkor
Malabsorption
Major causes of deficiency
Tropical sprue; gluten-induced enteropathy in children and adults; and in association with dermatitis herpetiformis, specific malabsorption of folate, intestinal megaloblastosis caused by severe cobalamin or folate deficiency
Minor causes of deficiency
Extensive jejunal resection, Crohn's disease, partial gastrectomy, congestive heart failure, Whipple's disease, scleroderma, amyloid, diabetic enteropathy, systemic bacterial infection, lymphoma, salazopyrine
Excess utilization or loss
Physiologic
Pregnancy and lactation, prematurity
Pathologic
Hematologic diseases: chronic hemolytic anemias, sickle cell anemia, thalassemia major, myelofibrosis
Malignant diseases: carcinoma, lymphoma, leukemia, myeloma
Inflammatory diseases: tuberculosis, Crohn's disease, psoriasis, exfoliative dermatitis, malaria
Metabolic disease: homocystinuria
Excess urinary loss: congestive heart failure, active liver disease
Hemodialysis, peritoneal dialysis
Antifolate drugs[b]
Anticonvulsant drugs (phenytoin, primidone, barbiturates), sulphasalazine
Nitrofurantoin, tetracycline, antituberculosis (less well documented)
Mixed causes
Liver diseases, alcoholism, intensive care units

[a]In severely folate-deficient patients with causes other than those listed under Dietary, poor dietary intake is often present.
[b]Drugs inhibiting dihydrofolate reductase are discussed in the text.

adopted, the prevalence of folate deficiency has dropped dramatically and is now almost restricted to high-risk groups with increased folate needs. Nutritional folate deficiency occurs in kwashiorkor and scurvy and in infants with repeated infections or those who are fed solely on goats' milk, which has a low folate content.

Malabsorption

Malabsorption of dietary folate occurs in tropical sprue and in gluten-induced enteropathy. In the rare congenital syndrome of selective malabsorption of folate due to mutation of the protein-coupled folate transporter (PCFT), there is an associated defect of folate transport into the cerebrospinal fluid, and these patients show megaloblastic anemia, which responds to physiologic doses of folic acid given parenterally but not orally. They also show mental retardation, convulsions, and other central nervous system abnormalities. Minor degrees of malabsorption may also occur after jejunal resection or partial gastrectomy, in Crohn's disease, and in systemic infections, but in these conditions, if severe deficiency occurs, it is usually largely due to poor nutrition. Malabsorption of folate has been described in patients receiving salazopyrine, cholestyramine, and triamterene.

Excess utilization or loss

Pregnancy

Folate requirements are increased by 200–300 μg to ~400 μg daily in a normal pregnancy, partly because of transfer of the vitamin to the fetus but mainly because of increased folate catabolism due to cleavage of folate coenzymes in rapidly proliferating tissues. Megaloblastic anemia due to this deficiency is prevented by prophylactic folic acid therapy. It occurred in 0.5% of pregnancies in the UK and other Western countries before prophylaxis with folic acid, but the incidence is much higher in countries where the general nutritional status is poor.

Prematurity

A newborn infant, whether full term or premature, has higher serum and red cell folate concentrations than does an adult. However, a newborn infant's demand for folate has been estimated to be up to 10 times that of adults on a weight basis, and the neonatal folate level falls rapidly to the lowest values at about 6 weeks of age. The falls are steepest and are liable to reach subnormal levels in premature babies, a number of whom develop megaloblastic anemia responsive to folic acid at about 4–6 weeks of age. This occurs particularly in the smallest babies (<1500 g birth weight) and those who have feeding difficulties or infections or have undergone multiple exchange transfusions. In these babies, prophylactic folic acid should be given.

Hematologic disorders

Folate deficiency frequently occurs in chronic hemolytic anemia, particularly in sickle cell disease, autoimmune hemolytic anemia, and congenital spherocytosis. In these and other conditions of increased cell turnover (e.g., myelofibrosis, malignancies), folate deficiency arises because it is not completely reutilized after performing coenzyme functions.

Inflammatory conditions

Chronic inflammatory diseases such as tuberculosis, rheumatoid arthritis, Crohn's disease, psoriasis, exfoliative dermatitis, bacterial endocarditis, and chronic bacterial infections cause deficiency by reducing the appetite and increasing the demand for folate. Systemic infections also may cause malabsorption of folate. Severe deficiency is virtually confined to the patients with the most active disease and the poorest diet.

Homocystinuria

This is a rare metabolic defect in the conversion of homocysteine to cystathionine. Folate deficiency occurring in most of these patients may be due to excessive utilization because of compensatory increased conversion of homocysteine to methionine.

Long-term dialysis

As folate is only loosely bound to plasma proteins, it is easily removed from plasma by dialysis. In patients with anorexia, vomiting, infections, and hemolysis, folate stores are particularly likely to become depleted. Routine folate prophylaxis is now given.

Congestive heart failure, liver disease

Excess urinary folate losses of >100 μg per day may occur in some of these patients. The explanation appears to be release of folate from damaged liver cells.

Antifolate drugs

A large number of people with epilepsy who are receiving long-term therapy with phenytoin or primidone, with or without barbiturates, develop low serum and red cell folate levels. The exact mechanism is unclear. Alcohol may also be a folate antagonist, as patients who are drinking spirits may develop megaloblastic anemia that will respond to normal quantities of dietary folate or to physiologic doses of folic acid only if alcohol is withdrawn. Macrocytosis of red cells is associated with chronic alcohol intake even when folate levels are normal. Inadequate folate intake is the major factor in the development of deficiency in spirit-drinking alcoholics. Beer is relatively folate-rich in some countries, depending on the technique used for brewing.

The drugs that inhibit DHF reductase include methotrexate, pyrimethamine, and trimethoprim. Methotrexate has the most powerful action against the human enzyme, whereas trimethoprim is most active against the bacterial enzyme and is likely to cause megaloblastic anemia only when used in conjunction with sulphamethoxazole in patients with preexisting folate or cobalamin deficiency. The activity of pyrimethamine is intermediate. The antidote to these drugs is folinic acid (5-formyl-THF).

Congenital abnormalities of folate metabolism

Some infants with congenital defects of folate enzymes (e.g., cyclohydrolase or methionine synthase) have had megaloblastic anemia.

DIAGNOSIS OF COBALAMIN AND FOLATE DEFICIENCIES

The diagnosis of cobalamin or folate deficiency has traditionally depended on the recognition of the relevant abnormalities in the peripheral blood and analysis of the blood levels of the vitamins.

Serum cobalamin

This is measured by an automated enzyme-linked immunosorbent assay (ELISA). Normal serum levels range from 118–148 pmol/L (160–200 ng/L) to ~738 pmol/L (1000 ng/L). In patients with megaloblastic anemia due to cobalamin deficiency, the level is usually <74 pmol/L (100 ng/L). In general, the more severe the deficiency, the lower the serum cobalamin level. In patients with spinal cord damage due to the deficiency, levels are very low even in the absence of anemia. Values between 74 and 148 pmol/L (100 and 200 ng/L) are regarded as borderline. They may occur, for instance, in pregnancy and in patients with megaloblastic anemia due to folate deficiency. They may also be due to heterozygous, homozygous, or compound heterozygous mutations of the gene *TCN1* that codes for HC (transcobalamin I). There is no clinical or hematologic abnormality. The serum cobalamin level is sufficiently robust, cost-effective, and most convenient to rule out cobalamin deficiency in the vast majority of patients suspected of having this problem.

Serum methylmalonate and homocysteine

In patients with cobalamin deficiency sufficient to cause anemia or neuropathy, the serum MMA level is raised. Sensitive methods for measuring MMA and homocysteine in serum have been introduced and recommended for the early diagnosis of cobalamin deficiency, even in the absence of hematologic abnormalities or subnormal levels of serum cobalamin. Serum MMA levels fluctuate, however, in patients with renal failure. Mildly elevated serum MMA and/or homocysteine levels occur in up to 30% of apparently healthy volunteers, with serum cobalamin levels up to 258 pmol/L (350 ng/L) and normal serum folate levels; 15% of elderly subjects, even with cobalamin levels >258 pmol/L (>350 ng/L), have this pattern of raised metabolite levels. These findings bring into question the exact cutoff points for normal MMA and homocysteine levels. It is also unclear at present whether these mildly raised metabolite levels have clinical consequences.

Serum homocysteine is raised in both early cobalamin and folate deficiency but may be raised in other conditions, e.g., chronic renal disease, alcoholism, smoking, pyridoxine deficiency, hypothyroidism, and therapy with steroids, cyclosporine, and other drugs.

Levels are also higher in serum than in plasma, in men than in premenopausal women, in women taking hormone replacement therapy or in oral contraceptive users, and in elderly persons and patients with several inborn errors of metabolism affecting enzymes in transsulfuration pathways of homocysteine metabolism. Thus, homocysteine levels are not used for diagnosis of cobalamin or folate deficiency.

Other tests

Studies of cobalamin absorption once were widely used, but difficulty in obtaining radioactive cobalamin and ensuring that IF preparations are free of viruses have made these tests obsolete. Tests to diagnose PA include serum gastrin, which is raised, and serum pepsinogen I, which is low in PA (90–92%) but also in other conditions. Tests for IF and parietal cell antibodies are also used as well as tests for individual intestinal diseases.

Serum folate

This is also measured by an ELISA technique. In most laboratories, the normal range is from 11 nmol/L (2 μg/L) to ~82 nmol/L (15 μg/L). The serum folate level is low in all folate-deficient patients. It also reflects recent diet. Because of this, serum folate may be low before there is hematologic or biochemical evidence of deficiency. Serum folate rises in severe cobalamin deficiency because of the block in conversion of MTHF to THF inside cells; raised levels have also been reported in the intestinal stagnant loop syndrome due to absorption of bacterially synthesized folate.

Red cell folate

The red cell folate assay is a valuable test of body folate stores. It is less affected than the serum assay by recent diet and traces of hemolysis. In normal adults, concentrations range from 880–3520 μmol/L (160–640 μg/L) of packed red cells. Subnormal levels occur in patients with megaloblastic anemia due to folate deficiency but also in nearly two-thirds of patients with severe cobalamin deficiency. False-normal results may occur if a folate-deficient patient has received a recent blood transfusion or if a patient has a raised reticulocyte count.

TREATMENT Megaloblastic Anemia

It is usually possible to establish which of the two deficiencies, folate or cobalamin, is the cause of the anemia and to treat only with the appropriate vitamin. In patients who enter the hospital severely ill, however, it may be necessary to treat with both vitamins in large doses once blood samples have been taken for cobalamin and folate assays and a bone marrow biopsy has been performed (if deemed necessary). Transfusion is usually unnecessary and inadvisable. If it is essential, packed red cells should be given slowly, 1 or 2 units only, with the usual treatment for heart failure if present. Potassium supplements have been recommended to obviate the danger of the hypokalemia but are not necessary. Occasionally, an excessive rise in platelets occurs after 1–2 weeks of therapy. Antiplatelet therapy, e.g., aspirin, should be considered if the platelet count rises to >800 × 10^9/L.

COBALAMIN DEFICIENCY It is usually necessary to treat patients who have developed cobalamin deficiency with lifelong regular cobalamin injections. In the UK, the form used is hydroxocobalamin; in the United States, cyanocobalamin. In a few instances, the underlying cause of cobalamin deficiency can be permanently corrected, e.g., fish tapeworm, tropical sprue, or an intestinal stagnant loop that is amenable to surgery. The indications for starting cobalamin therapy are a well-documented megaloblastic anemia or other hematologic abnormalities and neuropathy due to the deficiency. Patients with borderline serum cobalamin levels but no hematologic or other abnormality may be followed to make sure that the cobalamin deficiency does not progress (discussed later). If malabsorption of cobalamin or rises in serum MMA levels have been demonstrated, however, these patients also should be given regular maintenance cobalamin therapy. Cobalamin should be given routinely to all patients who have had a total gastrectomy or ileal resection. Patients who have undergone gastric reduction for control of obesity or who are receiving long-term treatment with proton pump inhibitors should be screened and, if necessary, given cobalamin replacement.

Replenishment of body stores should be complete with six 1000-μg IM injections of hydroxocobalamin given at 3- to 7-day intervals. More frequent doses are usually used in patients with cobalamin neuropathy, but there is no evidence that they produce a better response. Allergic reactions are rare and may require desensitization or antihistamine or glucocorticoid cover. For maintenance therapy, 1000 μg hydroxocobalamin IM once every 3 months is satisfactory. Because of the poorer retention of cyanocobalamin, protocols generally use higher and more frequent doses, e.g., 1000 μg IM monthly for maintenance treatment.

Because a small fraction of cobalamin can be absorbed passively through mucous membranes even when there is complete failure of physiologic IF-dependent absorption, large daily oral doses (1000–2000 μg) of cyanocobalamin have been used in PA for replacement and maintenance of normal cobalamin status in, e.g., food malabsorption of cobalamin. Sublingual therapy has also been proposed for those in whom injections are difficult because of a bleeding tendency and who may not tolerate oral therapy. If oral therapy is used, it is important to monitor compliance, particularly with elderly, forgetful patients.

For treatment of patients with subnormal serum B_{12} levels with a normal MCV and no hypersegmentation of neutrophils, a negative IF antibody test result in the absence of tests of B_{12} absorption is problematic. Some (perhaps 15%) cases may be due to TC I (HC) deficiency. Homocysteine and/or MMA measurements may help, but in the absence of these tests and with otherwise normal gastrointestinal function, repeat serum B_{12} assay after 6–12 months may help one decide whether to start cobalamin therapy.

FOLATE DEFICIENCY Oral doses of 5–15 mg folic acid daily are satisfactory, as sufficient folate is absorbed from these extremely large doses even in patients with severe malabsorption. The length of time therapy must be continued depends on the underlying disease. It is customary to continue therapy for about 4 months, when all folate-deficient red cells will have been eliminated and replaced by new folate-replete populations.

Before large doses of folic acid are given, cobalamin deficiency must be excluded and, if present, corrected; otherwise cobalamin neuropathy may develop despite a response of the anemia of cobalamin deficiency to folate therapy. Studies in the United States, however, suggest that there is no increase in the proportion of individuals with low serum cobalamin levels and no anemia since food fortification with folic acid, but it is unknown if there has been a change in incidence of cobalamin neuropathy.

Long-term folic acid therapy is required when the underlying cause of the deficiency cannot be corrected and the deficiency is likely to recur, e.g., in chronic dialysis or hemolytic anemias. It may also be necessary in gluten-induced enteropathy that does not respond to a gluten-free diet. When mild but chronic folate deficiency occurs, it is preferable to encourage improvement in the diet after correcting the deficiency with a short course of folic acid. In any patient receiving long-term folic acid therapy, it is important to measure the serum cobalamin level at regular (e.g., once-yearly) intervals to exclude the coincidental development of cobalamin deficiency.

Folinic Acid (5-Formyl-THF) This is a stable form of fully reduced folate. It is given orally or parenterally to overcome the toxic effects of methotrexate or other DHF reductase inhibitors.

PROPHYLACTIC FOLIC ACID In many countries, food is fortified with folic acid (in grain or flour) to prevent neural tube defects. It is also used in chronic dialysis patients and in parenteral feeds. Prophylactic folic acid has been used to reduce homocysteine levels to prevent cardiovascular disease, but further data are needed to assess the benefit for this and for cognitive function in the elderly.

Pregnancy Folic acid, 400 μg daily, should be given as a supplement before and throughout pregnancy. In women who have had a previous fetus with an NTD, 5 mg daily is recommended when pregnancy is contemplated and throughout the subsequent pregnancy.

Infancy and Childhood The incidence of folate deficiency is so high in the smallest premature babies during the first 6 weeks of life that folic acid (e.g., 1 mg daily) should be given routinely to those weighing <1500 g at birth and to larger premature babies who require exchange transfusions or develop feeding difficulties, infections, or vomiting and diarrhea.

The World Health Organization currently recommends routine supplementation with iron and folic acid in children in countries where iron deficiency is common and child mortality, largely due to infectious diseases, is high. However, some studies suggest that in areas where malaria rates are high, this approach may increase the incidence of severe illness and death. Even where malaria is rare, there appears to be no survival benefit.

MEGALOBLASTIC ANEMIA NOT DUE TO COBALAMIN OR FOLATE DEFICIENCY OR ALTERED METABOLISM

This may occur with many antimetabolic drugs (e.g., hydroxyurea, cytosine arabinoside, 6-mercaptopurine) that inhibit DNA replication. Antiviral nucleoside analogues used in treatment of HIV infection may also cause macrocytosis and megaloblastic marrow changes. In the rare disease orotic aciduria, two consecutive enzymes in purine synthesis are defective. The condition responds to therapy with uridine, which bypasses the block. In thiamine-responsive megaloblastic anemia, there is a genetic defect in the high-affinity thiamine transport (*SLC19A2*) gene. This causes defective RNA ribose synthesis through impaired activity of trans-ketolase, a thiamine-dependent enzyme in the pentose cycle. This leads to reduced nucleic acid production. It may be associated with diabetes mellitus and deafness and the presence of many ringed sideroblasts in the marrow. The explanation is unclear for megaloblastic changes in the marrow in some patients with acute myeloid leukemia and myelodysplasia.

CHAPTER 10

HEMOLYTIC ANEMIAS AND ANEMIA DUE TO ACUTE BLOOD LOSS

Lucio Luzzatto

DEFINITIONS

A finite life span is a distinct characteristic of red cells. Hence, a logical, time-honored classification of anemias is in three groups: (1) decreased production of red cells, (2) increased destruction of red cells, and (3) acute blood loss. Decreased production is covered in Chaps. 7, 9, and 11; increased destruction and acute blood loss are covered in this chapter.

All patients who are anemic as a result of either increased destruction or acute blood loss have two important elements in common: the anemia results from overconsumption of red cells from the peripheral blood, yet the supply of cells from the bone marrow (in the absence of coexisting marrow disease) is usually increased, as reflected by a reticulocytosis. On the other hand, physical loss of red cells from the bloodstream—which in most cases also means physical loss *from* the body—is fundamentally different from destruction of red cells *within* the body. Therefore, the clinical aspects and the pathophysiology of anemia in these two groups of patients are quite different, and they will be considered separately.

HEMOLYTIC ANEMIAS

With respect to primary etiology, anemias due to increased destruction of red cells, which we know as hemolytic anemias (HAs), may be *inherited* or *acquired* (**Table 10-1**). From the clinical point of view they may be more *acute* or more *chronic*, they may vary from mild to very severe, and the site of hemolysis may be predominantly *intravascular* or *extravascular*. With respect to mechanisms, HAs may be due to *intracorpuscular* causes or to *extracorpuscular* causes. But before reviewing the individual types of HA, it is appropriate to consider what they have in common.

GENERAL CLINICAL AND LABORATORY FEATURES

The clinical presentation of a patient with anemia is greatly influenced in the first place by whether the onset is abrupt or gradual, and HAs are no exception. A patient with autoimmune HA or with favism may be a medical emergency, whereas a patient with mild hereditary spherocytosis or with cold agglutinin disease may be diagnosed after years. This is due in large measure to the remarkable ability of the body to adapt to anemia when it is slowly progressing (Chap. 2).

TABLE 10-1

CLASSIFICATION OF HEMOLYTIC ANEMIAS*

	INTRACORPUSCULAR DEFECTS	EXTRACORPUSCULAR FACTORS
Hereditary	Hemoglobinopathies Enzymopathies Membrane-cytoskeletal defects	Familial (atypical) hemolytic uremic syndrome
Acquired	Paroxysmal nocturnal hemoglobinuria (PNH)	Mechanical destruction (microangiopathic) Toxic agents Drugs Infectious Autoimmune

*Hereditary causes correlate with intracorpuscular defects because these defects are due to inherited mutations. The one exception is PNH because the defect is due to an acquired somatic mutation. Similarly, acquired causes correlate with extracorpuscular factors because mostly these factors are exogenous. The one exception is familial hemolytic uremic syndrome (HUS; often referred to as atypical HUS) because here an inherited abnormality allows complement activation to be excessive, with bouts of production of membrane attack complex capable of destroying normal red cells.

TABLE 10-2

SOME COMMON FEATURES OF HEMOLYTIC DISORDERS

General examination	Jaundice, pallor
Other physical findings	Spleen may be enlarged; bossing of skull in severe congenital cases
Hemoglobin level	From normal to severely reduced
MCV, MCH	Usually increased
Reticulocytes	Increased
Bilirubin	Increased (mostly unconjugated)
LDH	Increased (up to 10× normal with intravascular hemolysis)
Haptoglobin	Reduced to absent (if hemolysis is part intravascular)

Abbreviations: LDH, lactate dehydrogenase; MCH, mean corpuscular hemoglobin; MCV, mean corpuscular volume.

What differentiates HAs from other anemias is that the patient has signs and symptoms arising directly from hemolysis (Table 10-2). At the clinical level, the main sign is *jaundice*; in addition, the patient may report discoloration of the urine. In many cases of HA, the spleen is enlarged because it is a preferential site of hemolysis, and in some cases, the liver may be enlarged as well. In all severe congenital forms of HA, there also may be skeletal changes due to overactivity of the bone marrow (although they are never as severe as they are in thalassemia).

The laboratory features of HA are related to hemolysis per se and the erythropoietic response of the bone marrow. Hemolysis regularly produces in the serum an increase in unconjugated bilirubin and aspartate transaminase (AST); urobilinogen will be increased in both urine and stool. If hemolysis is mainly intravascular, the telltale sign is hemoglobinuria (often associated with hemosiderinuria); in the serum, there is increased hemoglobin, lactate dehydrogenase (LDH) is increased, and haptoglobin is reduced. In contrast, the bilirubin level may be normal or only mildly elevated. The main sign of the erythropoietic response by the bone marrow is an increase in reticulocytes (Table 10-2), a test all too often neglected in the initial workup of a patient with anemia. Usually the increase will be reflected in both the percentage of reticulocytes (the more commonly quoted figure) and the absolute reticulocyte count (the more definitive parameter). The increased number of reticulocytes is associated with an increased mean corpuscular volume (MCV) in the blood count. On the blood smear, this is reflected in the presence of macrocytes; there is also polychromasia and sometimes one sees nucleated red cells. In most cases, a bone marrow aspirate is not necessary in the diagnostic workup; if it is done, it will show erythroid hyperplasia. In practice, once a HA is suspected, specific tests will usually be required for a definitive diagnosis of a specific type of HA.

GENERAL PATHOPHYSIOLOGY

The mature red cell is the product of a developmental pathway that brings the phenomenon of differentiation to an extreme. An orderly sequence of events produces synchronous changes whereby the gradual accumulation of a huge amount of hemoglobin in the cytoplasm (to a final level of 340 g/L, i.e., about 5 m*M*) goes hand in hand with the gradual loss of cellular organelles and of biosynthetic abilities. In the end, the erythroid cell undergoes a process that has features of apoptosis, including nuclear pyknosis and actual loss of the nucleus. However, the final result is more altruistic than suicidal; the cytoplasmic body, instead of disintegrating, is now able to provide oxygen to all cells in the human organism for some remaining 120 days of the red cell "life" span.

As a result of this unique process of differentiation and maturation, intermediary metabolism is drastically curtailed in mature red cells (Fig. 10-1); for instance, cytochrome-mediated oxidative phosphorylation has been lost with the loss of mitochondria (through a process of physiologic autophagy); therefore, there is no backup to anaerobic glycolysis for the production of adenosine triphosphate (ATP). Also the capacity of making protein has been lost with the loss of ribosomes. This places the cell's limited metabolic apparatus at risk because if any protein component deteriorates, it cannot be replaced, as it would be in most other cells, and in fact the activity of most enzymes gradually decreases as red cells age. Another consequence of the relative simplicity of red cells is that they have a very limited range of ways to manifest distress under hardship: in essence, any sort of metabolic failure will eventually lead either to structural damage to the membrane or to failure of the cation pump. In either case, the life span of the red cell is reduced, which is the definition of a *hemolytic disorder*. If the rate of red cell destruction exceeds the capacity of the bone marrow to produce more red cells, the hemolytic disorder will manifest as HA.

Thus, the essential pathophysiologic process common to all HAs is an increased red cell turnover. The gold standard for proving that the life span of red cells is reduced (compared with the normal value of about 120 days) is a *red cell survival* study, which can be carried out by labeling the red cells with ^{51}Cr and measuring residual radioactivity over several days or weeks; however, this classic test is now available in very few centers, and it is rarely necessary. If the hemolytic event is transient, it does not usually cause any long-term

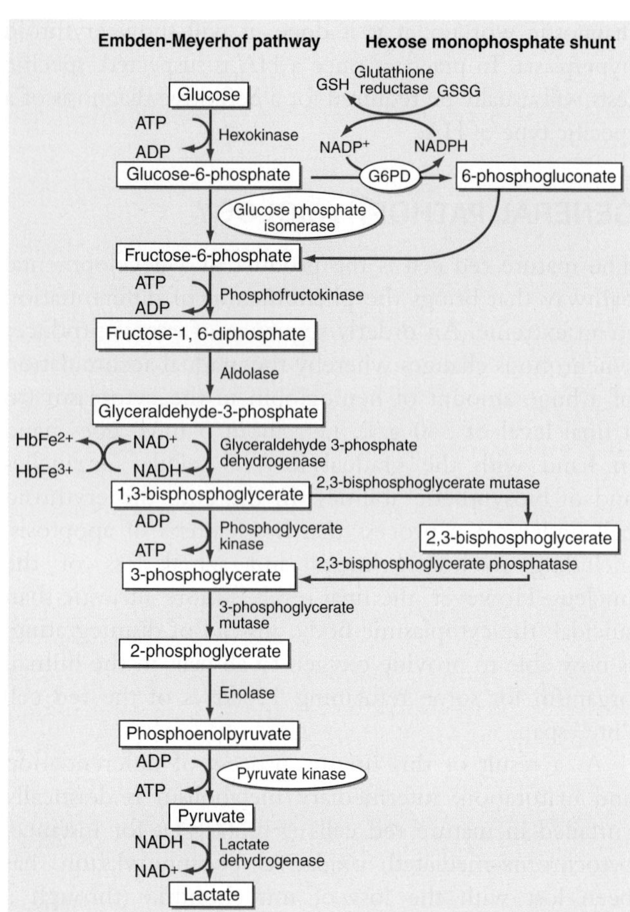

FIGURE 10-1

Red blood cell metabolism. The Embden-Meyerhof pathway (glycolysis) generates adenosine triphosphate (ATP) for energy and membrane maintenance. The generation of nicotinamide adenine dinucleotide phosphate (NADPH) maintains hemoglobin in a reduced state. The hexose monophosphate shunt generates nicotinamide adenine dinucleotide phosphate (NADPH) that is used to reduce glutathione, which protects the red cell against oxidant stress. Regulation of 2,3-bisphosphoglycerate levels is a critical determinant of oxygen affinity of hemoglobin. Enzyme deficiency states in order of prevalence: glucose-6-phosphate dehydrogenase (G6PD) > pyruvate kinase > glucose-6-phosphate isomerase > rare deficiencies of other enzymes in the pathway. The more common enzyme deficiencies are encircled. ADP, adenosine diphosphate.

consequences, except for an increased requirement for erythropoietic factors, particularly folic acid. However, if hemolysis is recurrent or persistent, the increased bilirubin production favors the formation of gallstones. If a considerable proportion of hemolysis takes place in the spleen, as is often the case, splenomegaly may become increasingly a feature, and hypersplenism may develop, with consequent neutropenia and/or thrombocytopenia.

The increased red cell turnover also has metabolic consequences. In normal subjects, the iron from effete red cells is very efficiently recycled by the body; however, with chronic intravascular hemolysis, the persistent hemoglobinuria will cause considerable iron loss, needing replacement. With chronic extravascular hemolysis the opposite problem, iron overload, is more common, especially if the patient needs frequent blood transfusions. Chronic iron overload will cause secondary hemochromatosis: this will cause damage particularly to the liver, eventually leading to cirrhosis, and to the heart muscle, eventually causing heart failure.

Compensated hemolysis versus hemolytic anemia

Red cell destruction is a potent stimulus for erythropoiesis, which is mediated by erythropoietin (EPO) produced by the kidney. This mechanism is so effective that in many cases the increased output of red cells from the bone marrow can fully balance an increased destruction of red cells. In such cases, we say that hemolysis is *compensated*. The pathophysiology of compensated hemolysis is similar to what we have just described, except there is no anemia. This notion is important from the diagnostic point of view because a patient with a hemolytic condition, even an inherited one, may present without anemia. It is also important from the point of view of management because compensated hemolysis may become "decompensated"—i.e., anemia may suddenly appear—in certain circumstances, for instance pregnancy, folate deficiency, or renal failure, interfering with adequate EPO production. Another general feature of chronic HAs is seen when any intercurrent condition, for instance, an acute infection, depresses erythropoiesis. When this happens, in view of the increased rate of red cell turnover, the effect will be predictably much more marked than in a person who does not have hemolysis. The most dramatic example is infection by parvovirus B19, which may cause a rather precipitous fall in hemoglobin, an occurrence sometimes referred to as *aplastic crisis*.

INHERITED HEMOLYTIC ANEMIAS

There are three essential components in the red cell: (1) hemoglobin, (2) the membrane–cytoskeleton complex, and (3) the metabolic machinery necessary to keep (1) and (2) in working order. Diseases caused by abnormalities of hemoglobin, or hemoglobinopathies, are covered in Chap. 8. Here we will deal with diseases of the other two components.

Hemolytic anemias due to abnormalities of the membrane-cytoskeleton complex

The detailed architecture of the red cell membrane is complex, but its basic design is relatively simple (Fig. 10-2). The lipid bilayer incorporates phospholipids

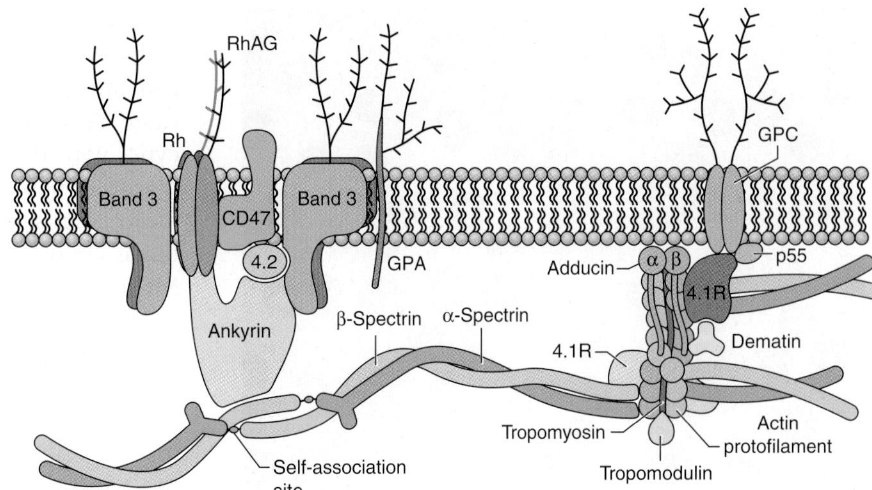

FIGURE 10-2
Diagram of red cell membrane-cytoskeleton. GPA, glycophorin A; GPC, glycophorin C; RhAG, Rh-associated glycoprotein (For explanation see text.) *(From N Young et al: Clinical Hematology. Copyright Elsevier, 2006; with permission.)*

and cholesterol, and it is spanned by a number of proteins that have their hydrophobic transmembrane domains embedded in the membrane. Most of these proteins have hydrophilic domains extending toward both the outside and the inside of the cell. Other proteins are tethered to the membrane through a glycosylphosphatidylinositol (GPI) anchor, and they have only an extracellular domain. These proteins are arranged roughly perpendicular to or lying across the membrane; they include ion channels, receptors for complement components, receptors for other ligands, and some of unknown function. The most abundant of these proteins are glycophorins and the so-called band 3, an anion transporter. The extracellular domains of many of these proteins are heavily glycosylated, and they carry antigenic determinants that correspond to blood groups. Underneath the membrane and tangential to it is a network of other proteins that make up the cytoskeleton: the main cytoskeletal protein is spectrin, the basic unit of which is a dimer of α-spectrin and β-spectrin. The membrane is physically linked to the cytoskeleton by a third set of proteins (including ankyrin and the so-called band 4.1 and band 4.2), which thus make these two structures intimately connected to each other.

The membrane–cytoskeleton complex is indeed so integrated that, not surprisingly, an abnormality of almost any of its components will be disturbing or disruptive, causing structural failure, which results ultimately in hemolysis. These abnormalities are almost invariably inherited mutations; thus, diseases of the membrane–cytoskeleton complex belong to the category of inherited HAs. Before the red cells lyse, they often exhibit more or less specific morphologic changes that alter the normal biconcave disk shape. Thus, the majority of the diseases in this group have been known for over a century as *hereditary spherocytosis* and *hereditary elliptocytosis*.

Hereditary spherocytosis (HS)

This is a relatively common type of HA, with an estimated frequency of at least 1 in 5000. Its identification is credited to Minkowksy and Chauffard, who at the end of the nineteenth century reported families in which HS was inherited as an autosomal dominant condition (Fig 10-3*A*). From this seminal work, HS came to be defined as an inherited form of HA associated with the presence of spherocytes in the peripheral blood. In addition, in vitro studies revealed that the red cells were abnormally susceptible to lysis in hypotonic media: indeed, the presence of *osmotic fragility* became the main diagnostic test for HS. Today we know that HS, thus defined, is genetically heterogeneous, i.e., it can arise from a variety of mutations in one of several genes (Table 10-3). Whereas classically the inheritance of HS is autosomal dominant (with the patients being heterozygous), some severe forms are instead autosomal recessive (with the patient being homozygous).

Clinical presentation and diagnosis

The spectrum of clinical severity of HS is broad. Severe cases may present in infancy with severe anemia, whereas mild cases may present in young adults or even later in life. In women, HS is sometimes first diagnosed when anemia is investigated during pregnancy. The main clinical findings are jaundice, an enlarged spleen, and often gallstones; indeed, it is often the finding of gallstones in a young person that triggers diagnostic investigations.

The variability in clinical manifestations that is observed among patients with HS is largely due to the different underlying molecular lesions (Table 10-3). Not only are mutations of several genes involved, but individual mutations of the same gene can also give very different clinical manifestations. In milder cases,

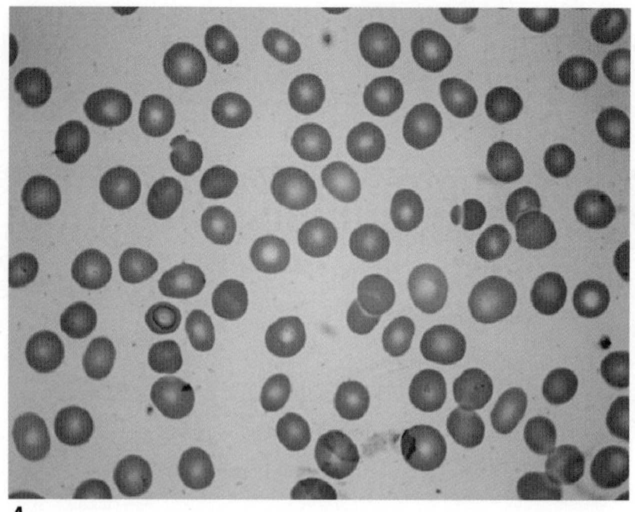

A

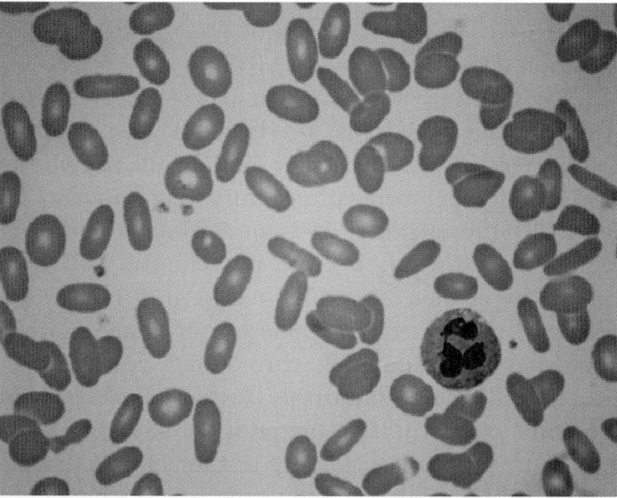

B

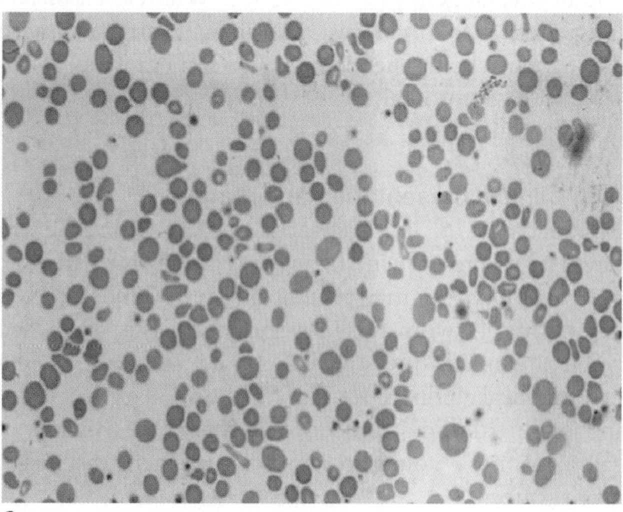

C

FIGURE 10-3

Peripheral blood smear from patients with membrane-cytoskeleton abnormalities. ***A.*** Hereditary spherocytosis. ***B.*** Hereditary elliptocytosis, heterozygote. ***C.*** Elliptocytosis, with both alleles of the α-spectrin gene mutated.

hemolysis is often compensated (discussed earlier), and this may cause variation in time, even in the same patient, because intercurrent conditions (e.g., infection) cause decompensation. The anemia is usually normocytic, with the characteristic morphology that gives the disease its name. A characteristic feature is an increase in mean corpuscular hemoglobin concentration (MCHC); this is almost the only condition in which an increased MCHC is seen.

When there is a family history (Fig. 10-3A), it is usually easy to suspect the diagnosis, but there may be no family history for at least two reasons. (1) The patient may have a de novo mutation, i.e., a mutation that has taken place in a germ cell of one of his or her parents or early after zygote formation. (2) The patient may have a recessive form of HS (Table 10-3). In most cases, the diagnosis can be made on the basis of red cell morphology and of a test for osmotic fragility, a modified version of which is called the "pink test." In some cases, a definitive diagnosis can be obtained only by molecular studies demonstrating a mutation in one of the genes underlying HS. This is usually carried out in laboratories with special expertise in this area.

TREATMENT Hereditary Spherocytosis

We don't have a causal treatment for HS; i.e., no way has yet been found to correct the basic defect in the membrane–cytoskeleton structure. However, it has been apparent for a long time that the spleen plays a special role in HS through a dual mechanism. On one hand, like in many other HAs, the spleen itself is a major site of destruction; on the other hand, transit through the splenic circulation makes the defective red cells more spherocytic and therefore accelerates their demise, even though lysis may take place elsewhere. For these reasons, splenectomy has long been regarded as a prime, almost obligatory, therapeutic measure in HS. Therefore, current guidelines (not evidence-based) are as follows. (1) Avoid splenectomy in mild cases. (2) Delay splenectomy until at least 4 years of age, after the risk of severe sepsis has peaked. (3) Antipneumococcal vaccination before splenectomy is imperative, whereas penicillin prophylaxis postsplenectomy is controversial. (4) There is no doubt that HS patients often may require cholecystectomy, in which case the practice has been to also carry out a splenectomy at the same time. Today the decision regarding this combined surgery should not be regarded as automatic; cholecystectomy is usually done via the laparoscopic approach, and splenectomy should be carried out if clinically indicated.

TABLE 10-3

INHERITED DISEASES OF THE RED CELL MEMBRANE–CYTOSKELETON

GENE	CHROMOSOMAL LOCATION	PROTEIN PRODUCED	DISEASE(S) WITH CERTAIN MUTATIONS (INHERITANCE)	COMMENTS
SPTA1	1q22-q23	α-Spectrin	HS (recessive)	Rare
			HE (dominant)	Mutations of this gene account for about 65% of HE. More severe forms may be due to coexistence of an otherwise silent mutant allele
SPTB	14q23-q24.1	β-Spectrin	HS (dominant)	Rare
			HE (dominant)	Mutations of this gene account for about 30% of HE, including some severe forms
ANK1	8p11.2	Ankyrin	HS (dominant)	May account for majority of HS
SLC4A1	17q21	Band 3 (anion channel)	HS (dominant)	Mutations of this gene may account for about 25% of HS
			Southeast Asia ovalocytosis (dominant)	Polymorphic mutation (deletion of 9 amino acids); clinically asymptomatic; protective against *Plasmodium falciparum*
			Stomatocytosis	Certain specific missense mutations shift protein function from anion exchanger to cation conductance
EPB41	1p33-p34.2	Band 4.1	HE (dominant)	Mutations of this gene account for about 5% of HE: mostly with prominent morphology but no hemolysis in heterozygotes; severe hemolysis in homozygotes
EPB42	15q15-q21	Band 4.2	HS (recessive)	Mutations of this gene account for about 3% of HS.
RHAG	6p21.1-p11	Rhesus antigen	Chronic nonspherocytic hemolytic anemia	Very rare; associated with total loss of all Rh antigens

Abbreviations: HE, hereditary elliptocytosis; HS, hereditary spherocytosis.

Hereditary elliptocytosis (HE)

HE is at least as heterogeneous as HS, both from the genetic point of view (Table 10-3) and from the clinical point of view. Again, it is the shape of the red cells that gives the name to these conditions, but there is no direct correlation between the elliptocytic morphology and clinical severity. In fact, some mild or even asymptomatic cases may have nearly 100% elliptocytes, whereas in severe cases, it is all sorts of bizarre poikilocytes that predominate. Clinical features and recommended management are similar to those outlined above for HS. Although the spleen may not have the specific role it has in HS, in severe cases, splenectomy may be beneficial. The prevalence of HE causing clinical disease is similar to that of HS. However, an asymptomatic form, referred to as Southeast Asia ovalocytosis, has a frequency of up to 7% in certain populations, presumably as a result of malaria selection.

Disorders of cation transport

These rare conditions with autosomal dominant inheritance are characterized by increased intracellular sodium in red cells, with concomitant loss of potassium: indeed, they are sometimes discovered through the incidental finding, in a blood test, of high serum K^+ (*pseudohyperkalemia*). In patients from some families, the cation transport disturbance is associated with gain of water: as a result, the red cells are overhydrated (low MCHC), and on a blood smear, the normally round-shaped central pallor is replaced by a linear-shaped central pallor, which has earned this disorder the name *stomatocytosis*. In patients from other families, the red cells are instead dehydrated (high MCHC), and their consequent rigidity has earned this disorder the name *xerocytosis*. In these disorders, one would suspect that the primary defect may be in a cation transporter. In most cases, this has not yet been demonstrated, but interestingly, certain missense mutations of the *SLC4A1* gene encoding band 3 (Table 10-3) give stomatocytosis. Hemolysis can vary from relatively mild to quite severe. From the practical point of view, it is important to know that splenectomy is contraindicated, as it has been followed in a majority of cases by severe thromboembolic complications.

Enzyme abnormalities

When there is an important defect in the membrane or in the cytoskeleton, hemolysis is a direct consequence of the fact that the very structure of the red cell is abnormal. Instead, when one of the enzymes is defective, the consequences will depend on the precise role of that enzyme in the metabolic machinery of the red cell, which, in first approximation, has two important functions: (1) to provide energy in the form of ATP and (2) to prevent oxidative damage to hemoglobin and to other proteins.

Abnormalities of the glycolytic pathway

Since red cells, in the course of their differentiation, have sacrificed not only their nucleus and their ribsomes but also their mitochondria, they rely exclusively on the anaerobic portion of the glycolytic pathway for producing energy in the form of ATP. Most of the ATP is required by the red cell for cation transport against a concentration gradient across the membrane. If this fails, due to a defect of any of the enzymes of the glycolytic pathway, the result will be hemolytic disease (**Table 10-4**).

Pyruvate kinase deficiency

Abnormalities of the glycolytic pathway are all inherited and all rare. Among them, deficiency of pyruvate kinase (PK) is the least rare, with an estimated prevalence of the order of 1:10,000. The clinical picture is that of an HA that often presents in a newborn with neonatal jaundice; the jaundice persists, and it is usually associated with a very high reticulocytosis. The anemia is of variable severity; sometimes it is so severe as to require regular blood transfusion treatment; sometimes it is mild, bordering on a nearly compensated hemolytic

TABLE 10-4

RED CELL ENZYME ABNORMALITIES CAUSING HEMOLYSIS

	ENZYME (ACRONYM)	CHROMOSOMAL LOCATION	PREVALENCE OF ENZYME DEFICIENCY (RANK)	CLINICAL MANIFESTATIONS EXTRA-RED CELL	COMMENTS
Glycolytic pathway	Hexokinase (HK)	10q22	Very rare		Other isoenzymes known
	Glucose 6-phosphate isomerase (G6PI)	19q31.1	Rare (4)*	NM, CNS	
	Phosphofructokinase (PFK)	12q13	Very rare	Myopathy	
	Aldolase	16q22-24	Very rare		
	Triose phosphate isomerase (TPI)	12p13	Very rare	CNS (severe), NM	
	Glyceraldehyde 3-phosphate dehydrogenase (GAPD)	12p13.31-p13.1	Very rare	Myopathy	
	Diphosphoglycerate mutase (DPGM)	7q31-q34	Very rare		Erythrocytosis rather than hemolysis
	Phosphoglycerate kinase (PGK)	Xq13	Very rare	CNS, NM	May benefit from splenectomy
	Pyruvate kinase (PK)	1q21	Rare (2)*		May benefit from splenectomy
Redox	Glucose 6-phosphate dehydrogenase (G6PD)	Xq28	Common (1)*	Very rarely granulocytes	In almost all cases only AHA from exogenous trigger
	Glutathione synthase	20q11.2	Very rare	CNS	
	γ-Glutamylcysteine synthase	6p12	Very rare	CNS	
	Cytochrome b5 reductase	22q13.31-qter	Rare	CNS	Methemoglobinemia rather than hemolysis
Nucleotide	Adenylate kinase (AK)	9q34.1	Very rare	CNS	
Metabolism	Pyrimidine 5′-nucleotidase (P5N)	3q11-q12	Rare (3)*		May benefit from splenectomy

*The numbers from (1) to (4) indicate the ranking order of these enzymopathies in terms of frequency.

Abbreviations: AHA, acquired hemolytic anemia; CNS, central nervous system: NM, neuromuscular manifestations.

disorder. As a result, the diagnosis may be delayed, and in some cases, it is made in young adults, for instance, in a woman, during her first pregnancy, when the anemia may get worse. In part, the delay in diagnosis is due to the fact that the anemia is remarkably well tolerated because the metabolic block at the last step in glycolysis causes an increase in bisphosphoglycerate (or DPG), a major effector of the hemoglobin–oxygen dissociation curve; thus, the oxygen delivery to the tissues is enhanced.

TREATMENT **Pryuvate Kinase Deficiency**

The management of PK deficiency is mainly supportive. In view of the marked increase in red cell turnover, oral folic acid supplements should be given constantly. Blood transfusion should be used as necessary, and iron chelation may have to be added if the blood transfusion requirement is high enough to cause iron overload. In these patients, who have more severe disease, splenectomy may be beneficial. There is a single case report of curative treatment of PK deficiency by bone marrow transplantation from an HLA-identical PK-normal sibling. This seems a viable option for severe cases when a sibling donor is available.

Other glycolytic enzyme abnormalities

All of these defects are rare to very rare (Table 10-4), and all cause HA with varying degrees of severity. It is not unusual for the presentation to be in the guise of severe neonatal jaundice, which may require exchange transfusion. If the anemia is less severe, it may present later in life, or it may even remain asymptomatic and be detected incidentally when a blood count is done for unrelated reasons. The spleen is often enlarged. When other systemic manifestations occur, they involve the central nervous system, sometimes entailing severe mental retardation (particularly in the case of triose phosphate isomerase deficiency), the neuromuscular system, or both. The *diagnosis* of HA is usually not difficult because of the triad of normomacrocytic anemia, reticulocytosis, and hyperbilirubinemia. Enzymopathies should be considered in the differential diagnosis of any chronic Coombs-negative HA. In most cases of glycolytic enzymopathies, the morphologic abnormalities of red cells characteristically seen in membrane disorders are conspicuous by their absence. A definitive diagnosis can be made only by demonstrating the deficiency of an individual enzyme by quantitative assays carried out in only a few specialized laboratories. If a particular molecular abnormality is already known in a family, then of course one could test directly for that at the DNA level, bypassing the need for enzyme assays.

Abnormalities of redox metabolism

G6PD deficiency

Glucose 6-phosphate dehydrogenase (G6PD) is a housekeeping enzyme critical in the redox metabolism of all aerobic cells (Fig. 10-1). In red cells, its role is even more critical because it is the only source of NADPH that directly and via glutathione (GSH) defends these cells against oxidative stress. G6PD deficiency is a prime example of an HA due to interaction between an intracorpuscular cause and an extracorpuscular cause because in the majority of cases, hemolysis is triggered by an exogenous agent. Although a decrease in G6PD activity is noted in most tissues of G6PD-deficient subjects, the decrease is less marked than in red cells, and it does not seem to have a clinical impact.

GENETIC CONSIDERATIONS

The G6PD gene is X-linked, and this has important implications. First, as males have only one G6PD gene (i.e., they are hemizygous for this gene), they must be either normal or G6PD-deficient. By contrast, females, having two G6PD genes, can be normal, deficient (homozygous), or intermediate (heterozygous). As a result of the phenomenon of X-chromosome inactivation, heterozygous females are genetic mosaics, with a highly variable ratio of G6PD-normal to G6PD-deficient cells and an equally variable degree of clinical expression: some heterozygotes can be just as affected as hemizygous males. The enzymatically active form of G6PD is either a dimer or a tetramer of a single protein subunit of 514 amino acids. G6PD-deficient subjects have been found invariably to have mutations in the coding region of the G6PD gene (Fig. 10-4). Almost all of some 150 different mutations known are single missense point mutations, entailing single amino acid replacements in the G6PD protein. In most cases, these

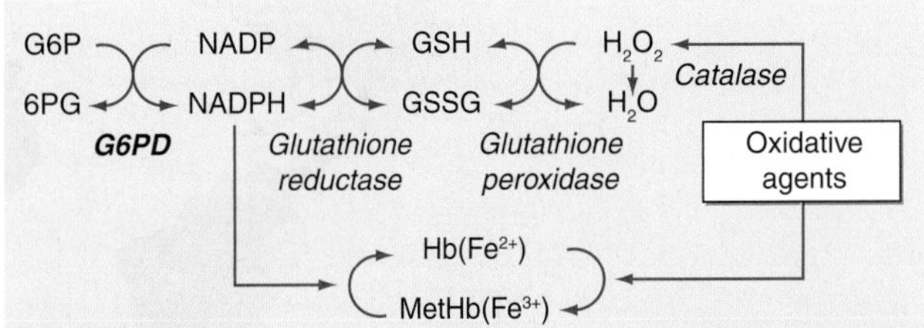

FIGURE 10-4

Diagram of redox metabolism in the red cell. G6P, glucose 6-phosphate; G6PD, glucose 6-phosphate dehydrogenase; GSH, reduced glutathione; GSSG, oxidized glutathione; Hb, hemoglobin; MetHb, methemoglobin; NADP, nicotinamide adenine dinucleotide phosphate; NADPH, reduced nicotinamide adenine dinucleotide phosphate, 6PG, 6-phosphogluconate.

mutations cause G6PD deficiency by decreasing the in vivo stability of the protein; thus, the physiologic decrease in G6PD activity that takes place with red cell aging is greatly accelerated. In some cases, an amino acid replacement can also affect the catalytic function of the enzyme.

Among these mutations, those underlying *chronic nonspherocytic hemolytic anemia* (CNSHA; see "Clinical Manifestations" below) are a discrete subset. This much more severe clinical phenotype can be ascribed in some cases to adverse qualitative changes (for instance, a decreased affinity for the substrate, glucose 6-phosphate) or simply to the fact that the enzyme deficit is more extreme because of a more severe instability of the enzyme. For instance, a cluster of mutations map at or near the dimer interface, and clearly they compromise severely the formation of the dimer.

Epidemiology

G6PD deficiency is widely distributed in tropical and subtropical parts of the world (Africa, Southern Europe, the Middle East, Southeast Asia, and Oceania) (Fig. 10-5) and wherever people from those areas have migrated. A conservative estimate is that at least 400 million people have a G6PD deficiency gene. In several of these areas, the frequency of a G6PD deficiency gene may be as high as 20% or more. It would be quite extraordinary for a trait that causes significant pathology to spread widely and reach high frequencies in many populations without conferring some biologic advantage. Indeed, G6PD is one of the best characterized examples of genetic polymorphisms in the human species. Clinical field studies and in vitro experiments strongly support the view that G6PD deficiency has been selected by *Plasmodium falciparum* malaria, by virtue of the fact that it confers a relative resistance against this highly lethal infection. Whether this protective effect is exerted mainly in hemizygous males or in females heterozygous for G6PD deficiency is still not quite clear. Different G6PD variants underlie G6PD deficiency in different parts of the world. Some of the more widespread variants are G6PD Mediterranean on the shores of that sea, in the Middle East, and in India; G6PD A in Africa and in Southern Europe; G6PD Vianchan and G6PD Mahidol in Southeast Asia; G6PD Canton in China; and G6PD Union worldwide. The heterogeneity of polymorphic G6PD variants is proof of their independent origin, and it supports the notion that they have been selected by a common environmental agent, in keeping with the concept of convergent evolution (Fig. 10-5).

Clinical manifestations

The vast majority of people with G6PD deficiency remain clinically asymptomatic throughout their lifetimes; however, all of them have an increased risk of developing neonatal jaundice (NNJ) and a risk of developing acute hemolytic anemia (AHA) when challenged by a number of oxidative agents. NNJ related to G6PD deficiency is very rarely present at birth. The peak incidence of clinical onset is between day 2 and day 3, and in most cases the anemia is not severe. However, NNJ can be very severe in some G6PD-deficient babies, especially in association with prematurity, infection, or environmental factors (such as naphthalene–camphor balls used in babies' bedding and clothing), and the risk of severe NNJ is also increased by the coexistence of a monoallelic or biallelic mutation in the uridyl transferase gene (*UGT1A1*; the same mutations are associated with Gilbert syndrome). If

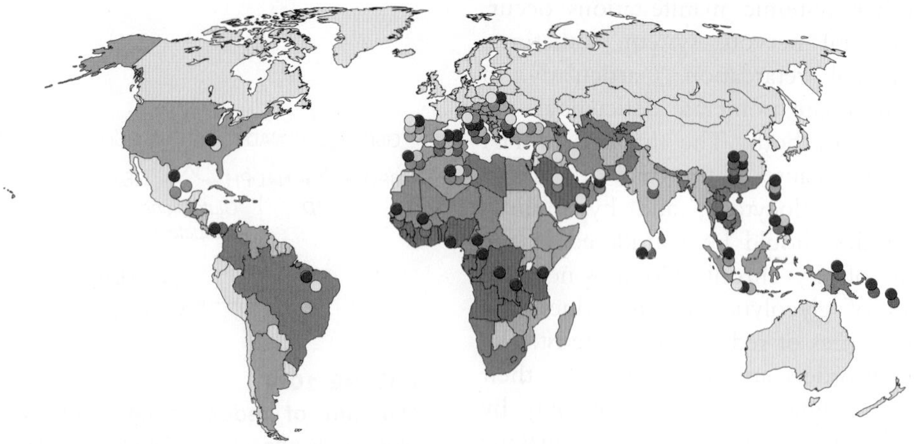

FIGURE 10-5
Epidemiology of G6PD deficiency throughout the world. The different shadings indicate increasingly high levels of prevalence, up to about 20%; the different colored symbols indicate individual genetic variants of G6PD, each one having a different mutation. (*From L Luzzatto et al, in C Scriver et al [eds]: The Metabolic & Molecular Bases of Inherited Disease, 8th ed. New York, McGraw-Hill, 2001.*)

TABLE 10-5

DRUGS THAT CARRY RISK OF CLINICAL HEMOLYSIS IN PERSONS WITH G6PD DEFICIENCY

	DEFINITE RISK	POSSIBLE RISK	DOUBTFUL RISK
Antimalarials	Primaquine Dapsone/chlorproguanil*	Chloroquine	Quinine
Sulphonamides/sulphones	Sulfamethoxazole Others Dapsone	Sulfasalazine Sulfadimidine	Sulfisoxazole Sulfadiazine
Antibacterial/antibiotics	Cotrimoxazole Nalidixic acid Nitrofurantoin Niridazole	Ciprofloxacin Norfloxacin	Chloramphenicol *p*-Aminosalicylic acid
Antipyretic/analgesics	Acetanilide Phenazopyridine	Acetylsalicylic acid high dose (>3 g/d)	Acetylsalicylic acid (<3 g/d) Acetaminophen Phenacetin
Other	Naphthalene Methylene blue	Vitamin K analogues Ascorbic acid >1 g Rasburicase	Doxorubicin Probenecid

*Marketed as Lapdap from 2003 to 2008.

inadequately managed, NNJ associated with G6PD deficiency can produce kernicterus and permanent neurologic damage.

AHA can develop as a result of three types of triggers: (1) fava beans, (2) infections, and (3) drugs (**Table 10-5**). Typically, a hemolytic attack starts with malaise, weakness, and abdominal or lumbar pain. After an interval of several hours to 2–3 days, the patient develops jaundice and often dark urine, due to hemoglobinuria. The onset can be extremely abrupt, especially with favism in children. The anemia is from moderate to extremely severe. It is usually normocytic and normochromic, and it is due partly to intravascular hemolysis. Hence, it is associated with hemoglobinemia, hemoglobinuria, high LDH, and low or absent plasma haptoglobin. The blood film shows anisocytosis, polychromasia, and spherocytes (**Fig. 10-6**). The most typical feature is the presence of bizarre poikilocytes, with red cells that appear to have unevenly distributed hemoglobin ("hemighosts") and red cells that appear to have had parts of them bitten away ("bite cells" or "blister cells"). A classical test, now rarely carried out, is supravital staining with methyl violet that, if done promptly, reveals the presence of Heinz bodies, consisting of precipitates of denatured hemoglobin and regarded as a signature of oxidative damage to red cells (except for the rare occurrence of an unstable hemoglobin). LDH is high and so is the unconjugated bilirubin, indicating that there is also extravascular hemolysis. The most serious threat from AHA in adults is the development of acute renal failure (this is exceedingly rare in children). Once the threat of acute anemia is over, and in the absence of comorbidity, full recovery from AHA associated with G6PD deficiency is the rule.

A very small minority of subjects with G6PD deficiency have *chronic nonspherocytic hemolytic anemia* (CNSHA) of variable severity. The patient is always a male, usually with a history of NNJ, who may present with anemia

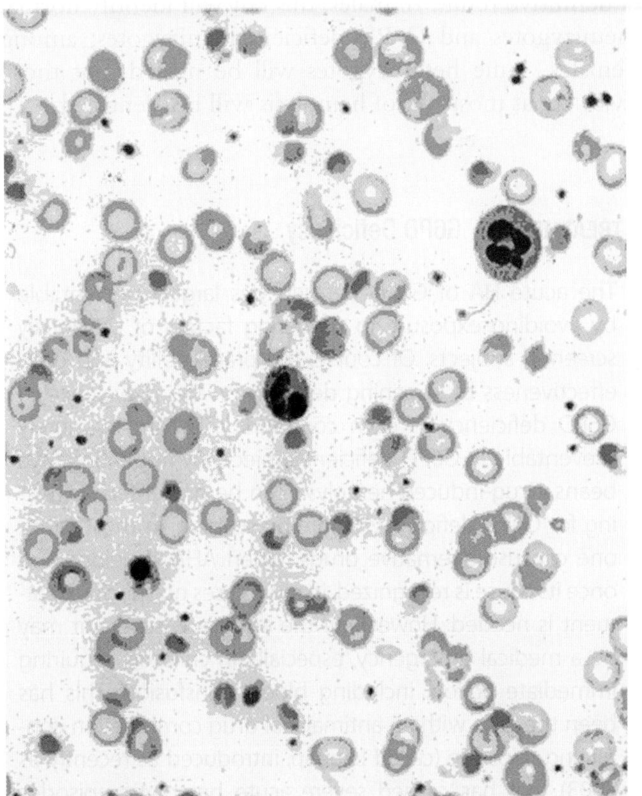

FIGURE 10-6

Peripheral blood smear from a 5-year-old G6PD-deficient boy with acute favism.

or unexplained jaundice or because of gallstones later in life. The spleen may be enlarged. The severity of anemia ranges in different patients from borderline to transfusion-dependent. The anemia is usually normo-macrocytic, with reticulocytosis. Bilirubin and LDH are increased. Although hemolysis is, by definition, chronic in these patients, they are also vulnerable to acute oxidative damage, and therefore the same agents that can cause acute HA in people with the ordinary type of G6PD deficiency will cause severe exacerbations in people with the severe form of G6PD deficiency. In some cases of CNSHA, the deficiency of G6PD is so severe in granulocytes that it becomes rate-limiting for their oxidative burst, with consequent increased susceptibility to some bacterial infections.

Laboratory diagnosis

The suspicion of G6PD deficiency can be confirmed by semiquantitative methods often referred to as screening tests, which are suitable for population studies and can correctly classify male subjects, in the steady state, as G6PD-normal or G6PD- deficient. However, in clinical practice, a diagnostic test is usually needed when the patient has had a hemolytic attack. This implies that the oldest, most G6PD-deficient red cells have been selectively destroyed, and young red cells, having higher G6PD activity, are being released into the circulation. Under these conditions, only a quantitative test can give a definitive result. In males, this test will identify normal hemizygotes and G6PD-deficient hemizygotes; among females, some heterozygotes will be missed, but those who are at most risk of hemolysis will be identified.

TREATMENT G6PD Deficiency

The acute HA of G6PD deficiency is largely preventable by avoiding exposure to triggering factors of previously screened subjects. Of course, the practicability and cost-effectiveness of screening depends on the prevalence of G6PD deficiency in each community. Favism is entirely preventable in G6PD-deficient subjects by not eating fava beans. Drug-induced hemolysis can be prevented by testing for G6PD deficiency before prescribing; in most cases, one can use alternative drugs. When AHA develops and once its cause is recognized, in most cases no specific treatment is needed. However, if the anemia is severe, it may be a medical emergency, especially in children, requiring immediate action, including blood transfusion. This has been the case with an antimalarial drug combination containing dapsone (called Lapdap, introduced as recently as 2003) that has caused severe acute hemolytic episodes in children with malaria in several African countries; after a few years, it was taken off the market. If there is acute renal failure, hemodialysis may be necessary, but if there is no previous kidney disease, recovery is the rule. The management of NNJ associated with G6PD deficiency is no different from that of NNJ due to other causes.

In cases with CNSHA, if the anemia is not severe, regular folic acid supplements and regular hematologic surveillance will suffice. It will be important to avoid exposure to potentially hemolytic drugs, and blood transfusion may be indicated when exacerbations occur, mostly in concomitance with intercurrent infection. In rare patients, regular blood transfusions may be required, in which case appropriate iron chelation should be instituted. Unlike in hereditary spherocytosis, there is no evidence of selective red cell destruction in the spleen; however, in practice, splenectomy has proven beneficial in severe cases.

Other abnormalities of the redox system

As mentioned earlier, GSH is a key player in the defense against oxidative stress. Inherited defects of GSH metabolism are exceedingly rare, but each one of them can give rise to chronic HA (Table 10-4). A rare, peculiar, usually self-limited severe HA of the first month of life, called *infantile poikilocytosis*, may be associated with deficiency of glutathione peroxidase (GSHPx) due not to an inherited abnormality but to transient nutritional deficiency of selenium, an element essential for the activity of GSHPx.

Pyrimidine 5′-nucleotidase (P5N) deficiency

P5N is a key enzyme in the catabolism of nucleotides arising from the degradation of nucleic acids that takes place in the final stages of erythroid cell maturation. How exactly its deficiency causes HA is not well understood, but a highly distinctive feature of this condition is a morphologic abnormality of the red cells known as *basophilic stippling*. The condition is rare, but it probably ranks third in frequency among red cell enzyme defects (after G6PD deficiency and PK deficiency). The anemia is lifelong, of variable severity, and may benefit from splenectomy.

Familial (atypical) hemolytic uremic syndrome (aHUS)

This phrase is used to designate a group of rare disorders, mostly affecting children, characterized by microangiopathic HA with presence of fragmented erythrocytes in the peripheral blood smear, thrombocytopenia (usually mild), and acute renal failure. (The word *atypical* is part of the phrase because it is the HUS caused by infection with *Escherichia coli* producing the Shiga toxin that is regarded as typical). The genetic basis of aHUS has been elucidated only recently. Studies of more than 100 families have revealed that family members who have developed HUS have mutations in any one of several genes encoding complement regulatory proteins: complement factor H (*CFH*), CD46 or membrane cofactor protein (*MCP*), complement factor I (*CFI*), complement component C3, complement factor B (*CFB*), and thrombomodulin. Thus, whereas all other inherited HAs are due to intrinsic red cell abnormalities, this group is unique in that hemolysis results from an inherited defect external to red cells (Table 10-1). Because the regulation of the complement cascade has considerable redundancy, in the steady state, any of the above abnormalities can be tolerated. However, when an intercurrent infection or some other trigger activates complement through the alternative pathway, the deficiency of one of the complement regulators becomes critical. Endothelial cells get damaged, especially in the kidney, and at the same time and partly as a result of this, there will be brisk hemolysis (thus, the more common Shiga toxin–related HUS can be regarded as a phenocopy of aHUS). aHUS is a severe disease with up to 15% mortality in the acute phase and up to 50% of cases progressing to end-stage renal disease. aHUS often undergoes spontaneous remission, and the best tested form of treatment is plasma exchange, which supplies the deficient complement regulator. Because the basis of aHUS is an inherited abnormality, it is not surprising that given exposure to an appropriate trigger, the syndrome will tend to recur: when it does, the prognosis is always serious. In some cases, kidney (and liver) transplantation has been carried out, but the role of these procedures is controversial.

ACQUIRED HEMOLYTIC ANEMIA

Mechanical destruction of red cells

Although red cells are characterized by the remarkable deformability that enables them to squeeze through capillaries narrower than themselves for thousands of times in their lifetimes, there are at least two situations in which they succumb to shear, if not to wear and tear. The result is intravascular hemolysis, resulting in hemoglobinuria. One situation is acute and self-inflicted, *march hemoglobinuria*. Why sometimes a marathon runner may develop this complication, whereas on another occasion this does not happen, we do not know (perhaps her or his footwear needs attention). A similar syndrome may develop after prolonged barefoot ritual dancing. The other situation is chronic and iatrogenic (it has been called *microangiopathic hemolytic anemia*); it takes place in patients with prosthetic heart valves, especially when paraprosthetic regurgitation is present. If the hemolysis consequent to mechanical trauma to the red cells is mild, and provided the supply of iron is adequate, it may be largely compensated. If more than mild anemia develops, reintervention to correct regurgitation may be required.

Toxic agents and drugs

A number of chemicals with oxidative potential, whether medicinal or not, can cause hemolysis even in people who are not G6PD-deficient (discussed earlier). Examples are hyperbaric oxygen (or 100% oxygen), nitrates, chlorates, methylene blue, dapsone, cisplatin, and numerous aromatic (cyclic) compounds. Other chemicals may be hemolytic through a nonoxidative, largely unknown mechanism; examples are arsine, stibine, copper, and lead. The HA caused by lead poisoning is characterized by basophilic stippling. It is in fact a phenocopy of that seen in P5N deficiency (discussed earlier), suggesting it is mediated at least in part by lead inhibiting this enzyme.

In these cases, hemolysis appears to be mediated by a direct chemical action on red cells. But drugs can cause hemolysis through at least two other mechanisms. (1) A drug can behave as a hapten and induce antibody production. In rare subjects, this happens, for instance, with penicillin. Upon a subsequent exposure, red cells are caught, as innocent bystanders, in the reaction between penicillin and antipenicillin antibodies. Hemolysis will subside as soon as penicillin administration is stopped. (2) A drug can trigger, perhaps through mimicry, the production of an antibody against a red cell antigen. The best known example is methyldopa, an antihypertensive agent no longer in use, which in a small fraction of patients stimulates the production of the Rhesus antibody anti-e. In patients who have this antigen, the anti-e is a true autoantibody, which would then cause an autoimmune HA (discussed later). Usually this would gradually subside when methyldopa was discontinued.

Severe intravascular hemolysis can be caused by the venom of certain snakes (cobras and vipers), and HA can also follow spider bites.

Infection

By far, the most frequent infectious cause of HA, in endemic areas, is malaria. In other parts of the world, the most frequent cause is probably Shiga toxin–producing *Escherichia coli* O157:H7, now recognized as the main etiologic agent of the hemolytic-uremic syndrome, more common in children than in adults. Life-threatening intravascular hemolysis, due to a toxin with lecithinase activity, occurs with *Clostridium perfringens* sepsis, particularly following open wounds or septic abortion or as a disastrous accident due to a contaminated blood unit. Occasionally, HA is seen, especially in children, with sepsis or endocarditis from a variety of organisms.

Autoimmune hemolytic anemia (AIHA)

Except for countries where malaria is endemic, AIHA is the most common form of *acquired hemolytic anemia*. In fact, not quite appropriately, the two phrases are sometimes used as synonymous.

Pathophysiology

AIHA is caused by an autoantibody directed against a red cell antigen, i.e., a molecule present on the surface of red cells. The autoantibody binds to the red cells. Once a red cell is coated by antibody, it will be destroyed by one or more mechanisms. In most cases the Fc portion of the antibody will be recognized by the Fc receptor of macrophages, and this will trigger erythrophagocytosis (Fig. 10-7). Thus, destruction of red cells will take place wherever macrophages are abundant, i.e., in the spleen, liver, and bone marrow. Because of the special anatomy of the spleen, it is particularly efficient in trapping antibody-coated red cells, and often this is the predominant site of red cell destruction. Although in severe cases even circulating monocytes can take part in this process, most of the phagocytosis-mediated red cell destruction takes place in the organs just mentioned, and it is therefore called *extravascular hemolysis*. In some cases, the nature of the antibody (usually an IgM antibody) is such that the antigen–antibody complex on the surface of red cells is able to activate complement (C). As a result, a large amount of membrane attack complex will form, and the red cells may be destroyed directly; this is known as *intravascular hemolysis*.

Clinical features

The onset of AIHA is very often abrupt and can be dramatic. The hemoglobin level can drop, within days, to as low as 4 g/dL; the massive red cell removal will produce jaundice; and sometimes the spleen is enlarged. When this triad is present, the suspicion of AIHA must be high. When hemolysis is (in part) intravascular, the telltale sign will be hemoglobinuria, which the patient may report or for which the physician must inquire and test. The diagnostic test for AIHA is the antiglobulin test worked out in 1945 by R. R. A. Coombs and known since by his name. The beauty of this test is that it directly detects the pathogenetic mediator of the disease, i.e., the presence of antibody on the red cells themselves. When the test result is positive, it clinches the diagnosis, and when it is negative, the diagnosis is unlikely. However, the sensitivity of the Coombs test varies depending on the technology that is used, and in doubtful cases, a repeat in a specialized lab is advisable; the term "Coombs-negative AIHA" is a last resort. In some cases, the autoantibody has a defined identity: it may be specific for an antigen belonging to the Rhesus system (it is often anti-e). In many cases, it is regarded as "unspecific" because it reacts with virtually all types of red cells.

As in autoimmune diseases in general, the real cause of AIHA remains obscure. However, from the clinical point of view, an important feature is that AIHA can appear to be isolated, or it can develop as part of a more general autoimmune disease, particularly systemic lupus erythematosus, of which sometimes it may be the first manifestation. Therefore, when AIHA is diagnosed, a full screen for autoimmune disease is imperative. In some cases, AIHA can be associated, on first presentation or subsequently, with autoimmune thrombocytopenia (Evans's syndrome).

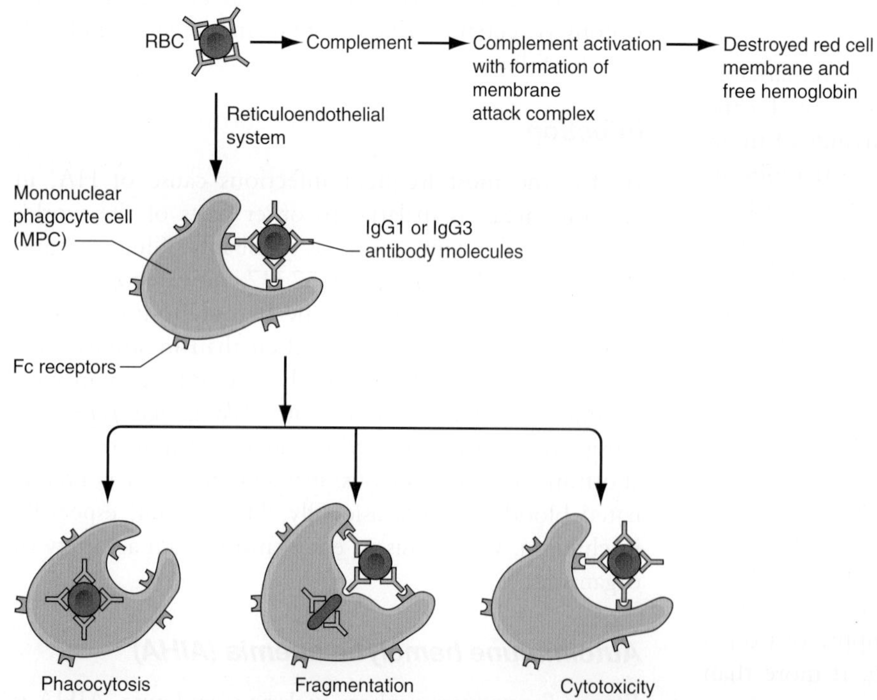

FIGURE 10-7
Mechanism of antibody-mediated immune destruction of red cells. *(From N Young et al: Clinical Hematology. Philadelphia, Elsevier, 2006; with permission.)*

TREATMENT Autoimmune Hemolytic Anemia

Severe acute AIHA can be a medical emergency. The immediate treatment almost invariably includes transfusion of red cells. This may pose a special problem because if the antibody involved is unspecific, all the blood units cross-matched will be incompatible. In these cases, it is often correct, paradoxically, to transfuse incompatible blood, the rationale being that the transfused red cells will be destroyed no less but no more than the patient's own red cells, but in the meantime the patient stays alive. Clearly, this rather unique situation requires good liaison and understanding between the clinical unit treating the patient and the blood transfusion/serology lab. Apart from emergency blood transfusion, the first-line treatment of AIHA is by using corticosteroids. In at least one-half of the cases, prednisone (1 mg/kg per day) will produce a remission promptly. Whereas some patients are then apparently cured, relapses are not uncommon. Although unfortunately most of the management of AIHA is not evidence-based, for patients who do not respond and for those who have relapsed (or who require more than 15 mg/d of prednisone to prevent relapse), it is highly recommended to consider a second-line treatment option, which might be either splenectomy or rituximab (anti-CD20). Splenectomy, although it does not cure the disease, can produce significant benefit by removing a major site of hemolysis, thus improving the anemia and/or reducing the need for other therapies (e.g., the dose of prednisone). Rituximab has emerged as a significant alternative to splenectomy because it can produce remissions in up to 80% of patients and it can be used repeatedly, even though progressive multifocal leukoencephalopathy is a dreaded if rare side effect. Azathioprine, cyclophosphamide, cyclosporine, and IV immunoglobulin have become third-line agents since the introduction of rituximab. In severe refractory cases, either auto- or allohematopoietic stem cell transplantation has been used, sometimes successfully.

Paroxysmal cold hemoglobinuria (PCH)

PCH is a rather rare form of AIHA occurring mostly in children, usually triggered by a viral infection, usually self-limited, and characterized by the involvement of the so-called Donath-Landsteiner antibody. In vitro this antibody has unique serologic features: it has anti-P specificity and it binds to red cells only at a low temperature (optimally at 4°C), but when the temperature is shifted to 37°C, lysis of red cells takes place in the presence of complement. Consequently, in vivo there is intravascular hemolysis, resulting in hemoglobinuria. Clinically, the differential diagnosis must include other causes of hemoglobinuria (Table 10-6), but the presence of the Donath-Landsteiner antibody will prove PCH. Active supportive treatment, including blood transfusion, is needed to control the anemia; subsequently, recovery is the rule.

Cold agglutinin disease (CAD)

This designation is used for a form of chronic AIHA that usually affects the elderly and has special clinical and pathologic features. First, the term *cold* refers to the fact that the autoantibody involved reacts with red cells poorly or not at all at 37°C, whereas it reacts strongly at lower temperatures.[1] As a result, hemolysis is more prominent the more the body is exposed to the cold. The antibody is usually IgM with an anti-I specificity (the I antigen is present on the red cells of almost everybody), and it may have a very high titer (1:100,000 or more has been observed). Second, the antibody is produced by an expanded clone of B lymphocytes, and sometimes its concentration in the plasma is high enough to show up as a spike in plasma protein electrophoresis, i.e., as a monoclonal gammopathy. Third, since the antibody is IgM, CAD is related to Waldenström macroglobulinemia (WM) (Chap. 17), although in most cases the other clinical features of this disease are not present. Thus, CAD must be regarded as a form of WM, i.e., as a low-grade mature B cell lymphoma that manifests at an earlier stage precisely because the unique biologic properties of the IgM that it produces give the clinical picture of chronic HA.

In mild forms of CAD, avoidance of exposure to cold may be all that is needed to enable the patient to have a reasonably comfortable quality of life, but in more severe forms, the management of CAD is not easy. Blood transfusion is not very effective because donor red cells are I-positive and will be rapidly removed. Immunosuppressive/cytotoxic treatment with azathioprine or cyclophosphamide can reduce the antibody titer, but clinical efficacy is limited and, in view of the chronic nature of the disease, the side effects may prove, in the long run, unacceptable. Unlike in AIHA, prednisone and splenectomy are ineffective. Plasma exchange is in theory a rational approach, but it is laborious and must be carried out at frequent intervals if it is to be beneficial. Since the advent of rituximab, the picture has changed significantly for those 60% of patients with CAD who respond to this agent. Given the long clinical course of CAD, it remains to be seen with what periodicity rituximab will need to be administered.

[1]In the past this type of antibody was called a cold antibody, and the antibodies causing the more common form of AIHA were called warm antibodies.

TABLE 10-6

DISEASES AND CLINICAL SITUATIONS WITH PREDOMINANTLY INTRAVASCULAR HEMOLYSIS

	ONSET OR TIME COURSE	MAIN MECHANISM	APPROPRIATE DIAGNOSTIC PROCEDURE	COMMENTS
Mismatched blood transfusion	Abrupt	Nearly always ABO incompatibility	Repeat cross-match	
Paroxysmal nocturnal hemoglobinuria (PNH)	Chronic with acute exacerbations	Complement (C)-mediated destruction of CD59(–) red cells	Flow cytometry to display a CD59(–) red cell population	Exacerbations due to C activation through any pathway
Paroxysmal cold hemoglobinuria (PCH)	Acute	Immune lysis of normal red cells	Test for Donath-Landsteiner antibody	Often triggered by viral infection
Septicemia	Very acute	Exotoxins produced by *Clostridium perfringens*	Blood cultures	Other organisms may be responsible
Microangiopathic	Acute or chronic	Red cell fragmentation	Red cell morphology on blood smear	Different causes ranging from endothelial damage to hemangioma to leaky prosthetic heart valve
March hemoglobinuria	Abrupt	Mechanical destruction	Targeted history taking	
Favism	Acute	Destruction of older fraction of G6PD-deficient red cells	G6PD assay	Triggered by ingestion of large dish of fava beans, but trigger can be infection or drug instead

Paroxysmal nocturnal hemoglobinuria (PNH)

PNH is an acquired chronic HA characterized by persistent intravascular hemolysis (Table 10-6) subject to recurrent exacerbations. In addition to hemolysis, there are often pancytopenia and a distinct tendency to venous thrombosis. This triad makes PNH a truly unique clinical condition. However, when not all of these three features are manifest on presentation, the diagnosis is often delayed, although it can be always made by appropriate laboratory investigations (discussed later).

PNH has about the same frequency in men and in women, and it is encountered in all populations throughout the world, but it is a rare disease. Its prevalence is estimated to be between 1 and 5 per million (it may be somewhat less rare in Southeast Asia and in the Far East). There is no evidence of inherited susceptibility. PNH has never been reported as a congenital disease, but it can present in small children or as late as in the seventies, although most patients are young adults.

Clinical features

The patient may seek medical attention because, one morning, she or he has "passed blood instead of urine" (Fig. 10-8). This distressing or frightening event may be regarded as the classical presentation; however, more frequently, this symptom is not noticed or is suppressed. Indeed, the patient often presents simply as a problem in the differential diagnosis of *anemia*, whether symptomatic or discovered incidentally. Sometimes the anemia is associated from the outset with neutropenia, thrombocytopenia, or both, thus signaling an element of bone marrow failure (discussed later). Some patients may present with recurrent attacks of severe abdominal pain, defying a specific diagnosis and eventually found

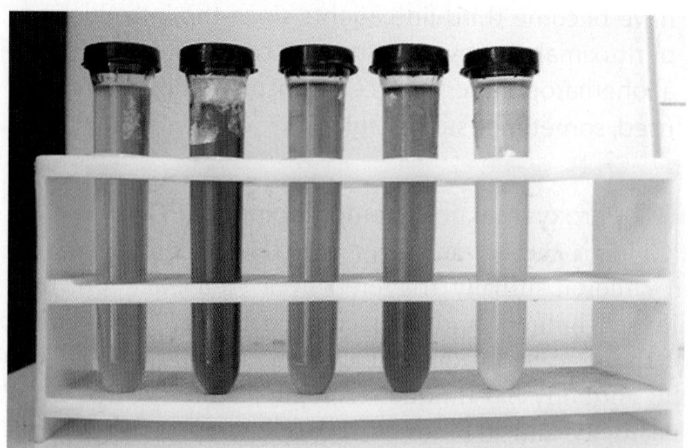

FIGURE 10-8

Consecutive urine samples from a patient with paroxysmal nocturnal hemoglobinuria. The variation in the severity of hemoglobinuria within hours is probably unique to this condition.

to be related to thrombosis. When thrombosis affects the hepatic veins, it may produce acute hepatomegaly and ascites, i.e., a full-fledged Budd-Chiari syndrome, which in the absence of liver disease ought to raise the suspicion of PNH.

The *natural history* of PNH can extend over decades. Without treatment, the median survival time is estimated to be about 8–10 years. In the past, the most common cause of death was venous thrombosis, followed by infection secondary to severe neutropenia and hemorrhage secondary to severe thrombocytopenia. PNH may evolve into aplastic anemia (AA), and PNH may manifest itself in patients who previously had AA. Rarely (estimated 1–2% of all cases), PNH may terminate in acute myeloid leukemia. On the other hand, full spontaneous recovery from PNH has been well documented, albeit rarely.

Laboratory investigations and diagnosis

The most consistent blood finding is anemia, which may range from mild to moderate to very severe. The anemia is usually normo-macrocytic, with unremarkable red cell morphology; if the MCV is high, it is usually largely accounted for by reticulocytosis, which may be quite marked (up to 20%, or up to 400,000/μL). The anemia may become microcytic if the patient is allowed to become iron-deficient as a result of chronic urinary blood loss through hemoglobinuria. Unconjugated bilirubin is mildly or moderately elevated, LDH is typically markedly elevated (values in the thousands are common), and haptoglobin is usually undetectable. All these findings make the diagnosis of HA compelling. Hemoglobinuria, the telltale sign of intravascular hemolysis (Table 10-6), may be overt in a random urine sample. If it is not, it may be helpful to obtain serial urine samples, since hemoglobinuria can vary dramatically from day to day and even from hour to hour (Fig. 10-8). The bone marrow is usually cellular, with marked to massive erythroid hyperplasia, often with mild to moderate dyserythropoietic features (these do not justify confusing PNH with myelodysplastic syndrome). At some stage of the disease, the marrow may become hypocellular or even frankly aplastic (discussed later).

The definitive diagnosis of PNH must be based on the demonstration that a substantial proportion of the patient's red cells have an increased susceptibility to complement (C), due to the deficiency on their surface of proteins (particularly CD59 and CD55) that normally protect the red cells from activated C. The sucrose hemolysis test is unreliable, and the acidified serum (Ham) test is carried out in few labs. The gold standard today is flow cytometry, which can be carried out on granulocytes as well as on red cells. A bimodal distribution of cells, with a discrete population that is CD59-, CD55-, is diagnostic of PNH. Usually this population is at least 5% of the total in the case of red cells and at least 20% of the total in the case of granulocytes.

Pathophysiology

Hemolysis in PNH is due to an intrinsic abnormality of the red cell, which makes it exquisitely sensitive to activated C, whether it is activated through the alternative pathway or through an antigen–antibody reaction (Fig. 10-9). The former mechanism is mainly responsible for intravascular hemolysis in PNH. The latter mechanism explains why the hemolysis can be dramatically exacerbated in the course of a viral or bacterial infection. Hypersusceptibility to C is due to deficiency of several protective membrane proteins, of which CD59 is the most important because it hinders the insertion into the membrane of C9 polymers. The molecular basis for the deficiency of these proteins has been pinpointed not to a defect in any of the respective genes, but rather to the shortage of a unique glycolipid molecule, glycosylphosphatidyl-inositol (GPI), which, through a peptide bond, anchors these proteins to the surface membrane of cells. The shortage of GPI is due in turn to a mutation in an X-linked gene, called *PIG-A*, required for an early step in GPI biosynthesis. In virtually every patient, the PIG-A mutation is different. This is not surprising, since these mutations are not inherited; rather, each one takes place de novo in a hematopoietic stem cell (i.e., they are somatic mutations). As a result, the patient's marrow is a mosaic of mutant and nonmutant cells, and the peripheral blood always contains both PNH cells and normal (non-PNH) cells. Thrombosis is one of the most immediately life-threatening complications of PNH and yet one of the least understood in its pathogenesis. It could be that deficiency of CD59 on the PNH platelet causes inappropriate platelet activation; however, other mechanisms are possible.

Bone marrow failure (BMF) and relationship between PNH and aplastic anemia (AA)

It is not unusual that patients with firmly established PNH have a previous history of well-documented AA. On the other hand, sometimes a patient with PNH becomes less hemolytic and more pancytopenic and ultimately has the clinical picture of AA. Since AA is probably an organ-specific autoimmune disease in which T cells cause damage to hematopoietic stem cells, the same may be true of PNH, with the specific proviso that the damage spares PNH stem cells. Skewing of the T cell repertoire in patients with PNH lends some support to this notion. In addition, there is evidence in mouse models that PNH stem cells do not expand when the rest of the bone marrow is normal, and by using high-sensitivity flow cytometry technology, very rare PNH cells harboring PIG-A mutations can be demonstrated in normal people. In view of these

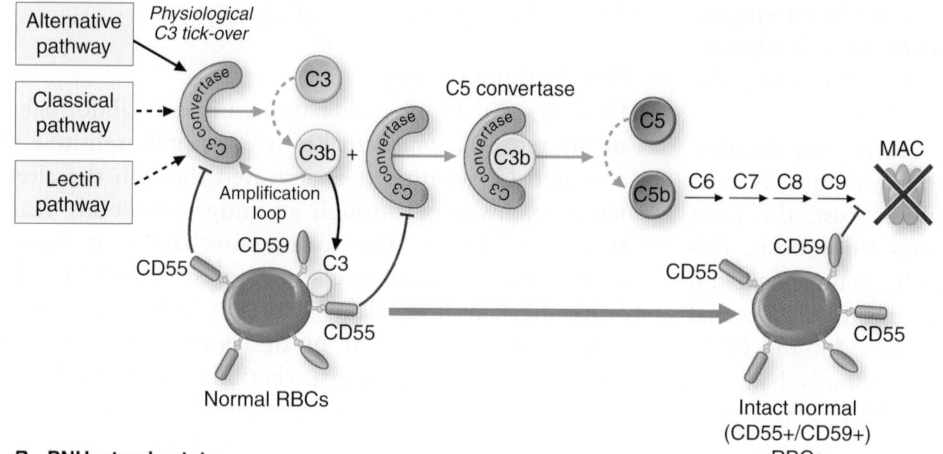

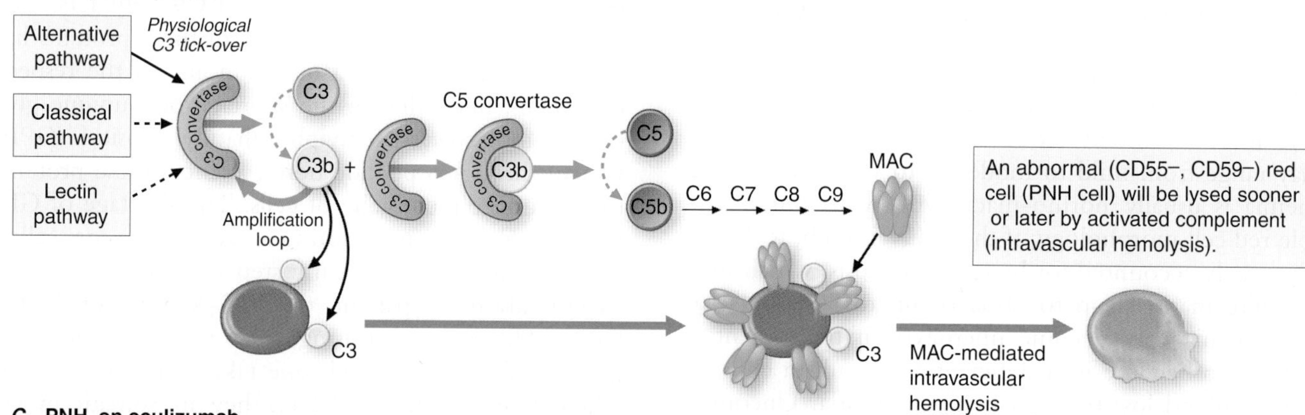

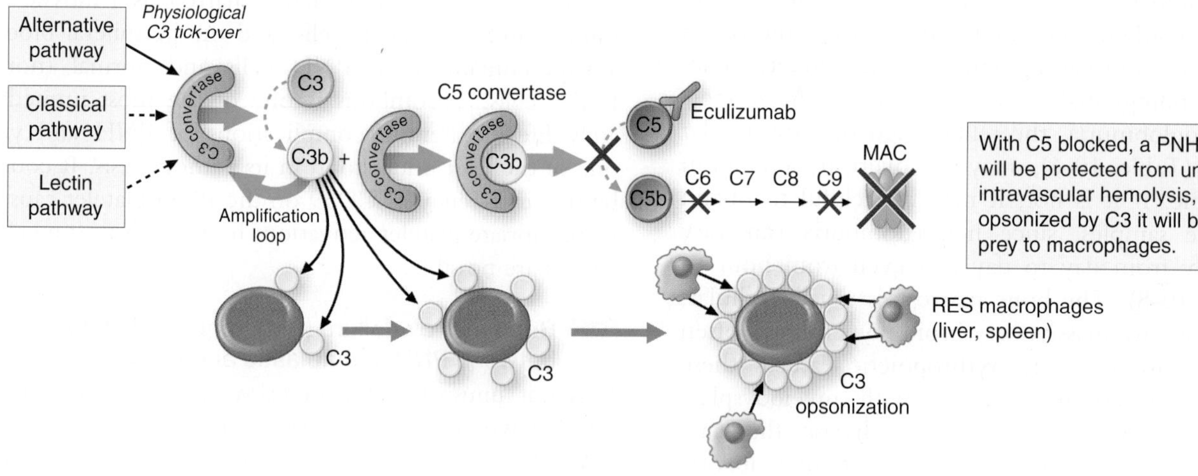

FIGURE 10-9

The complement cascade and the fate of red cells. ***A.*** Normal red cells are protected from complement activation and subsequent hemolysis by CD55 and CD59. These two proteins, being GPI-linked, are missing from the surface of PNH red cells as a result of a somatic mutation of the X-linked *PIG-A* gene that encodes a protein required for an early step of the GPI molecule biosynthesis. ***B.*** In the steady state, PNH erythrocytes suffer from spontaneous (tick-over) complement activation, with consequent intravascular hemolysis through formation of the membrane attack complex (MAC); when extra complement is activated through the classical pathway, an exacerbation of hemolysis will result. ***C.*** On eculizumab, PNH erythrocytes are protected from hemolysis from the inhibition of C5 cleavage; however, upstream complement activation may lead to C3 opsonization and possible extravascular hemolysis. GPI, glycosylphosphatidylinositol; PNH, paroxysmal nocturnal hemoglobinuria reticuloendothelial system. (*From L Luzzatto et al: Haematologica 95:523, 2010.*)

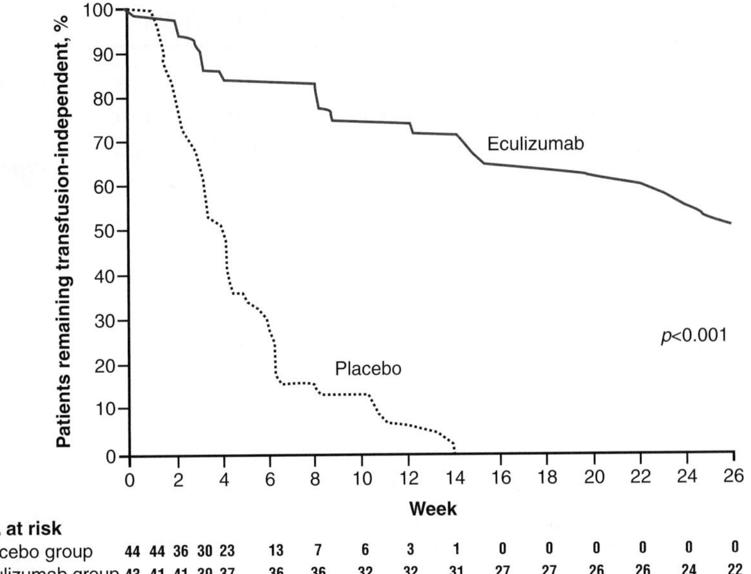

FIGURE 10-10
Therapeutic efficacy of an anti-C5 antibody on the anemia of paroxysmal nocturnal hemoglobinuria. *(From P Hillmen et al: N Engl J Med 355:1233, 2006; with permission.)*

facts, it seems that an element of BMF in PNH is the rule rather than the exception. An extreme view is that PNH is a form of AA in which BMF is masked by the massive expansion of the PNH clone that populates the patient's bone marrow. The mechanism whereby PNH stem cells escape the damage suffered by non-PNH stem cells is not yet known.

TREATMENT Paroxysmal Nocturnal Hemoglobinuria

Unlike other acquired HAs, PNH may be a lifelong condition; standard care was formerly supportive treatment only, including transfusion of filtered red cells[2] whenever necessary, which, for some patients, means quite frequently. Folic acid supplements (at least 3 mg/d) are mandatory, and the serum iron should be checked periodically and iron supplements administered as appropriate. Long-term glucocorticoids are not indicated because there is no evidence that they have any effect on chronic hemolysis; in fact, they are contraindicated because of their many dangerous side effects. A major advance in the management of PNH has been the development of a humanized monoclonal antibody, eculizumab, directed against the complement component C5. In an international, multicenter, placebo-controlled randomized trial of 87 patients (so far the only controlled therapeutic trial in PNH) who had been selected on grounds of having severe hemolysis making them transfusion-dependent, eculizumab proved effective and was licensed in 2007 (Fig. 10-10). By blocking the complement cascade downstream of C5, eculizumab abrogates complement-dependent intravascular hemolysis in all PNH patients, which in itself significantly improves their quality of life. One would expect that, as a result, the need for blood transfusion would be also abrogated, and this indeed is the case in about one-half of the patients, in many of whom there is also a rise in hemoglobin levels. In the remaining patients, the anemia remains sufficiently severe to require blood transfusion, apparently because of ongoing extravascular hemolysis of red cells opsonized by complement (C3) fragments. Based on its half-life, eculizumab must be administered intravenously every 14 days. The only form of treatment that currently can provide a definitive cure for PNH is allogeneic bone marrow transplantation (BMT). When an HLA-identical sibling is available, BMT should be offered to any young patient with severe PNH; the availability of eculizumab has probably decreased significantly the proportion of those who take up this option.

For patients with the PNH-AA syndrome, immunosuppressive treatment with antilymphocyte globulin (ALG or ATG) and cyclosporine A may be indicated. Although no formal trial has ever been conducted, this approach has helped particularly to relieve severe thrombocytopenia and/or neutropenia in patients in whom these were the main problem(s). By contrast, there is often little immediate effect on hemolysis. Any patient who has had venous thrombosis or who has a genetically determined thrombophilic state in addition to PNH should be on regular anticoagulant prophylaxis.

[2]Now that filters with excellent retention of white cells are routinely used, the traditional washing of red cells, aiming to avoid white cell reactions triggering hemolysis, is no longer necessary and is wasteful

ANEMIA DUE TO ACUTE BLOOD LOSS

Blood loss causes anemia by two main mechanisms. First, by the direct loss of red cells, and second, because if the loss of blood is protracted, it will gradually deplete the iron stores, eventually resulting in iron deficiency. The latter type of anemia is covered in Chap. 7. Here we are concerned with the former type, i.e., the *post-hemorrhagic anemia*, which follows *acute* blood loss. This can be *external* (as after trauma or obstetric hemorrhage) or *internal* (e.g., from bleeding in the gastrointestinal tract, rupture of the spleen, rupture of an ectopic pregnancy, subarachnoid hemorrhage). In any of these cases, i.e., after the sudden loss of a large amount of blood, there are three clinical or pathophysiologic stages. First, the dominant feature is hypovolemia, which poses a threat particularly to organs that normally have a high blood supply, such as the brain and the kidneys; therefore, loss of consciousness and acute renal failure are major threats. It is important to note that at this stage, an ordinary blood count will not show anemia, as the hemoglobin concentration is not affected. Second, as an emergency response, baroreceptors and stretch receptors will cause release of vasopressin and other peptides, and the body will shift fluid from the extravascular to the intravascular compartment, producing hemodilution; thus, the hypovolemia gradually converts to anemia. The degree of anemia will reflect the amount of blood lost: if after 3 days the hemoglobin is, say 7 g/dL, it means that about half of the entire blood volume had been lost. Third, provided bleeding does not continue, the bone marrow response will gradually ameliorate the anemia.

The diagnosis of acute posthemorrhagic anemia (APHA) is usually straighforward, but sometimes internal bleeding episodes—after a traumatic injury or otherwise—may not be immediately obvious, even when large. Whenever an abrupt fall in hemoglobin has taken place, whatever history is given by the patient, APHA should be suspected: supplementary history may have to be obtained by asking the appropriate questions, and appropriate investigations (e.g., a sonogram or an endoscopy) may have to be carried out.

TREATMENT Anemia Due to Acute Blood Loss

With respect to treatment, a two-pronged approach is imperative. (1) In many cases the blood lost needs to be replaced promptly. Unlike with many chronic anemias, when finding and correcting the cause of the anemia is the first priority and blood transfusion may not be even necessary because the body is adapted to the anemia, with acute blood loss the reverse is true; i.e., since the body is not adapted to the anemia, blood transfusion takes priority. (2) While the emergency is being confronted, it is imperative to stop the hemorrhage and to eliminate its source.

A special type of APHA is blood loss during and immediately after surgery, which can be substantial (for instance, up to 2 L in the case of a radical prostatectomy). Of course, with elective surgical procedures, the patient's own stored blood may be available (through preoperative autologous blood donation), and in any case, blood loss is carefully monitored. Since this blood loss is iatrogenic, ever more effort should be invested in optimizing transfusion management.

A Holy Grail of emergency medicine for a long time has been the idea of a blood substitute that would be universally available, suitable for all recipients, easy to store and to transport, safe, and as effective as blood itself. Two main paths have been pursued: (1) fluorocarbon synthetic chemicals that bind oxygen reversibly and (2) artificially modified hemoglobins, known as hemoglobin-based oxygen carriers (HBOCs). Although there are numerous anecdotal reports of the use of both approaches in humans and although HBOCs have reached the stage of phase II to III clinical trials, no "blood substitute" has yet become standard treatment.

CHAPTER 11
APLASTIC ANEMIA, MYELODYSPLASIA, AND RELATED BONE MARROW FAILURE SYNDROMES

Neal S. Young

The hypoproliferative anemias are normochromic, normocytic, or macrocytic and are characterized by a low reticulocyte count. Deficient production of red blood cells (RBCs) occurs with marrow damage and dysfunction, which may be secondary to infection, inflammation, and cancer. Hypoproliferative anemia is also a prominent feature of hematologic diseases that are described as bone marrow failure states; these include aplastic anemia, myelodysplastic syndrome (MDS), pure RBC aplasia (PRCA), and myelophthisis. Anemia in these disorders is often not a solitary or even the major hematologic finding. More frequent in bone marrow failure is pancytopenia: anemia, leukopenia, and thrombocytopenia. Low blood counts in the marrow failure diseases result from deficient hematopoiesis, as distinguished from blood count depression due to peripheral destruction of RBCs (hemolytic anemias), platelets (idiopathic thrombocytopenic purpura [ITP] or due to splenomegaly), and granulocytes (as in the immune leukopenias).

Hematopoietic failure syndromes are classified by dominant morphologic features of the bone marrow (Table 11-1). Although practical distinction among these syndromes usually is clear, they can occur secondary to other diseases, and some processes are so closely related that the diagnosis may be complex. Patients may seem to have two or three related diseases simultaneously, or one diagnosis may appear to evolve into another. Many of these syndromes share an immune-mediated mechanism of marrow destruction and some element of genomic instability resulting in a higher rate of malignant transformation. It is important that internists and general practitioners recognize the marrow failure syndromes, as their prognosis may be poor if the patient is untreated; effective therapies are often available but sufficiently complex in their choice and delivery so as to warrant the care of a hematologist or oncologist.

APLASTIC ANEMIA

DEFINITION

Aplastic anemia is pancytopenia with bone marrow hypocellularity. Acquired aplastic anemia is distinguished from iatrogenic marrow aplasia, marrow hypocellularity after intensive cytotoxic chemotherapy for cancer. Aplastic anemia can also be constitutional: the genetic diseases Fanconi's anemia and dyskeratosis congenita, although frequently associated with typical physical anomalies and the development of pancytopenia early in life, can also present as marrow failure in normal-appearing adults. Acquired aplastic anemia is often stereotypical in its manifestations, with the abrupt onset of low blood counts in a previously well young adult; seronegative hepatitis or a course of an incriminated medical drug may precede the onset. The diagnosis in these instances is uncomplicated. Sometimes blood count depression is moderate or incomplete, resulting in anemia, leukopenia, and thrombocytopenia in some combination. Aplastic anemia is related to both paroxysmal nocturnal hemoglobinuria (PNH; Chap. 10) and to MDS, and in some cases a clear distinction among these disorders may not be possible.

EPIDEMIOLOGY

The incidence of acquired aplastic anemia in Europe and Israel is two cases per million persons annually. In Thailand and China, rates of five to seven per million have been established. In general, men and women are affected with equal frequency, but the age distribution is biphasic, with the major peak in the teens and twenties and a second rise in older adults.

TABLE 11-1

DIFFERENTIAL DIAGNOSIS OF PANCYTOPENIA

Pancytopenia with Hypocellular Bone Marrow	
Acquired aplastic anemia	
Constitutional aplastic anemia (Fanconi's anemia, dyskeratosis congenita)	
Some myelodysplasia	
Rare aleukemic leukemia	
Some acute lymphoid leukemia	
Some lymphomas of bone marrow	
Pancytopenia with Cellular Bone Marrow	
Primary bone marrow diseases	Secondary to systemic diseases
Myelodysplasia	Systemic lupus erythematosus
Paroxysmal nocturnal hemoglobinuria	Hypersplenism
Myelofibrosis	B_{12}, folate deficiency
Some aleukemic leukemia	Overwhelming infection
Myelophthisis	Alcohol
Bone marrow lymphoma	Brucellosis
Hairy cell leukemia	Sarcoidosis
	Tuberculosis
	Leishmaniasis
Hypocellular Bone Marrow ± Cytopenia	
Q fever	
Legionnaires' disease	
Anorexia nervosa, starvation	
Mycobacterium	

ETIOLOGY

The origins of aplastic anemia have been inferred from several recurring clinical associations (Table 11-2); unfortunately, these relationships are not reliable in an individual patient and may not be etiologic. In addition, although most cases of aplastic anemia are idiopathic, little other than history separates these cases from those with a presumed etiology such as a drug exposure.

Radiation

Marrow aplasia is a major acute sequela of radiation. Radiation damages DNA; tissues dependent on active mitosis are particularly susceptible. Nuclear accidents can involve not only power plant workers but also employees of hospitals, laboratories, and industry (food sterilization, metal radiography, etc.), as well as innocents exposed to stolen, misplaced, or misused sources. Whereas the radiation dose can be approximated from the rate and degree of decline in blood counts, dosimetry by reconstruction of the exposure can help to estimate the patient's prognosis and protect medical personnel from contact with radioactive tissue and excreta. MDS and leukemia, but probably not aplastic anemia, are late effects of radiation.

TABLE 11-2

CLASSIFICATION OF APLASTIC ANEMIA AND SINGLE CYTOPENIAS

ACQUIRED	INHERITED
Aplastic Anemia	
Secondary	Fanconi's anemia
Radiation	Dyskeratosis congenita
Drugs and chemicals	Shwachman-Diamond syndrome
Regular effects	Reticular dysgenesis
Idiosyncratic reactions	Amegakaryocytic thrombocytopenia
Viruses	Familial aplastic anemias
Epstein-Barr virus (infectious mononucleosis)	Preleukemia (monosomy 7, etc.)
Hepatitis (non-A, non-B, non-C hepatitis)	Nonhematologic syndrome (Down, Dubowitz, Seckel)
Parvovirus B19 (transient aplastic crisis, PRCA)	
HIV-1 (AIDS)	
Immune diseases	
Eosinophilic fasciitis	
Hyperimmunoglobulinemia	
Thymoma/thymic carcinoma	
Graft-vs.-host disease in immunodeficiency	
Paroxysmal nocturnal hemoglobinuria	
Pregnancy	
Idiopathic	
Cytopenias	
PRCA (see Table 11-4)	Congenital PRCA (Diamond-Blackfan anemia)
Neutropenia/agranulocytosis	
Idiopathic	Kostmann's syndrome
Drugs, toxins	Shwachman-Diamond syndrome
Pure white cell aplasia	Reticular dysgenesis
Thrombocytopenia	
Drugs, toxins	Amegakaryocytic thrombocytopenia
Idiopathic amegakaryocytic	Thrombocytopenia with absent radii

Abbreviation: PRCA, pure RBC aplasia.

Chemicals

Benzene is a notorious cause of bone marrow failure: epidemiologic, clinical, and laboratory data link benzene to aplastic anemia, acute leukemia, and blood and marrow abnormalities. For leukemia, the incidence is correlated with cumulative exposure, but susceptibility must also be important, as only a minority of even heavily exposed workers develop myelotoxicity. The employment history is important, especially in industries where benzene is used for a secondary purpose, usually as a solvent. Benzene-related blood diseases have declined with regulation of industrial exposure. Although benzene is no longer generally available as a household solvent, exposure to its metabolites occurs in the normal diet and in the environment. The association between marrow failure and other chemicals is much less well substantiated.

Drugs

(Table 11-3) Many chemotherapeutic drugs have marrow suppression as a major toxicity; effects are dose dependent and occur in all recipients. In contrast, idiosyncratic reactions to a large and diverse group of drugs may lead to aplastic anemia without a clear dose-response relationship. These associations rested largely on accumulated case reports until a large international study in Europe in the 1980s quantitated drug relationships, especially for nonsteroidal analgesics, sulfonamides, thyrostatic drugs, some psychotropics, penicillamine, allopurinol, and gold. Association does not equal causation: a drug may have been used to treat the first symptoms of bone marrow failure (antibiotics for fever or the preceding viral illness) or provoked the first symptom of a preexisting disease (petechiae by nonsteroidal anti-inflammatory agents administered to a thrombocytopenic patient). In the context of total drug use, idiosyncratic reactions, although individually devastating, are rare events. Risk estimates are usually lower when determined in population-based studies; furthermore, the low absolute risk is also made more obvious: even a 10 or 20-fold increase in risk translates, in a rare disease, to but a handful of drug-induced aplastic anemia cases among hundreds of thousands of exposed persons.

TABLE 11-3

SOME DRUGS AND CHEMICALS ASSOCIATED WITH APLASTIC ANEMIA
Agents that regularly produce marrow depression as major toxicity in commonly employed doses or normal exposures:
Cytotoxic drugs used in cancer chemotherapy: *alkylating agents*, *antimetabolites*, *antimitotics*, some antibiotics
Agents that frequently but not inevitably produce marrow aplasia:
Benzene
Agents associated with aplastic anemia but with a relatively low probability:
Chloramphenicol
Insecticides
Antiprotozoals: *quinacrine* and chloroquine, mepacrine
Nonsteroidal anti-inflammatory drugs (including *phenylbutazone*, indomethacin, ibuprofen, sulindac, aspirin)
Anticonvulsants (*hydantoins*, *carbamazepine*, phenacemide, felbamate)
Heavy metals (*gold*, arsenic, bismuth, mercury)
Sulfonamides: some antibiotics, antithyroid drugs (methimazole, methylthiouracil, propylthiouracil), antidiabetes drugs (tolbutamide, chlorpropamide), carbonic anhydrase inhibitors (acetazolamide and methazolamide)
Antihistamines (*cimetidine*, chlorpheniramine)
D-Penicillamine
Estrogens (in pregnancy and in high doses in animals)
Agents whose association with aplastic anemia is more tenuous:
Other antibiotics (streptomycin, tetracycline, methicillin, mebendazole, trimethoprim/sulfamethoxazole, flucytosine)
Sedatives and tranquilizers (chlorpromazine, prochlorperazine, piperacetazine, chlordiazepoxide, meprobamate, methyprylon)
Allopurinol
Methyldopa
Quinidine
Lithium
Guanidine
Potassium perchlorate
Thiocyanate
Carbimazole

Note: Terms set in italic show the most consistent association with aplastic anemia.

Infections

Hepatitis is the most common preceding infection, and posthepatitis marrow failure accounts for approximately 5% of etiologies in most series. Patients are usually young men who have recovered from a bout of liver inflammation 1 to 2 months earlier; the subsequent pancytopenia is very severe. The hepatitis is seronegative (non-A, non-B, non-C) and possibly due to an as yet undiscovered infectious agent. Fulminant liver failure in childhood also follows seronegative hepatitis, and marrow failure occurs at a high rate in these patients. Aplastic anemia can rarely follow infectious mononucleosis. Parvovirus B19, the cause of transient aplastic crisis in hemolytic anemias and of some PRCAs (discussed later), does not usually cause generalized bone marrow failure. Mild blood count depression is frequent in the course of many viral and bacterial infections but resolves with the infection.

Immunologic diseases

Aplasia is a major consequence and the inevitable cause of death in transfusion-associated graft-versus-host disease (GVHD) that can occur after infusion of nonirradiated blood products to an immunodeficient recipient. Aplastic anemia is strongly associated with the rare collagen vascular syndrome eosinophilic fasciitis that is characterized by painful induration of subcutaneous tissues. Pancytopenia with marrow hypoplasia can also occur in systemic lupus erythematosus (SLE).

Pregnancy

Aplastic anemia very rarely may occur and recur during pregnancy and resolve with delivery or with spontaneous or induced abortion.

Paroxysmal nocturnal hemoglobinuria

An acquired mutation in the *PIG-A* gene in a hematopoietic stem cell is required for the development of PNH, but *PIG-A* mutations probably occur commonly in normal individuals. If the *PIG-A* mutant stem cell proliferates, the result is a clone of progeny deficient in glycosylphosphatidylinositol-linked cell surface membrane proteins (Chap. 10). Small clones of deficient cells can be detected by sensitive flow cytometry tests in approximately half of patients with aplastic anemia at the time of presentation (and PNH cells are also seen in MDS [discussed later]). Functional studies of bone marrow from PNH patients, even those with mainly hemolytic manifestations, show evidence of defective hematopoiesis. Patients with an initial clinical diagnosis of PNH, especially younger individuals, may later develop frank marrow aplasia and pancytopenia; patients with an initial diagnosis of aplastic anemia may have hemolytic PNH years after recovery of blood counts.

Constitutional disorders

Fanconi's anemia, an autosomal recessive disorder, manifests as congenital developmental anomalies, progressive pancytopenia, and an increased risk of malignancy. Chromosomes in Fanconi's anemia are peculiarly susceptible to DNA cross-linking agents, the basis for a diagnostic assay. Patients with Fanconi's anemia typically have short stature; café au lait spots; and anomalies involving the thumb, radius, and genitourinary tract. At least 12 different genetic defects (all but one with an identified gene) have been defined; the most common, type A Fanconi's anemia, is due to a mutation in *FANCA*. Most of the Fanconi's anemia gene products form a protein complex that activates FANCD2 by monoubiquitination to play a role in the cellular response to DNA damage and especially interstrand cross-linking.

Dyskeratosis congenita is characterized by mucous membrane leukoplasia, dystrophic nails, reticular hyperpigmentation, and the development of aplastic anemia in childhood. Dyskeratosis is due to mutations in genes of the telomere repair complex, which acts to maintain telomere length in replicating cells: the X-linked variety is due to mutations in the *DKC1* (*dyskerin*) gene; the more unusual autosomal dominant type is due to mutation in *TERC*, which encodes an RNA template, and *TERT*, which encodes the catalytic reverse transcriptase, telomerase. Mutations in TNF2, a component of the shelterin, proteins that bind the telomere DNA, also occur in dyskeratosis.

In Shwachman-Diamond syndrome, marrow failure is seen with pancreatic insufficiency and malabsorption; most patients have compound heterozygous mutations in *SBDS* that may affect marrow stroma function. Mutations in *TERT*, *TERC*, *TNF2*, and *SBDS* also can occur in patients with apparently acquired aplastic anemia. (*TERT* and *TERC* mutations also are etiologic in familial pulmonary fibrosis and in some hepatic cirrhosis.)

PATHOPHYSIOLOGY

Bone marrow failure results from severe damage to the hematopoietic cell compartment. In aplastic anemia, replacement of the bone marrow by fat is apparent in the morphology of the biopsy specimen (Fig. 11-1) and magnetic resonance imaging (MRI) of the spine. Cells bearing the CD34 antigen, a marker of early hematopoietic cells, are greatly diminished, and in functional studies, committed and primitive progenitor cells are virtually absent; in vitro assays have suggested that the stem cell pool is reduced to ≤1% of normal in severe disease at the time of presentation.

An intrinsic stem cell defect exists for the constitutional aplastic anemias: cells from patients with Fanconi's anemia exhibit chromosome damage and death on exposure to certain chemical agents. Telomeres are short in some patients with aplastic anemia, due to heterozygous mutations in genes of the telomere repair complex. Variable penetrance means that *TERT* and *TERC* mutations represent risk factors for marrow failure, as family members with the same mutations may have normal or only slight hematologic abnormalities but more subtle evidence of (compensated) hematopoietic insufficiency.

DRUG INJURY

Extrinsic damage to the marrow follows massive physical or chemical insults such as high doses of radiation and toxic chemicals. For the more common idiosyncratic reaction to modest doses of medical drugs, altered drug metabolism has been invoked as a likely mechanism. The metabolic pathways of many drugs and chemicals, especially if they are polar and have limited water solubility, involve enzymatic degradation to highly reactive electrophilic compounds; these intermediates are toxic because of their propensity to bind to cellular macromolecules. For example, derivative hydroquinones and quinolones are responsible for benzene-induced tissue injury. Excessive generation of toxic intermediates or failure to detoxify the intermediates may be genetically determined and apparent only on specific drug challenge; the complexity and specificity of the pathways imply multiple susceptibility loci and would provide an explanation for the rarity of idiosyncratic drug reactions.

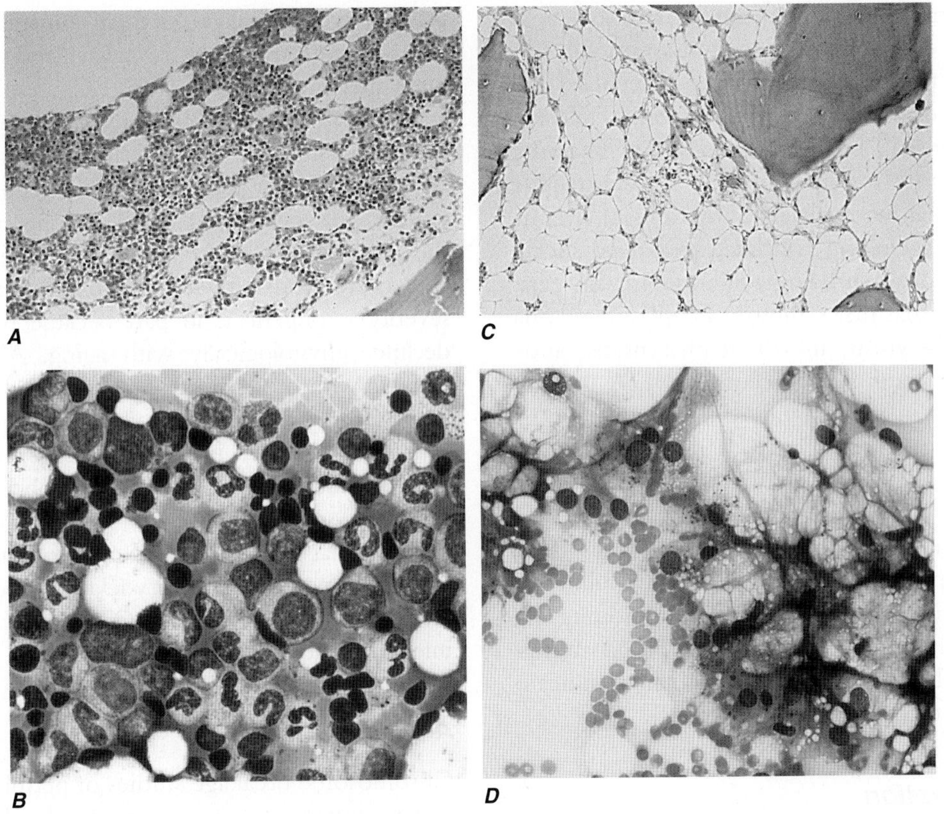

FIGURE 11-1
A. Normal bone marrow biopsy. ***B.*** Normal bone marrow aspirate smear. The marrow is normally 30 70% cellular, and there is a heterogeneous mix of myeloid, erythroid, and lymphoid cells. ***C.*** Aplastic anemia biopsy. ***D.*** Marrow smear in aplastic anemia. The marrow shows replacement of hematopoietic tissue by fat and only residual stromal and lymphoid cells.

Immune-mediated injury

The recovery of marrow function in some patients prepared for bone marrow transplantation with antilymphocyte globulin (ALO) first suggested that aplastic anemia might be immune mediated. Consistent with this hypothesis was the frequent failure of simple bone marrow transplantation from a syngeneic twin, without conditioning cytotoxic chemotherapy, which also argued both *against* simple stem cell absence as the cause and *for* the presence of a host factor producing marrow failure. Laboratory data support an important role for the immune system in aplastic anemia. Blood and bone marrow cells of patients can suppress normal hematopoietic progenitor cell growth, and removal of T cells from aplastic anemia bone marrow improves colony formation in vitro. Increased numbers of activated cytotoxic T cell clones are observed in aplastic anemia patients and usually decline with successful immunosuppressive therapy; cytokine measurements show a T_H1 immune response (interferon γ [IFN-γ] and tumor necrosis factor [TNF]). Interferon and induce Fas expression on CD34 cells, leading to apoptotic cell death; localization of activated T cells to bone marrow and local production of their soluble factors are probably important in stem cell destruction.

Early immune system events in aplastic anemia are not well understood. An oligoclonal, T cell response implies an antigenic stimulus. Many different exogenous antigens appear capable of initiating a pathologic immune response, but at least some of the T cells may recognize true self-antigens. The rarity of aplastic anemia despite common exposures (medicines, seronegative hepatitis) suggests that genetically determined features of the immune response can convert a normal physiologic response into a sustained abnormal autoimmune process, including polymorphisms in histocompatibility antigens, cytokine genes, and genes that regulate T cell polarization and effector function.

CLINICAL FEATURES

History

Aplastic anemia can appear with seeming abruptness or have a more insidious onset. Bleeding is the most common early symptom; a complaint of days to weeks of easy bruising, oozing from the gums, nose bleeds, heavy menstrual flow, and sometimes petechiae will have been noticed. With thrombocytopenia, massive hemorrhage is unusual, but small amounts of bleeding in the central nervous system can result in catastrophic intracranial or retinal hemorrhage. Symptoms of anemia are also frequent, including lassitude, weakness, shortness of breath, and a pounding sensation in the ears. Infection is an unusual first symptom in aplastic anemia (unlike in agranulocytosis, in which pharyngitis, anorectal infection, or frank sepsis occurs early). A striking feature of aplastic anemia is the restriction of symptoms to the hematologic system; patients often feel and look remarkably well despite drastically reduced blood counts. Systemic complaints and weight loss should point to other etiologies of pancytopenia. Prior drug use, chemical exposure, and preceding viral illnesses must often be elicited with repeated questioning. A family history of hematologic diseases or blood abnormalities and of pulmonary or liver fibrosis may indicate a constitutional etiology of marrow failure.

Physical examination

Petechiae and ecchymoses are typical, and retinal hemorrhages may be present. Pelvic and rectal examinations can often be deferred but, when performed, should be undertaken with great gentleness to avoid trauma; these often show bleeding from the cervical os and blood in the stool. Pallor of the skin and mucous membranes is common except in the most acute cases and those already transfused. Infection on presentation is unusual but may occur if the patient has been symptomatic for a few weeks. Lymphadenopathy and splenomegaly are highly atypical of aplastic anemia. Café au lait spots and short stature suggest Fanconi's anemia; peculiar nails and leukoplakia suggest dyskeratosis congenita.

LABORATORY STUDIES

Blood

The smear shows large erythrocytes and a paucity of platelets and granulocytes. Mean corpuscular volume (MCV) is commonly increased. Reticulocytes are absent or few, and lymphocyte numbers may be normal or reduced. The presence of immature myeloid forms suggests leukemia or MDS, nucleated RBCs suggest marrow fibrosis or tumor invasion, and abnormal platelets suggest either peripheral destruction, and or MDS.

Bone marrow

The bone marrow is usually readily aspirated but dilute on smear, and the fatty biopsy specimen may be grossly pale on withdrawal; a "dry tap" instead suggests fibrosis or myelophthisis. In severe aplasia, the smear of the aspirated specimen shows only RBCs, residual lymphocytes, and stromal cells; the biopsy (which should be >1 cm in length) is superior for determination of cellularity and shows mainly fat under the microscope, with hematopoietic cells occupying <25% of the marrow space; in the most serious cases, the biopsy is virtually 100% fat. The correlation between marrow cellularity and disease severity is imperfect, in part because marrow cellularity declines physiologically with aging. Additionally, some patients with moderate disease by blood counts will have empty iliac crest biopsies, while "hot spots" of hematopoiesis may be seen in severe cases. If an iliac crest specimen is inadequate, cells may also be obtained by aspiration from the sternum. Residual hematopoietic cells should have normal morphology, except for mildly megaloblastic erythropoiesis; megakaryocytes are invariably greatly reduced and usually absent. Granulomas may indicate an infectious etiology of the marrow failure.

Ancillary studies

Chromosome breakage studies of peripheral blood using diepoxybutane or mitomycin C should be performed on children and younger adults to exclude Fanconi's anemia. Very short telomere length (available commercially) strongly suggests the presence of a telomerase or shelterin mutation, which can be pursued by family studies and nucleotide sequencing. Chromosome studies of bone marrow cells are often revealing in MDS and should be negative in typical aplastic anemia. Flow cytometry offers a sensitive diagnostic test for PNH. Serologic studies may show evidence of viral infection, such as Epstein-Barr virus and HIV. Posthepatitis aplastic anemia is seronegative. The spleen size should be determined by computed tomography scanning or ultrasonography if the physical examination of the abdomen is unsatisfactory. MRI may be helpful to assess the fat content of a few vertebrae to distinguish aplasia from MDS.

Diagnosis

The diagnosis of aplastic anemia is usually straightforward, based on the combination of pancytopenia with a fatty bone marrow. Aplastic anemia is a disease of the young and should be a leading diagnosis in adolescents or young adults with pancytopenia. When pancytopenia is secondary, the primary diagnosis is usually obvious from either history or physical examination: the massive spleen of alcoholic cirrhosis, the history of metastatic cancer or SLE, or miliary tuberculosis on chest radiograph (Table 11-1).

Diagnostic problems can occur with atypical presentations and among related hematologic diseases.

Although pancytopenia is most common, some patients with bone marrow hypocellularity have depression of only one or two of three blood lines, with later progression to pancytopenia. The bone marrow in constitutional aplastic anemia is indistinguishable morphologically from the aspirate in acquired disease. The diagnosis can be suggested by family history, abnormal blood counts since childhood, or the presence of associated physical anomalies. Aplastic anemia may be difficult to distinguish from the hypocellular variety of MDS: MDS is favored by finding morphologic abnormalities, particularly of megakaryocytes and myeloid precursor cells, and typical cytogenetic abnormalities (discussed later).

Prognosis

The natural history of severe aplastic anemia is rapid deterioration and death. Provision first of RBC and later of platelet transfusions and effective antibiotics are of some benefit, but few patients show spontaneous recovery. The major prognostic determinant is the blood count. Historically, severe disease was defined by the presence of two of three parameters: absolute neutrophil count <500/μL, platelet count <20,000/μL, and corrected reticulocyte count <1% (or absolute reticulocyte count <60,000/μL). In the era of effective immunosuppressive therapies, absolute numbers of reticulocytes (>25,000/uL) and lymphocytes (>1000/uL) may be a better predictor of response to treatment and long-term outcome.

TREATMENT Aplastic Anemia

Severe acquired aplastic anemia can be cured by replacement of the absent hematopoietic cells (and the immune system) by stem cell transplant, or it can be ameliorated by suppression of the immune system to allow recovery of the patient's residual bone marrow function. Hematopoietic growth factors have limited usefulness, and glucocorticoids are of no value. Suspect exposures to drugs or chemicals should be discontinued; however, spontaneous recovery of severe blood count depression is rare, and a waiting period before beginning treatment may not be advisable unless the blood counts are only modestly depressed.

HEMATOPOIETIC STEM CELL TRANSPLANTATION This is the best therapy for a younger patient with a fully histocompatible sibling donor (Chap. 30). Human leukocyte antigen (HLA) typing should be ordered as soon as the diagnosis of aplastic anemia is established in a child or younger adult. In transplant candidates, transfusion of blood from family members should be avoided so as to prevent sensitization to histocompatibility antigens, but limited numbers of blood products probably do not greatly affect outcome. For allogeneic transplant from fully matched siblings, long-term survival rates for children are approximately 90%. Transplant morbidity and mortality rates are increased among adults, due mainly to the higher risk of chronic GVHD and serious infections.

Most patients do not have a suitable sibling donor. Occasionally, a full phenotypic match can be found within the family and serve as well. Far more available are other alternative donors, either unrelated but histocompatible volunteers or closely but not perfectly matched family members. High-resolution matching at HLA, as well as more effective conditioning regimens and GVHD prophylaxis, have led to improving survival rates in those patients who do proceed to alternative donor transplant, in some series approximating results with conventional sibling donors. Patients are at risk for late complications, especially a higher rate of cancer, if radiation is used as a component of conditioning.

IMMUNOSUPPRESSION The standard regimen of ATG in combination with cyclosporine induces hematologic recovery (independence from transfusion and a leukocyte count adequate to prevent infection) in 60–70% of patients. Children do especially well, while older adult patients often develop complications due to the presence of comorbidities. An early robust hematologic response correlates with long-term survival. Improvement in granulocyte number is generally apparent within 2 months of treatment. Most recovered patients continue to have some degree of blood count depression, the MCV remains elevated, and the bone marrow cellularity returns toward normal very slowly if at all. Relapse (recurrent pancytopenia) is frequent, often occurring as cyclosporine is discontinued; most, but not all, patients respond to reinstitution of immunosuppression, but some responders become dependent on continued cyclosporine administration. Development of MDS, with typical marrow morphologic or cytogenetic abnormalities, occurs in approximately 15% of treated patients, usually but not invariably associated with a return of pancytopenia, and some patients develop leukemia. A laboratory diagnosis of PNH can generally be made at the time of presentation of aplastic anemia by flow cytometry; recovered patients may have frank hemolysis if the PNH clone expands. Bone marrow examinations should be performed if there is an unfavorable change in blood counts.

Horse ATG and rabbit antilymphocyte globulin (ALG) are administered as intravenous infusions over 4 or 5 days, respectively. ATG binds to peripheral blood cells; therefore, platelet and granulocyte numbers may decrease further during active treatment. Serum sickness, a flulike illness with a characteristic cutaneous eruption and arthralgia, often develops approximately

10 days after initiating treatment. Methylprednisolone, 1 mg/kg per d for 2 weeks, can ameliorate the immune consequences of heterologous protein infusion. Excessive or extended glucocorticoid therapy is associated with avascular joint necrosis. Cyclosporine is administered orally at an initial high dose, with subsequent adjustment according to blood levels obtained every 2 weeks, rough levels should be between 150 and 200 ng/mL. The most important side effects are nephrotoxicity, hypertension, seizures, and opportunistic infections, especially *Pneumocystis carinii* (prophylactic treatment with monthly inhaled pentamidine is recommended).

Most patients with aplastic anemia lack a suitable marrow donor, and immunosuppression is the treatment of choice. Overall survival is equivalent with transplantation and immunosuppression. However, successful transplant cures marrow failure, whereas patients who recover adequate blood counts after immunosuppression remain at risk of relapse and malignant evolution. Because of excellent results in children and younger adults, allogeneic transplant should be performed if a suitable sibling donor is available. Increasing age and the severity of neutropenia are the most important factors weighing in the decision between transplant and immunosuppression in adults who have a matched family donor: older patients do better with ATG and cyclosporine, whereas transplant is preferred if granulocytopenia is profound. Some patients may prefer immunosuppression; transplant is used for failure to recover blood counts or occurrence of late complications.

Outcomes following both transplant and immunosuppression have improved with time. High doses of cyclophosphamide, without stem cell rescue, have been reported to produce durable hematologic recovery, without relapse or evolution to MDS, but this treatment can produce sustained severe fatal neutropenia, and response is often delayed.

OTHER THERAPIES The effectiveness of androgens has not been verified in controlled trials, but occasional patients will respond or even demonstrate blood count dependence on continued therapy. Sex hormones upregulate telomerase gene activity in vitro, possibly also their mechanism of action in improving marrow function. For patients with moderate disease or those with severe pancytopenia in whom immunosuppression has failed, a 3–4-month trial is appropriate. Hematopoietic growth factors (HGFs) are not recommended as initial therapy for severe aplastic anemia, and even their roles as adjuncts to immunosuppression are not clear.

SUPPORTIVE CARE Meticulous medical attention is required so that the patient may survive to benefit from definitive therapy or, having failed treatment, to maintain a reasonable existence in the face of pancytopenia. First and most important, infection in the presence of severe neutropenia must be aggressively treated by prompt institution of parenteral, broad-spectrum antibiotics, usually ceftazidime or a combination of an aminoglycoside, cephalosporin, and semisynthetic penicillin. Therapy is empirical and must not await results of culture, although specific foci of infection such as oropharyngeal or anorectal abscesses, pneumonia, sinusitis, and typhlitis (necrotizing colitis) should be sought on physical examination and with radiographic studies. When indwelling plastic catheters become contaminated, vancomycin should be added. Persistent or recrudescent fever implies fungal disease: *Candida* and *Aspergillus* are common, especially after several courses of antibacterial antibiotics. A major reason for the improved prognosis in aplastic anemia has been the development of better antifungal drugs and the timely institution of such therapy when infection is suspected. Granulocyte transfusions using granulocyte colony-stimulating factor (G-CSF)–mobilized peripheral blood may be effective in the treatment of overwhelming or refractory infections. Hand washing, the single best method of preventing the spread of infection, remains a neglected practice. Nonabsorbed antibiotics for gut decontamination are poorly tolerated and not of proven value. Total reverse isolation does not reduce mortality from infections.

Both platelet and erythrocyte numbers can be maintained by transfusion. Alloimmunization historically limited the usefulness of platelet transfusions and is now minimized by several strategies, including use of single donors to reduce exposure and physical or chemical methods to diminish leukocytes in the product; HLA-matched platelets are often effective in patients refractory to random donor products. Inhibitors of fibrinolysis such as aminocaproic acid have not been shown to relieve mucosal oozing; the use of low-dose glucocorticoids to induce "vascular stability" is unproven and not recommended. Whether platelet transfusions are better used prophylactically or only as needed remains unclear. Any rational regimen of prophylaxis requires transfusions once or twice weekly to maintain the platelet count >10,000/μL (oozing from the gut, and presumably also from other vascular beds, increases precipitously at counts <5000/μL). Menstruation should be suppressed either by oral estrogens or nasal follicle-stimulating hormone/luteinizing hormone (FSH/LH) antagonists. Aspirin and other nonsteroidal anti-inflammatory agents inhibit platelet function and must be avoided.

Red blood cells should be transfused to maintain a normal level of activity, usually at a hemoglobin value of 70 g/L (90 g/L if there is underlying cardiac or pulmonary disease); a regimen of 2 units every 2 weeks will replace normal losses in a patient without a functioning bone marrow. In chronic anemia, the iron chelators deferoxamine and deferasirox should be added at approximately the fiftieth transfusion to avoid secondary hemochromatosis.

PURE RBC APLASIA

Other, more restricted forms of marrow failure occur, in which only a single circulating cell type is affected and the marrow shows corresponding absence or decreased numbers of specific precursor cells: aregenerative anemia as in PRCA (discussed later), thrombocytopenia with amegakaryocytosis (Chap. 19), and neutropenia without marrow myeloid cells in agranulocytosis (Chap. 5). In general and in contrast to aplastic anemia and MDS, the unaffected lineages appear quantitatively and qualitatively normal. Agranulocytosis, the most frequent of these syndromes, is usually a complication of medical drug use (with agents similar to those related to aplastic anemia), either by a mechanism of direct chemical toxicity or by immune destruction. Agranulocytosis has an incidence similar to aplastic anemia but is especially frequent among older adults and in women. The syndrome should resolve with discontinuation of exposure, but significant mortality is attached to neutropenia in an older and often previously unwell patient. Both pure white cell aplasia (agranulocytosis without incriminating drug exposure) and amegakaryocytic thrombocytopenia are exceedingly rare and, like PRCA, appear to be due to destructive antibodies or lymphocytes and can respond to immunosuppressive therapies. In all the single-lineage failure syndromes, progression to pancytopenia or leukemia is unusual.

TABLE 11-4

CLASSIFICATION OF PURE RBC APLASIA

- Self-limited
  - Transient erythroblastopenia of childhood
  - Transient aplastic crisis of hemolysis (acute B19 parvovirus infection)
- Fetal red blood cell aplasia
  - Nonimmune hydrops fetalis (in utero B19 parvovirus infection)
- Hereditary pure RBC aplasia
  - Congenital pure RBC aplasia (Diamond-Blackfan syndrome)
- Acquired pure RBC aplasia
  - Thymoma and malignancy
    - Thymoma
    - Lymphoid malignancies (and more rarely other hematologic diseases)
    - Paraneoplastic to solid tumors
  - Connective tissue disorders with immunologic abnormalities
    - Systemic lupus erythematosus, juvenile rheumatoid arthritis, rheumatoid arthritis
    - Multiple endocrine gland insufficiency
  - Virus
    - Persistent B19 parvovirus, hepatitis, adult T cell leukemia virus, Epstein-Barr virus
  - Pregnancy
  - Drugs
    - Especially phenytoin, azathioprine, chloramphenicol, procainamide, isoniazid
    - Erythropoietin
- Idiopathic

DEFINITION AND DIFFERENTIAL DIAGNOSIS

PRCA is characterized by anemia, reticulocytopenia, and absent or rare erythroid precursor cells in the bone marrow. The classification of PRCA is shown in Table 11-4. In adults, PRCA is acquired. An identical syndrome can occur constitutionally: Diamond-Blackfan anemia, or congenital PRCA, is diagnosed at birth or in early childhood and often responds to glucocorticoid treatment; mutations in ribosomal RNA processing genes are etiologic. Temporary RBC failure occurs in transient aplastic crisis of hemolytic anemias due to acute parvovirus infection and in transient erythroblastopenia of childhood, which affects normal children.

CLINICAL ASSOCIATIONS AND ETIOLOGY

PRCA has important associations with immune system diseases. A small minority of cases occur with a thymoma. More frequently, RBC aplasia can be the major manifestation of large granular lymphocytosis or may occur in chronic lymphocytic leukemia. Some patients may be hypogammaglobulinemic. Infrequently (compared with agranulocytosis), PRCA can be due to an idiosyncratic drug reaction. Subcutaneous administration of erythropoietin (EPO) has provoked PRCA mediated by neutralizing antibodies.

Like aplastic anemia, PRCA results from diverse mechanisms. Antibodies to RBC precursors are frequently present in the blood, but T cell inhibition is probably the more common immune mechanism. Cytotoxic lymphocyte activity restricted by histocompatibility locus or specific for human T cell leukemia/lymphoma virus I—infected cells, as well as natural killer cell activity inhibitory of erythropoiesis, have been demonstrated in particularly well-studied individual cases.

PERSISTENT PARVOVIRUS B19 INFECTION

Chronic parvovirus infection is an important, treatable cause of PRCA. This common virus causes a benign exanthem of childhood (fifth disease) and a

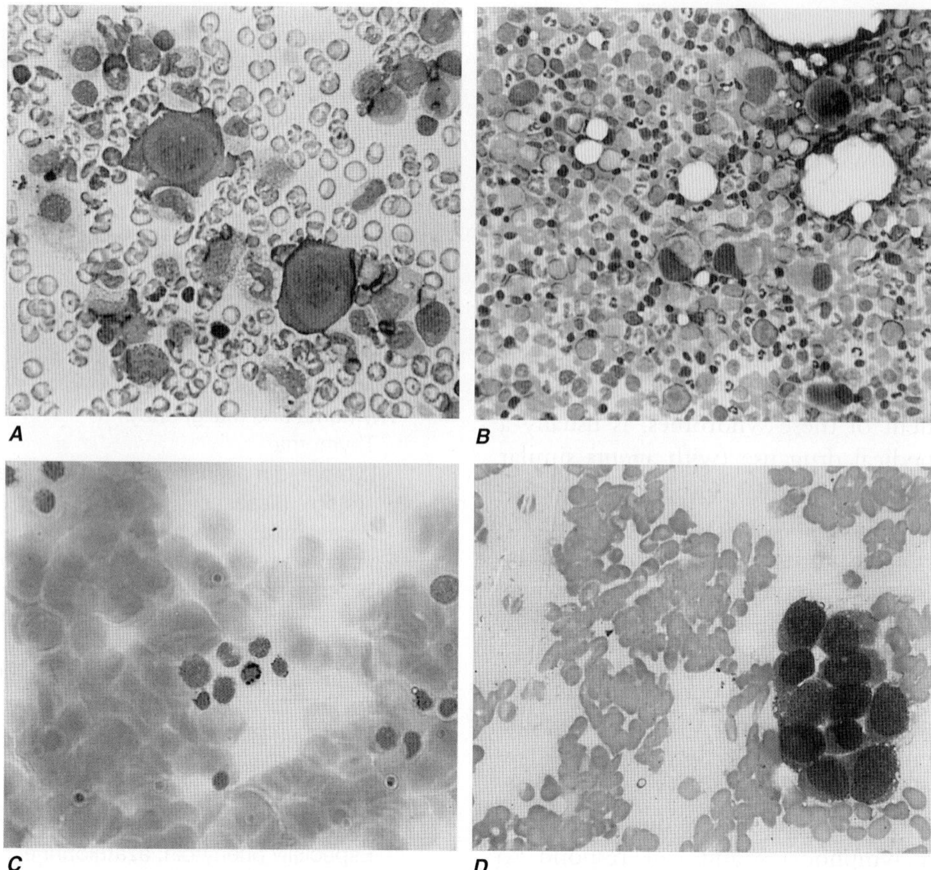

FIGURE 11-2

Pathognomonic cells in marrow failure syndromes. ***A.*** Giant pronormoblast, the cytopathic effect of B19 parvovirus infection of the erythroid progenitor cell. ***B.*** Uninuclear megakaryocyte and microblastic erythroid precursors typical of the 5q–myelodysplasia syndrome. ***C.*** Ringed sideroblast showing perinuclear iron granules. ***D.*** Tumor cells present on a touch preparation made from the marrow biopsy of a patient with metastatic carcinoma.

polyarthralgia/arthritis syndrome in adults. In patients with underlying hemolysis (or any condition that increases demand for RBC production), parvovirus infection can cause a transient aplastic crisis and an abrupt but temporary worsening of the anemia due to failed erythropoiesis. In normal individuals, acute infection is resolved by production of neutralizing antibodies to the virus, but in the setting of congenital, acquired, or iatrogenic immunodeficiency, persistent viral infection may occur. The bone marrow shows RBC aplasia and the presence of giant pronormoblasts (Fig. 11-2), which is the cytopathic sign of B19 parvovirus infection. Viral tropism for human erythroid progenitor cells is due to its use of erythrocyte P antigen as a cellular receptor for entry. Direct cytotoxicity of virus causes anemia if demands on erythrocyte production are high; in normal individuals, the temporary cessation of RBC production is not clinically apparent, and skin and joint symptoms are mediated by immune complex deposition.

TREATMENT Pure RBC Aplasia

History, physical examination, and routine laboratory studies may disclose an underlying disease or a drug exposure. Thymoma should be sought by radiographic procedures. Tumor excision is indicated, but anemia does not necessarily improve with surgery. The diagnosis of parvovirus infection requires detection of viral DNA sequences in the blood (IgG and IgM antibodies are commonly absent). The presence of erythroid colonies has been considered predictive of response to immunosuppressive therapy in idiopathic PRCA.

Red cell aplasia is compatible with long-term survival with supportive care alone: a combination of erythrocyte transfusions and iron chelation. For persistent B19 parvovirus infection, almost all patients respond to intravenous immunoglobulin therapy (e.g., 0.4 g/kg daily for 5 days), although relapse and retreatment may be expected, especially in patients with AIDS. The majority of patients with idiopathic PRCA respond favorably to immunosuppression. Most first receive a course of glucocorticoids. Also effective are cyclosporine, ATG, azathioprine, cyclophosphamide, and the monoclonal antibody daclizumab, an antibody to the high affinity IL-2 receptor. PRCA developing on EPO therapy should be treated with immunosuppression and withdrawal of EPO.

MYELODYSPLASIA

DEFINITION

Myelodysplasia or the MDSs are a heterogeneous group of hematologic disorders broadly characterized by cytopenias associated with a dysmorphic (or abnormal appearing) and usually cellular bone marrow and by consequent ineffective blood cell production. A clinically useful nosology of these entities was first developed by the French-American-British Cooperative Group in 1983. Five entities were defined: refractory anemia (RA), refractory anemia with ringed sideroblasts (RARS), refractory anemia with excess blasts (RAEB), refractory anemia with excess blasts in transformation (RAEB-t), and chronic myelomonocytic leukemia (CMML). The World Health Organization (WHO) classification (2002) recognized that the distinction between RAEB-t and acute myeloid leukemia is arbitrary and groups them together as acute leukemia, that CMML behaves as a myeloproliferative disease, and separated refractory anemias with dysmorphic change restricted to erythroid lineage from those with multilineage changes. In a revision, specific categories for unilineage dysplasias were added (Table 11-5).

The diagnosis of MDS may be a challenge, as sometimes subtle clinical and pathologic features must be distinguished in a usually older adult patient >70 years of age with comorbidities; furthermore, precise diagnostic categorization requires a hematopathologist knowledgeable in the latest classification scheme. Nonetheless, it is important that the internist and primary care physician be sufficiently familiar with MDS to expedite referral to a hematologist, both because many new therapies are now available to improve hematopoietic function and the judicious use of supportive care can improve the patient's quality of life.

EPIDEMIOLOGY

Idiopathic MDS is a disease of older adults; the mean age at onset is older than 70 years. There is a slight male preponderance. MDS is a relatively common form of bone marrow failure, with reported incidence rates of 35 to >100 per million persons in the general population and 120 to >500 per million in older adults. MDS is rare in children, but monocytic leukemia can be seen. Secondary or therapy-related MDS is not age related. Rates of MDS have increased over time, due to the recognition of the syndrome by physicians and the aging of the population.

ETIOLOGY AND PATHOPHYSIOLOGY

MDS is associated with environmental exposures such as radiation and benzene; other risk factors have been reported inconsistently. Secondary MDS occurs as a late toxicity of cancer treatment, usually with a combination of radiation and the radiomimetic alkylating agents such as busulfan, nitrosourea, or procarbazine (with a latent period of 5–7 years) or the DNA topoisomerase inhibitors (2 years). Both acquired aplastic anemia following immunosuppressive treatment and Fanconi's anemia can evolve into MDS.

MDS is a clonal hematopoietic stem cell disorder leading to impaired cell proliferation and differentiation. Cytogenetic abnormalities are found in approximately half of patients, and some of the same specific lesions are also seen in frank leukemia; aneuploidy is more frequent than translocations. Both presenting and evolving hematologic manifestations result from the accumulation of multiple genetic lesions: loss of tumor suppressor genes, activating oncogene mutations, or other harmful alterations. Cytogenetic abnormalities are not random (loss of all or part of 5, 7, and 20; trisomy of 8) and may be related to etiology (11q23 following topoisomerase II inhibitors); CMML is often associated with t(5;12) that creates a chimeric *tel-PDGFβ* gene. The type and number of cytogenetic abnormalities strongly correlate with the probability of leukemic transformation and survival. Mutations of N-*ras* (an oncogene), *p53* and *IRF-1* (tumor suppressor genes), *Bcl-2* (an antiapoptotic gene), and others have been reported in some patients but likely occur late in the sequence leading to leukemic transformation. Apoptosis of marrow cells is increased in early stage and low-risk categories of MDS, presumably due to these acquired genetic alterations or possibly to an overlaid immune response. An immune pathophysiology has been suggested for trisomy 8 MDS, which often responds clinically to immunosuppressive therapy. Such patients have T cell activity directed to the cytogenetically aberrant clone. Sideroblastic anemia may be related to mutations in mitochondrial genes; ineffective erythropoiesis and disordered iron metabolism are the functional consequences of the genetic alterations.

CLINICAL FEATURES

Anemia dominates the early course. Most symptomatic patients complain of the gradual onset of fatigue and weakness, dyspnea, and pallor, but at least half the

TABLE 11-5

WORLD HEALTH ORGANIZATION (WHO) CLASSIFICATION OF MYELODYSPLASTIC SYNDROMES AND NEOPLASMS

NAME	WHO ESTIMATED PROPORTION OF PATIENTS WITH MDS	PERIPHERAL BLOOD: KEY FEATURES	BONE MARROW: KEY FEATURES
Refractory cytopenias with unilineage dysplasia (RCUD):			
Refractory anemia (RA)	10-20%	Anemia <1% of blasts	Unilineage erythroid dysplasia (in ≥10% of cells) <5% blasts
Refractory neutropenia (RN)	<1%	Neutropenia <1% blasts	Unilineage granulocytic dysplasia <5% blasts
Refractory thrombocytopenia (RT)	<1%	Thrombocytopenia <1% blasts	Unilineage megakaryocytic dysplasia <5% blasts
Refractory anemia with ring sideroblasts (RARS)	3-11%	Anemia No blasts	Unilineage erythroid dysplasia ≥15% of erythroid precursors are ring sideroblasts <5% blasts
Refractory cytopenias with multilineage dysplasia (RCMD)	30%	Cytopenia(s) <1% blasts No Auer rods	Multilineage dysplasia ± ring sideroblasts <5% blasts No Auer rods
Refractory anemia with excess blasts, type 1 (RAEB-1)	40%	Cytopenia(s) <5% blasts No Auer rods	Unilineage or multilineage dysplasia
Refractory anemia with excess blasts, type 2 (RAEB-2)		Cytopenia(s) 5-19% blasts ± Auer rods	Unilineage or multilineage dysplasia 10-19% blasts ± Auer rods
MDS associated with isolated Del(5q) (Del(5q)	Uncommon	Anemia Normal or high platelet count <1% blasts	Isolated 5q31 chromosome deletion Anemia; hypolobated megakaryocytes <5% blasts
Childhood MDS, including refractory cytopenia of childhood (*provisional?*) (RCC)	<1 %	Pancytopenia	<5% marrow blasts for RCC Marrow usually hypocellular
MDS, unclassifiable (MDS-U)	?	Cytopenia ≤1% blasts	Does not fit other categories Dysplasia <5% blasts If no dysplasia, MDS-associated karyotype

Note: If peripheral blood blasts are 2–4%, the diagnosis is RAEB-1 even if marrow blasts are less than 5%. If Auer rods are present, the WHO considers the diagnosis RAEB-2 if the blast proportion is less than 20% (even if less than 10%), AML if at least 20% blasts. For all subtypes, peripheral blood monocytes are less than 1×10^9/L. Bicytopenia may be observed in RCUD subtypes, but pancytopenia with unilineage marrow dysplasia should be classified as MDS-U. Therapy-related MDS (t-MDS), whether due to alkylating agents, topoisomerase II (t-MDS/t-AML) in the WHO classification of AML and precursor lesions. The listing in this table excludes MDS/myeloproliferative neoplasm overlap categories, such as chronic myelomonocytic leukemia, juvenile myelomonocytic leukemia, and the provisional entity RARS with thrombocytosis.
Abbreviation: MDS, myelodysplastic syndrome.

patients are asymptomatic, and their MDS is discovered only incidentally on routine blood counts. Previous chemotherapy or radiation exposure is an important historic fact. Fever and weight loss should point to a myeloproliferative rather than myelodysplastic process. Children with Down syndrome are susceptible to MDS, and a family history may indicate a hereditary form of sideroblastic anemia or Fanconi's anemia.

The physical examination is remarkable for signs of anemia; approximately 20% of patients have splenomegaly. Some unusual skin lesions, including Sweet's syndrome (febrile neutrophilic dermatosis), occur with MDS. Autoimmune syndromes are not infrequent.

LABORATORY STUDIES

Blood

Anemia is present in the majority of cases, either alone or as part of bi- or pancytopenia; isolated neutropenia or thrombocytopenia is more unusual. Macrocytosis is common, and the smear may be dimorphic with a distinctive population of large red blood cells. Platelets are also large and lack granules. In functional studies, they may show marked abnormalities, and patients may have bleeding symptoms despite seemingly adequate numbers. Neutrophils are hypogranulated; have hyposegmented, ringed, or abnormally segmented nuclei; contain Döhle bodies; and may be functionally deficient. Circulating myeloblasts usually correlate with marrow blast numbers, and their quantitation is important for classification and prognosis. The total white blood cell (WBC) count is usually normal or low, except in chronic myelomonocytic leukemia. As in aplastic anemia, MDS can be associated with a clonal population of PNH cells.

Bone marrow

The bone marrow is usually normal or hypercellular, but in 20% of cases, it is sufficiently hypocellular to be confused with aplasia. No single characteristic feature of marrow morphology distinguishes MDS, but the following are commonly observed: dyserythropoietic changes (especially nuclear abnormalities) and ringed sideroblasts in the erythroid lineage; hypogranulation and hyposegmentation in granulocytic precursors, with an increase in myeloblasts; and megakaryocytes showing reduced numbers or disorganized nuclei. Megaloblastic nuclei associated with defective hemoglobinization in the erythroid lineage are common. The prognosis strongly correlates with the proportion of marrow blasts. Cytogenetic analysis and fluorescent in situ hybridization can identify chromosomal abnormalities.

DIFFERENTIAL DIAGNOSIS

Deficiencies of vitamin B_{12} or folate should be excluded by appropriate blood tests; vitamin B_6 deficiency can be assessed by a therapeutic trial of pyridoxine if the bone marrow shows ringed sideroblasts. Marrow dysplasia can be observed in acute viral infections, drug reactions, or chemical toxicity but should be transient. More difficult are the distinctions between hypocellular MDS and aplasia or between refractory anemia with excess blasts and early acute leukemia. The WHO considers the presence of 20% blasts in the marrow as the criterion that separates acute myeloid leukemia (AML) from MDS.

PROGNOSIS

The median survival varies greatly from years for patients with 5q- or sideroblastic anemia to a few months in refractory anemia with excess blasts or severe pancytopenia associated with monosomy 7; an International Prognostic Scoring System (IPSS; Table 11-6) assists in making predictions. Most patients die as a result of complications of pancytopenia and not due to leukemic transformation; perhaps one-third succumb to other diseases unrelated to their MDS. Precipitous worsening of pancytopenia, acquisition of new chromosomal abnormalities on serial cytogenetic determination, an increase in the number of blasts, and marrow fibrosis are all poor prognostic indicators. The outlook in therapy-related MDS, regardless of type, is extremely poor, and most patients progress within a few months to refractory AML.

TREATMENT Myelodysplasia

Historically, the therapy of MDS has been unsatisfactory. Only stem cell transplantation offers cure. Survival rates of 50% at 3 years have been reported, but older patients are particularly prone to develop treatment-related mortality and morbidity. Results of transplant

TABLE 11-6

INTERNATIONAL PROGNOSTIC SCORING SYSTEM (IPSS)

	SCORE VALUE				
PROGNOSTIC VARIABLE	**0**	**0.5**	**1**	**1.5**	**2**
Bone marrow blasts (%)	<5%	5–10%		11–20%	21–30%
Karyotype[a]	Good	Intermediate	Poor		
Cytopenia[b] (lineages affected)	0 or 1	2 or 3			
Risk Group Scores	**Score**				
Low	0				
Intermediate-1	0.5–1				
Intermediate-2	1.5–2				
High	≥2.5				

[a]Good, normal, -Y, del(5q), del (20q); poor, complex (≥3 abnormalities) or chromosome 7 abnormalities; intermediate, all other abnormalities.
[b]Cytopenias defined as Hb <100 g/L, platelet count <100,000/μL, absolute neutrophil count <1500/μL.

using matched unrelated donors are comparable, although most series contain younger and more highly selected cases. However, multiple new drugs have been approved for use in MDS. Several regimens appear to not only improve blood counts but to also delay the onset of leukemia and to improve survival. The choice of therapy and implementation of treatment are complicated and require hematologic expertise.

MDS has been regarded as particularly refractory to cytotoxic chemotherapy regimens but is probably no more resistant to effective treatment than AML in older adults, in whom drug toxicity is often fatal and remissions, if achieved, are brief.

Low doses of cytotoxic drugs have been administered for their "differentiating" potential, and from this experience has emerged drug therapies based on pyrimidine analogues. Azacitidine is directly cytotoxic but also inhibits DNA methylation, thereby altering gene expression; however, demethylation status has not correlated well with clinical effects. Azacitidine improves blood counts and survival in a minority of MDS patients compared with best supportive care. Azacitidine has been administered subcutaneously, daily for 7 days, at 4-week intervals, for at least four cycles before assessing for response. Decitabine is closely related to azacitidine and is more potent. Similar to azacitidine, approximately 20% of patients show responses in blood counts, with a duration of response of almost 1 year. Activity may be higher in more advanced MDS subtypes. Decitabine is administered by continuous intravenous infusion, every 8 hours for 3 days, in repeating cycles. The optimal dose regimens for both azacitidine and decitabine are still being determined in clinical research protocols. The major toxicity of both azacitidine and decitabine is myelosuppression, leading to worsened blood counts. Other symptoms associated with cancer chemotherapy frequently occur.

Lenalidomide, a thalidomide derivative with a more favorable toxicity profile, is particularly effective in reversing anemia in MDS patients with 5q- syndrome; not only do a high proportion of these patients become transfusion independent with normal or near-normal hemoglobin levels, but their cytogenetics also become normal. The drug has many biologic activities, and it is unclear which is critical for clinical efficacy. Lenalidomide is administered orally. Most patients improve within 3 months of initiating therapy. Toxicities include myelosuppression (worsening thrombocytopenia and neutropenia, necessitating blood count monitoring) and an increased risk of deep vein thrombosis and pulmonary embolism.

ATG and cyclosporine, as employed in aplastic anemia, also may produce sustained independence from transfusion and improve survival. Immunosuppression with ATG or, in more recent studies, the anti-CD52 monoclonal antibody Campath is especially effective in younger MDS patients (younger than age 60 years) with more favorable IPSS scores and who bear the histocompatability antigen HLA-DR15.

HGFs can improve blood counts but, as in most other marrow failure states, have been most beneficial to patients with the least severe pancytopenia. G-CSF treatment alone failed to improve survival in a controlled trial. EPO alone or in combination with G-CSF can improve hemoglobin levels, but mainly in those with low serum EPO levels who have no or only a modest need for transfusions, and retrospective analysis suggests improved survival with treatment

The same principles of supportive care described for aplastic anemia apply to MDS. Despite improvements in drug therapy, many patients will be anemic for years. RBC transfusion support should be accompanied by iron chelation to prevent secondary hemochromatosis.

MYELOPHTHISIC ANEMIAS

Fibrosis of the bone marrow (see Fig. 103-2), usually accompanied by a characteristic blood smear picture called *leukoerythroblastosis*, can occur as a primary hematologic disease, called *myelofibrosis* or *myeloid metaplasia* (Chap. 13), and as a secondary process, called *myelophthisis*. Myelophthisis, or secondary myelofibrosis, is reactive. Fibrosis can be a response to invading tumor cells, usually an epithelial cancer of breast, lung, a prostate origin or neuroblastoma. Marrow fibrosis may occur with infection of mycobacteria (both *Mycobacterium tuberculosis* and *Mycobacterium avium*), fungi, or HIV and in sarcoidosis. Intracellular lipid deposition in Gaucher's disease and obliteration of the marrow space related to absence of osteoclast remodeling in congenital osteopetrosis also can produce fibrosis. Secondary myelofibrosis is a late consequence of radiation therapy or treatment with radiomimetic drugs. Usually the infectious or malignant underlying processes are obvious. Marrow fibrosis can also be a feature of a variety of hematologic syndromes, especially chronic myeloid leukemia, multiple myeloma, lymphomas, myeloma, and hairy cell leukemia.

The pathophysiology has three distinct features: proliferation of fibroblasts in the marrow space (myelofibrosis); the extension of hematopoiesis into the long bones and into extramedullary sites, usually the spleen, liver, and lymph nodes (myeloid metaplasia); and ineffective erythropoiesis. The etiology of the fibrosis is unknown but most likely involves dysregulated production of growth factors: platelet-derived growth factor and transforming growth factor β have been implicated. Abnormal regulation of other hematopoietins would lead to localization of blood-producing cells in nonhematopoietic tissues and uncoupling of the usually balanced processes of stem cell proliferation and differentiation. Myelofibrosis is remarkable for pancytopenia despite very large numbers of circulating hematopoietic progenitor cells.

Anemia is dominant in secondary myelofibrosis, usually normocytic and normochromic. The diagnosis is suggested by the characteristic leukoerythroblastic smear (see Fig. 108-1). Erythrocyte morphology is highly abnormal, with circulating nucleated RBCs, teardrops, and shape distortions. WBC numbers are often elevated, sometimes mimicking a leukemoid reaction, with circulating myelocytes, promyelocytes, and myeloblasts. Platelets may be abundant and are often of giant size. An inability to aspirate the bone marrow, the characteristic "dry tap," can allow a presumptive diagnosis in the appropriate setting before the biopsy is decalcified.

The course of secondary myelofibrosis is determined by its etiology, usually a metastatic tumor or an advanced hematologic malignancy. Treatable causes must be excluded, especially tuberculosis and fungus. Transfusion support can relieve symptoms.

CHAPTER 12

TRANSFUSION BIOLOGY AND THERAPY

Jeffery S. Dzieczkowski ■ Kenneth C. Anderson

BLOOD GROUP ANTIGENS AND ANTIBODIES

The study of red blood cell (RBC) antigens and antibodies forms the foundation of transfusion medicine. Serologic studies initially characterized these antigens, but now the molecular composition and structure of many are known. Antigens, either carbohydrate or protein, are assigned to a blood group system based on the structure and similarity of the determinant epitopes. Other cellular blood elements and plasma proteins are also antigenic and can result in *alloimmunization*, the production of antibodies directed against the blood group antigens of another individual. These antibodies are called *alloantibodies*.

Antibodies directed against RBC antigens may result from "natural" exposure, particularly to carbohydrates that mimic some blood group antigens. Antibodies that occur via natural stimuli are usually produced by a T cell—independent response (thus, generating no memory) and are IgM isotypes. *Autoantibodies* (antibodies against autologous blood group antigens) arise spontaneously or as the result of infectious sequelae (e.g., from *Mycoplasma pneumoniae*) and are also often IgM. These antibodies are often clinically insignificant due to their low affinity for antigen at body temperature. However, IgM antibodies can activate the complement cascade and result in hemolysis. Antibodies that result from allogeneic exposure, such as transfusion or pregnancy, are usually IgG. IgG antibodies commonly bind to antigen at warmer temperatures and may hemolyze RBCs. Unlike IgM antibodies, IgG antibodies can cross the placenta and bind fetal erythrocytes bearing the corresponding antigen, resulting in hemolytic disease of the newborn, or *hydrops fetalis*.

Alloimmunization to leukocytes, platelets, and plasma proteins may also result in transfusion complications such as fevers and urticaria but generally does not cause hemolysis. Assay for these other alloantibodies is not routinely performed; however, they may be detected using special assays.

ABO ANTIGENS AND ANTIBODIES

The first blood group antigen system, recognized in 1900, was ABO, the most important in transfusion medicine. The major blood groups of this system are A, B, AB, and O. O type RBCs lack A or B antigens. These antigens are carbohydrates attached to a precursor backbone, may be found on the cellular membrane either as glycosphingolipids or glycoproteins, and are secreted into plasma and body fluids as glycoproteins. H substance is the immediate precursor on which the A and B antigens are added. This H substance is formed by the addition of fucose to the glycolipid or glycoprotein backbone. The subsequent addition of *N*-acetylgalactosamine creates the A antigen, while the addition of galactose produces the B antigen.

The genes that determine the A and B phenotypes are found on chromosome 9p and are expressed in a Mendelian codominant manner. The gene products are glycosyl transferases, which confer the enzymatic capability of attaching the specific antigenic carbohydrate. Individuals who lack the "A" and "B" transferases are phenotypically type "O," while those who inherit both transferases are type "AB." Rare individuals lack the H gene, which codes for fucose transferase, and cannot form H substance. These individuals are homozygous for the silent h allele (hh) and have Bombay phenotype (O_h).

The ABO blood group system is important because essentially all individuals produce antibodies to the ABH carbohydrate antigen that they lack. The naturally occurring anti-A and anti-B antibodies are termed *isoagglutinins*. Thus, type A individuals produce anti-B, while type B individuals make anti-A. Neither isoagglutinin is found in type AB individuals, while type O individuals produce both anti-A and anti-B. Thus, persons with type AB are "universal recipients" because they do not have antibodies against any ABO phenotype, while persons with type O blood can donate to essentially all recipients because their cells are not recognized by any ABO isoagglutinins. The rare individuals with Bombay phenotype produce antibodies to H substance (which is present on all red cells except those of hh phenotype) as well as to both A and B antigens and are therefore compatible only with other hh donors.

In most people, A and B antigens are secreted by the cells and are present in the circulation. Nonsecretors are susceptible to a variety of infections (e.g., *Candida albicans*, *Neisseria meningitidis*, *Streptococcus pneumoniae*, *Haemophilus influenzae*) as many organisms may bind to polysaccharides on cells. Soluble blood group antigens may block this binding.

Rh SYSTEM

The Rh system is the second most important blood group system in pretransfusion testing. The Rh antigens are found on a 30- to 32-kDa RBC membrane protein that has no defined function. Although >40 different antigens in the Rh system have been described, five determinants account for the vast majority of phenotypes. The presence of the D antigen confers Rh "positivity," while persons who lack the D antigen are Rh negative. Two allelic antigen pairs, E/e and C/c, are also found on the Rh protein. The three Rh genes, E/e, D, and C/c, are arranged in tandem on chromosome 1 and inherited as a haplotype, i.e., cDE or Cde. Two haplotypes can result in the phenotypic expression of two to five Rh antigens.

The D antigen is a potent alloantigen. About 15% of individuals lack this antigen. Exposure of these Rh-negative people to even small amounts of Rh-positive cells, by either transfusion or pregnancy, can result in the production of anti-D alloantibody.

OTHER BLOOD GROUP SYSTEMS AND ALLOANTIBODIES

More than 100 blood group systems are recognized, composed of more than 500 antigens. The presence or absence of certain antigens has been associated with various diseases and anomalies; antigens also act as receptors for infectious agents. Alloantibodies of importance in routine clinical practice are listed in Table 12-1.

Antibodies to *Lewis system* carbohydrate antigens are the most common cause of incompatibility during pretransfusion screening. The Lewis gene product is a fucosyl transferase and maps to chromosome 19. The antigen is not an integral membrane structure but is adsorbed to the RBC membrane from the plasma. Antibodies to Lewis antigens are usually IgM and cannot cross the placenta. Lewis antigens may be adsorbed onto tumor cells and may be targets of therapy.

I system antigens are also oligosaccharides related to H, A, B, and Le. I and i are not allelic pairs but are carbohydrate antigens that differ only in the extent of branching. The i antigen is an unbranched chain that is converted by the I gene product, a glycosyltransferase, into a branched chain. The branching process affects all the ABH antigens, which become progressively more branched in the first 2 years of life. Some patients with cold agglutinin disease or lymphomas can produce anti-I autoantibodies that cause RBC destruction. Occasional patients with mononucleosis or *Mycoplasma* pneumonia may develop cold agglutinins of either anti-I or anti-i specificity. Most adults lack i expression; thus, finding a donor for patients with anti-i is not difficult. Even though most adults express I antigen, binding is generally low at body temperature. Thus, administration of warm blood prevents isoagglutination.

The *P system* is another group of carbohydrate antigens controlled by specific glycosyltransferases. Its clinical significance is in rare cases of syphilis and viral infection that lead to paroxysmal cold hemoglobinuria. In these cases, an unusual autoantibody to P is produced that binds to

TABLE 12-1

RED BLOOD CELL BLOOD GROUP SYSTEMS AND ALLOANTIGENS

BLOOD GROUP SYSTEM	ANTIGEN	ALLOANTIBODY	CLINICAL SIGNIFICANCE
Rh (D, C/c, E/e)	RBC protein	IgG	HTR, HDN
Lewis (Le^a, Le^b)	Oligosaccharide	IgM/IgG	Rare HTR
Kell (K/k)	RBC protein	IgG	HTR, HDN
Duffy (Fy^a/Fy^b)	RBC protein	IgG	HTR, HDN
Kidd (Jk^a/Jk^b)	RBC protein	IgG	HTR (often delayed), HDN (mild)
I/i	Carbohydrate	IgM	None
MNSsU	RBC protein	IgM/IgG	Anti-M rare HDN, anti-S, -s, and -U HDN, HTR

Abbreviations: HDN, hemolytic disease of the newborn; HTR, hemolytic transfusion reaction; RBC, red blood cell.

RBCs in the cold and fixes complement upon warming. Antibodies with these biphasic properties are called *Donath-Landsteiner antibodies*. The P antigen is the cellular receptor of parvovirus B19 and also may be a receptor for *Escherichia coli* binding to urothelial cells.

The *MNSsU system* is regulated by genes on chromosome 4. M and N are determinants on glycophorin A, an RBC membrane protein, and S and s are determinants on glycophorin B. Anti-S and anti-s IgG antibodies may develop after pregnancy or transfusion and lead to hemolysis. Anti-U antibodies are rare but problematic; virtually every donor is incompatible because nearly all persons express U.

The *Kell* protein is very large (720 amino acids), and its secondary structure contains many different antigenic epitopes. The immunogenicity of Kell is third behind the ABO and Rh systems. The absence of the Kell precursor protein (controlled by a gene on X) is associated with acanthocytosis, shortened RBC survival, and a progressive form of muscular dystrophy that includes cardiac defects. This rare condition is called the *McLeod phenotype*. The K_x gene is linked to the 91-kDa component of the NADPH-oxidase on the X chromosome, deletion or mutation of which accounts for about 60% of cases of chronic granulomatous disease.

The *Duffy* antigens are codominant alleles, Fy^a and Fy^b, that also serve as receptors for *Plasmodium vivax*. More than 70% of persons in malaria-endemic areas lack these antigens, probably from selective influences of the infection on the population.

The *Kidd* antigens, Jk^a and Jk^b, may elicit antibodies transiently. A delayed hemolytic transfusion reaction that occurs with blood tested as compatible is often related to delayed appearance of anti-Jk^a.

PRETRANSFUSION TESTING

Pretransfusion testing of a potential recipient consists of the "type and screen." The "forward type" determines the ABO and Rh phenotype of the recipient's RBC by using antisera directed against the A, B, and D antigens. The "reverse type" detects isoagglutinins in the patient's serum and should correlate with the ABO phenotype, or forward type.

The alloantibody screen identifies antibodies directed against other RBC antigens. The alloantibody screen is performed by mixing patient serum with type O RBCs that contain the major antigens of most blood group systems and whose extended phenotype is known. The specificity of the alloantibody is identified by correlating the presence or absence of antigen with the results of the agglutination.

Cross-matching is ordered when there is a high probability that the patient will require a packed RBC (PRBC) transfusion. Blood selected for cross-matching must be ABO compatible and lack antigens for which the patient has alloantibodies. Nonreactive cross-matching confirms the absence of any major incompatibility and reserves that unit for the patient.

In the case of Rh-negative patients, every attempt must be made to provide Rh-negative blood components to prevent alloimmunization to the D antigen. In an emergency, Rh-positive blood can be safely transfused to an Rh-negative patient who lacks anti-D; however, the recipient is likely to become alloimmunized and produce anti-D. Rh-negative women of childbearing age who are transfused with products containing Rh-positive RBCs should receive passive immunization with anti-D (RhoGam or WinRho) to reduce or prevent sensitization.

BLOOD COMPONENTS

Blood products intended for transfusion are routinely collected as whole blood (450 mL) in various anticoagulants. Most donated blood is processed into components: PRBCs, platelets, and fresh-frozen plasma (FFP) or cryoprecipitate (Table 12-2). Whole blood is first separated into PRBCs and platelet-rich plasma by slow centrifugation. The platelet-rich plasma is then centrifuged at high speed to yield one unit of random donor (RD) platelets and one unit of FFP. Cryoprecipitate is produced by thawing FFP to precipitate the plasma proteins and then separated by centrifugation.

Apheresis technology is used for the collection of multiple units of platelets from a single donor. These single-donor apheresis platelets (SDAP) contain the equivalent of at least six units of RD platelets and have fewer contaminating leukocytes than pooled RD platelets.

Plasma may also be collected by apheresis. Plasma derivatives such as albumin, intravenous immunoglobulin, antithrombin, and coagulation factor concentrates are prepared from pooled plasma from many donors and are treated to eliminate infectious agents.

WHOLE BLOOD

Whole blood provides both oxygen-carrying capacity and volume expansion. It is the ideal component for patients who have sustained acute hemorrhage of ≤25% total blood volume loss. Whole blood is stored at 4°C to maintain erythrocyte viability, but platelet dysfunction and degradation of some coagulation factors occur. In addition, 2,3-bisphosphoglycerate levels fall over time, leading to an increase in the oxygen affinity of the hemoglobin and a decreased capacity to deliver oxygen to the tissues, a problem with all red cell storage. Fresh whole blood avoids these problems, but it is typically used only in emergency settings (i.e., military). Whole

TABLE 12-2

CHARACTERISTICS OF SELECTED BLOOD COMPONENTS

COMPONENT	VOLUME, mL	CONTENT	CLINICAL RESPONSE
PRBC	180–200	RBCs with variable leukocyte content and small amount of plasma	Increase hemoglobin 10 g/L and hematocrit 3%
Platelets	50–70	5.5×10^{10}/RD unit	Increase platelet count 5000–10,000/μL
	200–400	$\geq 3 \times 10^{11}$/SDAP product	CCI $\geq 10 \times 10^9$/L within 1 h and $\geq 7.5 \times 10^9$/L within 24 h posttransfusion
FFP	200–250	Plasma proteins—coagulation factors, proteins C and S, antithrombin	Increases coagulation factors about 2%
Cryoprecipitate	10–15	Cold-insoluble plasma proteins, fibrinogen, factor VIII, vWF	Topical fibrin glue; also 80 IU factor VIII

Abbreviations: CCI, corrected count increment; FFP, fresh-frozen plasma; PRBC, packed red blood cells; RBC, red blood cell; RD, random donor; SDAP, single-donor apheresis platelets; vWF, von Willebrand factor.

blood is not readily available, since it is routinely processed into components.

PACKED RED BLOOD CELLS

This product increases oxygen-carrying capacity in patients with anemia. Adequate oxygenation can be maintained with a hemoglobin content of 70 g/L in normovolemic patients without cardiac disease; however, comorbid factors may necessitate transfusion at a higher threshold. The decision to transfuse should be guided by the clinical situation and not by an arbitrary laboratory value. In the critical care setting, liberal use of transfusions to maintain near-normal levels of hemoglobin has not proven advantageous. In most patients requiring transfusion, levels of hemoglobin of 100 g/L are sufficient to keep oxygen supply from being critically low.

PRBCs may be modified to prevent certain adverse reactions. The majority of cellular blood products are now leukocyte reduced, and universal prestorage leukocyte reduction has been recommended. Prestorage filtration appears superior to bedside filtration as smaller amounts of cytokines are generated in the stored product. These PRBC units contain $<5 \times 10^6$ donor white blood cells (WBCs), and their use lowers the incidence of posttransfusion fever, cytomegalovirus (CMV) infections, and alloimmunization. Other theoretical benefits include less immunosuppression in the recipient and a lower risk of infections. Plasma, which may cause allergic reactions, can be removed from cellular blood components by washing.

PLATELETS

Thrombocytopenia is a risk factor for hemorrhage, and platelet transfusion reduces the incidence of bleeding. The threshold for prophylactic platelet transfusion is 10,000/μL. In patients without fever or infections, a threshold of 5000/μL may be sufficient to prevent spontaneous hemorrhage. For invasive procedures, 50,000/μL of platelets is the usual target level.

Platelets are given either as pools prepared RDs or as SDAPs from a single donor. In an unsensitized patient without increased platelet consumption (splenomegaly, fever, disseminated intravascular coagulation [DIC]), two units of transfused RD per square-meter body surface area (BSA) is anticipated to increase the platelet count by approximately 10,000/uL. Patients who have received multiple transfusions may be alloimmunized to many HLA- and platelet-specific antigens and have little or no increase in their posttransfusion platelet counts. Patients who may require multiple transfusions are best served by receiving SDAP and leukocyte-reduced components to lower the risk of alloimmunization.

Refractoriness to platelet transfusion may be evaluated using the corrected count increment (CCI):

$$\text{CCI} = \frac{\text{posttransfusion count}(/\mu\text{L}) - \text{pretransfusion count }(/\mu\text{L})}{\text{number of platelets transfused} \times 10^{-11}} \times \text{BSA }(\text{m}^2)$$

where BSA is body surface area measured in square meters. The platelet count performed 1 h after the transfusion is acceptable if the CCI is 10×10^9/mL, and after 18–24 h an increment of 7.5×10^9/mL is expected. Patients who have suboptimal responses are likely to have received multiple transfusions and have antibodies directed against class I HLA antigens. Refractoriness can be investigated by detecting anti-HLA antibodies in the recipient's serum. Patients who are sensitized will often react with 100% of the lymphocytes used for the HLA-antibody screen, and

HLA-matched SDAPs should be considered for those patients who require transfusion. Although ABO-identical HLA-matched SDAPs provide the best chance for increasing the platelet count, locating these products is difficult. Platelet cross-matching is available in some centers. Additional clinical causes for a low platelet CCI include fever, bleeding, splenomegaly, DIC, or medications in the recipient.

FRESH-FROZEN PLASMA

FFP contains stable coagulation factors and plasma proteins: fibrinogen, antithrombin, albumin, as well as proteins C and S. Indications for FFP include correction of coagulopathies, including the rapid reversal of warfarin; supplying deficient plasma proteins; and treatment of thrombotic thrombocytopenic purpura. FFP should not be routinely used to expand blood volume. FFP is an acellular component and does not transmit intracellular infections, e.g., CMV. Patients who are IgA-deficient and require plasma support should receive FFP from IgA-deficient donors to prevent anaphylaxis (discussed later).

CRYOPRECIPITATE

Cryoprecipitate is a source of fibrinogen, factor VIII, and von Willebrand factor (vWF). It is ideal for supplying fibrinogen to volume-sensitive patients. When factor VIII concentrates are not available, cryoprecipitate may be used since each unit contains approximately 80 units of factor VIII. Cryoprecipitate may also supply vWF to patients with dysfunctional (type II) or absent (type III) von Willebrand disease.

PLASMA DERIVATIVES

Plasma from thousands of donors may be pooled to derive specific protein concentrates, including albumin, intravenous immunoglobulin, antithrombin, and coagulation factors. In addition, donors who have high-titer antibodies to specific agents or antigens provide hyperimmune globulins, such as anti-D (RhoGam, WinRho), and antisera to hepatitis B virus (HBV), varicella-zoster virus, CMV, and other infectious agents.

ADVERSE REACTIONS TO BLOOD TRANSFUSION

Adverse reactions to transfused blood components occur despite multiple tests, inspections, and checks. Fortunately, the most common reactions are not life threatening, although serious reactions can present with mild symptoms and signs. Some reactions can be reduced or prevented by modified (filtered, washed, or irradiated) blood components. When an adverse reaction is suspected, the transfusion should be stopped and reported to the blood bank for investigation.

Transfusion reactions may result from immune and nonimmune mechanisms. Immune-mediated reactions are often due to preformed donor or recipient antibody; however, cellular elements may also cause adverse effects. Nonimmune causes of reactions are due to the chemical and physical properties of the stored blood component and its additives.

Transfusion-transmitted viral infections are increasingly rare due to improved screening and testing. As the risk of viral infection is reduced, the relative risk of other reactions increases, such as hemolytic transfusion reactions and sepsis from bacterially contaminated components. Pretransfusion quality assurance improvements further increase the safety of transfusion therapy. Infections, like any adverse transfusion reaction, must be brought to the attention of the blood bank for appropriate studies (Table 12-3).

TABLE 12-3

RISKS OF TRANSFUSION COMPLICATIONS

	FREQUENCY, EPISODES: UNIT
Reactions	
Febrile (FNHTR)	• 1–4:100
Allergic	• 1–4:100
Delayed hemolytic	• 1:1000
TRALI	• 1:5000
Acute hemolytic	• 1:12,000
Fatal hemolytic	• 1:100,000
Anaphylactic	• 1:150,000
Infections[a]	
Hepatitis B	• 1:220,000
Hepatitis C	• 1:1,800,000
HIV-1, -2	• 1:2,300,000
HTLV-I and -II	• 1:2,993,000
Malaria	• 1:4,000,000
Other complications	
RBC allosensitization	• 1:100
HLA allosensitization	• 1:10
Graft-vs.-host disease	Rare

[a]Infectious agents rarely associated with transfusion, theoretically possible or of unknown risk include West Nile virus, hepatitis A virus, parvovirus B-19, *Babesia microti* (babesiosis), *Borrelia burgdorferi* (Lyme disease), *Anaplasma phagocytophilum* (human granulocytic ehrlichiosis), *Trypanosoma cruzi* (Chagas disease), *Treponema pallidum*, and human herpesvirus-8.

Abbreviations: FNHTR, febrile nonhemolytic transfusion reaction; HTLV, human T lymphotropic virus; RBC, red blood cell; TRALI, transfusion-related acute lung injury.

IMMUNE-MEDIATED REACTIONS

Acute hemolytic transfusion reactions

Immune-mediated hemolysis occurs when the recipient has preformed antibodies that lyse donor erythrocytes. The ABO isoagglutinins are responsible for the majority of these reactions, although alloantibodies directed against other RBC antigens, i.e., Rh, Kell, and Duffy, may result in hemolysis.

Acute hemolytic reactions may present with hypotension, tachypnea, tachycardia, fever, chills, hemoglobinemia, hemoglobinuria, chest and/or flank pain, and discomfort at the infusion site. Monitoring the patient's vital signs before and during the transfusion is important to identify reactions promptly. When acute hemolysis is suspected, the transfusion must be stopped immediately, intravenous access maintained, and the reaction reported to the blood bank. A correctly labeled posttransfusion blood sample and any untransfused blood should be sent to the blood bank for analysis. The laboratory evaluation for hemolysis includes the measurement of serum haptoglobin, lactate dehydrogenase (LDH), and indirect bilirubin levels.

The immune complexes that result in RBC lysis can cause renal dysfunction and failure. Diuresis should be induced with intravenous fluids and furosemide or mannitol. Tissue factor released from the lysed erythrocytes may initiate DIC. Coagulation studies including prothrombin time (PT), activated partial thromboplastin time (aPTT), fibrinogen, and platelet count should be monitored in patients with hemolytic reactions.

Errors at the patient's bedside, such as mislabeling the sample or transfusing the wrong patient, are responsible for the majority of these reactions. The blood bank investigation of these reactions includes examination of the pre- and posttransfusion samples for hemolysis and repeat typing of the patient samples; direct antiglobulin test (DAT), sometimes called the *direct Coombs test*, of the posttransfusion sample; repeating the cross-matching of the blood component; and checking all clerical records for errors. DAT detects the presence of antibody or complement bound to RBCs in vivo.

Delayed hemolytic and serologic transfusion reactions

Delayed hemolytic transfusion reactions (DHTRs) are not completely preventable. These reactions occur in patients previously sensitized to RBC alloantigens who have a negative alloantibody screen result due to low antibody levels. When the patient is transfused with antigen-positive blood, an anamnestic response results in the early production of alloantibody that binds donor RBCs. The alloantibody is detectable 1–2 weeks following the transfusion, and the posttransfusion DAT may become positive due to circulating donor RBCs coated with antibody or complement. The transfused, alloantibody-coated erythrocytes are cleared by the reticuloendothelial system. These reactions are detected most commonly in the blood bank when a subsequent patient sample reveals a positive alloantibody screen or a new alloantibody in a recently transfused recipient.

No specific therapy is usually required, although additional RBC transfusions may be necessary. Delayed serologic transfusion reactions are similar to DHTR, as the DAT is positive and alloantibody is detected; however, RBC clearance is not increased.

Febrile nonhemolytic transfusion reaction

The most frequent reaction associated with the transfusion of cellular blood components is a febrile nonhemolytic transfusion reaction (FNHTR). These reactions are characterized by chills and rigors and a ≥1°C rise in temperature. FNHTR is diagnosed when other causes of fever in the transfused patient are ruled out. Antibodies directed against donor leukocyte and HLA antigens may mediate these reactions; thus, multiply transfused patients and multiparous women are believed to be at increased risk. Although anti-HLA antibodies may be demonstrated in the recipient's serum, investigation is not routinely done because of the mild nature of most FNHTR. The use of leukocyte-reduced blood products may prevent or delay sensitization to leukocyte antigens and thereby reduce the incidence of these febrile episodes. Cytokines released from cells within stored blood components may mediate FNHTR; thus, leukoreduction before storage may prevent these reactions.

Allergic reactions

Urticarial reactions are related to plasma proteins found in transfused components. Mild reactions may be treated symptomatically by temporarily stopping the transfusion and administering antihistamines (diphenhydramine, 50 mg orally or intramuscularly). The transfusion may be completed after the signs and/or symptoms resolve. Patients with a history of allergic transfusion reaction should be premedicated with an antihistamine. Cellular components can be washed to remove residual plasma for the extremely sensitized patient.

Anaphylactic reaction

This severe reaction presents after transfusion of only a few milliliters of the blood component. Symptoms and signs include difficulty breathing, coughing, nausea and vomiting, hypotension, bronchospasm, loss of consciousness, respiratory arrest, and shock. Treatment includes stopping the transfusion, maintaining vascular access, and administering epinephrine (0.5–1 mL of 1:1000 dilution subcutaneously). Glucocorticoids may be required in severe cases.

Patients who are IgA-deficient, <1% of the population, may be sensitized to this Ig class and are at risk for anaphylactic reactions associated with plasma transfusion. Individuals with severe IgA deficiency should therefore receive only IgA-deficient plasma and washed cellular blood components. Patients who have anaphylactic or repeated allergic reactions to blood components should be tested for IgA deficiency.

Graft-versus-host disease

Graft-versus-host disease (GVHD) is a frequent complication of allogeneic stem cell transplantation, in which lymphocytes from the donor attack and cannot be eliminated by an immunodeficient host. Transfusion-related GVHD is mediated by donor T lymphocytes that recognize host HLA antigens as foreign and mount an immune response, which is manifested clinically by the development of fever, a characteristic cutaneous eruption, diarrhea, and liver function abnormalities. GVHD can also occur when blood components that contain viable T lymphocytes are transfused to immunodeficient recipients or to immunocompetent recipients who share HLA antigens with the donor (e.g., a family donor). In addition to the aforementioned clinical features of GVHD, transfusion-associated GVHD (TA-GVHD) is characterized by marrow aplasia and pancytopenia. TA-GVHD is highly resistant to treatment with immunosuppressive therapies, including glucocorticoids, cyclosporine, antithymocyte globulin, and ablative therapy followed by allogeneic bone marrow transplantation. Clinical manifestations appear at 8–10 days, and death occurs at 3–4 weeks posttransfusion.

TA-GVHD can be prevented by irradiation of cellular components (minimum of 2500 cGy) before transfusion to patients at risk. Patients at risk for TA-GVHD include fetuses receiving intrauterine transfusions, selected immunocompetent (e.g., lymphoma patients) or immunocompromised recipients, recipients of donor units known to be from a blood relative, and recipients who have undergone marrow transplantation. Directed donations by family members should be discouraged (they are not less likely to transmit infection); lacking other options, the blood products from family members should always be irradiated.

Transfusion-related acute lung injury

Transfusion-related acute lung injury (TRALI) presents as acute respiratory distress, either during or within 6 h of transfusing the patient. The recipient develops symptoms of respiratory compromise and signs of noncardiogenic pulmonary edema, including bilateral interstitial infiltrates on chest x-ray. Treatment is supportive, and patients usually recover without sequelae. TRALI usually results from the transfusion of donor plasma that contains high-titer anti-HLA antibodies that bind recipient leukocytes. The leukocytes aggregate in the pulmonary vasculature and release mediators that increase capillary permeability. Testing the donor's plasma for anti-HLA antibodies can support this diagnosis. The implicated donors are frequently multiparous women, and transfusion of their plasma component should be avoided.

Posttransfusion purpura

This reaction presents as thrombocytopenia 7–10 days after platelet transfusion and occurs predominantly in women. Platelet-specific antibodies are found in the recipient's serum, and the most frequently recognized antigen is HPA-1a found on the platelet glycoprotein IIIa receptor. The delayed thrombocytopenia is due to the production of antibodies that react to both donor and recipient platelets. Additional platelet transfusions can worsen the thrombocytopenia and should be avoided. Treatment with intravenous immunoglobulin may neutralize the effector antibodies, or plasmapheresis can be used to remove the antibodies.

Alloimmunization

A recipient may become alloimmunized to a number of antigens on cellular blood elements and plasma proteins. Alloantibodies to RBC antigens are detected during pretransfusion testing, and their presence may delay finding antigen-negative cross-match-compatible products for transfusion. Women of childbearing age who are sensitized to certain RBC antigens (i.e., D, c, E, Kell, or Duffy) are at risk for bearing a fetus with hemolytic disease of the newborn. Matching for D antigen is the only pretransfusion selection test to prevent RBC alloimmunization.

Alloimmunization to antigens on leukocytes and platelets can result in refractoriness to platelet transfusions. Once alloimmunization has developed, HLA-compatible platelets from donors who share similar antigens with the recipient may be difficult to find. Hence, prudent transfusion practice is directed at preventing sensitization through the use of leukocyte-reduced cellular components, as well as limiting antigenic exposure by the judicious use of transfusions and use of SDAPs.

NONIMMUNOLOGIC REACTIONS

Fluid overload

Blood components are excellent volume expanders, and transfusion may quickly lead to volume overload. Monitoring the rate and volume of the transfusion and using a diuretic can minimize this problem.

Hypothermia

Refrigerated (4°C) or frozen (−18°C or below) blood components can result in hypothermia when rapidly infused. Cardiac dysrhythmias can result from exposing the sinoatrial node to cold fluid. Use of an in-line warmer will prevent this complication.

Electrolyte toxicity

RBC leakage during storage increases the concentration of potassium in the unit. Neonates and patients in renal failure are at risk for hyperkalemia. Preventive measures, such as using fresh or washed RBCs, are warranted for neonatal transfusions because this complication can be fatal.

Citrate, commonly used to anticoagulate blood components, chelates calcium and thereby inhibits the coagulation cascade. Hypocalcemia, manifested by circumoral numbness and/or tingling sensation of the fingers and toes, may result from multiple rapid transfusions. Because citrate is quickly metabolized to bicarbonate, calcium infusion is seldom required in this setting. If calcium or any other intravenous infusion is necessary, it must be given through a separate line.

Iron overload

Each unit of RBCs contains 200–250 mg of iron. Symptoms and signs of iron overload affecting endocrine, hepatic, and cardiac function are common after 100 units of RBCs have been transfused (total-body iron load of 20 g). Preventing this complication by using alternative therapies (e.g., erythropoietin) and judicious transfusion is preferable and cost effective. Chelating agents, such as deferoxamine and deferasirox, are available, but the response though is often suboptimal.

Hypotensive reactions

Transient hypotension may be noted among transfused patients who take angiotensin-converting enzyme (ACE) inhibitors. Since blood products contain bradykinin that is normally degraded by ACE, patients on ACE inhibitors may have increased bradykinin levels that cause hypotension in the recipient. The blood pressure typically returns to normal without intervention.

Immunomodulation

Transfusion of allogeneic blood is immunosuppressive. Multiply transfused renal transplant recipients are less likely to reject the graft, and transfusion may result in poorer outcomes in cancer patients and increase the risk of infections. Transfusion-related immunomodulation is thought to be mediated by transfused leukocytes. Leukocyte-depleted cellular products may cause less immunosuppression, though controlled data have not been obtained and are unlikely to be obtained as the blood supply becomes universally leukocyte-depleted.

INFECTIOUS COMPLICATIONS

The blood supply is initially screened by selecting healthy donors without high-risk lifestyles, medical conditions, or exposure to transmissible pathogens, such as intravenous drug use or visiting malaria endemic areas. Multiple tests performed on donated blood to detect the presence of infectious agents using nucleic acid amplification testing (NAT) or evidence of prior infections by testing for antibodies to pathogens further reduce the risk of transfusion-acquired infections.

Viral infections

Hepatitis C virus

Blood donations are tested for antibodies to HCV and HCV RNA. The risk of acquiring HCV through transfusion is now calculated to be approximately 1 in 2,000,000 units. Infection with HCV may be asymptomatic or lead to chronic active hepatitis, cirrhosis, and liver failure.

Human immunodeficiency virus type 1

Donated blood is tested for antibodies to HIV-1, HIV-1 p24 antigen, and HIV RNA using NAT. Approximately a dozen seronegative donors have been shown to harbor HIV RNA. The risk of HIV-1 infection per transfusion episode is 1 in 2 million. Antibodies to HIV-2 are also measured in donated blood. No cases of HIV-2 infection have been reported in the United States since 1992.

Hepatitis B virus

Donated blood is screened for HBV using assays for hepatitis B surface antigen (HbsAg). NAT testing is not practical because of slow viral replication and lower levels of viremia. The risk of transfusion-associated HBV infection is several times greater than for HCV. Vaccination of individuals who require long-term transfusion therapy can prevent this complication.

Other hepatitis viruses

Hepatitis A virus is rarely transmitted by transfusion; infection is typically asymptomatic and does not lead to chronic disease. Other transfusion-transmitted viruses—TTV, SEN-V, and GBV-C—do not cause chronic hepatitis or other disease states. Routine testing does not appear to be warranted.

West nile virus

Transfusion-transmitted WNV infections were documented in 2002. This RNA virus can be detected using NAT; routine screening began in 2003. WNV infections range in severity from asymptomatic to fatal, with the older population at greater risk.

Cytomegalovirus

This ubiquitous virus infects ≥50% of the general population and is transmitted by the infected "passenger" WBCs found in transfused PRBCs or platelet components. Cellular components that are leukocyte-reduced have a decreased risk of transmitting CMV, regardless of the serologic status of the donor. Groups at risk for CMV infections include immunosuppressed patients, CMV-seronegative transplant recipients, and neonates; these patients should receive leukocyte-depleted components or CMV seronegative products.

Human T lymphotropic virus (HTLV) type I

Assays to detect HTLV-I and -II are used to screen all donated blood. HTLV-I is associated with adult T cell leukemia/lymphoma and tropical spastic paraparesis in a small percentage of infected persons. The risk of HTLV-I infection via transfusion is 1 in 641,000 transfusion episodes. HTLV-II is not clearly associated with any disease.

Parvovirus B-19

Blood components and pooled plasma products can transmit this virus, the etiologic agent of erythema infectiosum, or fifth disease, in children. Parvovirus B-19 shows tropism for erythroid precursors and inhibits both erythrocyte production and maturation. Pure red cell aplasia, presenting either as acute aplastic crisis or chronic anemia with shortened RBC survival, may occur in individuals with an underlying hematologic disease, such as sickle cell disease or thalassemia (Chap. 11). The fetus of a seronegative woman is at risk for developing hydrops from this virus.

Bacterial contamination

The relative risk of transfusion-transmitted bacterial infection has increased as the absolute risk of viral infections has dramatically decreased.

Most bacteria do not grow well at cold temperatures; thus, PRBCs and FFP are not common sources of bacterial contamination. However, some gram-negative bacteria can grow at 1° to 6°C. *Yersinia*, *Pseudomonas*, *Serratia*, *Acinetobacter*, and *Escherichia* species have all been implicated in infections related to PRBC transfusion. Platelet concentrates, which are stored at room temperature, are more likely to contain skin contaminants such as gram-positive organisms, including coagulase-negative staphylococci. It is estimated that 1 in 1000—2000 platelet components is contaminated with bacteria. The risk of death due to transfusion-associated sepsis has been calculated at 1 in 17,000 for single-unit platelets derived from whole blood donation and 1 in 61,000 for apheresis product. Since 2004, blood banks have instituted methods to detect contaminated platelet components.

Recipients of transfusion contaminated with bacteria may develop fever and chills, which can progress to septic shock and DIC. These reactions may occur abruptly, within minutes of initiating the transfusion, or after several hours. The onset of symptoms and signs is often sudden and fulminant, which distinguishes bacterial contamination from an FNHTR. The reactions, particularly those related to gram-negative contaminants, are the result of infused endotoxins formed within the contaminated stored component.

When these reactions are suspected, the transfusion must be stopped immediately. Therapy is directed at reversing any signs of shock, and broad-spectrum antibiotics should be given. The blood bank should be notified to identify any clerical or serologic error. The blood component bag should be sent for culture and Gram stain.

Other infectious agents

Various parasites, including those causing malaria, babesiosis, and Chagas disease, can be transmitted by blood transfusion. Geographic migration and travel of donors shift the incidence of these rare infections. Other agents implicated in transfusion transmission include dengue, chikungunya virus, variant Creutzfeldt-Jakob disease, *Anaplasma phagocytophilum*, and yellow fever vaccine virus and the list will grow. Tests for some pathogens are available, such as *Trypanosoma cruzi*, but not universally required. These infections should be considered in transfused patients in the appropriate clinical setting.

ALTERNATIVES TO TRANSFUSION

Alternatives to allogeneic blood transfusions that avoid homologous donor exposures with attendant immunologic and infectious risks remain attractive. Autologous blood is the best option when transfusion is anticipated. However, the cost–benefit ratio of autologous transfusion remains high. No transfusion is a zero-risk event; clerical errors and bacterial contamination remain potential complications even with autologous transfusions. Additional methods of autologous transfusion in surgical patients include preoperative hemodilution, recovery of shed blood from sterile surgical sites, and postoperative drainage collection. Directed or designated donation from friends and family of the potential recipient has not been safer than volunteer donor component transfusions. Such directed donations may in fact place the recipient at higher risk for complications such as GVHD and alloimmunization.

Granulocyte and granulocyte-macrophage colony-stimulating factors are clinically useful to hasten leukocyte recovery in patients with leukopenia related to high-dose chemotherapy. Erythropoietin stimulates erythrocyte production in patients with anemia of chronic renal failure and other conditions, thus avoiding or reducing the need for transfusion. This hormone can also stimulate erythropoiesis in the autologous donor to enable additional donation.

SECTION IV

MYELOPROLIFERATIVE DISORDERS

CHAPTER 13

POLYCYTHEMIA VERA AND OTHER MYELOPROLIFERATIVE DISEASES

Jerry L. Spivak

The World Health Organization (WHO) classification of the chronic myeloproliferative diseases (MPDs) includes eight disorders, some of which are rare or poorly characterized (Table 13-1) but all of which share an origin in a multipotent hematopoietic progenitor cell; overproduction of one or more of the formed elements of the blood without significant dysplasia; a predilection to extramedullary hematopoiesis, myelofibrosis; and transformation at varying rates to acute leukemia. Within this broad classification, however, significant phenotypic heterogeneity exists. Some diseases such as chronic myeloid leukemia (CML), chronic neutrophilic leukemia (CNL), and chronic eosinophilic leukemia (CEL) express primarily a myeloid phenotype, while in others such as polycythemia vera (PV), primary myelofibrosis (PMF), and essential thrombocytosis (ET), erythroid or megakaryocytic hyperplasia predominates. The latter three disorders, in contrast to the former three, also appear capable of transforming into each other.

Such phenotypic heterogeneity has a genetic basis; CML is the consequence of the balanced translocation between chromosomes 9 and 22 (t[9;22][q34;11]), CNL has been associated with a t(15;19) translocation, and CEL occurs with a deletion or balanced translocations involving the *PDGFRα* gene. By contrast, to a greater or lesser extent, PV, PMF, and ET are characterized by expression of a *JAK2* mutation, V617F that causes constitutive activation of this tyrosine kinase that is essential for the function of the erythropoietin and thrombopoietin receptors but not the granulocyte colony-stimulating factor receptor. This essential distinction is also reflected in the natural history of CML, CNL, and CEL, which is usually measured in years, and their high rate of transformation into acute leukemia. By contrast, the natural history of PV, PMF, and ET is usually measured in decades, and transformation to acute leukemia is uncommon in the absence of exposure to mutagenic agents. This chapter, therefore, will focus only on PV, PMF, and ET because their clinical overlap is substantial but their clinical courses are distinctly different. Other chronic myeloproliferative disorders will be discussed in Chap. 14.

TABLE 13-1

WHO CLASSIFICATION OF CHRONIC MYELOPROLIFERATIVE DISORDERS
Chronic myeloid leukemia, bcr-abl–positive
Chronic neutrophilic leukemia
Chronic eosinophilic leukemia, not otherwise specified
Polycythemia vera
Primary myelofibrosis
Essential thrombocytosis
Mastocytosis
Myeloproliferative neoplasms, unclassifiable

POLYCYTHEMIA VERA

PV is a clonal disorder involving a multipotent hematopoietic progenitor cell in which phenotypically normal red cells, granulocytes, and platelets accumulate in the absence of a recognizable physiologic stimulus. The most common of the chronic myeloproliferative disorders, PV occurs in 2 per 100,000 persons, sparing no adult age group and increasing with age to rates as high as 18/100,000. Familial transmission occurs but is infrequent and women predominate among sporadic cases.

ETIOLOGY

The etiology of PV is unknown. Although nonrandom chromosome abnormalities such as 20q and trisomy 8 and

9 have been documented in up to 30% of untreated PV patients, unlike CML, no consistent cytogenetic abnormality has been associated with the disorder. However, a mutation in the autoinhibitory, pseudokinase domain of the tyrosine kinase JAK2—that replaces valine with phenylalanine (V617F), causing constitutive activation of the kinase—appears to have a central role in the pathogenesis of PV.

JAK2 is a member of an evolutionarily well-conserved, nonreceptor tyrosine kinase family and serves as the cognate tyrosine kinase for the erythropoietin and thrombopoietin receptors. It also functions as an obligate chaperone for these receptors in the Golgi apparatus and is responsible for their cell-surface expression. The conformational change induced in the erythropoietin and thrombopoietin receptors following binding to erythropoietin or thrombopoietin leads to JAK2 autophosphorylation, receptor phosphorylation, and phosphorylation of proteins involved in cell proliferation, differentiation, and resistance to apoptosis. Transgenic animals lacking *JAK2* die as embryos from severe anemia. Constitutive activation of JAK2 can explain the erythropoietin-independent erythroid colony formation, and the hypersensitivity of PV erythroid progenitor cells to erythropoietin and other hematopoietic growth factors, their resistance to apoptosis in vitro in the absence of erythropoietin, their rapid terminal differentiation, and their increase in Bcl-X_L expression, all of which are characteristic in PV.

Importantly, the *JAK2* gene is located on the short arm of chromosome 9, and loss of heterozygosity on chromosome 9p due to mitotic recombination is the most common cytogenetic abnormality in PV. The segment of 9p involved contains the *JAK2* locus; loss of heterozygosity in this region leads to homozygosity for the mutant *JAK2* V617F. More than 90% of PV patients express this mutation, as do approximately 50% of PMF and ET patients. Homozygosity for the mutation occurs in approximately 30% of PV patients and 60% of PMF patients; homozygosity is rare in ET. Over time, a portion of PV *JAK2* V617F heterozygotes become homozygotes due to mitotic recombination but usually not after 10 years of the disease. PV patients who do not express *JAK2* V617F are not clinically different from those who do, nor do *JAK2* V617F heterozygotes differ clinically from homozygotes. Interestingly, predisposition to acquire mutations in *JAK2* appears to be associated with a specific *JAK2* haplotype, GGCC. *JAK2* V617F is the basis for many of the phenotypic and biochemical characteristics of PV such as elevation of the leukocyte alkaline phosphatase (LAP) score; however, it cannot solely account for the entire PV phenotype and is probably not the initiating lesion in the three MPDs. First, some PV patients with the same phenotype and documented clonal disease lack this mutation. Second, ET and PMF patients have the same mutation but different clinical phenotypes. Third, familial PV can occur without the mutation even when other members of the same family express it. Fourth, not all the cells of the malignant clone express *JAK2* V617F. Fifth, *JAK2* V617F has been observed in patients with long-standing idiopathic erythrocytosis. Sixth, in some patients, *JAK2* V617F appears to be acquired after another mutation. Finally, in some *JAK2* V617F-positive PV or ET patients, acute leukemia can occur in a *JAK2* V617F–negative progenitor cell. However, while *JAK2* V617F alone may not be sufficient to cause PV, it is essential for the transformation of ET to PV, though not for its transformation to PMF.

CLINICAL FEATURES

Although splenomegaly may be the initial presenting sign in PV, most often the disorder is first recognized by the incidental discovery of a high hemoglobin or hematocrit. With the exception of aquagenic pruritus, no symptoms distinguish PV from other causes of erythrocytosis.

Uncontrolled erythrocytosis causes hyperviscosity, leading to neurologic symptoms such as vertigo, tinnitus, headache, visual disturbances, and transient ischemic attacks (TIAs). Systolic hypertension is also a feature of the red cell mass elevation. In some patients, venous or arterial thrombosis may be the presenting manifestation of PV. Any vessel can be affected, but cerebral, cardiac, or mesenteric vessels are most commonly involved. Intraabdominal venous thrombosis is particularly common in young women and may be catastrophic if a sudden and complete obstruction of the hepatic vein occurs. Indeed, PV should be suspected in any patient who develops hepatic vein thrombosis. Digital ischemia, easy bruising, epistaxis, acid-peptic disease, or gastrointestinal hemorrhage may occur due to vascular stasis or thrombocytosis. Erythema, burning, and pain in the extremities, a symptom complex known as erythromelalgia, is another complication of the thrombocytosis of PV due to increased platelet stickiness. Given the large turnover of hematopoietic cells, hyperuricemia with secondary gout, uric acid stones, and symptoms due to hypermetabolism can also complicate the disorder.

DIAGNOSIS

When PV presents with erythrocytosis in combination with leukocytosis, thrombocytosis, or both, the diagnosis is apparent. However, when patients present with an elevated hemoglobin or hematocrit alone or with thrombocytosis alone, the diagnostic evaluation is more complex because of the many diagnostic possibilities (Table 13-2). Furthermore, unless the hemoglobin level is ≤20 g/dL (hematocrit ≤60%), it is

TABLE 13-2

CAUSES OF ERYTHROCYTOSIS

Relative Erythrocytosis	
Hemoconcentration secondary to dehydration, diuretics, ethanol abuse, androgens or tobacco abuse	
Absolute Erythrocytosis	
Hypoxia	**Tumors**
Carbon monoxide intoxication	Hypernephroma
	Hepatoma
High oxygen-affinity hemoglobin	Cerebellar hemangioblastoma
High altitude	Uterine myoma
Pulmonary disease	Adrenal tumors
Right-to-left cardiac or vascular shunts	Meningioma
	Pheochromocytoma
Sleep apnea syndrome	**Drugs**
Hepatopulmonary syndrome	Androgens
Renal Disease	Recombinant erythropoietin
Renal artery stenosis	**Familial (with normal hemoglobin function)**
Focal sclerosing or membranous glomerulonephritis	Erythropoietin receptor mutation
Postrenal transplantation	
Renal cysts	VHL mutations (Chuvash polycythemia)
Bartter's syndrome	
	2,3-BPG mutation
	Polycythemia vera

Abbreviations: 2,3-BPG, 2,3-bisphosphoglycerate; VHL, von Hippel-Lindau.

not possible to distinguish true erythrocytosis from disorders causing plasma volume contraction. Uniquely in PV, in contrast to other causes for true erythrocytosis, an expanded plasma volume can mask the elevated red cell mass; thus, red cell mass and plasma volume determinations are mandatory to establish the presence of an absolute erythrocytosis and to distinguish this from relative erythrocytosis due to a reduction in plasma volume alone (also known as *stress* or *spurious erythrocytosis* or *Gaisböck's syndrome*). This is true even with the finding of *JAK2* V617F mutation because not every patient with PV expresses this mutation but patients without PV do. Figure 2-18 illustrates a diagnostic algorithm for the evaluation of suspected erythrocytosis.

After absolute erythrocytosis has been established, its cause must be determined. An elevated plasma erythropoietin level suggests either a hypoxic cause for erythrocytosis or autonomous erythropoietin production, in which case assessment of pulmonary function and an abdominal CT scan to evaluate renal and hepatic anatomy are appropriate. A normal erythropoietin level, however, does not exclude a secondary cause for erythrocytosis or PV. In PV, in contrast to hypoxic erythrocytosis, the arterial oxygen saturation is normal. However, a normal oxygen saturation does not exclude a high-affinity hemoglobin as a cause for erythrocytosis; documentation of previous hemoglobin levels and a family study are important in this regard.

Other laboratory studies that may aid in diagnosis include the red cell count, mean corpuscular volume, and red cell distribution width (RDW). Only three situations cause microcytic erythrocytosis: β-thalassemia trait, hypoxic erythrocytosis, and PV. With β-thalassemia trait the RDW is normal, whereas with hypoxic erythrocytosis and PV, the RDW is usually elevated due to iron deficiency. Today, an assay for *JAK2* V617F has superseded other tests for establishing the diagnosis of PV. Of course, in patients with associated acid-peptic disease, occult gastrointestinal bleeding may lead to presentation with hypochromic, microcytic anemia, masking the presence of PV.

A bone marrow aspirate and biopsy provide no specific diagnostic information since these may be normal or indistinguishable from ET or PMF, and unless there is a need to exclude some other disorder, these procedures need not be done. Although the presence of a cytogenetic abnormality such as trisomy 8 or 9 or 20q− in the setting of an expanded red cell mass supports a clonal etiology, no specific cytogenetic abnormality is associated with PV, and the absence of a cytogenetic marker does not exclude the diagnosis.

COMPLICATIONS

Many of the clinical complications of PV relate directly to the increase in blood viscosity associated with red cell mass elevation and indirectly to the increased turnover of red cells, leukocytes, and platelets with the attendant increase in uric acid and cytokine production. The latter appears to be responsible for constitutional symptoms, while peptic ulcer disease may be due to *Helicobacter pylori*, and the pruritus associated with this disorder may be a consequence of basophil activation by *JAK2* V617F. A sudden increase in spleen size can be associated with splenic infarction. Myelofibrosis appears to be part of the natural history of the disease but is a reactive, reversible process that does not itself impede hematopoiesis and by itself has no prognostic significance. In some patients, however, the myelofibrosis is accompanied by significant extramedullary hematopoiesis, hepatosplenomegaly, and transfusion-dependent anemia, which are manifestations of stem cell failure. The organomegaly can cause significant mechanical discomfort, portal hypertension, and progressive cachexia. Although the incidence of acute nonlymphocytic leukemia is increased in PV, the incidence of acute leukemia in patients not exposed to chemotherapy or radiation is low, and the development of leukemia is related to the development of extramedullary hematopoiesis, hepatosplenomegaly, and transfusion-dependent anemia or exposure to chemotherapy. Importantly, chemotherapy alone, including hydroxyurea, has been associated with acute leukemia that develops in *JAK2* V617F–negative stem cells. *Erythromelalgia* is a curious syndrome of unknown etiology associated with thrombocytosis, primarily involving the lower extremities and usually manifested by erythema, warmth, and pain of the affected appendage and occasionally digital infarction. It occurs with a variable frequency in MPD patients and is usually responsive to salicylates. Some of the central nervous system symptoms observed in patients with PV, such as ocular migraine, appear to represent a variant of erythromelalgia.

If left uncontrolled, erythrocytosis can lead to thrombosis involving vital organs such as the liver, heart, brain, or lungs. Patients with massive splenomegaly are particularly prone to thrombotic events because the associated increase in plasma volume masks the true extent of the red cell mass elevation as measured by the hematocrit or hemoglobin level. A "normal" hematocrit or hemoglobin level in a PV patient with massive splenomegaly should be considered indicative of an elevated red cell mass until proven otherwise.

TREATMENT Polycythemia Vera

PV is generally an indolent disorder, the clinical course of which is measured in decades, and its management should reflect its tempo. Thrombosis due to erythrocytosis is the most significant complication, and maintenance of the hemoglobin level at ≤140 g/L (14 g/dL; hematocrit <45%) in men and ≤120 g/L (12 g/dL; hematocrit <42%) in women is mandatory to avoid thrombotic complications. Phlebotomy serves initially to reduce hyperviscosity by bringing the red cell mass into the normal range. Periodic phlebotomies thereafter serve to maintain the red cell mass within the normal range and to induce a state of iron deficiency that prevents an accelerated reexpansion of the red cell mass. In most PV patients, once an iron-deficient state is achieved, phlebotomy is usually only required at 3-month intervals. Neither phlebotomy nor iron deficiency increases the platelet count relative to the effect of the disease itself, and thrombocytosis is not correlated with thrombosis in PV, in contrast to the strong correlation between erythrocytosis and thrombosis in this disease. The use of salicylates as a tonic against thrombosis in PV patients is not only potentially harmful if the red cell mass is not controlled by phlebotomy but is also an unproven remedy. Anticoagulants are only indicated when a thrombosis has occurred and can be difficult to monitor owing to the artifactual imbalance between the test tube anticoagulant and plasma that occurs when blood from these patients is assayed for prothrombin or partial thromboplastin activity if the red cell mass is substantially elevated. Asymptomatic hyperuricemia (<10 mg%) requires no therapy, but allopurinol should be administered to avoid further elevation of uric acid when chemotherapy is employed to reduce splenomegaly or leukocytosis or to treat pruritus. Generalized pruritus intractable to antihistamines or antidepressants such as doxepin can be a major problem in PV; interferon α (IFN-α), psoralens with ultraviolet light in the A range (PUVA) therapy, and hydroxyurea are other methods of palliation. Asymptomatic thrombocytosis requires no therapy unless the platelet count is sufficiently high to cause an acquired form of von Willebrand disease due to adsorption and proteolysis of high-molecular-weight von Willebrand factor (vWF) multimers by the expanded platelet mass. Symptomatic splenomegaly can be treated with IFN-α, although the drug can be associated with significant side effects when used chronically. Pegylated IFN-α produces complete remissions in PV patients, and its role in this disorder may be expanding. Anagrelide, a phosphodiesterase inhibitor, can reduce the platelet count and, if tolerated, is preferable to hydroxyurea because it lacks marrow toxicity and actually is protective against venous thrombosis. A reduction in platelet number may be necessary for the treatment of erythromelalgia or ocular migraine if salicylates are not effective or if the platelet count is sufficiently high to cause a hemorrhagic diathesis but only to the degree that symptoms are alleviated. Alkylating agents and radioactive sodium phosphate (^{32}P) are leukemogenic in PV, and their use should be avoided. If a cytotoxic agent must be used, hydroxyurea is preferred, but this drug does not prevent either thrombosis or myelofibrosis in this disorder, is itself leukemogenic, and should only be used for as short a time as possible. In some patients, massive splenomegaly unresponsive to reduction by therapy and associated with intractable weight loss will require splenectomy. In some patients with end-stage disease, pulmonary hypertension may develop due to fibrosis and extramedullary hematopoiesis. Allogeneic bone marrow transplantation may be curative in young patients. Several *JAK2* inhibitors are undergoing clinical trials; to date, these agents have been demonstrated to alleviate constitutional symptoms and to rapidly reduce spleen size without significant effects on blood counts or the *JAK2* V617F neutrophil allele burden, suggesting that they may at least have an important palliative role.

Most patients with PV can live long lives without functional impairment when their red cell mass is effectively managed with phlebotomy alone. Chemotherapy is never indicated to control the red cell mass unless venous access is inadequate.

PRIMARY MYELOFIBROSIS

Chronic PMF (other designations include idiopathic myelofibrosis, *agnogenic myeloid metaplasia*, or *myelofibrosis with myeloid metaplasia*) is a clonal disorder of a multipotent hematopoietic progenitor cell of unknown etiology characterized by marrow fibrosis, extramedullary hematopoiesis, and splenomegaly. PMF is the least common chronic MPD, and establishing this diagnosis in the absence of a specific clonal marker is difficult because myelofibrosis and splenomegaly are also features of both PV and CML. Furthermore, myelofibrosis and splenomegaly also occur in a variety of benign and malignant disorders (Table 13-3), many of which are amenable to specific therapies not effective in PMF. In contrast to the other chronic MPDs and so-called acute or malignant myelofibrosis, which can occur at any age, PMF primarily afflicts men in their sixth decade or later.

ETIOLOGY

The etiology of PMF is unknown. Nonrandom chromosome abnormalities such as 9p, 20q− 13q− trisomy 8 or 9, or partial trisomy 1q are common, but no cytogenetic abnormality specific to the disease has been identified. *JAK2* V617F is present in approximately 50% of PMF patients, and mutations in the thrombopoietin receptor *Mpl* occur in about 5%. The degree of myelofibrosis and the extent of extramedullary hematopoiesis are also not related. Fibrosis in this disorder is associated with overproduction of transforming growth factor β and tissue inhibitors of metalloproteinases, while osteosclerosis is associated with overproduction of osteoprotegerin, an osteoclast inhibitor. Marrow angiogenesis occurs due to increased production of vascular endothelial growth factor. Importantly, fibroblasts in PMF are polyclonal and not part of the neoplastic clone.

TABLE 13-3

DISORDERS CAUSING MYELOFIBROSIS

MALIGNANT	NONMALIGNANT
Acute leukemia (lymphocytic, myelogenous, megakaryocytic)	HIV infection
Chronic myeloid leukemia	Hyperparathyroidism
Hairy cell leukemia	Renal osteodystrophy
Hodgkin disease	Systemic lupus erythematosus
Idiopathic myelofibrosis	Tuberculosis
Lymphoma	Vitamin D deficiency
Multiple myeloma	Thorium dioxide exposure
Myelodysplasia	Gray platelet syndrome
Metastatic carcinoma	
Polycythemia vera	
Systemic mastocytosis	

CLINICAL FEATURES

No signs or symptoms are specific for PMF. Many patients are asymptomatic at presentation, and the disease is usually detected by the discovery of splenic enlargement and/or abnormal blood counts during a routine examination. However, in contrast to its companion MPDs, night sweats, fatigue, and weight loss are common presenting complaints. A blood smear will show the characteristic features of extramedullary hematopoiesis: teardrop-shaped red cells, nucleated red cells, myelocytes, and promyelocytes; myeloblasts may also be present (Fig. 13-1). Anemia, usually mild initially, is the rule, while the leukocyte and platelet counts are either normal or increased, but either can be depressed. Mild hepatomegaly may accompany the splenomegaly but is unusual in the absence of splenic enlargement; isolated lymphadenopathy should suggest another diagnosis. Both serum lactate dehydrogenase and alkaline phosphatase levels can be elevated. The LAP score can be low, normal, or high. Marrow is usually inaspirable due to the myelofibrosis (Fig. 13-2), and bone radiographs may reveal osteosclerosis. Exuberant extramedullary hematopoiesis can cause ascites; portal, pulmonary, or intracranial hypertension; intestinal or ureteral obstruction; pericardial tamponade; spinal cord compression; or skin nodules. Splenic enlargement can be sufficiently rapid to cause splenic infarction with fever and pleuritic chest pain. Hyperuricemia and secondary gout may ensue.

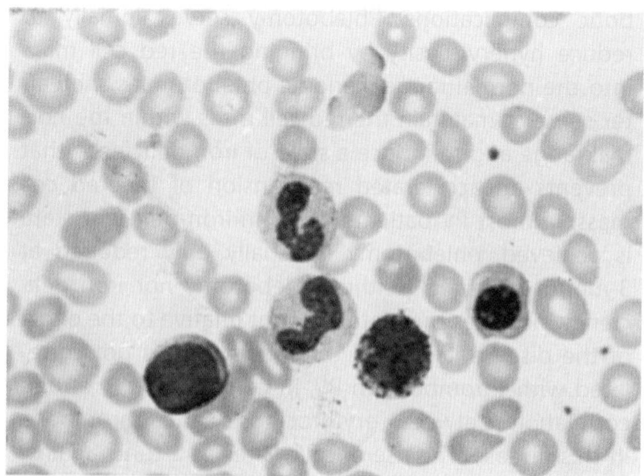

FIGURE 13-1

Teardrop-shaped red blood cells indicative of membrane damage from passage through the spleen, a nucleated red blood cell, and immature myeloid cells indicative of extramedullary hematopoiesis are noted. This peripheral blood smear is related to any cause of extramedullary hematopoiesis.

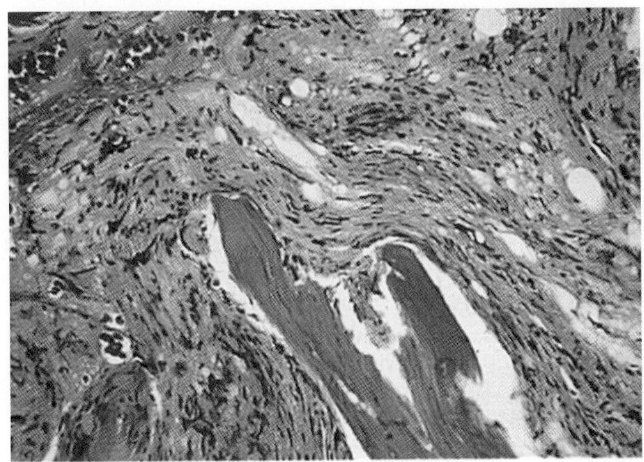

FIGURE 13-2

This marrow section shows the marrow cavity replaced by fibrous tissue composed of reticulin fibers and collagen. When this fibrosis is due to a primary hematologic process, it is called *myelofibrosis*. When the fibrosis is secondary to a tumor or a granulomatous process, it is called *myelophthisis*.

DIAGNOSIS

While the clinical picture described earlier is characteristic of PMF, all of the clinical features described can also be observed in PV or CML. Massive splenomegaly commonly masks erythrocytosis in PV, and reports of intraabdominal thromboses in PMF most likely represent instances of unrecognized PV. In some patients with PMF, erythrocytosis has developed during the course of the disease. Furthermore, since many other disorders have features that overlap with PMF but respond to distinctly different therapies, the diagnosis of PMF is one of exclusion, which requires that the disorders listed in Table 13-3 be ruled out. A diagnostic algorithm has been proposed but does not distinguish one disease causing myeloid metaplasia from another.

The presence of teardrop-shaped red cells, nucleated red cells, myelocytes, and promyelocytes establishes the presence of extramedullary hematopoiesis, while the presence of leukocytosis, thrombocytosis with large and bizarre platelets, and circulating myelocytes suggests the presence of an MPD as opposed to a secondary form of myelofibrosis (Table 13-3). Marrow is usually not aspirable due to increased marrow reticulin, but marrow biopsy will reveal a hypercellular marrow with trilineage hyperplasia and, in particular, increased numbers of megakaryocytes in clusters and with large, dysplastic nuclei. However, there are no characteristic morphologic abnormalities of the bone marrow that distinguish PMF from the other chronic MPDs. Splenomegaly due to extramedullary hematopoiesis may be sufficiently massive to cause portal hypertension and variceal formation. In some patients, exuberant extramedullary hematopoiesis can dominate the clinical picture. An intriguing feature of PMF is the occurrence of autoimmune abnormalities such as immune complexes, antinuclear antibodies, rheumatoid factor, or a positive Coombs' test result. Whether these represent a host reaction to the disorder or are involved in its pathogenesis is unknown. Cytogenetic analysis of blood is useful both to exclude CML and for prognostic purposes because complex karyotype abnormalities portend a poor prognosis in PMF. For unknown reasons, the number of circulating CD34+ cells is markedly increased in PMF (>15,000/μL) compared with the other chronic MPDs unless they too develop myeloid metaplasia.

Importantly, approximately 50% of PMF patients, similar to patients with its companion myeloproliferative disorders PV and ET, express the *JAK2* V617F mutation, often as homozygotes. Such patients had a poorer survival in one retrospective study but not in another, in which they were found to be older and to have higher hematocrits than patients who were *JAK2* V617F negative. Patients with an *MPL* mutation tend to be more anemic than those without this mutation.

COMPLICATIONS

Survival in PMF varies according to specific clinical features (Table 13-4) but is shorter than in patients with PV or ET. The natural history of PMF is one of increasing marrow failure with transfusion-dependent anemia and increasing organomegaly due to extramedullary hematopoiesis. As with CML, PMF can evolve from a chronic phase to an accelerated phase with constitutional symptoms and increasing marrow failure. About 10% of patients spontaneously transform to an aggressive form of acute leukemia for which therapy is usually ineffective. Important prognostic factors for disease acceleration include anemia; leukocytosis; thrombocytopenia, the presence of circulating myeloblasts, older age; the presence of complex cytogenetic abnormalities; and constitutional symptoms such as unexplained fever, night sweats, or weight loss.

TREATMENT Primary Myelofibrosis

No specific therapy exists for PMF. Anemia may be due to gastrointestinal blood loss, may be exacerbated by folic acid deficiency, and in rare instances, pyridoxine therapy has been effective. However, anemia is more often due to ineffective erythropoiesis uncompensated by extramedullary hematopoiesis in the spleen and liver. Neither recombinant erythropoietin nor androgens such as Danazol have proved consistently effective as therapy for the anemia. Erythropoietin may

TABLE 13-4

RISK STRATIFICATION FOR PRIMARY MYELOFIBROSIS

RISK FACTORS	FREQUENCY OF OCCURRENCE (%)
Age >65 years	45
Constitutional symptoms	26
Hemoglobin <10 g/dL	35
WBC count >25 × 109/L	10
Blood blasts >10%	36

Risk Groups	No. of Factors	Proportion of Patients (%)	Median Survival (years)
Low	0	22	11
Intermediate-1	1	29	8
Intermediate-2	2	28	4
High	≥3	21	2

Abbreviation: WBC, white blood cell.
Source: From F Cervantes et al: Blood 113:2895, 2009.

worsen splenomegaly and will be ineffective if the serum erythropoietin level is >125 mU/L. A red cell splenic sequestration study can establish the presence of hypersplenism, for which splenectomy is indicated. Splenectomy may also be necessary if splenomegaly impairs alimentation and should be performed before cachexia sets in. In this situation, splenectomy should not be avoided because of concern over rebound thrombocytosis, loss of hematopoietic capacity, or compensatory hepatomegaly. However, for unexplained reasons, splenectomy increases the risk of blastic transformation. Splenic irradiation is, at best, temporarily palliative and associated with a significant risk of neutropenia, infection, and operative hemorrhage. Allopurinol can control significant hyperuricemia, and hydroxyurea has proved useful for controlling organomegaly in some patients. The role of IFN-α is still undefined; its side effects are more pronounced in the older individuals who are usually affected by this disorder, and it should be used at lower doses. Glucocorticoids have been used to control constitutional symptoms and autoimmune complications and may ameliorate anemia alone or in combination with low-dose thalidomide (50–100 mg/d); such therapy may also palliate splenomegaly. Allogeneic bone marrow transplantation is the only curative treatment and should be considered in younger patients; reduced-intensity conditioning regimens may permit hematopoietic cell transplantation to be extended to older individuals. *JAK2* inhibitors have been effective in alleviating constitutional symptoms and splenomegaly in PMF patients and are currently used in phase III clinical trials. While their effects are reversible, these agents may offer a less toxic and more effective means of palliation in this disorder.

ESSENTIAL THROMBOCYTOSIS

Essential thrombocytosis (other designations include *essential thrombocythemia*, *idiopathic thrombocytosis*, *primary thrombocytosis*, and *hemorrhagic thrombocythemia*) is a clonal disorder of unknown etiology involving a multipotent hematopoietic progenitor cell manifested clinically by overproduction of platelets without a definable cause. ET is an uncommon disorder, with an incidence of 1–2/100,000 and a distinct female predominance. No clonal marker is available to consistently distinguish ET from the more common nonclonal, reactive forms of thrombocytosis (Table 13-5), making its diagnosis difficult. Once considered a disease of the elderly and responsible for significant morbidity due to hemorrhage or thrombosis, with the widespread use of electronic cell counters, it is now clear that ET can occur at any age in adults and often without symptoms or disturbances of hemostasis. There is an unexplained female predominance in contrast to PMF or the reactive forms of thrombocytosis in which no sex difference exists. Because no specific clonal marker is available, clinical criteria have been proposed to distinguish ET from the other chronic MPDs, which may also present with thrombocytosis but have differing prognoses and therapies (Table 13-5). These criteria do not establish clonality; therefore, they are truly useful only in identifying disorders such as CML, PV, or myelodysplasia, which can masquerade as ET, as opposed to actually establishing the presence of ET. Furthermore, as with "idiopathic" erythrocytosis, nonclonal benign forms of thrombocytosis exist (e.g., hereditary overproduction of thrombopoietin) that are not widely recognized because we currently lack adequate diagnostic tools. Approximately 50% of ET patients carry the *JAK2* V617F mutation, but its absence does not exclude the disorder.

TABLE 13-5

CAUSES OF THROMBOCYTOSIS

Tissue inflammation: collagen vascular disease, inflammatory bowel disease	Hemorrhage
Malignancy	Iron-deficiency anemia
Infection	Surgery
Myeloproliferative disorders: polycythemia vera, primary myelofibrosis, essential thrombocytosis, chronic myeloid leukemia	Rebound: correction of vitamin B_{12} or folate deficiency, post-ethanol abuse
Myelodysplastic disorders: 5q-syndrome, idiopathic refractory sideroblastic anemia	Hemolysis
Postsplenectomy or hyposplenism	Familial: thrombopoietin overproduction, constitutive Mpl activation

ETIOLOGY

Megakaryocytopoiesis and platelet production depend on thrombopoietin and its receptor *Mpl.* As in the case of early erythroid and myeloid progenitor cells, early megakaryocytic progenitors require the presence of interleukin 3 (IL-3) and stem cell factor for optimal proliferation in addition to thrombopoietin. Their subsequent development is also enhanced by the chemokine stromal cell–derived factor 1 (SDF-1). However, megakaryocyte maturation requires thrombopoietin.

Megakaryocytes are unique among hematopoietic progenitor cells because reduplication of their genome is endomitotic rather than mitotic. In the absence of thrombopoietin, endomitotic megakaryocytic reduplication and, by extension, the cytoplasmic development necessary for platelet production are impaired. Like erythropoietin, thrombopoietin is produced in both the liver and the kidneys, and an inverse correlation exists between the platelet count and plasma thrombopoietic activity. Like erythropoietin levels, plasma levels of thrombopoietin are controlled largely by the size of its progenitor cell pool. In contrast to erythropoietin, but like its myeloid counterparts, granulocyte- and granulocyte-macrophage colony-stimulating factors, thrombopoietin not only enhances the proliferation of its target cells but also enhances the reactivity of their end-stage product, the platelet. In addition to its role in thrombopoiesis, thrombopoietin also enhances the survival of multipotent hematopoietic stem cells.

The clonal nature of ET was established by analysis of glucose-6-phosphate dehydrogenase isoenzyme expression in patients hemizygous for this gene; by analysis of X-linked DNA polymorphisms in informative female patients; and by the expression in patients of nonrandom, although variable, cytogenetic abnormalities. Although thrombocytosis is its principal manifestation, like the other chronic MPDs, a multipotent hematopoietic progenitor cell is involved in ET. Furthermore, a number of families have been described in which ET was inherited, in one instance as an autosomal dominant trait. In addition to ET, PMF and PV have also been observed in some kindreds.

CLINICAL FEATURES

Clinically, ET is most often identified incidentally when a platelet count is obtained during the course of a routine medical evaluation. Occasionally, review of previous blood counts will reveal that an elevated platelet count was present but overlooked for many years. No symptoms or signs are specific for ET, but these patients can have hemorrhagic and thrombotic tendencies expressed as easy bruising for the former and microvascular occlusions for the latter such as erythromelalgia, ocular migraine, or TIAs. Physical examination is generally unremarkable except occasionally for mild splenomegaly. Massive splenomegaly is indicative of another MPD, in particular PV, PMF, or CML.

Anemia is unusual, but a mild neutrophilic leukocytosis is not. The blood smear is most remarkable for the number of platelets present, some of which may be very large. The large mass of circulating platelets may prevent the accurate measurement of serum potassium due to release of platelet potassium upon blood clotting. This type of hyperkalemia is a laboratory artifact and not associated with electrocardiographic abnormalities. Similarly, arterial oxygen measurements can be inaccurate unless thrombocythemic blood is collected on ice. The prothrombin and partial thromboplastin times are normal, while abnormalities of platelet function such as a prolonged bleeding time and impaired platelet aggregation can be present. However, despite much study, no platelet function abnormality is characteristic of ET, and no platelet function test predicts the risk of clinically significant bleeding or thrombosis.

The elevated platelet count may hinder marrow aspiration, but marrow biopsy usually reveals megakaryocyte hyperplasia and hypertrophy, as well as an overall increase in marrow cellularity. If marrow reticulin is increased, another diagnosis should be considered. The absence of stainable iron demands an explanation because iron deficiency alone can cause thrombocytosis, and absent marrow iron in the presence of marrow hypercellularity is a feature of PV. Nonrandom cytogenetic abnormalities occur in ET but are uncommon, and no specific or consistent abnormality is notable, even those involving chromosomes 3 and 1, in which the genes for thrombopoietin and its receptor *Mpl*, respectively, are located.

DIAGNOSIS

Thrombocytosis is encountered in a broad variety of clinical disorders (Table 13-5) in many of which production of cytokines is increased. The absolute level of the platelet count is not a useful diagnostic aid for distinguishing between benign and clonal causes of thrombocytosis. About 50% of ET patients express the *JAK2* V617F mutation. When *JAK2* V617F is absent, cytogenetic evaluation is mandatory to determine if the thrombocytosis is due to CML or a myelodysplastic disorder such as the 5q- syndrome. Because the bcr-abl translocation can be present in the absence of the Ph chromosome, and because bcr-abl reverse transcriptase polymerase chain reaction is associated with false-positive results, fluorescence in situ hybridization (FISH) analysis for bcr-abl is the preferred assay in patients with thrombocytosis in whom a cytogenetic study for the Ph chromosome is negative. Anemia and ringed sideroblasts are not features of ET, but they are features of idiopathic refractory sideroblastic anemia, and in some of these patients, the thrombocytosis occurs in association with *JAK2* V617F expression. Massive splenomegaly should suggest the presence of another MPD, and in this setting a red cell mass determination should be performed because splenomegaly can mask the presence of erythrocytosis. Importantly, what appears to be ET can evolve into PV or PMF after a period of many years, revealing the true nature of the underlying MPD. There is sufficient overlap of the *JAK2* V617F neutrophil allele burden between ET and PV that this cannot be used as a distinguishing diagnostic feature; only a red cell mass and plasma volume determination can distinguish PV from ET, and importantly in this regard, 64% of *JAK2* V617F–positive ET patients actually were found to have PV when red cell mass and plasma volume determinations were performed.

COMPLICATIONS

Perhaps no other condition in clinical medicine has caused otherwise astute physicians to intervene inappropriately more often than thrombocytosis, particularly if the platelet count is >1 × 10^6/μL. It is commonly believed that a high platelet count causes intravascular stasis and thrombosis; however, no controlled clinical study has ever established this association, and in patients younger than age 60 years, the incidence of thrombosis was not greater in patients with thrombocytosis than in age-matched control participants.

To the contrary, very high platelet counts are associated primarily with hemorrhage due to acquired von Willebrand disease. This is not meant to imply that an elevated platelet count cannot cause symptoms in an ET patient but rather that the focus should be on the patient, not the platelet count. For example, some of the most dramatic neurologic problems in ET are migraine-related and respond only to lowering of the platelet count, while other symptoms such as erythromelalgia respond simply to platelet cyclooxygenase 1 inhibitors such as aspirin or ibuprofen, without a reduction in platelet number. Still others may represent an interaction between an atherosclerotic vascular system and a high platelet count, and others may have no relationship to the platelet count whatsoever. Recognition that PV can present with thrombocytosis alone as well as the discovery of previously unrecognized causes of hypercoagulability (Chap. 21) make the older literature on the complications of thrombocytosis unreliable.

TREATMENT Essential Thrombocytosis

Survival of patients with ET is not different than for the general population. An elevated platelet count in an asymptomatic patient without cardiovascular risk factors requires no therapy. Indeed, before any therapy is initiated in a patient with thrombocytosis, the cause of symptoms must be clearly identified as due to the elevated platelet count. When the platelet count rises above 1 × 10^6/μL, a substantial quantity of high-molecular-weight von Willebrand multimers are removed from the circulation and destroyed by the enlarged platelet mass, resulting in an acquired form of von Willebrand's disease. This can be identified by a reduction in ristocetin cofactor activity. In this situation, aspirin could promote hemorrhage. Bleeding in this situation usually responds to ε-aminocaproic acid, which can be given prophylactically before and after elective surgery. Plateletpheresis is at best a temporary and inefficient remedy that is rarely required. Importantly, ET patients treated with ^{32}P or alkylating agents are at risk of developing acute leukemia without any proof of benefit; combining either therapy with hydroxyurea increases this risk. If platelet reduction is deemed necessary on the basis of symptoms refractory to salicylates alone, IFN-α, the quinazoline derivative anagrelide, or hydroxyurea can be used to reduce the platelet count, but none of these is uniformly effective nor without significant side effects. Hydroxyurea and aspirin are more effective than anagrelide and aspirin for prevention of TIAs but not more effective for the prevention of other types of arterial thrombosis and are actually less effective for venous thrombosis. The effectiveness of hydroxyurea in preventing TIAs is because it is an nitric oxide (NO) donor. Normalizing the platelet count also does not prevent either arterial or venous thrombosis. The risk of gastrointestinal bleeding is also higher when aspirin is combined with anagrelide.

As more clinical experience is acquired, ET appears more benign than previously thought. Evolution to acute leukemia is more likely to be a consequence of therapy than of the disease itself. In managing patients with thrombocytosis, the physician's first obligation is to do no harm.

SECTION V

HEMATOLOGIC MALIGNANCIES

CHAPTER 14

ACUTE AND CHRONIC MYELOID LEUKEMIA

Meir Wetzler ■ Guido Marcucci ■ Clara D. Bloomfield

The myeloid leukemias are a heterogeneous group of diseases characterized by infiltration of the blood, bone marrow, and other tissues by neoplastic cells of the hematopoietic system. In 2010, the estimated number of new myeloid leukemia cases in the United States was 17,200. These leukemias comprise a spectrum of malignancies that, untreated, range from rapidly fatal to slowly growing. Based on their untreated course, the myeloid leukemias have traditionally been designated acute or chronic.

ACUTE MYELOID LEUKEMIA

INCIDENCE

The incidence of acute myeloid leukemia (AML) is ~3.5 per 100,000 people per year, and the age-adjusted incidence is higher in men than in women (4.3 vs 2.9). AML incidence increases with age; it is 1.7 in individuals aged <65 years and 15.9 in those aged >65 years. The median age at diagnosis is 67 years.

ETIOLOGY

Heredity, radiation, chemical and other occupational exposures, and drugs have been implicated in the development of AML. No direct evidence suggests a viral etiology.

Heredity

Certain syndromes with somatic cell chromosome aneuploidy, such as trisomy 21 noted in Down syndrome, are associated with an increased incidence of AML. Inherited diseases with defective DNA repair, e.g., Fanconi anemia, Bloom syndrome, and ataxia-telangiectasia, are also associated with AML. Congenital neutropenia (Kostmann syndrome) is a disease with mutations in the granulocyte colony-stimulating factor (G-CSF) receptor and often neutrophil elastase that may evolve into AML. Myeloproliferative syndromes may also evolve into AML (Chap. 13). Germ-line mutations of CCAAT/enhancer-binding protein α (*CEBPA*), runt-related transcription factor 1 (*RUNX1*), and tumor protein p53 (*TP53*) have also been associated with a higher predisposition to AML in some series.

Radiation

High-dose radiation, like that experienced by survivors of the atomic bombs in Japan or nuclear reactor accidents, increases the risk of myeloid leukemias that peak 5–7 years after exposure. Therapeutic radiation alone seems to add little risk of AML but can increase the risk in people also exposed to alkylating agents.

Chemical and other exposures

Exposure to benzene, a solvent used in the chemical, plastic, rubber, and pharmaceutical industries, is associated with an increased incidence of AML. Smoking and exposure to petroleum products, paint, embalming fluids, ethylene oxide, herbicides, and pesticides have also been associated with an increased risk of AML.

Drugs

Anticancer drugs are the leading cause of therapy-associated AML. Alkylating agent–associated leukemias occur on average 4–6 years after exposure, and affected individuals have aberrations in chromosomes 5 and 7. Topoisomerase II inhibitor–associated leukemias occur 1–3 years after exposure, and affected individuals often have aberrations involving chromosome 11q23. Chloramphenicol, phenylbutazone, and, less commonly, chloroquine and methoxypsoralen can result in bone marrow failure that may evolve into AML.

CLASSIFICATION

The current categorization of AML uses the World Health Organization (WHO) classification (Table 14-1), which includes different biologically distinct groups based on clinical features and cytogenetic and molecular abnormalities in addition to morphology. In contrast to the previously used French-American-British (FAB) schema, the WHO classification places limited reliance on cytochemistry. Since some of the recent literature and some ongoing studies use the FAB classification, a description of this system is also provided in Table 14-1. A major difference between the WHO and FAB systems is the blast cutoff for a diagnosis of AML as opposed to myelodysplastic syndrome it is 20% in the WHO classification and 30% in the FAB. AML with 20–30% blasts as defined by the WHO classification can benefit from therapies for MDS (such as decitabine or 5-azacytidine) that were approved by the U.S. Food and Drug Administration (FDA) based on trials using the FAB criteria. Selected components of the WHO classification are outlined below.

Immunophenotype and relevance to the WHO classification

The immunophenotype of human leukemia cells can be studied by multiparameter flow cytometry after the cells are labeled with monoclonal antibodies to cell-surface antigens. This can be important for separating AML from acute lymphoblastic leukemia (ALL) and identifying some types of AML. For example, AML with minimal differentiation that is characterized by immature morphology and no lineage-specific cytochemical reactions may be diagnosed by flow-cytometric demonstration of the myeloid-specific antigens cluster designation (CD) 13 and/or 117. Similarly, acute megakaryoblastic leukemia can often be diagnosed only by expression of the platelet-specific antigens CD41 and/or CD61. While flow cytometry is useful, widely used, and in some cases essential for the diagnosis of AML, it is supportive only in establishing the different subtypes of AML through the WHO classification.

Clinical features and relevance to the WHO classification

The WHO classification considers clinical features in subdividing AML. For example, it identifies therapy-related AML as a separate entity that develops after therapy (e.g., alkylating agents, topoisomerase II inhibitors, ionizing radiation). It also identifies AML with myelodysplasia-related changes based in part on medical history of an antecedent MDS or

TABLE 14-1

AML CLASSIFICATION SYSTEMS

WORLD HEATH ORGANIZATION CLASSIFICATION[a]	
AML with recurrent genetic abnormalities	**Myeloid proliferations related to Down syndrome**
AML with t(8;21)(q22;q22);*RUNX1-RUNX1T1*[b]	Transient abnormal myelopoiesis
AML with inv(16)(pl3.1q22) or t(16;16)(p13.1;q22); *CBFB-MYH11*[b]	Myeloid leukemia associated with Down syndrome
Acute promyelocytic leukemia with t(15;17)(q22;q12); *PML-RARA*[b]	**Blastic plasmacytoid dendritic cell neoplasm**
AML with t(9;11)(p22;q23); *MLLT3-MLL*	**Acute leukemia of ambiguous lineage**
AML with t(6;9)(p23;q34); *DEK-NUP214*	Acute undifferentiated leukemia
AML with inv(3)(q21q26.2) or t(3;3)(q21;q26.2); *RPN1-EVI1*	Mixed phenotype acute leukemia with t(9;22)(q34;q11,20); *BCR-ABL11*
AML (megakaryoblastic) with t(1;22)(p13;q13); *RBM15-MKL1*	Mixed phenotype acute leukemia with t(v;11q23); *MLL* rearranged
Provisional entity: AML with mutated NPM1	Mixed phenotype acute leukemia, B/myeloid, NOS
Provisional entity: AML with mutated CEBPA	Mixed phenotype acute leukemia, T/myeloid, NOS*Provisional entity: Natural killer (NK)-cell lymphoblastic leukemia/lymphoma*
AML with myelodysplasia-related changes	**French-American-British (FAB) Classification**[c]
Therapy-related myeloid neoplasms	MO: Minimally differentiated leukemia
AML not otherwise specified	Ml: Myeloblastic leukemia without maturation
AML with minimal differentiation	M2: Myeloblastic leukemia with maturation
AML without maturation	M3: Hypergranular promyelocytic leukemia
AML with maturation	M4: Myelomonocytic leukemia
Acute myelomonocytic leukemia	M4Eo: Variant: Increase in abnormal marrow eosinophils
Acute monoblastic and monocytic leukemia	M5: Monocytic leukemia
Acute erythroid leukemia	M6: Erythroleukemia (DiGuglielmo's disease)
Acute megakaryoblastic leukemia	M7: Megakaryoblastic leukemia
Acute basophilic leukemia	
Acute panmyelosis with myelofibrosis	
Myeloid sarcoma	

[a]From SH Swerdlow et al (eds): *World Health Organization Classification of Tumours of Haematopoietic and Lymphoid Tissues.* Lyon, IARC Press, 2008.
[b]Diagnosis is AML regardless of blast count.
[c]From JM Bennett et al: Proposed revised criteria for the classification of acute myeloid leukemia. A report of the French-American-British Cooperative Group. Ann Intern Med 103:620, 1985.
Abbreviation: AML, acute myeloid leukemia.

myelodysplastic/myeloproliferative neoplasm. The clinical features likely contribute to the prognosis of AML and have therefore been included in the classification.

Genetic findings and relevance to the WHO classification

The WHO classification is the first AML classification to incorporate genetic (chromosomal and molecular) information. Indeed, AML is first subclassified based on the presence or absence of specific recurrent genetic abnormalities. For example, AML FAB M3 is now designated *acute promyelocytic leukemia* (APL) based on the presence of either the t(15;17)(q22;q12) cytogenetic rearrangement or the *PML-RARA* fusion product of the translocation. A similar approach is taken with regard to core binding factor (CBF) AML that is now designated based on the presence of t(8;21)(q22;q22) or inv(16)(p13q22) or the respective fusion products *RUNX1-RUNX1T1* and *CBFB-MYH11*. Thus, the WHO classification separates recurrent cytogenetic and/or molecular types of AML and forces the clinician to take the appropriate steps to correctly identify the entity and thus tailor treatment(s) accordingly.

Chromosomal analyses

Chromosomal analysis of the leukemic cell provides the most important pretreatment prognostic information in AML. The WHO classification incorporates cytogenetics in the AML classification by recognizing a category of AML with recurrent genetic abnormalities and a category of AML with myelodysplasia-related changes (Table 14-1). The latter category is diagnosed in part by AML with selected myelodysplasia-related cytogenetic abnormalities (e.g., complex karyotypes and unbalanced and balanced changes involving among others, chromosomes 5, 7, and 11). Only one cytogenetic abnormality has been invariably associated with specific morphologic features: t(15;17)(q22;q12) with APL. Other chromosomal abnormalities have been associated primarily with one morphologic/immunophenotypic group, including inv(16)(p13q22) with AML with abnormal bone marrow eosinophils; t(8;21)(q22;q22) with slender Auer rods, expression of CD19, and increased normal eosinophils; and t(9;11)(p22;q23) and other translocations involving 11q23 with monocytic features. Recurring chromosomal abnormalities in AML may also be associated with specific clinical characteristics. More commonly associated with younger age are t(8;21) and t(15;17) and with older age, del(5q) and del(7q). Myeloid sarcomas (see below) are associated with t(8;21), and disseminated intravascular coagulation (DIC) with t(15;17).

Molecular classification

Molecular study of many recurring cytogenetic abnormalities has revealed genes that may be involved in leukemogenesis; this information is increasingly being incorporated into the WHO classification. For instance, t(15;17) results in the fusion gene *PML-RARA* that encodes a chimeric protein, promyelocytic leukemia (Pml)–retinoic acid receptor α (Rarα), which is formed by the fusion of the retinoic acid receptor α (*RARA*) gene from chromosome 17, and the promyelocytic leukemia (*PML*) gene from chromosome 15. The *RARA* gene encodes a member of the nuclear hormone receptor family of transcription factors. After binding retinoic acid, *RARA* can promote expression of a variety of genes. The 15;17 translocation juxtaposes *PML* with *RARA* in a head-to-tail configuration that is under the transcriptional control of *PML*. Three different breakpoints in the *PML* gene lead to various fusion protein isoforms. The Pml-Rarα fusion protein tends to suppress gene transcription and blocks differentiation of the cells. Pharmacologic doses of the Rarα ligand, all-*trans*-retinoic acid (tretinoin), relieve the block and promote hematopoietic cell differentiation (see below). Similar examples of molecular subtypes of the disease included in the category of AML with recurrent genetic abnormalities are those characterized by the leukemogenic fusion genes *RUNX1-RUNX1T1*, *CBFB-MYH11*, *MLLT3-MLL*, and *DEK-NUP214*, resulting, respectively, from t(8;21), inv(16), t(9;11), and t(6;9)(p23;q34).

Two new provisional entities defined by the presence of gene mutations, rather than macroscopic chromosomal abnormalities, have been recently added to the category of AML with recurrent genetic abnormalities: *AML with mutated nucleophosmin* (*NPM1*) and *AML with mutated CEBPA*. AML with fms-related tyrosine kinase 3 (*FLT3*) mutations is not considered a distinct entity, although determining the presence of such mutations is recommended by WHO in patients with cytogenetically normal AML (CN-AML) because the relatively frequent *FLT3*-internal tandem duplication (ITD) carries a negative prognostic significance and therefore is clinically relevant **(Table 14-2)**. *FLT3* encodes a tyrosine kinase receptor important in the development of myeloid and lymphoid lineages. Activating mutations of *FLT3* are present in ~30% of adult AML patients due to ITD in the juxtamembrane domain or mutations of the activating loop of the kinase. Continuous activation of the *FLT3*-encoded protein provides increased proliferation and antiapoptotic signals to the myeloid progenitor cell. *FLT3*-ITD, the more common of the *FLT3* mutations, occurs preferentially in patients with CN-AML. The importance of identifying *FLT3*-ITD at diagnosis relates to the fact that it not only is useful in prognostication but also may predict response to specific treatment such as the tyrosine kinase inhibitors that are being tested in clinical trials.

Other molecular prognostic factors (Table 14-2) in AML include v-kit Hardy-Zuckerman 4 feline sarcoma viral oncogene homolog (*KIT*) mutations that are

TABLE 14-2

MOLECULAR PROGNOSTIC MARKERS IN ACUTE MYELOID LEUKEMIA

MARKER	MARKER LOCATION	PROGNOSTIC IMPACT
NPM1 mutation	5q35	Favorable
CEBPA mutation	19q13.1	Favorable
FLT3-ITD	13q12	Adverse
WT1 mutation	11p13	Adverse
KIT mutation	4q11-q12	Adverse
BAALC overexpression	8q22.3	Adverse
ERG overexpression	21q22.3	Adverse
MN1 overexpression	22q12.1	Adverse
EVI1 overexpression	3q26	Adverse

Abbreviations: AML, acute myeloid leukemia; ITD, internal tandem duplication.

found in 25–30% of t(8;21) or inv(16) patients. Others include Wilms' tumor 1 (*WT1*) mutations found in 10–13% of CN-AML and overexpression of genes such as brain and acute leukemia, cytoplasmic (*BAALC*), ets erythroblastosis virus E26 oncogene homologue (avian) (*ERG*), meningioma (disrupted in balanced translocation) 1 (*MN1*), and MDS1 and EVI1 complex locus (*MECOM*, also known as *EVI1*), which predict for poor outcome in CN-AML. The applicability of screening for these molecular aberrations to AML classification and clinical practice is being tested.

With progress in genomics technology including genomewide investigation of gene mutations and expression levels, additional aberrations are being discovered, underscoring the molecular heterogeneity of AML. The applicability of gene expression profiling to diagnosis and outcome prediction of cytogenetic and molecular subsets of AML patients and to clinical management of AML is under active investigation. MicroRNAs, naturally occurring noncoding RNAs, have been shown to regulate the expression of proteins involved in hematopoietic differentiation and survival pathways by degradation or translation inhibition of target coding RNAs. Deregulated expression levels of microRNAs have been shown to associate with specific cytogenetic and molecular subsets of AML and predict outcome in CN-AML. Finally, massive parallel sequencing of the whole genome from AML patients' blasts is revealing previously unrecognized mutations of genes that are involved in metabolic pathways that have not been previously hypothesized to be disrupted in AML, such as mutations in the isocitrate dehydrogenase 1 (NADP+), soluble (*IDH1*) and isocitrate dehydrogenase 2 (NADP+), and mitochondrial (*IDH2*) genes.

It is likely that once the biologic and clinical significance of these emerging genetic aberrations is understood, AML will be primarily classified molecularly to define specific entities and stratify patients to a corresponding, optimal targeting therapy.

CLINICAL PRESENTATION

Symptoms

Patients with AML most often present with nonspecific symptoms that begin gradually or abruptly and are the consequence of anemia, leukocytosis, leukopenia or leukocyte dysfunction, or thrombocytopenia. Nearly half have had symptoms for ≤3 months before the leukemia was diagnosed.

Half mention fatigue as the first symptom, but most complain of fatigue or weakness at the time of diagnosis. Anorexia and weight loss are common. Fever with or without an identifiable infection is the initial symptom in ~10% of patients. Signs of abnormal hemostasis (bleeding, easy bruising) are noted first in 5% of patients. On occasion, bone pain, lymphadenopathy, nonspecific cough, headache, or diaphoresis is the presenting symptom.

Rarely, patients may present with symptoms from a myeloid sarcoma that is a tumor mass consisting of myeloid blasts occurring at anatomic sites other than bone marrow. Sites involved are most commonly the skin, lymph node, gastrointestinal tract, soft tissue, and testis. This rare presentation, often characterized by chromosome aberrations (e.g., monosomy 7, trisomy 8, *MLL* rearrangement, inv[16], trisomy 4, t[8;21]) may precede or coincide with AML.

Physical findings

Fever, splenomegaly, hepatomegaly, lymphadenopathy, sternal tenderness, and evidence of infection and hemorrhage are often found at diagnosis. Significant gastrointestinal bleeding, intrapulmonary hemorrhage, or intracranial hemorrhage occur most often in APL. Bleeding associated with coagulopathy may also occur in monocytic AML and with extreme degrees of leukocytosis or thrombocytopenia in other morphologic subtypes. Retinal hemorrhages are detected in 15% of patients. Infiltration of the gingivae, skin, soft tissues, or the meninges with leukemic blasts at diagnosis is characteristic of the monocytic subtypes and those with 11q23 chromosomal abnormalities.

Hematologic findings

Anemia is usually present at diagnosis and can be severe. The degree varies considerably, irrespective of other hematologic findings, splenomegaly, or duration of symptoms. The anemia is usually normocytic normochromic. Decreased erythropoiesis often results in a reduced reticulocyte count, and red blood cell (RBC) survival is decreased by accelerated destruction. Active blood loss also contributes to the anemia.

The median presenting leukocyte count is about 15,000/μL. Between 25 and 40% of patients have counts <5000/μL, and 20% have counts >100,000/μL. Fewer than 5% have no detectable leukemic cells in the blood. The morphology of the malignant cell varies in different subsets. In AML, the cytoplasm often contains primary (nonspecific) granules, and the nucleus shows fine, lacy chromatin with one or more nucleoli characteristic of immature cells. Abnormal rod-shaped granules called Auer rods are not uniformly present, but when they are, myeloid lineage is virtually certain (Fig. 14-1). Poor neutrophil function may be noted functionally by impaired phagocytosis and migration and morphologically by abnormal lobulation and deficient granulation.

Platelet counts <100,000/μL are found at diagnosis in ~75% of patients, and about 25% have counts <25,000/μL. Both morphologic and functional platelet abnormalities can be observed, including large and bizarre shapes with abnormal granulation and an inability of platelets to aggregate or adhere normally to one another.

Pretreatment evaluation

When a diagnosis of AML is suspected, a rapid evaluation and initiation of appropriate therapy should follow (Table 14-3). In addition to clarifying the subtype of leukemia, initial studies should evaluate the overall functional integrity of the major organ systems, including the cardiovascular, pulmonary, hepatic, and renal systems. Factors that have prognostic significance, either for achieving complete remission (CR) or for predicting

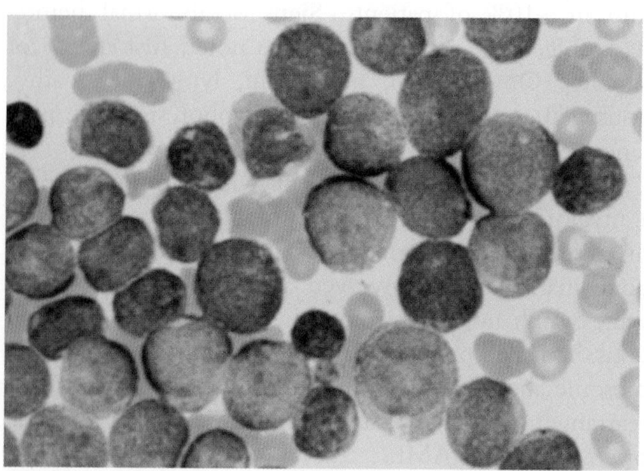

A

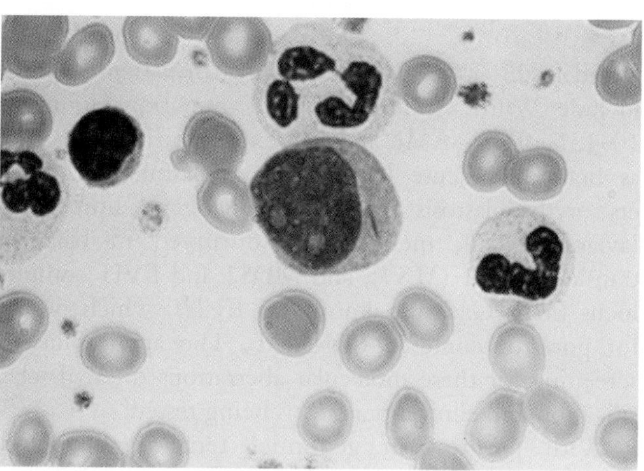

B

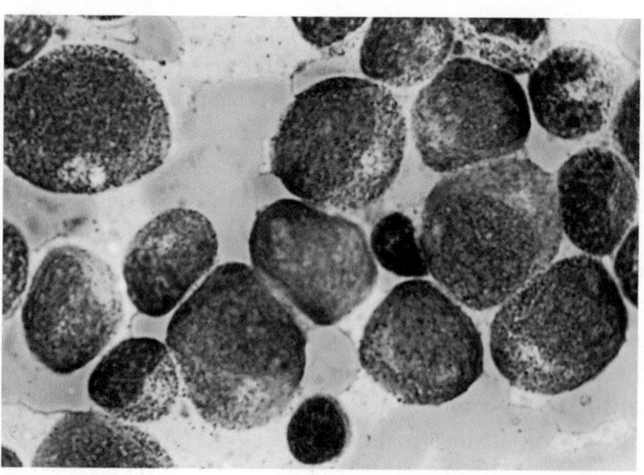

C

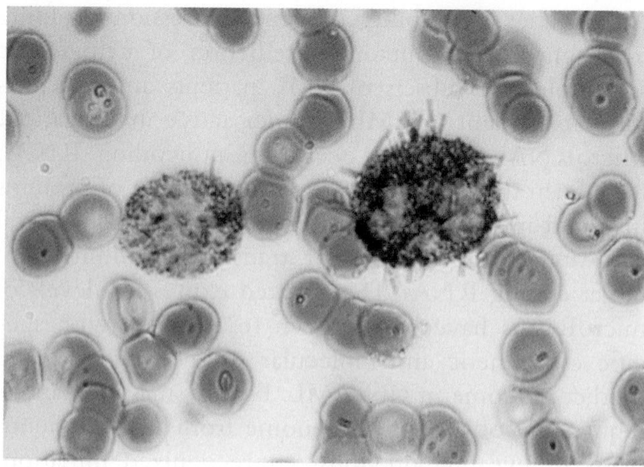

D

FIGURE 14-1

Morphology of AML cells. ***A.*** Uniform population of primitive myeloblasts with immature chromatin, nucleoli in some cells, and primary cytoplasmic granules. ***B.*** Leukemic myeloblast containing an Auer rod. ***C.*** Promyelocytic leukemia cells with prominent cytoplasmic primary granules. ***D.*** Peroxidase stain shows the dark blue color characteristic of peroxidase in granules in AML.

TABLE 14-3

INITIAL DIAGNOSTIC EVALUATION AND MANAGEMENT OF ADULT PATIENTS WITH ACUTE MYELOID LEUKEMIA

History
Increasing fatigue or decreased exercise tolerance (anemia)
Excess bleeding or bleeding from unusual sites (DIC, thrombocytopenia)
Fevers or recurrent infections (granulocytopenia)
Headache, vision changes, nonfocal neurologic abnormalities (CNS leukemia or bleeding)
Early satiety (splenomegaly)
Family history of AML (Fanconi, Bloom, or Kostmann syndromes or ataxia-telangiectasia)
History of cancer (exposure to alkylating agents, radiation, topoisomerase II inhibitors)
Occupational exposures (radiation, benzene, petroleum products, paint, smoking, pesticides)
Physical Examination
Performance status (prognostic factor)
Ecchymosis and oozing from IV sites (DIC, possible acute promyelocytic leukemia)
Fever and tachycardia (signs of infection)
Papilledema, retinal infiltrates, cranial nerve abnormalities (CNS leukemia)
Poor dentition, dental abscesses
Gum hypertrophy (leukemic infiltration, most common in monocytic leukemia)
Skin infiltration or nodules (leukemia infiltration, most common in monocytic leukemia)
Lymphadenopathy, splenomegaly, hepatomegaly
Back pain, lower extremity weakness (spinal granulocytic sarcoma, most likely in t[8;21] patients)
Laboratory and Radiologic Studies
CBC with manual differential cell count
Chemistry tests (electrolytes, creatinine, BUN, calcium, phosphorus, uric acid, hepatic enzymes, bilirubin, LDH, amylase, lipase)
Clotting studies (prothrombin time, partial thromboplastin time, fibrinogen, D-dimer)
Viral serologies (CMV, HSV-1, varicella-zoster)
RBC type and screen
HLA typing for potential allogeneic HSCT
Bone marrow aspirate and biopsy (morphology, cytogenetics, flow cytometry, molecular studies for *NPM1* and *CEBPA* mutations and *FLT3*-ITD)
Cryopreservation of viable leukemia cells
Echocardiogram or heart scan
PA and lateral chest radiograph
Placement of central venous access device
Interventions for Specific Patients
Dental evaluation (for those with poor dentition)
Lumbar puncture (for those with symptoms of CNS involvement)
Screening spine MRI (for patients with back pain, lower extremity weakness, paresthesias)
Social work referral for patient and family psychosocial support
Counseling for All Patients
Provide patient with information regarding their disease, financial counseling, and support group contacts

Abbreviations: AML, acute myeloid leukemia; BUN, blood urea nitrogen; CBC, complete blood count; CMV, cytomegalovirus; CNS, central nervous system; DIC, disseminated intravascular coagulation; HLA, human leukocyte antigen; HSCT, hematopoietic stem cell transplant; HSV, herpes simplex virus; LDH, lactate dehydrogenase; MRI, magnetic resonance imaging; PA, posteroanterior; RBC, red blood cell.

the duration of CR, should also be assessed before initiating treatment, including cytogenetics and molecular markers (at least *NMP1* and *CEBPA* mutations and *FLT3*-ITD in CN-AML). Leukemic cells should be obtained from all patients and cryopreserved for future use as new tests and therapeutics become available. All patients should be evaluated for infection.

Most patients are anemic and thrombocytopenic at presentation. Replacement of the appropriate blood components, if necessary, should begin promptly. Because qualitative platelet dysfunction or the presence of an infection may increase the likelihood of bleeding, evidence of hemorrhage justifies the immediate use of platelet transfusion, even if the platelet count is only moderately decreased.

About 50% of patients have a mild to moderate elevation of serum uric acid at presentation. Only 10% have marked elevations, but renal precipitation of uric acid and the nephropathy that may result is a serious but uncommon complication. The initiation of chemotherapy may aggravate hyperuricemia, and patients are usually started immediately on allopurinol and hydration at diagnosis. Rasburicase (recombinant uric oxidase) is also useful for treating uric acid nephropathy and often can normalize the serum uric acid level within hours with a single dose of treatment. The presence of high concentrations of lysozyme, a marker for monocytic differentiation, may be etiologic in renal tubular dysfunction, which could worsen other renal problems that arise during the initial phases of therapy.

PROGNOSTIC FACTORS

Many factors influence the likelihood of entering CR, the length of CR, and the curability of AML. CR is defined after examination of both blood and bone marrow. The blood neutrophil count must be ≥1000/μL and the platelet count ≥100,000/μL. Hemoglobin concentration is not considered in determining CR. Circulating blasts should be absent. While rare blasts may be detected in the blood during marrow regeneration, they should disappear on successive studies. The bone marrow should contain <5% blasts, and Auer rods should be absent. Extramedullary leukemia should not be present.

For patients in morphologic CR, immunophenotyping to detect minute populations of blasts, reverse transcriptase polymerase chain reaction (RT-PCR) to detect AML-associated molecular abnormalities, and either metaphase cytogenetics or interphase cytogenetics by fluorescence in situ hybridization (FISH) to detect AML-associated cytogenetic aberrations are currently being investigated to assess whether residual disease that has clinical significance is present following treatment. Detection of minimal residual disease may become a reliable discriminator between patients in CR who do or do not require additional and/or alternative therapies. In APL, detection of the *PML-RARA* fusion gene transcript by RT-PCR in bone marrow and/or blood during CR predicts relapse, and this assay is being routinely used in the clinic to anticipate clinical relapse and initiate timely salvage treatment. In other types of AML, the clinical relevance of minimal residual disease requires further investigation.

Age at diagnosis is among the most important risk factors. Advancing age is associated with a poorer prognosis, in part because of its influence on the patient's ability to survive induction therapy. Age also influences outcome because AML in older patients differs biologically. The leukemic cells in elderly patients more commonly express the multidrug resistance 1 (MDR1) efflux pump that conveys resistance to natural product–derived agents such as the anthracyclines (see below). With each successive decade of age, a greater proportion of patients have more resistant disease. Chronic and intercurrent diseases impair tolerance to rigorous therapy; acute medical problems at diagnosis reduce the likelihood of survival. Performance status, independent of age, also influences ability to survive induction therapy and thus respond to treatment.

A prolonged symptomatic interval with cytopenias preceding diagnosis or a history of an antecedent hematologic disorder is another pretreatment clinical feature associated with a lower CR rate and shorter survival time. The CR rate is lower in patients who have had anemia, leukopenia, and/or thrombocytopenia for >3 months before the diagnosis of AML compared with those without such a history. Responsiveness to chemotherapy declines as the duration of the antecedent disorder(s) increases. AML developing after treatment with cytotoxic agents for other malignancies is usually difficult to treat successfully.

A high presenting leukocyte count in some series is an independent prognostic factor for attaining a CR. Among patients with hyperleukocytosis (>100,000/μL), early central nervous system bleeding and pulmonary leukostasis contribute to poor outcome with initial therapy.

Chromosome findings at diagnosis are currently the most important independent prognostic factor. Patients with t(15;17) have a very good prognosis (approximately 85% cured), and those with t(8;21) and inv(16) a good prognosis (approximately 55% cured), while those with no cytogenetic abnormality have a moderately favorable outcome (approximately 40% cured). Patients with a complex karyotype, t(6;9), inv(3), or -7 have a very poor prognosis.

For patients lacking prognostic cytogenetic abnormalities, such as those with CN-AML, outcome prediction utilizes molecular genetic abnormalities. *NPM1* mutations without concurrent presence of *FLT3*-ITD, and *CEBPA* mutations, especially if concurrently present in two different alleles, have been shown to predict favorable outcome, whereas *FLT3*-ITD predicts a poor outcome. Given the prognostic importance of *NPM1* and *CEBPA* mutations and *FLT3*-ITD, molecular assessment of these genes at diagnosis have been incorporated in AML management guidelines by the National Comprehensive Cancer Network (NCCN) and the European Leukemia Net (ELN). Other molecular aberrations (Table 14-2) may in the future be utilized for prognostication.

In addition to pretreatment variables such as age, leukocyte count, and cytogenetics and/or molecular genetic aberrations, several treatment factors correlate with prognosis in AML, including, most importantly, achievement of CR. In addition, patients who achieve CR after one induction cycle have longer CR durations than those requiring multiple cycles.

TREATMENT Acute Myeloid Leukemia

Treatment of a newly diagnosed patient with AML is usually divided into two phases, induction and postremission management (Fig. 14-2). The initial goal is to quickly induce CR. When CR is obtained, further therapy must be used to prolong survival and achieve cure. The initial induction treatment and subsequent postremission therapy are often chosen based on the patient's age. Intensifying therapy with traditional chemotherapy agents such as cytarabine and anthracyclines in younger patients (<60 years) appears to increase the cure rate of AML. In older patients the benefit of intensive therapy is controversial; novel therapies are being pursued.

INDUCTION CHEMOTHERAPY The most commonly used CR induction regimens (for patients other than those with APL) consist of combination chemotherapy with cytarabine and an anthracycline. Cytarabine is a cell cycle S-phase–specific antimetabolite that becomes phosphorylated intracellularly to an active triphosphate form that interferes with DNA synthesis. Anthracyclines are DNA intercalators. Their primary mode of action is thought to be inhibition of topoisomerase II, leading to DNA breaks. Cytarabine is usually administered as a continuous intravenous infusion for 7 days. Anthracycline therapy generally consists of daunorubicin intravenously on days 1, 2, and 3 (the 7 and 3 regimen). Treatment with idarubicin for 3 days in conjunction with cytarabine by 7-day continuous infusion is at least as effective as daunorubicin in younger patients. The addition of etoposide may improve the CR duration. When combined with cytarabine in a 7 and 3 regimen,

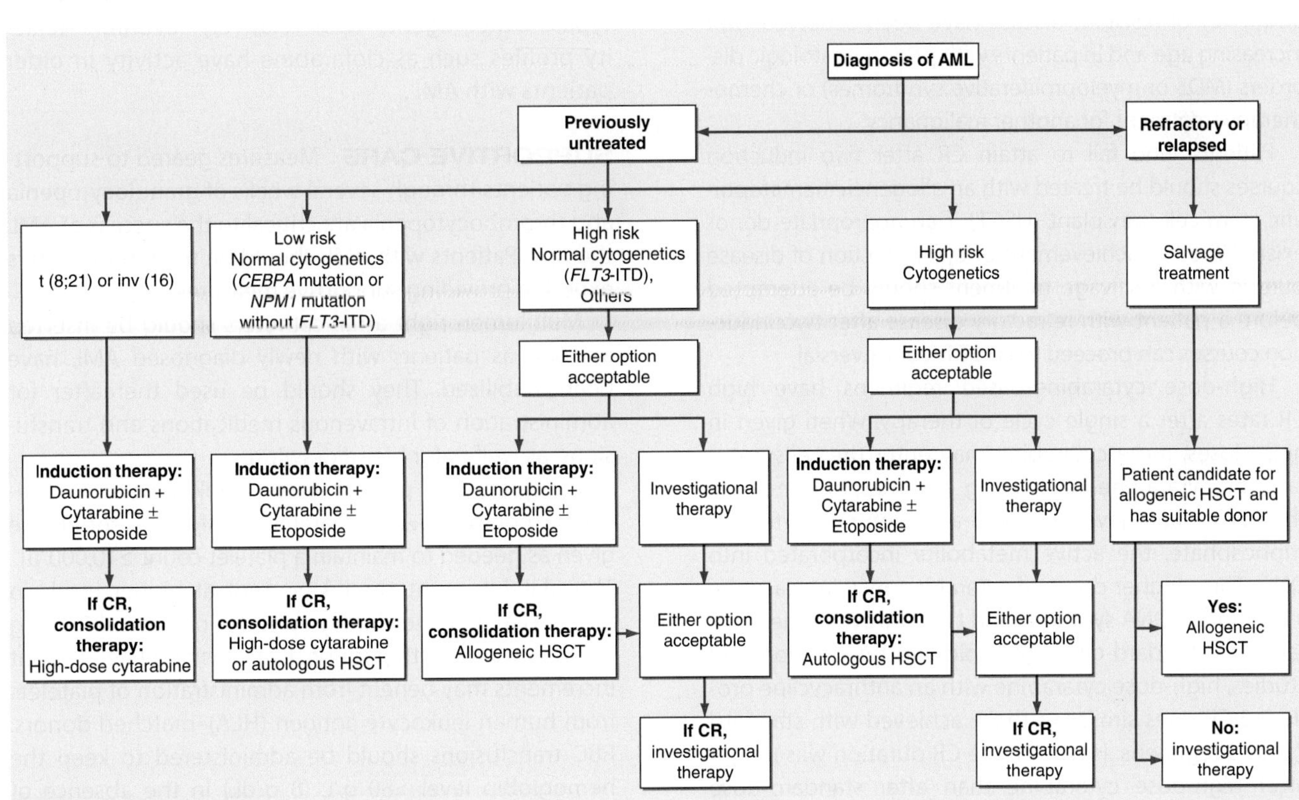

FIGURE 14-2

Flow chart for the therapy of newly diagnosed acute myeloid leukemia (AML). For all forms of AML except acute promyelocytic leukemia (APL), standard therapy includes a 7-day continuous infusion of cytarabine (100–200 mg/m^2 per day) and a 3-day course of daunorubicin (60–90 mg/m^{2}per day) with or without 3 days of etoposide (only with daunorubicin 60 mg/m^2 per day) or novel therapies based on their predicted risk of relapse (i.e., risk-stratified therapy). Idarubicin (12–13 mg/m^2 per day) could be used in place of daunorubicin (not shown). Patients who achieve complete remission undergo postremission consolidation therapy, including sequential courses of high-dose cytarabine, autologous hematopoietic stem cell transplant (HSCT), allogeneic HSCT, or novel therapies, based on their predicted risk of relapse (i.e., risk-stratified therapy). Patients with APL (see text for treatment) usually receive tretinoin together with anthracycline-based chemotherapy for remission induction and then arsenic trioxide followed by consolidation with anthracycline-based chemotherapy and possibly maintenance with tretinoin. The role of cytarabine in APL induction and consolidation is controversial.

a higher dose of anthracycline (i.e., daunorubicin 90 mg/m^2) improves outcome compared with a lower dose (i.e., daunorubicin 45 mg/m^2).

After induction chemotherapy, if persistence of leukemia is documented, the patient is usually retreated with cytarabine and an anthracycline in doses similar to those given initially, but for 5 and 2 days, respectively. Our recommendation, however, is to consider changing therapy in this setting.

With the 7 and 3 cytarabine/daunorubicin regimen outlined above, 65–75% of adults with de novo AML younger than age 60 years achieve CR. Two-thirds achieve CR after a single course of therapy, and one-third require two courses. About 50% of patients who do not achieve CR have a drug-resistant leukemia, and 50% do not achieve CR because of fatal complications of bone marrow aplasia or impaired recovery of normal stem cells. A higher induction treatment–related mortality rate and frequency of resistant disease have been observed with increasing age and in patients with prior hematologic disorders (MDS or myeloproliferative syndromes) or chemotherapy treatment for another malignancy.

Patients who fail to attain CR after two induction courses should be treated with an allogeneic hematopoietic stem cell transplant (HSCT) if an appropriate donor exists. Whether achievement of cytoreduction of disease burden with a salvage treatment should be attempted before a patient with refractory disease after two induction courses can proceed to HSCT is controversial.

High-dose cytarabine-based regimens have high CR rates after a single cycle of therapy. When given in high doses, more cytarabine may enter the cells; saturate the cytarabine-inactivating enzymes; and increase the intracellular levels of 1-β-d-arabinofuranylcytosine-triphosphate, the active metabolite incorporated into DNA. Thus, higher doses of cytarabine may increase the inhibition of DNA synthesis and thereby overcome resistance to standard-dose cytarabine. In two randomized studies, high-dose cytarabine with an anthracycline produced CR rates similar to those achieved with standard 7 and 3 regimens. However, the CR duration was longer after high-dose cytarabine than after standard-dose cytarabine.

The hematologic toxicity of high-dose cytarabine-based induction regimens has typically been greater than that associated with 7 and 3 regimens. Toxicity with high-dose cytarabine includes myelosuppression, pulmonary toxicity, and significant and occasionally irreversible cerebellar toxicity. All patients treated with high-dose cytarabine must be closely monitored for cerebellar toxicity. Full cerebellar testing should be performed before each dose, and further high-dose cytarabine should be withheld if evidence of cerebellar toxicity develops. This toxicity occurs more commonly in patients with renal impairment and in those older than age 60 years. The increased toxicity observed with high-dose cytarabine has limited the use of this therapy in elderly AML patients.

Because of the negative impact of age on outcome when treatment with conventional chemotherapy is administered, clinical trials in elderly patients have focused on new agents or alternative approaches such as reduced-intensity allogeneic HSCT. Among these, one promising therapy is decitabine, a nucleoside analogue that inhibits DNA methyltransferase, reverses aberrant DNA methylation, and subsequently induces transcription of otherwise silenced tumor suppressor genes in AML cells. Interestingly, this effect on inhibiting DNA methyltransferase occurs at a much lower dose than previously used with this agent to produce a cytotoxic effect in AML. Low-dose decitabine yields complete responses in older patients with AML, including those with unfavorable karyotypes. Other agents with relatively favorable toxicity profiles such as clofarabine have activity in older patients with AML.

SUPPORTIVE CARE Measures geared to supporting patients through several weeks of granulocytopenia and thrombocytopenia are critical to the success of AML therapy. Patients with AML should be treated in centers expert in providing supportive measures.

Multilumen right atrial catheters should be inserted as soon as patients with newly diagnosed AML have been stabilized. They should be used thereafter for administration of intravenous medications and transfusions, as well as for blood drawing.

Adequate and prompt blood bank support is critical to therapy of AML. Platelet transfusions should be given as needed to maintain a platelet count ≥10,000/μL. The platelet count should be kept at higher levels in febrile patients and during episodes of active bleeding or DIC. Patients with poor posttransfusion platelet count increments may benefit from administration of platelets from human leukocyte antigen (HLA)–matched donors. RBC transfusions should be administered to keep the hemoglobin level >80 g/L (8 g/dL) in the absence of active bleeding, DIC, or congestive heart failure, which require higher hemoglobin levels. Blood products leukodepleted by filtration should be used to avert or delay alloimmunization as well as febrile reactions. Blood products should also be irradiated to prevent transfusion associated graft-versus-host disease (GVHD). Cytomegalovirus (CMV)-negative blood products should be used for CMV-seronegative patients who are potential candidates for allogeneic HSCT. Leukodepleted products are also effective for these patients if CMV-negative products are not available.

Infectious complications remain the major cause of morbidity and death during induction and postremission chemotherapy for AML. Antibacterial (i.e., quinolones) and antifungal (e.g, fluconazole, posaconazole) prophylaxis in the absence of fever is likely to be beneficial. For patients who are herpes simplex virus– or varicella zoster–seropositive, antiviral prophylaxis should be initiated.

Fever develops in most patients with AML, but infections are documented in only half of febrile patients. Early initiation of empirical broad-spectrum antibacterial and antifungal antibiotics has significantly reduced the number of patients dying of infectious complications (Chap. 29). An antibiotic regimen adequate to treat gram-negative organisms should be instituted at the onset of fever in a granulocytopenic patient after clinical evaluation, including a detailed physical examination with inspection of the indwelling catheter exit site and a perirectal examination, as well as procurement of cultures and radiographs aimed at documenting the source of fever. Specific antibiotic regimens should be based on antibiotic sensitivity data obtained from the institution at which the patient is being treated. Acceptable regimens for empiric antibiotic therapy include monotherapy with imipenem–cilastin, meropenem, piperacillin–tazobactam, or an extended-spectrum antipseudomonal cephalosporin (cefepime or ceftazidime); an aminoglycoside in combination with an antipseudomonal penicillin (e.g., piperacillin); an aminoglycoside in combination with an extended-spectrum antipseudomonal cephalosporin; and ciprofloxacin in combination with an antipseudomonal penicillin. Aminoglycosides should be avoided if possible in patients with renal insufficiency. Empirical vancomycin should be initiated in neutropenic patients with catheter-related infections, blood cultures positive for gram-positive bacteria before final identification and susceptibility testing, hypotension or shock, and increased risk for viridans group streptococcal bacteremia.

Caspofungin (or similar echinocandin) or liposomal amphotericin B should be considered for antifungal treatment if fever persists 4–7 days following initiation of empiric antibiotic therapy in a patient who has received fluconazole prophylaxis. Voriconazole has also been shown to be equivalent in efficacy and less toxic than amphotericin B. Antibacterial and antifungal antibiotics should be continued until patients are no longer neutropenic regardless of whether a specific source has been found for the fever.

Recombinant hematopoietic growth factors have been incorporated into clinical trials in AML. These trials have been designed to lower the infection rate after chemotherapy. Both G-CSF and granulocyte-macrophage colony-stimulating factor (GM-CSF) have reduced the median time to neutrophil recovery. This accelerated rate of neutrophil recovery, however, has not generally translated into significant reductions in infection rates or shortened hospitalizations. In most randomized studies, both G-CSF and GM-CSF have failed to improve the CR rate, disease-free survival, or overall survival. Although receptors for both G-CSF and/or GM-CSF are present on AML blasts, therapeutic efficacy is neither enhanced nor inhibited by these agents. The use of growth factors as supportive care for AML patients is controversial. We favor their use in elderly patients with complicated courses, those receiving intensive postremission regimens, patients with uncontrolled infections, and those participating in clinical trials.

TREATMENT OF PROMYELOCYTIC LEUKEMIA Tretinoin is an oral drug that induces the differentiation of leukemic cells bearing the t(15;17). APL is responsive to cytarabine and daunorubicin, but about 10% of patients treated with these drugs die from DIC induced by the release of granule components by dying tumor cells. Tretinoin does not produce DIC but produces another complication called the APL differentiation syndrome. Occurring within the first 3 weeks of treatment, it is characterized by fever, fluid retention, dyspnea, chest pain, pulmonary infiltrates, pleural and pericardial effusions, and hypoxemia. The syndrome is related to adhesion of differentiated neoplastic cells to the pulmonary vasculature endothelium. Glucocorticoids, chemotherapy, and/or supportive measures can be effective for management of the APL differentiation syndrome. Temporary discontinuation of tretinoin is necessary in cases of severe APL differentiation syndrome (i.e., patients developing renal failure or requiring admission to the intensive care unit due to respiratory distress). The mortality rate of this syndrome is about 10%.

Tretinoin (45 mg/m^2 per day orally until remission is documented) plus concurrent anthracycline-based chemotherapy appears to be among the most effective treatments for APL, leading to CR rates of 90–95%. The addition of cytarabine, although not demonstrated to increase the CR rate, seemingly decreases the risk for relapse. Following achievement of CR, patients should receive at least two cycles of anthracycline-based chemotherapy.

Given the progress made in APL, resulting in high cure rates, the goals are to identify patients with very low risk of relapse where attempts are being made to decrease the amount of therapy administered and to identify patients at greatest risk of relapse in order to develop new approaches to increase cure.

Arsenic trioxide has significant antileukemic activity and is being explored as part of initial treatment in clinical trials of APL. In a randomized trial, arsenic trioxide improved outcome if utilized after achievement of CR and before consolidation therapy with anthracycline-based chemotherapy. Additionally, studies combining arsenic trioxide with tretinoin in the absence of chemotherapy are ongoing and preliminarily have shown promise in those patients "unfit" to receive chemotherapy. Furthermore, combinations of arsenic trioxide, tretinoin, and/or chemotherapy and/or gemtuzumab ozogamicin, a monoclonal CD33 antibody linked to the cytotoxic agent calicheamicin, have shown favorable response in high-risk APL patients (i.e., those presenting with a leukocyte count ≥10,000/μL) at diagnosis. Patients receiving arsenic trioxide are at risk of APL differentiation syndrome, especially when it is administered during induction or salvage treatment after disease relapse. In addition, arsenic trioxide may prolong the QT interval, increasing the risk of cardiac arrhythmias.

Assessment of residual disease by RT-PCR amplification of the t(15;17) chimeric gene product *PML-RARA* following the final cycle of chemotherapy is an important step in the management of APL patients. Disappearance of the signal is associated with long-term disease-free survival; its persistence documented by two consecutive tests performed 2 weeks apart invariably predicts relapse. Sequential monitoring of RT-PCR for t(15;17) is now considered standard for postremission monitoring of APL.

Patients who continue in molecular remission may benefit from maintenance therapy with tretinoin. Patients in molecular, cytogenetic, or clinical relapse should be salvaged with arsenic trioxide; it produces meaningful responses in up to 85% of patients and can be followed by HSCT.

POSTREMISSION THERAPY Induction of a durable first CR is critical to long-term disease-free survival in AML. However, without further therapy, virtually all patients experience relapse. Once relapse has occurred, AML is generally curable only by HSCT.

Postremission therapy is designed to eradicate residual leukemic cells to prevent relapse and prolong survival. Postremission therapy in AML is often based on age (younger than ages 55–65 years and older than ages 55–65 years). For younger patients, most studies include intensive chemotherapy and allogeneic or autologous HSCT. High-dose cytarabine is more effective than standard-dose cytarabine. The Cancer and Leukemia Group B (CALGB), for example, compared the duration of CR in patients randomly assigned postremission to four cycles of high (3 g/m^2, every 12 hours on days 1, 3, and 5), intermediate (400 mg/m^2 for 5 days by continuous infusion), or standard (100 mg/m^2 per day for 5 days by continuous infusion) doses of cytarabine. A dose-response effect for cytarabine in patients with AML who were aged ≤60 years was demonstrated. High-dose cytarabine significantly prolonged CR and increased the fraction cured in patients with favorable (t[8;21] and inv[16]) and normal cytogenetics, but it had no significant effect on patients with other abnormal karyotypes. For older patients, exploration of attenuated intensive therapy that includes either chemotherapy or reduced-intensity allogeneic HSCT has been pursued. Postremission therapy is a setting for introduction of new agents (Table 14-4).

Allogeneic HSCT is used in patients ages <70–75 years with an HLA-compatible donor who have high-risk cytogenetics. In patients with CN-AML and high-risk molecular features such as *FLT3*-ITD, allogeneic HSCT is best applied in the context of clinical trials, as the impact of aggressive therapy on outcome is unknown. Relapse following allogeneic HSCT occurs in only a small fraction of patients, but treatment-related toxicity is relatively high; complications include venoocclusive disease, GVHD, and infections. Autologous HSCT can be administered in young and older patients and uses the same preparative regimens. Patients subsequently

TABLE 14-4

SELECTED NEW AGENTS UNDER STUDY FOR THE TREATMENT OF ADULTS WITH ACUTE MYELOID LEUKEMIA

CLASS OF DRUGS	EXAMPLES OF AGENTS IN CLASS
Tyrosine kinase inhibitors	PKC412, MLN518, SU11248, CHIR-258, imatinib (STI571, Gleevec), dasatinib, AMN107
Demethylating agents	Decitabine, 5-azacytidine
Histone deacetylase inhibitors	Suberoylanilide hydroxamic acid (SAHA), MS275, LBH589, valproic acid
Heavy metals	Arsenic trioxide
Farnesyl transferase inhibitors	R115777, SCH66336
HSP-90 antagonists	17-allylaminogeldanamycin (17-AAG), DMAG, or derivatives
Cell cycle inhibitors	Flavopiridol, CYC202 (R-Roscovitine), SNS-032
Nucleoside analogues	Clofarabine, troxacitabine
Humanized antibodies	Anti-CD33 (SGN33), anti-KIR
Toxin-conjugated antibodies	Gemtuzumab ozogamicin
Proteasome inhibitors	Bortezomib
Aurora inhibitors	AZD1152, MLN-8237, AT9283
Immunomodulatory	Lenalidomide, IL-2, histamine dihydrochloride

Abbreviations: AML, acute myeloid leukemia; IL-2, interleukin-2.

receive their own stem cells collected while in remission. The toxicity is relatively low with autologous HSCT (5% mortality rate), but the relapse rate is higher than with allogeneic HSCT due to the absence of the graft-versus-leukemia (GVL) effect seen with allogeneic HSCT and possible contamination of the autologous stem cells with residual tumor cells. Purging tumor from the autologous stem cells has not lowered the relapse rate with autologous HSCT.

Randomized trials comparing intensive chemotherapy and autologous and allogeneic HSCT have shown an improved duration of remission with allogeneic HSCT compared with autologous HSCT or chemotherapy alone. However, overall survival is generally not different; the improved disease control with allogeneic HSCT is erased by the increase in fatal toxicity. While stem cells were previously harvested from the bone marrow, virtually all efforts currently collect these from the blood following mobilization regimens. Prognostic factors may help select patients in first CR for whom transplant is most effective.

Our approach includes allogeneic HSCT if feasible in first CR for patients with high-risk karyotypes (Fig. 14-2). Patients with CN-AML who have other poor risk factors (e.g., an antecedent hematologic disorder, or failure to attain remission with a single induction course) and patients lacking a favorable genotype (e.g., patients who do not have *CEBPA* mutations or *NPM1* mutations without *FLT3*-ITD) are also potential candidates. If a suitable HLA donor does not exist, investigational therapeutic approaches are considered. As *FLT3*-ITD can be targeted with emerging novel inhibitors, patients with this molecular abnormality should be considered for clinical trials with these agents whenever possible. New transplant strategies, including reduced-intensity HSCT, are being explored for consolidation of high-risk AML patients (Chap. 30). Patients with t(8;21) and inv(16) are treated with repetitive doses of high-dose cytarabine, which offers a high frequency of cure without the morbidity of transplant. In AML patients with t(8;21) and inv(16), those with *KIT* mutations, who have a worse prognosis, may be considered for novel investigational studies.

Autologous HSCT is generally applied to AML patients only in the context of a clinical trial or when the risk of repetitive intensive chemotherapy represents a higher risk than the autologous HSCT (e.g., in patients with severe platelet alloimmunization).

RELAPSE Once relapse occurs, patients are rarely cured with further standard-dose chemotherapy. Patients eligible for allogeneic HSCT should receive transplants expeditiously at the first sign of relapse. Long-term disease-free survival is approximately the same (30–50%) with allogeneic HSCT in first relapse or in second remission. Autologous HSCT rescues about 20% of relapsed patients with AML who have chemosensitive disease. The most important factors predicting response at relapse are the length of the previous CR, whether initial CR was achieved with one or two courses of chemotherapy, and the type of postremission therapy.

Because of the poor outcome of patients in early first relapse (<12 months), it is justified (for patients without HLA-compatible donors) to explore innovative approaches, such as new drugs or immunotherapies (Table 14-4). Patients with longer first CRs (>12 months) generally relapse with drug-sensitive disease and have a higher chance of attaining a CR. However, cure is uncommon, and treatment with novel approaches should be considered if allogeneic HSCT is not possible. New agents that may have clinical activity in AML are needed, and many are being tested in clinical trials (Table 14-4).

For elderly patients (age >60 years) for whom clinical trials are not available, gemtuzumab ozogamicin is another alternative. The CR rate with this agent is ~30%. However, its effectiveness in early relapsing (<6 months) or refractory AML patients is limited, possibly due to calicheamicin being a potent MDR1 substrate. Toxicity, including myelosuppression, infusion toxicity, and venoocclusive disease, can be observed with gemtuzumab ozogamicin. Pretreatment with glucocorticoids can diminish many of the associated infusion reactions. Studies are examining this treatment in combination with chemotherapy for both young and older patients with previously untreated AML. This agent has been withdrawn from the U.S. market at the request of the U.S. FDA due to concerns about the product's safety and clinical benefit as shown in trials subsequent to those leading to its accelerated approval.

CHRONIC MYELOID LEUKEMIA

INCIDENCE

The incidence of chronic myeloid leukemia (CML) is 1.5 per 100,000 people per year, and the age-adjusted incidence is higher in men than in women (1.9 vs 1.1). The incidence of CML increases slowly with age until the middle forties, when it starts to rise rapidly. The incidence of CML for females decreased slightly (1.8%) between 1994 and 2006 compared with 1975–1994.

DEFINITION

The diagnosis of CML is established by identifying a clonal expansion of a hematopoietic stem cell possessing a reciprocal translocation between chromosomes 9 and 22. This translocation results in the head-to-tail fusion of the breakpoint cluster region (*BCR*) gene on chromosome 22q11 with the *ABL1* (named after the abelson murine leukemia virus) gene located on chromosome 9q34. Untreated, the disease is characterized by the inevitable transition from a chronic phase to an accelerated phase and on to blast crisis in a median time of 4 years.

ETIOLOGY

No clear correlation with exposure to cytotoxic drugs has been found, and no evidence suggests a viral etiology. In the pre-imatinib era, cigarette smoking accelerated the progression to blast crisis and therefore adversely affected survival in CML. Atomic bomb survivors had an increased incidence; the development of a CML cell mass of 10,000/μL took 6.3 years. No increase in CML incidence was found in the survivors of the Chernobyl accident, suggesting that only large doses of radiation can induce CML.

PATHOPHYSIOLOGY

The product of the fusion gene resulting from the t(9;22) plays a central role in the development of CML. This chimeric gene is transcribed into a hybrid *BCR-ABL1* mRNA in which exon 1 of *ABL1* is replaced by variable numbers of 5′ *BCR* exons. Bcr-Abl fusion proteins, p210*BCR-ABL1*, are produced that contain NH_2-terminal domains of Bcr and the COOH-terminal domains of Abl. A rare breakpoint, occurring within the 3′ region of the *BCR* gene, yields a fusion protein of 230 kDa, $p230^{BCR\text{-}ABL1}$. Bcr-Abl fusion proteins can transform hematopoietic progenitor cells in vitro. Furthermore, reconstituting lethally irradiated mice with bone marrow cells infected with retrovirus carrying the gene encoding the $p210^{BCR\text{-}ABL1}$ leads to the development of a myeloproliferative syndrome resembling CML in 50% of the mice. Specific antisense oligomers to the *BCR-ABL1* junction inhibit the growth of t(9;22)-positive leukemic cells without affecting normal colony formation.

The mechanism(s) by which $p210^{BCR\text{-}ABL1}$ promotes the transition from the benign state to the fully malignant one is still unclear. Messenger RNA for *BCR-ABL1* can occasionally be detected in normal individuals. However, attachment of the *BCR* sequences to *ABL1* results in three critical functional changes: (1) the Abl protein becomes constitutively active as a tyrosine kinase (TK) enzyme, activating downstream kinases that prevent apoptosis; (2) the DNA-protein-binding activity of Abl is attenuated; and (3) the binding of Abl to cytoskeletal actin microfilaments is enhanced.

Disease progression

The events associated with transition to the acute phase, a common occurrence in the pre-imatinib era, were extensively studied. Chromosomal instability of the malignant clone resulting, for example, in the acquisition of an additional t(9;22), trisomy 8, or 17p- (*TP*53 loss) is a basic feature of CML. Acquisition of these additional genetic and/or molecular abnormalities is critical to the phenotypic transformation. Heterogeneous structural alterations of the *TP53* gene, as well as structural alterations and lack of protein production of the retinoblastoma 1 (*RB1*) gene and the catalytic component of telomerase, have been associated with disease progression in a subset of patients. Rare patients show alterations in the rat sarcoma viral oncogene homologue (*RAS*). Sporadic reports also document the presence of an altered v-myc myelocytomatosis viral oncogene homologue (avian) (*MYC*) gene. Progressive de novo DNA methylation at the *BCR-ABL1* locus and hypomethylation of the *LINE-1* retrotransposon promoter herald blastic transformation. Further, interleukin 1β may be involved in the progression of CML to the blastic phase. In addition, functional inactivation of the tumor suppressor protein phosphatase A2 may be required for blastic transformation. Finally, CML that develops resistance to imatinib is at an increased risk of progressing to accelerated or blast crisis. Multiple pathways to disease transformation exist, but the exact timing and relevance of each remain unclear.

CLINICAL PRESENTATION

Symptoms

The clinical onset of the chronic phase is generally insidious. Accordingly, some patients are diagnosed, while still asymptomatic, during health-screening tests; other patients present with fatigue, malaise, and weight loss or have symptoms resulting from splenic enlargement, such as early satiety and left upper quadrant pain or mass. Less common are features related to granulocyte or platelet dysfunction, such as infections, thrombosis, or bleeding. Occasionally, patients present with leukostatic manifestations due to severe leukocytosis or thrombosis such as vasoocclusive disease, cerebrovascular accidents, myocardial infarction, venous thrombosis, priapism, visual disturbances, and pulmonary insufficiency. Patients with $p230^{BCR\text{-}ABL1}$-positive CML have a more indolent course.

Progression of CML is associated with worsening symptoms. Unexplained fever, significant weight loss, increasing dose requirement of the drugs controlling the disease, bone and joint pain, bleeding, thrombosis, and infections suggest transformation into accelerated or blastic phases. Less than 10–15% of newly diagnosed patients present with accelerated disease or with de novo blastic phase CML.

Physical findings

Minimal to moderate splenomegaly is the most common physical finding; mild hepatomegaly is found occasionally. Persistent splenomegaly despite continued therapy is a sign of disease acceleration. Lymphadenopathy and myeloid sarcomas are unusual except late in the course of the disease; when they are present, the prognosis is poor.

Hematologic findings

Elevated white blood cell (WBC) counts, with increases in both immature and mature granulocytes, are present at diagnosis. Usually <5% circulating blasts and <10% blasts and promyelocytes are noted, with the majority of cells being myelocytes, metamyelocytes, and band forms. Cycling of the counts may be observed in patients followed without treatment. Platelet counts are almost always elevated at diagnosis, and a mild degree of normocytic normochromic anemia is present. Leukocyte alkaline phosphatase is low in CML cells. Phagocytic functions are usually normal at diagnosis and remain normal during the chronic phase. Histamine production secondary to basophilia is increased in later stages, causing pruritus, diarrhea, and flushing.

At diagnosis, bone marrow cellularity is increased, with an increased myeloid-to-erythroid ratio. The marrow blast percentage is generally normal or slightly elevated. Marrow or blood basophilia, eosinophilia, and monocytosis may be present. While collagen fibrosis in the marrow is unusual at presentation, significant degrees of reticulin stain–measured fibrosis are noted in about half of the patients.

Disease acceleration is defined by the development of increasing degrees of anemia unaccounted for by bleeding or therapy; cytogenetic clonal evolution; or blood or marrow blasts between 10 and 20%, blood or marrow basophils ≥20%, or platelet count <100,000/μL. *Blast crisis* is defined as acute leukemia, with blood or marrow blasts ≥20%. Hyposegmented neutrophils may appear (Pelger-Huët anomaly). Blast cells can be classified as myeloid, lymphoid, erythroid, or undifferentiated, based on morphologic, cytochemical, and immunologic features. Occurrence of de novo blast crisis or following imatinib therapy is rare.

Chromosomal findings

The cytogenetic hallmark of CML, found in 90–95% of patients, is the t(9;22)(q34;q11.2). Originally, this was recognized by the presence of a shortened chromosome 22 (22q-), designated as the *Philadelphia chromosome*, that arises from the reciprocal t(9;22). Some patients may have complex translocations (designated as *variant translocations*) involving three, four, or five chromosomes (usually including chromosomes 9 and 22). However, the molecular consequences of these changes are similar to those resulting from the typical t(9;22). All patients should have evidence of the translocation molecularly or by cytogenetics or FISH to make a diagnosis of CML.

PROGNOSTIC FACTORS

The clinical outcome of patients with CML is variable. Before imatinib mesylate, death was expected in 10% of patients within 2 years and in about 20% yearly thereafter, and the median survival time was ~4 years. Therefore, several prognostic models that identify different risk groups in CML were developed. The most commonly used staging systems have been derived from multivariate analyses of prognostic factors. The *Sokal index* identified percentage of circulating blasts, spleen size, platelet count, age, and cytogenetic clonal evolution as the most important prognostic indicators. This system was developed based on chemotherapy-treated patients. The *Hasford system* was developed based on interferon (IFN) α–treated patients. It identified percentage of circulating blasts, spleen size, platelet count, age, and percentage of eosinophils and basophils as the most important prognostic indicators. This system differs from the Sokal index by ignoring clonal evolution and incorporating percentage of eosinophils and basophils. When applied to a data set of 272 patients treated with IFN-α, the Hasford system was better than the Sokal score for predicting survival time; it identified more low-risk patients but left only a small number of cases in the high-risk group. Preliminary results suggest that both the Sokal and the Hasford systems are applicable to imatinib-treated patients.

TREATMENT Chronic Myeloid Leukemia

The therapy of CML is changing rapidly because we have a proven curative treatment (allogeneic transplantation) that has significant toxicity and a new targeted treatment (imatinib) with outstanding outcome based on 8-year follow-up data. We recommend starting with TK inhibitors and reserving allogeneic transplantation for those who develop imatinib resistance.

At present, the goal of therapy in CML is to achieve prolonged, durable, nonneoplastic, nonclonal hematopoiesis, which entails the eradication of any residual cells containing the *BCR-ABL1* transcript. Hence, the goal is complete molecular remission and cure. A proposed imatinib treatment algorithm for the newly diagnosed CML patient is presented in Table 14-5.

TABLE 14-5

IMATINIB TREATMENT MILESTONES FOR NEWLY DIAGNOSED CHRONIC MYELOID LEUKEMIA PATIENTS

	NCCN[a]		ELN[b]	
TIME (MONTHS)	**EXPECTED[c]**	**FAILURE[d]**	**SUBOPTIMAL[e]**	**FAILURE[d]**
3	Complete hematologic remission[f]	No complete hematologic remission	Minor cytogenetic remission	No cytogenetic remission; new mutations
6	Any cytogenetic remission	No cytogenetic remission	Partial cytogenetic remission	Minimal cytogenetic remission[g]; new mutations
12	Complete[h] or partial[i] cytogenetic remission	Minor[j] or no cytogenetic remission	Less than major molecular response	Less than partial cytogenetic remission; new mutations
18	Complete cytogenetic remission	Partial, minor, or no cytogenetic remission		
Anytime	Loss of previously achieved hematologic, cytogenetic, or molecular remission; new mutations[d]			

[a]National Comprehensive Cancer Network.
[b]European Leukemia Net.
[c]Denotes that at the indicated milestone, patients should stay on the same dose.
[d]Denotes that at the indicated milestones, for patients on 400 mg/d, one can either increase the dose to a maximum of 600–800 mg, as tolerated, or probably switch to another tyrosine kinase inhibitor.
[e]Denotes that the patients may still have substantial long-term benefit from continuing a specific treatment, but chances are reduced, and therefore these patients may be eligible for alternative treatments.
[f]Complete hematologic remission, white blood cell count <10,000/μL, normal morphology, hemoglobin and platelet counts, and disappearance of splenomegaly.
[g]Minimal cytogenetic remission, 66–95% bone marrow metaphases with t(9;22).
[h]Complete cytogenetic remission, no bone marrow metaphases with t(9;22).
[i]Partial cytogenetic remission, 1–35% bone marrow metaphases with t(9;22).
[j]Minor cytogenetic remission, 36–85% bone marrow metaphases with t(9;22).

IMATINIB MESYLATE Imatinib mesylate (Gleevec) functions through competitive inhibition at the ATP-binding site of the Abl kinase in the inactive conformation, which leads to inhibition of tyrosine phosphorylation of proteins involved in Bcr-Abl signal transduction. It shows specificity for Bcr-Abl, the receptor for platelet-derived growth factor, and Kit TK. Imatinib induces apoptosis in cells expressing Bcr-Abl.

In newly diagnosed CML, imatinib (400 mg/d) is more effective than IFN-α and cytarabine. The complete hematologic remission rate of patients treated with imatinib was 95% compared with 56% in patients treated with IFN-α and cytarabine. Similarly, the complete cytogenetic remission rate at 18 months was 76% with imatinib compared with 15% with IFN-α and cytarabine. The rate of complete cytogenetic remission in imatinib-treated patients differed by Sokal score: the rate in those with low-risk disease was 89% compared with 82% for patients with intermediate-risk disease and 69% for those with high-risk disease.

All imatinib-treated patients who achieved major molecular remission (26%), defined as ≥3 log reduction in *BCR-ABL1* transcript level at 18 months compared with pretreatment level, were progression-free at 5 years. The progression-free survival (PFS) at 5 years for patients achieving complete cytogenetic remission but less pronounced molecular remission is 98%. The 5-year PFS for patients not achieving complete cytogenetic remission at 18 months was 87%. These results have led to a consensus that molecular responses can be used as a treatment goal in CML. Specific milestones have been developed for chronic-phase CML patients (Table 14-5). They differ between the Americans (NCCN) and the Europeans (ELN), with more strict milestones by the latter. For example, in the NCCN milestones, chronic-phase CML patients who do not achieve any cytogenetic remission following 6 months of imatinib should be offered other treatment approaches, but in the ELN milestones, the same recommendation is offered following 3 months of imatinib treatment. We favor the ELN approach and expect the NCCN milestones to align with the ELN ones in the very near future.

Progression to accelerated or blastic phases of the disease was noted in 3% of patients treated with imatinib compared with 8.5% of patients treated with IFN-α and cytarabine during the first year. Over time, the annual incidence of disease progression on imatinib decreased gradually to <1% during the fourth year and beyond, and no patient who achieved major molecular response by 12 months progressed to the accelerated or blastic phases of the disease.

Treatment is currently recommended for life unless patients are enrolled in a clinical trial with a specific question of treatment discontinuation. An early trial evaluating the effect of imatinib discontinuation after at least 2 years of complete molecular remission revealed molecular relapse in 6 of 12 patients. Interestingly, 6 of 10 patients who were treated with IFN-α before imatinib maintained molecular remission, while both patients who were not exposed to IFN-α relapsed. These results raised the hypothesis that IFN-α may have a protective effect against relapse, possibly by eradicating the leukemia-initiating cells. This hypothesis is supported by the randomized trial comparing imatinib with imatinib plus IFN-α; preliminary results from this trial revealed better major molecular response for the combination, although a significant number of patients discontinued IFN-α treatment during the first year due to toxicity. Finally, a recent IFN-α maintenance study, following imatinib discontinuation, demonstrated maintained molecular remission in 15 (75%) of 20 patients. IFN's mechanism of action in this situation is unclear.

Imatinib is administered orally. The main side effects are fluid retention, nausea, muscle cramps, diarrhea, and skin rashes. The management of these side effects is usually supportive. Myelosuppression is the most common hematologic side effect. Myelosuppression, while rare, may require holding drug and/or growth factor support. Doses <300 mg/d seem ineffective and may lead to development of resistance.

Four mechanisms of resistance to imatinib have been described to date. These are (1) gene amplification, (2) mutations at the kinase site, (3) enhanced expression of multidrug exporter proteins, and (4) alternative signaling pathways functionally compensating for the imatinib-sensitive mechanisms. All four mechanisms are being targeted in clinical trials.

BCR-ABL1 gene amplification and decreased intracellular imatinib concentrations are addressed by intensifying the therapy with higher (≤800 mg/d) imatinib doses. Three randomized trials have been published so far. The first randomized study compared 400 mg/d with 800 mg/d in newly diagnosed CML patients and revealed improved major molecular responses at 3, 6, and 9 months but similar results at 12 months. A similar study comparing 600 mg/d with 800 mg/d showed a borderline benefit for the higher dose based on both cytogenetic and major molecular responses at 12 months, while a third study concentrating only on high-risk (Sokal) patients failed to show any significant difference between 400 mg/d and 800 mg/d at 12 months. All of these studies have too short follow-up times to evaluate dosing effect on survival.

Mutations at the kinase domain occur in approximately half of imatinib-resistant chronic-phase cases and even more frequently in the more advanced phases of the disease. These mutations are being targeted by novel TK inhibitors that have a different conformation than imatinib, demonstrating activity against most imatinib-resistant mutations. Nilotinib (Tasigma), similar to imatinib, binds to the kinase domain in the inactive conformation. Dasatinib (Sprycel) binds to the kinase domain in the open conformation and inhibits the SRC (sarcoma) family of kinases, addressing the last mechanism of resistance. CML with the T315I mutation is resistant to imatinib, nilotinib, and dasatinib. In addition, nilotinib is also resistant to E255K/V and Y253F/H, and dasatinib is also resistant to X299L and F317L.

Dasatinib is approved by the FDA at a dose of 100 mg/d for the treatment of all stages of CML with resistance or intolerance to prior therapy, including imatinib. Nilotinib is approved by the FDA at a dose of 400 mg twice daily for the treatment of chronic- and accelerated-phase CML with resistance or intolerance to prior therapy, including imatinib. Both are oral agents dasatinib is given once daily while daily, and nilotinib is given twice daily with food restrictions before and after dosing. Their toxicity profiles are similar to that of imatinib with small but significant differences. Dasatinib causes pleural effusions in 22% of patients, with 7% developing grade 3–4 toxicity. Nilotinib was associated with sudden death in 6 of approximately 550 CML patients. A suspected relationship to nilotinib was reported in two of these cases and led to a requirement for additional cardiac monitoring while using this drug. A randomized trial in chronic-phase imatinib-resistant CML patients showed superiority of switching to dasatinib over increasing imatinib to 800 mg/d. Finally, randomized trials have demonstrated that either nilotinib or dasatinib is more effective than imatinib as first-line treatment in newly diagnosed chronic-phase CML patients in time to complete hematologic and cytogenetic remission and major molecular response at 1 year and led to their approval for the first line setting. Similar results are likely with bosutinib, another Src and Abl TK inhibitor. These studies are expanding the armamentarium for newly diagnosed CML patients.

These new agents have already changed the treatment algorithm of CML. For example, patients who do not achieve any cytogenetic remission at 6 months (or 3 months by ELN) on imatinib are now offered dasatinib, nilotinib, or HSCT. IFN-α is FDA approved for CML but is only offered if all other options have failed.

The encouraging results with imatinib have led clinicians to offer it as first-line therapy for newly diagnosed CML patients, including those who otherwise would have benefited from transplant (e.g., young patients with a matched sibling donor). Prior exposure to imatinib does not affect transplant outcome. Similar data, in smaller series, were also described for dasatinib and nilotinib treatment before HSCT. However, delaying HSCT for high-risk patients (Sokal/Hasford criteria) may result in disease progression. HSCT after disease progression is associated with poorer outcome. Therefore, we recommend close monitoring of TK inhibitors response in these patients.

NEW AGENTS Several new agents are now in development for CML with T315I and patients who fail all currently available TK inhibitors. These include omacetaxine, XL228, FTY720, AP24534, DCC-2036, PH-739358, and sorafenib (Table 14-6).

ALLOGENEIC HSCT Allogeneic HSCT is complicated by early mortality owing to the transplant procedure. Outcome of HSCT depends on multiple factors, including (1) the patient (e.g., age and phase of disease); (2) the type of donor (e.g., syngeneic [monozygotic twins] or HLA-compatible allogeneic, related or unrelated); (3) the preparative regimen (myeloablative or reduced-intensity); (4) GVHD; and (5) posttransplantation treatment.

Posttransplantation Treatment Posttransplant *BCR-ABL1* transcript levels have served as early predictors for hematologic relapse following HSCT. These should facilitate risk-adapted approaches with immunosuppression or TK inhibitor(s) or a combination of the two. Donor leukocyte infusions (without any preparative chemotherapy or GVHD prophylaxis) can induce hematologic and cytogenetic remissions in patients with CML who have relapsed after allogeneic HSCT but carry the risk of significant GVHD.

Imatinib can control CML that has recurred after allogeneic HSCT but is sometimes associated with myelosuppression and recurrence of severe GVHD. Imatinib after allogeneic HSCT is being studied for prevention of relapse in patients with advanced disease at the time of transplantation (i.e., patients at high risk for relapse), patients undergoing reduced-intensity transplants, or patients with slow reduction of *BCR-ABL1* message following transplantation. Imatinib has also been combined with donor lymphocytes to induce rapid molecular remissions in CML patients with disease relapse after allogeneic HSCT. Of interest are studies with newer TK inhibitors following transplantation for imatinib-resistant CML.

TABLE 14-6

NOVEL AGENTS FOR BCR-ABL WITH T315I AND PATIENTS WHO FAILED ALL CURRENTLY AVAILABLE TYROSINE KINASE INHIBITORS

AGENT	MECHANISM OF ACTION
Omacetaxine (formerly known as homoharringtonine)	Protein translation inhibitor
XL228	Dual Src/Abl inhibitor with potential effect against T315I mutation
FTY720 (also known as fingolimod)	Activation of protein phosphatase 2A that is essential for *ABL1*-mediated leukemogenesis
AP24534	Pan-Bcr-Abl inhibitor that inhibits T315I
DCC-2036	Non–ATP-competitive Abl inhibition, avoids the steric clash with T315I mutation
PH-739358	Aurora kinase inhibitor that is also active against T315I mutation
Sorafenib	Raf kinase inhibitor that downregulates down stream Bcr-Abl targets

INTERFERON Before imatinib, when allogeneic HSCT was not feasible, IFN-α therapy was the treatment of choice. Only longer follow-up of patients treated with imatinib will prove whether IFN-α will still have a role in the treatment of CML. Its mode(s) of action in CML is still unknown.

CHEMOTHERAPY Initial management of patients with chemotherapy is currently reserved for rapid lowering of WBC counts, reduction of symptoms, and reversal of symptomatic splenomegaly. Hydroxyurea, a ribonucleotide reductase inhibitor, induces rapid disease control. The initial dose is 1–4 g/d; the dose should be halved with each 50% reduction of the leukocyte count. Unfortunately, cytogenetic remissions with hydroxyurea are uncommon. Busulphan, an alkylating agent that acts on early progenitor cells, has a more prolonged effect. However, we do not recommend its use because of its serious side effects, which include unexpected, and occasionally fatal, myelosuppression in 5–10% of patients; pulmonary, endocardial, and marrow fibrosis; and an Addison-like wasting syndrome.

AUTOLOGOUS HSCT Autologous HSCT could potentially cure CML if cells are collected at complete molecular remission. However, since patients who achieve this degree of response do not relapse, this treatment modality has been abandoned by most groups.

LEUKAPHERESIS AND SPLENECTOMY Intensive leukapheresis may control the blood counts in chronic-phase CML; however, it is expensive and cumbersome. It is useful in emergencies in which leukostasis-related complications, such as pulmonary failure or cerebrovascular accidents, are likely. It may also have a role in the treatment of pregnant women, in whom it is important to avoid potentially teratogenic drugs.

Splenectomy was used in CML in the past because of the suggestion that evolution to the acute phase might occur in the spleen. However, this does not appear to be the case, and splenectomy is now reserved for symptomatic relief of painful splenomegaly unresponsive to imatinib or chemotherapy or for significant anemia or thrombocytopenia associated with hypersplenism. Splenic radiation is used rarely to reduce the size of the spleen.

MINIMAL RESIDUAL DISEASE The kinetics of *BCR-ABL1* transcript elimination is currently replacing qualitative detection of the *BCR-ABL1* message as an index of tumor burden despite a lack of standard acceptable methodology. A consensus panel has proposed ways to harmonize the different methods and to use a conversion factor so that individual laboratories will be able to express *BCR-ABL1* transcript levels on an agreed upon scale.

Slow reduction of *BCR-ABL1* transcripts following HSCT correlates with the possibility of hematologic relapse. However, the definition of "slow reduction" depends on the preparative regimen (reduced-intensity vs fully myeloablative) and the selection of time points to measure the transcript levels. While persistent RT-PCR positivity at 6 months was regarded as an indication for additional therapy in the past, current studies utilize periods between engraftment and day 100 for evaluating the clearance rate of *BCR-ABL1* transcripts and recommending additional therapies. Large trials with longer follow-up are needed to establish consensus guidelines.

The randomized trial of imatinib versus IFN-α and cytarabine was the first to establish the concept of $\log_{10}$ reduction of *BCR-ABL1* transcript from a standardized baseline for untreated patients. This measurement unit was developed instead of either the transcript numbers expressed per microgram of leukocyte RNA or the ratio of *BCR-ABL1* to a housekeeping gene on a log scale. In this randomized trial, patients who achieved ≥3 log reduction of *BCR-ABL1* message had an extremely low probability of relapse, with a median follow-up of 96 months.

These studies also established the value and convenience of using peripheral blood instead of bone marrow testing as a means to assess disease status in patients who achieve complete cytogenetic responses. However, one still needs to consider following CML patients in complete cytogenetic remission and at least major molecular remission with occasional cytogenetic bone marrow testing. This should be performed if they develop cytopenia late in the treatment course as such patients are at risk of developing cytogenetic aberrations, especially monosomy 7, in t(9;22)-negative cells and secondary MDS/AML. Other aberrations in the t(9;22)-negative cells are frequently transient, and their clinical significance is unclear. Development of secondary MDS/AML is rare.

TREATMENT OF BLAST CRISIS Treatments for primary blast crisis, including imatinib, are generally ineffective. Only 52% of patients treated with imatinib achieved hematologic remission (21% complete hematologic remission), and the median overall survival time was 6.6 months. Patients who achieve complete hematologic remission or whose disease returns to a second chronic phase should be considered for allogeneic HSCT. Other approaches include induction chemotherapy tailored to the phenotype of the blast cell followed by TK inhibitors with or without additional chemotherapy and HSCT. Blast crisis following initial therapy with imatinib carries a dismal prognosis even if the patient is treated with dasatinib or nilotinib.

CHAPTER 15

MALIGNANCIES OF LYMPHOID CELLS

Dan L. Longo

Malignancies of lymphoid cells range from the most indolent to the most aggressive human malignancies. These cancers arise from cells of the immune system at different stages of differentiation, resulting in a wide range of morphologic, immunologic, and clinical findings. Insights on the normal immune system have allowed a better understanding of these sometimes confusing disorders.

Some malignancies of lymphoid cells almost always present as leukemia (i.e., primary involvement of bone marrow and blood), while others almost always present as lymphomas (i.e., solid tumors of the immune system). However, other malignancies of lymphoid cells can present as either leukemia or lymphoma. In addition, the clinical pattern can change over the course of the illness. This change is more often seen in a patient who seems to have a lymphoma and then develops the manifestations of leukemia over the course of the illness.

BIOLOGY OF LYMPHOID MALIGNANCIES: CONCEPTS OF THE WORLD HEALTH ORGANIZATION CLASSIFICATION OF LYMPHOID MALIGNANCIES

The classification of lymphoid cancers evolved steadily throughout the twentieth century. The distinction between leukemia and lymphoma was made early, and separate classification systems were developed for each. Leukemias were first divided into acute and chronic subtypes based on average survival. Chronic leukemias were easily subdivided into those of lymphoid or myeloid origin based on morphologic characteristics. However, a spectrum of diseases that were formerly all called *chronic lymphoid leukemia* has become apparent (Table 15-1). The acute leukemias were usually malignancies of blast cells with few identifying characteristics. When cytochemical stains became available, it was possible to divide these objectively into myeloid malignancies and acute leukemias of lymphoid cells. Acute leukemias of lymphoid cells have been subdivided based on morphologic characteristics by the French-American-British (FAB) group (Table 15-2). Using this system, lymphoid malignancies of small uniform blasts (e.g., typical childhood acute lymphoblastic leukemia) were called L1, lymphoid malignancies with larger and more variable size cells were called L2, and lymphoid malignancies of uniform cells with basophilic and sometimes vacuolated cytoplasm were called L3 (e.g., typical Burkitt's lymphoma cells). Acute leukemias of lymphoid cells have also been subdivided based on immunologic (i.e., T cell vs. B cell) and cytogenetic abnormalities (Table 15-2). Major cytogenetic subgroups include the t(9;22) (e.g., Philadelphia chromosome–positive acute lymphoblastic

TABLE 15-1

LYMPHOID DISORDERS THAT CAN PRESENT AS "CHRONIC LEUKEMIA" AND BE CONFUSED WITH TYPICAL B CELL CHRONIC LYMPHOID LEUKEMIA

Follicular lymphoma	Prolymphocytic leukemia (B cell or T cell)
Splenic marginal zone lymphoma	Lymphoplasmacytic lymphoma
Nodal marginal zone lymphoma	Sézary's syndrome
Mantle cell lymphoma	Smoldering adult T cell leukemia/lymphoma
Hairy cell leukemia	

TABLE 15-2

CLASSIFICATION OF ACUTE LYMPHOID LEUKEMIA (ALL)

IMMUNOLOGIC SUBTYPE	% OF CASES	FAB SUBTYPE	CYTOGENETIC ABNORMALITIES
Pre-B ALL	75	L1, L2	t(9;22), t(4;11), t(1;19)
T cell ALL	20	L1, L2	14q11 or 7q34
B cell ALL	5	L3	t(8;14), t(8;22), t(2;8)

Abbreviation: FAB, French-American-British classification.

TABLE 15-3

WORLD HEALTH ORGANIZATION CLASSIFICATION OF LYMPHOID MALIGNANCIES

B CELL	T CELL	HODGKIN'S DISEASE
Precursor B cell neoplasm	Precursor T cell neoplasm	Nodular lymphocyte-predominant Hodgkin's disease
Precursor B lymphoblastic leukemia/ lymphoma (precursor B cell acute lymphoblastic leukemia)	**Precursor T lymphoblastic lymphoma/leukemia (precursor T cell acute lymphoblastic leukemia)**	
Mature (peripheral) B cell neoplasms	Mature (peripheral) T cell neoplasms	Classical Hodgkin's disease
B cell chronic lymphocytic leukemia/ small lymphocytic lymphoma	T cell prolymphocytic leukemia	Nodular sclerosis Hodgkin's disease
B cell prolymphocytic leukemia	T cell granular lymphocytic leukemia	Lymphocyte-rich classic Hodgkin's disease
Lymphoplasmacytic lymphoma	Aggressive NK cell leukemia	Mixed-cellularity Hodgkin's disease
Splenic marginal zone B cell lymphoma (± villous lymphocytes)	Adult T cell lymphoma/leukemia (HTLV-I+)	Lymphocyte-depletion Hodgkin's disease
Hairy cell leukemia	Extranodal NK/T cell lymphoma, nasal type	
Plasma cell myeloma/plasmacytoma	Enteropathy-type T cell lymphoma	
Extranodal marginal zone B cell lymphoma of MALT type	Hepatosplenic γδ T cell lymphoma	
Mantle cell lymphoma	Subcutaneous panniculitis-like T cell lymphoma	
Follicular lymphoma	**Mycosis fungoides/Sézary's syndrome**	
Nodal marginal zone B cell lymphoma (± monocytoid B cells)	Anaplastic large cell lymphoma, primary cutaneous type	
Diffuse large B cell lymphoma	**Peripheral T cell lymphoma, not otherwise specified**	
Burkitt's lymphoma/Burkitt's cell leukemia	**Angioimmunoblastic T cell lymphoma**	
	Anaplastic large cell lymphoma, primary systemic type	

Note: Malignancies in bold occur in at least 1% of patients.
Abbreviations: HTLV, human T cell lymphotropic virus; MALT, mucosa-associated lymphoid tissue; NK, natural killer.
Source: Adapted from NL Harris et al: J Clin Oncol 17:3835, 1999.

leukemia) and the t(8;14) found in the L3 or Burkitt's leukemia.

Non-Hodgkin's lymphomas were separated from Hodgkin's disease by recognition of the Sternberg-Reed cells early in the twentieth century. The histologic classification for non-Hodgkin's lymphomas has been one of the most contentious issues in oncology. Imperfect morphologic systems were supplanted by imperfect immunologic systems, and poor reproducibility of diagnosis has hampered progress. In 1999, the World Health Organization (WHO) classification of lymphoid malignancies was devised through a process of consensus development among international leaders in hematopathology and clinical oncology. The WHO classification takes into account morphologic, clinical, immunologic, and genetic information and attempts to divide non-Hodgkin's lymphomas and other lymphoid malignancies into clinical/pathologic entities that have clinical and therapeutic relevance. This system is presented in Table 15-3. This system is clinically relevant and has a higher degree of diagnostic accuracy than those used previously. The possibilities for subdividing lymphoid malignancies are extensive. However, Table 15-3 presents in bold malignancies that occur in at least 1% of patients. Specific lymphoma subtypes are dealt with later in the chapter.

GENERAL ASPECTS OF LYMPHOID MALIGNANCIES

ETIOLOGY AND EPIDEMIOLOGY

The relative frequency of the various lymphoid malignancies is shown in Fig. 15-1. Chronic lymphoid leukemia (CLL) is the most prevalent form of leukemia in Western

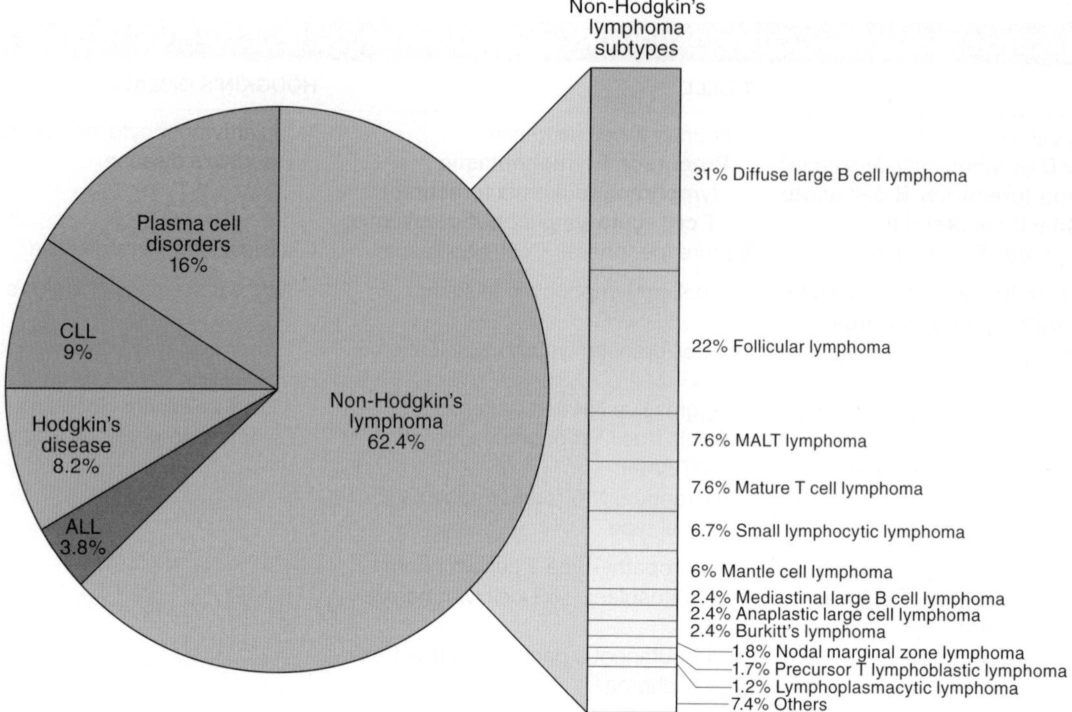

FIGURE 15-1

Relative frequency of lymphoid malignancies. ALL, acute lymphoid leukemia; CLL, chronic lymphoid leukemia; MALT, mucosa-associated lymphoid tissue.

countries. It occurs most frequently in older adults and is exceedingly rare in children. In 2010, 14,990 new cases were diagnosed in the United States, but because of the prolonged survival associated with this disorder, the total prevalence is many times higher. CLL is more common in men than in women and more common in whites than in blacks. This is an uncommon malignancy in Asia. The etiologic factors for typical CLL are unknown.

In contrast to CLL, acute lymphoid leukemias (ALLs) are predominantly cancers of children and young adults. The L3 or Burkitt's leukemia occurring in children in developing countries seems to be associated with infection by the Epstein-Barr virus (EBV) in infancy. However, the explanation for the etiology of more common subtypes of ALL is much less certain. Childhood ALL occurs more often in higher socioeconomic subgroups. Children with trisomy 21 (Down syndrome) have an increased risk for childhood ALL as well as acute myeloid leukemia (AML). Exposure to high-energy radiation in early childhood increases the risk of developing T cell ALL.

The etiology of ALL in adults is also uncertain. ALL is unusual in middle-aged adults but increases in incidence in the elderly. However, AML is still much more common in older patients. Environmental exposures, including certain industrial exposures, exposure to agricultural chemicals, and smoking, might increase the risk of developing ALL as an adult. ALL was diagnosed in 5330 persons and AML in 12,330 persons in the United States in 2010.

The preponderance of evidence suggests that Hodgkin's disease is of B cell origin. The incidence of Hodgkin's disease appears fairly stable, with 8490 new cases diagnosed in 2010 in the United States. Hodgkin's disease is more common in whites than in blacks and more common in males than in females. A bimodal distribution of age at diagnosis has been observed, with one peak incidence occurring in patients in their twenties and the other in those in their eighties. Some of the late age peak may be attributed to confusion among entities with similar appearance such as anaplastic large cell lymphoma and T cell–rich B cell lymphoma. Patients in the younger age groups diagnosed in the United States largely have the nodular sclerosing subtype of Hodgkin's disease. Elderly patients, patients infected with HIV and patients in developing countries more commonly have mixed-cellularity Hodgkin's disease or lymphocyte-depleted Hodgkin's disease. Infection by HIV is a risk factor for developing Hodgkin's disease. In addition, an association between infection by EBV and Hodgkin's disease has been suggested. A monoclonal or oligoclonal proliferation of EBV-infected cells in 20–40% of the patients with Hodgkin's disease has led to proposals for this virus having an etiologic role in Hodgkin's disease. However, the matter is not settled definitively.

For unknown reasons, non-Hodgkin's lymphomas increased in frequency in the United States at the rate of 4% per year and increased 2–8% per year globally between 1950 and the late 1990s. The rate of increase in the past few years seems to be decreasing. About 65,540 new cases of non-Hodgkin's lymphoma were diagnosed in the United States in 2010 and nearly 360,000 cases worldwide. Non-Hodgkin's lymphomas are more frequent in the elderly and more frequent in men. Patients with both primary and secondary immunodeficiency states are predisposed to developing non-Hodgkin's lymphomas. These include patients with HIV infection; patients who have undergone organ transplantation; and patients with inherited immune deficiencies, the sicca syndrome, and rheumatoid arthritis.

The incidence of non-Hodgkin's lymphomas and the patterns of expression of the various subtypes differ geographically. T cell lymphomas are more common in Asia than in Western countries, while certain subtypes of B cell lymphomas such as follicular lymphoma are more common in Western countries. A specific subtype of non-Hodgkin's lymphoma known as the angiocentric nasal T/natural killer (NK) cell lymphoma has a striking geographic occurrence, being most frequent in Southern Asia and parts of Latin America. Another subtype of non-Hodgkin's lymphoma associated with infection by human T cell lymphotropic virus (HTLV) I is seen particularly in southern Japan and the Caribbean.

A number of environmental factors have been implicated in the occurrence of non-Hodgkin's lymphoma, including infectious agents, chemical exposures, and medical treatments. Several studies have demonstrated an association between exposure to agricultural chemicals and an increased incidence in non-Hodgkin's lymphoma. Patients treated for Hodgkin's disease can develop non-Hodgkin's lymphoma; it is unclear whether this is a consequence of the Hodgkin's disease or its treatment. However, a number of non-Hodgkin's lymphomas are associated with infectious agents (Table 15-4). HTLV-I infects T cells and leads directly to the development of adult T cell lymphoma (ATL) in a small percentage of infected patients. The cumulative lifetime risk of developing lymphoma in an infected patient is 2.5%. The virus is transmitted by infected lymphocytes ingested by nursing babies of infected mothers, bloodborne transmission, or sexually. The median age of patients with ATL is ~56 years, emphasizing the long latency. HTLV-I is also the cause of tropical spastic paraparesis, a neurologic disorder that occurs somewhat more frequently than lymphoma and with shorter latency and usually from transfusion-transmitted virus.

EBV is associated with the development of Burkitt's lymphoma in Central Africa and the occurrence of aggressive non-Hodgkin's lymphomas in immunosuppressed patients in Western countries. The majority of primary central nervous system (CNS) lymphomas are associated with EBV. EBV infection is strongly associated with the occurrence of extranodal nasal T/NK cell lymphomas in Asia and South America. Infection with HIV predisposes to the development of aggressive B cell non-Hodgkin's lymphoma. This may be through overexpression of interleukin 6 (IL-6) by infected macrophages. Infection of the stomach by the bacterium *Helicobacter pylori* induces the development of gastric MALT (mucosa-associated lymphoid tissue) lymphomas. This association is supported by evidence that patients treated with antibiotics to eradicate *H. pylori* have regression of their MALT lymphoma. The bacterium does not transform lymphocytes to produce the lymphoma; instead, a vigorous immune response is made to the bacterium, and the chronic antigenic stimulation leads to the neoplasia. MALT lymphomas of the skin may be related to *Borrelia* sp. infections, those of the eyes to *Chlamydophila psittaci*, and those of the small intestine to *Campylobacter jejuni*.

Chronic hepatitis C virus infection has been associated with the development of lymphoplasmacytic lymphoma. Human herpesvirus 8 is associated with primary effusion lymphoma in HIV-infected persons and multicentric Castleman's disease, a diffuse lymphadenopathy associated with systemic symptoms of fever, malaise, and weight loss.

In addition to infectious agents, a number of other diseases or exposures may predispose to developing lymphoma (Table 15-5).

TABLE 15-4

INFECTIOUS AGENTS ASSOCIATED WITH THE DEVELOPMENT OF LYMPHOID MALIGNANCIES

INFECTIOUS AGENT	LYMPHOID MALIGNANCY
Epstein-Barr virus	Burkitt's lymphoma Post–organ transplant lymphoma Primary CNS diffuse large B cell lymphoma Hodgkin's disease Extranodal NK/T cell lymphoma, nasal type
HTLV-I	Adult T cell leukemia/lymphoma
HIV	Diffuse large B cell lymphoma Burkitt's lymphoma
Hepatitis C virus	Lymphoplasmacytic lymphoma
Helicobacter pylori	Gastric MALT lymphoma
Human herpesvirus 8	Primary effusion lymphoma Multicentric Castleman's disease

Abbreviations: CNS, central nervous system; HIV, human immunodeficiency virus; HTLV, human T cell lymphotropic virus; MALT, mucosa-associated lymphoid tissue; NK, natural killer.

TABLE 15-5

DISEASES OR EXPOSURES ASSOCIATED WITH INCREASED RISK OF DEVELOPMENT OF MALIGNANT LYMPHOMA

Inherited immunodeficiency disease	Autoimmune disease
Klinefelter's syndrome	Sjögren's syndrome
Chédiak-Higashi syndrome	Celiac sprue
Ataxia-telangiectasia syndrome	Rheumatoid arthritis and systemic lupus erythematosus
Wiskott-Aldrich syndrome	Chemical or drug exposures
Common variable immunodeficiency disease	Phenytoin
Acquired immunodeficiency diseases	Dioxin, phenoxy herbicides
Iatrogenic immunosuppression	Radiation
HIV-1 infection	Prior chemotherapy and radiation therapy
Acquired hypogammaglobulinemia	

IMMUNOLOGY

All lymphoid cells are derived from a common hematopoietic progenitor that gives rise to lymphoid, myeloid, erythroid, monocyte, and megakaryocyte lineages. Through the ordered and sequential activation of a series of transcription factors, the cell first becomes committed to the lymphoid lineage and then gives rise to B and T cells. About 75% of all lymphoid leukemias and 90% of all lymphomas are of B cell origin. A cell becomes committed to B cell development when it begins to rearrange its immunoglobulin genes. The sequence of cellular changes, including changes in cell-surface phenotype, that characterizes normal B cell development is shown in Fig. 15-2. A cell becomes committed to T cell differentiation upon migration to the thymus and rearrangement of T cell antigen receptor genes. The sequence of the events that characterize T cell development is depicted in Fig. 15-3.

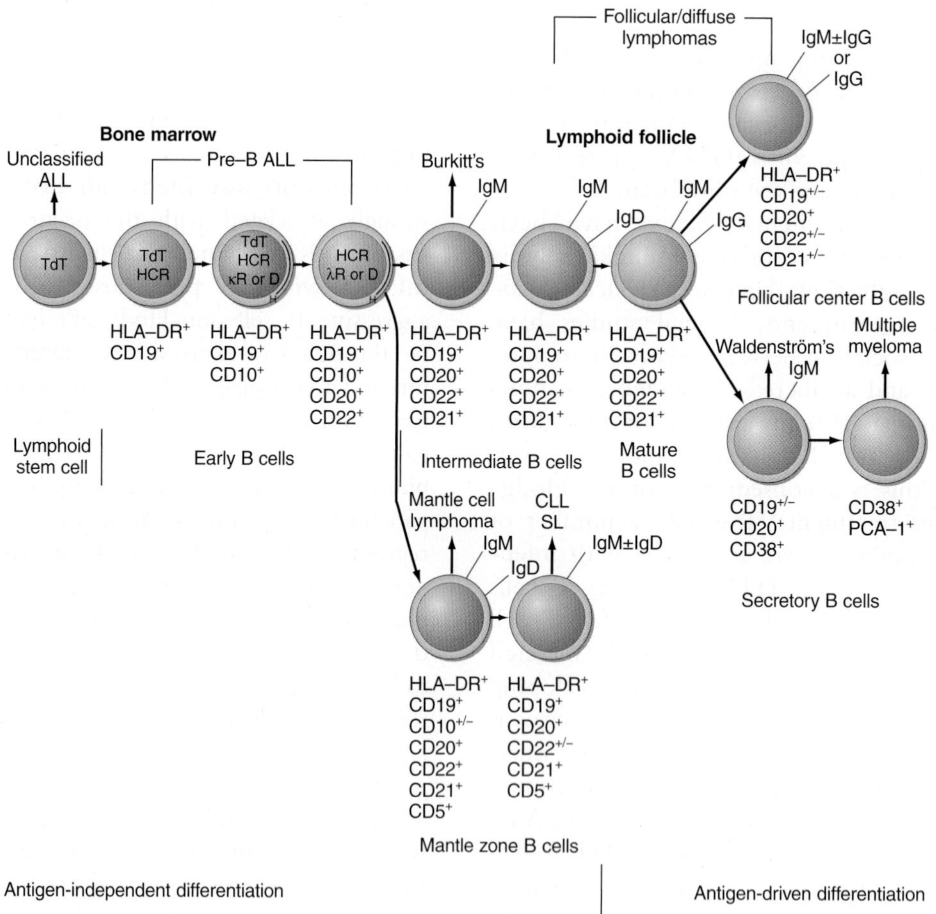

FIGURE 15-2

Pathway of normal B cell differentiation and relationship to B cell lymphomas. HLA-DR, CD10, CD19, CD20, CD21, CD22, CD5, and CD38 are cell markers used to distinguish stages of development. Terminal transferase (TdT) is a cellular enzyme. Immunoglobulin heavy chain gene rearrangement (HCR) and light chain gene rearrangement or deletion (κR or D, λR or D) occur early in B cell development. The approximate normal stage of differentiation associated with particular lymphomas is shown. ALL, acute lymphoid leukemia; CLL, chronic lymphoid leukemia; SL, small lymphocytic lymphoma.

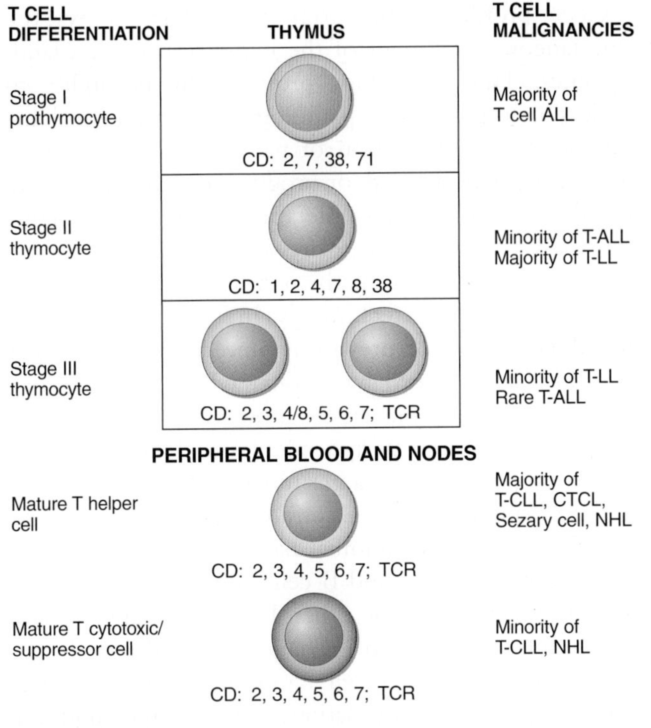

FIGURE 15-3

Pathway of normal T cell differentiation and relationship to T cell lymphomas. CD1, CD2, CD3, CD4, CD5, CD6, CD7, CD8, CD38, and CD71 are cell markers used to distinguish stages of development. T cell antigen receptors (TCR) rearrange in the thymus, and mature T cells emigrate to nodes and peripheral blood. ALL, acute lymphoid leukemia; CTCL, cutaneous T cell lymphoma; NHL, non-Hodgkin's lymphoma; T-ALL, T cell ALL; T-CLL, T cell chronic lymphoid leukemia; T-LL, T cell lymphoblastic lymphoma.

Although lymphoid malignancies often retain the cell-surface phenotype of lymphoid cells at particular stages of differentiation, this information is of little consequence. The so-called stage of differentiation of a malignant lymphoma does not predict its natural history. For example, the clinically most aggressive lymphoid leukemia is Burkitt's leukemia, which has the phenotype of a mature follicle center IgM-bearing B cell. Leukemias bearing the immunologic cell-surface phenotype of more primitive cells (e.g., pre-B ALL, CD10+) are less aggressive and more amenable to curative therapy than the "more mature" appearing Burkitt's leukemia cells. Furthermore, the apparent stage of differentiation of the malignant cell does not reflect the stage at which the genetic lesions that gave rise to the malignancy developed. For example, follicular lymphoma has the cell-surface phenotype of a follicle center cell, but its characteristic chromosomal translocation, the t(14;18), which involves juxtaposition of the antiapoptotic *bcl-2* gene next to the immunoglobulin heavy chain gene (see below), had to develop early in ontogeny as an error in the process of immunoglobulin gene rearrangement. Why the subsequent steps that led to transformation became manifest in a cell of follicle center differentiation is not clear.

The major value of cell-surface phenotyping is to aid in the differential diagnosis of lymphoid tumors that appear similar by light microscopy. For example, benign follicular hyperplasia may resemble follicular lymphoma; however, the demonstration that all the cells bear the same immunoglobulin light chain isotype strongly suggests the mass is a clonal proliferation rather than a polyclonal response to an exogenous stimulus.

Malignancies of lymphoid cells are associated with recurring genetic abnormalities. While specific genetic abnormalities have not been identified for all subtypes of lymphoid malignancies, it is presumed that they exist. Genetic abnormalities can be identified at a variety of levels including gross chromosomal changes (i.e., translocations, additions, or deletions); rearrangement of specific genes that may or may not be apparent from cytogenetic studies; and overexpression, underexpression, or mutation of specific oncogenes. Altered expression or mutation of specific proteins is particularly important. Many lymphomas contain balanced chromosomal translocations involving the antigen receptor genes; immunoglobulin genes on chromosomes 2, 14, and 22 in B cells; and T cell antigen receptor genes on chromosomes 7 and 14 in T cells. The rearrangement of chromosome segments to generate mature antigen receptors must create a site of vulnerability to aberrant recombination. B cells are even more susceptible to acquiring mutations during their maturation in germinal centers; the generation of antibody of higher affinity requires the introduction of mutations into the variable region genes in the germinal centers. Other nonimmunoglobulin genes, e.g., *bcl-6*, may acquire mutations as well.

In the case of diffuse large B cell lymphoma, the translocation t(14;18) occurs in ~30% of patients and leads to overexpression of the *bcl-2* gene found on chromosome 18. Some other patients without the translocation also overexpress the BCL-2 protein. This protein is involved in suppressing apoptosis—i.e., the mechanism of cell death most often induced by cytotoxic chemotherapeutic agents. A higher relapse rate has been observed in patients whose tumors overexpress the BCL-2 protein, but not in patients whose lymphoma cells show only the translocation. Thus, particular genetic mechanisms have clinical ramifications.

Table 15-6 presents the best documented translocations and associated oncogenes for various subtypes of lymphoid malignancies. In some cases, such as the association of the t(14;18) in follicular lymphoma, the t(2;5) in anaplastic large T/null cell lymphoma, the t(8;14) in Burkitt's lymphoma, and the t(11;14) in mantle cell lymphoma, the great majority of tumors in patients with these diagnoses display these abnormalities. In other types of lymphoma in which a minority of the patients

TABLE 15-6

CYTOGENETIC TRANSLOCATION AND ASSOCIATED ONCOGENES OFTEN SEEN IN LYMPHOID MALIGNANCIES

DISEASE	CYTOGENETIC ABNORMALITY	ONCOGENE
CLL/small lymphocytic lymphoma	t(14;15)(q32;q13)	—
MALT lymphoma	t(11;18)(q21;q21)	API2/MALT, BCL-10
Precursor B cell acute lymphoid leukemia	t(9;22)(q34;q11) or variant t(4;11) (q21;q23)	BCR/ABL AF4, ALLI
Precursor acute lymphoid leukemia	t(9;22) t(1;19) t(17;19) t(5;14)	BCR, ABL E2A, PBX HLF, E2A HOX11L2, CTIP2
Mantle cell lymphoma	t(11;14)(q13;q32)	BCL-1, IgH
Follicular lymphoma	t(14;18)(q32;q21)	BCL-2, IgH
Diffuse large cell lymphoma	t(3;-)(q27;-)[a] t(17;-)(p13;-)	BCL-6 p53
Burkitt's lymphoma, Burkitt's leukemia	t(8;-)(q24;-)[a]	C-MYC
CD30+ Anaplastic large cell lymphoma	t(2;5)(p23;q35)	ALK
Lymphoplasmacytoid lymphoma	t(9;14)(p13;q32)	PAX5, IgH

[a]Numerous sites of translocation may be involved with these genes.
Abbreviations: CLL, chronic lymphoid leukemia; IgH, immunoglobulin heavy chain; MALT, mucosa-associated lymphoid tissue.

have tumors expressing specific genetic abnormalities, the defects may have prognostic significance. No specific genetic abnormalities have been identified in Hodgkin's disease other than aneuploidy.

In typical B cell CLL, trisomy 12 conveys a poorer prognosis. In ALL in both adults and children, genetic abnormalities have important prognostic significance. Patients whose tumor cells display the t(9;22) and translocations involving the *MLL* gene on chromosome 11q23 have a much poorer outlook than patients who do not have these translocations. Other genetic abnormalities that occur frequently in adults with ALL include the t(4;11) and the t(8;14). The t(4;11) is associated with younger age, female predominance, high white blood cell (WBC) counts, and L1 morphology. The t(8;14) is associated with older age, male predominance, frequent CNS involvement, and L3 morphology. Both are associated with a poor prognosis. In childhood ALL, hyperdiploidy has been shown to have a favorable prognosis.

Gene profiling using array technology allows the simultaneous assessment of the expression of thousands of genes. This technology provides the possibility to identify new genes with pathologic importance in lymphomas, the identification of patterns of gene expression with diagnostic and/or prognostic significance, and the identification of new therapeutic targets. Recognition of patterns of gene expression is complicated and requires sophisticated mathematical techniques. Early successes using this technology in lymphoma include the identification of previously unrecognized subtypes of diffuse large B cell lymphoma whose gene expression patterns resemble either those of follicular center B cells or activated peripheral blood B cells. Patients whose lymphomas have a germinal center B cell pattern of gene expression have a considerably better prognosis than those whose lymphomas have a pattern resembling activated peripheral blood B cells. This improved prognosis is independent of other known prognostic factors. Similar information is being generated in follicular lymphoma and mantle cell lymphoma. The challenge remains to provide information from such techniques in a clinically useful time frame.

APPROACH TO THE PATIENT: Lymphoid Cell Malignancies

Regardless of the type of lymphoid malignancy, the initial evaluation of the patient should include performance of a careful history and physical examination. These will help confirm the diagnosis, identify manifestations of the disease that might require prompt attention, and aid in the selection of further studies to optimally characterize the patient's status to allow the best choice of therapy. It is difficult to overemphasize the importance of a carefully done history and physical examination. They might provide observations that lead to reconsidering the diagnosis, provide hints at etiology, clarify the stage, and allow the physician to establish rapport with the patient that will make it possible to develop and carry out a therapeutic plan.

For patients with ALL, evaluation is usually completed after a complete blood count, chemistry studies reflecting major organ function, a bone marrow biopsy with genetic and immunologic studies, and a lumbar puncture. The latter is necessary to rule out occult CNS involvement. At this point, most patients would be ready to begin therapy. In ALL, the prognosis depends on the genetic characteristics of the tumor, the patient's age, the WBC count, and the patient's overall clinical status and major organ function.

In CLL, the patient evaluation should include a complete blood count, chemistry tests to measure major organ function, serum protein electrophoresis, and a bone marrow biopsy. However, some physicians believe that the diagnosis would not always require a bone marrow biopsy. Patients often have imaging studies of the chest and abdomen looking for pathologic lymphadenopathy. Patients with typical B cell CLL can be subdivided into three major prognostic groups. Patients with only blood and bone marrow involvement by leukemia but no lymphadenopathy, organomegaly, or signs of bone marrow failure have the best prognosis. Those with lymphadenopathy and organomegaly have an intermediate prognosis, and patients with bone marrow failure, defined as hemoglobin <100 g/L (10 g/dL) or platelet count <100,000/μL, have the worst prognosis. The pathogenesis of the anemia or thrombocytopenia is important to discern. The prognosis is adversely affected when either or both of these abnormalities are due to progressive marrow infiltration and loss of productive marrow. However, either or both may be due to autoimmune phenomena or to hypersplenism that can develop during the course of the disease. These destructive mechanisms are usually completely reversible (glucocorticoids for autoimmune disease; splenectomy for hypersplenism) and do not influence disease prognosis.

Two popular staging systems have been developed to reflect these prognostic groupings (Table 15-7).

TABLE 15-7

STAGING OF TYPICAL B CELL LYMPHOID LEUKEMIA

STAGE	CLINICAL FEATURES	MEDIAN SURVIVAL, YEARS
Rai System		
0: Low risk	Lymphocytosis only in blood and marrow	>10
I: Intermediate risk	Lymphocytosis + lymphadenopathy	>7
II: Intermediate risk	Lymphocytosis + lymphadenopathy + splenomegaly ± hepatomegaly	
III: High risk	Lymphocytosis + anemia	1.5
IV: High risk	Lymphocytosis + thrombocytopenia	
Binet System		
A	Fewer than three areas of clinical lymphadenopathy; no anemia or thrombocytopenia	>10
B	Three or more involved node areas; no anemia or thrombocytopenia	7
C	Hemoglobin ≤10 g/dL and/or platelets <100,000/μL	2

Patients with typical B cell CLL can have their course complicated by immunologic abnormalities, including autoimmune hemolytic anemia, autoimmune thrombocytopenia, and hypogammaglobulinemia. Patients with hypogammaglobulinemia benefit from regular (monthly) γ globulin administration. Because of expense, γ globulin is often withheld until the patient experiences a significant infection. These abnormalities do not have a clear prognostic significance and should not be used to assign a higher stage.

Two other features may be used to assess prognosis in B cell CLL, but neither has yet been incorporated into a staging classification. At least two subsets of CLL have been identified based on the cytoplasmic expression of ZAP-70; expression of this protein, which is usually expressed in T cells, identifies a subgroup with a poorer prognosis. A less powerful subsetting tool is CD38 expression. CD38+ tumors tend to have a poorer prognosis than CD38– tumors.

The initial evaluation of a patient with Hodgkin's disease or non-Hodgkin's lymphoma is similar. In both situations, the determination of an accurate anatomic stage is an important part of the evaluation. Staging is done using the Ann Arbor staging system originally developed for Hodgkin's disease (Table 15-8).

Evaluation of patients with Hodgkin's disease typically includes a complete blood count; erythrocyte sedimentation rate; chemistry studies reflecting major organ function; computed tomography scans of the chest, abdomen, and pelvis; and a bone marrow biopsy. Neither a positron emission tomography (PET) scan nor a gallium scan is absolutely necessary for primary staging, but one performed at the completion of therapy allows evaluation of persisting radiographic abnormalities, particularly of the mediastinum. Knowing that the PET scan or gallium scan is abnormal before treatment can help in this assessment. In most cases, these studies allow assignment of anatomic stage and the development of a therapeutic plan.

In patients with non-Hodgkin's lymphoma, the same evaluation described for patients with Hodgkin's disease is usually carried out. In addition, serum levels of lactate dehydrogenase (LDH) and β_2-microglobulin and serum protein electrophoresis are often included in the evaluation. Anatomic stage is assigned in the same manner as used for Hodgkin's disease. However, the prognosis of patients with non-Hodgkin's lymphoma is best assigned using the International Prognostic Index (IPI) (Table 15-9). This is a powerful predictor of outcome in all subtypes of non-Hodgkin's lymphoma. Patients are assigned an IPI score based on the presence or absence of five adverse prognostic factors and may have none or all five of these adverse prognostic factors. Figure 15-4 shows the prognostic significance of this score in 1300 patients with all types of non-Hodgkin's lymphoma.

TABLE 15-8

THE ANN ARBOR STAGING SYSTEM FOR HODGKIN'S DISEASE

STAGE	DEFINITION
I	Involvement of a single lymph node region or lymphoid structure (e.g., spleen, thymus, Waldeyer's ring)
II	Involvement of two or more lymph node regions on the same side of the diaphragm (the mediastinum is a single site; hilar lymph nodes should be considered "lateralized" and, when involved on both sides, constitute stage II disease)
III	Involvement of lymph node regions or lymphoid structures on both sides of the diaphragm
III_1	Subdiaphragmatic involvement limited to spleen, splenic hilar nodes, celiac nodes, or portal nodes
III_2	Subdiaphragmatic involvement includes paraaortic, iliac, or mesenteric nodes plus structures in III_1
IV	Involvement of extranodal site(s) beyond that designated as "E" More than one extranodal deposit at any location Any involvement of liver or bone marrow
A	No symptoms
B	Unexplained weight loss of >10% of the body weight during the 6 months before staging investigation Unexplained, persistent, or recurrent fever with temperatures >38°C during the previous month Recurrent drenching night sweats during the previous month
E	Localized, solitary involvement of extralymphatic tissue, excluding liver and bone marrow

With the addition of rituximab to CHOP (cyclophosphamide, doxorubicin, vincristine, and prednisone), treatment outcomes have improved and the original IPI has lost some of its discrimination power. A revised IPI has been proposed that better predicts outcome of rituximab plus chemotherapy-based programs (Table 15-9). CT scans are routinely used in the evaluation of patients with all subtypes of non-Hodgkin's lymphoma, but PET and gallium scans are much more useful in aggressive subtypes such as diffuse large B cell lymphoma than in more indolent subtypes such as follicular lymphoma or small lymphocytic lymphoma. While the IPI does divide patients with follicular lymphoma into subsets with distinct prognoses, the distribution of such patients is skewed toward lower risk categories. A follicular lymphoma–specific IPI (FLIPI) has been proposed that replaces performance status with hemoglobin level (<120 g/L [<12 g/dL]) and number of extranodal sites with number of nodal sites (more than four). Low risk (zero or one factor) was assigned to 36% of patients, intermediate risk (two factors) to 37%, and poor risk (more than two factors) to 27% of patients.

TABLE 15-9

INTERNATIONAL PROGNOSTIC INDEX FOR NON-HODGKIN'S LYMPHOMA

Five clinical risk factors:	
Age ≥ 60 years	
Serum lactate dehydrogenase levels elevated	
Performance status ≥2 (ECOG) or ≤70 (Karnofsky)	
Ann Arbor stage III or IV	
>1 site of extranodal involvement	
Patients are assigned a number for each risk factor they have	
Patients are grouped differently based on the type of lymphoma	
For diffuse large B cell lymphoma:	
0, 1 factor = low risk:	35% of cases; 5-year survival, 73%
2 factors = low-intermediate risk:	27% of cases; 5-year survival, 51%
3 factors = high-intermediate risk:	22% of cases; 5-year survival, 43%
4, 5 factors = high risk:	16% of cases; 5-year survival, 26%
For diffuse large B cell lymphoma treated with R-CHOP:	
0 factor = very good:	10% of cases; 5-year survival, 94%
1, 2 factors = good:	45% of cases; 5-year survival, 79%
3, 4, 5 factors = poor:	45% of cases; 5-year survival, 55%

Abbreviations: ECOG, Eastern Cooperative Oncology Group; R-CHOP, rituximab, cyclophosphamide, doxorubicin, vincristine, prednisone.

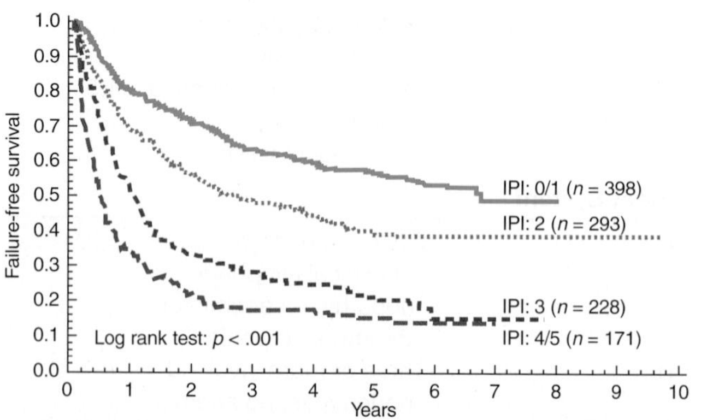

FIGURE 15-4

Relationship of International Prognostic Index (IPI) to survival. Kaplan-Meier survival curves for 1300 patients with various kinds of lymphoma stratified according to the IPI.

CLINICAL FEATURES, TREATMENT, AND PROGNOSIS OF SPECIFIC LYMPHOID MALIGNANCIES

PRECURSOR B CELL NEOPLASMS

Precursor B cell lymphoblastic leukemia/lymphoma

The most common cancer in childhood is B cell ALL. Although this disorder can also present as a lymphoma in either adults or children, presentation as lymphoma is rare.

The malignant cells in patients with precursor B cell lymphoblastic leukemia are most commonly of pre–B cell origin. Patients typically present with signs of bone marrow failure such as pallor, fatigue, bleeding, fever, and infection related to peripheral blood cytopenias. Peripheral blood counts regularly show anemia and thrombocytopenia but might show leukopenia, a normal leukocyte count, or leukocytosis based largely on the number of circulating malignant cells (Fig. 15-5). Extramedullary sites of disease are frequently involved in patients who present with leukemia, including lymphadenopathy, hepato- or splenomegaly, CNS disease, testicular enlargement, and/or cutaneous infiltration.

The diagnosis is usually made by bone marrow biopsy, which shows infiltration by malignant lymphoblasts. Demonstration of a pre–B cell immunophenotype (Fig. 15-2) and, often, characteristic cytogenetic abnormalities (Table 15-6) confirm the diagnosis. An adverse prognosis in patients with precursor B cell ALL is predicted by a very high WBC count, the presence of symptomatic CNS disease, and unfavorable cytogenetic abnormalities. For example, t(9;22), frequently found in adults with B cell ALL, has been associated with a very poor outlook. The bcr/abl kinase inhibitors have improved the prognosis.

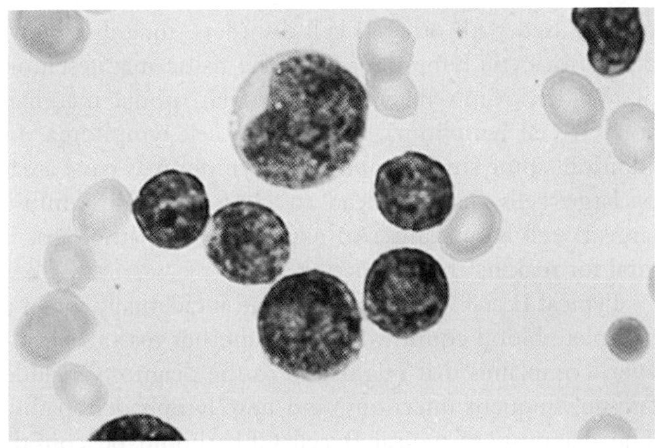

FIGURE 15-5
Acute lymphoblastic leukemia. The cells are heterogeneous in size and have round or convoluted nuclei, a high nuclear/cytoplasmic ratio, and absence of cytoplasmic granules.

TREATMENT Precursor B Cell Lymphoblastic Leukemia

The treatment of patients with precursor B cell ALL involves remission induction with combination chemotherapy, a consolidation phase that includes administration of high-dose systemic therapy and treatment to eliminate disease in the CNS, and a period of continuing therapy to prevent relapse and effect cure. The overall cure rate in children is 90%, while ~50% of adults are long-term disease-free survivors. This reflects the high proportion of adverse cytogenetic abnormalities seen in adults with precursor B cell ALL.

Precursor B cell lymphoblastic lymphoma is a rare presentation of precursor B cell lymphoblastic malignancy. These patients often have a rapid transformation to leukemia and should be treated as though they had presented with leukemia. The few patients who present with the disease confined to lymph nodes have a high cure rate.

MATURE (PERIPHERAL) B CELL NEOPLASMS

B cell chronic lymphoid leukemia/small lymphocytic lymphoma

B cell CLL/small lymphocytic lymphoma represents the most common lymphoid leukemia, and when presenting as a lymphoma, it accounts for ~7% of non-Hodgkin's lymphomas. Presentation can be as either leukemia or lymphoma. The major clinical characteristics of B cell CLL/small lymphocytic lymphoma are presented in Table 15-10.

The diagnosis of typical B cell CLL is made when an increased number of circulating lymphocytes (i.e., $>4 \times 10^9$/L and usually $>10 \times 10^9$/L) is found (Fig. 15-6) that are monoclonal B cells expressing the CD5 antigen. Finding bone marrow infiltration by the same cells confirms the diagnosis. The peripheral blood smear in such patients typically shows many "smudge" or "basket" cells, nuclear remnants of cells damaged by the physical shear stress of making the blood smear. If cytogenetic studies are performed, trisomy 12 is found in 25–30% of patients. Abnormalities in chromosome 13 are also seen.

If the primary presentation is lymphadenopathy and a lymph node biopsy is performed, pathologists usually have little difficulty in making the diagnosis of small lymphocytic lymphoma based on morphologic findings and immunophenotype. However, even in these patients, 70–75% will be found to have bone marrow involvement, and circulating monoclonal B lymphocytes are often present.

The differential diagnosis of typical B cell CLL is extensive (Table 15-1). Immunophenotyping will eliminate the T cell disorders and can often help sort out

TABLE 15-10

CLINICAL CHARACTERISTICS OF PATIENTS WITH COMMON TYPES OF NON-HODGKIN'S LYMPHOMAS (NHL)

DISEASE	MEDIAN AGE, YEARS	FREQUENCY IN CHILDREN	% MALE	STAGE I/II VS III/IV, %	B SYMPTOMS, %	BONE MARROW INVOLVEMENT, %	GASTROINTESTINAL TRACT INVOLVEMENT, %	% SURVIVING 5 YEARS
B cell chronic lymphocytic leukemia/small lymphocytic lymphoma	65	Rare	53	9 vs 91	33	72	3	51
Mantle cell lymphoma	63	Rare	74	20 vs 80	28	64	9	27
Extranodal marginal zone B cell lymphoma of MALT type	60	Rare	48	67 vs 33	19	14	50	74
Follicular lymphoma	59	Rare	42	33 vs 67	28	42	4	72
Diffuse large B cell lymphoma	64	~25% of childhood NHL	55	54 vs 46	33	16	18	46
Burkitt's lymphoma	31	~30% of childhood NHL	89	62 vs 38	22	33	11	45
Precursor T cell lymphoblastic lymphoma	28	~40% of childhood NHL	64	11 vs 89	21	50	4	26
Anaplastic large T/null cell lymphoma	34	Common	69	51 vs 49	53	13	9	77
Peripheral T cell non-Hodgkin's lymphoma	61	~5% of childhood NHL	55	20 vs 80	50	36	15	25

Abbreviation: MALT, mucosa-associated lymphoid tissue.

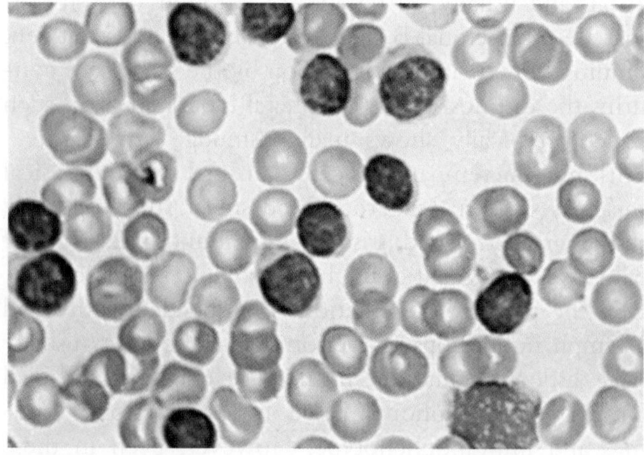

FIGURE 15-6

Chronic lymphocytic leukemia. The peripheral white blood cell count is high due to increased numbers of small, well-differentiated, normal-appearing lymphocytes. The leukemia lymphocytes are fragile, and substantial numbers of broken, smudged cells are usually also present on the blood smear.

other B cell malignancies. For example, only mantle cell lymphoma and typical B cell CLL are usually CD5 positive. Typical B cell small lymphocytic lymphoma can be confused with other B cell disorders, including lymphoplasmacytic lymphoma (i.e., the tissue manifestation of Waldenström's macroglobulinemia), nodal marginal zone B cell lymphoma, and mantle cell lymphoma. In addition, some small lymphocytic lymphomas have areas of large cells that can lead to confusion with diffuse large B cell lymphoma. An expert hematopathologist is vital for making this distinction.

Typical B cell CLL is often found incidentally when a complete blood count is done for another reason. However, complaints that might lead to the diagnosis include fatigue, frequent infections, and new lymphadenopathy. The diagnosis of typical B cell CLL should be considered in a patient presenting with an autoimmune hemolytic anemia or autoimmune thrombocytopenia. B cell CLL has also been associated with red cell aplasia. When this disorder presents as lymphoma, the most common

TABLE 15-11

STAGING EVALUATION FOR NON-HODGKIN'S LYMPHOMA

Physical examination
Documentation of B symptoms
Laboratory evaluation
  Complete blood counts
  Liver function tests
  Uric acid
  Calcium
  Serum protein electrophoresis
  Serum β_2-microglobulin
  Chest radiograph
CT scan of abdomen, pelvis, and usually chest
Bone marrow biopsy
Lumbar puncture in lymphoblastic, Burkitt's, and diffuse large B cell lymphoma with positive marrow biopsy results
Gallium scan (SPECT) or PET scan in large cell lymphoma

Abbreviations: CT, computed tomography; PET, positron emission tomography; SPECT, single photon emission computed tomography.

abnormality is asymptomatic lymphadenopathy, with or without splenomegaly. The staging systems predict prognosis in patients with typical B cell CLL (Table 15-7). The evaluation of a new patient with typical B cell CLL/small lymphocytic lymphoma will include many of the studies **(Table 15-11)** that are used in patients with other non-Hodgkin's lymphomas. In addition, particular attention needs to be given to detecting immune abnormalities such as autoimmune hemolytic anemia, autoimmune thrombocytopenia, hypogammaglobulinemia, and red cell aplasia. Molecular analysis of immunoglobulin gene sequences in CLL has demonstrated that about half the patients have tumors expressing mutated immunoglobulin genes and half have tumors expressing unmutated or germ-line immunoglobulin sequences. Patients with unmutated immunoglobulins tend to have a more aggressive clinical course and are less responsive to therapy. Unfortunately, immunoglobulin gene sequencing is not routinely available. CD38 expression is said to be low in the better-prognosis patients expressing mutated immunoglobulin and high in poorer-prognosis patients expressing unmutated immunoglobulin, but this test has not been confirmed as a reliable means of distinguishing the two groups. ZAP-70 expression correlates with the presence of unmutated immunoglobulin genes, but the assay is not yet standardized and widely available.

TREATMENT B Cell Chronic Lymphoid Leukemia/Small Lymphocytic Lymphoma

Patients whose presentation is typical B cell CLL with no manifestations of the disease other than bone marrow involvement and lymphocytosis (i.e., Rai stage 0 and Binet stage A; Table 15-7) can be followed without specific therapy for their malignancy. These patients have a median survival >10 years, and some will never require therapy for this disorder. If the patient has an adequate number of circulating normal blood cells and is asymptomatic, many physicians would not initiate therapy for patients in the intermediate stage of the disease manifested by lymphadenopathy and/or hepatosplenomegaly. However, the median survival for these patients is ~7 years, and most will require treatment in the first few years of follow-up. Patients who present with bone marrow failure (i.e., Rai stage III or IV or Binet stage C) will require initial therapy in almost all cases. These patients have a serious disorder with a median survival time of only 1.5 years. It must be remembered that immune manifestations of typical B cell CLL should be managed independently of specific antileukemia therapy. For example, glucocorticoid therapy for autoimmune cytopenias and γ globulin replacement for patients with hypogammaglobulinemia should be used whether or not antileukemia therapy is given.

Patients who present primarily with lymphoma and have low IPI scores have a 5-year survival of ~75%, but those with high IPI scores have a 5-year survival of <40% and are more likely to require early therapy.

The most common treatments for patients with typical B cell CLL/small lymphocytic lymphoma have been chlorambucil or fludarabine, alone or in combination. Chlorambucil can be administered orally with few immediate side effects, while fludarabine is administered IV and is associated with significant immune suppression. However, fludarabine is by far the more active agent and is the only drug associated with a significant incidence of complete remission. The combination of rituximab (375–500 mg/m^2 day 1), fludarabine (25 mg/m^2 days 2–4 on cycle 1 and 1–3 in subsequent cycles), and cyclophosphamide (250 mg/m^2 with fludarabine) achieves complete responses in 69% of patients, and those responses are associated with molecular remissions in half of the cases. Half of patients experience grade III or IV neutropenia. For young patients presenting with leukemia requiring therapy, regimens containing fludarabine are the treatment of choice. Because fludarabine is an effective second-line agent in patients with tumors unresponsive to chlorambucil, the latter agent is often chosen in elderly patients who require therapy. Bendamustine, an alkylating agent structurally related to nitrogen mustard, is highly effective and is vying with fludarabine as the primary treatment of choice. Patients who present with lymphoma (rather than leukemia) are also highly responsive to bendamustine, and some patients will receive a combination chemotherapy regimen used in other lymphomas such as CVP (cyclophosphamide, vincristine, and prednisone) or CHOP (cyclophosphamide, doxorubicin, vincristine, and prednisone) plus rituximab. Alemtuzumab (anti-CD52) is an antibody with activity in the disease, but it kills both B and T cells and is associated with more immune compromise than rituximab. Young patients with this disease can be candidates for bone marrow transplantation. Allogeneic bone marrow transplantation can be curative but is associated with a significant treatment-related mortality rate. Mini-transplants using immunosuppressive rather than myeloablative doses of preparative drugs are being studied (Chap. 30). The use of autologous transplantation in patients with this disorder has been discouraging.

Extranodal marginal zone B cell lymphoma of MALT type

Extranodal marginal zone B cell lymphoma of MALT type (MALT lymphoma) makes up ~8% of non-Hodgkin's lymphomas. This small cell lymphoma presents in extranodal sites. It was previously considered a small lymphocytic lymphoma or sometimes a pseudolymphoma. The recognition that the gastric presentation of this lymphoma was associated with *H. pylori* infection was an important step in recognizing it as a separate entity. The clinical characteristics of MALT lymphoma are presented in Table 15-10.

The diagnosis of MALT lymphoma can be made accurately by an expert hematopathologist based on a characteristic pattern of infiltration of small lymphocytes that are monoclonal B cells and CD5 negative. In some cases, transformation to diffuse large B cell lymphoma occurs, and both diagnoses may be made in the same biopsy. The differential diagnosis includes benign lymphocytic infiltration of extranodal organs and other small cell B cell lymphomas.

MALT lymphoma may occur in the stomach, orbit, intestine, lung, thyroid, salivary gland, skin, soft tissues, bladder, kidney, and CNS. It may present as a new mass, be found on routine imaging studies, or be associated with local symptoms such as upper abdominal discomfort in gastric lymphoma. Most MALT lymphomas are gastric in origin. At least two genetic forms of gastric MALT exist: one (accounting for ~50% of cases) characterized by t(11;18)(q21;q21) that juxtaposes the amino terminal of the *API2* gene with the carboxy terminal of the *MALT1* gene creating an API2/MALT1 fusion product, and the other characterized by multiple sites of genetic instability including trisomies of chromosomes 3, 7, 12, and 18. About 95% of gastric MALT lymphomas are associated with *H. pylori* infection, and those that are do not usually express t(11;18). The t(11;18) usually results in activation of NF-κB, which acts as a survival factor for the cells. Lymphomas with t(11;18) translocations are genetically stable and do not evolve to diffuse large B cell lymphoma. By contrast, t(11;18)-negative MALT lymphomas often acquire *BCL6* mutations and progress to aggressive histology lymphoma. MALT lymphomas are localized to the organ of origin in ~40% of cases and to the organ and regional lymph nodes in ~30% of patients. However, distant metastasis can occur, particularly with transformation to diffuse large B cell lymphoma. Many patients who develop this lymphoma will an autoimmune or inflammatory process such as Sjögren's syndrome (salivary gland MALT), Hashimoto's thyroiditis (thyroid MALT), *Helicobacter* gastritis (gastric MALT), *C. psittaci* conjunctivitis (ocular MALT), or *Borrelia* skin infections (cutaneous MALT).

Evaluation of patients with MALT lymphoma follows the pattern (Table 15-11) for staging a patient with non-Hodgkin's lymphoma. In particular, patients with gastric lymphoma need to have studies performed to document the presence or absence of *H. pylori* infection. Endoscopic studies including ultrasound can help define the extent of gastric involvement. Most patients with MALT lymphoma have a good prognosis, with a 5-year survival rate of ~75%. In patients with a low IPI score, the 5-year survival rate is ~90%, while it drops to ~40% in patients with a high IPI score.

TREATMENT Mucosa-Associated Lymphoid Tissue Lymphoma

MALT lymphoma is often localized. Patients with gastric MALT lymphomas who are infected with *H. pylori* can achieve remission in the 80% of cases with eradication of the infection. These remissions can be durable, but molecular evidence of persisting neoplasia is not infrequent. After *H. pylori* eradication, symptoms generally improve quickly but molecular evidence of persistent disease may be present for 12–18 months. Additional therapy is not indicated unless progressive disease is documented. Patients with more extensive disease or progressive disease are most often treated with single-agent chemotherapy such as chlorambucil. Combination regimens that include rituximab are also highly effective. Coexistent diffuse large B cell lymphoma must be treated with combination chemotherapy (see later discussion). The additional acquired mutations that mediate the histologic progression also convey *Helicobacter* independence to the growth.

Mantle cell lymphoma

Mantle cell lymphoma makes up ~6% of all non-Hodgkin's lymphomas. This lymphoma was previously placed in a number of other subtypes. Its existence was confirmed by the recognition that these lymphomas have a characteristic chromosomal translocation, t(11;14), between the immunoglobulin heavy chain gene on chromosome 14 and the *bcl-1* gene on chromosome 11, and regularly overexpress the BCL-1 protein, also known as cyclin D1. Table 15-10 shows the clinical characteristics of mantle cell lymphoma.

The diagnosis of mantle cell lymphoma can be made accurately by an expert hematopathologist. As with all subtypes of lymphoma, an adequate biopsy is important. The differential diagnosis of mantle cell lymphoma includes other small cell B cell lymphomas. In particular, mantle cell lymphoma and small lymphocytic lymphoma share a characteristic expression of CD5. Mantle cell lymphoma usually has a slightly indented nucleus.

The most common presentation of mantle cell lymphoma is with palpable lymphadenopathy, frequently accompanied by systemic symptoms. The median age is 63 years and men are affected four times as commonly as women. Approximately 70% of patients will have stage IV disease at the time of diagnosis, with frequent bone marrow and peripheral blood involvement. Of the extranodal organs that can be involved, gastrointestinal involvement is particularly important to recognize. Patients who present with lymphomatosis polyposis in the large intestine usually have mantle cell lymphoma. Table 15-11 outlines the evaluation of patients with mantle cell lymphoma. Patients who present with gastrointestinal tract involvement often have Waldeyer's ring involvement and vice versa. The 5-year survival rate for all patients with mantle cell lymphoma is ~25%, with only occasional patients who present with a high IPI score surviving 5 years and ~50% of patients with a low IPI score surviving 5 years.

TREATMENT Mantle Cell Lymphoma

Current therapies for mantle cell lymphoma are evolving. Patients with localized disease might be treated with combination chemotherapy followed by radiotherapy; however, these patients are exceedingly rare. For the usual presentation with disseminated disease, standard lymphoma treatments have been unsatisfactory, with the minority of patients achieving complete remission. Aggressive combination chemotherapy regimens followed by autologous or allogeneic bone marrow transplantation are frequently offered to younger patients. For the occasional elderly, asymptomatic patient, observation followed by single-agent chemotherapy might be the most practical approach. An intensive combination chemotherapy regimen originally used in the treatment of acute leukemia, HyperC-VAD (cyclophosphamide, vincristine, doxorubicin, dexamethasone, cytarabine, and methotrexate), in combination with rituximab, seems to be associated with better response rates, particularly in younger patients. Alternating two regimens, HyperC-VAD with rituximab added (R-HyperC-VAD) and rituximab plus high-dose methotrexate and cytarabine, can achieve complete responses in >80% of patients and 8-year survival rate of 56%, comparable to regimens employing high-dose therapy and autologous hematopoietic stem cell transplantation. Bortezomib, temsirolimus, and bendamustine are single agents that induce transient partial responses in a minority of patients and are being added to primary combinations.

Follicular lymphoma

Follicular lymphomas make up 22% of non-Hodgkin's lymphomas worldwide and at least 30% of non-Hodgkin's lymphomas diagnosed in the United States. This type of lymphoma can be diagnosed accurately on morphologic findings alone and has been the diagnosis in the majority of patients in therapeutic trials for "low-grade" lymphoma in the past. The clinical characteristics of follicular lymphoma are presented in Table 15-10.

Evaluation of an adequate biopsy by an expert hematopathologist is sufficient to make a diagnosis of follicular lymphoma. The tumor is composed of small cleaved and large cells in varying proportions organized in a follicular pattern of growth (Fig. 15-7). Confirmation of B cell immunophenotype and the existence of the t(14;18) and abnormal expression of BCL-2 protein are confirmatory. The major differential diagnosis is between lymphoma and reactive follicular hyperplasia. The coexistence of diffuse large B cell lymphoma must be considered. Patients with follicular lymphoma are

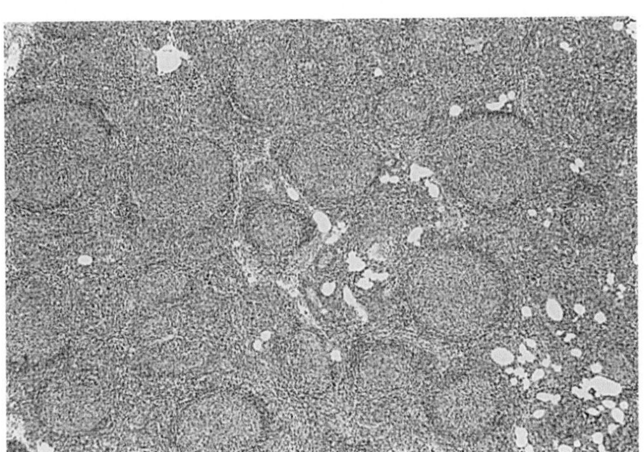

FIGURE 15-7

Follicular lymphoma. The normal nodal architecture is effaced by nodular expansions of tumor cells. Nodules vary in size and contain predominantly small lymphocytes with cleaved nuclei along with variable numbers of larger cells with vesicular chromatin and prominent nucleoli.

often subclassified into those with predominantly small cells, those with a mixture of small and large cells, and those with predominantly large cells. While this distinction cannot be made simply or very accurately, these subdivisions do have prognostic significance. Patients with follicular lymphoma with predominantly large cells have higher proliferative fractions, progress more rapidly, and have shorter overall survival times with simple chemotherapy regimens.

The most common presentation for follicular lymphoma is with new, painless lymphadenopathy. Multiple sites of lymphoid involvement are typical, and unusual sites such as epitrochlear nodes are sometimes seen. However, essentially any organ can be involved, and extranodal presentations do occur. Most patients do not have fevers, sweats, or weight loss, and an IPI score of 0 or 1 is found in ~50% of patients. Fewer than 10% of patients have a high (i.e., 4 or 5) IPI score. The staging evaluation for patients with follicular lymphoma should include the studies included in Table 15-11.

TREATMENT Follicular Lymphoma

Follicular lymphoma is one of the malignancies most responsive to chemotherapy and radiotherapy. In addition, tumors in as many as 25% of the patients undergo spontaneous regression—usually transient—without therapy. In an asymptomatic patient, no initial treatment and watchful waiting can be an appropriate management strategy and is particularly likely to be adopted for older patients with advanced-stage disease. For patients who do require treatment, single-agent chlorambucil or cyclophosphamide or combination chemotherapy with CVP or CHOP are most frequently used. With adequate treatment, 50–75% of patients will achieve a complete remission. While most patients relapse (median response duration is ~2 years), at least 20% of complete responders will remain in remission for >10 years. For the rare patient (15%) with localized follicular lymphoma, involved field radiotherapy produces long-term disease-free survival in the majority.

A number of therapies have been shown to be active in the treatment of patients with follicular lymphoma. These include cytotoxic agents such as fludarabine, biologic agents such as interferon α, monoclonal antibodies with or without radionuclides, and lymphoma vaccines. In patients treated with a doxorubicin-containing combination chemotherapy regimen, interferon α given to patients in complete remission seems to prolong survival, but interferon toxicities can affect quality of life. The monoclonal antibody rituximab can cause objective responses in 35–50% of patients with relapsed follicular lymphoma, and radiolabeled antibodies appear to have response rates well in excess of 50%. The addition of rituximab to CHOP and other effective combination chemotherapy programs is beginning to show prolonged overall survival and a decreased risk of histologic progression. Complete remissions can be noted in 85% or more of patients treated with R-CHOP, and median remission durations can exceed 6 or 7 years. Maintenance intermittent rituximab therapy can prolong remissions even further, though it is not completely clear that overall survival is prolonged. Some trials with tumor vaccines have been encouraging. Both autologous and allogeneic hematopoietic stem cell transplantation yield high complete response rates in patients with relapsed follicular lymphoma, and long-term remissions can occur in 40% or more of patients.

Patients with follicular lymphoma with a predominance of large cells have a shorter survival when treated with single-agent chemotherapy but seem to benefit from receiving an anthracycline-containing combination chemotherapy regimen plus rituximab. When their disease is treated aggressively, the overall survival for such patients is no lower than for patients with other follicular lymphomas, and the failure-free survival is superior.

Patients with follicular lymphoma have a high rate of histologic transformation to diffuse large B cell lymphoma (5–7% per year). This is recognized ~40% of the time during the course of the illness by repeat biopsy and is present in almost all patients at autopsy. This transformation is usually heralded by rapid growth of lymph nodes—often localized—and the development of systemic symptoms such as fevers, sweats, and weight loss. Although these patients have a poor prognosis, aggressive combination chemotherapy regimens can sometimes cause a complete remission in the diffuse large B cell lymphoma, at times leaving the patient with persisting follicular lymphoma. With more frequent use of R-CHOP to treat follicular lymphoma at diagnosis, it appears that the rate of histologic progression is decreasing.

Diffuse large B cell lymphoma

Diffuse large B cell lymphoma is the most common type of non-Hodgkin's lymphoma, representing approximately one-third of all cases. This lymphoma makes up the majority of cases in previous clinical trials of "aggressive" or "intermediate-grade" lymphoma. Table 15-10 shows the clinical characteristics of diffuse large B cell lymphoma.

The diagnosis of diffuse large B cell lymphoma can be made accurately by an expert hematopathologist (**Fig. 15-8**). Cytogenetic and molecular genetic studies are not necessary for diagnosis, but some evidence

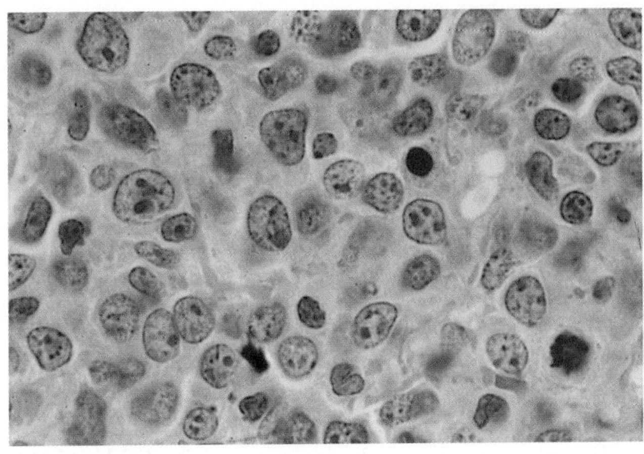

FIGURE 15-8

Diffuse large B cell lymphoma. The neoplastic cells are heterogeneous but predominantly large cells with vesicular chromatin and prominent nucleoli.

has accumulated that patients whose tumors overexpress the BCL-2 protein might be more likely to relapse than others. Patients with prominent mediastinal involvement are sometimes diagnosed as a separate subgroup having primary mediastinal diffuse large B cell lymphoma. This latter group of patients has a younger median age (i.e., 37 years) and a female predominance (66%). Subtypes of diffuse large B cell lymphoma, including those with an immunoblastic subtype and tumors with extensive fibrosis, are recognized by pathologists but do not appear to have important independent prognostic significance.

Diffuse large B cell lymphoma can present as either primary lymph node disease or at extranodal sites. More than 50% of patients will have some site of extranodal involvement at diagnosis, with the most common sites being the gastrointestinal tract and bone marrow, each being involved in 15–20% of patients. Essentially any organ can be involved, making a diagnostic biopsy imperative. For example, diffuse large B cell lymphoma of the pancreas has a much better prognosis than pancreatic carcinoma but would be missed without biopsy. Primary diffuse large B cell lymphoma of the brain is being diagnosed with increasing frequency. Other unusual subtypes of diffuse large B cell lymphoma such as pleural effusion lymphoma and intravascular lymphoma have been difficult to diagnose and associated with a very poor prognosis.

Table 15-11 shows the initial evaluation of patients with diffuse large B cell lymphoma. After a careful staging evaluation, ~50% of patients will be found to have stage I or II disease, and ~50% will have widely disseminated lymphoma. Bone marrow biopsy shows involvement by lymphoma in ~15% of cases, with marrow involvement by small cells more frequent than by large cells.

TREATMENT Diffuse Large B Cell Lymphoma

The initial treatment of all patients with diffuse large B cell lymphoma should be with a combination chemotherapy regimen. The most popular regimen in the United States is CHOP plus rituximab, although a variety of other anthracycline-containing combination chemotherapy regimens appear to be equally efficacious. Patients with stage I or nonbulky stage II disease can be effectively treated with three to four cycles of combination chemotherapy with or without subsequent involved field radiotherapy. The need for radiation therapy is unclear. Cure rates of 70–80% in stage II disease and 85–90% in stage I disease can be expected.

For patients with bulky stage II, stage III, or stage IV disease, six to eight cycles of CHOP plus rituximab are usually administered. A large randomized trial showed the superiority of CHOP combined with rituximab over CHOP alone in elderly patients. A frequent approach would be to administer four cycles of therapy and then reevaluate. If the patient has achieved a complete remission after four cycles, two more cycles of treatment might be given and then therapy discontinued. Using this approach, 70–80% of patients can be expected to achieve a complete remission, and 50–70% of complete responders will be cured. The chances for a favorable response to treatment are predicted by the IPI. In fact, the IPI was developed based on the outcome of patients with diffuse large B cell lymphoma treated with CHOP-like regimens. For the 35% of patients with a low IPI score of 0–1, the 5-year survival rate is >70%, while for the 20% of patients with a high IPI score of 4–5, the 5-year survival rate is ~20%. The addition of rituximab to CHOP has improved each of these numbers by ~15%. A number of other factors, including molecular features of the tumor, levels of circulating cytokines and soluble receptors, and other surrogate markers, have been shown to influence prognosis. However, they have not been validated as rigorously as the IPI and have not been uniformly applied clinically.

Because a number of patients with diffuse large B cell lymphoma are either initially refractory to therapy or relapse after apparently effective chemotherapy, 30–40% of patients will be candidates for salvage treatment at some point. Alternative combination chemotherapy regimens can induce complete remission in as many as 50% of these patients, but long-term disease-free survival is seen in ≤10%. Autologous bone marrow transplantation is superior to salvage chemotherapy at usual doses and leads to long-term disease-free survival in ~40% of patients whose lymphomas remain chemotherapy-sensitive after relapse.

Burkitt's lymphoma/leukemia

Burkitt's lymphoma/leukemia is a rare disease in adults in the United States, making up <1% of non-Hodgkin's lymphomas, but it makes up ~30% of childhood non-Hodgkin's lymphoma. Burkitt's leukemia, or L3 ALL, makes up a small proportion of childhood and adult acute leukemias. Table 15-10 shows the clinical features of Burkitt's lymphoma.

Burkitt's lymphoma can be diagnosed morphologically by an expert hematopathologist with a high degree of accuracy. The cells are homogeneous in size and shape (Fig. 15-9). Demonstration of a very high proliferative fraction and the presence of the t(8;14) or one of its variants, t(2;8) (*c-myc* and the λ light chain gene) or t(8;22) (*c-myc* and the κ light chain gene), can be confirmatory. Burkitt's cell leukemia is recognized by the typical monotonous mass of medium-sized cells with round nuclei, multiple nucleoli, and basophilic cytoplasm with cytoplasmic vacuoles. Demonstration of surface expression of immunoglobulin and one of the above-noted cytogenetic abnormalities is confirmatory.

Three distinct clinical forms of Burkitt's lymphoma are recognized: endemic, sporadic, and immunodeficiency-associated. Endemic and sporadic Burkitt's lymphomas occur frequently in children in Africa, and the sporadic form occurs in Western countries. Immunodeficiency-associated Burkitt's lymphoma is seen in patients with HIV infection.

Pathologists sometimes have difficulty distinguishing between Burkitt's lymphoma and diffuse large B cell lymphoma. In the past, a separate subgroup of non-Hodgkin's lymphoma intermediate between the two was recognized. When tested, this subgroup could not be diagnosed accurately. Distinction between the two major types of B cell aggressive non-Hodgkin's lymphoma can sometimes be made based on the extremely high proliferative fraction seen in patients with Burkitt's lymphoma (i.e., essentially 100% of tumor cells are in cycle) caused by *c-myc* deregulation.

Most patients in the United States with Burkitt's lymphoma present with peripheral lymphadenopathy or an intraabdominal mass. The disease is rapidly progressive and has a propensity to metastasize to the CNS. Initial evaluation should always include an examination of cerebrospinal fluid to rule out metastasis in addition to the other staging evaluations noted in Table 15-11. When the diagnosis of Burkitt's lymphoma is suspected, a diagnosis must be made promptly and staging evaluation must be accomplished expeditiously. This is the most rapidly progressive human tumor, and any delay in initiating therapy can adversely affect the patient's prognosis.

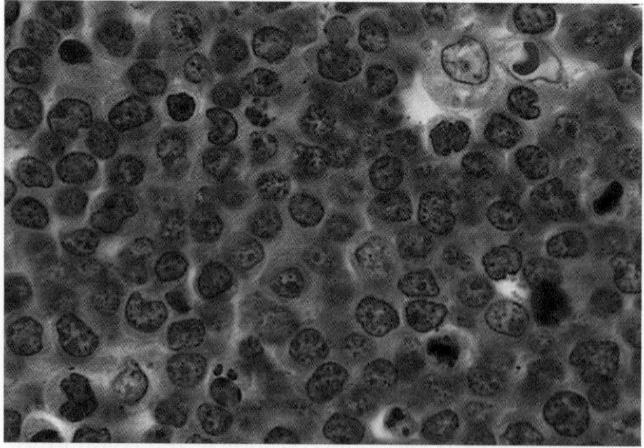

FIGURE 15-9
Burkitt's lymphoma. The neoplastic cells are homogeneous, medium-sized B cells with frequent mitotic figures, a morphologic correlate of high growth fraction. Reactive macrophages are scattered through the tumor, and their pale cytoplasm in a background of blue-staining tumor cells give the tumor a so-called starry sky appearance.

TREATMENT Burkitt's Lymphoma

Treatment of Burkitt's lymphoma in both children and adults should begin within 48 h of diagnosis and involves the use of intensive combination chemotherapy regimens incorporating high doses of cyclophosphamide. Prophylactic therapy to the CNS is mandatory. Burkitt's lymphoma was one of the first cancers shown to be curable by chemotherapy. Today, cure can be expected in 70–80% of both children and young adults when effective therapy is administered precisely. Salvage therapy has been generally ineffective in patients failing the initial treatment, emphasizing the importance of the initial treatment approach.

Other B cell lymphoid malignancies

B cell prolymphocytic leukemia involves blood and marrow infiltration by large lymphocytes with prominent nucleoli. Patients typically have high WBC counts, splenomegaly, and minimal lymphadenopathy. The chances for a complete response to therapy are poor.

Hairy cell leukemia is a rare disease that presents predominantly in older males. Typical presentation involves pancytopenia, although occasional patients will have a leukemic presentation. Splenomegaly is usual. The malignant cells appear to have "hairy" projections on light and electron microscopy and show a characteristic staining pattern with tartrate-resistant acid phosphatase. Bone marrow is typically not able to be aspirated, and biopsy shows a pattern of fibrosis with diffuse infiltration by the malignant cells. Patients with this disorder are prone to unusual infections, including infection by

Mycobacterium avium intracellulare, and to vasculitic syndromes. Hairy cell leukemia is responsive to chemotherapy with interferon α, pentostatin, or cladribine, with the latter being the usually preferred treatment. Clinical complete remissions with cladribine occur in the majority of patients, and long-term disease-free survival is frequent.

Splenic marginal zone lymphoma involves infiltration of the splenic white pulp by small, monoclonal B cells. This is a rare disorder that can present as leukemia as well as lymphoma. Definitive diagnosis is often made at splenectomy, which is also an effective therapy. This is an extremely indolent disorder, but when chemotherapy is required, the most usual treatment has been chlorambucil.

Lymphoplasmacytic lymphoma is the tissue manifestation of Waldenström's macroglobulinemia (Chap. 17). This type of lymphoma has been associated with chronic hepatitis C virus infection, and an etiologic association has been proposed. Patients typically present with lymphadenopathy, splenomegaly, bone marrow involvement, and occasionally peripheral blood involvement. The tumor cells do not express CD5. Patients often have a monoclonal IgM protein, high levels of which can dominate the clinical picture with the symptoms of hyperviscosity. Treatment of lymphoplasmacytic lymphoma can be aimed primarily at reducing the abnormal protein, if present, but will usually also involve chemotherapy. Chlorambucil, fludarabine, and cladribine have been utilized. The median 5-year survival rate for patients with this disorder is ~60%.

Nodal marginal zone lymphoma, also known as *monocytoid B cell lymphoma*, represents ~1% of non-Hodgkin's lymphomas. This lymphoma has a slight female predominance and presents with disseminated disease (i.e., stage III or IV) in 75% of patients. Approximately one-third of patients have bone marrow involvement, and a leukemic presentation occasionally occurs. The staging evaluation and therapy should use the same approach as used for patients with follicular lymphoma. Approximately 60% of the patients with nodal marginal zone lymphoma will survive 5 years after diagnosis.

PRECURSOR T CELL MALIGNANCIES

Precursor T cell lymphoblastic leukemia/lymphoma

Precursor T cell malignancies can present either as ALL or as an aggressive lymphoma. These malignancies are more common in children and young adults, with males more frequently affected than females.

Precursor T cell ALL can present with bone marrow failure, although the severity of anemia, neutropenia, and thrombocytopenia is often less than in precursor B cell ALL. These patients sometimes have very high WBC counts, a mediastinal mass, lymphadenopathy, and hepatosplenomegaly. Precursor T cell lymphoblastic lymphoma is most often found in young men presenting with a large mediastinal mass and pleural effusions. Both presentations have a propensity to metastasize to the CNS, and CNS involvement is often present at diagnosis.

TREATMENT Precursor T Cell Lymphoblastic Leukemia/Lymphoma

Children with precursor T cell ALL seem to benefit from very intensive remission induction and consolidation regimens. The majority of patients treated in this manner can be cured. Older children and young adults with precursor T cell lymphoblastic lymphoma are also often treated with "leukemia-like" regimens. Patients who present with localized disease have an excellent prognosis. However, advanced age is an adverse prognostic factor. Adults with precursor T cell lymphoblastic lymphoma who present with high LDH levels or bone marrow or CNS involvement are often offered bone marrow transplantation as part of their primary therapy.

MATURE (PERIPHERAL) T CELL DISORDERS

Mycosis fungoides

Mycosis fungoides is also known as *cutaneous T cell lymphoma*. This lymphoma is more often seen by dermatologists than internists. The median age of onset is in the midfifties, and the disease is more common in males and in blacks.

Mycosis fungoides is an indolent lymphoma with patients often having several years of eczematous or dermatitic skin lesions before the diagnosis is finally established. The skin lesions progress from patch stage to plaque stage to cutaneous tumors. Early in the disease, biopsies are often difficult to interpret, and the diagnosis may only become apparent by observing the patient over time. In advanced stages, the lymphoma can spread to lymph nodes and visceral organs. Patients with this lymphoma may develop generalized erythroderma and circulating tumor cells, called *Sézary's syndrome*.

Rare patients with localized early-stage mycosis fungoides can be cured with radiotherapy, often total-skin electron beam irradiation. More advanced disease has been treated with topical glucocorticoids, topical nitrogen mustard, phototherapy, psoralen with ultraviolet A (PUVA), extracorporeal photopheresis, retinoids (bexarotene), electron beam radiation, interferon, antibodies, fusion toxins, histone deacetylase inhibitors, and systemic cytotoxic therapy. Unfortunately, these treatments are palliative.

Adult T cell lymphoma/leukemia

Adult T cell lymphoma/leukemia is one manifestation of infection by the HTLV-I retrovirus. Patients can be infected through transplacental transmission, mother's milk, blood transfusion, and sexual transmission of the virus. Patients who acquire the virus from their mother through breast milk are most likely to develop lymphoma, but the risk is still only 2.5%, and the latency period averages 55 years. Nationwide testing for HTLV-I antibodies and the aggressive implementation of public health measures could theoretically lead to the disappearance of adult T cell lymphoma/leukemia. Tropical spastic paraparesis, another manifestation of HTLV-I infection, occurs after a shorter latency (1–3 years) and is most common in individuals who acquire the virus during adulthood from transfusion or sex.

The diagnosis of adult T cell lymphoma/leukemia is made when an expert hematopathologist recognizes the typical morphologic picture, a T cell immunophenotype (i.e., CD4 positive), and the presence in serum of antibodies to HTLV-I. Examination of the peripheral blood will usually reveal characteristic, pleomorphic abnormal CD4-positive cells with indented nuclei, which have been called "flower" cells (Fig. 15-10).

A subset of patients have a smoldering clinical course and long survival, but most patients present with an aggressive disease manifested by lymphadenopathy, hepatosplenomegaly, skin infiltration, pulmonary infiltrates, hypercalcemia, lytic bone lesions, and elevated LDH levels. The skin lesions can be papules, plaques, tumors, and ulcerations. Lung lesions can be either tumor or opportunistic infection in light of the underlying immunodeficiency in the disease. Bone marrow involvement is not usually extensive, and anemia and thrombocytopenia are not usually prominent. Although treatment with combination chemotherapy regimens can result in objective responses, true complete remissions are unusual, and the median survival time of patients is ~7 months. A small phase II study reported a high response rate with interferon plus zidovudine and arsenic trioxide.

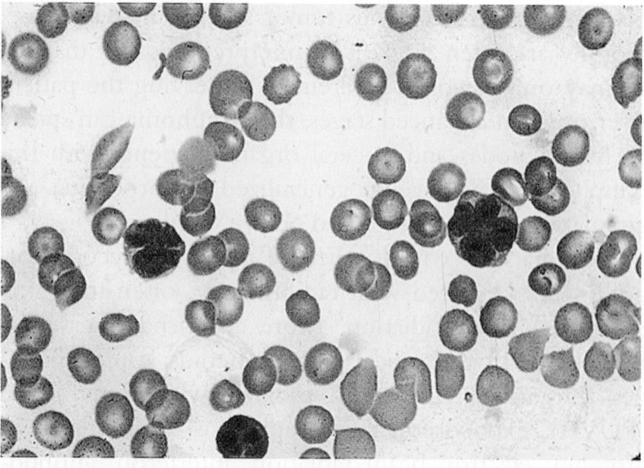

FIGURE 15-10
Adult T cell leukemia/lymphoma. Peripheral blood smear showing leukemia cells with typical "flower-shaped" nucleus.

Anaplastic large T/null cell lymphoma

Anaplastic large T/null cell lymphoma was previously usually diagnosed as undifferentiated carcinoma or malignant histiocytosis. Discovery of the CD30 (Ki-1) antigen and the recognition that some patients with previously unclassified malignancies displayed this antigen led to the identification of a new type of lymphoma. Subsequently, discovery of the t(2;5) and the resultant frequent overexpression of the anaplastic lymphoma kinase (ALK) protein confirmed the existence of this entity. This lymphoma accounts for ~2% of all non-Hodgkin's lymphomas. Table 15-10 shows the clinical characteristics of patients with anaplastic large T/null cell lymphoma.

The diagnosis of anaplastic large T/null cell lymphoma is made when an expert hematopathologist recognizes the typical morphologic picture and a T cell or null cell immunophenotype with CD30 positivity. Documentation of the t(2;5) and/or overexpression of ALK protein confirm the diagnosis. Some diffuse large B cell lymphomas can also have an anaplastic appearance but have the same clinical course or response to therapy as other diffuse large B cell lymphomas.

Patients with anaplastic large T/null cell lymphoma are typically young (median age, 33 years) and male (~70%). Some 50% of patients present in stage I/II and the remainder with more extensive disease. Systemic symptoms and elevated LDH levels are seen in about half of patients. Bone marrow and the gastrointestinal tract are rarely involved, but skin involvement is frequent. Some patients with disease confined to the skin have a different and more indolent disorder that has been termed *cutaneous anaplastic large T/null cell lymphoma* and might be related to lymphomatoid papulosis.

TREATMENT Anaplastic Large T/Null Cell Lymphoma

Treatment regimens appropriate for other aggressive lymphomas, such as diffuse large B cell lymphoma, should be utilized in patients with anaplastic large T/null cell lymphoma, with the exception that the B cell-specific antibody, rituximab, is omitted. Surprisingly, given the anaplastic appearance, this disorder has the best survival rate of any aggressive lymphoma. The 5-year survival is >75%. While traditional prognostic factors such as the IPI predict treatment outcome, overexpression of the ALK protein is an important prognostic factor, with patients overexpressing this protein having a superior treatment outcome. The ALK inhibitor crizotinib appears highly active as well.

Peripheral T cell lymphoma

The peripheral T cell lymphomas make up a heterogeneous morphologic group of aggressive neoplasms that share a mature T cell immunophenotype. They represent ~7% of all cases of non-Hodgkin's lymphoma. A number of distinct clinical syndromes are included in this group of disorders. Table 15-10 shows the clinical characteristics of patients with peripheral T cell lymphoma.

The diagnosis of peripheral T cell lymphoma, or any of its specific subtypes, requires an expert hematopathologist, an adequate biopsy, and immunophenotyping. Most peripheral T cell lymphomas are CD4+, but a few will be CD8+, both CD4+ and CD8+, or have an NK cell immunophenotype. No characteristic genetic abnormalities have yet been identified, but translocations involving the T cell antigen receptor genes on chromosomes 7 or 14 may be detected. The differential diagnosis of patients suspected of having peripheral T cell lymphoma includes reactive T cell infiltrative processes. In some cases, demonstration of a monoclonal T cell population using T cell receptor gene rearrangement studies will be required to make a diagnosis.

The initial evaluation of a patient with a peripheral T cell lymphoma should include the studies in Table 15-11 for staging patients with non-Hodgkin's lymphoma. Unfortunately, patients with peripheral T cell lymphoma usually present with adverse prognostic factors, with >80% of patients having IPI scores ≥2 and >30% having IPI scores ≥4. As this would predict, peripheral T cell lymphomas are associated with a poor outcome, and only 25% of the patients survive 5 years after diagnosis. Treatment regimens are the same as those used for diffuse large B cell lymphoma (omitting rituximab), but patients with peripheral T cell lymphoma have a poorer response to treatment. Because of this poor treatment outcome, hematopoietic stem cell transplantation is often considered early in the care of young patients.

A number of specific clinical syndromes are seen in the peripheral T cell lymphomas. *Angioimmunoblastic T cell lymphoma* is one of the more common subtypes, making up ~20% of T cell lymphomas. These patients typically present with generalized lymphadenopathy, fever, weight loss, skin rash, and polyclonal hypergammaglobulinemia. In some cases, it is difficult to separate patients with a reactive disorder from those with true lymphoma.

Extranodal T/NK cell lymphoma of nasal type has also been called *angiocentric lymphoma* and was previously termed *lethal midline granuloma*. This disorder is more frequent in Asia and South America than in the United States and Europe. EBV is thought to play an etiologic role. Although most frequent in the upper airway, it can also involve other organs. The course is aggressive, and patients frequently have the hemophagocytic syndrome. When marrow and blood involvement occur, distinction between this disease and leukemia might be difficult. Some patients will respond to aggressive combination chemotherapy regimens, but the overall outlook is poor.

Enteropathy-type intestinal T cell lymphoma is a rare disorder that occurs in patients with untreated gluten-sensitive enteropathy. Patients are frequently wasted and sometimes present with intestinal perforation. The prognosis is poor. *Hepatosplenic γδ T cell lymphoma* is a systemic illness that presents with sinusoidal infiltration of the liver, spleen, and bone marrow by malignant T cells. Tumor masses generally do not occur. The disease is associated with systemic symptoms and is often difficult to diagnose. Treatment outcome is poor. *Subcutaneous panniculitis-like T cell lymphoma* is a rare disorder that is often confused with panniculitis. Patients present with multiple subcutaneous nodules, which progress and can ulcerate. Hemophagocytic syndrome is common. Response to therapy is poor. The development of the hemophagocytic syndrome (profound anemia, ingestion of erythrocytes by monocytes and macrophages) in the course of any peripheral T cell lymphoma is generally associated with a fatal outcome.

HODGKIN'S DISEASE

Classical Hodgkin's disease

Hodgkin's disease occurs in 8000 patients in the United States each year, and the disease does not appear to be increasing in frequency. Most patients present with palpable lymphadenopathy that is nontender; in most patients, these lymph nodes are in the neck, supraclavicular area, and axilla. More than half the patients will have mediastinal adenopathy at diagnosis, and this is sometimes the initial manifestation. Subdiaphragmatic presentation of Hodgkin's disease is unusual and more common in older males. One-third of patients present with fevers, night sweats, and/or weight loss—B symptoms in the Ann Arbor staging classification (Table 15-8). Occasionally, Hodgkin's disease can present as a fever of unknown origin. This is more common in older patients who are found to have mixed-cellularity Hodgkin's disease in an abdominal site. Rarely, the fevers persist for days to weeks followed by afebrile intervals and then recurrence of the fever. This pattern is known as *Pel-Ebstein fever*.

Hodgkin's disease can occasionally present with unusual manifestations. These include severe and unexplained itching, cutaneous disorders such as erythema nodosum and ichthyosiform atrophy, paraneoplastic cerebellar degeneration and other distant effects on the CNS, nephrotic syndrome, immune hemolytic anemia and thrombocytopenia, hypercalcemia, and pain in lymph nodes on alcohol ingestion.

The diagnosis of Hodgkin's disease is established by review of an adequate biopsy specimen by an expert hematopathologist. In the United States, most patients have nodular sclerosing Hodgkin's disease, with a minority of patients having mixed-cellularity Hodgkin's disease. Lymphocyte-predominant and lymphocyte-depleted Hodgkin's disease are rare. Mixed-cellularity Hodgkin's disease or lymphocyte-depletion Hodgkin's disease are seen more frequently in patients infected by HIV (Fig. 15-11). Hodgkin's disease is a tumor characterized by rare neoplastic cells of B cell origin (immunoglobulin genes are rearranged but not expressed) in a tumor mass that is largely polyclonal inflammatory infiltrate, probably a reaction to cytokines produced by the tumor cells. The differential diagnosis of a lymph node biopsy suspicious for Hodgkin's disease includes inflammatory processes, mononucleosis, non-Hodgkin's lymphoma, phenytoin-induced adenopathy, and non-lymphomatous malignancies.

The staging evaluation for a patient with Hodgkin's disease would typically include a careful history and physical examination; complete blood count; erythrocyte sedimentation rate; serum chemistry studies including LDH; chest radiograph; CT scan of the chest, abdomen, and pelvis; and bone marrow biopsy. Many patients would also have a PET scan or a gallium scan. Although rarely utilized, a bipedal lymphangiogram can be helpful. PET and gallium scans are most useful to document remission. Staging laparotomies were once popular for most patients with Hodgkin's disease but are now done rarely because of an increased reliance on systemic rather than local therapy.

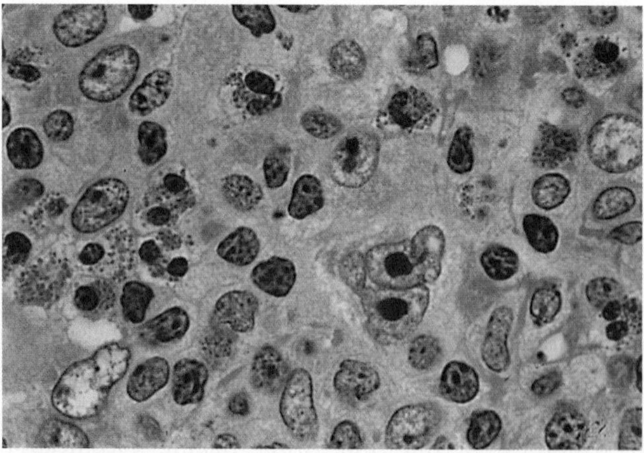

FIGURE 15-11
Mixed-cellularity Hodgkin's disease. A Reed-Sternberg cell is present near the center of the field; this is a large cell with a bilobed nucleus and prominent nucleoli giving an "owl's eyes" appearance. The majority of the cells are normal lymphocytes, neutrophils, and eosinophils that form a pleomorphic cellular infiltrate.

TREATMENT Classical Hodgkin's Disease

Patients with localized Hodgkin's disease are cured >90% of the time. In patients with good prognostic factors, extended-field radiotherapy has a high cure rate. Increasingly, patients with all stages of Hodgkin's disease are treated initially with chemotherapy. Patients with localized or good-prognosis disease receive a brief course of chemotherapy followed by radiotherapy to sites of node involvement. Patients with more extensive disease or those with B symptoms receive a complete course of chemotherapy. The most popular chemotherapy regimens used in Hodgkin's disease include doxorubicin, bleomycin, vinblastine, and dacarbazine (ABVD) and mechlorethamine, vincristine, procarbazine, and prednisone (MOPP) or combinations of the drugs in these two regimens. Today, most patients in the United States receive ABVD, but a weekly chemotherapy regimen administered for 12 weeks called *Stanford V* is becoming increasingly popular, but it includes radiation therapy, which has been associated with life-threatening late toxicities such as premature coronary artery disease and second solid tumors. In Europe, a high-dose regimen called *BEACOPP* incorporating alkylating agents has become popular and might have a better response rate in very high-risk patients. Long-term disease-free survival in patients with advanced disease can be achieved in >75% of patients who lack systemic symptoms and in 60–70% of patients with systemic symptoms.

Patients who relapse after primary therapy of Hodgkin's disease can frequently still be cured. Patients who relapse after initial treatment with only radiotherapy have excellent outcomes when treated with chemotherapy. Patients who relapse after an effective chemotherapy regimen are usually not curable with subsequent chemotherapy administered at standard doses. However, patients with long initial remissions can be an exception to this rule. Autologous bone marrow transplantation can cure half of patients who fail effective chemotherapy regimens.

Because of the very high cure rate in patients with Hodgkin's disease, long-term complications have become a major focus for clinical research. In fact, in some series of patients with early-stage disease, more patients died from late complications of therapy than from Hodgkin's disease itself. This is particularly true in patients with localized disease. The most serious late side effects include second malignancies and cardiac injury. Patients are at risk for the development of acute leukemia in the first 10 years after treatment with combination chemotherapy regimens that contain alkylating agents plus radiation therapy. The risk for development of acute leukemia appears to be greater after MOPP-like regimens than with ABVD. The risk of development of acute leukemia after treatment for Hodgkin's disease is also related to the number of exposures to potentially leukemogenic agents (i.e., multiple treatments after relapse) and the age of the patient being treated, with those aged >60 years at particularly high risk. The development of carcinomas as a complication of treatment for Hodgkin's disease has become a major problem. These tumors usually occur ≥10 years after treatment and are associated with use of radiotherapy. For this reason, young women treated with thoracic radiotherapy for Hodgkin's disease should institute screening mammograms 5–10 years after treatment, and all patients who receive thoracic radiotherapy for Hodgkin's disease should be discouraged from smoking. Thoracic radiation also accelerates coronary artery disease, and patients should be encouraged to minimize risk factors for coronary artery disease such as smoking and elevated cholesterol levels. Cervical radiation therapy increases the risk of carotid atherosclerosis and stroke.

A number of other late side effects from the treatment of Hodgkin's disease are well known. Patients who receive thoracic radiotherapy are at very high risk for the eventual development of hypothyroidism and should be observed for this complication; intermittent measurement of thyrotropin should be made to identify the condition before it becomes symptomatic. Lhermitte's syndrome occurs in ~15% of patients who receive thoracic radiotherapy. This syndrome is manifested by an "electric shock" sensation into the lower extremities on flexion of the neck. Infertility is a concern for all patients undergoing treatment for Hodgkin's disease. In both women and men, the risk of permanent infertility is age-related, with younger patients more likely to recover fertility. In addition, treatment with ABVD rather than MOPP increases the chances to retain fertility.

Nodular lymphocyte-predominant Hodgkin's disease

Nodular lymphocyte-predominant Hodgkin's disease is now recognized as an entity distinct from classical Hodgkin's disease. Previous classification systems recognized that biopsies from a subset of patients diagnosed as having Hodgkin's disease contained a predominance of small lymphocytes and rare Reed-Sternberg cells (Fig. 15-11). A subset of these patients have tumors with nodular growth pattern and a clinical course that varied from that of patients with classical Hodgkin's disease. This is an unusual clinical entity and represents <5% of cases of Hodgkin's disease.

Nodular lymphocyte-predominant Hodgkin's disease has a number of characteristics that suggest its relationship to non-Hodgkin's lymphoma. These include a clonal proliferation of B cells and a distinctive immunophenotype; tumor cells express J chain and display CD45 and epithelial membrane antigen (EMA) and do not express two markers normally found on Reed-Sternberg cells, CD30 and CD15. This lymphoma tends to have a chronic, relapsing course and sometimes transforms to diffuse large B cell lymphoma.

The treatment of patients with nodular lymphocyte-predominant Hodgkin's disease is controversial. Some clinicians favor no treatment and merely close follow-up. In the United States, most physicians will treat localized disease with radiotherapy and disseminated disease with regimens utilized for patients with classical Hodgkin's disease. Regardless of the therapy utilized, most series report a long-term survival rate of >80%.

LYMPHOMA-LIKE DISORDERS

The most common condition that pathologists and clinicians might confuse with lymphoma is reactive, atypical lymphoid hyperplasia. Patients might have localized or disseminated lymphadenopathy and might have the systemic symptoms characteristic of lymphoma. Underlying causes include a drug reaction to phenytoin or carbamazepine. Immune disorders such as rheumatoid arthritis and lupus erythematosus, viral infections such as cytomegalovirus and EBV, and bacterial infections such as cat-scratch disease may cause adenopathy (Chap. 4). In the absence of a definitive diagnosis after initial biopsy, continued follow-up, further testing, and repeated biopsies, if necessary, are the appropriate approach rather than instituting therapy.

Specific conditions that can be confused with lymphoma include *Castleman's disease*, which can present with localized or disseminated lymphadenopathy; some patients have systemic symptoms. The disseminated form is often accompanied by anemia and polyclonal hypergammaglobulinemia, and the condition has been associated with overproduction of IL-6 possibly produced by human herpesvirus 8. Patients with localized disease can be treated effectively with local therapy, while the initial treatment for patients with disseminated disease is usually with systemic glucocorticoids. IL-6-directed therapy is being developed.

Sinus histiocytosis with massive lymphadenopathy (Rosai-Dorfman's disease) usually presents with bulky lymphadenopathy in children or young adults. The disease is usually nonprogressive and self-limited, but patients can manifest autoimmune hemolytic anemia.

Lymphomatoid papulosis is a cutaneous lymphoproliferative disorder that is often confused with anaplastic large cell lymphoma involving the skin. The cells of lymphomatoid papulosis are similar to those seen in lymphoma and stain for CD30, and T cell receptor gene rearrangements are sometimes seen. However, the condition is characterized by waxing and waning skin lesions that usually heal, leaving small scars. In the absence of effective communication between the clinician and the pathologist regarding the clinical course in the patient, this disease will be misdiagnosed. Since the clinical picture is usually benign, misdiagnosis is a serious mistake.

ACKNOWLEDGMENT

James Armitage was a coauthor of this chapter in prior editions of Harrison's Principles of Internal Medicine, and substantial material from those editions has been included here.

CHAPTER 16

LESS COMMON HEMATOLOGIC MALIGNANCIES

Dan L. Longo

The most common lymphoid malignancies are discussed in Chap. 15, myeloid leukemias in Chap. 14, myelodysplastic syndromes in Chap. 11, and myeloproliferative syndromes in Chap. 13. This chapter will focus on the more unusual forms of hematologic malignancy. The diseases discussed here are listed in Table 16-1. Each of these entities accounts for less than 1% of hematologic neoplasms.

LYMPHOID MALIGNANCIES

Precursor B cell and precursor T cell neoplasms are discussed in Chap. 15. All the lymphoid tumors discussed here are mature B cell or T cell, natural killer (NK) cell neoplasms.

MATURE B CELL NEOPLASMS

B cell prolymphocytic leukemia (B-PLL)

This is a malignancy of medium-sized (about twice the size of a normal small lymphocyte), round lymphocytes with a prominent nucleolus and light blue cytoplasm on Wright's stain. It dominantly affects the blood, bone marrow, and spleen and usually does not cause adenopathy. The median age of affected patients is 70 years, and men are more often affected than women (male:female ratio is 1.6). This entity is distinct from chronic lymphoid leukemia (CLL) and does not develop as a consequence of that disease.

The clinical presentation is generally from symptoms of splenomegaly or incidental detection of an elevated white blood cell (WBC) count. The clinical course can be rapid. The cells express surface IgM (with or without IgD) and typical B cell markers (CD19, CD20, CD22). CD23 is absent, and about one-third of cases express CD5. The CD5 expression along with the presence of the t(11;14) translocation in 20% of cases leads to confusion in distinguishing B-PLL from the leukemic form of mantle cell lymphoma. No reliable criteria for the distinction have emerged. About half of patients have mutation or loss of p53, and deletions have been noted in 11q23 and 13q14. Nucleoside analogues such as fludarabine and cladribine and combination chemotherapy (cyclophosphamide, doxorubicin, vincristine, prednisone, or CHOP) have produced responses. CHOP plus rituximab may be more effective than CHOP alone, but the disease is sufficiently rare that large series have not been reported. Splenectomy can produce palliation of symptoms but appears to have little or no impact on the course of the disease.

Splenic marginal zone lymphoma (SMZL)

This tumor of mainly small lymphocytes originates in the marginal zone of the spleen white pulp, grows to efface the germinal centers and mantle, and invades the red pulp. Splenic hilar nodes, bone marrow, and peripheral blood may be involved. The circulating tumor cells have short surface villi and are called *villous lymphocytes*. Table 16-2 shows differences in tumor cells of a number of neoplasms of small lymphocytes that aid in the differential diagnosis. SMZL cells express surface immunoglobulin and CD20 but are negative for CD5, CD10, and CD103.

The median age of patients with SMZL is the mid fifties, and men and women are equally represented. Patients present with incidental or symptomatic splenomegaly or incidental detection of lymphocytosis in the peripheral blood with villous lymphocytes. Autoimmune anemia or thrombocytopenia may be present. The immunoglobulin produced by these cells contains somatic mutations that reflect transit through a germinal

TABLE 16-1

UNUSUAL LYMPHOID AND MYELOID MALIGNANCIES

Lymphoid
Mature B cell neoplasms
B cell prolymphocytic leukemia
Splenic marginal zone lymphoma
Hairy cell leukemia
Nodal marginal zone B cell lymphoma
Mediastinal large B cell lymphoma
Intravascular large B cell lymphoma
Primary effusion lymphoma
Lymphomatoid granulomatosis
Mature T cell and NK cell neoplasms
T cell prolymphocytic leukemia
T cell large granular lymphocytic leukemia
Aggressive NK cell leukemia
Extranodal NK/T cell lymphoma, nasal type
Enteropathy-type T cell lymphoma
Hepatosplenic T cell lymphoma
Subcutaneous panniculitis-like T cell lymphoma
Blastic NK cell lymphoma
Primary cutaneous CD30+ T cell lymphoma
Angioimmunoblastic T cell lymphoma
Myeloid
Chronic neutrophilic leukemia
Chronic eosinophilic leukemia/hypereosinophilic syndrome
Histiocytic and Dendritic Cell Neoplasms
Histiocytic sarcoma
Langerhans cell histiocytosis
Langerhans cell sarcoma
Interdigitating dendritic cell sarcoma
Follicular dendritic cell sarcoma
Mast Cells
Mastocytosis
Cutaneous mastocytosis
Systemic mastocytosis
Mast cell sarcoma
Extracutaneous mastocytoma

center, and ongoing mutations suggest that the mutation machinery has remained active. About 40% of patients have either deletions or translocations involving 7q21, the site of the *CDK6* gene. The genetic lesions typically found in extranodal marginal zone lymphomas (e.g., trisomy 3 and t[11;18]) are uncommon in SMZL.

The clinical course of disease is generally indolent. Long remissions can be seen after splenectomy. A small fraction of patients undergo histologic progression to diffuse large B cell lymphoma with a concomitant change to a more aggressive natural history. Experience with combination chemotherapy in SMZL is limited.

Hairy cell leukemia

Hairy cell leukemia is a tumor of small lymphocytes with oval nuclei, abundant cytoplasm, and distinctive membrane projections (hairy cells). Patients have splenomegaly and diffuse bone marrow involvement. While some circulating cells are noted, the clinical picture is dominated by symptoms from the enlarged spleen and pancytopenia. The mechanism of the pancytopenia is not completely clear and may be mediated by both inhibitory cytokines and marrow replacement. The marrow has an increased level of reticulin fibers; indeed, hairy cell leukemia is a common cause of inability to aspirate bone marrow or so-called "dry tap" (Table 16-3). Monocytopenia is profound and may explain a predisposition to atypical mycobacterial infection that is observed clinically. The tumor cells have strong expression of CD22, CD25, and CD103; soluble CD25 level in serum is an excellent tumor marker for disease activity. The cells also express tartrate-resistant acid phosphatase. The immunoglobulin genes are rearranged and mutated, indicating the influence of a germinal center. No specific cytogenetic abnormality has been found, but most cases contain the activating BRAF mutation V600E.

TABLE 16-2

IMMUNOPHENOTYPE OF TUMORS OF SMALL LYMPHOCYTES

	CD5	CD20	CD43	CD10	CD103	SIG	CYCLIND1
Follicular lymphoma	neg	pos	pos	pos	neg	pos	neg
Chronic lymphoid leukemia	pos	pos	pos	neg	neg	pos	neg
B cell prolymphocytic leukemia	pos	pos	pos	neg	neg	pos	pos
Mantle cell lymphoma	pos	pos	pos	neg	neg	pos	pos
Splenic marginal zone lymphoma	neg	pos	neg	neg	neg	pos	neg
Hairy cell leukemia	neg	pos	?	neg	pos	pos	neg

Abbreviations: neg, negative; pos, positive.

TABLE 16-3

DIFFERENTIAL DIAGNOSIS OF "DRY TAP"—INABILITY TO ASPIRATE BONE MARROW

Dry taps occur in about 4% of attempts and are associated with:	
Metastatic carcinoma infiltration	17%
Chronic myeloid leukemia	15%
Myelofibrosis	14%
Hairy cell leukemia	10%
Acute leukemia	10%
Lymphomas, Hodgkin's disease	9%
Normal marrow	Rare

The median age of affected patients is the mid fifties, and the male:female ratio is 5:1. Treatment options are numerous. Splenectomy is often associated with prolonged remission. Nucleosides including cladribine and deoxycoformycin are highly active but are also associated with further immunosuppression and can increase the risk of certain opportunistic infections. However, after brief courses of these agents, patients usually obtain very durable remissions during which immune function spontaneously recovers. Interferon α is also an effective therapy but is not as effective as nucleosides.

Nodal marginal zone B cell lymphoma

This rare node-based disease bears an uncertain relationship with extranodal marginal zone lymphomas, which are often mucosa-associated and are called mucosa-associated lymphoid tissue or MALT lymphomas, and splenic marginal zone lymphomas. Patients may have localized or generalized adenopathy. The neoplastic cell is a marginal zone B cell with monocytoid features and has been called monocytoid B cell lymphoma in the past. Up to one-third of patients may have extranodal involvement, and involvement of the lymph nodes can be secondary to the spread of a mucosal primary lesion. In authentic nodal primaries, the cytogenetic abnormalities associated with MALT lymphomas (trisomy 3 and t[11;18]) are very rare. The clinical course is indolent. Patients often respond to combination chemotherapy, though remissions have not been durable. Few patients have received CHOP plus rituximab, which is likely to be an effective approach to management.

Mediastinal (thymic) large B cell lymphoma

This entity was originally considered a subset of diffuse large B cell lymphoma; however, additional study has identified it as a distinct entity with its own characteristic clinical, genetic, and immunophenotypic features. This is a disease that can be bulky in size but usually remains confined to the mediastinum. It can be locally aggressive, including progressing to produce a superior vena cava obstruction syndrome or pericardial effusion. About one-third of patients develop pleural effusions, and 5–10% can disseminate widely to kidney, adrenal, liver, skin, and even brain. The disease affects women more often than men (male:female ratio is 1:2–3), and the median age is 35–40 years.

The tumor is composed of sheets of large cells with abundant cytoplasm accompanied by variable, but often abundant, fibrosis. It is distinguished from nodular sclerosing Hodgkin's disease by the paucity of normal lymphoid cells and the absence of lacunar variants of Reed-Sternberg cells. However, more than one-third of the genes that are expressed to a greater extent in primary mediastinal large B cell lymphoma than in usual diffuse large B cell lymphoma are also overexpressed in Hodgkin's disease, suggesting a possible pathogenetic relationship between the two entities that affect the same anatomic site. Tumor cells may overexpress *MAL*. The genome of tumor cells is characterized by frequent chromosomal gains and losses. The tumor cells in mediastinal large B cell lymphoma express CD20, but surface immunoglobulin, and HLA class I and class II molecules may be absent or incompletely expressed. Expression of lower levels of class II HLA identifies a subset with poorer prognosis. The cells are CD5 and CD10 negative but may show light staining with anti-CD30. The cells are CD45 positive, unlike cells of classical Hodgkin's disease.

MACOP-B and R-CHOP are effective treatments, achieving 5-year survival rates of 75–87%. A role for mediastinal radiation therapy has not been definitively demonstrated, but it is frequently used, especially in patients whose mediastinal area remains positron emission tomography avid after four to six cycles of chemotherapy.

Intravascular large B cell lymphoma

This is an extremely rare form of diffuse large B cell lymphoma characterized by the presence of lymphoma in the lumen of small vessels, particularly capillaries. It is also known as malignant angioendotheliomatosis or angiotropic large cell lymphoma. It is sufficiently rare that no consistent picture has emerged to define a clinical syndrome or its epidemiologic and genetic features. It is thought to remain inside vessels because of a defect in adhesion molecules and homing mechanisms, an idea supported by scant data suggesting absence of expression of β-1 integrin and intercellular adhesion molecule 1. Patients commonly present with symptoms of small vessel occlusion, skin lesions, or neurologic symptoms. The tumor cell clusters can promote thrombus formation. In general, the clinical course is aggressive, and the disease is poorly responsive to therapy. Often a diagnosis is not made until very late in the course of the disease.

Primary effusion lymphoma

This entity is another variant of diffuse large B cell lymphoma that presents with pleural effusions, usually without apparent tumor mass lesions. It is most common in the setting of immune deficiency disease, especially AIDS, and is caused by human herpes virus 8 (HHV-8)/Kaposi's sarcoma herpes virus (KSHV). It is also known as body cavity–based lymphoma. Some patients have been previously diagnosed with Kaposi's sarcoma. It can also occur in the absence of immunodeficiency in elderly men of Mediterranean heritage, similar to Kaposi's sarcoma but even less common.

The malignant effusions contain cells positive for HHV-8/KSHV, and many are also co-infected with Epstein-Barr virus (EBV). The cells are large with large nuclei and prominent nucleoli that can be confused with Reed-Sternberg cells. The cells express CD20 and CD79a (immunoglobulin-signaling molecule), though they often do not express immunoglobulin. Some cases aberrantly express T cell markers such as CD3 or rearranged T cell receptor genes. No characteristic genetic lesions have been reported, but gains in chromosome 12 and X material have been seen, similar to other HIV-associated lymphomas. The clinical course is generally characterized by rapid progression and death within 6 months.

Lymphomatoid granulomatosis

This is an angiocentric, angiodestructive lymphoproliferative disease comprised by neoplastic EBV-infected monoclonal B cells accompanied and outnumbered by a polyclonal reactive T cell infiltrate. The disease is graded based on histologic features such as cell number and atypia in the B cells. It is most often confused with extranodal NK–T cell lymphoma, nasal type, which can also be angiodestructive and is EBV related. The disease usually presents in adults (male > female) as a pulmonary infiltrate. Involvement is often entirely extranodal and can include kidney (32%), liver (29%), skin (25%), and brain (25%). The disease often but not always occurs in the setting of immune deficiency.

The disease can be remitting and relapsing in nature or can be rapidly progressive. The course is usually predicted by the histologic grade. The disease is highly responsive to combination chemotherapy and is curable in most cases. Some investigators have claimed that low-grade disease (grade I and II) can be treated with interferon α.

MATURE T CELL AND NATURAL KILLER CELL NEOPLASMS

T cell prolymphocytic leukemia

This is an aggressive leukemia of medium-sized prolymphocytes involving the blood, marrow, nodes, liver, spleen, and skin. It accounts for 1–2% of all small lymphocytic leukemias. Most patients present with elevated WBC count (often >100,000/μL), hepatosplenomegaly, and adenopathy. Skin involvement occurs in 20%. The diagnosis is made from a peripheral blood smear, which shows cells about 25% larger than those in small lymphocytes, with cytoplasmic blebs and nuclei that may be indented. The cells express T cell markers such as CD2, CD3, and CD7; two-thirds of patients have cells that are CD4+ and CD8–, and 25% have cells that are CD4+ and CD8+. T cell receptor β chains are clonally rearranged. In 80% of patients, inversion of chromosome 14 occurs between q11 and q32. Ten percent have t(14;14) translocations that bring the T cell receptor alpha/beta gene locus into juxtaposition with oncogenes *TCL1* and *TCL1b* at 14q32.1. Chromosome 8 abnormalities are also common. Deletions in the *ATM* gene are also noted.

The course of the disease is generally rapid, with a median survival time of about 12 months. Responses have been seen with the anti-CD52 antibody, nucleoside analogs, and CHOP chemotherapy. Small numbers of patients with T cell prolymphocytic leukemia have also been treated with high-dose therapy and allogeneic bone marrow transplantation after remission has been achieved with conventional-dose therapy.

T cell large granular lymphocytic leukemia

T cell large granular lymphocytic leukemia (LGL leukemia) is characterized by increases in the number of LGLs in the peripheral blood (2000–20,000/μL) often accompanied by severe neutropenia with or without concomitant anemia. Patients may have splenomegaly and frequently have evidence of systemic autoimmune disease, including rheumatoid arthritis, hypergammaglobulinemia, autoantibodies, and circulating immune complexes. Bone marrow involvement is mainly interstitial in pattern, with fewer than 50% lymphocytes on differential count. Usually the cells express CD3, T cell receptors, and CD8; NK-like variants may be CD3–. The leukemic cells often express Fas and Fas ligand.

The course of the disease is generally indolent and dominated by the neutropenia. Paradoxically, immunosuppressive therapy with cyclosporine, methotrexate, or cyclophosphamide plus glucocorticoids can produce an increase in granulocyte counts. Nucleosides have been used anecdotally. Occasionally the disease can accelerate to a more aggressive clinical course.

Aggressive natural killer cell leukemia

NK neoplasms are very rare, and they may follow a range of clinical courses from very indolent to highly aggressive. They are more common in Asians than whites, and the cells frequently harbor a clonal EBV episome. The peripheral blood WBC count is usually not greatly elevated, but abnormal large lymphoid cells with granular cytoplasm are noted. The aggressive form is characterized by symptoms of fever and laboratory abnormalities of pancytopenia. Hepatosplenomegaly is common; node involvement less so. Patients may have hemophagocytosis, coagulopathy, or multiorgan failure. Serum levels of Fas ligand are elevated.

The cells express CD2 and CD56 and do not have rearranged T cell receptor genes. Deletions involving chromosome 6 are common. The disease can be rapidly progressive. Some forms of NK neoplasms are more indolent. They tend to be discovered incidentally with LGL lymphocytosis and do not manifest the fever and hepatosplenomegaly characteristic of the aggressive leukemia. The cells are also CD2 and CD56 positive, but they do not contain clonal forms of EBV and are not accompanied by pancytopenia or autoimmune disease.

Extranodal natural killer/T cell lymphoma, nasal type

Similar to lymphomatoid granulomatosis, extranodal NK/T cell lymphoma tends to be an angiocentric and angiodestructive lesion, but the malignant cells are not B cells. In most cases, they are CD56+ EBV-infected cells; occasionally they are CD56– EBV-infected cytotoxic T cells. They are most commonly found in the nasal cavity. Historically, this illness was called lethal midline granuloma, polymorphic reticulosis, and angiocentric immunoproliferative lesion. This form of lymphoma is prevalent in Asia, Mexico, and Central and South America; it affects males more commonly than females. When it spreads beyond the nasal cavity, it may affect soft tissue, the gastrointestinal tract, or the testis. In some cases, hemophagocytic syndrome may influence the clinical picture. Patients may have B symptoms. Many of the systemic manifestations of disease are related to the production of cytokines by the tumor cells and the cells responding to their signals. Deletions and inversions of chromosome 6 are common.

Many patients with extranodal NK/T cell lymphoma, nasal type, particularly those with localized disease, have excellent antitumor responses with combination chemotherapy regimens. Radiation therapy is often used after completion of chemotherapy. Four risk factors have been defined, including B symptoms, advanced stage, elevated lactate dehydrogenase, and regional lymph node involvement. Patient survival is linked to the number of risk factors: 5-year survival is 81% for 0 risk factors, 64% for 1, 32% for 2, and 7% for 3 or 4. Combination regimens without anthracyclines have been touted as superior to CHOP, but data are sparse. High-dose therapy with stem cell transplantation has been used but its role is unclear.

Enteropathy-type T cell lymphoma

Enteropathy-type T cell lymphoma is a rare complication of long-standing celiac disease. It most commonly occurs in the jejunum or the ileum. In adults, the lymphoma may be diagnosed at the same time as celiac disease, but the suspicion is that the celiac disease was a longstanding precursor to the development of lymphoma. The tumor usually presents as multiple ulcerating mucosal masses but may also produce a dominant exophytic mass or multiple ulcerations. The tumor expresses CD3 and CD7 nearly always and may or may not express CD8. The normal-appearing lymphocytes in the adjacent mucosa often have a similar phenotype to the tumor. Most patients have the HLA genotype associated with celiac disease, HLA DQA1*0501 or DQB1*0201.

The prognosis of this form of lymphoma is typically (median survival is 7 months) poor, but some patients have a good response to CHOP chemotherapy. Patients who respond can develop bowel perforation from responding tumor. If the tumor responds to treatment, recurrence may develop elsewhere in the celiac disease–affected small bowel.

Hepatosplenic T cell lymphoma

Hepatosplenic T cell lymphoma is a malignancy derived from T cells expressing the gamma/delta T cell antigen receptor that affects mainly the liver and fills the sinusoids with medium-size lymphoid cells. When the spleen is involved, dominantly the red pulp is infiltrated. It is a disease of young people, especially young people with an underlying immunodeficiency or with an autoimmune disease that demands immunosuppressive therapy. The use of thiopurine and infliximab is particularly common in the history of patients with this disease. The cells are CD3+ and usually CD4- and CD8-negative. The cells may contain isochromosome 7q, often together with trisomy 8. The lymphoma has an aggressive natural history. Combination chemotherapy may induce remissions, but most patients relapse. Median survival time is about 2 years. The tumor does not appear to respond to reversal of immunosuppressive therapy.

Subcutaneous panniculitis-like T cell lymphoma

Subcutaneous panniculitis-like T cell lymphoma involves multiple subcutaneous collections of neoplastic T cells that are usually cytotoxic cells in phenotype (i.e., contain perforin and granzyme B and express CD3 and CD8). The rearranged T cell receptor is usually alpha/beta-derived but occasionally the gamma/delta receptors are involved, particularly in the setting of immunosuppression. The cells are negative for EBV.

Patients may have a hemophagocytic syndrome in addition to the skin infiltration; fever and hepatosplenomegaly may also be present. Nodes are generally not involved. Patients frequently respond to combination chemotherapy, including CHOP. When the disease is progressive, the hemophagocytic syndrome can be a component of a fulminant downhill course. Effective therapy can reverse the hemophagocytic syndrome.

Blastic NK cell lymphoma

The neoplastic cells express NK cell markers, especially CD56, and are CD3 negative. They are large blastic-appearing cells and may produce a leukemia picture, but the dominant site of involvement is the skin. Morphologically, the cells are similar to the neoplastic cells in acute lymphoid and myeloid leukemia. No characteristic chromosomal abnormalities have been described. The clinical course is rapid, and the disease is largely unresponsive to typical lymphoma treatments.

Primary cutaneous CD30+ T cell lymphoma

This tumor involves the skin and is composed of cells that appear similar to the cells of anaplastic T cell lymphoma. Among cutaneous T cell tumors, about 25% are CD30+ anaplastic lymphomas. If dissemination to lymph nodes occurs, it is difficult to distinguish between the cutaneous and systemic forms of the disease. The tumor cells are often CD4+, and the cells contain granules that are positive for granzyme B and perforin in 70% of cases. The typical t(2;5) of anaplastic T cell lymphoma is absent; indeed, its presence should prompt a closer look for systemic involvement and a switch to a diagnosis of anaplastic T cell lymphoma. This form of lymphoma has sporadically been noted as a rare complication of silicone on saline breast implants. Cutaneous CD30+ T cell lymphoma often responds to therapy. Radiation therapy can be effective, and surgery can also produce long-term disease control. The 5-year survival rate exceeds 90%.

Angioimmunoblastic T cell lymphoma

Angioimmunoblastic T cell lymphoma is a systemic disease that accounts for about 15% of all T cell lymphomas. Patients frequently have fever; advanced stage, diffuse adenopathy; hepatosplenomegaly; skin rash; polyclonal hypergammaglobulinemia; and a wide range of autoantibodies, including cold agglutinins, rheumatoid factor, and circulating immune complexes. Patients may have edema, arthritis, pleural effusions, and ascites. The nodes contain a polymorphous infiltrate of neoplastic T cells and nonneoplastic inflammatory cells together with proliferation of high endothelial venules and follicular dendritic cells. The most common chromosomal abnormalities are trisomy 3, trisomy 5, and an extra X chromosome. Aggressive combination chemotherapy can induce regressions. The underlying immune defects make conventional lymphoma treatments more likely to produce infectious complications.

MYELOID MALIGNANCIES

CHRONIC NEUTROPHILIC LEUKEMIA

Chronic neutrophilic leukemia is a rare myeloproliferative disorder that may be confused with the much more common chronic myeloid leukemia. Patients present with increased peripheral blood neutrophil counts (>25,000/μL) and hepatosplenomegaly, but unlike those with chronic myeloid leukemia, no Philadelphia chromosome or *BCR/ABL* fusion gene is detectable, and immature forms comprise less than 10% of circulating white blood cells. The diagnosis is one of exclusion. One must rule out leukemoid reactions and other myeloproliferative and myelodysplastic syndromes. No morphologic dysplasia of myeloid precursors is present. Some patients with chronic neutrophilic leukemia appear to have an underlying plasma cell disorder, but the relationship between the entities is not defined. In the vast majority of patients, cytogenetic analysis results are normal. The disease course is variable from 1 to 20 years or more. A small number of patients may develop acute leukemia or myelodysplasia. Most have progressive marrow replacement with myeloid cells and crowding out of red cell and platelet precursors. Hydroxyurea can control the WBC count, but this is generally unnecessary even at counts >100,000/μL because, unlike the cells of acute leukemia, the cells of chronic neutrophilic leukemia are not invasive and not likely to cause leukostasis. Patients do not respond to splenectomy, and no therapy has been shown to alter the natural history of the disease.

CHRONIC EOSINOPHILIC LEUKEMIA/ HYPEREOSINOPHILIC SYNDROME

The diagnostic criteria for chronic eosinophilic leukemia/hypereosinophilic syndrome are provided in **Table 16-4**. The presence of eosinophilia is critical, defined as eosinophils ≥1500/μL in blood, increased marrow eosinophils, and myeloblasts <20% in blood or marrow for at least 6 months in the absence of other symptoms requiring more immediate treatment. The eosinophilic disorders are much more common in men than women (9:1). Patients may be totally asymptomatic and have the eosinophilia detected incidentally in routine blood work, or they may have any of a myriad of symptoms, including fever, fatigue, cough, edema, shortness of breath, central nervous system (CNS)

TABLE 16-4

DIAGNOSIS OF CHRONIC EOSINOPHILIC LEUKEMIA AND HYPEREOSINOPHILIC SYNDROME

Required: Persistent eosinophilia ≥1500/μL in blood, increased marrow eosinophils, and myeloblasts <20% in blood or marrow.

1. Exclude all causes of reactive eosinophilia: allergy, parasites, infection, pulmonary disease (e.g., hypersensitivity pneumonitis, Loeffler's syndrome), and collagen vascular diseases
2. Exclude primary neoplasms associated with secondary eosinophilia: T cell lymphomas, Hodgkin's disease, acute lymphoid leukemia, mastocytosis
3. Exclude other primary myeloid neoplasms that may involve eosinophils: chronic myeloid leukemia, acute myeloid leukemia with inv(16) or t(16;16)(p13;q22), other myeloproliferative syndromes, and myelodysplasia
4. Exclude T cell reaction with increased interleukin 5 or other cytokine production

If these entities have been excluded and no evidence documents a clonal myeloid disorder, the diagnosis is hypereosinophilic syndrome.

If these entities have been excluded and the myeloid cells show a clonal chromosome abnormality or some other evidence of clonality and blast cells are present in the peripheral blood (>2%) or are increased in the marrow (but <20%), the diagnosis is chronic eosinophilic leukemia.

dysfunction, muscle aches and pains, itching, abdominal pain, diarrhea, peripheral neuropathy, or rheumatologic findings. The key diagnostic issue is distinguishing clonal eosinophilia, a neoplastic proliferation of eosinophils, from the many entities and drug exposures that can cause secondary eosinophilia. Because of the paucity of markers of eosinophil clonality, the diagnosis tends to be one of exclusion.

The first condition to rule out is eosinophilia accompanying a *FIP1L1-PDGFRA*–associated myeloproliferative disorder. If a mutation is noted in the peripheral blood, patients are treated with imatinib, which inhibits the platelet-derived growth factor receptor activated in this condition. If mutation is absent, a bone marrow analysis is done with cytogenetics looking for a 5q33 (*PDGFRB*), 4q12 (*PDGFRA*), or 8p11.2 (*FGFR1*) translocation. These clonal eosinophilias are part of the clinical picture of myeloid malignancies involving these genes. The platelet-derived growth factor (PDGF) receptor abnormalities predict a favorable response to imatinib, whereas the fibroblast growth factor receptor abnormality is associated with chemotherapy-refractory disease.

If these genetic lesions are absent, peripheral blood lymphocytes are studied for immunophenotype and T cell receptor gene rearrangements. The presence of clonal lymphocytes makes the diagnosis of lymphocyte variant hypereosinophilia and implies a cytokine-driven process. If the peripheral blood T cells are normal, one is left with chronic eosinophilic leukemia/hypereosinophilic syndrome as the diagnosis, and these two related entities are distinguished mainly by peripheral blood and bone marrow blast counts. If the peripheral blood has >2% blasts and the marrow has >5% blasts, chronic eosinophilic leukemia is the diagnosis; if the peripheral blood has <2% blasts and the marrow has <5% blasts, the diagnosis is hypereosinophilic syndrome.

The heart, lungs, and CNS are the organ systems often most affected by eosinophil-mediated tissue damage. Patients should have chest radiographs, echocardiography, and troponin level measured to assess lung and cardiac involvement. In the absence of abnormalities in the PDGF receptors, asymptomatic patients can be observed. When treatment is indicated based on symptoms, glucocorticoids are the initial treatment. Hydroxyurea, interferon α, cladribine, and cyclosporine have also been used. The anti–interleukin 5 antibody mepolizumab is being tested. Responses are noted but are not durable. Anti-CD52 antibody (alemtuzumab) has also produced responses but is profoundly immunosuppressive.

HISTIOCYTIC AND DENDRITIC CELL NEOPLASMS

Tumors derived from histiocytes or dendritic cells are exceedingly rare. Through the past century, a number of disorders have been labeled initially as histiocytic disorders, but upon further study with newer analytic tools, the origin has been found to be nonhistiocytic; often, rare T cell disorders such as anaplastic large cell lymphoma were initially thought to be derived from histiocytes. Histiocytes and macrophages are not cell types that routinely circulate; therefore, neoplasms derived from them tend to produce localized tumor masses in the site of origin. The range of markers that characterize these cells is not as broad as those available for lymphocyte subsets. However, the four main types of macrophages and dendritic cells have some distinguishing features. Langerhans cells are bone marrow–derived and reside in the skin; their main function is to present antigen to T cells. They are major histocompatibility class (MHC) class II, Fc receptor, and S100 protein positive; they express CD4 and CD1a, and they are not phagocytosing cells. They contain distinctive morphologic features such as Birbeck granules, rod or tennis racket–shaped structures of uncertain function. Interdigitating dendritic cells are also bone marrow–derived antigen-presenting cells, and they can be in any tissue. They are MHC class II and S100 positive but do not express other known markers. Follicular dendritic cells appear to be derived from a mesenchymal stem cell and reside in lymph node follicles; they present antigen to B cells. They are CD21 and CD35 positive and CD68 and CD45 negative. Macrophages are also CD21 and CD38 positive, but they express CD68 and are phagocytic and express lysozyme.

HISTIOCYTIC SARCOMA

This is a tumor of histiocytes or macrophages that may present as a solitary mass with or without systemic symptoms of fever and weight loss. The tumor is composed of sheets of large cells effacing the tissue architecture. The cells resemble the cells of diffuse large B cell lymphoma, but they do not express lymphocyte markers and are CD68, lysozyme, CD11c, and CD14 positive. The tumor is not highly responsive to treatment, and the natural history is usually aggressive.

LANGERHANS CELL HISTIOCYTOSIS

Langerhans cell histiocytosis is a disease of childhood that has been called histiocytosis X, Letterer-Siwe disease, Hand-Schuller-Christian disease, and eosinophilic granuloma. Patients with Langerhans cell histiocytosis are at increased risk for acute lymphoid leukemia or other lymphoid malignancy. Three clinical syndromes are recognized. Solitary bone lesions, particularly those involving the skull, femur, pelvis, or ribs, are frequently called eosinophilic granuloma. The presence of multiple lesions affecting a single tissue, most often bone, is called Hand-Schuller-Christian disease. The presence of multiple lesions in multiple organs, including bones, skin, liver, spleen, and nodes, is called Letterer-Siwe disease. The characteristic Birbeck granules are pathognomonic but only visible on electron microscopy. The clinical course tends to be inversely related to the number of lesions. Patients with solitary lesions may progress to multiple lesion and multiorgan involvement in 10% of cases; however, most patients respond to chemotherapy. Long-term survival is seen in 70–90% of cases.

LANGERHANS CELL SARCOMA

Langerhans cell sarcoma is distinguished from Langerhans cell histiocytosis by the presence of a high degree of cellular atypia; it can arise de novo or progress from prior Langerhans cell histiocytosis. The natural history is more aggressive, but the disease is responsive to treatment, and the long-term survival rate is about 50%.

INTERDIGITATING DENDRITIC CELL SARCOMA

Interdigitating dendritic cell sarcoma is a proliferation of spindle- to ovoid-shaped cells that usually present in lymph nodes but also can form skin nodules. The initial mass is usually asymptomatic, but fatigue, fever, or night sweats may accompany the lesion. The cells express S100 and are negative for follicular dendritic cell markers such as CD21 and CD35. The clinical course is variable. Localized disease is curable with local therapy.

FOLLICULAR DENDRITIC CELL SARCOMA

Follicular dendritic cell sarcoma is a tumor of follicular dendritic cells that originates in lymph nodes in about two-thirds of cases, usually cervical nodes. Extranodal sites may also be involved. The presentation is usually a slow-growing painless mass. The microscopic anatomy of the tumor is similar to that of the interdigitating dendritic cell tumors, but the tumor cells express different markers (i.e., they are CD21 and CD35 positive and negative for CD1a). The tumor is typically indolent and can be controlled with surgery. There is no clear role for radiation therapy or chemotherapy.

MASTOCYTOSIS

Mastocytosis is a proliferation and accumulation of mast cells in one or more organ systems. In about 80% of cases, only the skin is involved. In the other 20%, the skin and at least one other organ system are involved.

CUTANEOUS MASTOCYTOSIS

Three major variants of cutaneous mastocytosis are described: (1) urticaria pigmentosa, the most common form, is a maculopapular pigmented rash affecting the papillary dermis; (2) diffuse cutaneous mastocytosis, occurring rarely but almost entirely in children, does not produce the maculopapular rash; instead, the skin is relatively smooth but may be red or thickened and on biopsy have infiltration in the papillary and reticular dermis with mast cells; (3) mastocytoma of skin, a single lesion, most often on the trunk or wrist, in which a tumor mass composed of mast cells forms.

SYSTEMIC MASTOCYTOSIS

Clinical manifestations of systemic mastocytosis may be mediated either by the infiltration of organs with mast cells or the release of mediators from the mast cells, including proteases, histamine, eicosanoids, or heparin. The signs and symptoms can be grouped into the following categories: (1) constitutional symptoms (fatigue, fever, weight loss, sweats), (2) skin manifestations of mast cell infiltration (pruritus, urticaria, rash, dermatographism), (3) mediator-related symptoms (abdominal pain, flushing, syncope, hypertension, headache, tachycardia, diarrhea), and (4) bone-related symptoms (fracture, pain, arthralgia). Patients may have splenomegaly, anemia, and either increases or decreases in platelet count and white blood cell count. Bone marrow involvement is common and can progress to crowd out normal hematopoietic elements. Eosinophilia can be seen to such a marked degree that a primary eosinophilic disorder is suspected. Serum tryptase is a useful marker for mast cell mass. Tryptase levels >20 ng/mL indicate the presence of systemic mastocytosis. Tryptase levels tend to be <15 ng/mL in cutaneous mastocytosis.

In the Mayo Clinic series, 40% of patients with systemic mastocytosis had an associated myeloid neoplasm; in about 45% of these patients, the associated tumor was a myeloproliferative syndrome; in 29%, it was chronic myelomonocytic leukemia and in 23%, it was a myelodysplastic syndrome. Eosinophilia was noted in about one-third of the patients with an associated myeloid neoplasm. The median survival time for patients with systemic mastocytosis and another myeloid neoplasm was about 2 years.

In the absence of a myeloid neoplasm, systemic mastocytosis can have an indolent or an aggressive clinical course. Patients who follow a more indolent course do not have high levels of tryptase or bone marrow mastocytosis, no dysplasia, no hepatosplenomegaly, no skeletal involvement, normal blood counts, and no symptoms of malabsorption with weight loss. Such patients comprised 46% of the Mayo Clinic experience and had a median survival time of 16+ years.

By contrast, about 12% of the Mayo Clinic patients with systemic mastocytosis had an aggressive course. They often had anemia and thrombocytopenia, B symptoms, and hepatosplenomegaly. Their median survival time was about 3.5 years.

However, many of these patients were diagnosed and treated before it became widely known that the majority of patients with systemic mastocytosis have activating mutations of c-KIT, most notably *KIT*D816V. KIT is one of the kinases that are inhibited by imatinib, but this mutation is relatively resistant to its effects. The second- and third-generation inhibitors have not been tested. Interferon α produces response in about half of patients, and the responses last about 1 year. Hydroxyurea may unpack the marrow sufficiently to restore hematopoiesis. Median responses last 2.5 years. Cladribine produced responses in 55% of patients, with responses lasting about 1 year, and is a reasonable first-line therapy.

MAST CELL SARCOMA/LEUKEMIA

Mast cell sarcoma is very rare but consists of a destructive tumor mass composed of atypical-looking immature mast cells. They may appear de novo or in the setting of systemic mastocytosis as a solitary mass that is growing unusually fast compared with other involved sites. When the bone marrow becomes >50% mast cells, one may see circulating mast cells accounting for >10% of the WBC count. This finding permits a diagnosis of mast cell leukemia.

EXTRACUTANEOUS MASTOCYTOMA

These rare tumors of normal-appearing mast cells often present in the lung. The treatment experience is anecdotal.

CHAPTER 17

PLASMA CELL DISORDERS

Nikhil C. Munshi ■ Dan L. Longo ■ Kenneth C. Anderson

The *plasma cell disorders* are monoclonal neoplasms related to each other by virtue of their development from common progenitors in the B lymphocyte lineage. Multiple myeloma (MM), Waldenström's macroglobulinemia, primary amyloidosis (Chap. 18), and the heavy chain diseases comprise this group and may be designated by a variety of synonyms such as *monoclonal gammopathies*, *paraproteinemias*, *plasma cell dyscrasias*, and *dysproteinemias*. Mature B lymphocytes destined to produce IgG bear surface immunoglobulin molecules of both M and G heavy chain isotypes with both isotypes having identical idiotypes (variable regions). Under normal circumstances, maturation to antibody-secreting plasma cells and their proliferation is stimulated by exposure to the antigen for which the surface immunoglobulin is specific; however, in the plasma cell disorders, the control over this process is lost. The clinical manifestations of all the plasma cell disorders relate to the expansion of the neoplastic cells, to the secretion of cell products (immunoglobulin molecules or subunits, lymphokines), and to some extent to the host's response to the tumor.

There are three categories of structural variation among immunoglobulin molecules that form antigenic determinants, and these are used to classify immunoglobulins. *Isotypes* are determinants that distinguish among the main classes of antibodies of a given species and are the same in all normal individuals of that species. Therefore, isotypic determinants are, by definition, recognized by antibodies from a distinct species (heterologous sera) but not by antibodies from the same species (homologous sera). There are five heavy chain isotypes (M, G, A, D, E) and two light chain isotypes (κ, λ). *Allotypes* are distinct determinants that reflect regular small differences between individuals of the same species in the amino acid sequences of otherwise similar immunoglobulins. These differences are determined by allelic genes; by definition, they are detected by antibodies made in the same species. *Idiotypes* are the third category of antigenic determinants. They are unique to the molecules produced by a given clone of antibody-producing cells. Idiotypes are formed by the unique structure of the antigen-binding portion of the molecule.

Antibody molecules are composed of two heavy chains (~50,000 mol wt) and two light chains (~25,000 mol wt). Each chain has a constant portion (limited amino acid sequence variability) and a variable region (extensive sequence variability). The light and heavy chains are linked by disulfide bonds and are aligned so that their variable regions are adjacent to one another. This variable region forms the antigen recognition site of the antibody molecule; its unique structural features form a particular set of determinants, or idiotypes, that are reliable markers for a particular clone of cells because each antibody is formed and secreted by a single clone. Each chain is specified by distinct genes, synthesized separately, and assembled into an intact antibody molecule after translation. Because of the mechanics of the gene rearrangements necessary to specify the immunoglobulin variable regions (VDJ joining for the heavy chain, VJ joining for the light chain), a particular clone rearranges only one of the two chromosomes to produce an immunoglobulin molecule of only one light chain isotype and only one allotype (allelic exclusion). After exposure to antigen, the variable region may become associated with a new heavy chain isotype (class switch). Each clone of cells performs these sequential gene arrangements in a unique way. This results in each clone producing a unique immunoglobulin molecule. In most plasma cells, light chains are synthesized in slight excess, secreted as free light chains, and are cleared by the kidney, but <10 mg of such light chains is excreted per day.

Electrophoretic analysis permits separation of components of the serum proteins (Fig. 17-1). The immunoglobulins move heterogeneously in an electric field and form a broad peak in the gamma region.

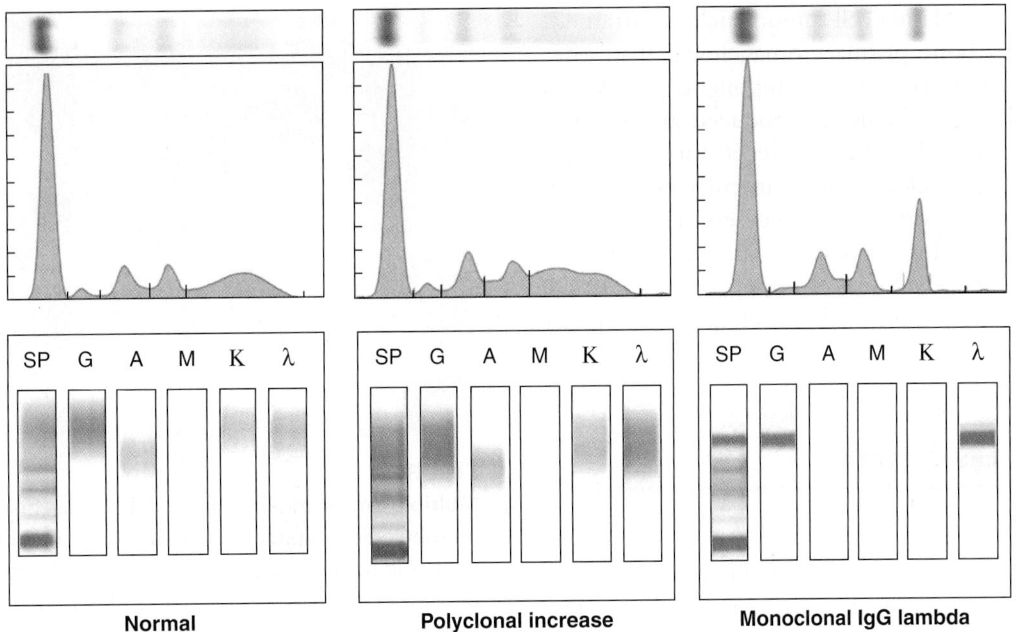

FIGURE 17-1

Representative patterns of serum electrophoresis and immunofixation. The upper panels represent agarose gel, middle The panel are the densitometric tracing of the gel, and lower panels are immunofixation patterns. The panel on the left illustrates the normal pattern of serum protein on electrophoresis. Since there are many different immunoglobulins in the serum, their differing mobilities in an electric field produce a broad peak. In conditions associated with increases in polyclonal immunoglobulin, the broad peak is more prominent (middle panel). In monoclonal gammopathies, the predominance of a product of a single cell produces a "church spire" sharp peak, usually in the γ globulin region (right panel). The immunofixation (lower panel) identifies the type of immunoglobulin. For example, normal and polyclonal increase in immunoglobulins produce no distinct bands; however, the right panel shows distinct bands in IgG and lambda protein lanes, confirming the presence of IgG lambda monoclonal protein.*(Courtesy of Dr. Neal I. Lindeman; with permission.)*

The γ globulin region of the electrophoretic pattern is usually increased in the sera of patients with plasma cell tumors. There is a sharp spike in this region called an *M component* (M for monoclonal). Less commonly, the M component may appear in the β_2 or α_2 globulin region. The monoclonal antibody must be present at a concentration of at least 5 g/L (0.5 g/dL) to be accurately quantitated by this method. This corresponds to ~10^9 cells producing the antibody. Confirmation that such an M component is truly monoclonal and the type of immunoglobulin is determined by immunoelectrophoresis that reveals a single heavy and/or light chain type. Hence immunoelectrophoresis and electrophoresis provide qualitative and quantitative assessment of the M component, respectively. Once the presence of an M component has been confirmed, electrophoresis provides the more practical information for managing patients with monoclonal gammopathies. In a given patient, the amount of M component in the serum is a reliable measure of the tumor burden. This makes the M component an excellent tumor marker, yet it is not specific enough to be used to screen asymptomatic patients. In addition to the plasma cell disorders, M components may be detected in other lymphoid neoplasms such as chronic lymphocytic leukemia and lymphomas of B or T cell origin; nonlymphoid neoplasms such as chronic myeloid leukemia, breast cancer, and colon cancer; a variety of nonneoplastic conditions such as cirrhosis, sarcoidosis, parasitic diseases, Gaucher disease, and pyoderma gangrenosum; and a number of autoimmune conditions, including rheumatoid arthritis, myasthenia gravis, and cold agglutinin disease. At least two very rare skin diseases—lichen myxedematosus, or papular mucinosis, and necrobiotic xanthogranuloma—are associated with a monoclonal gammopathy. In papular mucinosis, highly cationic IgG is deposited in the dermis of patients. This organ specificity may reflect the specificity of the antibody for some antigenic component of the dermis. Necrobiotic xanthogranuloma is a histiocytic infiltration of the skin, usually of the face, that produces red or yellow nodules that can enlarge to plaques. Some 10% progress to myeloma. Five percent of patients with sensory motor neuropathy are associated with monoclonal protein.

The nature of the M component is variable in plasma cell disorders. It may be an intact antibody molecule of any heavy chain subclass, or it may be an altered antibody or fragment. Isolated light or heavy chains may be produced. In some plasma cell tumors such as extramedullary or solitary bone plasmacytomas, fewer than one-third of patients will have an M component. In ~20% of myelomas, only light chains are produced and in most cases are secreted in the urine as Bence Jones proteins. The frequency of myelomas of a particular heavy chain class is roughly proportional to the serum concentration, and therefore IgG myelomas are more common than IgA and IgD myelomas. In approximately 1% of patients with myeloma, biclonal or triclonal gammopathy is observed.

MULTIPLE MYELOMA

DEFINITION

Multiple myeloma represents a malignant proliferation of plasma cells derived from a single clone. The tumor, its products, and the host response to it result in a number of organ dysfunctions and symptoms, including bone pain or fracture, renal failure, susceptibility to infection, anemia, hypercalcemia, and occasionally clotting abnormalities, neurologic symptoms, and manifestations of hyperviscosity.

ETIOLOGY

The cause of myeloma is not known. Myeloma occurred with increased frequency in those exposed to the radiation of nuclear warheads in World War II after a 20-year latency. Myeloma has been seen more commonly than expected among farmers, wood workers, leather workers, and those exposed to petroleum products. A variety of chromosomal alterations with prognostic significance has been found in patients with myeloma; 13q14 deletions, 17p13 deletions, and translocations t(11;14)(q13;q32) and t(4;14)(p16;q32) predominate, and evidence is strong that errors in switch recombination—the genetic mechanism to change antibody heavy chain isotype—participate in the transformation process. However, no common molecular pathogenetic pathway has yet emerged. The neoplastic event in myeloma may involve cells earlier in B cell differentiation than the plasma cell. Interleukin (IL)-6 may play a role in driving myeloma cell proliferation. It remains difficult to distinguish benign from malignant plasma cells on the basis of morphologic criteria in all but a few cases (Fig. 17-2).

INCIDENCE AND PREVALENCE

An estimated 20,180 new cases of myeloma were diagnosed in 2010, and 10,650 people died from the disease in the United States. Myeloma increases in incidence with age. The median age at diagnosis is 70 years; it is

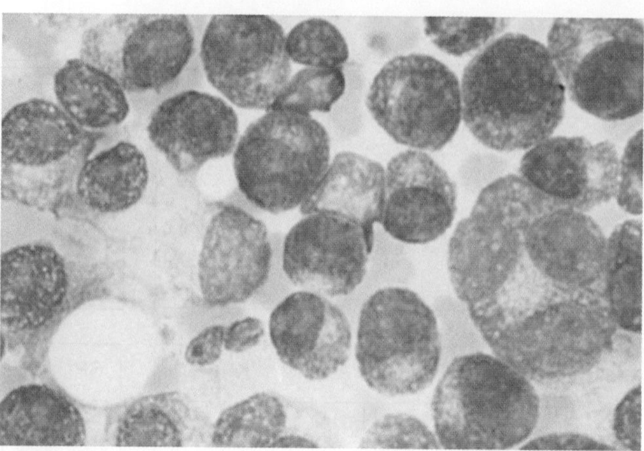

FIGURE 17-2
Multiple myeloma (marrow). The cells bear characteristic morphologic features of plasma cells, round or oval cells with eccentric nuclei composed of coarsely clumped chromatin, a densely basophilic cytoplasm, and a perinuclear clear zone containing the Golgi apparatus. Binucleate and multinucleate malignant plasma cells can be seen.

uncommon before age 40 years. Males are more commonly affected than females, and blacks have nearly twice the incidence of whites. Myeloma accounts for ~1% of all malignancies in whites and 2% in blacks and 13% of all hematologic cancers in whites and 33% in blacks.

GLOBAL CONSIDERATIONS

The incidence of myeloma is highest in African Americans and Pacific islanders; intermediate in Europeans and North American whites; and lowest in developing countries, including Asia. The higher incidence in more developed countries may result from the combination of a longer life expectancy and more frequent medical surveillance. The incidence of MM (MM) in other ethnic groups, including native Hawaiians, female Hispanics, American Indians from New Mexico, and Alaskan natives, is higher relative to U.S. whites in the same geographic area. Chinese and Japanese populations have a lower incidence than whites. Immunoproliferative small intestinal disease with alpha heavy chain disease is most prevalent in the Mediterranean area. Despite these differences in prevalence, the characteristics, response to therapy, and prognosis of myeloma are similar worldwide.

PATHOGENESIS AND CLINICAL MANIFESTATIONS (TABLE 17-1)

MM cells bind via cell-surface adhesion molecules to bone marrow stromal cells (BMSCs) and extracellular matrix (ECM), which triggers MM cell growth, survival,

TABLE 17-1

CLINICAL FEATURES OF MULTIPLE MYELOMA

CLINICAL FINDING	UNDERLYING CAUSE AND PATHOGENETIC MECHANISM
Hypercalcemia, osteoporosis, pathologic fractures, lytic bone lesions, bone pain	Tumor expansion, production of osteoclast activating factor by tumor cells, osteoblast inhibitory factors
Renal failure	Hypercalcemia, light chain deposition, amyloidosis, urate nephropathy, drug toxicity (nonsteroidal anti-inflammatory agents, bisphosphonates), contrast dye
Easy fatigue/anemia	Bone marrow infiltration, production of inhibitory factors, hemolysis, decreased red cell production, decreased erythropoietin levels
Recurrent infections	Hypogammaglobulinemia, low CD4 count, decreased neutrophil migration
Neurologic symptoms	Hyperviscosity, cryoglobulinemia, amyloid deposits, hypercalcemia, nerve compression, antineuronal antibody, POEMS syndrome, therapy-related toxicity
Nausea and vomiting	Renal failure, hypercalcemia
Bleeding/clotting disorder	Interference with clotting factors, antibody to clotting factors, amyloid damage of endothelium, platelet dysfunction, antibody coating of platelet, therapy-related hypercoagulable defects

Abbreviation: POEMS, polyneuropathy, organomegaly, endocrinopathy, multiple myeloma, and skin changes.

drug resistance, and migration in the bone marrow milieu (Fig. 17-3). These effects are due both to direct MM cell–BMSC binding and to induction of various cytokines, including IL-6, insulin-like growth factor type I (IGF-I), vascular endothelial growth factor (VEGF), and stromal cell–derived growth factor (SDF)-1α. Growth, drug resistance, and migration are mediated via Ras/Raf/mitogen-activated protein kinase, PI3-K/Akt, and protein kinase C signaling cascades, respectively.

Bone pain is the most common symptom in myeloma, affecting nearly 70% of patients. The pain usually involves the back and ribs, and unlike the pain of metastatic carcinoma, which often is worse at night, the pain of myeloma is precipitated by movement. Persistent localized pain in a patient with myeloma usually signifies a pathologic fracture. The bone lesions of myeloma are caused by the proliferation of tumor cells, activation of osteoclasts that destroy bone, and suppression of osteoblasts that form new bone. The increased osteoclast activity is mediated by osteoclast activating factors (OAF) made by the myeloma cells (OAF activity can be mediated by several cytokines, including IL-1, lymphotoxin, VEGF, receptor activator of NF-κB [RANK] ligand, macrophage inhibitory factor [MIP]-1α, and tumor necrosis factor [TNF]). The bone lesions are lytic in nature and are rarely associated with osteoblastic new bone formation due to their suppression by dickhoff-1 (DKK-1) produced by myeloma cells. Therefore, radioisotopic bone scanning is less useful in diagnosis than is plain radiography. The bony lysis results in substantial mobilization of calcium from bone, and serious acute and chronic complications of hypercalcemia may dominate the clinical picture (see below). Localized bone lesions may expand to the point that mass lesions may be palpated, especially on the skull (Fig. 17-4), clavicles, and sternum, and the collapse of vertebrae may lead to spinal cord compression.

The next most common clinical problem in patients with myeloma is susceptibility to bacterial infections. The most common infections are pneumonias and pyelonephritis, and the most frequent pathogens are *Streptococcus pneumoniae*, *Staphylococcus aureus*, and *Klebsiella pneumoniae* in the lungs and *Escherichia coli* and other gram-negative organisms in the urinary tract. In ~25% of patients, recurrent infections are the presenting features, and >75% of patients will have a serious infection at some time in their course. The susceptibility to infection has several contributing causes. First, patients with myeloma have diffuse hypogammaglobulinemia if the M component is excluded. The hypogammaglobulinemia is related to both decreased production and increased destruction of normal antibodies. Moreover, some patients generate a population of circulating regulatory cells in response to their myeloma that can suppress normal antibody synthesis. In the case of IgG myeloma, normal IgG antibodies are broken down more rapidly than normal because the catabolic rate for IgG antibodies varies directly with the serum concentration. The large M component results in fractional catabolic rates of 8–16% instead of the normal 2%. These patients have very poor antibody responses, especially to polysaccharide antigens such as those on bacterial cell walls. Most measures of T cell function in myeloma are normal, but a subset of CD4+ cells may be decreased. Granulocyte lysozyme content is low, and granulocyte migration is not as rapid as normal in patients with myeloma, probably the result of a tumor product. There are also a variety of abnormalities in complement functions in myeloma patients. All these factors contribute to the immune deficiency of these patients. Some commonly used therapeutic agents, e.g., dexamethasone, suppress immune responses and increase susceptibility to infection.

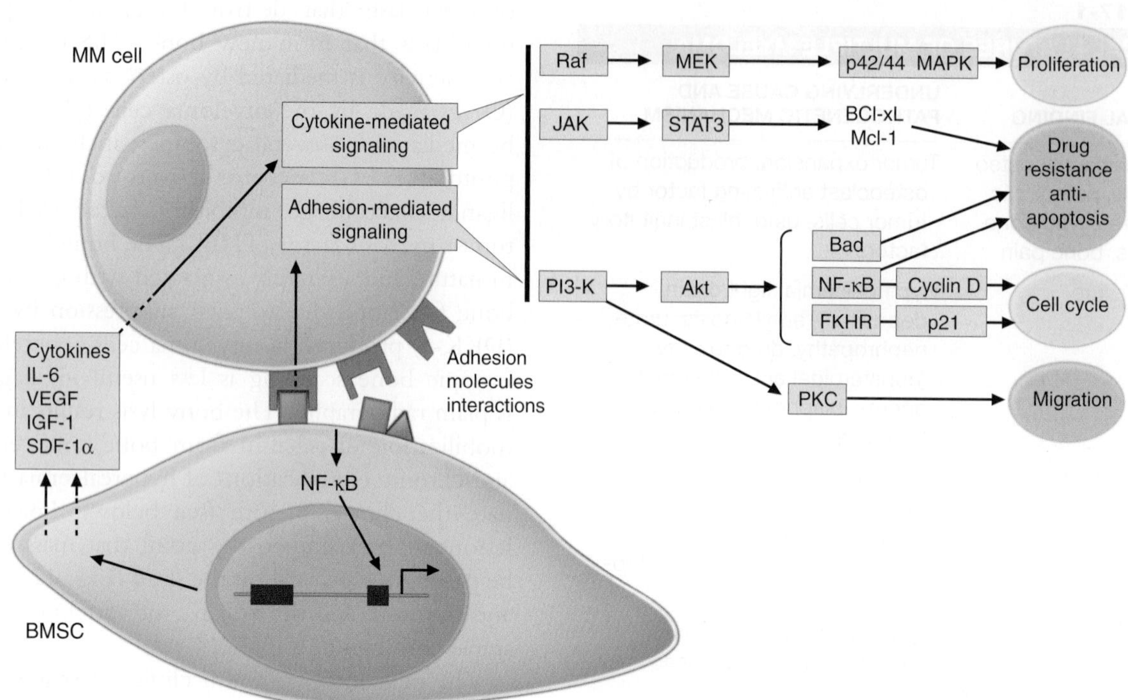

FIGURE 17-3

Pathogenesis of multiple myeloma. Multiple myeloma cells interact with bone marrow stromal cells and extracellular matrix proteins via adhesion molecules, triggering adhesion-mediated signaling as well as cytokine production. This triggers cytokine-mediated signaling that provides growth, survival, and antiapoptotic effects as well as development of drug resistance. HSP, heparin sulfate proteoglycan.

Renal failure occurs in nearly 25% of myeloma patients, and some renal pathology is noted in more than 50%. Many factors contribute to this. Hypercalcemia is the most common cause of renal failure. Glomerular deposits of amyloid, hyperuricemia, recurrent infections, frequent use of nonsteroidal anti-inflammatory agents for pain control, use of iodinated contrast dye for imaging, bisphosphonate use, and occasional infiltration of the kidney by myeloma cells all may contribute to renal dysfunction. However, tubular damage associated with the excretion of light chains is almost always present. Normally, light chains are filtered, reabsorbed in the tubules, and catabolized. With the increase in the amount of light chains presented to the tubule, the tubular cells become overloaded with these proteins, and tubular damage results either directly from light chain toxic effects or indirectly from the release of intracellular lysosomal enzymes. The earliest manifestation of this tubular damage is the adult Fanconi syndrome (a type 2 proximal renal tubular acidosis), with loss of glucose and amino acids, as well as defects in the ability of the kidney to acidify and concentrate the urine. The proteinuria is not accompanied by hypertension, and the protein is nearly all light chains. Generally, very little albumin is in the urine because glomerular function is usually normal. When the glomeruli are involved, nonselective proteinuria is also observed. Patients with myeloma also have a decreased anion gap (i.e., $Na^+ - [Cl^- + HCO_3^-]$) because the M component is cationic, resulting in retention of chloride. This is often accompanied by hyponatremia that is thought to be artificial

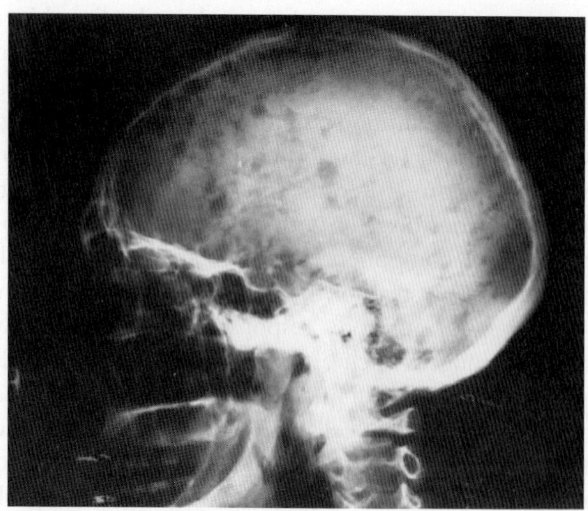

FIGURE 17-4

Bony lesions in multiple myeloma (MM). The skull demonstrates the typical "punched-out" lesions characteristic of MM. The lesion represents a purely osteolytic lesion with little or no osteoblastic activity. *(Courtesy of Dr. Geraldine Schechter; with permission.)*

(pseudohyponatremia) because each volume of serum has less water as a result of the increased protein. Renal dysfunction due to light chain deposition disease, light chain cast nephropathy, and amyloidosis is partially reversible with effective therapy. Myeloma patients are susceptible to developing acute renal failure if they become dehydrated.

Normocytic and normochromic anemia occurs in ~80% of myeloma patients. It is usually related to the replacement of normal marrow by expanding tumor cells, to the inhibition of hematopoiesis by factors made by the tumor, and to reduced production of erythropoietin by the kidney. In addition, mild hemolysis may contribute to the anemia. A larger than expected fraction of patients may have megaloblastic anemia due to either folate or vitamin B_{12} deficiency. Granulocytopenia and thrombocytopenia are very rare except when therapy-induced. Clotting abnormalities may be seen due to the failure of antibody-coated platelets to function properly or to the interaction of the M component with clotting factors I, II, V, VII, or VIII. Deep venous thrombosis is also observed with use of thalidomide or lenalidomide in combination with dexamethasone. Raynaud's phenomenon and impaired circulation may result if the M component forms cryoglobulins, and hyperviscosity syndromes may develop depending on the physical properties of the M component (most common with IgM, IgG3, and IgA paraproteins). Hyperviscosity is defined on the basis of the relative viscosity of serum compared with water. Normal relative serum viscosity is 1.8 (i.e., serum is normally almost twice as viscous as water). Symptoms of hyperviscosity occur at a level greater than 4 centipoise (cP), which is usually reached at paraprotein concentrations of ~40 g/L (4 g/dL) for IgM, 50 g/L (5 g/dL) for IgG3, and 70 g/L (7 g/dL) for IgA.

Although neurologic symptoms occur in a minority of patients, they may have many causes. Hypercalcemia may produce lethargy, weakness, depression, and confusion. Hyperviscosity may lead to headache, fatigue, visual disturbances, and retinopathy. Bony damage and collapse may lead to cord compression, radicular pain, and loss of bowel and bladder control. Infiltration of peripheral nerves by amyloid can be a cause of carpal tunnel syndrome and other sensorimotor mono- and polyneuropathies. Neuropathy associated with monoclonal gammopathy of undetermined significance (MGUS) and myeloma is more frequently sensory than motor neuropathy and is associated with IgM more than other isotypes. Sensory neuropathy is also a side effect of thalidomide and bortezomib therapy.

Many of the clinical features of myeloma, e.g., cord compression, pathologic fractures, hyperviscosity, sepsis, and hypercalcemia, can present as medical emergencies. Despite the widespread distribution of plasma cells in the body, tumor expansion is dominantly within bone and bone marrow and, for reasons unknown, rarely causes enlargement of spleen, lymph nodes, or gut-associated lymphatic tissue.

DIAGNOSIS AND STAGING

The classic triad of myeloma is marrow plasmacytosis (>10%), lytic bone lesions, and a serum and/or urine M component. Bone marrow plasma cells are CD138+ and monoclonal. The most important differential diagnosis in patients with myeloma involves their separation from individuals with MGUS or smoldering multiple myeloma (SMM). MGUS are vastly more common than myeloma, occurring in 1% of the population older than age 50 years and in up to 10% of individuals older than age 75 years. The diagnostic criteria for MGUS, SMM, and myeloma are described in Table 17-2. When bone marrow cells are exposed to radioactive thymidine in order to quantitate dividing cells, patients with MGUS always have a labeling index <1%, whereas patients with myeloma always have a labeling index >1%. Although ~1% per year of patients with MGUS go on to develop myeloma, all myeloma is preceded by MGUS. Non-IgG subtype, abnormal kappa/lambda free light chain ratio, and serum M protein >15 g/L (1.5 g/dL) are associated with a higher incidence of progression of MGUS to myeloma. The features responsible for higher risk of progression from smoldering myeloma to MM are bone marrow plasmacytosis >30%, abnormal kappa/lambda free light chain ratio, and serum M protein >30 g/L (3 g/dL). Typically, patients with MGUS and smoldering myeloma require no therapy. There are two important variants of myeloma, solitary bone plasmacytoma and extramedullary plasmacytoma. These lesions are associated with an M component in <30% of the cases, they may affect younger individuals, and both are associated with median survivals of ≥10 years. Solitary bone plasmacytoma is a single lytic bone lesion without marrow plasmacytosis. Extramedullary plasmacytomas usually involve the submucosal lymphoid tissue of the nasopharynx or paranasal sinuses without marrow plasmacytosis. Both tumors are highly responsive to local radiation therapy. If an M component is present, it should disappear after treatment. Solitary bone plasmacytomas may recur in other bony sites or evolve into myeloma. Extramedullary plasmacytomas rarely recur or progress.

The clinical evaluation of patients with myeloma includes a careful physical examination searching for tender bones and masses. Chest and bone radiographs may reveal lytic lesions or diffuse osteopenia. Magnetic resonance imaging offers a sensitive means to document extent of bone marrow infiltration and cord or root compression in patients with pain syndromes. A complete blood count with differential may reveal anemia. Erythrocyte sedimentation rate is elevated. Rare patients (~2%) may

TABLE 17-2

DIAGNOSTIC CRITERIA FOR MULTIPLE MYELOMA, MYELOMA VARIANTS, AND MONOCLONAL GAMMOPATHY OF UNDETERMINED SIGNIFICANCE

Monoclonal Gammopathy of Undetermined Significance (MGUS)
M protein in serum <30 g/L Bone marrow clonal plasma cells <10% No evidence of other B cell proliferative disorders No myeloma-related organ or tissue impairment (no end-organ damage, including bone lesions)[a]
Asymptomatic Myeloma (Smoldering Myeloma)
M protein in serum ≥30 g/L *and/or* Bone marrow clonal plasma cells ≥10% No myeloma-related organ or tissue impairment (no end-organ damage, including bone lesions)[a] or symptoms
Symptomatic Multiple Myeloma
M protein in serum and/or urine Bone marrow (clonal) plasma cells[b] or plasmacytoma Myeloma-related organ or tissue impairment (end-organ damage, including bone lesions)
Nonsecretory Myeloma
No M protein in serum and/or urine with immunofixation Bone marrow clonal plasmacytosis ≥10% or plasmacytoma Myeloma-related organ or tissue impairment (end-organ damage, including bone lesions)[a]
Solitary Plasmacytoma of Bone
No M protein in serum and/or urine[c] Single area of bone destruction due to clonal plasma cells Bone marrow not consistent with multiple myeloma Normal skeletal survey (and MRI of spine and pelvis if done) No related organ or tissue impairment (no end-organ damage other than solitary bone lesion)[a]

[a]Myeloma-related organ or tissue impairment (end organ damage) (ROTI): calcium levels increased: serum calcium >0.25 mmol/L above the upper limit of normal or >2.75 mmol/L; renal insufficiency: creatinine >173 mmol/L; anemia: hemoglobin 2 g/dL below the lower limit of normal or hemoglobin <10 g/dL; bone lesions: lytic lesions or osteoporosis with compression fractures (magnetic resonance imaging [MRI] or computed tomography may clarify); other: symptomatic hyperviscosity, amyloidosis, recurrent bacterial infections (>2 episodes in 12 months).

[b]If flow cytometry is performed, most plasma cells (>90%) will show a "neoplastic" phenotype.

[c]A small M component may sometimes be present.

have plasma cell leukemia with >2000 plasma cells/μL. This may be seen in disproportionate frequency in IgD (12%) and IgE (25%) myelomas. Serum calcium, urea nitrogen, creatinine, and uric acid levels may be elevated. Protein electrophoresis and measurement of serum immunoglobulins and free light chains are useful for detecting and characterizing M spikes, supplemented by immunoelectrophoresis, which is especially sensitive for identifying low concentrations of M components not detectable by protein electrophoresis. A 24-h urine specimen is necessary to quantitate Bence Jones protein excretion. Serum alkaline phosphatase is usually normal even with extensive bone involvement because of the absence of osteoblastic activity. It is also important to quantitate serum β_2-microglobulin (see later discussion).

The serum M component will be IgG in 53% of patients, IgA in 25%, and IgD in 1%; 20% of patients will have only light chains in serum and urine. Dipsticks for detecting proteinuria are not reliable at identifying light chains, and the heat test for detecting Bence Jones protein is falsely negative in ~50% of patients with light chain myeloma. Fewer than 1% of patients have no identifiable M component; these patients usually have light chain myeloma in which renal catabolism has made the light chains undetectable in the urine. In most of these patients, light chains can now be detected by serum free light chain assay. IgD myeloma may also present as light chain myeloma. About two-thirds of patients with serum M components also have urinary light chains. The light chain isotype may have an impact on survival. Patients secreting lambda light chains have a significantly shorter overall survival than those secreting kappa light chains. Whether this is due to some genetically important determinant of cell proliferation or because lambda light chains are more likely to cause renal damage and form amyloid than are kappa light chains is unclear. The heavy chain isotype may have an impact on patient management as well. About half of patients with IgM paraproteins develop hyperviscosity compared with only 2–4% of patients with IgA and IgG M components. Among IgG myelomas, the IgG3 subclass has the highest tendency to form both concentration- and temperature-dependent aggregates, leading to hyperviscosity and cold agglutination at lower serum concentrations.

The staging systems for patients with myeloma (Table 17-3) are functional systems for predicting survival and are based on a variety of clinical and laboratory tests, unlike the anatomic staging systems for solid tumors. The Durie-Salmon staging system used previously has been found not to predict prognosis after

TABLE 17-3

INTERNATIONAL STAGING SYSTEM

	STAGE[a]	MEDIAN SURVIVAL, MONTHS
β_2M < 3.5, alb ≥ 3.5	I (28%)	62
β_2M < 3.5, alb < 3.5 *or* β_2M = 3.5–5.5	II (39%)	44
β_2M > 5.5	III (33%)	29

[a](#), % patients presenting at each stage.

Abbreviations: alb, serum albumin in g/Dl; β_2M, serum β_2-microglobulin in mg/L.

treatment with high-dose therapy or the novel targeted therapies that have emerged.

Serum β_2-microglobulin is the single most powerful predictor of survival and can substitute for staging. β_2-Microglobulin is a protein of 11,000 mol wt with homologies to the constant region of immunoglobulins that is the light chain of the class I major histocompatibility antigens (HLA-A, -B, -C) on the surface of every cell. Patients with β_2-microglobulin levels <0.004 g/L have a median survival of 43 months, and those with levels >0.004 g/L only 12 months. Serum β_2-microglobulin and albumin levels are the basis for a three-stage International Staging System (ISS) (Table 17-3). It is also believed that once the diagnosis of myeloma is firm, histologic features of atypia may also exert an influence on prognosis. High labeling index and high levels of lactate dehydrogenase are also associated with poor prognosis.

Other factors that may influence prognosis are the presence and number of cytogenetic abnormalities; hypodiploidy; chromosome 13q and 17p deletion; translocations t(4;14) and t(14;16); circulating plasma cells; performance status; as well as serum levels of soluble IL-6 receptor, C-reactive protein, hepatocyte growth factor, C-terminal cross-linked telopeptide of collagen I, transforming growth factor (TGF)-β, and syndecan-1. Microarray profiling and comparative genomic hybridization have formed the basis for RNA- and DNA-based prognostic staging systems, respectively. The ISS system is the most widely used method of assessing prognosis (Table 17-3).

TREATMENT Multiple Myeloma

About 10% of patients with myeloma will have an indolent course (smoldering myeloma) demonstrating only very slow progression of disease over many years. Such patients only require antitumor therapy when the disease becomes symptomatic with development of anemia, hypercalcemia, progressive lytic bone lesions, renal dysfunction, a progressive rise in serum myeloma protein levels and/or Bence Jones proteinuria, or recurrent infections. Patients with solitary bone plasmacytomas and extramedullary plasmacytomas may be expected to enjoy prolonged disease-free survival after local radiation therapy to a dose of around 40 Gy. There is a low incidence of occult marrow involvement in patients with solitary bone plasmacytoma. Such patients are usually detected because their serum M component falls slowly or disappears initially only to return after a few months. These patients respond well to systemic therapy.

Patients with symptomatic and/or progressive myeloma require therapeutic intervention. In general, such therapy is of two sorts: systemic therapy to control the progression of myeloma and symptomatic supportive care to prevent serious morbidity from the complications of the disease. Therapy can significantly prolong survival and improve the quality of life for myeloma patients.

The initial standard treatment for newly diagnosed myeloma is dependent on whether or not the patient is a candidate for high-dose chemotherapy with autologous stem cell transplant.

In patients who are transplant candidates, alkylating agents such as melphalan should be avoided since they damage stem cells, leading to a decreased ability to collect stem cells for autologous transplant. Newer agents combined with pulsed glucocorticoids have now become standard of care as induction therapy in newly diagnosed patients. Two phase II studies have combined thalidomide with dexamethasone as initial therapy for newly diagnosed MM in transplant candidates and reported rapid responses in two-thirds of patients while allowing for successful harvesting of peripheral blood stem cells for transplantation. A randomized phase III trial showed significantly higher response rates for thalidomide (200 mg PO qhs) plus dexamethasone (40 mg for 4 days every 2 weeks) compared with dexamethasone alone, setting the stage for use of this combination as standard therapy in newly diagnosed patients. Importantly, novel agents bortezomib, a proteasome inhibitor, and lenalidomide, an immunomodulatory derivative of thalidomide, have similarly been combined with dexamethasone and obtained high response rates (>80%) without compromising stem cell collection for transplantation. Their superior toxicity profile with improved efficacy has made them the preferred agents for induction therapy. Efforts to improve the fraction of patients responding and the degree of response have involved adding agents to the treatment program. Combination of lenalidomide, bortezomib, and dexamethasone achieves close to a 100% response rate, and other similar three-drug combinations (bortezomib, thalidomide, and dexamethasone or bortezomib, cyclophosphamide, and dexamethasone) achieve a >90% response rate. Initial therapy is continued until maximal cytoreduction.

In patients who are not transplant candidates, besides the options available for transplant candidates, therapy consisting of intermittent pulses of an alkylating agent, melphalan with prednisone, has been utilized. The usual doses of melphalan/prednisone (MP) are melphalan, 0.25 mg/kg per day, and prednisone, 1 mg/kg per day for 4 days. Doses may need adjustment due to unpredictable absorption and based on marrow tolerance. However, a number of studies have combined novel agents with MP combination and reported superior response and survival outcome. In patients

>65 years old, combining thalidomide with MP (MPT) obtains higher response rates and overall survival compared with MP alone. Similarly, significantly improved response (71 vs 35%) and overall survival (3-year survival 72 vs 59%) were observed with combination of bortezomib with MP compared with MP alone. Lenalidomide added to MP followed by lenalidomide maintenance also prolonged progression-free survival compared with MP alone. These combinations of novel agents with MP also achieve high complete response rates (MPT ~15%; MPV ~30%, MPR ~20%, and MP ~2–4%). Patients responding to therapy generally have a prompt and gratifying reduction in bone pain, hypercalcemia, and anemia and often have fewer infections. Improvement in the serum M component may lag behind the symptomatic improvement. The fall in M component depends on the rate of tumor kill and the fractional catabolic rate of immunoglobulin, which in turn depends on the serum concentration (for IgG). Light chain excretion, with a functional half-life of ~6 h, may fall within the first week of treatment. Since urine light chain levels may relate to renal tubular function, they are not a reliable measure of tumor cell kill; however, improvements in serum free light chain measurement are often seen sooner. Although patients may not achieve complete remission, clinical responses may last long periods of time. The important feature of the level of the M protein is not how far or how fast it falls but the rate of its increase after therapy.

Randomized studies comparing standard-dose therapy to high-dose melphalan therapy (HDT) with hematopoietic stem cell support have shown that HDT can achieve high overall response rates and prolonged progression-free and overall survival; however, few, if any, patients are cured. Although complete responses are rare (<5%) with standard-dose chemotherapy, HDT achieves 25–40% complete responses. In randomized studies, HDT produced better median event-free survival in four of five studies, higher complete response rate in four of five trials, and better overall survival in three of five studies. A randomized study failed to show any significant difference in overall survival between early transplant after induction therapy versus delayed transplant at relapse. These data allow an option to delay transplant, especially with the availability of more agents and combinations. Two successive HDTs (tandem transplants) are more effective than single HDT in the subset of patients who do not achieve a complete or very good partial response to the first transplant. Allogeneic transplants may also produce high response rates, but treatment-related mortality may be as high as 40%. Nonmyeloablative allogeneic transplantation is now under evaluation to reduce toxicity while permitting an immune graft-vs-myeloma effect.

Oral prednisone maintenance therapy was effective in a single trial after standard-dose chemotherapy. Maintenance therapy prolongs remissions following standard-dose regimens as well as HDT. Thalidomide administered post-HDT prolongs relapse-free survival. Phase III studies have demonstrated improved outcome in patients receiving lenalidomide compared with placebo as maintenance therapy after HDT, and another phase III study showed prolonged progression-free survival after MP lenalidomide and lenalidomide maintenance therapy in nontransplant candidates.

Relapsed myeloma can be treated with novel agents, including lenalidomide and/or bortezomib. These agents target not only the tumor cell but also the tumor cell–bone marrow interaction and the bone marrow milieu. These agents in combination with dexamethasone can achieve up to 60% partial responses and 10–15% complete responses in patients with relapsed disease. The combination of bortezomib and liposomal doxorubicin is active in relapsed myeloma. Thalidomide, if not used as initial therapy, can achieve responses in refractory cases. High-dose melphalan and stem cell transplant, if not used earlier, also have activity in patients with refractory disease.

The median overall survival time of patients with myeloma is 7–8 years, with subsets of younger patients surviving more than 10 years. The major causes of death are progressive myeloma, renal failure, sepsis, and therapy-related myelodysplasia. Nearly a quarter of patients die of myocardial infarction, chronic lung disease, diabetes, or stroke—all intercurrent illnesses related more to the age of the patient group than to the tumor.

Supportive care directed at the anticipated complications of the disease may be as important as primary antitumor therapy. The hypercalcemia generally responds well to bisphosphonates, glucocorticoid therapy, hydration, and natriuresis. Calcitonin may add to the inhibitory effects of glucocorticoids on bone resorption. Bisphosphonates (e.g., pamidronate 90 mg or zoledronate 4 mg once a month) reduce osteoclastic bone resorption and preserve performance status and quality of life and decrease bone-related complications and may also have antitumor effects. Osteonecrosis of the jaw and renal dysfunction can occur in a minority of cases. Treatments aimed at strengthening the skeleton, such as fluorides, calcium, and vitamin D, with or without androgens, have been suggested but are not of proven efficacy. Iatrogenic worsening of renal function may be prevented by maintaining a high fluid intake to prevent dehydration and to help excrete light chains and calcium. In the event of acute renal failure, plasmapheresis is ~10 times more effective at clearing light chains than peritoneal dialysis; however, its role in reversing renal failure remains controversial. Importantly, reducing the protein load by effective antitumor therapy with agents such as bortezomib may result in functional improvement. Urinary tract infections should be watched for and treated early. Plasmapheresis may be the treatment of choice for hyperviscosity syndromes. Although pneumococcus is a dreaded pathogen in myeloma patients, pneumococcal polysaccharide vaccines may not elicit an antibody response. Prophylactic administration of IV γ globulin preparations is used in the setting of recurrent serious infections. Chronic oral antibiotic prophylaxis is probably not warranted. Patients developing neurologic symptoms in the lower extremities, severe localized back pain, or problems with bowel and bladder control may need emergency MRI and radiation therapy for cord compression. Most bone lesions respond to analgesics and chemotherapy, but certain painful lesions may respond most promptly to localized radiation. The anemia associated with myeloma may respond to erythropoietin along with hematinics (iron, folate, cobalamin). The pathogenesis of the anemia should be established and specific therapy instituted when possible.

WALDENSTRÖM'S MACROGLOBULINEMIA

In 1948, Waldenström described a malignancy of lymphoplasmacytoid cells that secreted IgM. In contrast to myeloma, the disease was associated with lymphadenopathy and hepatosplenomegaly, but the major clinical manifestation was the hyperviscosity syndrome. The disease resembles the related diseases chronic lymphocytic leukemia, myeloma, and lymphocytic lymphoma. It originates from a post–germinal center B cell that has undergone somatic mutations and antigenic selection in the lymphoid follicle and has the characteristics of an IgM-bearing memory B cell. Waldenström's macroglobulinemia and IgM myeloma follow a similar clinical course, but therapeutic options are different. The diagnosis of IgM myeloma is usually reserved for patients with lytic bone lesions and predominant infiltration with CD138+ plasma cells in the bone marrow. Such patients are at greater risk of pathologic fractures than patients with Waldenström's macroglobulinemia.

The cause of macroglobulinemia is unknown. The disease is similar to myeloma in being slightly more common in men and occurring with an increased incidence with age (median, 64 years). There have been reports that the IgM in some patients with macroglobulinemia may have specificity for myelin-associated glycoprotein (MAG), a protein that has been associated with demyelinating disease of the peripheral nervous system and may be lost earlier and to a greater extent than the better known myelin basic protein in patients with multiple sclerosis. Sometimes patients with macroglobulinemia develop a peripheral neuropathy, and half of these patients are positive for anti-MAG antibody. The neuropathy may precede the appearance of the neoplasm. There is speculation that the whole process begins with a viral infection that may elicit an antibody response that cross-reacts with a normal tissue component.

Similar to myeloma, the disease involves the bone marrow, but unlike myeloma, it does not cause bone lesions or hypercalcemia. Bone marrow shows >10% infiltration with lymphoplasmacytic cells (surface IgM+, CD19+, CD20+, and CD22+, rarely CD5+, but CD10− and CD23−) with an increase in number of mast cells. Similar to myeloma, M component is present in the serum in excess of 30 g/L (3 g/dL), but unlike myeloma, the size of the IgM paraprotein results in little renal excretion, and only ~20% of patients excrete light chains. Therefore, renal disease is not common. The light chain isotype is kappa in 80% of the cases. Patients present with weakness, fatigue, and recurrent infections, similar to myeloma patients, but epistaxis, visual disturbances, and neurologic symptoms such as peripheral neuropathy, dizziness, headache, and transient paresis are much more common in macroglobulinemia. Physical examination reveals adenopathy and hepatosplenomegaly, and ophthalmoscopic examination may reveal vascular segmentation and dilation of the retinal veins characteristic of hyperviscosity states. Patients may have a normocytic, normochromic anemia, but rouleaux formation and a positive Coombs' test result are much more common than in myeloma. Malignant lymphocytes are usually present in the peripheral blood. About 10% of macroglobulins are cryoglobulins. These are pure M components and are not the mixed cryoglobulins seen in rheumatoid arthritis and other autoimmune diseases. Mixed cryoglobulins are composed of IgM or IgA complexed with IgG, for which they are specific. In both cases, Raynaud's phenomenon and serious vascular symptoms precipitated by the cold may occur, but mixed cryoglobulins are not commonly associated with malignancy. Patients suspected of having a cryoglobulin based on history and physical examination should have their blood drawn into a warm syringe and delivered to the laboratory in a container of warm water to avoid errors in quantitating the cryoglobulin.

TREATMENT Waldenström's Macroglobulinemia

Control of serious hyperviscosity symptoms such as an altered state of consciousness or paresis can be achieved acutely by plasmapheresis because 80% of the IgM paraprotein is intravascular. The median survival is ~50 months, similar to that of MM. However, many individuals with Waldenström's macroglobulinemia have indolent disease that does not require therapy. Pretreatment parameters including older age, male sex, general symptoms, and cytopenias define a high-risk population. Fludarabine (25 mg/m^2 per day for 5 days every 4 weeks) or cladribine (0.1 mg/kg per day for 7 days every 4 weeks) are highly effective single agents. About 80% of patients respond to chemotherapy, and their median survival time is >3 years. Rituximab (anti-CD20) can produce responses alone or combined with chemotherapy. As in MM, the introduction of novel agents such as bortezomib, bendamustine, and lenalidomide has improved patient outcome.

POEMS SYNDROME

The features of this syndrome are *p*olyneuropathy, *o*rganomegaly, *e*ndocrinopathy, *M*M, and *s*kin changes (POEMS). Patients usually have a severe, progressive sensorimotor polyneuropathy associated with sclerotic bone lesions from myeloma. Polyneuropathy occurs in ~1.4% of myelomas, but the POEMS syndrome is only a rare subset of that group. Unlike typical myeloma, hepatomegaly and lymphadenopathy occur in about two-thirds of patients, and splenomegaly is seen in one-third. The lymphadenopathy frequently resembles Castleman's disease histologically, a condition that has been linked to IL-6 overproduction. The endocrine manifestations include amenorrhea in women and impotence and gynecomastia in men. Hyperprolactinemia due to loss of normal inhibitory control by the hypothalamus may be associated with other central nervous system manifestations such as papilledema and elevated cerebrospinal fluid pressure and protein. Type 2 diabetes mellitus occurs in about one-third of patients. Hypothyroidism and adrenal insufficiency are occasionally noted. Skin changes are diverse: hyperpigmentation, hypertrichosis, skin thickening, and digital clubbing. Other manifestations include peripheral edema, ascites, pleural effusions, fever, and thrombocytosis. Not all the components of POEMS syndrome may be present initially.

The pathogenesis of the disease is unclear, but high circulating levels of the proinflammatory cytokines IL-1, IL-6, VEGF, and TNF have been documented, and levels of the inhibitory cytokine TGF-β are lower than expected. Treatment of the myeloma may result in an improvement in the other disease manifestations.

Patients are often treated similarly to those with myeloma. Plasmapheresis does not appear to be of benefit in POEMS syndrome. Patients presenting with isolated sclerotic lesions may have resolution of neuropathic symptoms after local therapy for plasmacytoma with radiotherapy. Similar to MM, novel agents as well as high-dose therapy with autologous stem cell transplant have been pursued in selected patients and have been associated with prolonged progression-free survival.

HEAVY CHAIN DISEASES

The heavy chain diseases are rare lymphoplasmacytic malignancies. Their clinical manifestations vary with the heavy chain isotype. Patients have absence of light chain and secrete a defective heavy chain that usually has an intact Fc fragment and a deletion in the Fd region. Gamma, alpha, and mu heavy chain diseases have been described, but no reports of delta or epsilon heavy chain diseases have appeared. Molecular biologic analysis of these tumors has revealed structural genetic defects that may account for the aberrant chain secreted.

GAMMA HEAVY CHAIN DISEASE (FRANKLIN'S DISEASE)

This disease affects individuals of widely different age groups and countries of origin. It is characterized by lymphadenopathy, fever, anemia, malaise, hepatosplenomegaly, and weakness. It is frequently associated with autoimmune diseases, especially rheumatoid arthritis. Its most distinctive symptom is palatal edema, resulting from involvement of nodes in Waldeyer's ring, and this may progress to produce respiratory compromise. The diagnosis depends on the demonstration of an anomalous serum M component (often <20 g/L [<2 g/dL]) that reacts with anti-IgG but not anti–light chain reagents. *The M component is typically present in both serum and urine.* Most of the paraproteins have been of the γ_1 subclass, but other subclasses have been seen. The patients may have thrombocytopenia, eosinophilia, and nondiagnostic bone marrow that may show increased numbers of lymphocytes or plasma cells that do not stain for light chain. Patients usually have a rapid downhill course and die of infection; however, some patients have survived 5 years with chemotherapy. Therapy is indicated when symptomatic and involves chemotherapeutic combinations used in low-grade lymphoma. Rituximab has also been reported to show efficacy.

ALPHA HEAVY CHAIN DISEASE (SELIGMANN'S DISEASE)

This is the most common of the heavy chain diseases. It is closely related to a malignancy known as *Mediterranean lymphoma*, a disease that affects young persons in parts of the world where intestinal parasites are common, such as the Mediterranean, Asia, and South America. The disease is characterized by an infiltration of the lamina propria of the small intestine with lymphoplasmacytoid cells that secrete truncated alpha chains. Demonstrating alpha heavy chains is difficult because the alpha chains tend to polymerize and appear as a smear instead of a sharp peak on electrophoretic profiles. Despite the polymerization, hyperviscosity is not a common problem in alpha heavy chain disease. Without J chain–facilitated dimerization, viscosity does not increase dramatically. Light chains are absent from serum and urine. The patients present with chronic diarrhea, weight loss, and malabsorption and have extensive mesenteric and paraaortic adenopathy. Respiratory tract involvement occurs rarely. Patients may vary widely in their clinical course. Some may develop diffuse aggressive histologies of malignant lymphoma. Chemotherapy may produce long-term remissions. Rare patients appear to have responded to antibiotic therapy, raising the question of the etiologic role of antigenic stimulation, perhaps by some chronic intestinal infection. Chemotherapy plus antibiotics may be more effective than chemotherapy alone. Immunoproliferative small-intestinal disease (IPSID) is recognized as an infectious pathogen–associated human lymphoma that has association with *Campylobacter jejuni*. It involves mainly the proximal small intestine resulting in malabsorption, diarrhea, and abdominal pain. IPSID is associated with excessive plasma cell differentiation and produces truncated alpha heavy chain proteins lacking the light chains as well as the first constant domain. Early-stage IPSID responds to antibiotics (30–70% complete remission). Most untreated IPSID patients progress to lymphoplasmacytic and immunoblastic lymphoma. Patients not responding to antibiotic therapy are considered for treatment with combination chemotherapy used to treat low-grade lymphoma.

MU HEAVY CHAIN DISEASE

The secretion of isolated mu heavy chains into the serum appears to occur in a very rare subset of patients with chronic lymphocytic leukemia. The only features that may distinguish patients with mu heavy chain disease are the presence of vacuoles in the malignant lymphocytes and the excretion of kappa light chains in the urine. The diagnosis requires ultracentrifugation or gel filtration to confirm the nonreactivity of the paraprotein with the light chain reagents because some intact macroglobulins fail to interact with these serums. The tumor cells seem to have a defect in the assembly of light and heavy chains because they appear to contain both in their cytoplasm. There is no evidence that such patients should be treated differently from other patients with chronic lymphocytic leukemia (Chap. 15).

CHAPTER 18

AMYLOIDOSIS

David C. Seldin ■ Martha Skinner

GENERAL PRINCIPLES

Amyloidosis is the term for diseases caused by the extracellular deposition of insoluble polymeric protein fibrils in tissues and organs. These diseases are a subset of a growing group of disorders attributed to misfolding of proteins. Among these are Alzheimer's disease and other neurodegenerative diseases; transmissible prion diseases; and genetic diseases caused by mutations that lead to misfolding, aggregation, and protein loss of function, such as certain of the cystic fibrosis mutations. Amyloid fibrils share a common β-pleated sheet structural conformation that confers unique staining properties. The term *amyloid* was coined by the pathologist Rudolf Virchow around 1854, who thought such deposits were cellulose-like under the microscope.

Amyloid diseases are defined by the biochemical nature of the protein in the fibril deposits and are classified according to whether they are systemic or localized, acquired or inherited, and by their clinical patterns **(Table 18-1)**. The accepted nomenclature is *AX*, where *A* indicates amyloidosis and *X* represents the protein in the fibril. *AL* is amyloid composed of immunoglobulin light chains (LCs) and has been called *primary systemic amyloidosis*; it arises from a clonal B cell disorder and may be associated with myeloma or lymphoma. *AF* groups the *familial amyloidoses*, most commonly due to mutations in transthyretin, the transport protein for thyroid hormone and retinol-binding protein. *AA* amyloid is composed of the acute-phase reactant serum amyloid A protein, occurs in the setting of chronic inflammatory or infectious diseases, and has been termed *secondary amyloidosis*. $A\beta_2M$ is amyloid composed of β_2-microglobulin and occurs in individuals with end-stage renal disease (ESRD) of long duration. *Aβ* is the most common form of localized amyloidosis. Aβ is deposited in the brain in Alzheimer's disease and is derived from abnormal proteolytic processing of the amyloid precursor protein (APP).

Diagnosis and treatment of the amyloidoses rest upon the pathologic diagnosis of amyloid deposits and immunohistochemical or biochemical identification of amyloid type **(Fig. 18-1)**. In the systemic amyloidoses, the involved organs can be biopsied, but amyloid deposits may be found in any tissue of the body. Historically, blood vessels of the gingiva or rectal mucosa were examined, but the most easily accessible tissue, positive in more than 80% of patients with systemic amyloidosis, is fat. After local anesthesia, needle aspiration of fat from the abdominal wall can be expelled onto a slide and stained, avoiding even a minor surgical procedure. If the results for this material is negative, biopsy of kidney, heart, liver, or gastrointestinal tract can be considered. The regular β-sheet structure of amyloid deposits exhibits a unique green birefringence by polarized light microscopy when stained with Congo red dye; the 10-nm-diameter fibrils can be seen directly by electron microscopy of paraformaldehyde-fixed tissue. Once amyloid is found, the protein type must be determined, usually by immunohistochemistry, immunoelectron microscopy, or extraction and biochemical analysis by mass spectrometry or other technique. Careful evaluation of the patient's history, physical findings, and clinical presentation, including age and ethnic origin, organ system involvement, underlying diseases, and family history, can provide helpful clues to the type of amyloid.

The mechanisms of fibril formation and tissue toxicity remain controversial. Factors that contribute to fibrillogenesis include variant or unstable protein structure; extensive β-sheet conformation of the precursor protein; proteolytic processing of the precursor protein; association with components of the serum or extracellular matrix (e.g., amyloid P-component, apolipoprotein E, or glycosaminoglycans); and local physical properties, including pH of the tissue. Monomeric proteins appear to go through an oligomeric aggregation step and then form higher order polymers. Once the polymers reach a critical size, they become insoluble and deposit in

TABLE 18-1

AMYLOID FIBRIL PROTEINS AND THEIR CLINICAL SYNDROMES

TERM	PRECURSOR	CLINICAL SYNDROME	CLINICAL INVOLVEMENT
	Systemic Amyloidoses		
AL	Immunoglobulin light chain	Primary or myeloma associated[a]	Any
AH	Immunoglobulin heavy chain	Primary or myeloma associated (rare)	Any
AA	Serum amyloid A protein	Secondary; reactive[b]	Renal, any
Aβ_2M	β_2-Microglobulin	Hemodialysis associated	Synovial membrane, bone
ATTR	Transthyretin	Familial (mutant) Senile systemic (wild type)	Cardiac, peripheral and autonomic nerves
AApoAI	Apolipoprotein AI	Familial	Hepatic, renal
AApoAII	Apolipoprotein AII	Familial	Renal
AGel	Gelsolin	Familial	Corneas, cranial nerves, renal
AFib	Fibrinogen Aα	Familial	Renal
ALys	Lysozyme	Familial	Renal
ALECT2	Leukocyte chemotactic factor 2	?	Renal
	Localized Amyloidoses		
Aβ	Amyloid β protein	Alzheimer's disease; Down syndrome	CNS
ACys	Cystatin C	Cerebral amyloid angiopathy	CNS, vascular
APrP	Prion protein	Spongiform encephalopathies	CNS
AIAPP	Islet amyloid polypeptide (amylin)	Diabetes associated	Pancreas
ACal	Calcitonin	Medullary carcinoma of the thyroid	Thyroid
AANF	Atrial natriuretic factor	Age related	Cardiac atria
APro	Prolactin	Endocrinopathy	Pituitary

[a]Localized deposits can occur in skin, conjunctiva, urinary bladder, and tracheobronchial tree.
[b] Secondary to chronic inflammation or infection or to a hereditary periodic fever syndrome, e.g., familial Mediterranean fever.
Abbreviation: CNS, central nervous system.

extracellular tissue sites as fibrils. These large macromolecular deposits interfere with organ function and, due to cellular uptake of oligomeric amyloid precursors, may be toxic to target cells.

The clinical syndromes of the amyloidoses are associated with relatively nonspecific alterations in routine laboratory tests. Blood counts are usually normal, although the erythrocyte sedimentation rate is frequently elevated. Patients with renal involvement will usually have proteinuria, which can be as much as 30 g/d, producing hypoalbuminemia that can be profound. Patients with cardiac involvement will often have elevation of brain natriuretic peptide (BNP), pro-BNP, and troponin. These can be useful for monitoring disease activity and have been proposed as prognostic factors; they can be falsely elevated in the presence of renal insufficiency. Patients with liver involvement, even when it is advanced, usually develop cholestasis with an elevated alkaline phosphatase but minimal elevation of the transaminases and preservation of synthetic function. In AL amyloidosis, endocrinopathies can occur, with laboratory testing demonstrating hypothyroidism, hypoadrenalism, or even hypopituitarism. None of these findings are specific for amyloidosis. Thus, a diagnosis of amyloidosis rests upon a tissue biopsy that, after Congo red staining, shows "apple-green" birefringence on polarization microscopy.

AL AMYLOIDOSIS

ETIOLOGY AND INCIDENCE

AL amyloidosis is most frequently caused by a clonal expansion of plasma cells in the bone marrow that secrete a monoclonal immunoglobulin LC that deposits as amyloid fibrils in tissues. It may be purely serendipitous whether the clonal plasma cells produce a LC that misfolds and leads to AL amyloidosis or folds properly, allowing the cells to inexorably expand over time and develop into multiple

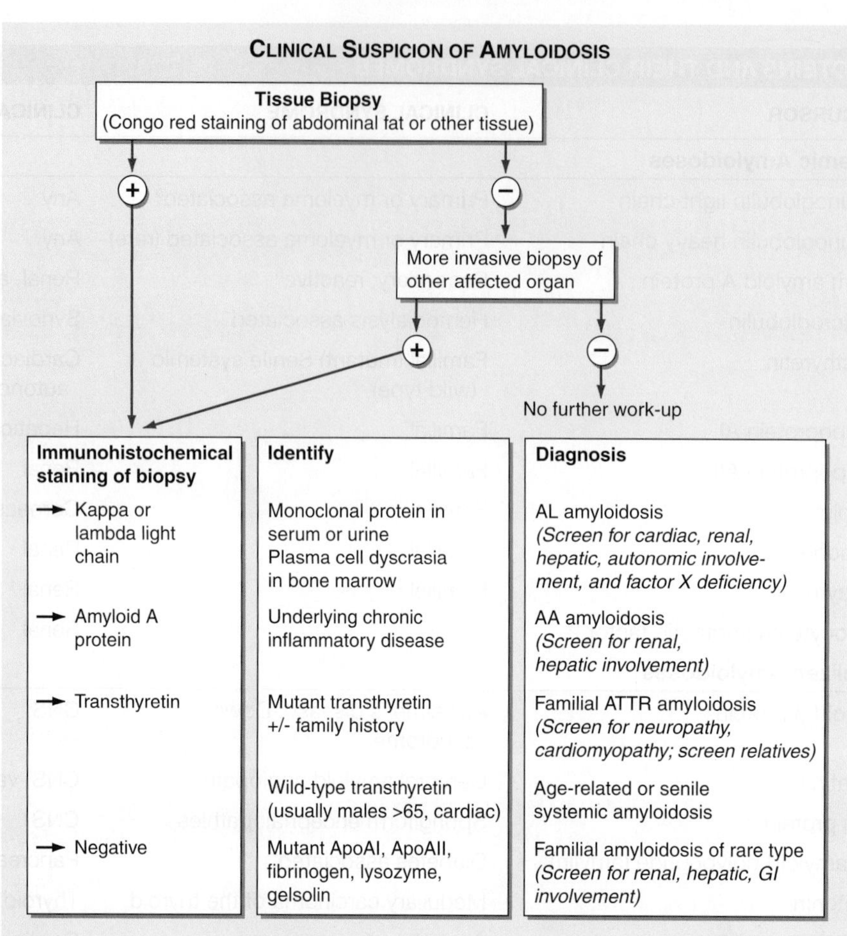

FIGURE 18-1

Algorithm for the diagnosis of amyloidosis and determination of type: Clinical suspicion: unexplained nephropathy, cardiomyopathy, neuropathy, enteropathy, arthropathy, and macroglossia. ApoAI, apolipoprotein AI; ApoAII, apolipoprotein AII; GI, gastrointestinal.

myeloma (Chap. 17). It is also possible that the two processes have diverse molecular etiologies. AL amyloidosis can occur with multiple myeloma or other B lymphoproliferative diseases, including non-Hodgkin's lymphoma (Chap. 15) and Waldenström's macroglobulinemia (Chap. 17). AL amyloidosis is the most common type of systemic amyloidosis in North America. Its incidence has been estimated at 4.5 per 100,000; however, ascertainment continues to be inadequate, and the true incidence may be much higher. AL amyloidosis, like other plasma cell diseases, usually occurs after age 40 years and is often rapidly progressive and fatal if untreated.

PATHOLOGY AND CLINICAL FEATURES OF AL AMYLOIDOSIS

Amyloid deposits are usually widespread in AL amyloidosis and can be present in the interstitium of any organ outside of the central nervous system. The amyloid fibril deposits are composed of intact 23-kDa monoclonal Ig LCs or smaller fragments, 11–18 kDa in size, representing the variable (V) region alone, or the V region and a portion of the constant (C) region. Although all kappa and lambda LC subtypes have been identified in AL amyloid fibrils, lambda subtypes predominate. The lambda 6 subtype appears to have unique structural properties that predispose it to fibril formation, often in the kidney.

AL amyloidosis is usually a rapidly progressive disease that presents with a pleiotropic set of clinical syndromes, recognition of which is key to initiating appropriate workup. Nonspecific symptoms of fatigue and weight loss are common; however, the diagnosis is rarely considered until symptoms referable to a specific organ develop. The kidneys are the most frequently affected organ, in 70–70% of patients. Renal amyloidosis is usually manifested as proteinuria, often in the nephrotic range and associated with significant hypoalbuminemia, secondary hypercholesterolemia, and edema or anasarca. In some patients, tubular rather than glomerular deposition of amyloid can produce azotemia without significant proteinuria.

The heart is the second most commonly affected organ, in 50–50% of patients, and the leading cause of death. Early on, the electrocardiogram may show low voltage in the limb leads, with a pseudo-infarct pattern. Eventually, the echocardiogram will display concentrically thickened ventricles and diastolic dysfunction, leading to a restrictive cardiomyopathy; systolic function is preserved until late in the disease. A "sparkly" appearance is usually not seen using modern high-resolution echocardiography equipment. Cardiac magnetic resonance imaging can show an increased wall thickness and a characteristic subendocardial enhancement with gadolinium. Nervous system symptoms include a peripheral sensory neuropathy and/or autonomic dysfunction with gastrointestinal motility disturbances (early satiety, diarrhea, constipation) and orthostatic hypotension. Macroglossia, with an enlarged, indented, or immobile tongue, is pathognomonic of AL amyloidosis but is seen only in ~10% of patients. Liver involvement causes cholestasis and hepatomegaly. The spleen is frequently involved, and there may be functional hyposplenism in the absence of significant splenomegaly. Many patients have "easy bruising" due to amyloid deposits in capillaries or to deficiency of clotting factor X, which can bind to amyloid fibrils; cutaneous ecchymoses appear, particularly around the eyes, giving the "raccoon-eye" sign. Other findings include nail dystrophy, alopecia, and amyloid arthropathy with thickening of synovial membranes in the wrists and shoulders (Fig. 18-2). The presence of a multisystem illness or general fatigue along with any of these clinical syndromes should prompt a workup for amyloidosis.

DIAGNOSIS

Identification of the underlying B lymphoproliferative process and clonal LC is key to the diagnosis of AL amyloidosis. The serum protein electrophoresis (SPEP) and urine protein electrophoresis (UPEP) are NOT useful screening tests if AL amyloidosis is suspected because the clonal LC or whole immunoglobulin, unlike in multiple myeloma, is often not present in sufficient quantity in the serum to produce a monoclonal "M-spike" or in the urine to cause LC (Bence Jones) proteinuria. However, more than 90% of patients have a serum or urine monoclonal LC or whole immunoglobulin that can be detected by immunofixation electrophoresis of serum (SIFE) or urine (UIFE) (Fig. 18-3*A*). Assaying for free immunoglobulin LCs circulating in the serum unbound to heavy chains using commercially available nephelometric (FreeLite©) assay demonstrates an elevation and abnormal free kappa:lambda ratio in more than 75% of patients. Examining the ratio as well as the absolute amount is essential, because in renal insufficiency LC clearance is reduced, and both types of LCs will be elevated. In addition, an increased percentage of plasma cells in the bone marrow, typically 5–30% of nucleated cells, is noted in about 90% of patients. Kappa or lambda clonality can be demonstrated by flow cytometry, immunohistochemical staining, or in situ hybridization for LC mRNA (Fig. 18-3*B*).

A monoclonal serum protein by itself is not diagnostic of amyloidosis, since monoclonal gammopathy of uncertain significance (MGUS) is common in older patients (Chap. 17). However, when MGUS is present in patients with biopsy-proven amyloidosis, the AL type should be strongly suspected. Similarly, patients thought to have "smoldering myeloma" because of modest elevation of bone marrow plasma cells should be screened for AL amyloidosis if they have evidence of organ dysfunction. Accurate typing is essential for appropriate treatment. Immunohistochemical staining of the amyloid deposits is useful if they bind one light chain antibody in preference to the other; some AL deposits bind many antisera nonspecifically. Immunoelectron microscopy is more reliable, and mass-spectrometry-based microsequencing of small amounts of protein extracted from fibril deposits can also be done. In ambiguous cases, other forms of amyloidosis should be thoroughly excluded with appropriate genetic and other testing.

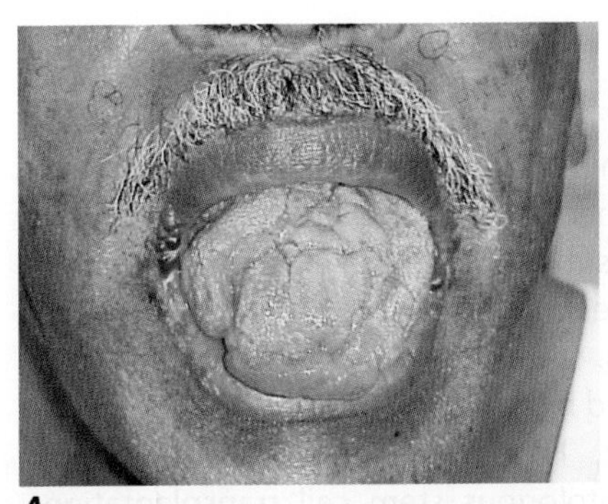
A

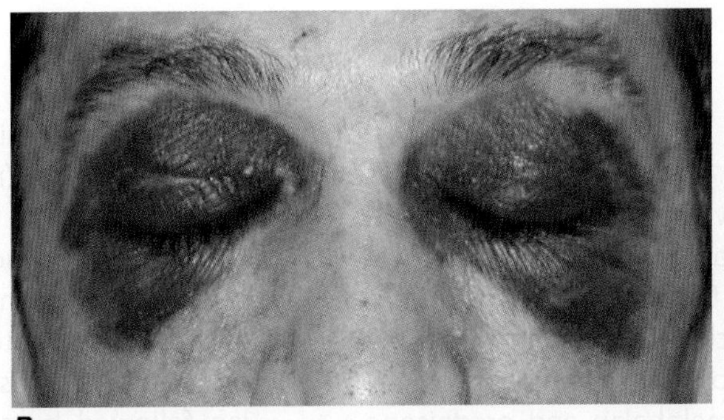
B

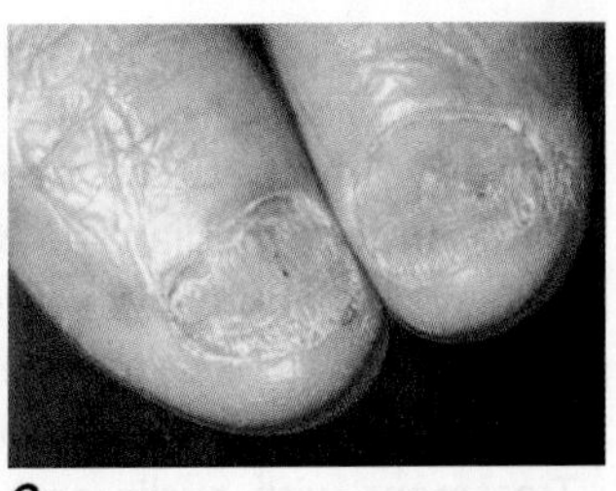
C

FIGURE 18-2
Clinical signs of AL amyloidosis. *A.* Macroglossia. ***B.*** Periorbital ecchymoses. ***C.*** Fingernail dystrophy.

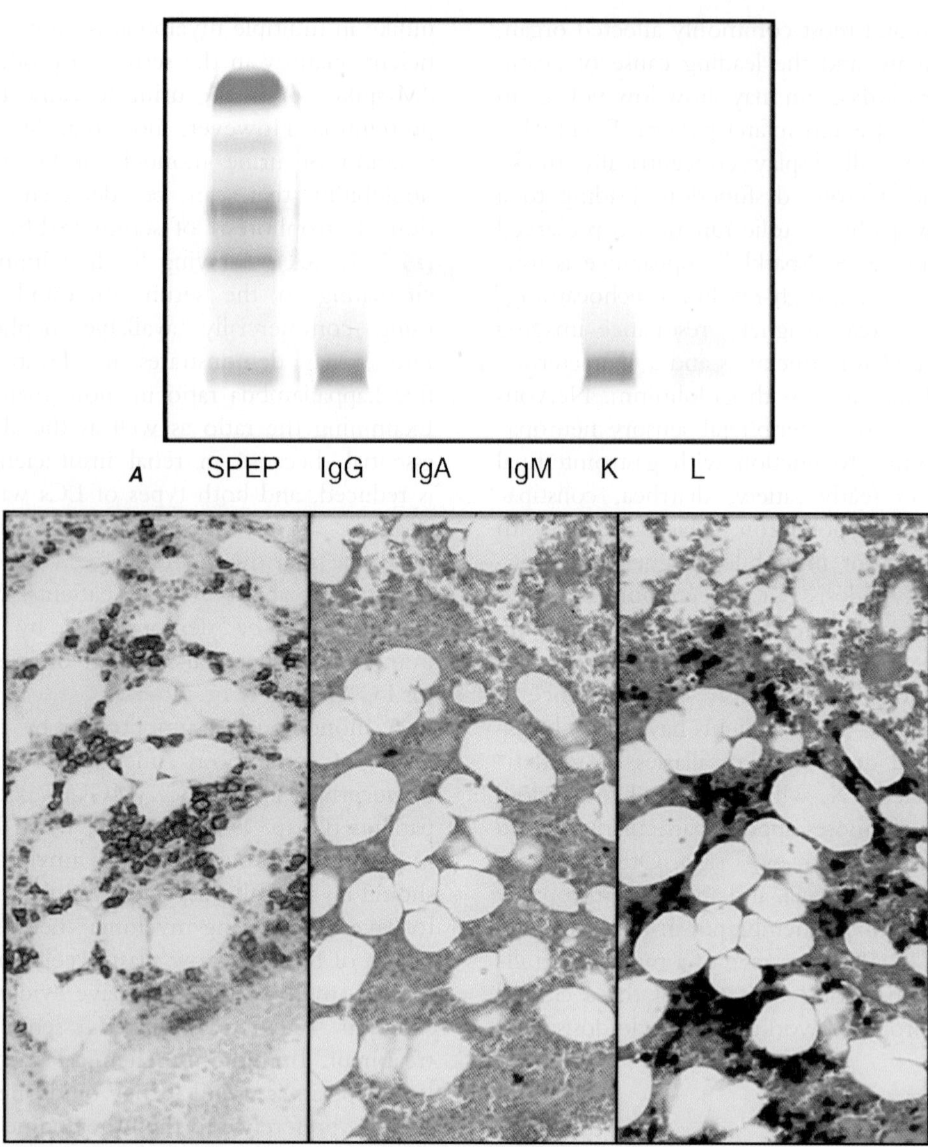

FIGURE 18-3

Laboratory features of AL amyloidosis. ***A.*** Serum immunofixation electrophoresis reveals an IgGκ monoclonal protein in this example; the serum protein electrophoresis is often normal. ***B.*** Bone marrow biopsy sections from another patient, stained with antibody to CD138 (syndecan, highly expressed on plasma cells) by immunohistochemistry (left panel). The middle and right panels are stained using in situ hybridization with fluorescein-tagged probes (Ventana Medical Systems) binding to κ and λ mRNA, respectively, in plasma cells. SPEP, serum protein electrophoresis. (*Photomicrograph courtesy of C. O'Hara; with permission*.)

TREATMENT AL Amyloidosis

Extensive multisystem involvement typifies AL amyloidosis, and the median survival time with no treatment is usually only about 1–2 years from the time of diagnosis. Current therapies target the clonal bone marrow plasma cells using approaches employed for multiple myeloma. Treatment with cyclic oral melphalan and prednisone can decrease the plasma cell burden but produces complete hematologic remission in only a few percent of patients and minimal organ responses and improvement in survival (median, 2 years), and it is no longer widely used. The substitution of dexamethasone for prednisone produces a higher response rate and more durable remissions, although dexamethasone is not always well tolerated by patients with significant edema or cardiac disease. High-dose intravenous melphalan followed by autologous stem cell transplantation (HDM/SCT) produces complete hematologic responses in about 40% of treated patients, as measured by complete loss (CR) of clonal plasma cells in the bone marrow and disappearance of the monoclonal LC by IFE and assay for free LCs. Hematologic responses can be followed in the subsequent 6–12 months by improvement in organ function and quality of life. The CRs after HDM/SCT appear to be more durable than those seen in multiple myeloma, with remissions continuing in some patients beyond 15 years without additional treatment. Unfortunately, only about half of AL amyloidosis patients are eligible for such aggressive treatment, and even at specialized treatment centers, the peritransplant mortality rate is higher than for other hematologic diseases because of impaired organ function. Amyloid cardiomyopathy, poor nutritional status, impaired performance status, and multiple-organ disease contribute to excess morbidity and mortality. The bleeding diathesis due to adsorption of clotting factor X to amyloid fibrils also confers high mortality during myelosuppressive therapy; however, this syndrome occurs in only a few percent of patients. The single randomized multicenter trial comparing oral melphalan and dexamethasone with HDM/SCT to date failed to show a benefit to dose-intensive treatment, although the transplant-related mortality rate in this study was very high.

For patients with impaired cardiac function or arrhythmias due to amyloid involvement of the myocardium, the median survival time is only about 6 months without treatment, and stem cell mobilization and high-dose chemotherapy are dangerous. In these patients, cardiac transplantation can be performed followed by treatment with HDM/SCT to prevent amyloid deposition in the transplanted heart or other organs.

Recently, novel agents have been investigated for treatment of plasma cell diseases. The immunomodulators thalidomide and lenalidomide have activity; lenalidomide is well tolerated in doses lower than those used for myeloma and, in combination with dexamethasone, produces complete hematologic remissions and improvement in organ function. The proteasome inhibitor bortezomib has also been found to be effective in single- and multicenter trials. Combination therapy trials are now under development, and studies are examining the as yet unproven role of induction and maintenance treatment. Clinical trials are essential for improving therapy for this rare disease.

Supportive care is important for patients with any type of amyloidosis. For nephrotic syndrome, diuretics and supportive stockings can ameliorate edema; angiotensin-converting enzyme inhibitors should be used with caution and have not been shown to slow renal disease progression. Congestive heart failure due to amyloid cardiomyopathy is also best treated with diuretics; it is important to note that digitalis, calcium channel blockers, and beta blockers are relatively contraindicated as they can interact with amyloid fibrils and produce heart block and worsening heart failure. Amiodarone has been used for atrial and ventricular arrhythmias. Automatic implantable defibrillators have reduced effectiveness due to the thickened myocardium, but they can benefit some patients. Atrial ablation is an effective approach for atrial fibrillation. For conduction abnormalities, ventricular pacing may be indicated. Atrial contractile dysfunction is common in amyloid cardiomyopathy and is an indication for anticoagulation even in the absence of atrial fibrillation. Autonomic neuropathy can be treated with α agonists such as midodrine to support the blood pressure; gastrointestinal dysfunction may respond to motility or bulk agents. Nutritional supplementation, either orally or parenterally, is also important.

In localized AL, amyloid deposits can be produced by clonal plasma cells infiltrating local sites in the airways, bladder, skin, or lymph nodes (Table 18-1). Deposits may respond to surgical intervention or radiation therapy; systemic treatment is generally not appropriate. Patients should be referred to a center familiar with management of these rare manifestations of amyloidosis.

AA AMYLOIDOSIS

ETIOLOGY AND INCIDENCE

AA amyloidosis can occur in association with almost any chronic inflammatory state (e.g., rheumatoid arthritis, inflammatory bowel disease, familial Mediterranean fever or other periodic fever syndromes) or chronic infections such as tuberculosis or subacute bacterial endocarditis. In the United States and Europe, AA amyloidosis has become less common, occurring in <2% of patients with these diseases, presumably because of advances in anti-inflammatory and antimicrobial therapies. It has also been described in association with Castleman's disease, and patients with AA amyloidosis should have computed tomography to look for such tumors, as well as serologic and microbiologic studies. AA amyloidosis can also be seen without any identifiable underlying disease. AA is the only type of systemic amyloidosis that occurs in children.

PATHOLOGY AND CLINICAL FEATURES

Deposits are more limited in AA amyloidosis than in AL amyloidosis; they usually begin in the kidneys. Hepatomegaly, splenomegaly, and autonomic neuropathy can also occur as the disease progresses; cardiomyopathy occurs albeit rarely. However, the symptoms and signs cannot be reliably distinguished from those of AL amyloidosis. AA amyloid fibrils are usually composed of an 8-kDa, 76-amino-acid *N*-terminal portion of a 12-kDa precursor protein, serum amyloid A (SAA). SAA is an acute-phase apoprotein synthesized in the liver and transported by high-density lipoprotein, HDL3, in the plasma. Several years of an underlying inflammatory disease causing chronic elevation of SAA usually precedes fibril formation, although infections can lead to AA deposition more rapidly.

TREATMENT AA Amyloidosis

The primary therapy in AA amyloidosis is treatment of the underlying inflammatory or infectious disease. Treatment that suppresses or eliminates the inflammation or infection also decreases the SAA protein concentration. For familial Mediterranean fever, colchicine in a dose of 1.2–1.8 mg/d is the appropriate treatment. Colchicine has not been helpful for AA amyloidosis of other causes or for other amyloidoses. TNF and IL-1 antagonists can also be effective in syndromes related to cytokine elevation. For this disease, there is also a fibril-specific agent. Eprodisate was designed to interfere with the interaction of AA amyloid protein with glycosaminoglycans in tissues and prevent or disrupt fibril formation. This drug is well tolerated and delays progression of AA renal disease, regardless of the underlying inflammatory process. Eprodisate is awaiting U.S. Food and Drug Administration approval.

AF AMYLOIDOSIS

The familial amyloidoses are autosomal dominant diseases in which a variant plasma protein forms amyloid deposits beginning in midlife. These diseases are rare, with an estimated incidence of <1 per 100,000 in the United States, although there are isolated areas of Portugal, Sweden, and Japan, where founder effects have led to a much higher incidence of the disease. The most common form of AF is caused by mutation of the abundant plasma protein transthyretin (TTR, also known as *prealbumin*). More than 100 TTR mutations are known, and most are associated with ATTR amyloidosis. One variant, V122I, has a carrier frequency that may be as high as 4% in the African-American population and is associated with late-onset cardiac amyloidosis. The actual incidence and penetrance of disease in the African-American population is the subject of ongoing research, but it would be wise to consider this in the differential diagnosis of African-American patients who present with concentric cardiac hypertrophy and evidence of diastolic dysfunction, particularly in the absence of a history of hypertension. Even wild-type TTR can form fibrils, leading to so-called senile systemic amyloidosis (SSA) in older patients. It can be found in up to 25% of autopsies in patients older than age 80 years, and it can produce a clinical syndrome of amyloid cardiomyopathy that is similar to that occurring in younger patients carrying a mutant TTR. Other familial amyloidoses, caused by variant apolipoproteins AI or AII, gelsolin, fibrinogen Aα, or lysozyme, are reported in only a few families worldwide. New amyloidogenic serum proteins continue to be identified periodically, including recently the leukocyte chemotactic factor LECT2.

In ATTR and in other forms of familial amyloidosis, the variant structure of the precursor protein is the key factor in fibril formation. The role of aging is intriguing, since patients born with the variant proteins do not have clinically apparent disease until middle age despite the lifelong presence of the abnormal protein. Further evidence of an age-related "trigger" is the occurrence of SSA in the elderly caused by the deposition of fibrils derived from normal TTR.

CLINICAL FEATURES AND DIAGNOSIS

AF amyloidosis has a variable presentation but is usually consistent within affected kindreds with the same mutant protein. A family history makes AF more likely, but many patients present sporadically with new mutations. ATTR usually presents as a syndrome of familial amyloidotic polyneuropathy or familial amyloidotic cardiomyopathy. Peripheral neuropathy usually begins as a lower-extremity sensory and motor neuropathy and progresses to the upper extremities. Autonomic neuropathy is manifest by gastrointestinal symptoms of diarrhea with weight loss and orthostatic hypotension. Patients with TTR V30M, the most common mutation, have normal echocardiographic findings but may have conduction defects and require a pacemaker. Patients with TTR T60A and several other mutations have myocardial thickening similar to that caused by AL amyloidosis, although heart failure is less common, and the prognosis is better. Vitreous opacities caused by amyloid deposits are pathognomonic of ATTR amyloidosis.

Typical syndromes associated with other forms of AF include renal amyloidosis with mutant fibrinogen, lysozyme, or apolipoproteins; hepatic amyloidosis with apolipoprotein AI; and amyloidosis of cranial nerves and cornea with gelsolin. Patients with AF amyloidosis can present with clinical syndromes that mimic those of patients with AL, and AF carriers can develop AL, or conversely, AF patients can develop MGUS. Thus, it is important to screen for both plasma cell disorders and for mutations in some patients with amyloidosis. Variant TTR proteins can usually be detected by isoelectric focusing, but DNA sequencing is now standard for diagnosis of ATTR and the other AF mutations.

TREATMENT ATTR Amyloidosis

Without intervention, survival after ATTR disease onset is 5–15 years. Orthotopic liver transplantation removes the major source of variant TTR production and replaces it with a source of normal TTR; it also arrests disease progression and leads to improvement in autonomic and peripheral neuropathy in some patients. Cardiomyopathy often does not improve, and in some patients, it can worsen after liver transplantation, perhaps due to deposition of wild-type TTR as seen in SSA. Compounds have been identified that stabilize TTR in a nonpathogenic tetrameric conformation in vitro and are undergoing clinical testing in multicenter trials.

Aβ_2M AMYLOIDOSIS

Aβ_2M amyloidosis is composed of β_2-microglobulin, the invariant chain of class I human leukocyte antigens, and produces rheumatologic manifestations in patients on long-term hemodialysis. β_2-Microglobulin is excreted by the kidneys, and levels become elevated in ESRD. The molecular mass of β_2M is 11.8 kDa, above the cutoff of some dialysis membranes. The incidence of this disease appears to be declining with newer high-flow dialysis techniques.

Aβ_2M amyloidosis usually presents with carpal tunnel syndrome, persistent joint effusions, spondyloarthropathy, or cystic bone lesions. Carpal tunnel syndrome is often the first symptom of disease. In the past, persistent joint effusions accompanied by mild discomfort were seen in up to 50% of patients on dialysis for more than 12 years. Involvement is bilateral, and large joints (shoulders, knees, wrists, and hips) are more frequently affected. The synovial fluid is noninflammatory, and β_2M amyloid can be found if the sediment is stained with Congo red. Although less common, visceral β_2M amyloid deposits do occasionally occur in the gastrointestinal tract, heart, tendons, and subcutaneous tissues of the buttocks. There is no specific therapy for Aβ_2M amyloidosis, but cessation of dialysis after renal allografting may lead to symptomatic improvement.

SUMMARY

A diagnosis of amyloidosis should be considered in patients with unexplained nephropathy, cardiomyopathy (particularly with diastolic dysfunction), neuropathy (either peripheral or autonomic), enteropathy, or the pathognomonic soft tissue findings of macroglossia or periorbital ecchymoses. Pathologic identification of amyloid fibrils can be made using Congo red staining of aspirated abdominal fat or of an involved organ biopsy specimen. Accurate typing using a combination of immunologic, biochemical, and genetic testing is essential to choosing the appropriate therapy (see algorithm for workup, Fig. 18-1). Tertiary referral centers can provide specialized diagnostic techniques and access to clinical trials for patients with these rare diseases.

SECTION VI

DISORDERS OF HEMOSTASIS

CHAPTER 19

DISORDERS OF PLATELETS AND VESSEL WALL

Barbara Konkle

Hemostasis is a dynamic process in which the platelet and the blood vessel wall play key roles. Platelets become activated upon adhesion to von Willebrand factor (vWF) and collagen in the exposed subendothelium after injury. Platelet activation is also mediated through shear forces imposed by blood flow itself, particularly in areas where the vessel wall is diseased, and is also affected by the inflammatory state of the endothelium. The activated platelet surface provides the major physiologic site for coagulation factor activation, which results in further platelet activation and fibrin formation. Genetic and acquired influences on the platelet and vessel wall, as well as on the coagulation and fibrinolytic systems, determine whether normal hemostasis or bleeding or clotting symptoms will result.

THE PLATELET

Platelets are released from the megakaryocyte, likely under the influence of flow in the capillary sinuses. The normal blood platelet count is 150,000–450,000/μL. The major regulator of platelet production is the hormone thrombopoietin (TPO), which is synthesized in the liver. Synthesis is increased with inflammation and specifically by interleukin 6. TPO binds to its receptor on platelets and megakaryocytes, by which it is removed from the circulation. Thus, a reduction in platelet and megakaryocyte mass increases the level of TPO, which then stimulates platelet production. Platelets circulate with an average life span of 7 to 10 days. Approximately one-third of the platelets reside in the spleen, and this number increases in proportion to splenic size, although the platelet count rarely decreases to <40,000/μL as the spleen enlarges. Platelets are physiologically very active but are anucleate and thus have limited capacity to synthesize new proteins.

Normal vascular endothelium contributes to preventing thrombosis by inhibiting platelet function (Chap. 3). When vascular endothelium is injured, these inhibitory effects are overcome, and platelets adhere to the exposed intimal surface primarily through vWF, a large multimeric protein present in both plasma and in the extracellular matrix of the subendothelial vessel wall. Platelet adhesion results in the generation of intracellular signals that lead to activation of the platelet glycoprotein (Gp) IIb/IIIa ($\alpha_{IIb}\beta_3$) receptor and resultant platelet aggregation.

Activated platelets undergo release of their granule contents, which include nucleotides, adhesive proteins, growth factors, and procoagulants that serve to promote platelet aggregation and blood clot formation and influence the environment of the forming clot. During platelet aggregation, additional platelets are recruited to the site of injury, leading to the formation of an occlusive platelet thrombus. The platelet plug is stabilized by the fibrin mesh that develops simultaneously as the product of the coagulation cascade.

THE VESSEL WALL

Endothelial cells line the surface of the entire circulatory tree, totaling $1–6 \times 10^{13}$ cells, enough to cover a surface area equivalent to about six tennis courts. The endothelium is physiologically active, controlling vascular permeability, flow of biologically active molecules and nutrients, blood cell interactions with the vessel wall, the inflammatory response, and angiogenesis.

The endothelium normally presents an antithrombotic surface (Chap. 3) but rapidly becomes prothrombotic when stimulated, which promotes coagulation, inhibits fibrinolysis, and activates platelets. In many cases, endothelium-derived vasodilators are also platelet inhibitors (e.g., nitric oxide) and, conversely, endothelium-derived vasoconstrictors (e.g., endothelin) can also be

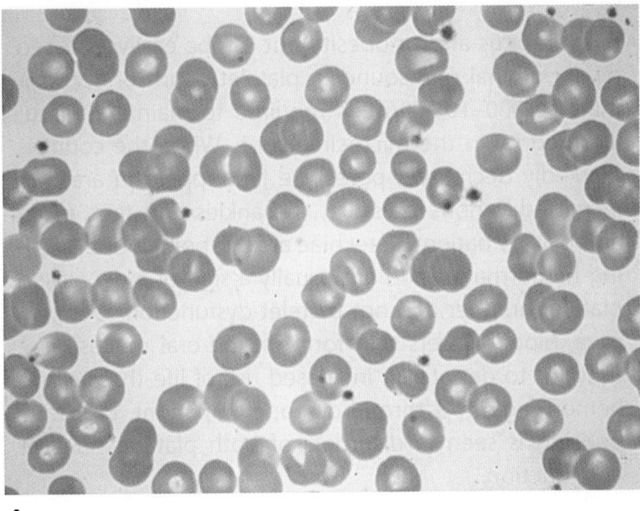

A

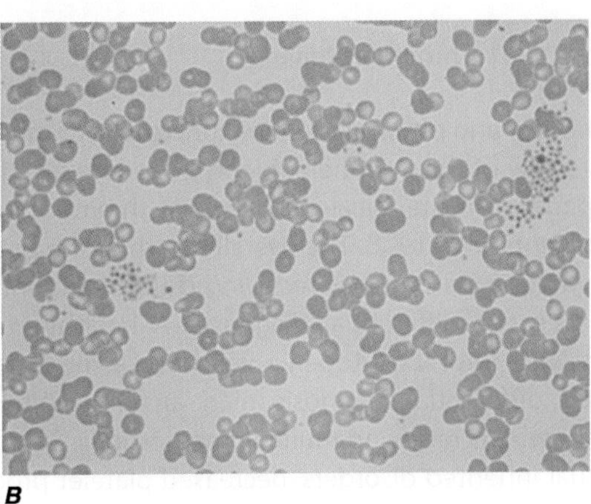

B

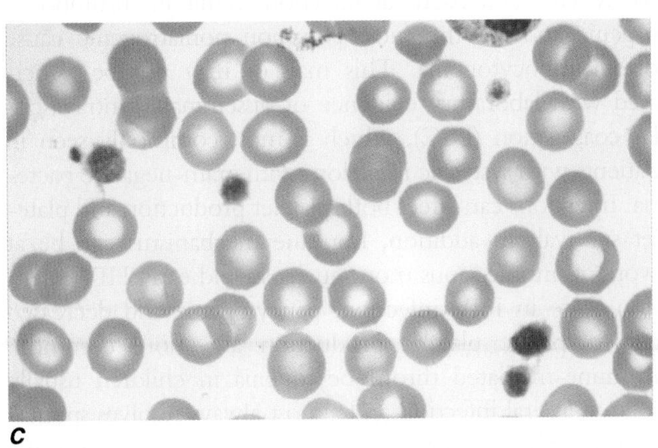

C

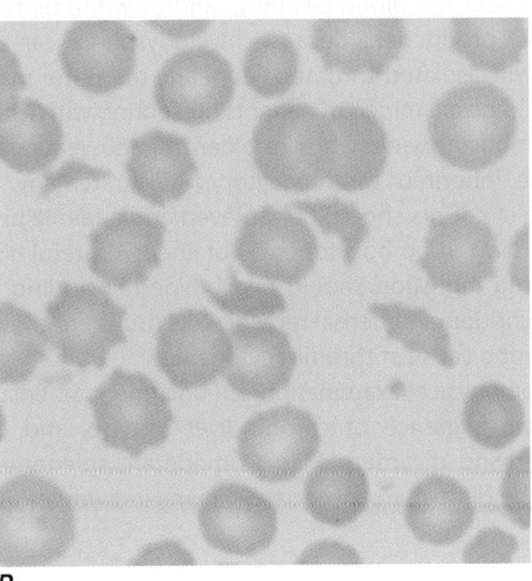

D

FIGURE 19-1
Photomicrographs of peripheral blood smears: *A.* Normal peripheral blood. ***B.*** Platelet clumping in pseudothrombocytopenia. ***C.*** Abnormal large platelet in autosomal dominant macrothrombocytopenia. ***D.*** Schistocytes and decreased platelets in microangiopathic hemolytic anemia.

platelet activators. The net effect of vasodilation and inhibition of platelet function is to promote blood fluidity, whereas the net effect of vasoconstriction and platelet activation is to promote thrombosis. Thus, blood fluidity and hemostasis is regulated by the balance of antithrombotic/prothrombotic and vasodilatory/vasoconstrictor properties of endothelial cells.

DISORDERS OF PLATELETS

THROMBOCYTOPENIA

Thrombocytopenia results from one or more of three processes: (1) decreased bone marrow production; (2) sequestration, usually in an enlarged spleen; and/or (3) increased platelet destruction. Disorders of production may be either inherited or acquired. In evaluating a patient with thrombocytopenia, a key step is to review the peripheral blood smear and to first rule out "pseudothrombocytopenia," particularly in a patient without an apparent cause for the thrombocytopenia. Pseudothrombocytopenia (Fig. 19-1*B*) is an in vitro artifact resulting from platelet agglutination via antibodies (usually IgG but also IgM and IgA) when the calcium content is decreased by blood collection in ethylenediamine tetraacetic (EDTA) (the anticoagulant present in tubes [purple top] used to collect blood for complete blood counts [CBCs]). If a low platelet count is obtained in EDTA-anticoagulated blood, a blood smear should be evaluated and a platelet count determined in blood collected into sodium citrate (blue top tube) or heparin (green top tube), or a smear of freshly obtained unanticoagulated blood, such as from a finger stick, can be examined.

APPROACH TO THE PATIENT Thrombocytopenia

The history and physical examination, results of the CBC, and review of the peripheral blood smear are all critical components in the initial evaluation of thrombocytopenic patients (Fig. 19-2). The overall health of the patient and whether he or she is receiving drug treatment will influence the differential diagnosis. A healthy young adult with thrombocytopenia will have a much more limited differential diagnosis than an ill hospitalized patient who is receiving multiple medications. Except in unusual inherited disorders, decreased platelet production usually results from bone marrow disorders that also affect red blood cell (RBC) and/or white blood cell (WBC) production. Because myelodysplasia can present with isolated thrombocytopenia, the bone marrow should be examined in patients presenting with isolated thrombocytopenia who are older than 60 years of age. While inherited thrombocytopenia is rare, any prior platelet counts should be retrieved and a family history regarding thrombocytopenia obtained. A careful history of drug ingestion should be obtained, including nonprescription and herbal remedies, as drugs are the most common cause of thrombocytopenia.

The physical examination can document an enlarged spleen, evidence of chronic liver disease, and other underlying disorders. Mild to moderate splenomegaly may be difficult to appreciate in many individuals due to body habitus and/or obesity but can be easily assessed by abdominal ultrasound. A platelet count of approximately 5000–10,000/μL is required to maintain vascular integrity in the microcirculation. When the count is markedly decreased, petechiae first appear in areas of increased venous pressure, the ankles and feet, in an ambulatory patient. Petechiae are pin-point, nonblanching hemorrhages and are usually a sign of a decreased platelet number and not platelet dysfunction. Wet purpura, blood blisters that form on the oral mucosa, are thought to denote an increased risk of life-threatening hemorrhage in a thrombocytopenic patient. Excessive bruising is seen in disorders of both platelet number and function.

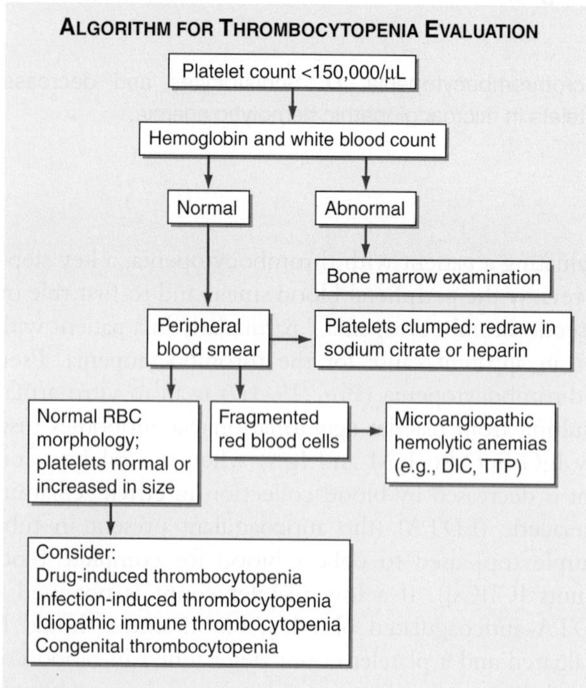

FIGURE 19-2

Algorithm for evaluating the thrombocytopenic patient. DIC, disseminated intravascular coagulation; RBC, red blood cell; TTP, thrombotic thrombocytopenic purpura.

Infection-induced thrombocytopenia

Many viral and bacterial infections result in thrombocytopenia and are the most common noniatrogenic cause of thrombocytopenia. This may or may not be associated with laboratory evidence of disseminated intravascular coagulation (DIC), which is most commonly seen in patients with systemic infections with gram-negative bacteria. Infections can affect both platelet production and platelet survival. In addition, immune mechanisms can be at work, as in infectious mononucleosis and early HIV infection. Late in HIV infection, pancytopenia and decreased and dysplastic platelet production are more common. Immune-mediated thrombocytopenia in children usually follows a viral infection and almost always resolves spontaneously. This association of infection with immune thrombocytopenic purpura (ITP) is less clear in adults.

Bone marrow examination is often requested for evaluation of occult infections. A study evaluating the role of bone marrow examination in fever of unknown origin in HIV-infected patients found that for 86% of patients, the same diagnosis was established by less-invasive techniques, notably blood culture. In some instances, however, the diagnosis can be made earlier; thus, a bone marrow examination and culture is recommended when the diagnosis is needed urgently or when other, less invasive methods have been unsuccessful.

Drug-induced thrombocytopenia

Many drugs have been associated with thrombocytopenia. A predictable decrease in platelet count occurs after treatment with many chemotherapeutic drugs due to bone marrow suppression (Chap. 28). Other, commonly used drugs that cause isolated thrombocytopenia are listed in Table 19-1, but all drugs should be suspect in a patient with thrombocytopenia without an apparent cause and should be stopped or substituted if possible. A helpful website, Platelets on the Internet (*http://www.ouhsc.edu/platelets/index.html*), lists drugs and supplements reported to have caused thrombocytopenia

TABLE 19-1

DRUGS REPORTED AS DEFINITELY OR PROBABLY CAUSING ISOLATED THROMBOCYTOPENIA[a]	
Abciximab	Ibuprofen
Acetaminophen	Iopanoic acid
Aminoglutethimide	Levamisole
Aminosalicylic acid	Linezolid
Amiodarone	Meclofenamate
Amphotericin B	Methicillin
Ampicillin	Methyldopa
Carbamazepine	Nalidixic acid
Chlorpropamide	Naproxen
Danazol	Oxyphenbutazone
Captopril	Phenytoin
Cimetidine	Piperacillin
Diatrizoate meglumine (Hypaque Meglumine®)	Procainamide
Diclofenac	Quinine
Digoxin	Quinidine
Dipyridamole	Rifampin
Eptifibatide	Simvastatin
Ethambutol	Sulfa-containing drugs
Famotidine	Tamoxifen
Fluconazole	Tirofiban
Furosemide	Trimethoprim–sulfamethoxazole
Glyburide	Valproic acid
Gold	Vancomycin
Hydrochlorothiazide	
Imipenem/cilastatin	

[a]Reported in ≥2 patients
Source: Data from http://www.ouhsc.edu/platelets/index.html.

and the level of evidence supporting the association. Although not as well studied, herbal and over-the-counter preparations may also result in thrombocytopenia and should be discontinued in patients who are thrombocytopenic.

Classic drug-dependent antibodies are antibodies that react with specific platelet surface antigens, and result in thrombocytopenia only when the drug is present. Many drugs are capable of inducing these antibodies, but for some reason, they are more common with quinine and sulfonamides. Drug-dependent antibody binding can be demonstrated by laboratory assays, showing antibody binding in the presence of, but not without, the drug present in the assay. The thrombocytopenia typically occurs after a period of initial exposure (median length, 21 days) or upon reexposure and usually resolves in 7–10 days after drug withdrawal. The thrombocytopenia caused by the platelet GpIIbIIIa inhibitory drugs, such as abciximab, differs in that it may occur within 24 h of initial exposure. This appears to be due to the presence of naturally occurring antibodies that cross-react with the drug bound to the platelet.

Heparin-induced thrombocytopenia

Drug-induced thrombocytopenia due to heparin differs from that seen with other drugs in two major ways. (1) The thrombocytopenia is not usually severe, with nadir counts rarely <20,000/μL. (2) Heparin-induced thrombocytopenia (HIT) is not associated with bleeding and, in fact, markedly increases the risk of thrombosis. HIT results from antibody formation to a complex of the platelet-specific protein platelet factor 4 (PF4) and heparin. The antiheparin/PF4 antibody can activate platelets through the FcγRIIa receptor and activate monocytes and endothelial cells. Many patients exposed to heparin develop antibodies to heparin/PF4 but do not appear to have adverse consequences. A fraction of those who develop antibodies will develop HIT, and a portion of those (≤50%) will develop thrombosis (HITT).

HIT can occur after exposure to low-molecular-weight heparin (LMWH) as well as unfractionated heparin (UFH), although it is about 10 times more common with the latter. Most patients develop HIT after exposure to heparin for 5–14 days (Fig. 19-3). It occurs before 5 days in those who were exposed to heparin in the prior few weeks or months (<~100 days) and have circulating antiheparin/PF4 antibodies. Rarely, thrombocytopenia and thrombosis begin several days after all heparin has been stopped (termed *delayed-onset HIT*). The 4 Ts have been recommended to be used in a diagnostic algorithm for HIT: *t*hrombocytopenia,

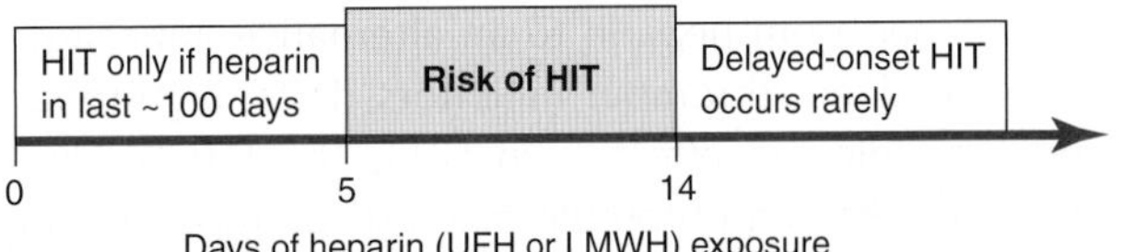

FIGURE 19-3
Time course of heparin-induced thrombocytopenia (HIT) development after heparin exposure. The timing of development after heparin exposure is a critical factor in determining the likelihood of HIT in a patient. HIT occurs early after heparin exposure in the presence of preexisting heparin/platelet factor 4 (PF4) antibodies, which disappear from circulation by ~100 days following an exposure. Rarely, HIT may occur later after heparin exposure (termed delayed-onset HIT). In this setting, heparin/PF4 antibody testing is usually markedly positive. HIT can occur after exposure to either unfractionated heparin (UFH) or low-molecular-weight heparin (LMWH).

timing of platelet count drop, *thrombosis* and other sequelae such as localized skin reactions, and other causes of thrombocytopenia not evident. A new scoring model based on broad expert opinion (the HIT Expert Probability [HEP] Score) has improved operating characteristics and should provide better utility as a scoring system.

Laboratory testing for HIT

HIT (anti-heparin/PF4) antibodies can be detected using two types of assays. The most widely available is an enzyme-linked immunoassay (ELISA) with PF4/polyanion complex as the antigen. Since many patients develop antibodies but do not develop clinical HIT, the test has a low specificity for the diagnosis of HIT. This is especially true in patients who have undergone cardiopulmonary bypass surgery, in which approximately 50% of patients develop these antibodies postoperatively. IgG-specific ELISAs increase specificity but may decrease sensitivity. The other assay is a platelet activation assay, which measures the ability of the patient's serum to activate platelets in the presence of heparin in a concentration-dependent manner. This test has lower sensitivity but higher specificity than ELISA. However, HIT remains a clinical diagnosis.

TREATMENT Heparin-Induced Thrombocytopenia

Early recognition is key in treatment of HIT, with prompt discontinuation of heparin and use of alternative anticoagulants. Thrombosis is a common complication of HIT, even after heparin discontinuation, and can occur in both the venous and arterial systems. Patients with higher anti-heparin/PF4 antibody titers have a higher risk of thrombosis. In patients diagnosed with HIT, imaging studies to evaluate the patient for thrombosis (at least lower extremity duplex Dopplers) are recommended. Patients requiring anticoagulation should be switched from heparin to an alternative anticoagulant. The direct thrombin inhibitors (DTIs) argatroban and lepirudin are effective in HITT. The DTI bivalirudin and the antithrombin-binding pentasaccharide fondaparinux are also effective but not yet approved by the U.S. Food and Drug Administration (FDA) for this indication. Danaparoid, a mixture of glycosoaminoglycans with anti-Xa activity, has been used extensively for the treatment of HITT; it is no longer available in the United States but is in other countries. HIT antibodies cross-react with LMWH, and these preparations should not be used in the treatment of HIT.

Because of the high rate of thrombosis in patients with HIT, anticoagulation should be strongly considered, even in the absence of thrombosis. In patients with thrombosis, patients can be transitioned to warfarin, with treatment usually for 3–6 months. In patients without thrombosis, the duration of anticoagulation needed is undefined. An increased risk of thrombosis is present for at least 1 month after diagnosis; however, most thromboses occur early, and whether thrombosis occurs later if the patient is initially anticoagulated is unknown. Options include continuing anticoagulation until a few days after platelet recovery or for 1 month. Introduction of warfarin alone in the setting of HIT or HITT may precipitate thrombosis, particularly venous gangrene, presumably due to clotting activation and severely reduced levels of proteins C and S. Warfarin therapy, if started, should be overlapped with a DTI or fonda parinux and started after resolution of the thrombocytopenia and lessening of the prothrombotic state.

Immune thrombocytopenic purpura

ITP (also termed *idiopathic thrombocytopenic purpura*) is an acquired disorder in which there is immune-mediated destruction of platelets and possibly inhibition of platelet release from the megakaryocyte. In children, it is usually an acute disease, most commonly following an infection, and with a self-limited course. In adults, it usually runs a more chronic course. ITP is termed *secondary* if it is associated with an underlying disorder; autoimmune disorders, particularly systemic lupus erythematosus (SLE), and infections, such as HIV and hepatitis C, are common causes. The association of ITP with *Helicobacter pylori* infection is unclear.

ITP is characterized by mucocutaneous bleeding and a low, often very low, platelet count, with an otherwise normal peripheral blood cells and smear. Patients usually present either with ecchymoses and petechiae or with thrombocytopenia incidentally found on a routine CBC. Mucocutaneous bleeding, such as oral mucosa, gastrointestinal, or heavy menstrual bleeding, may be present. Rarely, life-threatening, including central nervous system, bleeding can occur. Wet purpura (blood blisters in the mouth) and retinal hemorrhages may herald life-threatening bleeding.

Laboratory testing in ITP

Laboratory testing for antibodies (serologic testing) is usually not helpful due to the low sensitivity and specificity of the current tests. Bone marrow examination can be reserved for older adults (usually >60 years) or those who have other signs or laboratory abnormalities not explained by ITP, or in patients who do not respond to initial therapy. The peripheral blood smear may show large platelets, with otherwise normal morphology. Depending on the bleeding history, iron deficiency anemia may be present.

Laboratory testing is performed to evaluate for secondary causes of ITP and should include testing for

HIV infection and hepatitis C (and other infections if indicated); serologic testing for SLE, serum protein electrophoresis, and immunoglobulin levels to potentially detect hypogammaglobulinemia; selective testing for IgA deficiency or monoclonal gammopathies; and, if anemia is present, direct antiglobulin testing (Coombs test) to rule out combined autoimmune hemolytic anemia with ITP (Evans syndrome).

TREATMENT Immune Thrombocytopenic Purpura

The treatment of ITP utilizes drugs that decrease reticuloendothelial uptake of the antibody-bound platelet, decrease antibody production, and/or increase platelet production. The diagnosis of ITP does not necessarily mean that treatment must be instituted. Patients with platelet counts greater than 30,000/μL appear not to have increased mortality related to the thrombocytopenia.

Initial treatment in patients without significant bleeding symptoms, severe thrombocytopenia (<5000/μL), or signs of impending bleeding (such as retinal hemorrhage or large oral mucosal hemorrhages) can be instituted as an outpatient using single agents. Traditionally, this has been prednisone at 1 mg/kg, although Rh_0(D) immune globulin therapy (WinRho SDF) at 50–75 μg/kg is also being used in this setting. Rh_0(D) immune globulin must be used only in Rh-positive patients as the mechanism of action is production of limited hemolysis, with antibody-coated cells "saturating" the Fc receptors, inhibiting Fc receptor function. Monitoring patients for 8 h postinfusion is now advised by the FDA because of the rare complication of severe intravascular hemolysis. Intravenous gamma globulin (IVIgG), which is pooled, primarily IgG antibodies, also blocks the Fc receptor system, but appears to work primarily through different mechanism(s). IVIgG has more efficacy than anti-Rh_0(D) in postsplenectomized patients. IVIgG is dosed at 2 g/kg total, given in divided doses over 2–5 days. Side effects are usually related to the volume of infusion and infrequently include aseptic meningitis and renal failure. All immunoglobulin preparations are derived from human plasma and undergo treatment for viral inactivation.

For patients with severe ITP and/or symptoms of bleeding, hospital admission and combined-modality therapy is given using high-dose glucocorticoids with IVIgG or anti-Rh_0D therapy, and, as needed, additional immunosuppressive agents. Rituximab, an anti-CD20 (B cell) antibody, has shown efficacy in the treatment of refractory ITP.

Splenectomy has been used for treatment of patients who relapse after glucocorticoids are tapered. Splenectomy remains an important treatment option; however, more patients than previously thought will go into a remission over time. Observation, if the platelet count is high enough, or intermittent treatment with anti-Rh_0(D) or IVIgG may be a reasonable approach to see if the ITP will resolve. Vaccination against encapsulated organisms (especially pneumococcus but also meningococcus and *Haemophilus influenzae*, depending on patient age and potential exposure) is recommended before splenectomy. Accessory spleen(s) are a very rare cause of relapse.

Thrombopoietin receptor agonists are now available for the treatment of ITP. This approach stems from the finding that many patients with ITP do not have increased TPO levels, as was previously hypothesized. TPO levels reflect megakaryocyte mass, which is usually normal in ITP. TPO levels are not increased in the setting of platelet destruction. Two agents, one administered subcutaneously (romiplostim) and another orally (eltrombopag), have shown response in many patients with refractory ITP. Roles for these agents in ITP treatment are not fully defined, but given the chronicity of treatment, they are generally reserved for patients with refractory disease

Inherited thrombocytopenia

Thrombocytopenia is rarely inherited, either as an isolated finding or as part of a syndrome, and may be inherited in an autosomal dominant, autosomal recessive, or X-linked pattern. Many forms of autosomal dominant thrombocytopenia are now known to be associated with mutations in the nonmuscle myosin heavy chain *MYH9* gene. Interestingly, these include the May-Hegglin anomaly and Sebastian, Epstein's, and Fechtner syndromes, all of which have distinct distinguishing features. A common feature of these disorders is large platelets (Fig. 19-1*C*). Autosomal recessive disorders include congenital amegakaryocytic thrombocytopenia, thrombocytopenia with absent radii, and Bernard Soulier syndrome. The latter is primarily a functional platelet disorder due to absence of GPIb-IX-V, the vWF adhesion receptor. X-linked disorders include Wiskott-Aldrich syndrome and a dyshematopoietic syndrome resulting from a mutation in GATA-1, an important transcriptional regulator of hematopoiesis.

THROMBOTIC THROMBOCYTOPENIC PURPURA AND HEMOLYTIC UREMIC SYNDROME

Thrombotic thrombocytopenic microangiopathies are a group of disorders characterized by thrombocytopenia, a microangiopathic hemolytic anemia evident by fragmented RBCs (Fig. 19-1*D*) and laboratory evidence of hemolysis, and microvascular thrombosis. They include thrombotic thrombocytopenic purpura and hemolytic uremic syndrome (HUS), as well as syndromes complicating bone marrow transplantation, certain medications and infections, pregnancy, and vasculitis. In DIC, while thrombocytopenia and microangiopathy are seen, a coagulopathy predominates, with consumption of clotting factors and fibrinogen resulting in an elevated prothrombin time (PT), and often activated partial thromboplastin time (aPTT). The PT and aPTT are characteristically normal in TTP or HUS.

Thrombotic thrombocytopenic purpura

TTP and HUS were previously considered overlap syndromes. However, in the past few years, the pathophysiology of inherited and idiopathic TTP has become better understood and clearly differs from HUS. TTP was first described in 1924 by Eli Moschcowitz and characterized by a pentad of findings that include microangiopathic hemolytic anemia, thrombocytopenia, renal failure, neurologic findings, and fever. The full-blown syndrome is less commonly seen now, probably due to earlier diagnosis. The introduction of treatment with plasma exchange markedly improved the prognosis in patients, with a decrease in the mortality rate from 85–100% to 10–30%.

The pathogenesis of inherited (Upshaw-Schulman syndrome) and idiopathic TTP is related to a deficiency of, or antibodies to, the metalloprotease ADAMTS13, that cleaves vWF. vWF is normally secreted as ultra-large multimers, which are then cleaved by ADAMTS13. The persistence of ultra-large vWF molecules is thought to contribute to pathogenic platelet adhesion and aggregation (Fig. 19-4). This defect alone, however, is not sufficient to result in TTP as individuals with a congenital absence of ADAMTS13 develop TTP only episodically. Additional provocative factors have not been defined. The level of ADAMTS13 activity, as well as antibodies, can now be detected by laboratory assays. However, assays with sufficient sensitivity and specificity to direct clinical management have yet to be clearly defined.

Idiopathic TTP appears to be more common in women than in men. No geographic or racial distribution has been defined. TTP is more common in patients with HIV infection and in pregnant women. TTP in pregnancy is not clearly related to ADAMTS13. Medication-related microangiopathic hemolytic anemia may be secondary to antibody formation (ticlopidine and possibly clopidogrel) or direct endothelial toxicity (cyclosporine, mitomycin C, tacrolimus, quinine), although this is not always so clear, and fear of withholding treatment, as well as lack of other treatment alternatives, results in broad application of plasma exchange. However, withdrawal or reduction in dose of endothelial toxic agents usually decreases the microangiopathy.

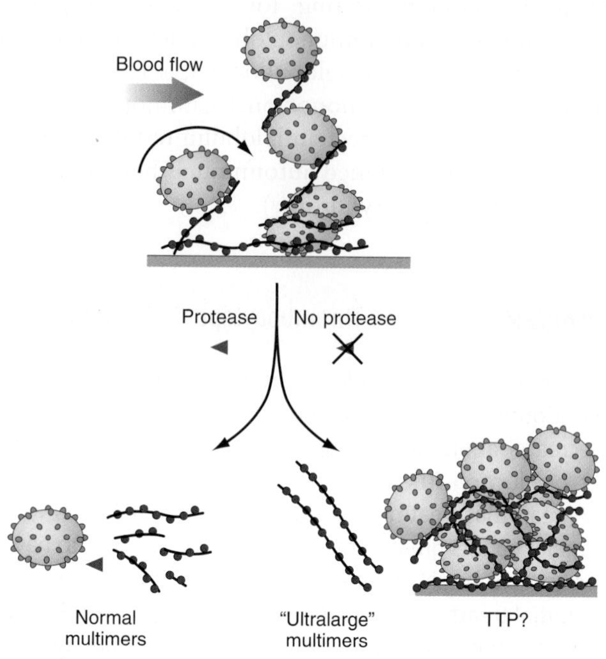

FIGURE 19-4
Pathogenesis of thrombotic thrombocytopenic purpura (TTP). Normally, the ultra-high-molecular-weight multimers of von Willebrand factor (VWF) produced by the endothelial cells are processed into smaller multimers by a plasma metalloproteinase called ADAMTS13. In TTP, the activity of the protease is inhibited, and the ultra-high-molecular-weight multimers of VWF initiate platelet aggregation and thrombosis.

TREATMENT Thrombotic Thrombocytopenic Purpura

TTP is a devastating disease if not diagnosed and treated promptly. In patients presenting with new thrombocytopenia, with or without evidence of renal insufficiency and other elements of classic TTP, laboratory data should be obtained to rule out DIC and to evaluate for evidence of microangiopathic hemolytic anemia. Findings to support the TTP diagnosis include an increased lactate dehydrogenase and indirect bilirubin, decreased haptoglobin, and increased reticulocyte count with a negative direct antiglobulin test result. The peripheral smear should be examined for evidence of schistocytes (Fig. 19-1*D*). Polychromasia is usually also present due to the increased number of young red blood cells, and nucleated RBCs are often present, which is thought to be due to infarction in the microcirculatory system of the bone marrow.

Plasma exchange remains the mainstay of treatment of TTP. ADAMTS13 antibody-mediated TTP (idiopathic TTP) appears to respond best to plasma exchange. Plasma exchange is continued until the platelet count is normal and signs of hemolysis are resolved for at least 2 days. While never evaluated in clinical trial, the use of glucocorticoids seems a reasonable approach but should only be used as an adjunct to plasma exchange. Additionally, other immunomodulatory therapies have been reported to be successful in refractory or relapsing TTP, including rituximab, vincristine, cyclophosphamide, and splenectomy. The role of rituximab in the treatment of this disorder needs to be defined. A significant relapse rate is noted, 25–45% within 30 days of initial "remission" and 12–40% with late relapses. Relapses may be more frequent in patients with severe ADAMTS13 deficiency at presentation.

Hemolytic uremic syndrome

HUS is a syndrome characterized by acute renal failure, microangiopathic hemolytic anemia, and thrombocytopenia. It is seen predominantly in children and in most cases is preceded by an episode of diarrhea, often hemorrhagic in nature. *Escherichia coli* O157:H7 is the most frequent, although not only, etiologic serotype. HUS not associated with diarrhea (termed *DHUS*) is more heterogeneous in presentation and course. Some children who develop DHUS have been found to have mutations in genes encoding factor H, a soluble complement regulator, and membrane cofactor protein that is mainly expressed in the kidney.

TREATMENT Hemolytic Uremic Syndrome

Treatment of HUS is primarily supportive. In D^+HUS, many (~40%) children require at least some period of support with dialysis; however, the overall mortality rate is <5%. In D^-HUS, the mortality rate is higher, approximately 26%. Plasma infusion or plasma exchange has not been shown to alter the overall course. ADAMTS13 levels are generally reported to be normal in HUS, although occasionally they have been reported to be decreased. As ADAMTS13 assays improve, they may help in defining a subset that better fit a TTP diagnosis, and may respond to plasma exchange.

THROMBOCYTOSIS

Thrombocytosis is almost always due to (1) iron deficiency; (2) inflammation, cancer, or infection (reactive thrombocytosis); or (3) an underlying myeloproliferative process (essential thrombocythemia or polycythemia vera [Chap. 13]) or, rarely, the 5q- myelodysplastic process (Chap. 11). Patients presenting with an elevated platelet count should be evaluated for underlying inflammation or malignancy, and iron deficiency should be ruled out. Thrombocytosis in response to acute or chronic inflammation has not been associated with an increased thrombotic risk. In fact, patients with markedly elevated platelet counts (>1.5 million), usually seen in the setting of a myeloproliferative disorder, have an increased risk of bleeding. This appears to be due, at least in part, to acquired von Willebrand disease (VWD) due to platelet-vWF adhesion and removal.

QUALITATIVE DISORDERS OF PLATELET FUNCTION

Inherited disorders of platelet function

Inherited platelet function disorders are thought to be relatively rare, although the prevalence of mild disorders of platelet function is unclear, in part because our testing for such disorders is suboptimal. Rare qualitative disorders include the autosomal recessive disorders Glanzmann's thrombasthenia (absence of the platelet GpIIb–IIIa receptor) and Bernard Soulier syndrome (absence of the platelet GpIb-IX-V receptor). Both are inherited in an autosomal recessive fashion and present with bleeding symptoms in childhood.

Platelet storage pool disorder (SPD) is the classic autosomal dominant qualitative platelet disorder. This results from abnormalities of platelet granule formation. It is also seen as a part of inherited disorders of granule formation, such as Hermansky-Pudlak syndrome. Bleeding symptoms in SPD are variable but often are mild. The most common inherited disorders of platelet function are disorders that prevent normal secretion of granule content. Few of the abnormalities have been dissected at the molecular level, but these are likely due to multiple abnormalities. They are usually described as *secretion defects*. Bleeding symptoms are usually mild in nature.

TREATMENT Inherited Disorders of Platelet Dysfunction

Bleeding symptoms or prevention of bleeding in patients with severe platelet dysfunction frequently requires platelet transfusion. Care is taken to limit the risk of alloimmunization by limiting exposure using apheresis leuko-depleted platelets for transfusion. Platelet disorders associated with milder bleeding symptoms frequently respond to desmopressin (1-deamino-8-D-arginine vasopressin [DDAVP]). DDAVP increases plasma vWF and FVIII levels; it may also have a direct effect on platelet function. Particularly for mucosal bleeding symptoms, antifibrinolytic therapy (epsilon-aminocaproic acid or tranexamic acid) is used alone or in conjunction with DDAVP or platelet therapy.

Acquired disorders of platelet function

Acquired platelet dysfunction is common, usually due to medications, either intentionally as with antiplatelet therapy or unintentionally as with high-dose penicillins. Acquired platelet dysfunction occurs in uremia. This is likely multifactorial, but the resultant effect is defective adhesion and activation. The platelet defect is improved most by dialysis but may also be improved by increasing the hematocrit to 27–32%, giving DDAVP (0.3 μg/kg), or use of conjugated estrogens. Platelet dysfunction also occurs with cardiopulmonary bypass due to the effect of the artificial circuit on platelets, and bleeding symptoms respond to platelet transfusion. Platelet dysfunction seen with underlying hematologic disorders can result from nonspecific interference by circulating paraproteins or intrinsic platelet defects in myeloproliferative and myelodysplastic syndromes.

VON WILLEBRAND DISEASE

VWD is the most common inherited bleeding disorder. Estimates from laboratory data suggest a prevalence of approximately 1%, but data based on symptomatic individuals suggest that it is closer to 0.1% of the population. vWF serves two roles: (1) as the major adhesion molecule that tethers the platelet to the exposed subendothelium and (2) as the binding protein for FVIII, resulting in significant prolongation of the FVIII half-life in circulation. The platelet-adhesive function of vWF is critically dependent on the presence of large vWF multimers, while FVIII binding is not. Most of the symptoms of VWD are "platelet-like" except in more severe VWD when the FVIII is low enough to produce symptoms similar to those found in FVIII deficiency (hemophilia A).

VWD has been classified into three major types, with four subtypes of type 2 (**Table 19-2; Fig. 19-5**). By far the most common type of VWD is type 1 disease, with a parallel decrease in vWF protein, vWF function, and FVIII levels, accounting for at least 80% of cases. Patients have predominantly mucosal bleeding symptoms, although postoperative bleeding can also be seen. Bleeding symptoms are very uncommon in infancy and usually manifest later in childhood with excessive bruising and epistaxis. Since these symptoms occur commonly in childhood, the clinician should particularly note bruising at sites unlikely to be traumatized and/or prolonged epistaxis requiring medical attention. Menorrhagia is a common manifestation of VWD. Menstrual bleeding resulting in anemia should warrant an evaluation for VWD and, if the result is negative, functional platelet disorders. Frequently, mild type 1 VWD first manifests with dental extractions, particularly wisdom tooth extraction, or tonsillectomy.

Not all patients with low vWF levels have bleeding symptoms. Whether patients bleed or not will depend on the overall hemostatic balance they have inherited, along with environmental influences and the type of hemostatic challenges they experience. Although the inheritance of VWD is autosomal, many factors modulate both vWF levels and bleeding symptoms. These have not all been defined but include blood type, thyroid hormone status, race, stress, exercise, and hormonal (both endogenous and exogenous) influences. Patients with type O blood have vWF protein levels of approximately half that of patients with AB blood type; in fact, the normal range for patients with type O blood overlaps that which has been considered diagnostic for VWD. A mildly decreased vWF level should perhaps be viewed more as a risk factor for bleeding than as an actual disease.

Patients with type 2 VWD have functional defects; thus, the vWF antigen measurement is significantly higher than the test of function. For types 2A, 2B, and 2M, vWF activity is decreased, measured as ristocetin cofactor or collagen-binding activity. In type 2A VWD, the impaired function is due either to increased susceptibility to cleavage by ADAMTS13, resulting in loss of intermediate- and high-molecular-weight multimers or to decreased secretion of these multimers by the cell. Type 2B VWD results from gain of function mutations that result in increased spontaneous binding of vWF to platelets in circulation, with subsequent clearance

TABLE 19-2

LABORATORY DIAGNOSIS OF VON WILLEBRAND DISEASE

TYPE	APTT	VWF ANTIGEN	VWF ACTIVITY	FVIII ACTIVITY	MULTIMER
1	Nl or ↑	↓	↓	↓	Normal distribution, decreased in quantity
2A	Nl or ↑	↓	↓↓	↓	Loss of high- and intermediate-MW multimers
2B[a]	Nl or ↑	↓	↓↓	↓	Loss of high-MW multimers
2M	Nl or ↑	↓	↓↓	↓	Normal distribution, decreased in quantity
2N	↑↑	Nl or ↓[b]	Nl or ↓[b]	↓↓	Normal distribution
3	↑↑	↓↓	↓↓	↓↓	Absent

[a]Usually also decreased platelet count.

[b]For type 2N, in the homozygous state, FVIII is very low; in the heterozygous state, only seen in conjunction with type 1 VWD.

Abbreviations: aPTT, activated partial thromboplastin time; F, factor; MW, molecular weight; Nl, normal; VWF, von Willebrand factor.

Type 1

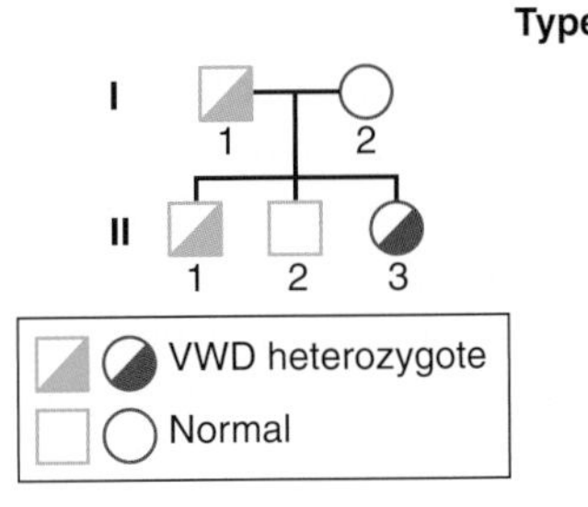

	II-1 VWD	II-2 Normal
VIII	↓	N
VWF:Ag	↓	N
VWF:RCof	↓	N
RIPA	↓or N	N
Multimer pattern		

Type 2A

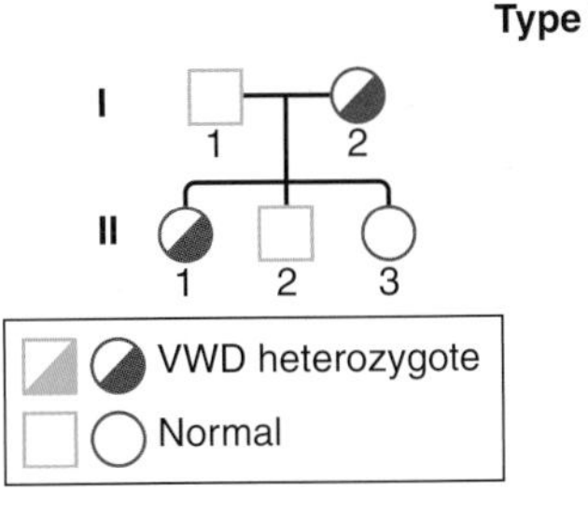

	II-1 VWD	II-2 Normal
VIII	↓	N
VWF:Ag	↓	N
VWF:RCof	↓↓	N
RIPA	↓↓	N
Multimer pattern		

Type 2B

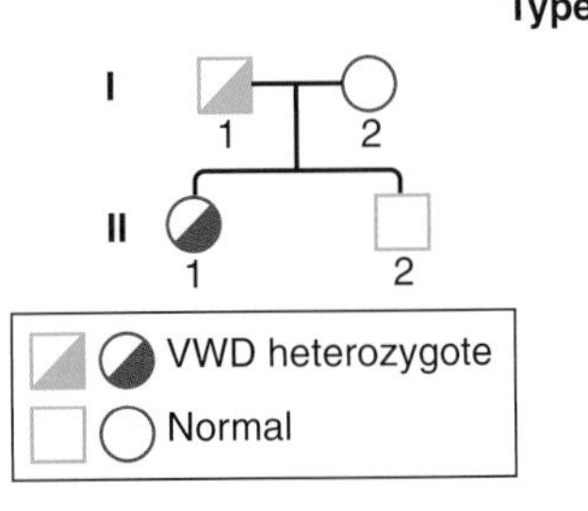

	II-1 VWD	II-2 Normal
VIII	↓	N
VWF:Ag	↓	N
VWF:RCof	↓↓	N
RIPA	↑	N
Multimer pattern		

FIGURE 19-5

Pattern of inheritance and laboratory findings in von Willebrand disease. The assays of platelet function include a coagulation assay of factor VIII bound and carried by von Willebrand factor (VWF), abbreviated VIII; immunoassay of total VWF protein (VWF:Ag); bioassay of the ability of patient plasma to support ristocetin-induced agglutination of normal platelets (VWF:RCoF); and ristocetin-induced aggregation of patient platelets, abbreviated RIPA. The multimer pattern illustrates the protein bands present when plasma is electrophoresed in a polyacrylamide gel. The II-1 and II-2 columns refer to the phenotypes of the second-generation offspring.

of this complex by the reticuloendothelial system. The resulting vWF in the patients' plasma lacks the highest-molecular-weight multimers, and the platelet count is usually modestly reduced. Type 2M occurs as a consequence of a group of mutations that cause dysfunction of the molecule but do not affect multimer structure.

Type 2N VWD is due to mutations in vWF that preclude binding of FVIII. As FVIII is stabilized by binding to vWF, the FVIII in patients with type 2N VWD has a very short half-life, and the FVIII level is markedly decreased. This is sometimes termed *autosomal hemophilia*. Type 3 VWD, or severe VWD, describes patients with virtually no vWF protein and FVIII levels <10%. Patients experience mucosal and joint postoperative symptoms as well as other bleeding symptoms. Some patients with type 3 VWD, particularly those with large vWF gene deletions, are at risk of developing antibodies to infused vWF.

Acquired VWD is a rare disorder, most commonly seen in patients with underlying lymphoproliferative disorders, including monoclonal gammopathies of underdetermined significance (MGUS), multiple myeloma, and Waldenström's macroglobulinemia. It is seen most commonly in the setting of MGUS and should be suspected in patients, particularly elderly patients, with a new onset of severe mucosal bleeding symptoms. Laboratory evidence of acquired VWD is found in some patients with aortic valvular disease. Heyde's syndrome (aortic stenosis with gastrointestinal bleeding) is attributed to the presence of angiodysplasia of the gastrointestinal tract in patients with aortic stenosis. However, the shear stress on blood passing through the stenotic aortic valve appears to produce a change in vWF, making it susceptible to serum proteases. Consequently, large multimer forms are lost, leading to an acquired type 2 VWD but return when the stenotic valve is replaced.

TREATMENT von Willebrand Disease

The mainstay of treatment for type 1 VWD is DDAVP, which results in release of vWF and FVIII from endothelial stores. DDAVP can be given intravenously or by a high concentration intranasal spray (1.5 mg/mL). The peak activity when given intravenously is approximately 30 minutes, while it is 2 h when given intranasally. The usual dose is 0.3 μg/kg intravenously or 2 squirts (1 in each nostril) for patients >50 kg (1 squirt for those <50 kg). It is recommended that patients with VWD be tested with DDAVP to assess their response before using it. In patients who respond well (increase in values of two- to fourfold), it can be used for procedures with a minor to moderate risk of bleeding. Depending on the procedure, additional doses may be needed; it is usually given every 12–24 h. Less frequent dosing may result in less tachyphylaxis, which occurs when synthesis cannot compensate for the released stores. The major side effect of DDAVP is hyponatremia due to decreased free water clearance. This occurs most commonly in the very young and the very old, but fluid restriction should be advised for all patients for the 24 h following each dose.

Some patients with types 2A and 2M VWD respond to DDAVP such that it can be used for minor procedures. For the other subtypes, for type 3 disease, and for major procedures requiring longer periods of normal hemostasis, vWF replacement can be given. Virally inactivated vWF-containing factor concentrates are thought to be safer than cryoprecipitate as the replacement product.

Antifibrinolytic therapy using either ε-aminocaproic acid or tranexamic acid is an important therapy, either alone or in an adjunctive capacity, particularly for the prevention or treatment of mucosal bleeding. These agents are particularly useful in prophylaxis for dental procedures, with DDAVP for dental extractions and tonsillectomy, menorrhagia, and prostate procedures. It is contraindicated in the setting of upper urinary tract bleeding due to the risk of ureteral obstruction.

DISORDERS OF THE VESSEL WALL

The vessel wall is an integral part of hemostasis, and separation of a fluid phase is artificial, particularly in disorders such as TTP or HIT that clearly involve the endothelium as well. Inflammation localized to the vessel wall, such as vasculitis, or inherited connective tissue disorders are abnormalities inherent to the vessel wall.

METABOLIC AND INFLAMMATORY DISORDERS

Acute febrile illnesses may result in vascular damage. This can result from immune complexes containing viral antigens or the viruses themselves. Certain pathogens, such as the rickettsiae causing Rocky Mountain spotted fever, replicate in endothelial cells and damage them. Vascular purpura may occur in patients with polyclonal gammopathies but more commonly in those with monoclonal gammopathies, including Waldenström's macroglobulinemia, multiple myeloma, and cryoglobulinemia. Patients with mixed cryoglobulinemia develop a more extensive maculopapular rash due to immune complex–mediated damage to the vessel wall.

Patients with scurvy (vitamin C deficiency) develop painful episodes of perifollicular skin bleeding as well as more systemic bleeding symptoms. Vitamin C is needed to synthesize hydroxyproline, an essential constituent of collagen. Patients with Cushing's syndrome or on chronic glucocorticoid therapy develop skin bleeding and easy bruising due to atrophy of supporting connective tissue. A similar phenomenon is seen with aging; following minor trauma, blood spreads superficially under the epidermis. This has been termed *senile purpura*. It is most common on skin that has been previously damaged by sun exposure.

Henoch-Schönlein, or anaphylactoid, purpura is a distinct, self-limited type of vasculitis that occurs in children and young adults. Patients have an acute inflammatory reaction with IgA and complement components in capillaries, mesangial tissues, and small arterioles, leading to increased vascular permeability and localized hemorrhage. The syndrome is often preceded by an upper respiratory infection, commonly with streptococcal pharyngitis, or is triggered by drug or food allergies. Patients develop a purpuric rash on the extensor surfaces of the arms and legs, usually accompanied by polyarthralgias or arthritis, abdominal pain, and hematuria from focal glomerulonephritis. All coagulation test results are normal but renal impairment may occur. Glucocorticoids can provide symptomatic relief but do not alter the course of the illness.

INHERITED DISORDERS OF THE VESSEL WALL

Patients with inherited disorders of the connective tissue matrix, such as Marfan's syndrome, Ehlers-Danlos syndrome, and pseudoxanthoma elasticum, frequently report easy bruising. Inherited vascular abnormalities can result in increased bleeding. This is notably seen in hereditary hemorrhagic telangiectasia (HHT, or Osler-Weber-Rendu disease), a disorder in which abnormal telangiectatic capillaries result in frequent bleeding episodes, primarily from the nose and gastrointestinal tract. Arteriovenous malformation (AVM) in the lung, brain, and liver may also occur in HHT. The telangiectasia can often be visualized on the oral and nasal mucosa. Signs and symptoms develop over time. Epistaxis begins, on average, at the age of 12 years and occurs in >95% of affected individuals by middle age. Two genes involved in the pathogenesis are *eng* (endoglin) on chromosome 9q33-34 (so-called HHT type 1), associated with pulmonary AVM in 40% of cases, and *alk1* (activin-receptor-like kinase 1*1*) on chromosome 12q13, associated with a much lower risk of pulmonary AVM.

ACKNOWLEDGMENT

Robert Handin, MD, contributed this chapter in the 16th edition of Harrison's Principles of Internal Medicine and some materials from his chapter are included here.

CHAPTER 20

COAGULATION DISORDERS

Valder R. Arruda ■ Katherine A. High

Deficiencies of coagulation factors have been recognized for centuries. Patients with genetic deficiencies of plasma coagulation factors exhibit life-long recurrent bleeding episodes into joints, muscles, and closed spaces, either spontaneously or following an injury. The most common inherited factor deficiencies are the hemophilias, X-linked diseases caused by deficiency of factor (F) VIII (hemophilia A) or factor IX (FIX, hemophilia B). Rare congenital bleeding disorders due to deficiencies of other factors, including FII (prothrombin), FV, FVII, FX, FXI, FXIII, and fibrinogen, are commonly inherited in an autosomal recessive manner (Table 20-1). Advances in characterization of the molecular bases of clotting factor deficiencies have contributed to better understanding of the disease phenotypes and may eventually allow more targeted therapeutic approaches through the development of small molecules, recombinant proteins, or cell and gene-based therapies.

Commonly used tests of hemostasis provide the initial screening for clotting factor activity (Fig. 20-1), and disease phenotype often correlates with the level of clotting activity. An isolated abnormal prothrombin time (PT) suggests FVII deficiency, whereas a prolonged activated partial thromboplastin time (aPTT) indicates most commonly hemophilia or FXI deficiency (Fig. 20-1). The prolongation of both PT and aPTT suggests deficiency of FV, FX, FII, or fibrinogen abnormalities. The addition of the missing factor at a range of doses to the subject's plasma will correct the abnormal clotting times; the result is expressed as a percentage of the activity observed in normal subjects.

Acquired deficiencies of plasma coagulation factors are more frequent than congenital disorders; the most common disorders include hemorrhagic diathesis of liver disease, disseminated intravascular coagulation (DIC), and vitamin K deficiency. In these disorders, blood coagulation is hampered by the deficiency of more than one clotting factor, and the bleeding episodes are the result of perturbation of both primary (coagulation) and secondary (e.g., platelet and vessel wall interactions) hemostasis.

The development of antibodies to coagulation plasma proteins, clinically termed *inhibitors*, is a relatively rare disease that often affects hemophilia A or B and FXI-deficient patients on repetitive exposure to the missing protein to control bleeding episodes. Inhibitors also occur among subjects without genetic deficiency of clotting factors (e.g., in the postpartum setting as a manifestation of underlying autoimmune or neoplastic disease or idiopathically). Rare cases of inhibitors to thrombin or FV have been reported in patients receiving topical bovine thrombin preparation as a local hemostatic agent in complex surgeries. The diagnosis of inhibitors is based on the same tests as those used to diagnose inherited plasma coagulation factor deficiencies. However, the addition of the missing protein to the plasma of a subject with an inhibitor does not correct the abnormal aPTT and/or PT test results. This is the major laboratory difference between deficiencies and inhibitors. Additional tests are required to measure the specificity of the inhibitor and its titer.

The treatment of these bleeding disorders often requires replacement of the deficient protein using recombinant or purified plasma-derived products or fresh-frozen plasma (FFP). Therefore, it is imperative to arrive at a proper diagnosis to optimize patient care without unnecessary exposure to suboptimal treatment and the risks of bloodborne disease.

HEMOPHILIA

PATHOGENESIS AND CLINICAL MANIFESTATIONS

Hemophilia is an X-linked recessive hemorrhagic disease due to mutations in the *F8* gene (hemophilia A or classic hemophilia) or *F9* gene (hemophilia B). The disease affects 1 in 10,000 males worldwide, in all ethnic

TABLE 20-1

GENETIC AND LABORATORY CHARACTERISTICS OF INHERITED COAGULATION DISORDERS

CLOTTING FACTOR DEFICIENCY	INHERITANCE	PREVALENCE IN GENERAL POPULATION	LABORATORY ABNORMALITY[a] aPTT	PT	TT	MINIMUM HEMOSTATIC LEVELS	TREATMENT	PLASMA HALF-LIFE
Fibrinogen	AR	1 in 1,000,000	+	+	+	100 mg/dL	Cryoprecipitate	2–4 d
Prothrombin	AR	1 in 2,000,000	+	+	–	20–30%	FFP/PCC	3–4 d
Factor V	AR	1 in 1,000,000	+/–	+/–	–	15–20%	FFP	36 h
Factor VII	AR	1 in 500,000	–	+	–	15–20%	FFP/PCC	4–6 h
Factor VIII	X-linked	1 in 5,000	+	–	–	30%	FVIII concentrates	8–12 h
Factor IX	X-linked	1 in 30,000	+	–	–	30%	FIX concentrates	18–24 h
Factor X	AR	1 in 1,000,000	+/–	+/–	–	15–20%	FFP/PCC	40–60 h
Factor XI	AR	1 in 1,000,000	+	–	–	15–20%	FFP	40–70 h
Factor XII	AR	ND	+	–	–	[b]	[b]	60 h
HK	AR	ND	+	–	–	[b]	[b]	150 h
Prekallikrein	AR	ND	+	–	–	[b]	[b]	35 h
Factor XIII	AR	1 in 2,000,000	–	–	+/–	2–5%	Cryoprecipitate	11–14 d

[a]Values within normal range (–) or prolonged (+).
[b]No risk for bleeding; treatment is not indicated.
Abbreviations: aPTT, activated partial thromboplastin time; AR, autosomal recessive; FFP, fresh-frozen plasma; HK, high-molecular-weight kininogen; ND, not determined; PCC, prothrombin complex concentrates; PT, prothrombin time; TT, thrombin time.

groups; hemophilia A represents 80% of all cases. Male subjects are clinically affected; women, who carry a single mutated gene, are generally asymptomatic. Family history of the disease is absent in ~30% of cases, and in these cases, 80% of the mothers are carriers of the de novo mutated allele. More than 500 different mutations have been identified in the *F8* or *F9* genes of patients with hemophilia A or B, respectively. One of the most common hemophilia A mutations results from an inversion of the intron 22 sequence, and it is present in 40% of cases of severe hemophilia A. Advances in molecular diagnosis now permit precise identification of mutations, allowing accurate diagnosis of women carriers of the hemophilia gene in affected families.

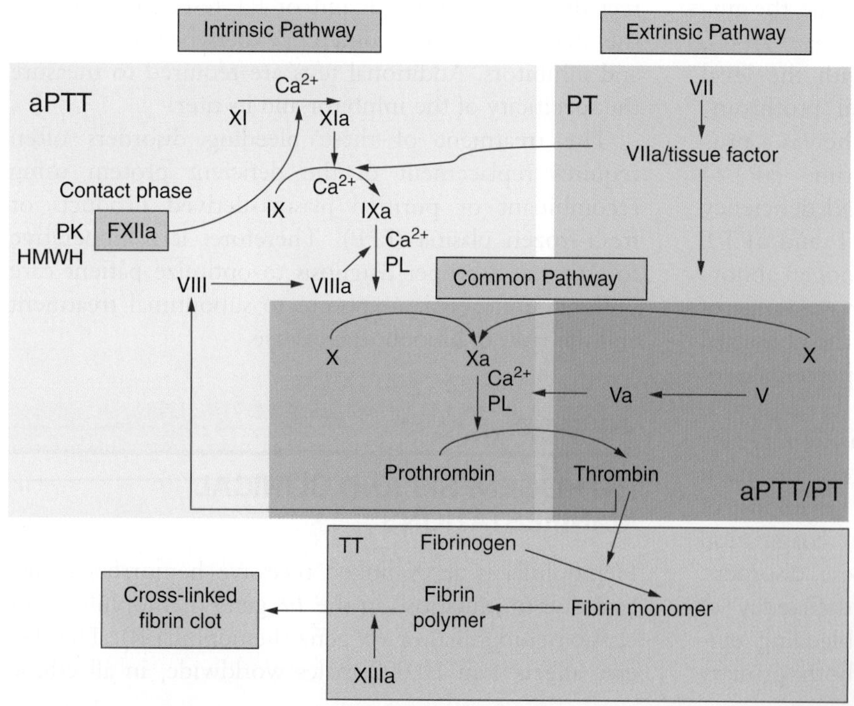

FIGURE 20-1

Coagulation cascade and laboratory assessment of clotting factor deficiency by activated partial prothrombin time (aPTT), prothrombin time (PT), and thrombin time (TT).

Clinically, hemophilia A and hemophilia B are indistinguishable. The disease phenotype correlates with the residual activity of FVIII or FIX and can be classified as severe (<1%), moderate (1–5%), or mild (6–30%). In the severe and moderate forms, the disease is characterized by bleeding into the joints (hemarthrosis), soft tissues, and muscles after minor trauma or even spontaneously. Patients with mild disease experience infrequent bleeding that is usually secondary to trauma. Among those with residual FVIII or FIX activity >25% of normal, the disease is discovered only by bleeding after major trauma or during routine presurgery laboratory tests. Typically, the global tests of coagulation show only an isolated prolongation of the aPTT assay. Patients with hemophilia have normal bleeding times and platelet counts. The diagnosis is made after specific determination of FVIII or FIX clotting activity.

Early in life, bleeding may present after circumcision or rarely as intracranial hemorrhages. The disease is more evident when children begin to walk or crawl. In the severe form, the most common bleeding manifestations are the recurrent hemarthroses, which can affect every joint but mainly the knees, elbows, ankles, shoulders, and hips. Acute hemarthroses are painful, and clinical signs are local swelling and erythema. To avoid pain, the patient may adopt a fixed position, which leads eventually to muscle contractures. Very young children unable to communicate verbally show irritability and a lack of movement of the affected joint. Chronic hemarthroses are debilitating, with synovial thickening and synovitis in response to the intraarticular blood. After a joint has been damaged, recurrent bleeding episodes result in the clinically recognized "target joint," which then establishes a vicious cycle of bleeding, resulting in progressive joint deformity that in critical cases requires surgery as the only therapeutic option. Hematomas into the muscle of distal parts of the limbs may lead to external compression of arteries, veins, or nerves that can evolve to a compartment syndrome.

Bleeding into the oropharyngeal spaces, central nervous system (CNS), or the retroperitoneum is life threatening and requires immediate therapy. Retroperitoneal hemorrhages can accumulate large quantities of blood with formation of masses with calcification and inflammatory tissue reaction (pseudotumor syndrome) and also result in damage to the femoral nerve. Pseudotumors can also form in bones, especially the long bones of the lower limbs. Hematuria is frequent among hemophilia patients, even in the absence of genitourinary pathology. It is often self-limited and may not require specific therapy.

TREATMENT Hemophilia

Without treatment, people with severe hemophilia have a limited life expectancy. Advances in the blood fractionation industry during World War II resulted in the realization that plasma could be used to treat hemophilia, but the volumes required to achieve even modest elevation of circulating factor levels limit the utility of plasma infusion as an approach to disease management. The discovery in the 1960s that the cryoprecipitate fraction of plasma was enriched for FVIII, and the eventual purification of FVIII and FIX from plasma led to the introduction of home infusion therapy with factor concentrates in the 1970s. The availability of factor concentrates resulted in a dramatic improvement in life expectancy and quality of life for people with severe hemophilia. However, the contamination of the blood supply with hepatitis viruses and subsequently HIV resulted in widespread transmission of these bloodborne infections within the hemophilia population; complications of HIV and of hepatitis C are now the leading causes of death among U.S. adults with severe hemophilia. The introduction of viral inactivation steps in the preparation of plasma-derived products in the mid-1980s greatly reduced the risk of HIV and hepatitis, and the risks were further reduced by the successful production of recombinant FVIII and FIX proteins, both licensed in the 1990s. It is uncommon for hemophilic patients born after 1985 to have contracted either hepatitis or HIV, and for these individuals, life expectancy is in the range of age 65 years.

Factor replacement therapy for hemophilia can be provided either in response to a bleeding episode or as a prophylactic treatment. Primary prophylaxis is defined as a strategy for maintaining the missing clotting factor at levels ~1% or higher on a regular basis in order to prevent bleeds, especially the onset of hemarthroses. Hemophilic boys receiving regular infusions of FVIII (3 days/week) or FIX (2 days/week) can reach puberty without detectable joint abnormalities.

Prophylaxis has become gradually more common in young patients. The Centers for Disease Control and Prevention reported that 51% of children with severe hemophilia who are younger than age 6 years receive prophylaxis, increasing considerably from 33% in 1995. Although highly recommended, the high cost and difficulties in accessing peripheral veins in young patients and the potential infectious and thrombotic risks of long-term central vein catheters are important limiting factors for many patients.

General considerations regarding the treatment of bleeds in hemophilia include (1) the need to begin the treatment as soon as possible because symptoms often precede objective evidence of bleeding; because of the superior efficacy of early therapeutic intervention, classic symptoms of bleeding into the joint in a reliable patient, headaches, or automobile or other accidents require prompt replacement and further laboratory investigation, and (2) the need to avoid drugs that hamper platelet function, such as aspirin or aspirin-containing drugs; to control pain, drugs such as ibuprofen or propoxyphene are preferred.

Factor VIII and FIX are dosed in units. One unit is defined as amount of FVIII (100 ng/mL) or FIX (5 μg/mL) in 1 mL of normal plasma. One unit of FVIII per kilogram of body weight increases the plasma FVIII level by 2%. One can calculate the dose needed to increase FVIII levels to 100% in a 70-kg severe hemophilia patient (<1%) using the simple formula below. Thus, 3500 units of FVIII will raise the circulating level to 100%.

$$\text{FVIII dose (IU)} = \text{Target FVIII levels} - \text{FVIII baseline levels} \times \text{body weight (kg)} \times 0.5\ \text{unit/kg}$$

The doses for FIX replacement are different from those for FVIII because FIX recovery postinfusion is usually only 50% of the predicted value. Therefore, the formula for FIX replacement is

$$\text{FIX dose (IU)} = \text{Target FIX levels} - \text{FIX baseline levels} \times \text{body weight (kg)} \times 1\ \text{unit/kg}$$

The FVIII half-life of 8–12 h requires injections twice a day to maintain therapeutic levels, whereas FIX's half-life is longer, ~24 h, so that once-a-day injection is sufficient. In specific situations such as postsurgery, continuous infusion of factor may be desirable because of its safety in achieving sustained factor levels at a lower total cost.

Cryoprecipitate is enriched with FVIII protein (each bag contains ~80 IU of FVIII) and was commonly used for the treatment of hemophilia A decades ago; it is still in use in some developing countries, but because of the risk of bloodborne diseases, this product should be avoided in hemophilia patients when factor concentrates are available.

Mild bleeds such as uncomplicated hemarthroses or superficial hematomas require initial therapy with factor levels of 30–50%. Additional doses to maintain levels of 15–25% for 2 or 3 days are indicated for severe hemarthroses, especially when these episodes affect the "target joint." Large hematomas, or bleeds into deep muscles, require factor levels of 50% or even higher if the clinical symptoms do not improve, and factor replacement may be required for a period of 1 week or longer. The control of serious bleeds, including those that affect the oropharyngeal spaces, CNS, and the retroperitoneum, requires sustained protein levels of 50–100% for 7–10 days. Prophylactic replacement for surgery is aimed at achieving normal factor levels (100%) for a period of 7–10 days; replacement can then be tapered depending on the extent of the surgical wounds. Oral surgery is associated with extensive tissue damage that usually requires factor replacement for 1–3 days coupled with oral antifibrinolytic drugs.

NONTRANFUSION THERAPY IN HEMOPHILIA

DDAVP (1-Amino-8-D-Arginine Vasopressin)

DDAVP is a synthetic vasopressin analog that causes a transient rise in FVIII and von Willebrand factor (vWF), but not FIX, through a mechanism involving release from endothelial cells. Patients with moderate or mild hemophilia A should be tested to determine if they respond to DDAVP before a therapeutic application. DDAVP at doses of 0.3 μg/kg body weight, over a 20-min period, is expected to raise FVIII levels by two- to threefold over baseline, peaking between 30 and 60 min postinfusion. DDAVP does not improve FVIII levels in severe hemophilia A patients, since there are no stores to release. Repeated dosing of DDAVP results in tachyphylaxis, since the mechanism is an increase in release rather than de novo synthesis of FVIII and vWF. More than three consecutive doses become ineffective, and if further therapy is indicated, FVIII replacement is required to achieve hemostasis.

Antifibrinolytic Drugs Bleeding in the gums and gastrointestinal tract and during oral surgery requires the use of oral antifibrinolytic drugs such as ε-aminocaproic acid (EACA) or tranexamic acid to control local hemostasis. The duration of the treatment depending on the clinical indication is 1 week or longer. Tranexamic acid is given at doses of 25 mg/kg three to four times a day. EACA treatment requires a loading dose of 200 mg/kg (maximum of 10 g) followed by 100 mg/kg per dose (maximum 30 g/d) every 6 h. These drugs are not indicated to control hematuria because of the risk of formation of an occlusive clot in the lumen of genitourinary tract structures.

COMPLICATIONS

Inhibitor Formation The formation of alloantibodies to FVIII or FIX is currently the major complication of hemophilia treatment. The prevalence of inhibitors to FVIII is estimated to be between 5 and 10% of all cases and ~20% of severe hemophilia A patients. Inhibitors to FIX are detected in only 3–5% of all hemophilia B patients. The high-risk group for inhibitor formation includes severe deficiency (>80% of all cases of inhibitors), familial history of inhibitor, African descent, mutations in the FVIII or FIX gene resulting in deletion of large coding regions, or gross gene rearrangements. Inhibitors usually appear early in life, at a median of 2 years of age, and after 10 cumulative days of exposure. However, intensive replacement therapy such as for major surgery, intracranial bleeding, or trauma increases the risk of inhibitor formation for patients of all ages that requires close laboratory monitoring in the following weeks.

The clinical diagnosis of an inhibitor is suspected when patients do not respond to factor replacement at therapeutic doses. Inhibitors increase both morbidity and mortality in hemophilia. Because early detection of an inhibitor is critical to a successful correction of the bleeding or to eradication of the antibody, most hemophilia centers perform annual screening for inhibitors. The laboratory test required to confirm the presence of an inhibitor is an aPTT with a mix (with normal plasma). In most hemophilia patients, a 1:1 mix with normal plasma completely corrects the aPTT. In inhibitor patients, the aPTT on a 1:1 mix is abnormally prolonged because the inhibitor neutralizes the FVIII clotting activity of the normal plasma. The Bethesda assay uses a similar principle and defines the specificity of the inhibitor and its titer. The results are expressed in Bethesda units (BU), in which 1 BU is the amount of antibody that neutralizes 50% of the FVIII or FIX present in normal plasma after 2 h of incubation at 37°C. Clinically, inhibitor patients are classified as low responders or high responders, which provides guidelines for optimal therapy. Therapy for inhibitor patients has two goals, the control of acute bleeding episodes and the eradication of the inhibitor. For the control of bleeding episodes, low responders, those with titer <5 BU, respond well to high doses of human or porcine FVIII (50–100 U/kg), with minimal or no increase in the inhibitor titers. However, high-responder patients, those with initial inhibitor titer >10 BU or an anamnestic response in the antibody titer to >10 BU even if low titer initially, do not respond to FVIII or FIX concentrates. The control of bleeding episodes in high-responder patients can be achieved by using concentrates enriched for prothrombin, FVII, FIX, FX (prothrombin complex concentrates [PCCs] or activated PCCs), and more recently by recombinant activated factor VII (FVIIa) (Fig. 20-1). The rates of therapeutic success have been higher for FVIIa than for PCC or aPCC. For eradication of the inhibitory antibody, immunosuppression alone is not effective. The most effective strategy is the immune tolerance induction (ITI) based on daily infusion of missing protein until the inhibitor disappears, typically requiring periods longer than 1 year, with success rates in the range of 60%. The management of patients with severe hemophilia A and inhibitors resistant to ITI is challenging. The use of anti-CD20 monoclonal antibody (rituximab) combined with FVIII was thought to be effective. Although this therapy may reduce the inhibitor titers, sustained eradication is uncommon and may require two to three infusions weekly of FVIII concentrates.

Infectious Diseases Hepatitis C viral (HCV) infection is the major cause of morbidity and the second leading cause of death in hemophilia patients exposed to older clotting factor concentrates. The vast majority of young patients treated with plasma-derived products from 1970 to 1985 became infected with HCV. It has been estimated that >80% of patients older than 20 years of age were HCV antibody positive as of 2006. The comorbidity of the underlying liver disease in hemophilia patients is clear when these individuals require invasive procedures; correction of both genetic and acquired (secondary to liver disease) deficiencies may be needed. Infection with HIV also swept the population of patients using plasma-derived concentrates 2 decades ago. Co-infection of HCV and HIV, present in almost 50% of hemophilia patients, is an aggravating factor for the evolution of liver disease. The response to HCV antiviral therapy in hemophilia is restricted to <30% of patients and even poorer among those with both HCV and HIV infection. End-stage liver disease requiring organ transplantation may be curative for both the liver disease and for hemophilia.

Emerging Clinical Problems in Aging Hemophilia Patients There has been continuous improvement of the management of hemophilia since the increase in the population of adults living beyond middle age in the developing world. The life expectancy of a patient with severe hemophilia is only ~10 years shorter than the general male population. In patients with mild or moderate hemophilia, life expectancy is approaching that of the male population without coagulopathy. Elderly hemophilia patients have different problems compared with the younger generation; they have more severe arthropathy and chronic pain due to suboptimal treatment and high rates of HCV and/or HIV infections.

Early data indicate that death from coronary artery disease is lower in hemophilia patients than the general male population. The underlying hypocoagulability probably provides a protective effect against thrombus formation, but it does not prevent the development of atherogenesis. Similar to the general population, these patients are exposed to cardiovascular risk factors such as older age, obesity, and smoking. Moreover, physical inactivity, hypertension, and chronic renal disease are commonly observed in hemophilia patients. In HIV patients on combined antiretroviral therapy, there may be a further increase in the risk of cardiovascular disease. Therefore, these patients should be carefully considered for preventive and therapeutic approaches to minimize the risk of cardiovascular disease.

Excessive replacement therapy should be avoided, and it is prudent to slowly infuse factor concentrates. Continuous infusion of clotting factor is preferable to bolus dosing in patients with cardiovascular risk factors undergoing invasive procedures. The management of an acute ischemic event and coronary revascularization should include the collaboration of hematologists and internists. The early assumption that hemophilia would protect against occlusive vascular disease may change in this aging population.

Cancer is a common cause of death in aging hemophilia patients as they are at risk for HIV- and HCV-related malignancies. Hepatocellular carcinoma (HCC) is the most prevalent primary liver cancer and a common cause of death in HIV-negative patients. The recommendations for cancer screening for the general population should be the same for age-matched hemophilia patients. Among those with high-risk HCV, a semiannual or annual ultrasound and α fetoprotein is recommended for HCC. Screening for urogenital neoplasm in the presence of hematuria or hematochezia may be delayed due to the underlying bleeding disease, thus preventing early intervention. Multidisciplinary interaction should facilitate the attempts to ensure optimal cancer prevention and treatment recommendations for those with hemophilia.

Management of Carriers of Hemophilia Usually hemophilia carriers, with factor levels of ~50% of normal, have not been considered to be at risk for bleeding. However, a wide range of values (22–116%) have been reported due to random inactivation of the X chromosomes (*lyonization*). Therefore, it is important to measure the factor level of carriers to recognize those at risk of bleeding and to optimize preoperative and postoperative management. During pregnancy, both FVIII and FIX levels increase gradually until delivery. FVIII levels increase approximately two- to threefold compared with nonpregnant women, whereas a FIX increase is less pronounced. After delivery, there is a rapid fall in the pregnancy-induced rise of maternal clotting factor levels. This represents an imminent risk of bleeding that can be prevented by infusion of factor concentrate to levels of 50–70% for 3 days in the setting of vaginal delivery and up to 5 days for cesarean section. In mild cases, the use of DDAVP and/or antifibrinolytic drugs is recommended.

FACTOR XI DEFICIENCY

Factor XI is a zymogen of an active serine protease (FIXa) in the intrinsic pathway of blood coagulation that activates FIX (Fig. 20-1). There are two pathways for the formation of FXIa. In an aPTT-based assay, the protease is the result of activation by FXIIa in conjunction with high-molecular-weight kininogen and kallikrein. In vivo data suggest that thrombin is the physiologic activator of FXI. The generation of thrombin by the tissue-factor/factor VIIa pathway activates FXI on the platelet surface that contributes to additional thrombin generation after the clot has formed and thus augments resistance to fibrinolysis through a thrombin-activated fibrinolytic inhibitor (TAFI).

Factor XI deficiency is a rare bleeding disorder that occurs in the general population at a frequency of one in a million. However, the disease is highly prevalent among Ashkenazi and Iraqi Jewish populations, reaching a frequency of 6% as heterozygotes and 0.1 to 0.3% as homozygotes. More than 65 mutations in the FXI gene have been reported, whereas fewer mutations (two to three) are found among affected Jewish populations.

Normal FXI clotting activity levels range from 70 to 150 U/dL. In heterozygous patients with moderate deficiency, FXI ranges from 20 to 70 U/dL, whereas in homozygous or double heterozygote patients, FXI levels are <1–20 U/dL. Patients with FXI levels <10% of normal have a high risk of bleeding, but the disease phenotype does not always correlate with residual FXI clotting activity. A family history is indicative of the risk of bleeding in the propositus. Clinically, the presence of mucocutaneous hemorrhages such as bruises, gum bleeding, epistaxis, hematuria, and menorrhagia are common, especially following trauma. This hemorrhagic phenotype suggests that tissues rich in fibrinolytic activity are more susceptible to FXI deficiency. Postoperative bleeding is common but not always present, even among patients with very low FXI levels.

FXI replacement is indicated in patients with severe disease required to undergo a surgical procedure. A negative history of bleeding complications following invasive procedures does not exclude the possibility of an increased risk for hemorrhage.

TREATMENT Factor XI Deficiency

The treatment of FXI deficiency is based on the infusion of FFP at doses of 15 to 20 mL/kg to maintain trough levels ranging from 10 to 20%. Because FXI has a half-life of 40–70 h, the replacement therapy can be given on alternate days. The use of antifibrinolytic drugs is beneficial to control bleeds, with the exception of hematuria or bleeds in the bladder. The development of an FXI inhibitor was observed in 10% of severely FXI-deficient patients who received replacement therapy. Patients with severe FXI deficiency who develop inhibitors usually do not bleed spontaneously. However, bleeding following a surgical procedure or trauma can be severe. In these patients, FFP and FXI concentrates should be avoided. The use of PCC/aPCC or recombinant activated FVII has been effective.

RARE BLEEDING DISORDERS

Collectively, the inherited disorders resulting from deficiencies of clotting factors other than FVIII, FIX, and FXI (Table 20-1) represent a group of rare bleeding diseases. The bleeding symptoms in these patients vary from asymptomatic (dysfibrinogenemia or FVII deficiency) to life-threatening (FX or FXIII deficiency). There is no pathognomonic clinical manifestation that suggests one specific disease, but overall, in contrast to hemophilia, hemarthrosis is a rare event, and bleeding in the mucosal tract or after umbilical cord clamping is common. Individuals heterozygous for plasma coagulation deficiencies are often asymptomatic. The laboratory assessment for the specific deficient factor following screening with general coagulation tests (Table 20-1) will define the diagnosis.

Replacement therapy using FFP or prothrombin complex concentrates (containing prothrombin, FVII, FIX, and FX) provides adequate hemostasis in response to bleeds or as prophylactic treatment. The use of PCC should be carefully monitored and avoided in patients with underlying liver disease or those at high risk for thrombosis because of the risk of disseminated intravascular coagulopathy.

FAMILIAL MULTIPLE COAGULATION DEFICIENCIES

There are several bleeding disorders characterized by the inherited deficiency of more than one plasma coagulation factor. To date, the genetic defects in two of these diseases have been characterized, and they provide new insights into the regulation of hemostasis by gene-encoding proteins outside blood coagulation.

Combined deficiency of FV and FVIII

Patients with combined FV and FVIII deficiency exhibit ~5% of residual clotting activity of each factor. Interestingly, the disease phenotype is a mild bleeding tendency, often following trauma. An underlying mutation has been identified in the endoplasmic reticulum/Golgi intermediate compartment (ERGIC-53) gene, a mannose-binding protein localized in the Golgi apparatus that functions as a chaperone for both FV and FVIII. In other families, mutations in the multiple coagulation factor deficiency 2 (MCFD2) gene have been defined; this gene encodes a protein that forms a Ca^{2+}–dependent complex with ERGIC-53 and provides cofactor activity in the intracellular mobilization of both FV and FVIII.

Multiple deficiencies of vitamin K–dependent coagulation factors

Two enzymes involved in vitamin K metabolism have been associated with combined deficiency of all vitamin K–dependent proteins, including the procoagulant proteins prothrombin, VII, IX, and X and the anticoagulant proteins C and S. Vitamin K is a fat-soluble vitamin that is a cofactor for carboxylation of the gamma carbon of the glutamic acid residues in

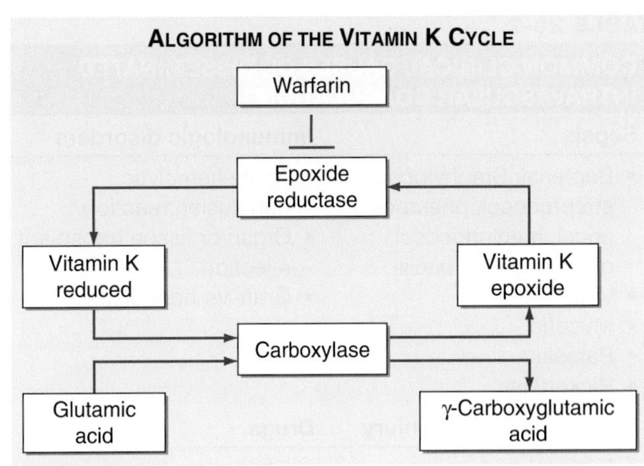

FIGURE 20-2
The vitamin K cycle. Vitamin K is a cofactor for the formation of γ-carboxyglutamic acid residues on coagulation proteins. Vitamin K–dependent γ-glutamylcarboxylase, the enzyme that catalyzes the vitamin K epoxide reductase, regenerates reduced vitamin K. Warfarin blocks the action of the reductase and competitively inhibits the effects of vitamin K.

the vitamin K–dependent factors, a critical step for calcium and phospholipid binding of these proteins (Fig. 20-2). The enzymes γ-glutamylcarboxylase and epoxide reductase are critical for the metabolism and regeneration of vitamin K. Mutations in the genes encoding the gamma-carboxylase (GGCX) or vitamin K epoxide reductase complex 1 (VKORC1) result in defective enzymes and thus in vitamin K–dependent factors with reduced activity, varying from 1 to 30% of normal. The disease phenotype is characterized by mild to severe bleeding episodes present from birth. Some patients respond to high doses of vitamin K. For severe bleeding, replacement therapy with FFP or PCC may be necessary for achieving full hemostatic control.

DISSEMINATED INTRAVASCULAR COAGULATION

Disseminated intravascular coagulation (DIC) is a clinicopathologic syndrome characterized by widespread intravascular fibrin formation in response to excessive blood protease activity that overcomes the natural anticoagulant mechanisms. There are several underlying pathologies associated with DIC (Table 20-2).

The most common causes are bacterial sepsis, malignant disorders such as solid tumors and acute promyelocytic leukemia, and obstetric causes. DIC is diagnosed in almost half of pregnant women with abruptio placentae or with amniotic fluid embolism. Trauma, particularly to the brain, can also result in DIC. The exposure of blood to phospholipids from damaged tissue, hemolysis, and endothelial damage are all contributing factors to the development of DIC in this setting. Purpura fulminans is a severe form of DIC

TABLE 20-2

COMMON CLINICAL CAUSES OF DISSEMINATED INTRAVASCULAR COAGULATION

Sepsis	Immunologic disorders
• Bacterial: Staphylococci, streptococci, pneumococci, meningococci, gram-negative bacilli • Viral • Mycotic • Parasitic • Rickettsial	• Acute hemolytic transfusion reaction • Organ or tissue transplant rejection • Graft-vs-host disease
Trauma and tissue injury	**Drugs**
• Brain injury (gunshot) • Extensive burns • Fat embolism • Rhabdomyolysis	• Fibrinolytic agents • Aprotinin • Warfarin (especially in neonates with protein C deficiency) • Prothrombin complex concentrates • Recreational drugs (amphetamines)
Vascular disorders	**Envenomation**
• Giant hemangiomas (Kasabach-Merritt syndrome) • Large vessel aneurysms (e.g., aorta)	• Snake • Insects
Obstetric complications	**Liver disease**
• Abruptio placentae • Amniotic-fluid embolism • Dead fetus syndrome • Septic abortion	• Fulminant hepatic failure • Cirrhosis • Fatty liver of pregnancy
Cancer	**Miscellaneous**
• Adenocarcinoma (prostate, pancreas, etc.) • Hematologic malignancies (acute promyelocytic leukemia)	• Shock • Respiratory distress syndrome • Massive transfusion

resulting from thrombosis of extensive areas of the skin; it affects predominantly young children following viral or bacterial infection, particularly those with inherited or acquired hypercoagulability due to deficiencies of the components of the protein C pathway. Neonates homozygous for protein C deficiency also present high risk for purpura fulminans with or without thrombosis of large vessels.

The central mechanism of DIC is the uncontrolled generation of thrombin by exposure of the blood to pathologic levels of tissue factor (Fig. 20-3). Simultaneous suppression of physiologic anticoagulant mechanisms and abnormal fibrinolysis further accelerate the process. Together, these abnormalities contribute to systemic fibrin deposition in small and midsize vessels. The duration and intensity of the fibrin deposition can compromise the blood supply of many organs, especially the lung, kidney, liver, and brain, with consequent organ failure. The sustained activation of coagulation results in consumption of clotting factors and platelets, which in turn leads to systemic bleeding. This is further aggravated by secondary hyperfibrinolysis. Studies in animals demonstrate that the fibrinolytic system is indeed suppressed at the time of maximal activation of coagulation. Interestingly, in patients with acute promyelocytic leukemia, a severe hyperfibrinolytic state often occurs in addition to the coagulation activation. The release of several proinflammatory cytokines such as interleukin 6 and tumor necrosis factor α play central roles in mediating the coagulation defects in DIC and symptoms associated with systemic inflammatory response syndrome (SIRS).

Clinical manifestations of DIC are related to the magnitude of the imbalance of hemostasis, the underlying disease, or both. The most common findings are bleeding ranging from oozing from venipuncture sites, petechiae, and ecchymoses to severe hemorrhage from the gastrointestinal tract or lung or into the CNS. In chronic DIC, the bleeding symptoms are discrete and restricted to skin or mucosal surfaces. The hypercoagulability of DIC manifests as the occlusion of vessels in the microcirculation and resulting organ failure. Thrombosis of large vessels and cerebral embolism can also occur. Hemodynamic complications and shock are common among patients with acute DIC. The mortality rate ranges from 30 to >80% depending on the underlying disease, the severity of the DIC, and the age of the patient.

The diagnosis of clinically significant DIC is based on the presence of clinical and/or laboratory abnormalities of coagulation or thrombocytopenia. The laboratory diagnosis of DIC should prompt a search for the underlying disease if it is not already apparent. There is no single test that establishes the diagnosis of DIC. The laboratory investigation should include coagulation tests (aPTT, PT, thrombin time [TT]) and markers of fibrin degradation products (FDPs) in addition to platelet and red cell count and analysis of the blood smear. These tests should be repeated over a period of 6–8 hours because an initially mild abnormality can change dramatically in patients with severe DIC.

Common findings include the prolongation of PT and/or aPTT, platelet counts $\leq 100{,}000/\mu L^3$ or a rapid decline in platelet numbers, the presence of schistocytes (fragmented red cells) in the blood smear, and elevated levels of FDP. The most sensitive test for DIC is the FDP level. DIC is an unlikely diagnosis in the presence of normal levels of FDP. The D-dimer test is more specific for detection of fibrin—but not fibrinogen—degradation products and indicates that the cross-linked fibrin has been digested by plasmin. Because fibrinogen has a prolonged half-life, plasma levels diminish

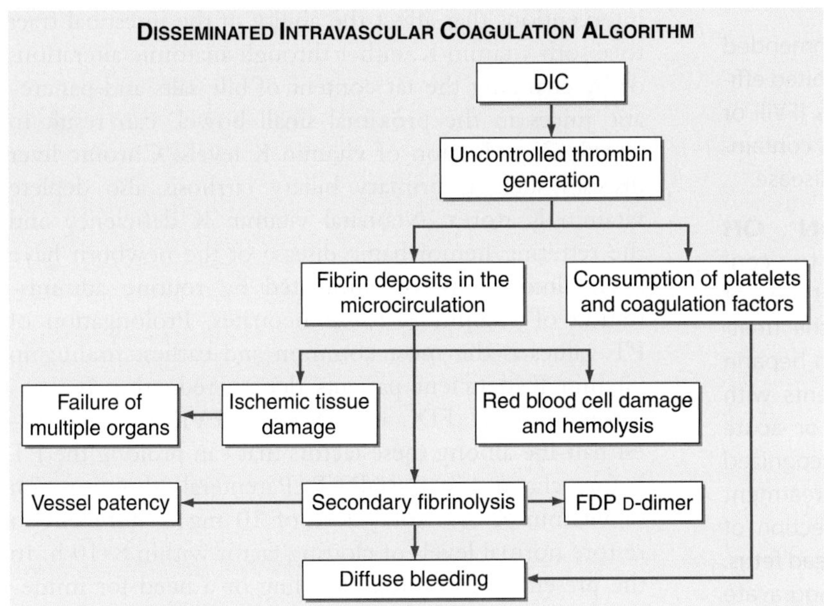

FIGURE 20-3
The pathophysiology of disseminated intravascular coagulation (DIC). Interactions between coagulation and fibrinolytic pathways result in bleeding and thrombosis in the microcirculation in patients with DIC. FDP, fibrin degradation product.

acutely only in severe cases of DIC. High-grade DIC is also associated with levels of antithrombin III or plasminogen activity <60% of normal.

Chronic DIC

Low-grade, compensated DIC can occur in clinical situations including giant hemangioma, metastatic carcinoma, or the dead fetus syndrome. Plasma levels of FDP or D-dimers are elevated. aPTT, PT, and fibrinogen values are within the normal range or high. Mild thrombocytopenia or normal platelet counts are also common findings. Red cell fragmentation is often detected but at a lower degree than in acute DIC.

Differential diagnosis

The differential diagnosis between DIC and severe liver disease is challenging and requires serial measurements of the laboratory parameters of DIC. Patients with severe liver disease are at risk for bleeding and manifest laboratory features including thrombocytopenia (due to platelet sequestration, portal hypertension, or hypersplenism), decreased synthesis of coagulation factors and natural anticoagulants, and elevated levels of FDP due to reduced hepatic clearance. However, in contrast to DIC, these laboratory parameters in liver disease do not change rapidly. Other important differential findings include the presence of portal hypertension or other clinical or laboratory evidence of an underlying liver disease.

Microangiopathic disorders such as thrombotic thrombocytopenic purpura present an acute clinical onset of illness accompanied by thrombocytopenia, red cell fragmentation, and multiorgan failure. However, there is no consumption of clotting factors or hyperfibrinolysis.

TREATMENT Disseminated Intravascular Coagulation

The morbidity and mortality associated with DIC are primarily related to the underlying disease rather than the complications of the DIC. The control or elimination of the underlying cause should therefore be the primary concern. Patients with severe DIC require control of hemodynamic parameters, respiratory support, and sometimes invasive surgical procedures. Attempts to treat DIC without accompanying treatment of the causative disease are likely to fail.

MANAGEMENT OF HEMORRHAGIC SYMPTOMS The control of bleeding in DIC patients with marked thrombocytopenia (platelet counts <10,000–20,000/μL^3) and low levels of coagulation factors will require replacement therapy. The PT (>1.5 times the normal) provides a good indicator of the severity of the clotting factor consumption. Replacement with FFP is indicated (1 unit of FFP increases most coagulation factors by 3% in an adult without DIC). Low levels of fibrinogen (<100 mg/dL) or brisk hyperfibrinolysis will require infusion of cryoprecipitate (plasma fraction enriched for fibrinogen, FVIII, and vWF). The replacement of 10 U of cryoprecipitate for every 2–3 U of FFP is sufficient to correct the hemostasis. The transfusion scheme must be adjusted according to the patient's clinical and laboratory evolution. Platelet concentrates at a dose of 1–2 U/10 kg body weight are sufficient for most DIC patients with severe thrombocytopenia.

Clotting factor concentrates are not recommended for control of bleeding in DIC because of the limited efficacy afforded by replacement of single factors (FVIII or FIX concentrates), and the high risk of products containing traces of aPCCs that further aggravate the disease.

REPLACEMENT OF COAGULATION OR FIBRINOLYSIS INHIBITORS Drugs to control coagulation such as heparin, ATIII concentrates, or antifibrinolytic drugs have all been tried in the treatment of DIC. Low doses of continuous infusion heparin (5–10 U/kg per h) may be effective in patients with low-grade DIC associated with solid tumor or acute promyelocytic leukemia or in a setting with recognized thrombosis. Heparin is also indicated for the treatment of purpura fulminans during the surgical resection of giant hemangiomas and during removal of a dead fetus. In acute DIC, the use of heparin is likely to aggravate bleeding. To date, the use of heparin in patients with severe DIC has no proven survival benefit.

The use of antifibrinolytic drugs, EACA, or tranexamic acid, to prevent fibrin degradation by plasmin may reduce bleeding episodes in patients with DIC and confirmed hyperfibrinolysis. However, these drugs can increase the risk of thrombosis, and concomitant use of heparin is indicated. Patients with acute promyelocytic leukemia or those with chronic DIC associated with giant hemangiomas are among the few patients who may benefit from this therapy.

The use of protein C concentrates to treat purpura fulminans associated with acquired protein C deficiency or meningococcemia has been proven efficacious. The results from the replacement of ATIII in early-phase studies are promising but require further study.

VITAMIN K DEFICIENCY

Vitamin K–dependent proteins are a heterogenous group, including clotting factor proteins and also proteins found in bone, lung, kidney, and placenta. Vitamin K mediates posttranslational modification of glutamate residues to γ-carboxylglutamate, a critical step for the activity of vitamin K–dependent proteins for calcium binding and proper assembly to phospholipid membranes (Fig. 20-2). Inherited deficiency of the functional activity of the enzymes involved in vitamin K metabolism, notably the GGCX or VKORC1 (see earlier discussion), results in bleeding disorders. The amount of vitamin K in the diet is often limiting for the carboxylation reaction; thus, recycling of the vitamin K is essential to maintain normal levels of vitamin K–dependent proteins. In adults, low dietary intake alone is seldom reason for severe vitamin K deficiency but may become common in association with the use of broad-spectrum antibiotics. Disease or surgical interventions that affect the ability of the intestinal tract to absorb vitamin K, either through anatomic alterations or by changing the fat content of bile salts and pancreatic juices in the proximal small bowel, can result in significant reduction of vitamin K levels. Chronic liver diseases such as primary biliary cirrhosis also deplete vitamin K stores. Neonatal vitamin K deficiency and the resulting hemorrhagic disease of the newborn have been almost entirely eliminated by routine administration of vitamin K to all neonates. Prolongation of PT values is the most common and earliest finding in vitamin K–deficient patients due to reduction in prothrombin, FVII, FIX, and FX levels. FVII has the shortest half-life among these factors that can prolong the PT before changes in the aPTT. Parenteral administration of vitamin K at a total dose of 10 mg is sufficient to restore normal levels of clotting factor within 8–10 h. In the presence of ongoing bleeding or a need for immediate correction before an invasive procedure, replacement with FFP or PCC is required. The latter should be avoided in patients with severe underlying liver disorders due to a high risk of thrombosis. The reversal of excessive anticoagulant therapy with warfarin or warfarin-like drugs can be achieved by minimal doses of vitamin K (1 mg orally or by intravenous injection) for asymptomatic patients. This strategy can diminish the risk of bleeding while maintaining therapeutic anticoagulation for an underlying prothrombotic state.

In patients with life-threatening bleeds, the use of recombinant factor VIIa in nonhemophilia patients on anticoagulant therapy has been shown to be effective at restoring hemostasis rapidly, allowing emergency surgical intervention. However, patients with underlying vascular disease, vascular trauma and other comorbidities are at risk for thromboembolic complications that affect both arterial and venous systems. Thus, the use of factor VIIa in this setting is limited to administration of low doses given for only a limited number of injections. Close monitoring for vascular complications is highly indicated.

COAGULATION DISORDERS ASSOCIATED WITH LIVER FAILURE

The liver is central to hemostasis because it is the site of synthesis and clearance of most procoagulant and natural anticoagulant proteins and of essential components of the fibrinolytic system. Liver failure is associated with a high risk of bleeding due to deficient synthesis of procoagulant factors and enhanced fibrinolysis. Thrombocytopenia is common in patients with liver disease and may be due to congestive splenomegaly (hypersplenism) or immune-mediated shortened platelet lifespan (primary biliary cirrhosis). In addition, several anatomic abnormalities secondary to

TABLE 20-3

COAGULATION DISORDERS AND HEMOSTASIS IN LIVER DISEASE

Bleeding
Portal hypertension
Esophageal varices
Thrombocytopenia
Splenomegaly
Chronic or acute DIC
Decreased synthesis of clotting factors
Hepatocyte failure
Vitamin K deficiency
Systemic fibrinolysis
DIC
Dysfibrinogenemia
Thrombosis
Decreased synthesis of coagulation inhibitors: protein C, protein S, antithrombin
Hepatocyte failure
Vitamin K deficiency (protein C, protein S)
Failure to clear activated coagulation proteins (DIC)
Dysfibrinogenemia
Iatrogenic: Transfusion of prothrombin complex concentrates
Antifibrinolytic agents: EACA, tranexamic acid

Abbreviations: DIC, disseminated intravascular coagulation; EACA, ε-aminocaproic acid.

underlying liver disease further promote the occurrence of hemorrhage (Table 20-3). Dysfibrinogenemia is a relatively common finding in patients with liver disease due to impaired fibrin polymerization. The development of DIC concomitant to chronic liver disease is not uncommon and may enhance the risk for bleeding. Laboratory evaluation is mandatory for an optimal therapeutic strategy, either to control ongoing bleeding or to prepare patients with liver disease for invasive procedures. Typically, these patients present with prolonged PT, aPTT, and TT depending on the degree of liver damage, thrombocytopenia, and normal or slight increase of FDP. Fibrinogen levels are diminished only in fulminant hepatitis, decompensated cirrhosis, or advanced liver disease or in the presence of DIC. The presence of prolonged TT and normal fibrinogen and FDP levels suggest dysfibrinogenemia. FVIII levels are often normal or elevated in patients with liver failure, and decreased levels suggest superimposing DIC. Because FV is only synthesized in the hepatocyte and is not a vitamin K–dependent protein, reduced levels of FV may be an indicator of hepatocyte failure. Normal levels of FV and low levels of FVII suggest vitamin K deficiency. Vitamin K levels may be reduced in patients with liver failure due to compromised storage in hepatocellular disease, changes in bile acids, or cholestasis that can diminish the absorption of vitamin K. Replacement of vitamin K may be desirable (10 mg given by slow intravenous injection) to improve hemostasis.

Treatment with FFP is the most effective to correct hemostasis in patients with liver failure. Infusion of FFP (5–10 mL/kg; each bag contains ~200 mL) is sufficient to ensure 10–20% of normal levels of clotting factors but not correction of PT or aPTT. Even high doses of FFP (20 mL/kg) do not correct the clotting times in all patients. Monitoring for clinical symptoms and clotting times will determine if repeated doses are required 8–12 h after the first infusion. Platelet concentrates are indicated when platelet counts are <10,000–20,000/μL^3 to control an ongoing bleed or immediately before an invasive procedure if counts are <50,000/μL^3. Cryoprecipitate is indicated only when fibrinogen levels are less than 100 mg/mL; dosing is six bags for a 70-kg patient daily. Prothrombin complex concentrate infusion in patients with liver failure should be avoided due to the high risk of thrombotic complications. The safety of the use of antifibrinolytic drugs to control bleeding in patients with liver failure is not yet well defined and should be avoided.

Liver disease and thromboembolism

The clinical bleeding phenotype of hemostasis in patients with stable liver disease is often mild or even asymptomatic. However, as the disease progresses, the hemostatic balance is less stable and more easily disturbed than in healthy individuals. Furthermore, the hemostatic balance is compromised by comorbid complications such as infections and renal failure (Fig. 20-4). Based on the clinical bleeding complications in patients with cirrhosis and laboratory evidence of hypocoagulation such as a prolonged PT/aPTT, it has long been assumed that these patients are protected against thrombotic disease. Cumulative clinical experience, however, has demonstrated that these patients are at risk for thrombosis, especially those with advanced liver disease. Although hypercoagulability could explain the occurrence of venous thrombosis, according to Virchow's triad, hemodynamic changes and damaged vasculature may also be a contributing factor, and both processes may potentially also occur in patients with liver disease. Liver-related thrombosis, in particular, thrombosis of the portal and mesenteric veins, is common in patients with advanced cirrhosis. Hemodynamic changes such as decreased portal flow and evidence that inherited thrombophilia may enhance the risk for portal vein thrombosis in patients with cirrhosis suggest that hypercoagulability may play a role as well. Patients with liver disease develop deep vein thrombosis and pulmonary embolism at appreciable rates (ranging from 0.5–1.9%). The implication of these findings is relevant

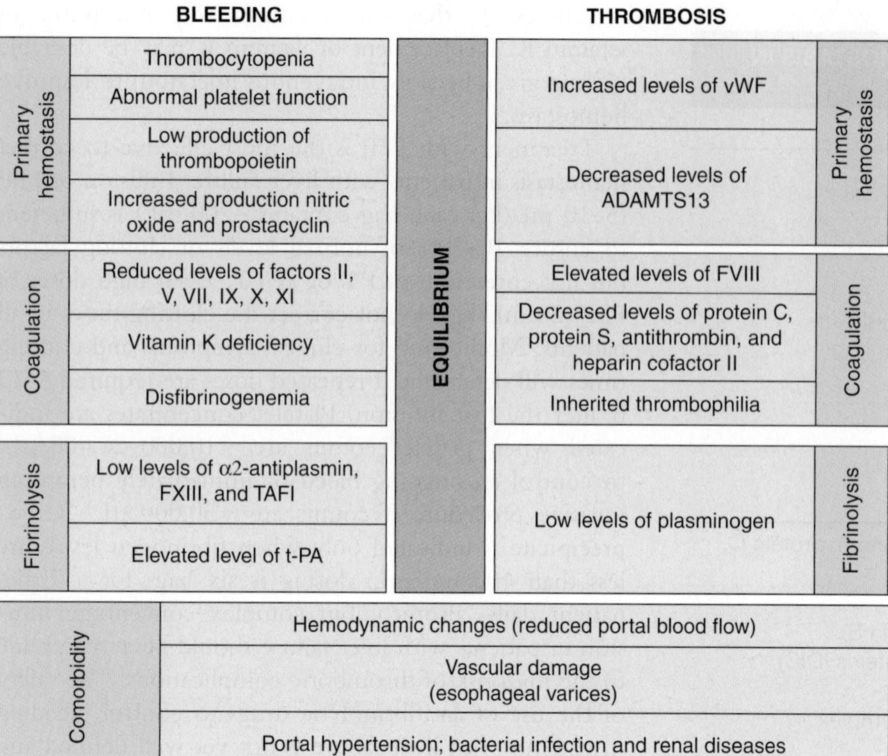

BLEEDING
THROMBOSIS
EQUILIBRIUM
Primary hemostasis
Thrombocytopenia
Abnormal platelet function
Low production of thrombopoietin
Increased production nitric oxide and prostacyclin
Coagulation
Reduced levels of factors II, V, VII, IX, X, XI
Vitamin K deficiency
Disfibrinogenemia
Fibrinolysis
Low levels of α2-antiplasmin, FXIII, and TAFI
Elevated level of t-PA
Increased levels of vWF
Decreased levels of ADAMTS13
Primary hemostasis
Elevated levels of FVIII
Decreased levels of protein C, protein S, antithrombin, and heparin cofactor II
Inherited thrombophilia
Coagulation
Low levels of plasminogen
Fibrinolysis
Comorbidity
Hemodynamic changes (reduced portal blood flow)
Vascular damage (esophageal varices)
Portal hypertension; bacterial infection and renal diseases

FIGURE 20-4

Balance of hemostasis in liver disease. TAFI, thrombin-activated fibriolytic inhibitor; t-PA, tissue plasminogen activator; vWF, von Willebrand factor.

to the erroneous exclusion of thrombosis in patients with advanced liver disease, even in the presence of prolongation of routine clotting times, and caution should be advised on overcorrection of these laboratory abnormalities.

ACQUIRED INHIBITORS OF COAGULATION FACTORS

An acquired inhibitor is an immune-mediated disease characterized by the presence of an autoantibody against a specific clotting factor. FVIII is the most common target of antibody formation, but inhibitors to prothrombin, FV, FIX, FX, and FXI are also reported. The disease occurs predominantly in older adults (median age of 60 years) but occasionally in pregnant or postpartum women with no previous history of bleeding. In 50% of the patients with inhibitors, no underlying disease is identified at the time of diagnosis. In the remaining, the causes are automminune diseases, malignancies (lymphomas, prostate cancer), dermatologic diseases, and pregnancy. Bleeding episodes occur commonly in soft tissues, in the gastrointestinal or urinary tracts, and on the skin. In contrast to hemophilia, hemarthrosis is rare in these patients. Retroperitoneal hemorrhages and other life-threatening bleeding may appear suddenly. The overall mortality rate in untreated patients ranges from 8 to 22%, and most deaths occur within the first few weeks after presentation. The diagnosis is based on the prolonged aPTT with normal PT and TT. The aPTT remains prolonged after mixture of the test plasma with equal amounts of pooled normal plasma for 2 h at 37°C. The Bethesda assay using FVIII-deficient plasma as performed for inhibitor detection in hemophilia will confirm the diagnosis. Major bleeding is treated with high doses of human or porcine FVIII, PCC/PCCa, or recombinant FVIIa. High-dose intravenous gamma globulin and anti-CD20 monoclonal antibody have been reported to be effective in patients with autoantibodies to FVIII. In contrast to hemophilia, inhibitors in nonhemophilia patients are sometimes responsive to prednisone alone or in association with cytotoxic therapy (e.g., cyclophosphamide).

Topical plasma-derived bovine and human thrombin are commonly used in the United States and worldwide. These effective hemostatic sealants are used during major surgery such as for cardiovascular, thoracic, neurologic, pelvic, and trauma indications, as well as in the setting of extensive burns. The development of antibody formation to the xenoantigen or its contaminant (bovine clotting protein) has the potential to show cross-reactivity with human clotting factors that may hamper their function and induce bleeding.

Clinical features of these antibodies include bleeding from a primary hemostatatic defect or coagulopathy that sometimes can be life threatening. The clinical diagnosis of these acquired coagulopathies is often complicated by the fact that the bleeding episodes may be detectable during or immediately following major surgery that could be assumed to be due to the procedure itself.

Notably, the risk of this complication is further increased by repeated exposure to topical thrombin preparations. Thus, a careful medical history of previous surgical interventions that may have occurred even decades earlier is critical to assessing risk.

The laboratory abnormalities are reflected by combined prolongation of the aPTT and PT that often fail to improve by transfusion of FFP and vitamin K. The abnormal laboratory tests cannot be corrected by mixing a test with equal parts of normal plasma that denotes the presence of inhibitory antibodies. The diagnosis of a specific antibody is obtained by the determination of the residual activity of human FV or other suspected human clotting factor. There are no commercially available assays specific for bovine thrombin coagulopathy.

There are no established treatment guidelines. Platelet transfusions have been utilized as a source of FV replacement for patients with FV inhibitors. Frequent injections of FFP and vitamin K supplementation may function as a co-adjuvant rather than an effective treatment of the coagulopathy itself. Experience with recombinant FVIIa as a bypass agent is limited, and outcomes have been generally poor. Specific treatments to eradicate the antibodies based on immunosuppression with steroids, intravenous immunoglobulin, or serial plasmapheresis have been sporadically reported. Patients should be advised to avoid any topical thrombin sealant in the future.

Recently, novel plasma-derived and recombinant human thrombin preparations for topical hemostasis have been approved by the Food and Drug Administration. These preparations have demonstrated hemostatic efficacy with reduced immunogenicity compared with the first generation of bovine thrombin products.

The presence of lupus anticoagulant can be associated with venous or arterial thrombotic disease. However, bleeding has also been reported in lupus anticoagulant; it is due to the presence of antibodies to prothrombin, which results in hypoprothrombinemia. Both disorders show a prolonged PTT that does not correct on mixing. To distinguish acquired inhibitors from lupus anticoagulant, note that the dilute Russell's viper venom test and the hexagonal-phase phospholipids test results will be negative in patients with an acquired inhibitor and positive in patients with lupus anticoagulants. Moreover, lupus anticoagulant interferes with the clotting activity of many factors (FVIII, FIX, FXII, FXI), whereas acquired inhibitors are specific to a single factor.

CHAPTER 21

ARTERIAL AND VENOUS THROMBOSIS

Jane E. Freedman ■ Joseph Loscalzo

OVERVIEW OF THROMBOSIS

GENERAL OVERVIEW

Thrombosis is defined as "hemostasis in the wrong place,"[1] and it is a major cause of morbidity and mortality in a wide range of arterial and venous diseases and patient populations. In 2009 in the United States, an estimated 785,000 people had a new coronary thrombotic event, and about 470,000 had a recurrent ischemic episode. Each year, approximately 795,000 people have a new or recurrent stroke. Annually, more than 200,000 new cases of venous thromboembolism are found; 30% of these individuals die within 30 days, with one-fifth having sudden death due to pulmonary embolism.

In the nondiseased state, physiologic hemostasis reflects a delicate interplay between factors that promote and inhibit blood clotting, favoring the former. This response is crucial as it prevents uncontrolled hemorrhage and exsanguination following injury. In specific settings, the same processes that regulate normal hemostasis can cause pathological thrombosis, leading to arterial or venous occlusion. Importantly, many commonly used therapeutic interventions may also alter the thrombotic–hemostatic balance adversely.

Hemostasis and thrombosis primarily involve the interplay among three factors: the vessel wall, coagulation proteins, and platelets. Many prevalent acute vascular diseases are due to thrombus formation within a vessel, including myocardial infarction, thrombotic cerebrovascular events, and venous thrombosis. Although the end result is vessel occlusion and tissue ischemia, the pathophysiologic processes governing these pathologies have similarities as well as distinct differences. While many of the pathways regulating thrombus formation are similar to those that regulate hemostasis, the processes triggering thrombosis and, often, perpetuating the thrombus are distinct. In venous thrombosis, primary hypercoagulable states reflecting defects in the proteins governing coagulation and/or fibrinolysis or secondary hypercoagulable states involving abnormalities of blood vessels and blood flow lead to thrombosis. By contrast, arterial thrombosis is highly dependent on the state of the vessel wall, the platelet, and factors related to blood flow.

ARTERIAL THROMBOSIS

OVERVIEW OF ARTERIAL THROMBOSIS

In arterial thrombosis, the platelet and abnormalities of the vessel wall typically play a key role in vessel occlusion. Arterial thrombus forms via a series of sequential steps in which platelets adhere to the vessel wall, additional platelets are recruited, and thrombin is activated. The regulation of platelet adhesion, activation, aggregation, and recruitment will be described in detail later in the chapter. In addition, while the primary function of platelets is regulation of hemostasis, our understanding of their role in other processes, such as immunity and inflammation, continues to grow.

ARTERIAL THROMBOSIS AND VASCULAR DISEASE

Arterial thrombosis is a major cause of morbidity and mortality both in the United States and, increasingly, worldwide. Coronary heart disease is estimated to cause about one of every five deaths in the United States. In addition to the 785,000 Americans who will have a new coronary event, an additional 195,000 silent first myocardial infarctions are projected to occur annually. Each year, about 795,000 people experience a new or recurrent stroke, although not all are caused by thrombotic occlusion of the vessel. Approximately 610,000 strokes are first events and 185,000 are recurrent events; it is estimated that 1 of every 18 deaths in the United States is due to stroke.

[1]Macfarlane RG. Haemostasis: Introduction. Brit Med Bull 33:183, 1977.

THE PLATELET

Many processes in platelets have parallels with other cell types, such as the presence of specific receptors and signaling pathways; however, unlike most cells, platelets lack a nucleus and are unable to adapt to changing biologic settings by altered gene transcription. Platelets sustain limited protein synthetic capacity from megakaryocyte-derived mRNA. Most of the molecules needed to respond to various stimuli, however, are maintained in storage granules and membrane compartments.

Platelets are disc-shaped, very small, anucleate cells (1–5 μm in diameter) that circulate in the blood at concentrations of 200–400,000/μL, with an average lifespan of 7–10 days. Platelets are derived from megakaryocytes, polyploidal hematopoietic cells found in the bone marrow. The primary regulator of platelet formation is thrombopoietin (TPO). The precise mechanism by which megakaryocytes produce and release fully formed platelets is unclear, but the process likely involves formation of proplatelets, pseudopod-like structures generated by the evagination of the cytoplasm from which platelets bud. Platelet granules are synthesized in megakaryocytes before thrombopoiesis and contain an array of prothrombotic, proinflammatory, and antimicrobial mediators. The two major types of platelet granules, alpha and dense, are distinguished by their size, abundance, and content. Alpha-granules contain soluble coagulation proteins, adhesion molecules, growth factors, integrins, cytokines, and inflammatory modulators. Platelet dense–granules are smaller than alpha-granules and less abundant. While alpha-granules contain proteins that may be more important in the inflammatory response, dense-granules contain high concentrations of small molecules, including adenosine diphosphate (ADP) and serotonin, that influence platelet aggregation.

Platelet adhesion

(See Fig. 21-1) The formation of a thrombus is initiated by the adherence of platelets to the damaged vessel wall. Damage exposes subendothelial components responsible for triggering platelet reactivity, including collagen; von Willebrand factor; fibronectin; and other adhesive proteins, such as vitronectin and thrombospondin. The hemostatic response may vary, depending on the extent of damage, the specific proteins exposed, and flow conditions. Certain proteins are expressed on the platelet surface that subsequently regulate collagen-induced platelet adhesion, particularly under flow conditions, and include glycoprotein (Gp) IV, GpVI, and the integrin $\alpha_2\beta_1$. The platelet GpIb-IX-V complex adhesive receptor is central

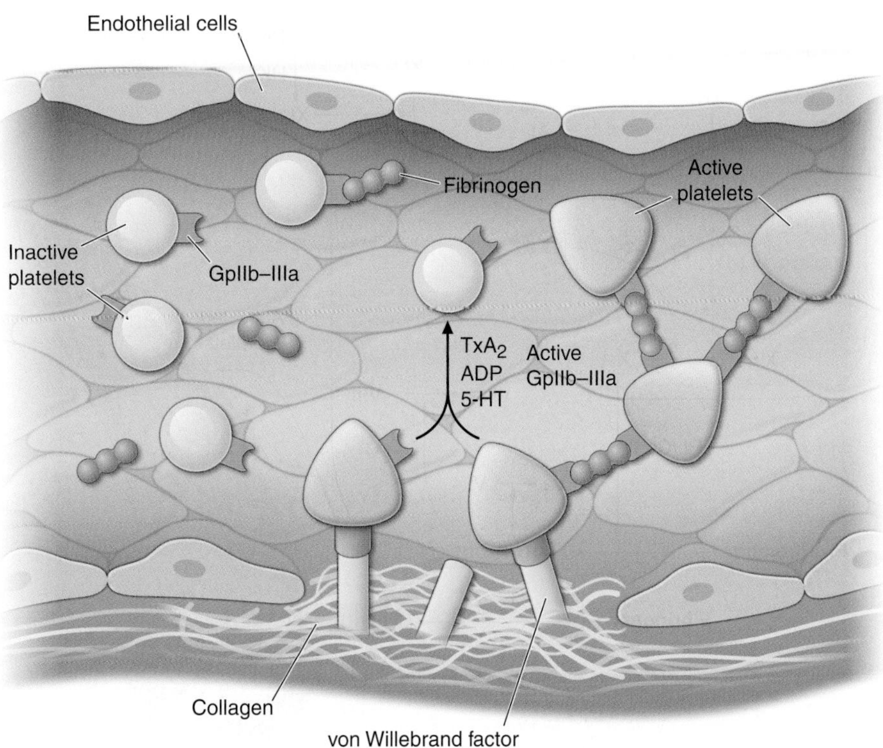

FIGURE 21-1

Platelet activation and thrombosis. Platelets circulate in an inactive form in the vasculature. Damage to the endothelium and/or external stimuli activates platelets that adhere to the exposed subendothelial von Willebrand factor and collagen. This adhesion leads to activation of the platelet, shape change, and the synthesis and release of thromboxane A_2 (TxA_2), serotonin (5-HT), and adenosine diphosphate (ADP). Platelet stimuli causes conformational change in the platelet integrin glycoprotein (Gp)IIb/IIIa receptor leading to the high-affinity binding of fibrinogen and the formation of a stable platelet thrombus.

both to platelet adhesion and to the initiation of platelet activation. Damage to the blood vessel wall exposes subendothelial von Willebrand factor and collagen to the circulating blood. The GpIb-IX-V complex binds to the exposed von Willebrand factor, causing platelets to adhere (Fig. 21-1). In addition, the engagement of the GpIb-IX-V complex with ligand induces signaling pathways that lead to platelet activation. von Willebrand factor–bound GpIb-IX-V promotes a calcium-dependent conformational change in the GpIIb/IIIa receptor, transforming it from an inactive low-affinity state to an active high-affinity receptor for fibrinogen.

Platelet activation

The activation of platelets is controlled by a variety of surface receptors that regulate various functions in the activation process. Platelet receptors are stimulated by a wide variety of agonists and adhesive proteins that result in variable degrees of activation. In general terms, the stimulation of platelet receptors triggers two specific processes: (1) activation of internal signaling pathways that lead to further platelet activation and granule release and (2) the capacity of the platelet to bind to other adhesive proteins/platelets. Both of these processes contribute to the formation of a thrombus.

Many families and subfamilies of receptors are found on platelets that regulate a variety of platelet functions. These include the seven transmembrane receptor family, which is the main agonist-stimulated receptor family. Several seven transmembrane receptors are found on platelets, including the ADP receptors, prostaglandin receptors, lipid receptors, and chemokine receptors. Receptors for thrombin comprise the major seven transmembrane receptors found on platelets. Among this last group, the first identified was the protease activation receptor 1 (PAR1). The PAR class of receptors has a distinct mechanism of activation that involves specific cleavage of the N-terminus of thrombin, which, in turn, acts as a ligand for the receptor. Other PARs are present on platelets, including PAR2 (not activated by thrombin) and PAR4. Adenosine receptors are responsible for transduction of ADP-induced signaling events, which are initiated by the binding of ADP to purinergic receptors on the platelet surface. There are several distinct ADP receptors, classified as $P2X_1$, $P2Y_1$, and $P2Y_{12}$ (Fig. 21-2). The activation of both the $P2Y_{12}$ and $P2Y_1$ receptors is essential for ADP-induced platelet

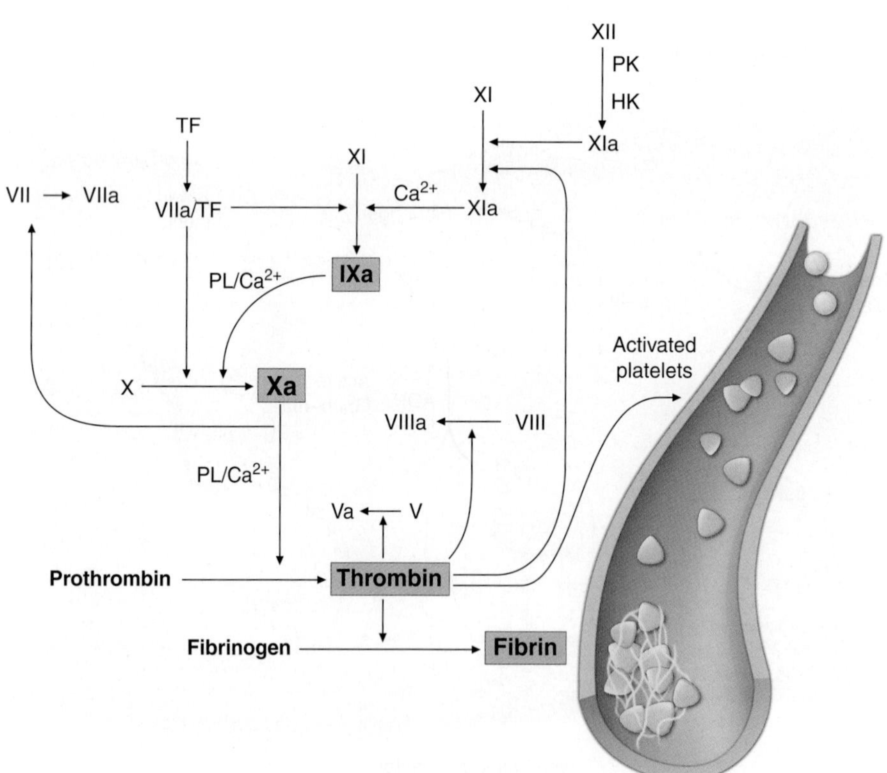

FIGURE 21-2

Summary of the coagulation pathways. Specific coagulation factors ("a" indicates activated form) are responsible for the conversion of soluble plasma fibrinogen into insoluble fibrin. This process occurs via a series of linked reactions in which the enzymatically active product subsequently converts the downstream inactive protein into an active serine protease. In addition, the activation of thrombin leads to stimulation of platelets. HK, high-molecular-weight kininogen; PK, prekallikrein; TF, tissue factor.

aggregation. The thienopyridine derivatives clopidogrel and prasugrel are clinically utilized inhibitors of ADP-induced platelet aggregation.

Platelet aggregation

Activation of platelets results in a rapid series of signal transduction events, including tyrosine kinase, serine/threonine kinase, and lipid kinase activation. In unstimulated platelets, the major platelet integrin GpIIb–IIIa is maintained in an inactive conformation and functions as a low-affinity adhesion receptor for fibrinogen. This integrin is unique as it is only expressed on platelets. After stimulation, the interaction between fibrinogen and GpIIb–IIIa forms intercellular connections between platelets leading to the formation of a platelet aggregate (Fig. 21-1). A calcium-sensitive conformational change in the extracellular domain of GpIIb–IIIa enables the high-affinity binding of soluble plasma fibrinogen as a result of a complex network of inside-out signaling events. The GpIIb–IIIa receptor serves as a bidirectional conduit with GpIIb–IIIa–mediated signaling (outside-in) occurring immediately after the binding of fibrinogen. This leads to additional intracellular signaling that further stabilizes the platelet aggregate and transforms platelet aggregation from a reversible to an irreversible process (inside-out).

THE ROLE OF PLATELETS AND THROMBOSIS IN INFLAMMATION

Inflammation plays an important role during the acute thrombotic phase of acute coronary syndromes. Patients with acute coronary syndromes have not only increased interactions between platelets (homotypic aggregates) but also increased interactions between platelets and leukocytes (heterotypic aggregates) detectable in circulating blood. These latter aggregates form when platelets are activated and adhere to circulating leukocytes. Platelets bind via P-selectin (CD62P) expressed on the surface of activated platelets to the leukocyte receptor, P-selectin glycoprotein ligand 1 (PSGL-1). This association leads to increased expression of CD11b/CD18 (Mac-1) on leukocytes, which itself supports interactions with platelets partially via bivalent fibrinogen linking this integrin with its platelet surface counterpart, GpIIb–IIIa. Platelet surface P-selectin also induces the expression of tissue factor on monocytes, which promotes fibrin formation.

In addition to platelet–monocyte aggregates, the immunomodulator, soluble CD40 ligand (CD40L or CD154), also reflects a link between thrombosis and inflammation. The CD40 ligand is a trimeric transmembrane protein of the tumor necrosis factor family and, with its receptor CD40, is an important contributor to the inflammatory process leading both to thrombosis and atherosclerosis. While many immunologic and vascular cells have been found to express CD40 and/or CD40 ligand, in platelets, CD40 ligand is rapidly translocated to the surface after stimulation and is upregulated in the newly formed thrombus. The surface-expressed CD40 ligand is cleaved from the platelet to generate a soluble fragment (soluble CD40 ligand).

Links have also been established among platelets, infection, immunity, and inflammation. Bacterial infections are associated with a transient increase in the risk of acute thrombotic events, such as acute myocardial infarction and stroke. In addition, platelets contribute significantly to the pathophysiology and high mortality rates of sepsis. The expression, functionality, and signaling pathways of toll-like receptors (TLRs) have been established in platelets. Stimulation of platelet TLR2 directly activates the platelet's thrombotic and inflammatory responses, and live bacteria induce a proinflammatory response in platelets in a TLR2-dependent manner, suggesting a mechanism by which specific bacteria and bacterial components can directly activate platelet-dependent thrombosis.

GENETICS OF ARTERIAL THROMBOSIS

Some studies have associated arterial thrombosis with genetic variants (Table 21-2*A*); however, in the area of genetic variability and platelet function, studies have primarily dealt with pharmacogenetics, the field of pharmacology dealing with the interindividual variability in drug response based on genetic determinants (Table 21-1). This focus has been driven by the wide variability among individuals in terms of response to antithrombotic drugs and the lack of a common explanation for this variance. The best described is the issue of "aspirin resistance," although heterogeneity for other antithrombotics (e.g.,

TABLE 21-1

GENETIC VARIATION AND PHARMACOGENETIC RESPONSES TO PLATELET INHIBITORS

POTENTIAL GENE ALTERED	TARGET THERAPEUTIC CLASS	SPECIFIC DRUG
P2Y1 and *P2Y12* *CYP2C19*, *CYP3A4*, *CYP3A5*	ADP receptor inhibitors	Clopidogrel, prasugrel
COX1, *COX2*	Cyclooxygenase inhibitors	Aspirin
PIA1/A2	Receptor inhibitors:	Abciximab, eptifibatide, tirofiban
INTB3, *GpIbA*	GpIIb–IIIa receptor inhibitors	

Abbreviations: ADP, adenosine diphosphate; Gp, glycoprotein.

TABLE 21-2

HERITABLE CAUSES OF ARTERIAL AND VENOUS THROMBOSIS

Arterial Thrombosis
Platelet Receptors
β3 and α2 integrins
P_IA2 polymorphism
Fc(γ)RIIA
GpIV T13254C polymorphism
GpIb
Thrombin receptor PAR-1-5061 → D
Redox Enzymes
Plasma glutathione peroxidase
H2 promoter haplotype
Endothelial nitric oxide synthase
−786T/C, −922A/G, −1468T/A
Paraoxonase
−107T allele, 192R allele
Homocysteine
Cystathionine β-synthase 833T → C
5,10-Methylene tetrahydrofolate reductase (MTHFR) 677C → T
Venous Thrombosis
Procoagulant Proteins
Fibrinogen
−455G/A, −854G/A
Prothrombin (20210G → A)
Protein C Anticoagulant Pathway
Factor V Leiden: 1691G → A (Arg506Gln)
Thrombomodulin 1481C → T (Ala455Val)
Fibrinolytic Proteins with Known Polymorphisms
Tissue plasminogen activator (tPA)
7351C/T, 20 099T/C in exon 6, 27 445T/A in intron 10
Plasminogen activator inhibitor (PAI-1)
4G/5G insertion/deletion polymorphism at position −675
Homocysteine
Cystathionine β-synthase 833T → C
5,10-Methylene tetrahydrofolate reductase (MTHFR) 677C → T

clopidogrel) has also been extensively examined. Primarily, platelet-dependent genetic determinants have been defined at the level of drug effect, drug compliance, and drug metabolism. Many candidate platelet genes have been studied for their interaction with antiplatelet and antithrombotic agents.

Many patients have an inadequate response to the inhibitory effects of aspirin. Heritable factors contribute to the variability; however, ex vivo tests of residual platelet responsiveness after aspirin administration have not provided firm evidence for a pharmacogenetic interaction between aspirin and cyclooxygenase 1 or other relevant platelet receptors. As such, currently, there is no clinical indication for genotyping to optimize aspirin's antiplatelet efficiency. For the platelet P2Y12 receptor inhibitor clopidogrel, additional data suggest that genetics may affect the drug's responsiveness and utility. The responsible genetic variant appears not to be the expected P2Y12 receptor but an enzyme responsible for drug metabolism. Clopidogrel is a prodrug, and liver metabolism by specific cytochrome P450 enzymes is required for activation. The genes encoding the CYP-dependent oxidative steps are polymorphic, and carriers of specific alleles of the CYP2C19 and CYP3A4 loci have increased platelet aggregability. Increased platelet activity has also been specifically associated with the CYP2C19*2 allele, which causes loss of platelet function in select patients. As these are common genetic variants, this observation has been shown to be clinically relevant in large studies.

VENOUS THROMBOSIS

OVERVIEW OF VENOUS THROMBOSIS

Coagulation is the process by which thrombin is activated and soluble plasma fibrinogen is converted into insoluble fibrin. These steps account for both normal hemostasis and the pathophysiologic processes influencing the development of venous thrombosis. The primary forms of venous thrombosis are deep-vein thrombosis (DVT) in the extremities and the subsequent embolization to the lungs (pulmonary embolism), referred to together as venous thromboembolic disease. Venous thrombosis occurs due to heritable causes (Table 21-2*B*) and acquired causes (Table 21-3).

DEEP-VEIN THROMBOSIS AND PULMONARY EMBOLISM

More than 200,000 new cases of venous thromboembolism occur each year. Of these patients, 30% die within 30 days and one-fifth experience sudden death owing to pulmonary embolism; 30% go on to develop recurrent venous thromboembolism within 10 years. Data from the Athereroscerosis Risk in Communities

TABLE 21-3

ACQUIRED CAUSES OF VENOUS THROMBOSIS

Surgery
Neurosurgery
Major abdominal surgery
Malignancy
Antiphospholipid syndrome
Other
Trauma
Pregnancy
Long-haul travel
Obesity
Oral contraceptives or hormone replacement
Myeloproliferative disorders
Polycythemia vera

study reported a 9% 28-day fatality rate from DVT and a 15% fatality rate from pulmonary embolism. Pulmonary embolism in the setting of cancer has a 25% fatality rate. The mean incidence of first DVT in the general population is 5 per 10,000 person-years; the incidence is similar in males and females and increases dramatically with age from 2 to 3 per 10,000 person-years at 30–49 years of age to 20 at 70–79 years of age.

OVERVIEW OF THE COAGULATION CASCADE AND ITS ROLE IN VENOUS THROMBOSIS

Coagulation is defined as the formation of fibrin by a series of linked enzymatic reactions in which each reaction product converts the subsequent inactive zymogen into an active serine protease (Fig. 21-2). This coordinated sequence is called the *coagulation cascade* and is a key mechanism for regulating hemostasis. Central to the function of the coagulation cascade is the principle of amplification: owing to a series of linked enzymatic reactions, a small stimulus can lead to much greater quantities of fibrin, the end product that prevents hemorrhage at the site of vascular injury.

The coagulation cascade is primarily initiated by vascular injury, exposing tissue factor to blood components (Fig. 21-2). Tissue factor may also be found in bloodborne cell-derived microparticles and, under pathophysiologic conditions, in leukocytes or platelets. Plasma factor VII (FVII) is the ligand for and is activated (FVIIa) by binding to tissue factor exposed at the site of vessel damage. The binding of FVII/VIIa to tissue factor activates the downstream conversion of factor X (FX) to active FX (FXa). In an alternative reaction, the FVII/FVIIa–tissue factor complex initially converts FIX to FIXa, which then activates FX in conjunction with its cofactor factor VIII (FVIIIa). Factor Xa with its cofactor FVa converts prothrombin to thrombin, which then converts soluble plasma fibrinogen to insoluble fibrin, leading to clot or thrombus formation. Thrombin also activates FXIII to FXIIIa, a transglutaminase that covalently cross-links and stabilizes the fibrin clot.

Several antithrombotic factors also regulate coagulation; these include antithrombin, tissue factor pathway inhibitor (TFPI), heparin cofactor II, and protein C/protein S. Under normal conditions, these factors limit the production of thrombin to prevent the perpetuation of coagulation and thrombus formation. Typically, after the clot has caused occlusion at the damaged site and begins to expand toward adjacent uninjured vessel segments, the anticoagulant reactions governed by the normal endothelium become pivotal in limiting the extent of this hemostatically protective clot.

RISK FACTORS FOR VENOUS THROMBOSIS

The risk factors for venous thrombosis are primarily related to hypercoagulability, which can be genetic (Table 21-2) or acquired or due to immobilization and venous stasis. Independent predictors for recurrence include increasing age, obesity, malignant neoplasm, and acute extremity paresis. Often, multiple risk factors are present in a single individual. Significant risk is incurred by major orthopedic, abdominal, or neurologic surgeries. Moderate risk is promoted by prolonged bedrest; certain types of cancer, pregnancy, hormone replacement therapy, or oral contraceptive use; and other sedentary conditions such as long-distance plane travel. It has been reported that the risk of developing a venous thromboembolic event doubles after air travel lasting 4 h, although the absolute risk remains low (1 in 6000). The relative risk of venous thromboembolism among pregnant or postpartum women is 4.3, and the overall incidence (absolute risk) is 199.7 per 100,000 woman-years.

GENETICS OF VENOUS THROMBOSIS

(See Table 21-2) Less common causes of venous thrombosis are those due to genetic variants. These abnormalities include loss-of-function mutations of endogenous anticoagulants as well as gain-of-function mutations of procoagulant proteins. Heterozygous antithrombin deficiency and homozygosity of the factor V Leiden mutation significantly increase the risk of venous thrombosis. While homozygous protein C or protein S deficiencies are rare and may lead to fatal purpura fulminans, heterozygous deficiencies are associated with a moderate risk of thrombosis. Activated protein C impairs coagulation by proteolytic degradation of FVa. Patients resistant to the activity of activated protein C may have a point mutation in the FV gene located on chromosome 1, a mutant denoted factor V Leiden. Mildly increased risk has been attributed to elevated levels of procoagulant factors, as well as low levels of TFPI. Polymorphisms of methylene tetrahydrofolate reductase as well as hyperhomocysteinemia have been shown to be independent risk factors for venous thrombosis, as well as arterial vascular disease; however, many of the initial descriptions of genetic variants and their associations with thromboembolism are being questioned in larger, more current studies.

FIBRINOLYSIS AND THROMBOSIS

Specific abnormalities in the fibrinolytic system have been associated with enhanced thrombosis. Factors such as elevated levels of tissue plasminogen activator (tPA) and plasminogen activator inhibitor type 1 (PAI-1) have been associated with decreased fibrinolytic activity and an increased risk of arterial thrombotic disease. Specific genetic variants have been associated with decreased fibrinolytic activity, including the 4G/5G insertion/deletion polymorphism in the (plasminogen activator type 1) PAI-1 gene. Additionally, the 311-bp Alu insertion/deletion in tPA's intron 8 has been associated with enhanced thrombosis; although genetic abnormalities have not been associated consistently with altered function or tPA levels, raising questions about the relevant pathophysiologic mechanism. Thrombin-activatable fibrinolysis inhibitor (TAFI) is a carboxypeptidase that regulates fibrinolysis; elevated plasma TAFI levels have been associated with an increased risk of both DVT and cardiovascular disease.

The metabolic syndrome also is accompanied by altered fibrinolytic activity. This syndrome, which comprises abdominal fat (central obesity), altered glucose and insulin metabolism, dyslipidemia, and hypertension, has been associated with atherothrombosis. The mechanism for enhanced thrombosis appears to be due both to altered platelet function and to a procoagulant and hypofibrinolytic state. One of the most frequently documented prothrombotic abnormalities reported in this syndrome is an increase in plasma levels of PAI-1.

THE DISTINCTION BETWEEN ARTERIAL AND VENOUS THROMBOSIS

Although there is overlap, venous and arterial thrombosis are initiated differently, and clot formation progresses by somewhat distinct pathways. In the setting of stasis or states of hypercoagulability, venous thrombosis is activated with the initiation of the coagulation cascade primarily due to exposure of tissue factor; this leads to the formation of thrombin and the subsequent conversion of fibrinogen to fibrin. In the artery, thrombin formation also occurs, but thrombosis is primarily promoted by the adhesion of platelets to an injured vessel and stimulated by exposed extracellular matrix (Figs. 21-1 and 21-2). There is wide variation in individual responses to vascular injury, an important determinant of which is the predisposition an individual has to arterial or venous thrombosis. This concept has been supported indirectly in prothrombotic animal models in which there is poor correlation between the propensity to develop venous versus arterial thrombosis.

Despite considerable progress in understanding the role of hypercoagulable states in venous thromboembolic disease, the contribution of hypercoagulability to arterial vascular disease is much less well understood. While specific thrombophilic conditions, such as factor V Leiden and the prothrombin G20210A mutation, are risk factors for DVT, pulmonary embolism, and other venous thromboembolic events, their contribution to arterial thrombosis is less well defined. In fact, to the contrary, many of these thrombophilic factors have not been found to be clinically important risk factors for arterial thrombotic events, such as acute coronary syndromes.

Clinically, although the pathophysiology is distinct, arterial and venous thrombosis do share common risk factors, including age, obesity, cigarette smoking, diabetes mellitus, arterial hypertension, hyperlipidemia, and metabolic syndrome. Select genetic variants, including those of the glutathione peroxidase gene, have also been associated with arterial and venous thrombo-occlusive disease. Importantly, arterial and venous thrombosis may both be triggered by pathophysiologic stimuli responsible for activating inflammatory and oxidative pathways.

The diagnosis and management of DVT and pulmonary embolus are discussed in Chap. 22.

Acknowledgment

The authors would like to thank Hannah Iafrati for her assistance with the figures.

CHAPTER 22

PULMONARY THROMBOEMBOLISM

Samuel Z. Goldhaber

EPIDEMIOLOGY

Venous thromboembolism (VTE), which encompasses deep-vein thrombosis (DVT) and pulmonary embolism, is one of the three major cardiovascular causes of death along with myocardial infarction and stroke. VTE can cause death from pulmonary embolism or, among survivors, chronic thromboembolic pulmonary hypertension and postphlebitic syndrome. The U.S. Surgeon General has declared that pulmonary embolism is the most common preventable cause of death among hospitalized patients. Medicare has labeled PE and DVT occurring after total hip or knee replacement as unacceptable "never events" and no longer reimburses hospitals for the incremental expenses associated with treating this postoperative complication. New nonprofit organizations have begun educating health care professionals and the public on the medical consequences of VTE along with risk factors and warning signs.

Between 100,000 and 300,000 VTE-related deaths occur annually in the United States. Mortality rates and length of hospital stay are decreasing as charges for hospital care increase. Approximately three of four symptomatic VTE events occur in the community, and the remainder are hospital acquired. Approximately 14 million hospitalized patients are at moderate to high risk for VTE in the United States annually: 6 million major surgery patients and 8 million medical patients with comorbidities such as heart failure, cancer, and stroke. The prophylaxis paradigm has changed from voluntary to mandatory compliance with guidelines to prevent VTE among hospitalized patients. With an estimated 370,000 pulmonary embolism-related deaths annually in Europe, the projected direct cost for VTE-associated care exceeds 3 billion euros per year. In Japan, as the lifestyle becomes more westernized, the rate of VTE appears to be increasing.

The long-term effects of nonfatal VTE lower the quality of life. Chronic thromboembolic pulmonary hypertension is often disabling and causes breathlessness. A late effect of DVT is *postphlebitic syndrome*, which eventually occurs in more than half of DVT patients. Postphlebitic syndrome (also known as *postthrombotic syndrome* or *chronic venous insufficiency*) is a delayed complication of DVT that causes the venous valves of the leg to become incompetent and exude interstitial fluid. Patients complain of chronic ankle or calf swelling and leg aching, especially after prolonged standing. In its most severe form, postphlebitic syndrome causes skin ulceration, especially in the medial malleolus of the leg. There is no effective medical therapy for this condition.

Prothrombotic states

Thrombophilia contributes to the risk of venous thrombosis. The two most common autosomal dominant genetic mutations are factor V Leiden, which causes resistance to activated protein C (which inactivates clotting factors V and VIII), and the prothrombin gene mutation, which increases the plasma prothrombin concentration (Chaps. 3 and 21). Antithrombin, protein C, and protein S are naturally occurring coagulation inhibitors. Deficiencies of these inhibitors are associated with VTE but are rare. Hyperhomocysteinemia can increase the risk of VTE, but lowering the homocysteine level with folate, vitamin B_6, or vitamin B_{12} does not reduce the incidence of VTE. Antiphospholipid antibody syndrome is the most common acquired cause of thrombophilia and is associated with venous or arterial thrombosis. Other common predisposing factors include cancer, systemic arterial hypertension, chronic obstructive pulmonary disease, long-haul air travel, air pollution, obesity, cigarette smoking, eating large amounts of red meat, oral contraceptives, pregnancy, postmenopausal hormone replacement, surgery, and trauma.

PATHOPHYSIOLOGY

Embolization

When venous thrombi are dislodged from their site of formation, they embolize to the pulmonary arterial circulation or, paradoxically, to the arterial circulation through a patent foramen ovale or atrial septal defect. About half of patients with pelvic vein thrombosis or proximal leg DVT develop pulmonary embolism, which is often asymptomatic. Isolated calf vein thrombi pose a much lower risk of pulmonary embolism but are the most common source of paradoxical embolism. These tiny thrombi can traverse a patent foramen ovale or atrial septal defect, unlike larger, more proximal leg thrombi. With increased use of chronic indwelling central venous catheters for hyperalimentation and chemotherapy, as well as more frequent insertion of permanent pacemakers and internal cardiac defibrillators, upper extremity venous thrombosis is becoming a more common problem. These thrombi rarely embolize and cause pulmonary embolism.

Physiology

The most common gas exchange abnormalities are hypoxemia (decreased arterial Po_2) and an increased alveolar-arterial O_2 tension gradient, which represents the inefficiency of O_2 transfer across the lungs. Anatomic dead space increases because breathed gas does not enter gas exchange units of the lung. Physiologic dead space increases because ventilation to gas exchange units exceeds venous blood flow through the pulmonary capillaries.

Other pathophysiologic abnormalities include the following:

1. *Increased pulmonary vascular resistance* due to vascular obstruction or platelet secretion of vasoconstricting neurohumoral agents such as serotonin. Release of vasoactive mediators can produce ventilation–perfusion mismatching at sites remote from the embolus, thereby accounting for a potential discordance between a small pulmonary embolism and a large alveolar-arterial O_2 gradient.
2. *Impaired gas exchange* due to increased alveolar dead space from vascular obstruction, hypoxemia from alveolar hypoventilation relative to perfusion in the nonobstructed lung, right-to-left shunting, and impaired carbon monoxide transfer due to loss of gas exchange surface
3. *Alveolar hyperventilation* due to reflex stimulation of irritant receptors
4. *Increased airway resistance* due to constriction of airways distal to the bronchi
5. *Decreased pulmonary compliance* due to lung edema, lung hemorrhage, or loss of surfactant

Right-ventricular dysfunction

Progressive right heart failure is the usual cause of death from pulmonary embolism. As pulmonary vascular resistance increases, right ventricular (RV) wall tension rises and causes further RV dilation and dysfunction. RV contraction continues even after the left ventricle (LV) starts relaxing at end-systole. Consequently, the interventricular septum bulges into and compresses an intrinsically normal LV. Diastolic LV impairment develops, attributable to septal displacement, and results in reduced LV distensibility and impaired LV filling during diastole. Increased RV wall tension also compresses the right coronary artery, diminishes subendocardial perfusion, limits myocardial oxygen supply, and may precipitate myocardial ischemia and RV infarction. Underfilling of the LV may lead to a fall in LV cardiac output and systemic arterial pressure, thereby provoking myocardial ischemia due to compromised coronary artery perfusion. Eventually, circulatory collapse and death may ensue.

DIAGNOSIS

Clinical evaluation

VTE mimics other illnesses, and pulmonary embolism is known as "the great masquerader," making diagnosis difficult. Occult pulmonary embolism is especially hard to detect when it occurs concomitantly with overt heart failure or pneumonia. In such circumstances, clinical improvement often fails to occur despite standard medical treatment of the concomitant illness. This scenario is a clinical clue to the possible coexistence of pulmonary embolism.

For patients who have DVT, the most common history is a cramp in the lower calf that persists for several days and becomes more uncomfortable as time progresses. For patients who have pulmonary embolism, the most common history is unexplained breathlessness.

In evaluating patients with possible VTE, the initial task is to decide on the clinical likelihood of the disorder. Patients with a low likelihood of DVT or a low to moderate likelihood of pulmonary embolism can undergo initial diagnostic evaluation with D-dimer testing alone (see "Blood tests") without obligatory imaging tests (Fig. 22-1). If the D-dimer is abnormally elevated, imaging tests are the next step.

Point score methods are useful for estimating the clinical likelihood of DVT and PE (Table 22-1).

Clinical syndromes

The differential diagnosis is critical because not all leg pain is due to DVT and not all dyspnea is due to

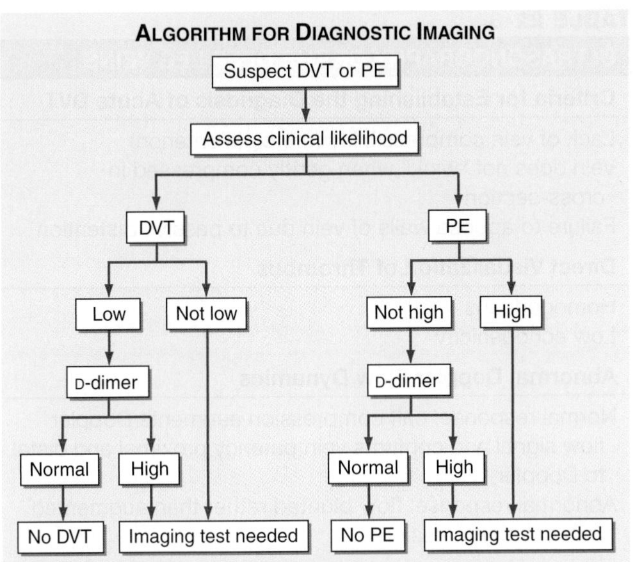

FIGURE 22-1

How to decide whether diagnostic imaging is needed. For assessment of clinical likelihood, see Table 22-1. DVT, deep-vein thrombosis; PE, pulmonary embolism.

pulmonary embolism (Table 22-2). Sudden, severe calf discomfort suggests a ruptured Baker's cyst. Fever and chills usually herald cellulitis rather than DVT, although DVT may be present concomitantly. Physical findings, if present at all, may consist only of mild palpation discomfort in the lower calf. Massive DVT is much easier to recognize. The patient presents with marked thigh swelling and tenderness during palpation of the common femoral vein. In extreme cases, patients are unable to walk or may require a cane, crutches, or a walker.

TABLE 22-1

CLINICAL DECISION RULES

Low Clinical Likelihood of DVT if Point Score Is Zero or Less; Moderate-Likelihood Score Is 1 to 2; High-Likelihood Score Is 3 or Greater

CLINICAL VARIABLE	SCORE
Active cancer	1
Paralysis, paresis, or recent cast	1
Bedridden for >3 days; major surgery <12 weeks	1
Tenderness along distribution of deep veins	1
Entire leg swelling	1
Unilateral calf swelling >3 cm	1
Pitting edema	1
Collateral superficial nonvaricose veins	1
Alternative diagnosis at least as likely as DVT	−2

High Clinical Likelihood of PE if Point Score Exceeds 4

CLINICAL VARIABLE	SCORE
Signs and symptoms of DVT	3.0
Alternative diagnosis less likely than PE	3.0
Heart rate >100/min	1.5
Immobilization >3 days; surgery within 4 weeks	1.5
Prior PE or DVT	1.5
Hemoptysis	1.0
Cancer	1.0

Abbreviations: DVT, deep-vein thrombosis; PE, pulmonary embolism.

TABLE 22-2

DIFFERENTIAL DIAGNOSIS

DVT
- Ruptured Baker's cyst
- Cellulitis
- Postphlebitic syndrome/venous insufficiency

PE
- Pneumonia, asthma, chronic obstructive pulmonary disease
- Congestive heart failure
- Pericarditis
- Pleurisy: "viral syndrome," costochondritis, musculoskeletal discomfort
- Rib fracture, pneumothorax
- Acute coronary syndrome
- Anxiety

Abbreviations: DVT, deep-vein thrombosis; PE, pulmonary embolism.

If the leg is diffusely edematous, DVT is unlikely. More probable is an acute exacerbation of venous insufficiency due to postphlebitic syndrome. Upper extremity venous thrombosis may present with asymmetry in the supraclavicular fossa or in the circumference of the upper arms. A prominent superficial venous pattern may be evident on the anterior chest wall.

Patients with *massive PE* present with systemic arterial hypotension and usually have anatomically widespread thromboembolism. Those with *moderate to large PE* have RV hypokinesis on echocardiography but normal systemic arterial pressure. Patients with *small to moderate PE* have both normal right heart function and normal systemic arterial pressure. They have an excellent prognosis with adequate anticoagulation.

The presence of *pulmonary infarction* usually indicates a small PE but one that is exquisitely painful because it lodges peripherally, near the innervation of pleural nerves. Pleuritic chest pain is more common with small, peripheral emboli. However, larger, more central PEs can occur concomitantly with peripheral pulmonary infarction.

Nonthrombotic PE may be easily overlooked. Possible etiologies include fat embolism after pelvic or long bone fracture, tumor embolism, bone marrow, and air embolism. Cement embolism and bony fragment embolism can occur after total hip or knee replacement. Intravenous drug users may inject themselves with a wide array of substances that can embolize such as hair, talc, and cotton. *Amniotic fluid embolism* occurs when fetal membranes leak or tear at the placental margin. Pulmonary edema in this syndrome probably is due to alveolar capillary leakage.

Dyspnea is the most common symptom of PE, and tachypnea is the most common sign. Dyspnea, syncope, hypotension, or cyanosis indicates a massive PE, whereas pleuritic pain, cough, or hemoptysis often suggests a small embolism situated distally near the pleura. On physical examination, young and previously healthy individuals may appear anxious but otherwise seem well, even with an anatomically large PE. They may have dyspnea only with moderate exertion. They often lack "classic" signs such as tachycardia, low-grade fever, neck vein distention, and an accentuated pulmonic component of the second heart sound. Sometimes paradoxical bradycardia occurs.

Nonimaging diagnostic modalities

Nonimaging tests are best utilized in combination with clinical likelihood assessment of DVT or PE (Fig. 22-1).

Blood tests

The quantitative *plasma D-dimer enzyme-linked immunosorbent assay (ELISA)* rises in the presence of DVT or PE because of the breakdown of fibrin by plasmin. Elevation of D-dimer indicates endogenous although often clinically ineffective thrombolysis. The sensitivity of the D-dimer is >80% for DVT (including isolated calf DVT) and >95% for PE. The D-dimer is less sensitive for DVT than for PE because the DVT thrombus size is smaller. The D-dimer is a useful "rule out" test. More than 95% of patients with a normal (<500 ng/mL) D-dimer do not have PE. The D-dimer assay is not specific. Levels increase in patients with myocardial infarction, pneumonia, sepsis, cancer, and the postoperative state and those in the second or third trimester of pregnancy. Therefore, D-dimer rarely has a useful role among hospitalized patients because levels are frequently elevated due to systemic illness.

Contrary to classic teaching, *arterial blood gases* lack diagnostic utility for PE even though both P_{O_2} and P_{CO_2} often decrease. Among patients suspected of having PE, neither the room air arterial P_{O_2} nor calculation of the alveolar–arterial O_2 gradient can reliably differentiate or triage patients who actually have PE at angiography.

Elevated cardiac biomarkers

Serum troponin and plasma heart-type fatty acid–binding protein levels increase because of RV microinfarction. Myocardial stretch results in elevation of brain natriuretic peptide or N-terminal or amino-terminal-pro-brain natriuretic peptide. Elevated cardiac biomarkers predict an increase in major complications and mortality from PE.

Electrocardiogram

The most frequently cited abnormality, in addition to sinus tachycardia, is the S1Q3T3 sign: an S wave in lead I, a Q wave in lead III, and an inverted T wave in lead III. This finding is relatively specific but insensitive. Perhaps the most common abnormality is T-wave inversion in leads V_1 to V_4.

TABLE 22-3

ULTRASONOGRAPHY OF THE DEEP LEG VEINS

Criteria for Establishing the Diagnosis of Acute DVT
Lack of vein compressibility (principal criterion) Vein does not "wink" when gently compressed in cross-section Failure to appose walls of vein due to passive distention
Direct Visualization of Thrombus
Homogeneous Low echogenicity
Abnormal Doppler Flow Dynamics
Normal response: calf compression augments Doppler flow signal and confirms vein patency proximal and distal to Doppler Abnormal response: flow blunted rather than augmented with calf compression

Abbreviation: DVT, deep-vein thrombosis.

Noninvasive imaging modalities

Venous ultrasonography

Ultrasonography of the deep-venous system (Table 22-3) relies on loss of vein compressibility as the primary criterion for DVT. When a normal vein is imaged in cross-section, it readily collapses with gentle manual pressure from the ultrasound transducer. This creates the illusion of a "wink." With acute DVT, the vein loses its compressibility because of passive distention by acute thrombus. The diagnosis of acute DVT is even more secure when thrombus is directly visualized. It appears homogeneous and has low echogenicity (Fig. 22-2). The vein itself often appears mildly dilated, and collateral channels may be absent.

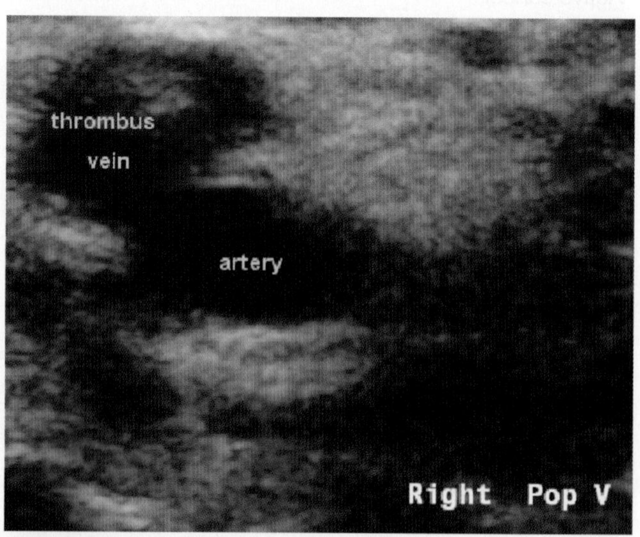

FIGURE 22-2

Acute popliteal deep-vein thrombosis on venous ultrasound in a 56-year-old man receiving chemotherapy for lung cancer.

Venous flow dynamics can be examined with Doppler imaging. Normally, manual calf compression causes augmentation of the Doppler flow pattern. Loss of normal respiratory variation is caused by an obstructing DVT or by any obstructive process within the pelvis. Because DVT and PE are so closely related and are both treated with anticoagulation (see "Treatment Deep-Vein Thrombosis") confirmed DVT is usually an adequate surrogate for PE. In contrast, normal venous ultrasound findings do not exclude PE. About half of patients with PE have no imaging evidence of DVT, probably because the clot already has embolized to the lung or is in the pelvic veins, where ultrasonography is usually inadequate. In patients without DVT, the ultrasound examination may identify other reasons for leg discomfort, such as a Baker's cyst (also known as a popliteal or synovial cyst) or a hematoma. For patients with a technically poor or nondiagnostic venous ultrasound, one should consider alternative imaging modalities for DVT, such as computed tomography (CT) and magnetic resonance imaging (MRI).

Chest radiography

A normal or nearly normal chest radiograph often occurs in PE. Well-established abnormalities include focal oligemia (Westermark's sign), a peripheral wedged-shaped density above the diaphragm (Hampton's hump), and an enlarged right descending pulmonary artery (Palla's sign).

Chest CT

CT of the chest with intravenous contrast is the principal imaging test for the diagnosis of PE (Fig. 22-3). Multidetector-row spiral CT acquires all chest images with ≤1 mm of resolution during a short breath hold. This generation of CT scanners can image small peripheral emboli. Sixth-order branches can be visualized with resolution superior to that of conventional invasive contrast pulmonary angiography. The CT scan also obtains excellent images of the RV and LV and can be used for risk stratification along with its use as a diagnostic tool. In patients with PE, RV enlargement on chest CT indicates an increased likelihood of death within the next 30 days compared with PE patients who have a normal RV size on chest CT. When imaging is continued below the chest to the knee, pelvic and proximal leg DVT also can be diagnosed by CT scanning. In patients without PE, the lung parenchymal images may establish alternative diagnoses not apparent on chest x-ray that explain the presenting symptoms and signs such as pneumonia, emphysema, pulmonary fibrosis, pulmonary mass, and aortic pathology. Sometimes asymptomatic early-stage lung cancer is diagnosed incidentally.

Lung scanning

Lung scanning has become a second-line diagnostic test for PE used mostly for patients who cannot tolerate intravenous contrast. Small particulate aggregates of albumin labeled with a gamma-emitting radionuclide are injected intravenously and are trapped in the pulmonary capillary bed. The perfusion scan defect indicates absent or decreased blood flow, possibly due to PE. Ventilation scans, obtained with a radiolabeled inhaled gas such as xenon or krypton, improve the specificity of the perfusion scan. Abnormal ventilation scans indicate abnormal nonventilated lung, thereby providing possible explanations for perfusion defects other than acute PE, such as asthma and chronic obstructive pulmonary disease. A high-probability scan for PE is defined as one that indicates two or more segmental perfusion defects in the presence of normal ventilation.

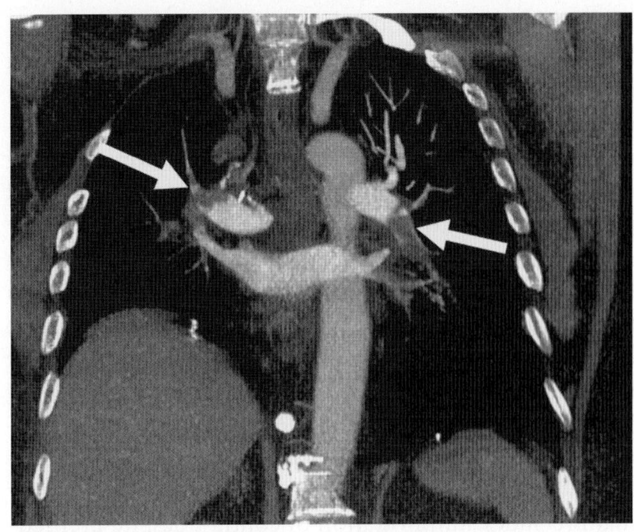

FIGURE 22-3
Large bilateral proximal pulmonary embolism on a coronal chest computed tomography image in a 54-year-old man with lung cancer and brain metastases. He had developed a sudden onset of chest heaviness and shortness of breath while at home. There are filling defects in the main and segmental pulmonary arteries bilaterally (*white arrows*). Only the left upper lobe segmental artery is free of thrombus.

The diagnosis of PE is very unlikely in patients with normal and nearly normal scans but is about 90% certain in patients with high-probability scans. Unfortunately, most patients have nondiagnostic scans, and fewer than half of patients with angiographically confirmed PE have a high probability scan. As many as 40% of patients with a high clinical suspicion for PE and "low-probability" scans do, in fact, have PE at angiography.

Magnetic resonance (contrast enhanced)

When ultrasound is equivocal, magnetic resonance (MR) venography with gadolinium contrast is an excellent imaging modality to diagnose DVT. MRI should be considered for suspected VTE patients with renal insufficiency or contrast dye allergy. MR pulmonary angiography may detect large proximal PE but is not reliable for smaller segmental and subsegmental PE.

Echocardiography

Echocardiography is *not* a reliable diagnostic imaging tool for acute PE because most patients with PE have normal echocardiographic findings. However, echocardiography is a very useful diagnostic tool for detecting conditions that may mimic PE, such as acute myocardial infarction, pericardial tamponade, and aortic dissection.

Transthoracic echocardiography rarely images thrombus directly. The best-known indirect sign of PE on transthoracic echocardiography is McConnell's sign: hypokinesis of the RV free wall with normal motion of the RV apex.

One should consider transesophageal echocardiography when CT scanning facilities are not available or when a patient has renal failure or severe contrast allergy that precludes administration of contrast despite premedication with high-dose steroids. This imaging modality can identify saddle, right main, or left main PE.

Invasive diagnostic modalities

Pulmonary angiography

Chest CT with contrast (see earlier discussion) has virtually replaced invasive pulmonary angiography as a diagnostic test. Invasive catheter-based diagnostic testing is reserved for patients with technically unsatisfactory chest CTs and those in whom an interventional procedure such as catheter-directed thrombolysis or embolectomy is planned. A definitive diagnosis of PE depends on visualization of an intraluminal filling defect in more than one projection. Secondary signs of PE include abrupt occlusion ("cut-off") of vessels; segmental oligemia or avascularity; a prolonged arterial phase with slow filling; and tortuous, tapering peripheral vessels.

Contrast phlebography

Venous ultrasonography has virtually replaced contrast phlebography as the diagnostic test for suspected DVT.

Integrated diagnostic approach

An integrated diagnostic approach (Fig. 22-1) streamlines the workup of suspected DVT and PE (Fig. 22-4).

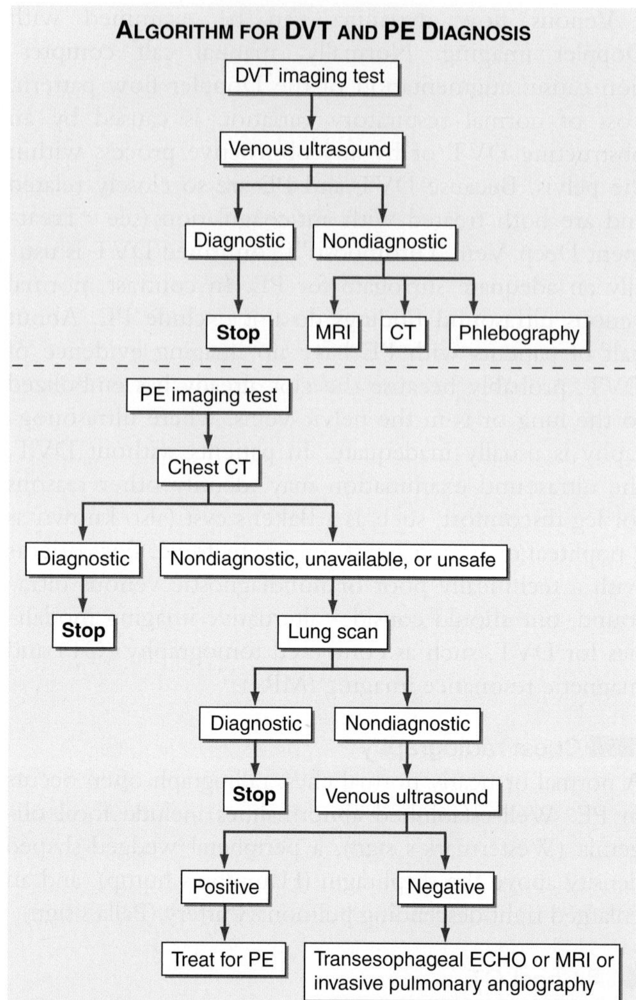

FIGURE 22-4

Imaging tests to diagnose deep-vein thrombosis (DVT) and pulmonary embolism (PE). CT, computed tomography; ECHO, echocardiography; MR, magnetic resonance imaging.

TREATMENT Deep-Vein Thrombosis

PRIMARY THERAPY VERSUS SECONDARY PREVENTION *Primary therapy* consists of clot dissolution with thrombolysis or removal of PE by embolectomy. Anticoagulation with heparin and warfarin or placement of an inferior vena caval filter constitutes *secondary prevention* of recurrent PE rather than primary therapy.

RISK STRATIFICATION Rapid and accurate risk stratification is critical in determining the optimal treatment strategy. The presence of hemodynamic instability, RV dysfunction, RV enlargement, or elevation of the troponin level due to RV microinfarction can identify high-risk patients. RV hypokinesis on echocardiography, RV enlargement on chest CT, and troponin elevation predict an increased mortality rate from PE.

Primary therapy should be reserved for patients at high risk of an adverse clinical outcome. When RV function remains normal in a hemodynamically stable patient, a good clinical outcome is highly likely with anticoagulation alone (Fig. 22-5).

TREATMENT Massive Pulmonary Embolism

ANTICOAGULATION Anticoagulation is the foundation for successful treatment of DVT and PE (Table 22-4). Immediately effective anticoagulation is

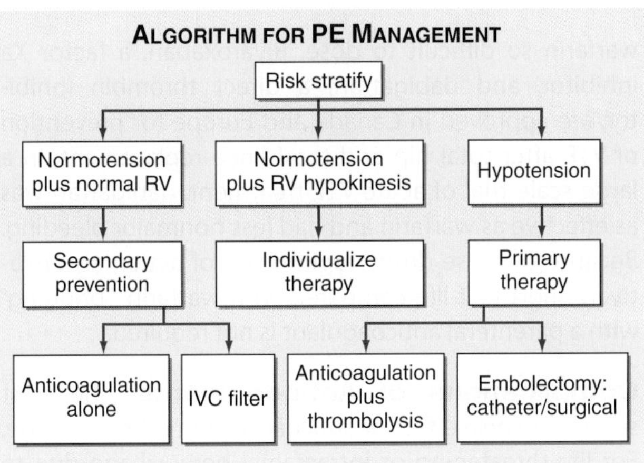

FIGURE 22-5

Acute management of pulmonary embolism (PE). IVC, inferior vena cava; RV, right ventricle/ventricular.

initiated with a parenteral drug: unfractionated heparin (UFH), low-molecular-weight heparin (LMWH), or fondaparinux. One should use a direct thrombin inhibitor—argatroban, lepirudin, or bivalirudin—in patients with proven or suspected heparin-induced thrombocytopenia (HIT). Parenteral agents are continued as a transition or "bridge" to stable, long-term anticoagulation with a vitamin K antagonist (exclusively warfarin in the United States). Warfarin requires 5–7 days to achieve a therapeutic effect. During that period, one should overlap the parenteral and oral agents. After 5–7 days of anticoagulation, residual thrombus begins to endothelialize in the vein or pulmonary artery. However, anticoagulants do *not* directly dissolve thrombus that already exists.

TABLE 22-4

ANTICOAGULATION OF VENOUS THROMBOEMBOLISM

Immediate Parenteral Anticoagulation
Unfractionated heparin, bolus and continuous infusion, to achieve aPTT two to three times the upper limit of the laboratory normal, *or*
Enoxaparin 1 mg/kg twice daily with normal renal function, *or* Dalteparin 200 U/kg once daily or 100 U/kg twice daily, with normal renal function, *or*
Tinzaparin 175 U/kg once daily with normal renal function, *or*
Fondaparinux weight-based once daily; adjust for impaired renal function
Warfarin Anticoagulation
Usual start dose is 5 mg
Titrate to INR, target 2.0–3.0
Continue parenteral anticoagulation for a minimum of 5 days and until two sequential INR values, at least 1 day apart, achieve the target INR range.

Abbreviations: aPTT, activated partial thromboplastin time; INR, international normalized ratio.

Unfractionated Heparin UFH anticoagulates by binding to and accelerating the activity of antithrombin, thus preventing additional thrombus formation and permitting endogenous fibrinolytic mechanisms to lyse clot that already has formed. UFH is dosed to achieve a target activated partial thromboplastin time (aPTT) that is 2–3 times the upper limit of the laboratory normal. This is usually equivalent to an aPTT of 60–80 s. For UFH, a typical intravenous bolus is 5000–10,000 units followed by a continuous infusion of 1000–1500 U/h. Nomograms based on a patient's weight may assist in adjusting the dose of heparin. The most popular nomogram utilizes an initial bolus of 80 U/kg followed by an initial infusion rate of 18/kg per hour.

The major advantage of UFH is its short half-life. This is especially useful if the patient may undergo an invasive procedure such as embolectomy. The major disadvantage of UFH is that achieving the target aPTT is empirical and may require repeated blood sampling and heparin dose adjustment every 4–6 hours. Furthermore, patients are at risk of developing HIT.

Low-Molecular-Weight Heparins These fragments of UFH exhibit less binding to plasma proteins and endothelial cells and consequently have greater bioavailability, a more predictable dose response, and a longer half-life than does UFH. No monitoring or dose adjustment is needed unless the patient is markedly obese or has chronic kidney disease.

There are two commonly used LMWH preparations in the United States: enoxaparin and dalteparin. *Enoxaparin* is approved as a bridge to warfarin for VTE. *Dalteparin* is also approved as monotherapy without warfarin for symptomatic VTE patients with cancer at a dose of 200 U/kg once daily for 30 days followed by 150 U/kg once daily for months 2–6. These weight-adjusted LMWH doses must be reduced in patients with chronic kidney disease because the kidneys metabolize LMWH.

Fondaparinux Fondaparinux, an anti-Xa pentasaccharide, is administered as a once-daily subcutaneous injection in a prefilled syringe to treat DVT and PE as a "bridge" to warfarin. No laboratory monitoring is required. Patients weighing <50 kg receive 5 mg, patients weighing 50–100 kg receive 7.5 mg, and patients weighing >100 kg receive 10 mg. Fondaparinux is synthesized in a laboratory and, unlike LMWH or UFH, is not derived from animal products. It does not cause HIT. The dose must be adjusted downward for patients with renal dysfunction because the kidneys metabolize the drug.

Warfarin This vitamin K antagonist prevents carboxylation activation of coagulation factors II, VII, IX, and X. The full effect of warfarin requires at least 5 days even if the prothrombin time (PT), used for monitoring, becomes elevated more rapidly. If warfarin is initiated as monotherapy during an acute thrombotic illness, a paradoxical exacerbation of hypercoagulability can increase the likelihood of thrombosis rather than prevent it. Overlapping UFH, LMWH, or fondaparinux with warfarin for at least 5 days can counteract the early procoagulant effect of unopposed warfarin.

Warfarin Dosing In an average-size adult, warfarin usually is initiated in a dose of 5 mg. Doses of 7.5 or 10 mg can be used in obese or large-framed young patients who are otherwise healthy. Patients who are malnourished or who have received prolonged courses of antibiotics are probably deficient in vitamin K and should receive smaller initial doses of warfarin, such as 2.5 mg. The PT is standardized by calculating the international normalized ratio (INR), which assesses the anticoagulant effect of warfarin (Chap. 3). The target INR is usually 2.5, with a range of 2.0–3.0.

The warfarin dose is titrated to achieve the target INR. Proper dosing is difficult because hundreds of drug–drug and drug–food interactions affect warfarin metabolism. Variables such as increasing age and comorbidities such as systemic illness reduce the required warfarin dose. Pharmacogenomics may provide more precise initial dosing of warfarin, especially for patients who require unusually large or small doses. *CYP2C9* variant alleles impair the hydroxylation of S-warfarin, thereby lowering the dose requirement. Variants in the gene encoding the vitamin K epoxide reductase complex 1 (*VKORC1*) can predict whether patients require low, moderate, or high warfarin doses. Nevertheless, more than half of warfarin dosing variability is caused by clinical factors such as age, sex, weight, concomitant drugs, and comorbid illnesses.

Nomograms have been developed (*www.warfarindosing.org*) to help clinicians initiate warfarin dosing based on clinical information and, if available, pharmacogenetic data. However, most practitioners utilize empirical dosing with an "educated guess." Centralized anticoagulation clinics have improved the efficacy and safety of warfarin dosing. Patients maintain a therapeutic INR more often if they self-monitor their INR with a home point-of-care fingerstick machine rather than obtaining a coagulation laboratory INR. The patient subgroup with the best results self-adjusts warfarin doses as well as self-tests INRs.

Novel Anticoagulants Novel oral anticoagulants are administered in a fixed dose, establish effective anticoagulation within hours of administration, require no laboratory coagulation monitoring, and have few of the drug–drug or drug–food interactions that make warfarin so difficult to dose. Rivaroxaban, a factor Xa inhibitor, and dabigatran, a direct thrombin inhibitor, are approved in Canada and Europe for prevention of VTE after total hip and total knee replacement. In a large-scale trial of acute VTE treatment, dabigatran was as effective as warfarin and had less nonmajor bleeding. Because of these drugs' rapid onset of action and relatively short half-life compared with warfarin, "bridging" with a parenteral anticoagulant is not required.

Complications of Anticoagulants The most serious adverse effect of anticoagulation is hemorrhage. For life-threatening or intracranial hemorrhage due to heparin or LMWH, protamine sulfate can be administered. There is no specific antidote for bleeding caused by fondaparinux or direct thrombin inhibitors.

Major bleeding from warfarin is best managed with prothrombin complex concentrate. With non–life-threatening bleeding in a patient who can tolerate large volume, fresh-frozen plasma can be used. Recombinant human coagulation factor VIIa (rFVIIa), approved by the U.S. Food and Drug Administration (FDA) for bleeding in hemophilia, is an off-label option to manage catastrophic bleeding from warfarin. For minor bleeding or to manage an excessively high INR in the absence of bleeding, oral vitamin K may be administered.

HIT and osteopenia are far less common with LMWH than with UFH. Thrombosis due to HIT should be managed with a direct thrombin inhibitor: argatroban for patients with renal insufficiency and lepirudin for patients with hepatic failure. In the setting of percutaneous coronary intervention, one should administer bivalirudin.

During pregnancy, warfarin should be avoided if possible because of warfarin embryopathy, which is most common with exposure during the sixth through twelfth weeks of gestation. However, women can take warfarin postpartum and breast feed safely. Warfarin can also be administered safely during the second trimester.

Duration of Hospital Stay Acute DVT patients with good family and social support, a permanent residence, telephone service, and no hearing or language impairment often can be managed as outpatients. They, a family member, or a visiting nurse must administer a parenteral anticoagulant. Warfarin dosing can be titrated to the INR and adjusted on an outpatient basis.

Acute PE patients, who traditionally have required hospital stays of 5–7 days for intravenous heparin as a "bridge" to warfarin, can be considered for abbreviated hospitalization if they have a reliable support system at home and an excellent prognosis. Criteria include clinical stability, absence of chest pain or shortness of breath, normal RV size and function, and normal levels of cardiac biomarkers.

Duration of Anticoagulation Patients with PE after surgery, trauma, or estrogen exposure (from oral contraceptives, pregnancy, or postmenopausal therapy) ordinarily have a low rate of recurrence after 3–6 months of anticoagulation. For DVT isolated to an upper extremity or calf that has been provoked by surgery, trauma, estrogen, or an indwelling central venous catheter or pacemaker, 3 months of anticoagulation suffices. For provoked proximal leg DVT or PE, 3–6 months of anticoagulation is sufficient. For patients with cancer and VTE, the consensus is to prescribe 3–6 months of LMWH as monotherapy without warfarin and to continue anticoagulation indefinitely unless the patient is rendered cancer-free. However, there is uncertainty whether subsequent anticoagulation should continue with LMWH or whether the patient should be prescribed warfarin.

Among patients with idiopathic, unprovoked VTE, the recurrence rate is high after cessation of anticoagulation. VTE that occurs during long-haul air travel is considered unprovoked. It appears that unprovoked VTE is often a chronic illness, with latent periods between flares of recurrent episodes. American College of Chest Physicians (ACCP) guidelines recommend considering anticoagulation for an indefinite duration with a target INR between 2 and 3 for patients with idiopathic VTE. An alternative approach after the first 6 months of anticoagulation is to reduce the intensity of anticoagulation and to lower the target INR range to between 1.5 and 2.

Counterintuitively, the presence of genetic mutations such as heterozygous factor V Leiden and prothrombin gene mutation do not appear to increase the risk of recurrent VTE. However, patients with moderate or high levels of anticardiolipin antibodies probably warrant indefinite-duration anticoagulation even if the initial VTE was provoked by trauma or surgery.

INFERIOR VENA CAVAL (IVC) FILTERS The two principal indications for insertion of an IVC filter are (1) active bleeding that precludes anticoagulation and (2) recurrent venous thrombosis despite intensive anticoagulation. Prevention of recurrent PE in patients with right heart failure who are not candidates for fibrinolysis and prophylaxis of extremely high-risk patients are "softer" indications for filter placement. The filter itself may fail by permitting the passage of small- to medium-size clots. Large thrombi may embolize to the pulmonary arteries via collateral veins that develop. A more common complication is caval thrombosis with marked bilateral leg swelling.

Paradoxically, by providing a nidus for clot formation, filters double the DVT rate over the ensuing 2 years after placement. Retrievable filters can now be placed for patients with an anticipated temporary bleeding disorder or for patients at temporary high risk of PE, such as individuals undergoing bariatric surgery who have a history of perioperative PE. The filters can be retrieved up to several months after insertion unless thrombus forms and is trapped within the filter. The retrievable filter becomes permanent if it remains in place or if, for technical reasons such as rapid endothelialization, it cannot be removed.

MAINTAINING ADEQUATE CIRCULATION For patients with massive PE and hypotension, one should administer 500 mL of normal saline. Additional fluid should be infused with extreme caution because excessive fluid administration exacerbates RV wall stress, causes more profound RV ischemia, and worsens LV compliance and filling by causing further interventricular septal shift toward the LV. Dopamine and dobutamine are first-line inotropic agents for treatment of PE-related shock. There should be a low threshold for initiating these pressors. Often, a "trial-and-error" approach works best; one should consider norepinephrine, vasopressin, or phenylephrine.

FIBRINOLYSIS Successful fibrinolytic therapy rapidly reverses right heart failure and may result in a lower rate of death and recurrent PE by (1) dissolving much of the anatomically obstructing pulmonary arterial thrombus; (2) preventing the continued release of serotonin and other neurohumoral factors that exacerbate pulmonary hypertension; and (3) lysing much of the source of the thrombus in the pelvic or deep leg veins, thereby decreasing the likelihood of recurrent PE.

The preferred fibrinolytic regimen is 100 mg of recombinant tissue plasminogen activator administered as a continuous peripheral intravenous infusion over 2 hours. Patients appear to respond to fibrinolysis for up to 14 days after the PE has occurred.

Contraindications to fibrinolysis include intracranial disease, recent surgery, and trauma. The overall major bleeding rate is about 10%, including a 1–3% risk of intracranial hemorrhage. Careful screening of patients for contraindications to fibrinolytic therapy is the best way to minimize bleeding risk.

The only FDA-approved indication for PE fibrinolysis is massive PE. For patients with preserved systolic blood pressure and submassive PE with moderate or severe RV dysfunction, ACCP guidelines for fibrinolysis recommend individual patient risk assessment of the thrombotic burden versus the bleeding risk.

PULMONARY EMBOLECTOMY The risk of intracranial hemorrhage with fibrinolysis has prompted a renaissance of surgical embolectomy. More prompt referral before the onset of irreversible cardiogenic shock and multisystem organ failure and improved surgical technique have resulted in a high survival rate. A possible alternative to open surgical embolectomy is catheter embolectomy. New-generation catheters are under development.

PULMONARY THROMBOENDARTERECTOMY Chronic thromboembolic pulmonary hypertension occurs in 2–4% of acute PE patients. Therefore, PE patients who have initial pulmonary hypertension (usually diagnosed with Doppler echocardiography) should be followed up at about 6 weeks with a repeat echocardiogram to determine whether pulmonary arterial pressure has normalized. Patients impaired by dyspnea due to chronic thromboembolic pulmonary hypertension should be considered for pulmonary thromboendarterectomy, which, if successful, can markedly reduce, and at times even cure pulmonary hypertension. The operation requires median sternotomy, cardiopulmonary bypass, deep hypothermia, and periods of hypothermic circulatory arrest. The mortality rate at experienced centers is approximately 5%.

EMOTIONAL SUPPORT Patients with VTE may feel overwhelmed when they learn that they are susceptible to recurrent PE or DVT. They worry about the health of their families and the genetic implications of their illness. Those who are advised to discontinue warfarin after 3–6 months of therapy may feel especially vulnerable. At Brigham and Woman's Hospital, a physician-nurse–facilitated PE support group has been maintained for patients and has met monthly for more than 15 years.

PREVENTION OF POSTPHLEBITIC SYNDROME Daily use of below-knee 30- to 40–mm Hg vascular compression stockings will halve the rate of developing postphlebitic syndrome. These stockings should be prescribed as soon as DVT is diagnosed and should be fitted carefully to maximize their benefit. When patients are in bed, the stockings need not be worn.

PREVENTION OF VENOUS THROMBOEMBOLISM

Prophylaxis (**Table 22-5**) is of paramount importance because VTE is difficult to detect and poses a profound medical and economic burden. Computerized reminder systems can increase the use of preventive measures and at Brigham and Women's Hospital have reduced the symptomatic VTE rate by more than 40%. Patients who have undergone total hip or knee replacement or cancer surgery will benefit from extended pharmacologic prophylaxis for a total of 4–5 weeks.

TABLE 22-5

PREVENTION OF VENOUS THROMBOEMBOLISM

CONDITION	PROPHYLAXIS STRATEGY
High-risk general surgery	Mini-UFH *or* LMWH
Thoracic surgery	Mini-UFH + IPC
Cancer surgery, including gynecologic cancer surgery	LMWH, consider 1 month of prophylaxis
Total hip replacement, total knee replacement, hip fracture surgery	LMWH; fondaparinux (a pentasaccharide) 2.5 mg SC once daily *or* (except for total knee replacement) warfarin (target INR, 2.5); rivaroxaban or dalteparin in countries where it is approved
Neurosurgery	IPC
Neurosurgery for brain tumor	Mini-UFH *or* LMWH + IPC + predischarge venous ultrasonography
Benign gynecologic surgery	Mini-UFH
Medically ill patients	Mini-UFH *or* LMWH
Anticoagulation contraindicated	IPC
Long-haul air travel	Consider LMWH for very high-risk patients

Abbreviations: IPC, intermittent pneumatic compression devices; LMWH, low-molecular-weight heparin, typically in the United States enoxaparin, 40 mg once daily, or dalteparin, 2500 or 5000 units once daily; mini-UFH, mini-dose unfractionated heparin, 5000 units subcutaneously twice (less effective) or three times daily (more effective).

CHAPTER 23

ANTIPLATELET, ANTICOAGULANT, AND FIBRINOLYTIC DRUGS

Jeffrey I. Weitz

Arterial and venous thromboses are major causes of morbidity and mortality rates. Arterial thrombosis is the most common cause of acute myocardial infarction (MI), ischemic stroke, and limb gangrene, whereas deep-vein thrombosis (DVT) leads to pulmonary embolism (Pulmonary Embolism), which can be fatal, and to the postphlebitic syndrome. Most arterial thrombi are superimposed on disrupted atherosclerotic plaque because plaque rupture exposes thrombogenic material in the plaque core to the blood. This material then triggers platelet aggregation and fibrin formation, which results in the generation of a platelet-rich thrombus that can temporarily or permanently occlude blood flow. In contrast to arterial thrombi, venous thrombi rarely form at sites of obvious vascular disruption. Although they can develop after surgical trauma to veins or secondary to indwelling venous catheters, venous thrombi usually originate in the valve cusps of the deep veins of the calf or in the muscular sinuses, where they are triggered by stasis. Sluggish blood flow in these veins reduces the oxygen supply to the avascular valve cusps. Endothelial cells lining these valve cusps become activated and express adhesion molecules on their surface. Tissue factor–bearing leukocytes and microparticles adhere to these activated cells and induce coagulation. Local thrombus formation is exacerbated by reduced clearance of activated clotting factors as a result of impaired blood flow. If the thrombi extend into more proximal veins of the leg, thrombus fragments can dislodge, travel to the lungs, and produce a Pulmonary Embolism.

Arterial and venous thrombi are composed of platelets and fibrin, but the proportions differ. Arterial thrombi are rich in platelets because of the high shear in the injured arteries. In contrast, venous thrombi, which form under low shear conditions, contain relatively few platelets and are predominantly composed of fibrin and trapped red cells. Because of the predominance of platelets, arterial thrombi appear white, whereas venous thrombi are red in color, reflecting the trapped red cells.

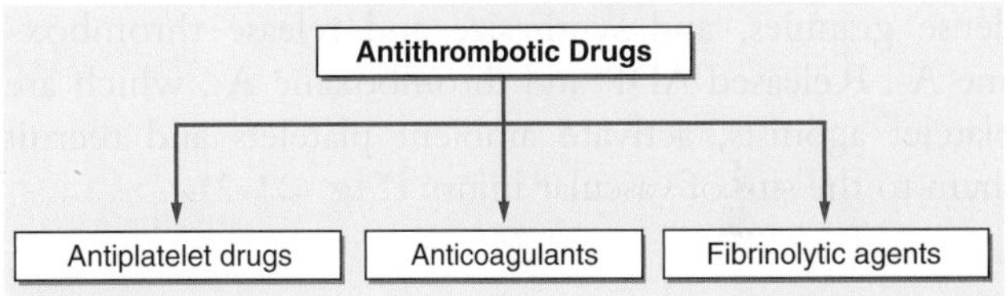

FIGURE 23-1
Classification of antithrombotic drugs.

Antithrombotic drugs are used for prevention and treatment of thrombosis. Targeting the components of thrombi, these agents include (1) antiplatelet drugs, (2) anticoagulants, and (3) fibrinolytic agents (Fig. 23-1). With the predominance of platelets in arterial thrombi, strategies to inhibit or treat arterial thrombosis focus mainly on antiplatelet agents, although, in the acute setting, they often include anticoagulants and fibrinolytic agents. Anticoagulants are the mainstay of prevention and treatment of venous thromboembolism (VTE) because fibrin is the predominant component of venous thrombi. Antiplatelet drugs are less effective than anticoagulants in this setting because of the limited platelet content of venous thrombi. Fibrinolytic therapy is used in selected patients with (VTE). For example, patients with massive or submassive Pulmonary Embolism can benefit from systemic or catheter-directed fibrinolytic therapy. The latter can also be used as an adjunct to anticoagulants for treatment of patients with extensive iliofemoral-vein thrombosis.

ANTIPLATELET DRUGS

ROLE OF PLATELETS IN ARTERIAL THROMBOSIS

In healthy vasculature, circulating platelets are maintained in an inactive state by nitric oxide (NO) and prostacyclin released by endothelial cells lining the blood vessels. In addition, endothelial cells also express CD39 on their surfaces, a membrane-associated ecto-adenosine diphosphatase (ADPase) that degrades adenosine diphosphate (ADP) released from activated platelets. When the vessel wall is damaged, release of these substances is impaired, and subendothelial matrix is exposed. Platelets adhere to exposed collagen via $\alpha_2\beta_1$ and glycoprotein (Gp)V1 and to von Willebrand factor (vWF) via GpIbα and GpIIb/IIIa ($\alpha_{IIb}\beta_3$)—receptors that are constitutively expressed on the platelet surface. Adherent platelets undergo a change in shape, secrete ADP from their dense granules, and synthesize and release thromboxane A_2. Released ADP and thromboxane A_2, which are platelet agonists, activate ambient platelets and recruit them to the site of vascular injury (Fig. 23-2).

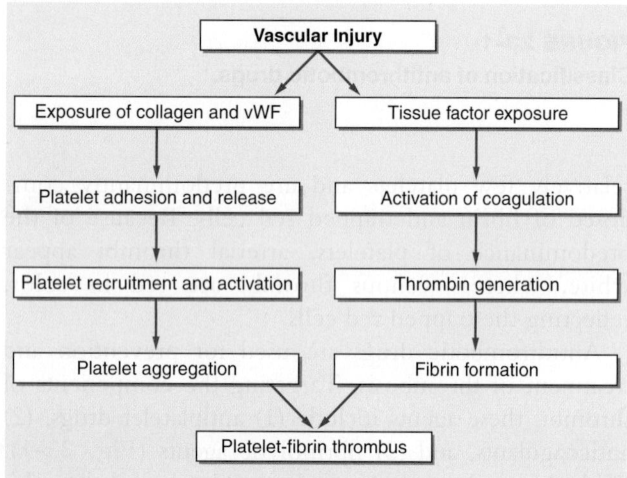

FIGURE 23-2

Coordinated role of platelets and the coagulation system in thrombogenesis. Vascular injury simultaneously triggers platelet activation and aggregation and activation of the coagulation system. Platelet activation is initiated by exposure of subendothelial collagen and von Willebrand factor (vWF), onto which platelets adhere. Adherent platelets become activated and release adenosine diphosphate and thromboxane A_2, platelet agonists that activate ambient platelets and recruit them to the site of injury. When platelets are activated, glycoprotein IIb/IIIa on their surfaces undergoes a conformational change that enables it to ligate fibrinogen and mediate platelet aggregation. Coagulation is triggered by tissue factor exposed at the site of injury. Tissue factor triggers thrombin generation. As a potent platelet agonist, thrombin amplifies platelet recruitment to the site of injury. Thrombin also converts fibrinogen to fibrin, and the fibrin strands then weave the platelet aggregates together to form a platelet–fibrin thrombus.

Disruption of the vessel wall also exposes tissue factor–expressing cells to the blood. Tissue factor initiates coagulation. Activated platelets potentiate coagulation by binding clotting factors and supporting the assembly of activation complexes that enhance thrombin generation. In addition to converting fibrinogen to fibrin, thrombin also serves as a potent platelet agonist and recruits more platelets to the site of vascular injury.

When platelets are activated, GpIIb/IIIa, the most abundant receptor on the platelet surface, undergoes a conformational change that enables it to bind fibrinogen and, under high shear conditions, vWF. Divalent fibrinogen or multivalent vWF molecules bridge adjacent platelets together to form platelet aggregates. Fibrin strands, generated through the action of thrombin, then weave these aggregates together to form a platelet–fibrin mesh.

Antiplatelet drugs target various steps in this process. The commonly used drugs include aspirin, thienopyridines (clopidogrel, prasugrel, and ticlopidine), dipyridamole, and GpIIb/IIIa antagonists.

ASPIRIN

The most widely used antiplatelet agent worldwide is aspirin. As a cheap and effective antiplatelet drug, aspirin serves as the foundation of most antiplatelet strategies.

Mechanism of action

Aspirin produces its antithrombotic effect by irreversibly acetylating and inhibiting platelet cyclooxygenase (COX)-1 (Fig. 23-3), a critical enzyme in the biosynthesis of thromboxane A_2. At high doses (~1 g/d), aspirin also inhibits COX-2, an inducible COX isoform found in endothelial cells and inflammatory cells. In endothelial cells, COX-2 initiates the synthesis of prostacyclin, a potent vasodilator and inhibitor of platelet aggregation.

Indications

Aspirin is widely used for secondary prevention of cardiovascular events in patients with coronary artery, cerebrovascular, or peripheral vascular disease. Compared with placebo, aspirin produces a 25% reduction in the risk of cardiovascular death, MI, or stroke. Aspirin is also used for primary prevention in patients whose estimated annual risk of MI is >1%, a point where its benefits are likely to outweigh harms. This includes patients older than age 40 years with two or more major risk factors for cardiovascular disease or those older than age 50 years with one or more such risk factors. Aspirin is equally effective in men and women. In men, aspirin mainly reduces the risk of MI, but in women, aspirin lowers the risk of stroke.

Dosages

Aspirin is usually administered at doses of 75–325 mg once daily. Higher doses of aspirin are not more effective than lower aspirin doses, and some analyses suggest reduced efficacy with higher doses. Because the

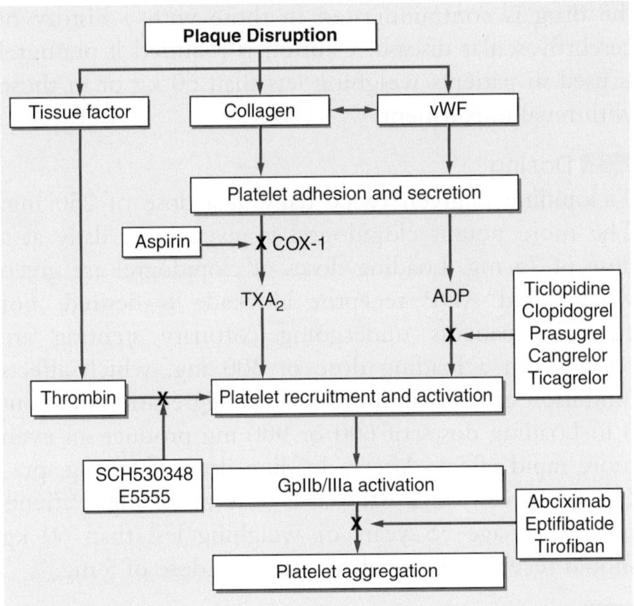

FIGURE 23-3

Site of action of antiplatelet drugs. Aspirin inhibits thromboxane A_2 (TXA_2) synthesis by irreversibly acetylating cyclooxygenase-1 (COX-1). Reduced TXA_2 release attenuates platelet activation and recruitment to the site of vascular injury. Ticlopidine, clopidogrel, and prasugrel irreversibly block $P2Y_{12}$, a key adenosine diphosphate (ADP) receptor on the platelet surface; cangrelor and ticagrelor are reversible inhibitors of $P2Y_{12}$. Abciximab, eptifibatide, and tirofiban inhibit the final common pathway of platelet aggregation by blocking fibrinogen and von Willebrand factor binding to activated glycoprotein (Gp) IIb/IIIa. SCH530348 and E5555 inhibit thrombin-mediated platelet activation by targeting protease-activated receptor-1 (PAR-1), the major thrombin receptor on human platelets.

side effects of aspirin are dose-related, daily aspirin doses of 75–100 mg are recommended for most indications. When rapid platelet inhibition is required, an initial aspirin dose of at least 160 mg should be given.

Side effects

Most common side effects are gastrointestinal and range from dyspepsia to erosive gastritis or peptic ulcers with bleeding and perforation. These side effects are dose-related. Use of enteric-coated or buffered aspirin in place of plain aspirin does not eliminate the risk of gastrointestinal side effects. The overall risk of major bleeding with aspirin is 1–3% per year. The risk of bleeding is increased when aspirin is given in conjunction with anticoagulants, such as warfarin. When dual therapy is used, low-dose aspirin should be given (75–100 mg/d). Eradication of *Helicobacter pylori* infection and administration of proton pump inhibitors may reduce the risk of aspirin-induced gastrointestinal bleeding in patients with peptic ulcer disease.

Aspirin should not be administered to patients with a history of aspirin allergy characterized by bronchospasm. This problem occurs in ~0.3% of the general population but is more common in those with chronic urticaria or asthma, particularly in individuals with nasal polyps or chronic rhinitis. Hepatic and renal toxicity are observed with aspirin overdose.

Aspirin resistance

Clinical aspirin resistance is defined as the failure of aspirin to protect patients from ischemic vascular events. This is not a helpful definition because it is made after the event occurs. Furthermore, it is not realistic to expect aspirin, which only blocks thromboxane A_2–induced platelet activation, to prevent all vascular events.

Aspirin resistance has also been described biochemically as failure of the drug to produce its expected inhibitory effects on tests of platelet function, such as thromboxane A_2 synthesis or arachidonic acid–induced platelet aggregation. However, the tests of platelet function used for diagnosis of biochemical aspirin resistance have not been well standardized. Furthermore, these tests are not proven to identify patients at risk of recurrent vascular events. In addition, resistance is not reversed by either giving higher doses of aspirin or adding other antiplatelet drugs. Thus, testing for aspirin resistance remains a research tool.

THIENOPYRIDINES

The thienopyridines include ticlopidine, clopidogrel, and prasugrel, drugs that target $P2Y_{12}$, a key ADP receptor on platelets.

Mechanism of action

The thienopyridines are structurally related drugs that selectively inhibit ADP-induced platelet aggregation by irreversibly blocking $P2Y_{12}$ (Fig. 23-3). Ticlopidine and clopidogrel are prodrugs that require metabolism by the hepatic cytochrome P450 (CYP) enzyme system to acquire activity. Consequently, when given in usual doses, their onset of action is delayed for several days. Although prasugrel also is a prodrug that requires metabolic activation, its onset of action is more rapid than that of ticlopidine or clopidogrel, and prasugrel produces greater and more predictable inhibition of ADP-induced platelet aggregation. These characteristics reflect the rapid and complete absorption of prasugrel from the gut and its more efficient activation pathways. Whereas nearly all of the absorbed prasugrel undergoes metabolic activation in the liver, only 15% of absorbed clopidogrel is activated; the remainder is inactivated by esterases.

Indications

Like aspirin, ticlopidine is more effective than placebo at reducing the risk of cardiovascular death, MI, and stroke in patients with atherosclerotic disease. Because of its delayed onset of action, ticlopidine is not recommended in patients with acute MI. Ticlopidine was used routinely as an adjunct to aspirin after coronary artery stenting and as an aspirin substitute in those intolerant to aspirin. Because clopidogrel is more potent than ticlopidine and has a better safety profile, clopidogrel has replaced ticlopidine.

When compared with aspirin in patients with recent ischemic stroke, MI, or peripheral arterial disease, clopidogrel reduced the risk of cardiovascular death, MI, and stroke by 8.7%. Therefore, clopidogrel is more effective than aspirin but is also more expensive. In some patients, clopidogrel and aspirin are combined to capitalize on their capacity to block complementary pathways of platelet activation. For example, the combination of aspirin plus clopidogrel is recommended for at least 4 weeks after implantation of a bare metal stent in a coronary artery and longer in those with a drug-eluting stent. Concerns about late in-stent thrombosis with drug-eluting stents have led some experts to recommend long-term use of clopidogrel plus aspirin for this indication.

The combination of clopidogrel and aspirin is also effective in patients with unstable angina. Thus, in 12,562 such patients, the risk of cardiovascular death, MI, or stroke was 9.3% in those randomized to the combination of clopidogrel and aspirin and 11.4% in those given aspirin alone. This 20% relative risk reduction with combination therapy was highly statistically significant. However, combining clopidogrel with aspirin increases the risk of major bleeding to about 2% per year. This bleeding risk persists even if the daily dose of aspirin is ≤100 mg. Therefore, the combination of clopidogrel and aspirin should only be used when there is a clear benefit. For example, this combination has not proven to be superior to clopidogrel alone in patients with acute ischemic stroke or to aspirin alone for primary prevention in those at risk for cardiovascular events.

Prasugrel was compared with clopidogrel in 13,608 patients with acute coronary syndromes who were scheduled to undergo a percutaneous coronary intervention. The incidence of the primary efficacy endpoint, a composite of cardiovascular death, MI, and stroke, was significantly lower with prasugrel than with clopidogrel (9.9% and 12.1%, respectively), mainly reflecting a reduction in the incidence of nonfatal MI. The incidence of stent thrombosis also was significantly lower with prasugrel than with clopidogrel (1.1% and 2.4%, respectively). However, these advantages were at the expense of significantly higher rates of fatal bleeding (0.4% and 0.1%, respectively) and life-threatening bleeding (1.4% and 0.9%, respectively) with prasugrel. Because patients older than age 75 years and those with a history of prior stroke or transient ischemic attack have a particularly high risk of bleeding, prasugrel should generally be avoided in older patients, and the drug is contraindicated in those with a history of cerebrovascular disease. Caution is required if prasugrel is used in patients weighing less than 60 kg or in those with renal impairment.

Dosing

Ticlopidine is given twice daily at a dose of 250 mg. The more potent clopidogrel is given once daily at a dose of 75 mg. Loading doses of clopidogrel are given when rapid ADP receptor blockade is desired. For example, patients undergoing coronary stenting are often given a loading dose of 300 mg, which affects inhibition of ADP-induced platelet aggregation in about 6 h. Loading doses of 600 or 900 mg produce an even more rapid effect. After a loading dose of 60 mg, prasugrel is given once daily at a dose of 10 mg. Patients older than age 75 years or weighing less than 60 kg should receive a lower daily prasugrel dose of 5 mg.

Side effects

The most common side effects of ticlopidine are gastrointestinal. More serious are the hematologic side effects, which include neutropenia, thrombocytopenia, and thrombotic thrombocytopenic purpura. These side effects usually occur within the first few months of starting treatment. Therefore, blood counts must be carefully monitored when initiating therapy with ticlopidine. Gastrointestinal and hematologic side effects are rare with clopidogrel and prasugrel.

Thienopyridine resistance

The capacity of clopidogrel to inhibit ADP-induced platelet aggregation varies among subjects. This variability reflects, at least in part, genetic polymorphisms in the CYP isoenzymes involved in the metabolic activation of clopidogrel. The most important of these is *CYP2C19*. Clopidogrel-treated patients with the loss-of-function *CYP2C19*2* allele exhibit reduced platelet inhibition compared with those with the wild-type *CYP2C19*1* allele and experience a higher rate of cardiovascular events. This is important because estimates suggest that up to 25% of whites, 30% of African Americans, and 50% of Asians carry the loss-of-function allele, which would render them resistant to clopidogrel. Even patients with the reduced function *CYP2C19*3*, **4*, or **5* alleles may derive less benefit from clopidogrel than those with the full-function *CYP2C19*1* allele. Concomitant administration of clopidogrel and proton pump inhibitors, which are inhibitors of *CYP2C19*, produces a small reduction in the inhibitory effects of clopidogrel on ADP-induced platelet aggregation. The extent to which this interaction increases the risk of cardiovascular events remains controversial.

In contrast to their effect on the metabolic activation of clopidogrel, *CYP2C19* polymorphisms appear to be less important determinants of the activation of prasugrel. Thus, no association was detected between the loss-of-function allele and decreased platelet inhibition or increased rate of cardiovascular events with prasugrel. The observation that genetic polymorphisms affecting clopidogrel absorption or metabolism influence clinical outcomes raises the possibilities that pharmacogenetic profiling may be useful to identify clopidogrel-resistant patients and that point-of-care assessment of the extent of clopidogrel-induced platelet inhibition may help detect patients at higher risk for subsequent cardiovascular events. It is unknown whether administration of higher doses of clopidogrel to such patients will overcome this resistance. Instead, prasugrel or newer $P2Y_{12}$ inhibitors may be better choices for these patients.

DIPYRIDAMOLE

Dipyridamole is a relatively weak antiplatelet agent on its own, but an extended-release formulation of dipyridamole combined with low-dose aspirin, a preparation known as *Aggrenox*, is used for prevention of stroke in patients with transient ischemic attacks.

Mechanism of action

By inhibiting phosphodiesterase, dipyridamole blocks the breakdown of cyclic adenosine monophosphate (AMP). Increased levels of cyclic AMP reduce intracellular calcium and inhibit platelet activation. Dipyridamole also blocks the uptake of adenosine by platelets and other cells. This produces a further increase in local cyclic AMP levels because the platelet adenosine A_2 receptor is coupled to adenylate cyclase (Fig. 23-4).

Dosing

Aggrenox is given twice daily. Each capsule contains 200 mg of extended-release dipyridamole and 25 mg of aspirin.

Side effects

Because dipyridamole has vasodilatory effects, it must be used with caution in patients with coronary artery disease. Gastrointestinal complaints, headache, facial flushing, dizziness, and hypotension can also occur. These symptoms often subside with continued use of the drug.

Indications

Dipyridamole plus aspirin was compared with aspirin or dipyridamole alone or with placebo in patients with an ischemic stroke or transient ischemic attack. The combination reduced the risk of stroke by 22.1% compared with aspirin and by 24.4% compared with dipyridamole. A second trial compared dipyridamole plus aspirin with aspirin alone for secondary prevention in patients with ischemic stroke. Vascular death, stroke, or MI occurred in 13% of patients given combination therapy and in 16% of those treated with aspirin alone. Based on these data, Aggrenox was often used for stroke prevention. Another trial randomized 20,332 patients with noncardioembolic ischemic stroke to either Aggrenox or clopidogrel. The primary efficacy endpoint of recurrent stroke occurred in 9.0% of those given Aggrenox and in 8.8% of patients treated with clopidogrel. Although this difference was not statistically significant, the study failed to meet the prespecified margin to claim noninferiority of Aggrenox relative to clopidogrel. These results have dampened enthusiasm for the use of Aggrenox.

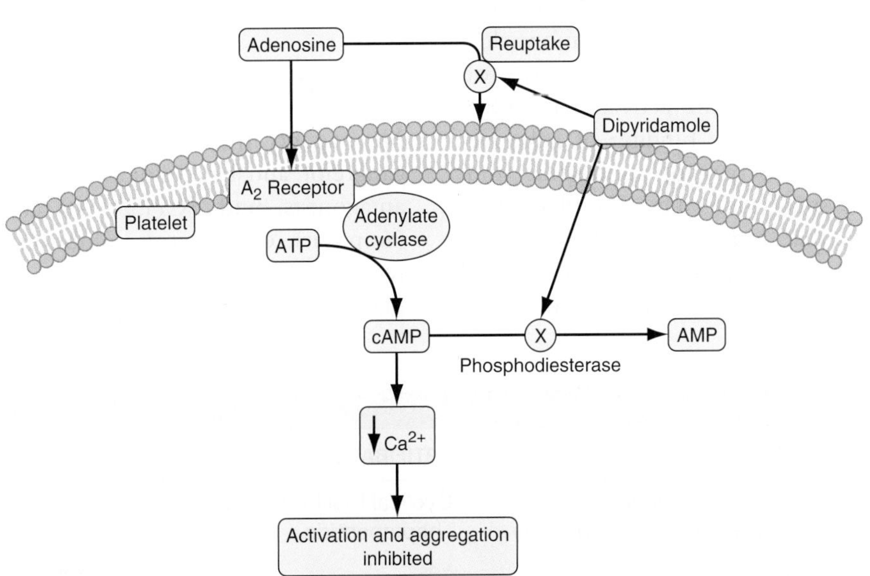

FIGURE 23-4

Mechanism of action of dipyridamole. Dipyridamole increases levels of cyclic adenosine monophosphate (AMP) in platelets by (1) blocking the reuptake of adenosine and (2) inhibiting phosphodiesterase-mediated cyclic AMP degradation. By promoting calcium uptake, cyclic AMP reduces intracellular levels of calcium. This, in turn, inhibits platelet activation and aggregation. ATP, adenosine triphosphate.

Because of its vasodilatory effects and the paucity of data supporting the use of dipyridamole in patients with symptomatic coronary artery disease, Aggrenox should not be used for stroke prevention in such patients. Clopidogrel is a better choice in this setting.

GLYCOPROTEIN IIB/IIIA RECEPTOR ANTAGONISTS

As a class, parenteral GpIIb/IIIa receptor antagonists have an established niche in patients with acute coronary syndromes. The three agents in this class are abciximab, eptifibatide, and tirofiban.

Mechanism of action

A member of the integrin family of adhesion receptors, GpIIb/IIIa is found on the surface of platelets and megakaryocytes. With about 80,000 copies per platelet, GpIIb/IIIa is the most abundant receptor. Consisting of a noncovalently linked heterodimer, GpIIb/IIIa is inactive on resting platelets. When platelets are activated, inside–outside signal transduction pathways trigger a conformational activation of the receptor. Once activated, GpIIb/IIIa binds adhesive molecules, such as fibrinogen and, under high shear conditions, vWF. Binding is mediated by the Arg-Gly-Asp (RGD) sequence found on the α chains of fibrinogen and on vWF and by the Lys-Gly-Asp (KGD) sequence located within a unique dodecapeptide domain on the γ chains of fibrinogen. Once bound, fibrinogen and/or vWF bridges adjacent platelets together to induce platelet aggregation.

Although abciximab, eptifibatide, and tirofiban all target the GpIIb/IIIa receptor, they are structurally and pharmacologically distinct (Table 23-1). Abciximab is a Fab fragment of a humanized murine monoclonal antibody directed against the activated form of GpIIb/IIIa. Abciximab binds to the activated receptor with high affinity and blocks the binding of adhesive molecules. In contrast to abciximab, eptifibatide and tirofiban are synthetic small molecules. Eptifibatide is a cyclic heptapeptide that binds GpIIb/IIIa because it incorporates the KGD motif, whereas tirofiban is a nonpeptidic tyrosine derivative that acts as an RGD mimetic. Abciximab has a long half-life and can be detected on the surface of platelets for up to 2 weeks. Eptifibatide and tirofiban have shorter half-lives.

In addition to targeting the GpIIb/IIIa receptor, abciximab also inhibits the closely related $\alpha_v\beta_3$ receptor, which binds vitronectin, and $\alpha_M\beta_2$, a leukocyte integrin. In contrast, eptifibatide and tirofiban are specific for GpIIb/IIIa. Inhibition of $\alpha_v\beta_3$ and $\alpha_M\beta_2$ may endow abciximab with anti-inflammatory and/or antiproliferative properties that extend beyond platelet inhibition.

Dosing

All of the GpIIb/IIIa antagonists are given as an intravenous (IV) bolus followed by an infusion. Because they are cleared by the kidneys, the doses of eptifibatide and tirofiban must be reduced in patients with renal insufficiency.

Side effects

In addition to bleeding, thrombocytopenia is the most serious complication. Thrombocytopenia is immune-mediated and is caused by antibodies directed against neoantigens on GpIIb/IIIa that are exposed upon antagonist binding. With abciximab, thrombocytopenia occurs in up to 5% of patients. Thrombocytopenia is severe in ~1% of these individuals. Thrombocytopenia is less common with the other two agents, occurring in ~1% of patients.

Indications

Abciximab and eptifibatide are used in patients undergoing percutaneous coronary interventions, particularly those with acute MI. Tirofiban is used in high-risk patients with unstable angina. Eptifibatide also can be used for this indication.

NEW ANTIPLATELET AGENTS

New agents in advanced stages of development include cangrelor and ticagrelor, direct-acting reversible $P2Y_{12}$ antagonists, and SCH530348 (vorapaxar) and E5555 (atopaxar), orally active inhibitors of protease-activated receptor 1 (PAR-1), the major thrombin receptor on platelets (Fig. 23-3). Cangrelor is an adenosine analogue

TABLE 23-1

FEATURES OF GLYCOPROTEIN IIB/IIIA ANTAGONISTS

FEATURE	ABCIXIMAB	EPTIFIBATIDE	TIROFIBAN
Description	Fab fragment of humanized mouse monoclonal antibody	Cyclical KGD-containing heptapeptide	Nonpeptidic RGD mimetic
Specific for GpIIb/IIIa	No	Yes	Yes
Plasma half-life	Short (min)	Long (2.5 h)	Long (2.0 h)
Platelet-bound half-life	Long (days)	Short (s)	Short (s)
Renal clearance	No	Yes	Yes

that binds reversibly to $P2Y_{12}$ and inhibits its activity. The drug has a half-life of 3–6 min and is given intravenously as a bolus followed by an infusion. When stopped, platelet function recovers within 60 min. Trials comparing cangrelor with placebo during percutaneous coronary interventions or comparing cangrelor with clopidogrel after such procedures revealed little or no advantages of cangrelor. Consequently, identification of a role for cangrelor requires additional studies.

Ticagrelor is an orally active, reversible inhibitor of $P2Y_{12}$. The drug is given twice daily and it not only has a more rapid onset and offset of action than clopidogrel but also produces greater and more predictable inhibition of ADP-induced platelet aggregation. When compared with clopidogrel in patients with acute coronary syndromes, ticagrelor produced a greater reduction in the primary efficacy endpoint, a composite of cardiovascular death, MI, and stroke at 1 year (9.8% and 11.7%, respectively; $p = .001$). This difference reflected a significantly greater reduction in cardiovascular death (4.0% and 5.1%, respectively; $p = .001$) and MI (5.8% and 6.9%, respectively; $p = .005$) with ticagrelor than with clopidogrel. Rates of stroke were similar with ticagrelor and clopidogrel (1.5% and 1.3%, respectively), and there were no differences in the rates of major bleeding. When minor bleeding was added to the major bleeding results, however, ticagrelor showed an increase relative to clopidogrel (16.1% and 14.6%, respectively; $p = 0.008$). Ticagrelor also was superior to clopidogrel in the acute coronary syndrome patients who underwent percutaneous coronary interventions or aortocoronary bypass surgery. Although not yet licensed, ticagrelor is the first new antiplatelet drug to demonstrate a greater reduction in cardiovascular death than clopidogrel in patients with acute coronary syndromes.

SCH530348, an orally active inhibitor of PAR-1, is under investigation as an adjunct to aspirin or aspirin plus clopidogrel. Two large phase III trials are underway. E5555, a second oral PAR-1 antagonist, is earlier in development.

ANTICOAGULANTS

There are both parenteral and oral anticoagulants. Currently available parenteral anticoagulants include heparin, low-molecular-weight heparin (LMWH), and fondaparinux, a synthetic pentasaccharide. The only available oral anticoagulants are the vitamin K antagonists, of which warfarin is the agent most often used in North America.

Dabigatran etexilate, an oral thrombin inhibitor, and rivaroxaban, an oral factor Xa inhibitor, are licensed in Europe and Canada for short-term thromboprophylaxis after elective hip or knee replacement surgery. Dabigatran etexilate was licensed in the United States and Canada as an alternative to warfarin for stroke prevention in patients with atrial fibrillation.

PARENTERAL ANTICOAGULANTS

Heparin

Heparin is a sulfated polysaccharide and is isolated from mammalian tissues rich in mast cells. Most commercial heparin is derived from porcine intestinal mucosa and is a polymer of alternating D-glucuronic acid and *N*-acetyl-D-glucosamine residues.

Mechanism of action

Heparin acts as an anticoagulant by activating antithrombin (previously known as antithrombin III) and accelerating the rate at which antithrombin inhibits clotting enzymes, particularly thrombin and factor Xa. Antithrombin, the obligatory plasma cofactor for heparin, is a member of the serine protease inhibitor (serpin) superfamily. Synthesized in the liver and circulating in plasma at a concentration of 2.6 ± 0.4 μM, antithrombin acts as a suicide substrate for its target enzymes.

To activate antithrombin, heparin binds to the serpin via a unique pentasaccharide sequence that is found on one-third of the chains of commercial heparin (Fig. 23-5). The remainder of the heparin chains that lack this pentasaccharide sequence have little or no anticoagulant activity. Once bound to antithrombin, heparin induces a conformational change in the reactive center loop of antithrombin that renders it more readily accessible to its target proteases. This conformational change enhances the rate at which antithrombin inhibits factor Xa by at least two orders of magnitude but has little effect on the rate of thrombin inhibition by antithrombin. To catalyze thrombin inhibition, heparin serves as a template that binds antithrombin and thrombin simultaneously. Formation of this ternary complex brings the enzyme in close apposition to the inhibitor, thereby promoting the formation of a stable covalent thrombin-antithrombin complex.

Only pentasaccharide-containing heparin chains composed of at least 18 saccharide units (which correspond to a molecular weight of 5400) are of sufficient length to bridge thrombin and antithrombin together. With a mean molecular weight of 15,000, and a range of 5000–30,000, almost all of the chains of unfractionated heparin are long enough to effect this bridging function. Consequently, by definition, heparin has equal capacity to promote the inhibition of thrombin and factor Xa by antithrombin and is assigned an anti-factor Xa to anti-factor IIa (thrombin) ratio of 1:1.

Heparin causes the release of tissue factor pathway inhibitor (TFPI) from the endothelium. A factor Xa–dependent inhibitor of tissue factor–bound factor

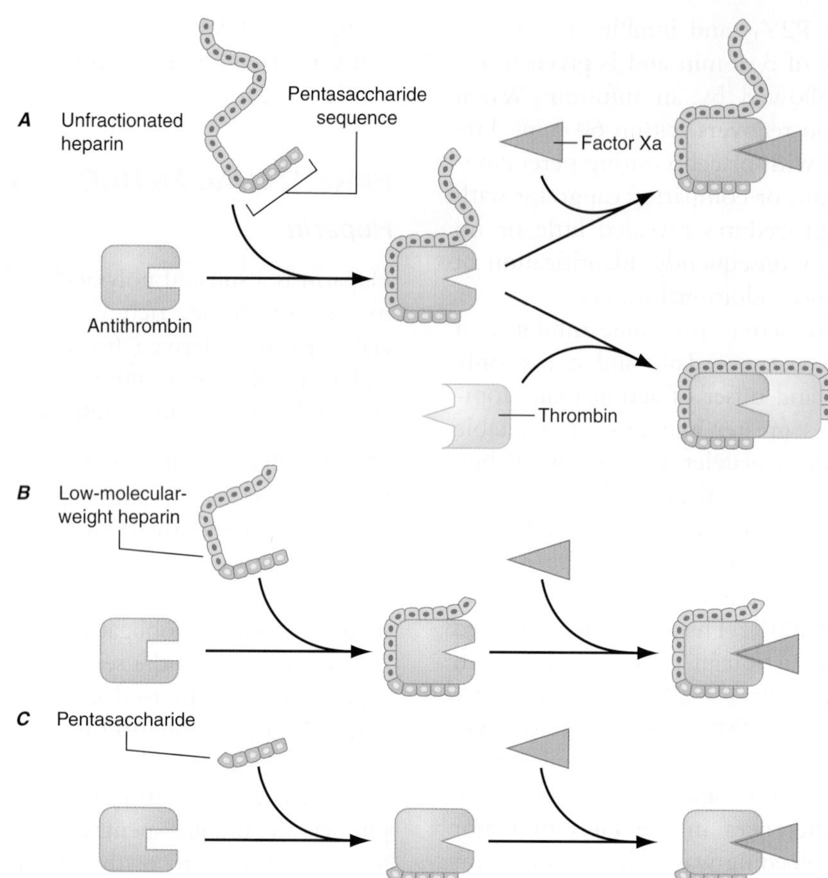

FIGURE 23-5

Mechanism of action of heparin, low-molecular-weight heparin (LMWH), and fondaparinux, a synthetic pentasaccharide. *A.* Heparin binds to antithrombin via its pentasaccharide sequence. This induces a conformational change in the reactive center loop of antithrombin that accelerates its interaction with factor Xa. To potentiate thrombin inhibition, heparin must simultaneously bind to antithrombin and thrombin. Only heparin chains composed of at least 18 saccharide units, which corresponds to a molecular weight of 5400, are of sufficient length to perform this bridging function. With a mean molecular weight of 15,000, all of the heparin chains are long enough to do this. ***B.*** LMWH has greater capacity to potentiate factor Xa inhibition by antithrombin than thrombin because, with a mean molecular weight of 4500–5000, at least half of the LMWH chains are too short to bridge antithrombin to thrombin. ***C.*** The pentasaccharide only accelerates factor Xa inhibition by antithrombin because the pentasaccharide is too short to bridge antithrombin to thrombin.

VIIa, TFPI may contribute to the antithrombotic activity of heparin. Longer heparin chains induce the release of more TFPI than shorter chains.

Pharmacology

Heparin must be given parenterally. It is usually administered subcutaneously (SC) or by continuous IV infusion. When used for therapeutic purposes, the IV route is most often employed. If heparin is given SC for treatment of thrombosis, the dose of heparin must be high enough to overcome the limited bioavailability associated with this method of delivery.

In the circulation, heparin binds to the endothelium and to plasma proteins other than antithrombin. Heparin binding to endothelial cells explains its dose-dependent clearance. At low doses, the half-life of heparin is short because it binds rapidly to the endothelium. With higher doses of heparin, the half-life is longer because heparin is cleared more slowly once the endothelium is saturated. Clearance is mainly extrarenal; heparin binds to macrophages, which internalize and depolymerize the long heparin chains and secrete shorter chains back into the circulation. Because of its dose-dependent clearance mechanism, the plasma half-life of heparin ranges from 30 to 60 min with bolus IV doses of 25 and 100 U/kg, respectively.

Once heparin enters the circulation, it binds to plasma proteins other than antithrombin, a phenomenon that reduces its anticoagulant activity. Some of the heparin-binding proteins found in plasma are acute-phase reactants whose levels are elevated in ill patients. Others, such as high-molecular-weight multimers of vWF, are released from activated platelets or endothelial cells. Activated platelets also release platelet factor 4 (PF4), a highly cationic protein that binds heparin with high affinity. The large amounts of PF4 found in the vicinity of platelet-rich arterial thrombi can neutralize the anticoagulant activity of heparin. This phenomenon may attenuate heparin's capacity to suppress thrombus growth.

Because the levels of heparin-binding proteins in plasma vary from person to person, the anticoagulant response to fixed or weight-adjusted doses of heparin is unpredictable. Consequently, coagulation monitoring is essential to ensure that a therapeutic response is obtained. This is particularly important when heparin is administered for treatment of established thrombosis because a subtherapeutic anticoagulant response may render patients at risk for recurrent thrombosis, whereas excessive anticoagulation increases the risk of bleeding.

Monitoring the anticoagulant effect

Heparin therapy can be monitored using the activated partial thromboplastin time (aPTT) or anti–factor Xa level. Although the aPTT is the test most often employed for this purpose, there are problems with this assay. aPTT reagents vary in their sensitivity to heparin, and the type of coagulometer used for testing can influence the results. Consequently, laboratories must establish a therapeutic aPTT range with each reagent-coagulometer combination by measuring the aPTT and anti–factor Xa level in plasma samples collected from heparin-treated patients. For most of the aPTT reagents and coagulometers in current use, therapeutic heparin levels are achieved with a two- to threefold prolongation of the aPTT.

Anti–factor Xa levels also can be used to monitor heparin therapy. With this test, therapeutic heparin levels range from 0.3 to 0.7 units/mL. Although this test is gaining in popularity, anti–factor Xa assays have yet to be standardized, and results can vary widely between laboratories.

Up to 25% of heparin-treated patients with VTE require >35,000 units/d to achieve a therapeutic aPTT. These patients are considered heparin resistant. It is useful to measure anti–factor Xa levels in heparin-resistant patients because many will have a therapeutic anti–factor Xa level despite a subtherapeutic aPTT. This dissociation in test results occurs because elevated plasma levels of fibrinogen and factor VIII, both of which are acute-phase proteins, shorten the aPTT but have no effect on anti–factor Xa levels. Heparin therapy in patients who exhibit this phenomenon is best monitored using anti–factor Xa levels instead of the aPTT. Patients with congenital or acquired antithrombin deficiency and those with elevated levels of heparin-binding proteins may also need high doses of heparin to achieve a therapeutic aPTT or anti–factor Xa level. If there is good correlation between the aPTT and the anti–factor Xa levels, either test can be used to monitor heparin therapy.

Dosing

For prophylaxis, heparin is usually given in fixed doses of 5000 units SC two or three times daily. With these low doses, coagulation monitoring is unnecessary. In contrast, monitoring is essential when the drug is given in therapeutic doses. Fixed-dose or weight-based heparin nomograms are used to standardize heparin dosing and to shorten the time required to achieve a therapeutic anticoagulant response. At least two heparin nomograms have been validated in patients with VTE and reduce the time required to achieve a therapeutic aPTT. Weight-adjusted heparin nomograms have also been evaluated in patients with acute coronary syndromes. After an IV heparin bolus of 5000 units or 70 units/kg, a heparin infusion rate of 12–15 units/kg per hour is usually administered. In contrast, weight-adjusted heparin nomograms for patients with VTE use an initial bolus of 5000 units or 80 units/kg followed by an infusion of 18 units/kg per hour. Thus, patients with VTE appear to require higher doses of heparin to achieve a therapeutic aPTT than do patients with acute coronary syndromes. This may reflect differences in the thrombus burden. Heparin binds to fibrin, and the fibrin content of extensive deep-vein thrombi is greater than that of small coronary thrombi.

Heparin manufacturers in North America have traditionally measured heparin potency in USP units, with 1 unit defined as the concentration of heparin that prevents 1 mL of citrated sheep plasma from clotting for 1 h after calcium addition. In contrast, manufacturers in Europe measure heparin potency with anti-Xa assays using an international heparin standard for comparison. Because of problems with heparin contamination with oversulfated chondroitin sulfate, which the USP assay system does not detect, North American heparin manufacturers now use the anti-Xa assay to assess heparin potency. Although use of international units in place of USP units results in a 10% reduction in heparin doses, this change is unlikely to affect patient care because heparin has been dosed in international units in Europe for many years. Furthermore, heparin monitoring ensures a therapeutic anticoagulant response in high-risk situations, such as cardiopulmonary bypass surgery or percutaneous coronary intervention.

Limitations

Heparin has pharmacokinetic and biophysical limitations (Table 23-2). The pharmacokinetic limitations reflect heparin's propensity to bind in a pentasaccharide-independent fashion to cells and plasma proteins. Heparin binding to endothelial cells explains its dose-dependent clearance, whereas binding to plasma proteins results

TABLE 23-2

PHARMACOKINETIC AND BIOPHYSICAL LIMITATIONS OF HEPARIN

LIMITATIONS	MECHANISM
Poor bioavailability at low doses	Binds to endothelial cells and macrophages
Dose-dependent clearance	Binds to macrophages
Variable anticoagulant response	Binds to plasma proteins whose levels vary from patient to patient
Reduced activity in the vicinity of platelet-rich thrombi	Neutralized by platelet factor 4 released from activated platelets
Limited activity against factor Xa incorporated in the prothrombinase complex and thrombin bound to fibrin	Reduced capacity of heparin–antithrombin complex to inhibit factor Xa bound to activated platelets and thrombin bound to fibrin

in a variable anticoagulant response and can lead to heparin resistance.

The biophysical limitations of heparin reflect the inability of the heparin–antithrombin complex to (1) inhibit factor Xa when it is incorporated into the prothrombinase complex, the complex that converts prothrombin to thrombin, and (2) to inhibit thrombin bound to fibrin. Consequently, factor Xa bound to activated platelets within platelet-rich thrombi has the potential to generate thrombin, even in the face of heparin. Once this thrombin binds to fibrin, it too is protected from inhibition by the heparin–antithrombin complex. Clot-associated thrombin can then trigger thrombus growth by locally activating platelets and amplifying its own generation through feedback activation of factors V, VIII, and XI. Further compounding the problem is the potential for heparin neutralization by the high concentrations of PF4 released from activated platelets within the platelet-rich thrombus.

Side effects

The most common side effect of heparin is bleeding. Other complications include thrombocytopenia, osteoporosis, and elevated levels of transaminases.

Bleeding

The risk of heparin-induced bleeding increases with higher heparin doses. Concomitant administration of drugs that affect hemostasis, such as antiplatelet or fibrinolytic agents, increases the risk of bleeding, as does recent surgery or trauma. Heparin-treated patients with serious bleeding can be given protamine sulfate to neutralize the heparin. Protamine sulfate, a mixture of basic polypeptides isolated from salmon sperm, binds heparin with high affinity, and the resultant protamine–heparin complexes are then cleared. Typically, 1 mg of protamine sulfate neutralizes 100 units of heparin. Protamine sulfate is given IV. Anaphylactoid reactions to protamine sulfate can occur, and drug administration by slow IV infusion is recommended to reduce the risk.

Thrombocytopenia

Heparin can cause thrombocytopenia. Heparin-induced thrombocytopenia (HIT) is an antibody-mediated process that is triggered by antibodies directed against neoantigens on PF4 that are exposed when heparin binds to this protein. These antibodies, which are usually of the IgG isotype, bind simultaneously to the heparin–PF4 complex and to platelet Fc receptors. Such binding activates the platelets and generates platelet microparticles. Circulating microparticles are prothrombotic because they express anionic phospholipids on their surfaces and can bind clotting factors and promote thrombin generation.

The clinical features of HIT are illustrated in Table 23-3. Typically, HIT occurs 5–14 days after initiation of heparin therapy, but it can manifest earlier if the patient has received heparin within the past 3 months. It is rare for the platelet count to fall below 100,000/μL in patients with HIT, and even a 50% decrease in the platelet count from the pretreatment value should raise the suspicion of HIT in those receiving heparin. HIT is more common in surgical patients than in medical patients and, like many autoimmune disorders, occurs more frequently in females than in males.

HIT can be associated with thrombosis, either arterial or venous. Venous thrombosis, which manifests as DVT and/or Pulmonary Embolism, is more common than arterial thrombosis. Arterial thrombosis can manifest as ischemic stroke or acute MI. Rarely, platelet-rich thrombi in the distal aorta or iliac arteries can cause critical limb ischemia.

TABLE 23-3

FEATURES OF HEPARIN-INDUCED THROMBOCYTOPENIA

FEATURES	DETAILS
Thrombocytopenia	Platelet count of ≤100,000/μL or a decrease in platelet count of ≥50%
Timing	Platelet count falls 5–10 days after starting heparin
Type of heparin	More common with unfractionated heparin than low-molecular-weight heparin
Type of patient	More common in surgical patients and patients with cancer than general medical patients; more common in women than in men
Thrombosis	Venous thrombosis more common than arterial thrombosis

TABLE 23-4

MANAGEMENT OF HEPARIN-INDUCED THROMBOCYTOPENIA

Stop all heparin.
Give an alternative anticoagulant, such as lepirudin, argatroban, bivalirudin, or fondaparinux.
Do not give platelet transfusions.
Do not give warfarin until the platelet count returns to its baseline level. If warfarin is administered, give vitamin K to restore the INR to normal.
Evaluate for thrombosis, particularly deep-vein thrombosis.

Abbreviation: INR, international normalized ratio.

The diagnosis of HIT is established using enzyme-linked assays to detect antibodies against heparin–PF4 complexes or with platelet activation assays. Enzyme-linked assays are sensitive but can be positive in the absence of any clinical evidence of HIT. The most specific diagnostic test is the serotonin release assay. This test is performed by quantifying serotonin release when washed platelets loaded with labeled serotonin are exposed to patient serum in the absence or presence of varying concentrations of heparin. If the patient's serum contains the HIT antibody, heparin addition induces platelet activation and serotonin release.

Management of HIT is outlined in Table 23-4. Heparin should be stopped in patients with suspected or documented HIT, and an alternative anticoagulant should be administered to prevent or treat thrombosis. The agents most often used for this indication are parenteral direct thrombin inhibitors, such as lepirudin, argatroban, or bivalirudin, or factor Xa inhibitors, such as fondaparinux.

Patients with HIT, particularly those with associated thrombosis, often have evidence of increased thrombin generation that can lead to consumption of protein C. If these patients are given warfarin without a concomitant parenteral anticoagulant to inhibit thrombin or thrombin generation, the further decrease in protein C levels induced by the vitamin K antagonist can trigger skin necrosis. To avoid this problem, patients with HIT should be treated with a direct thrombin inhibitor or fondaparinux until the platelet count returns to normal levels. At this point, low-dose warfarin therapy can be introduced, and the thrombin inhibitor can be discontinued when the anticoagulant response to warfarin has been therapeutic for at least 2 days.

Osteoporosis

Treatment with therapeutic doses of heparin for >1 month can cause a reduction in bone density. This complication has been reported in up to 30% of patients given long-term heparin therapy, and symptomatic vertebral fractures occur in 2–3% of these individuals.

Heparin causes bone loss both by decreasing bone formation and by enhancing bone resorption. Thus, heparin affects the activity of both osteoblasts and osteoclasts.

Elevated levels of transaminases

Therapeutic doses of heparin frequently cause modest elevation in the serum levels of hepatic transaminases, without a concomitant increase in the level of bilirubin. The levels of transaminases rapidly return to normal when the drug is stopped. The mechanism of this phenomenon is unknown.

Low-molecular-weight heparin

Consisting of smaller fragments of heparin, LMWH is prepared from unfractionated heparin by controlled enzymatic or chemical depolymerization. The mean molecular weight of LMWH is 5000, one-third the mean molecular weight of unfractionated heparin. LMWH has advantages over heparin (Table 23-5) and has replaced heparin for most indications.

Mechanism of action

Like heparin, LMWH exerts its anticoagulant activity by activating antithrombin. With a mean molecular weight of 5000, which corresponds to about 17 saccharide units, at least half of the pentasaccharide-containing chains of LMWH are too short to bridge thrombin to antithrombin (Fig. 23-5). However, these chains retain the capacity to accelerate factor Xa inhibition by antithrombin because this activity is largely the result of the conformational changes in antithrombin evoked by pentasaccharide binding. Consequently, LMWH catalyzes factor Xa inhibition by antithrombin more than thrombin inhibition. Depending on their unique

TABLE 23-5

ADVANTAGES OF LOW-MOLECULAR-WEIGHT HEPARIN OVER HEPARIN

ADVANTAGE	CONSEQUENCE
Better bioavailability and longer half-life after subcutaneous injection	Can be given subcutaneously once or twice daily for both prophylaxis and treatment
Dose-independent clearance	Simplified dosing
Predictable anticoagulant response	Coagulation monitoring is unnecessary in most patients
Lower risk of heparin-induced thrombocytopenia	Safer than heparin for short- or long-term administration
Lower risk of osteoporosis	Safer than heparin for extended administration

Abbreviation: LMWH, low-molecular-weight heparin.

molecular weight distributions, LMWH preparations have anti–factor Xa to anti–factor IIa ratios ranging from 2:1 to 4:1.

Pharmacology

Although usually given SC, LMWH also can be administered IV if a rapid anticoagulant response is needed. LMWH has pharmacokinetic advantages over heparin. These advantages reflect the fact that shorter heparin chains bind less avidly to endothelial cells, macrophages, and heparin-binding plasma proteins. Reduced binding to endothelial cells and macrophages eliminates the rapid, dose-dependent, and saturable mechanism of clearance that is a characteristic of unfractionated heparin. Instead, the clearance of LMWH is dose-independent, and its plasma half-life is longer. Based on measurement of anti–factor Xa levels, LMWH has a plasma half-life of ~4 h. LMWH is cleared almost exclusively by the kidneys, and the drug can accumulate in patients with renal insufficiency.

LMWH exhibits about 90% bioavailability after SC injection. Because LMWH binds less avidly to heparin-binding proteins in plasma than heparin, LMWH produces a more predictable dose response, and resistance to LMWH is rare. With a longer half-life and more predictable anticoagulant response, LMWH can be given SC once or twice daily without coagulation monitoring, even when the drug is given in treatment doses. These properties render LMWH more convenient than unfractionated heparin. Capitalizing on this feature, studies in patients with VTE have shown that home treatment with LMWH is as effective and safe as in-hospital treatment with continuous IV infusions of heparin. Outpatient treatment with LMWH streamlines care, reduces health care costs, and increases patient satisfaction.

Monitoring

In the majority of patients, LMWH does not require coagulation monitoring. If monitoring is necessary, anti–factor Xa levels must be measured because most LMWH preparations have little effect on the aPTT. Therapeutic anti–factor Xa levels with LMWH range from 0.5 to 1.2 units/mL when measured 3–4 h after drug administration. When LMWH is given in prophylactic doses, peak anti–factor Xa levels of 0.2–0.5 units/mL are desirable.

Indications for LMWH monitoring include renal insufficiency and obesity. LMWH monitoring in patients with a creatinine clearance of ≤50 mL/min is advisable to ensure that there is no drug accumulation. Although weight-adjusted LMWH dosing appears to produce therapeutic anti–factor Xa levels in patients who are overweight, this approach has not been extensively evaluated in those with morbid obesity. It may also be advisable to monitor the anticoagulant activity of LMWH during pregnancy because dose requirements can change, particularly in the third trimester. Monitoring should also be considered in high-risk settings, such as in patients with mechanical heart valves who are given LMWH for prevention of valve thrombosis, and when LMWH is used in treatment doses in infants or children.

Dosing

The doses of LMWH recommended for prophylaxis or treatment vary depending on the LMWH preparation. For prophylaxis, once-daily SC doses of 4000–5000 units are often used, whereas doses of 2500–3000 units are given when the drug is administered twice daily. For treatment of VTE, a dose of 150–200 units/kg is given if the drug is administered once daily. If a twice-daily regimen is employed, a dose of 100 units/kg is given. In patients with unstable angina, LMWH is given SC on a twice-daily basis at a dose of 100–120 units/kg.

Side effects

The major complication of LMWH is bleeding. Meta-analyses suggest that the risk of major bleeding is lower with LMWH than with unfractionated heparin. HIT and osteoporosis are less common with LMWH than with unfractionated heparin.

Bleeding

Like the situation with heparin, bleeding with LMWH is more common in patients receiving concomitant therapy with antiplatelet or fibrinolytic drugs. Recent surgery, trauma, or underlying hemostatic defects also increase the risk of bleeding with LMWH.

Although protamine sulfate can be used as an antidote for LMWH, protamine sulfate incompletely neutralizes the anticoagulant activity of LMWH because it only binds the longer chains of LMWH. Because longer chains are responsible for catalysis of thrombin inhibition by antithrombin, protamine sulfate completely reverses the anti–factor IIa activity of LMWH. In contrast, protamine sulfate only partially reverses the anti–factor Xa activity of LMWH because the shorter pentasaccharide-containing chains of LMWH do not bind to protamine sulfate. Consequently, patients at high risk for bleeding may be more safely treated with continuous IV unfractionated heparin than with SC LMWH.

Thrombocytopenia

The risk of HIT is about fivefold lower with LMWH than with heparin. LMWH binds less avidly to platelets and causes less PF4 release. Furthermore, with lower affinity for PF4 than heparin, LMWH is less likely to induce the conformational changes in PF4 that trigger the formation of HIT antibodies.

LMWH should not be used to treat HIT patients because most HIT antibodies exhibit cross-reactivity with LMWH. This in vitro cross-reactivity is not simply a laboratory phenomenon because there are case reports of thrombosis when HIT patients are treated with LMWH.

Osteoporosis

The risk of osteoporosis is lower with long-term LMWH than with heparin. For extended treatment, therefore, LMWH is a better choice than heparin because of the lower risk of osteoporosis and HIT.

Fondaparinux

A synthetic analogue of the antithrombin-binding pentasaccharide sequence, fondaparinux differs from LMWH in several ways (Table 23-6). Fondaparinux is licensed for thromboprophylaxis in general medical or surgical patients and in high-risk orthopedic patients and as an alternative to heparin or LMWH for initial treatment of patients with established VTE. The drug is not yet licensed in the United States as an alternative for heparin or LMWH in patients with acute coronary syndromes.

Mechanism of action

As a synthetic analogue of the antithrombin-binding pentasaccharide sequence found in heparin and LMWH, fondaparinux has a molecular weight of 1728. Fondaparinux binds only to antithrombin (Fig. 23-5) and is too short to bridge thrombin to antithrombin. Consequently, fondaparinux catalyzes factor Xa inhibition by antithrombin and does not enhance the rate of thrombin inhibition.

Pharmacology

Fondaparinux exhibits complete bioavailability after SC injection. With no binding to endothelial cells or plasma proteins, the clearance of fondaparinux is dose independent, and its plasma half-life is 17 h. The drug is given SC once daily. Because fondaparinux is cleared unchanged via the kidneys, it is contraindicated in patients with a creatinine clearance <30 mL/min and should be used with caution in those with a creatinine clearance <50 mL/min.

Fondaparinux produces a predictable anticoagulant response after administration in fixed doses because it does not bind to plasma proteins. The drug is given at a dose of 2.5 mg once daily for prevention of VTE. For initial treatment of established VTE, fondaparinux is given at a dose of 7.5 mg once daily. The dose can be reduced to 5 mg once daily for those weighing <50 kg and increased to 10 mg for those >100 kg. When given in these doses, fondaparinux is as effective as heparin or LMWH for initial treatment of patients with DVT or Pulmonary Embolism and produces similar rates of bleeding.

Fondaparinux is used at a dose of 2.5 mg once daily in patients with acute coronary syndromes. When this prophylactic dose of fondaparinux was compared with treatment doses of enoxaparin in patients with non–ST-segment elevation acute coronary syndromes, there was no difference in the rate of cardiovascular death, MI, or stroke at 9 days. However, the rate of major bleeding was 50% lower with fondaparinux than with enoxaparin, a difference that likely reflects the fact that the dose of fondaparinux was lower than that of enoxaparin. In acute coronary syndrome patients who require percutaneous coronary interventions, there is a risk of catheter thrombosis with fondaparinux unless adjunctive heparin is given.

TABLE 23-6

COMPARISON OF LOW-MOLECULAR-WEIGHT HEPARIN AND FONDAPARINUX

FEATURES	LMWH	FONDAPARINUX
Number of saccharide units	15–17	5
Catalysis of factor Xa inhibition	Yes	Yes
Catalysis of thrombin inhibition	Yes	No
Bioavailability after subcutaneous administration (%)	90	100
Plasma half-life (h)	4	17
Renal excretion	Yes	Yes
Induces release of TFPI	Yes	No
Neutralized by protamine sulfate	Partially	No

Abbreviation: LMWH, low-molecular-weight heparin; TFPI, tissue factor pathway inhibitor.

Side effects

Fondaparinux does not cause HIT because it does not bind to PF4. In contrast to LMWH, there is no cross-reactivity of fondaparinux with HIT antibodies. Consequently, fondaparinux appears to be effective for treatment of HIT patients, although large clinical trials supporting its use are lacking.

The major side effect of fondaparinux is bleeding. There is no antidote for fondaparinux. Protamine sulfate has no effect on the anticoagulant activity of fondaparinux because it fails to bind to the drug. Recombinant activated factor VII reverses the anticoagulant effects of fondaparinux in volunteers, but it is unknown whether this agent will control fondaparinux-induced bleeding.

Parenteral direct thrombin inhibitors

Heparin and LMWH are indirect inhibitors of thrombin because their activity is mediated by antithrombin. In contrast, direct thrombin inhibitors do not require a plasma cofactor; instead, these agents bind directly to thrombin and block its interaction with its substrates.

TABLE 23-7

COMPARISON OF THE PROPERTIES OF LEPIRUDIN, BIVALIRUDIN, AND ARGATROBAN

	LEPIRUDIN	BIVALIRUDIN	ARGATROBAN
Molecular mass	7000	1980	527
Site(s) of interaction with thrombin	Active site and exosite 1	Active site and exosite 1	Active site
Renal clearance	Yes	No	No
Hepatic metabolism	No	No	Yes
Plasma half-life (min)	60	25	45

Approved parenteral direct thrombin inhibitors include lepirudin, argatroban, and bivalirudin (Table 23-7). Lepirudin and argatroban are licensed for treatment of patients with HIT, whereas bivalirudin is approved as an alternative to heparin in patients undergoing percutaneous coronary interventions, including those with HIT.

Lepirudin

A recombinant form of hirudin, lepirudin is a bivalent direct thrombin inhibitor that interacts with both the active site and exosite 1, the substrate-binding site, on thrombin. For rapid anticoagulation, lepirudin is given by continuous IV infusion, but the drug can be given SC for thromboprophylaxis. Lepirudin has a plasma half-life of 60 min after IV infusion and is cleared by the kidneys. Consequently, lepirudin accumulates in patients with renal insufficiency. A high proportion of lepirudin-treated patients develop antibodies against the drug. Although these antibodies rarely cause problems, in a small subset of patients, they can delay lepirudin clearance and enhance its anticoagulant activity. Serious bleeding has been reported in some of these patients.

Lepirudin is usually monitored using the aPTT, and the dose is adjusted to maintain an aPTT that is 1.5–2.5 times the control. The aPTT is not an ideal test for monitoring lepirudin therapy because the clotting time plateaus with higher drug concentrations. Although the ecarin clotting time provides a better index of lepirudin dose than the aPTT, the ecarin clotting time has yet to be standardized.

Argatroban

A univalent inhibitor that targets the active site of thrombin, argatroban is metabolized in the liver. Consequently, this drug must be used with caution in patients with hepatic insufficiency. Argatroban is not cleared via the kidneys, so this drug is safer than lepirudin for HIT patients with renal insufficiency.

Argatroban is administered by continuous IV infusion and has a plasma half-life of ~45 min. The aPTT is used to monitor its anticoagulant effect, and the dose is adjusted to achieve an aPTT 1.5–3 times the baseline value, but not to exceed 100 s. Argatroban also prolongs the international normalized ratio (INR), a feature that can complicate the transitioning of patients to warfarin. This problem can be circumvented by using the levels of factor X to monitor warfarin in place of the INR. Alternatively, argatroban can be stopped for 2–3 h before INR determination.

Bivalirudin

A synthetic 20-amino-acid analogue of hirudin, bivalirudin is a divalent thrombin inhibitor. Thus, the N-terminal portion of bivalirudin interacts with the active site of thrombin, whereas its C-terminal tail binds to exosite 1, the substrate-binding domain on thrombin. Bivalirudin has a plasma half-life of 25 min, the shortest half-life of all the parenteral direct thrombin inhibitors. Bivalirudin is degraded by peptidases and is partially excreted via the kidneys. When given in high doses in the cardiac catheterization laboratory, the anticoagulant activity of bivalirudin is monitored using the activated clotting time. With lower doses, its activity can be assessed using the aPTT.

Studies comparing bivalirudin with heparin suggest that bivalirudin produces less bleeding. This feature plus its short half-life make bivalirudin an attractive alternative to heparin in patients undergoing percutaneous coronary interventions. Bivalirudin also has been used successfully in HIT patients who require percutaneous coronary interventions.

ORAL ANTICOAGULANTS

Current oral anticoagulant practice dates back almost 60 years to when the vitamin K antagonists were discovered as a result of investigations into the cause of hemorrhagic disease in cattle. Characterized by a decrease in prothrombin levels, this disorder is caused by ingestion of hay containing spoiled sweet clover. Hydroxycoumarin, which was isolated from bacterial contaminants in the hay, interferes with vitamin K metabolism, thereby causing a syndrome similar to vitamin K deficiency. Discovery of this compound provided the impetus for development of other vitamin K antagonists, including warfarin.

Warfarin

A water-soluble vitamin K antagonist initially developed as a rodenticide, warfarin is the coumarin derivative most often prescribed in North America. Like other vitamin K antagonists, warfarin interferes with the synthesis of the vitamin K–dependent clotting proteins, which include prothrombin (factor II) and factors VII, IX, and X. The synthesis of the vitamin K–dependent anticoagulant proteins, proteins C and S, is also reduced by vitamin K antagonists.

Mechanism of action

All of the vitamin K–dependent clotting factors possess glutamic acid residues at their N termini. A posttranslational modification adds a carboxyl group to the γ-carbon of these residues to generate γ-carboxyglutamic acid. This modification is essential for expression of the activity of these clotting factors because it permits their calcium-dependent binding to negatively charged phospholipid surfaces. The γ-carboxylation process is catalyzed by a vitamin K–dependent carboxylase. Thus, vitamin K from the diet is reduced to vitamin K hydroquinone by vitamin K reductase (Fig. 23-6). Vitamin K hydroquinone serves as a cofactor for the carboxylase enzyme, which in the presence of carbon dioxide replaces the hydrogen on the γ-carbon of glutamic acid residues with a carboxyl group. During this process, vitamin K hydroquinone is oxidized to vitamin K epoxide, which is then reduced to vitamin K by vitamin K epoxide reductase.

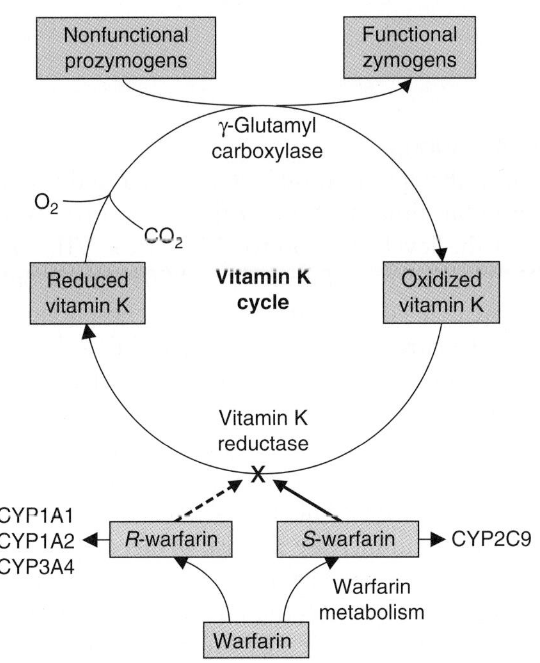

FIGURE 23-6

Mechanism of action of warfarin. A racemic mixture of *S*- and *R*-enantiomers, *S*-warfarin is most active. By blocking vitamin K epoxide reductase, warfarin inhibits the conversion of oxidized vitamin K into its reduced form. This inhibits vitamin K–dependent γ-carboxylation of factors II, VII, IX, and X because reduced vitamin K serves as a cofactor for a γ-glutamyl carboxylase that catalyzes the γ-carboxylation process, thereby converting prozymogens to zymogens capable of binding calcium and interacting with anionic phospholipid surfaces. S-warfarin is metabolized by *CYP2C9*. Common genetic polymorphisms in this enzyme can influence warfarin metabolism. Polymorphisms in the C1 subunit of vitamin K reductase (VKORC1) also can affect the susceptibility of the enzyme to warfarin-induced inhibition, thereby influencing warfarin dosage requirements.

Warfarin inhibits vitamin K epoxide reductase (VKOR), thereby blocking the γ-carboxylation process. This results in the synthesis of vitamin K–dependent clotting proteins that are only partially γ-carboxylated. Warfarin acts as an anticoagulant because these partially γ-carboxylated proteins have reduced or absent biologic activity. The onset of action of warfarin is delayed until the newly synthesized clotting factors with reduced activity gradually replace their fully active counterparts.

The antithrombotic effect of warfarin depends on a reduction in the functional levels of factor X and prothrombin, clotting factors that have half-lives of 24 and 72 h, respectively. Because of the delay in achieving an antithrombotic effect, initial treatment with warfarin is supported by concomitant administration of a rapidly acting parenteral anticoagulant, such as heparin, LMWH, or fondaparinux, in patients with established thrombosis or at high risk for thrombosis.

Pharmacology

Warfarin is a racemic mixture of *R* and *S* isomers. Warfarin is rapidly and almost completely absorbed from the gastrointestinal tract. Levels of warfarin in the blood peak about 90 min after drug administration. Racemic warfarin has a plasma half-life of 36–42 h, and more than 97% of circulating warfarin is bound to albumin. Only the small fraction of unbound warfarin is biologically active.

Warfarin accumulates in the liver, where the two isomers are metabolized via distinct pathways. *CYP2C9* mediates oxidative metabolism of the more active *S* isomer (Fig. 23-6). Two relatively common variants, *CYP2C9*2* and *CYP2C9*3*, encode an enzyme with reduced activity. Patients with these variants require lower maintenance doses of warfarin. Approximately 25% of whites have at least one variant allele of *CYP2C9*2* or *CYP2C9*3*, whereas those variant alleles are less common in African Americans and Asians (Table 23-8). Heterozygosity for *CYP2C9*2* or *CYP2C9*3* decreases the warfarin dose requirement by 20–30% relative to that required in subjects with the wild-type *CYP2C9*1/*1* alleles, whereas homozygosity for the *CYP2C9*2* or *CYP2C9*3* alleles reduces the warfarin dose requirement by 50–70%.

Consistent with their decreased warfarin dose requirement, subjects with at least one *CYP2C9* variant allele are at increased risk for bleeding. Compared with individuals with no variant alleles, the relative risks for warfarin-associated bleeding in *CYP2C9*2* or *CYP2C9*3* carriers are 1.91 and 1.77, respectively.

TABLE 23-8

FREQUENCIES OF *CYP2C9* GENOTYPES AND *VKORC1* HAPLOTYPES IN DIFFERENT POPULATIONS AND THEIR EFFECT ON WARFARIN DOSE REQUIREMENTS

	FREQUENCY, %			
GENOTYPE/HAPLOPTYE	WHITES	AFRICAN AMERICANS (A/A)	ASIANS (A)	DOSE REDUCTION COMPARED WITH WILD-TYPE
CYP2C9				
*1/*1	70	90	95	–
*1/*2	17	2	0	22
*1/*3	9	3	4	34
*2/*2	2	0	0	43
*2/*3	1	0	0	53
*3/*3	0	0	1	76
VKORC1				
Non-A/non-A	37	82	7	–
Non-A/A	45	12	30	26
A/A	18	6	63	50

Polymorphisms in *VKORC1* also can influence the anticoagulant response to warfarin. Several genetic variations of *VKORC1* are in strong linkage disequilibrium and have been designated as non-A haplotypes. *VKORC1* variants are more prevalent than variants of *CYP2C9*. Asians have the highest prevalence of *VKORC1* variants followed by whites and African Americans (Table 23-8). Polymorphisms in *VKORC1* likely explain 30% of the variability in warfarin dose requirements. Compared with *VKORC1* non-A/non-A homozygotes, the warfarin dose requirement decreases by 25 and 50% in A halotype heterozygotes and homozygotes, respectively. These findings prompted the Food and Drug Administration to amend the prescribing information for warfarin to indicate that lower initiation doses should be considered for patients with *CYP2C9* and *VKORC1* genetic variants. In addition to genotype data, other pertinent patient information has been incorporated into warfarin dosing algorithms. Although such algorithms help predict suitable warfarin doses, it remains unclear whether better dose identification improves patient outcome in terms of reducing hemorrhagic complications or recurrent thrombotic events.

In addition to genetic factors, the anticoagulant effect of warfarin is influenced by diet, drugs, and various disease states. Fluctuations in dietary vitamin K intake affect the activity of warfarin. A wide variety of drugs can alter absorption, clearance, or metabolism of warfarin. Because of the variability in the anticoagulant response to warfarin, coagulation monitoring is essential to ensure that a therapeutic response is obtained.

Monitoring

Warfarin therapy is most often monitored using the prothrombin time (PT), a test that is sensitive to reductions in the levels of prothrombin, factor VII, and factor X. The test is performed by adding thromboplastin, a reagent that contains tissue factor, phospholipid, and calcium, to citrated plasma and determining the time to clot formation. Thromboplastins vary in their sensitivity to reductions in the levels of the vitamin K–dependent clotting factors. Thus, less sensitive thromboplastins will trigger the administration of higher doses of warfarin to achieve a target PT. This is problematic because higher doses of warfarin increase the risk of bleeding.

The INR was developed to circumvent many of the problems associated with the PT. To calculate the INR, the patient's PT is divided by the mean normal PT, and this ratio is then multiplied by the international sensitivity index (ISI), an index of the sensitivity of the thromboplastin used for PT determination to reductions in the levels of the vitamin K–dependent clotting factors. Highly sensitive thromboplastins have an ISI of 1.0. Most current thromboplastins have ISI values that range from 1.0 to 1.4.

Although the INR has helped to standardize anticoagulant practice, problems persist. The precision of INR determination varies depending on reagent–coagulometer combinations. This leads to variability in the INR results. Also complicating INR determination is unreliable reporting of the ISI by thromboplastin manufacturers. Furthermore, every laboratory must establish the mean normal PT with each new batch of thromboplastin reagent. To accomplish this, the PT must be measured in fresh plasma samples from at least 20 healthy volunteers using the same coagulometer that is used for patient samples.

For most indications, warfarin is administered in doses that produce a target INR of 2.0–3.0. An exception is patients with mechanical heart valves, in whom a target INR of 2.5–3.5 is recommended. Studies in atrial fibrillation demonstrate an increased risk of cardioembolic stroke when the INR falls to <1.7 and an increase in bleeding with INR values >4.5. These findings highlight the fact that vitamin K antagonists have a narrow therapeutic window. In support of this concept, a study in patients receiving long-term warfarin therapy for unprovoked VTE demonstrated a higher rate of recurrent VTE with a target INR of 1.5–1.9 compared with a target INR of 2.0–3.0.

Dosing

Warfarin is usually started at a dose of 5–10 mg. Lower doses are used for patients with *CYP2C9* or *VKORC1* polymorphisms, which affect the pharmacodynamics or pharmacokinetics of warfarin and render patients more sensitive to the drug. The dose is then titrated to achieve the desired target INR. Because of its delayed onset of action, patients with established thrombosis or those at high risk for thrombosis are given concomitant treatment with a rapidly acting parenteral anticoagulant, such as heparin, LMWH, or fondaparinux. Initial prolongation of the INR reflects reduction in the functional levels of factor VII. Consequently, concomitant treatment with the parenteral anticoagulant should be continued until the INR has been therapeutic for at least 2 consecutive days. A minimum 5-day course of parenteral anticoagulation is recommended to ensure that the levels of prothrombin have been reduced into the therapeutic range with warfarin.

Because warfarin has a narrow therapeutic window, frequent coagulation monitoring is essential to ensure that a therapeutic anticoagulant response is obtained. Even patients with stable warfarin dose requirements should have their INR determined every 2–3 weeks. More frequent monitoring is necessary when new medications are introduced because so many drugs enhance or reduce the anticoagulant effects of warfarin.

Side effects

Like all anticoagulants, the major side effect of warfarin is bleeding. A rare complication is skin necrosis. Warfarin crosses the placenta and can cause fetal abnormalities. Consequently, warfarin should not be used during pregnancy.

Bleeding

At least half of the bleeding complications with warfarin occur when the INR exceeds the therapeutic range. Bleeding complications may be mild, such as epistaxis or hematuria, or more severe, such as retroperitoneal or gastrointestinal bleeding. Life-threatening intracranial bleeding can also occur.

To minimize the risk of bleeding, the INR should be maintained in the therapeutic range. In asymptomatic patients whose INR is between 3.5 and 4.5, warfarin should be withheld until the INR returns to the therapeutic range. If the INR is >4.5, a therapeutic INR can be achieved more rapidly by administration of low doses of sublingual vitamin K. A vitamin K dose of 1 mg is usually adequate for patients with an INR between 4.9 and 9, whereas 2–3 mg can be used for those with an INR >9. Higher doses of vitamin K can be administered if more rapid reversal of the INR is required or if the INR is excessively high. Although vitamin K administration results in a more rapid reduction in the INR compared with simply holding the warfarin, there is no evidence that vitamin K administration reduces the risk of hemorrhage.

Patients with serious bleeding need more aggressive treatment. These patients should be given 10 mg of vitamin K by slow IV infusion. Additional vitamin K should be given until the INR is in the normal range. Treatment with vitamin K should be supplemented with fresh-frozen plasma as a source of the vitamin K–dependent clotting proteins. For life-threatening bleeds or if patients cannot tolerate the volume load, prothrombin complex concentrates can be used.

Warfarin-treated patients who experience bleeding when their INR is in the therapeutic range require investigation into the cause of the bleeding. Those with gastrointestinal bleeding often have underlying peptic ulcer disease or a tumor. Similarly, investigation of hematuria or uterine bleeding in patients with a therapeutic INR may unmask a tumor of the genitourinary tract.

Skin necrosis

A rare complication of warfarin, skin necrosis usually is seen 2–5 days after initiation of therapy. Well-demarcated erythematous lesions form on the thighs, buttocks, breasts, or toes. Typically, the center of each lesion becomes progressively necrotic. Examination of skin biopsies taken from the border of these lesions reveals thrombi in the microvasculature.

Warfarin-induced skin necrosis is seen in patients with congenital or acquired deficiencies of protein C or protein S. Initiation of warfarin therapy in these patients produces a precipitous fall in plasma levels of proteins C or S, thereby eliminating this important anticoagulant pathway before warfarin exerts an antithrombotic effect through lowering of the functional levels of factor X and prothrombin. The resultant procoagulant state triggers thrombosis. Why the thrombosis is localized to the microvasculature of fatty tissues is unclear.

Treatment involves discontinuation of warfarin and reversal with vitamin K, if needed. An alternative anticoagulant, such as heparin or LMWH, should be given in patients with thrombosis. Protein C concentrates or recombinant activated protein C can be given to protein C–deficient patients to accelerate healing of the skin lesions; fresh-frozen plasma may be of value for those with protein S deficiency. Occasionally, skin grafting is necessary when there is extensive skin loss.

Because of the potential for skin necrosis, patients with known protein C or protein S deficiency require overlapping treatment with a parenteral anticoagulant when initiating warfarin therapy. Warfarin should be started in low doses in these patients, and the parenteral anticoagulant should be continued until the INR is therapeutic for at least 2–3 consecutive days.

Pregnancy

Warfarin crosses the placenta and can cause fetal abnormalities or bleeding. The fetal abnormalities include a characteristic embryopathy, which consists of nasal hypoplasia and stippled epiphyses. The risk of embryopathy is highest if warfarin is given in the first trimester of pregnancy. Central nervous system abnormalities can also occur with exposure to warfarin at any time during pregnancy. Finally, maternal administration of warfarin produces an anticoagulant effect in the fetus that can cause bleeding. This is of particular concern at delivery when trauma to the head during passage through the birth canal can lead to intracranial bleeding. Because of these potential problems, warfarin is contraindicated in pregnancy, particularly in the first and third trimesters. Instead, heparin, LMWH, or fondaparinux can be given during pregnancy for prevention or treatment of thrombosis.

Warfarin does not pass into the breast milk. Consequently, warfarin can safely be given to nursing mothers.

Special problems

Patients with a lupus anticoagulant or those who need urgent or elective surgery present special challenges. Although observational studies suggested that patients with thrombosis complicating the antiphospholipid antibody syndrome required higher intensity warfarin regimens to prevent recurrent thromboembolic events, two randomized trials showed that targeting an INR of 2.0–3.0 is as effective as higher intensity treatment and produces less bleeding. Monitoring warfarin therapy can be problematic in patients with antiphospholipid antibody syndrome if the lupus anticoagulant prolongs the baseline INR.

If patients receiving long-term warfarin treatment require an elective invasive procedure, warfarin can be stopped 5 days before the procedure to allow the INR to return to normal levels. Those at high risk for recurrent thrombosis can be bridged with once- or twice-daily SC injections of LMWH when the INR falls to <2.0. The last dose of LMWH should be given 12–24 h before the procedure, depending on whether LMWH is administered twice or once daily. After the procedure, treatment with warfarin can be restarted.

New oral anticoagulants

New oral anticoagulants that target thrombin or factor Xa are under development. These drugs have rapid onsets of action and half-lives that permit once- or twice-daily administration. Designed to produce a predictable level of anticoagulation, these new oral agents are given in fixed doses without routine coagulation monitoring. Therefore, these drugs are more convenient to administer than warfarin.

Dabigatran etexilate, an oral thrombin inhibitor, and rivaroxaban, an oral factor Xa inhibitor, are licensed in Europe and Canada for short-term thromboprophylaxis after elective hip or knee replacement surgery. Phase III trials with apixaban, another oral factor Xa inhibitor, also have been completed in patients undergoing major orthopedic surgery (Table 23-9).

The Randomized Evaluation of Long-Term Anticoagulation Therapy (RE-LY) trial shows the promise of these new agents for long-term indications. This trial compared two different dose regimens of dabigatran etexilate (110 mg or 150 mg twice daily) with warfarin (dose-adjusted to achieve an INR between 2 and 3) for stroke prevention in 18,113 patients with nonvalvular atrial fibrillation. The annual rates of the primary efficacy outcome, stroke or systemic embolism, were 1.7% with warfarin, 1.5% with the lower dose dabigatran regimen, and 1.1% with the higher dose regimen. Thus, the lower dose dabigatran regimen was noninferior to

TABLE 23-9

COMPARISON OF THE FEATURES OF NEW ORAL ANTICOAGULANTS IN ADVANCED STAGES OF DEVELOPMENT

FEATURES	RIVAROXABAN	APIXABAN	DABIGATRAN ETEXILATE
Target	Xa	Xa	IIa
Molecular weight	436	460	628
Prodrug	No	No	Yes
Bioavailability (%)	80	50	6
Time to peak (h)	3	3	2
Half-life (h)	9	9–14	12–17
Renal excretion (%)	65	25	80
Antidote	None	None	None

warfarin, while the higher dose regimen was superior. Annual rates of major bleeding were 3.4% with warfarin compared with 2.7% and 3.1% with the lower and higher dose dabigatran regimens, respectively. Thus, the lower dose dabigatran regimen was associated with significantly less major bleeding than warfarin, while the rate of major bleeding with the higher dose regimen was not significantly different from that with warfarin. Rates of intracerebral bleeding were significantly lower with both doses of dabigatran than with warfarin, as were rates of life-threatening bleeding. There was no evidence of hepatotoxicity with dabigatran.

Based on the results of the RE-LY trial, dabigatran etexilate has been licensed in the United States and Canada for stroke prevention in patients with atrial fibrillation. The 150 mg twice-daily dose of dabigatran is recommended for most patients. In the United States, a 75 mg twice-daily dose is recommended for patients with a creatinine clearance of 30 to 50 mL/min, while in Canada, the 110 mg twice-daily dose is recommended for those older than the age of 80 years and for patients at high risk of bleeding. The drug is contraindicated in patients with a creatinine clearance less than 15 mL/min.

Dabigatran etexilate also was compared with warfarin in 2539 patients with acute VTE. Patients were initially treated with heparin or LMWH and then randomized to a 6-month course of dabigatran (150 mg twice daily) or warfarin, which was dose-adjusted to achieve an INR of 2–3. The primary endpoint, a composite of recurrent VTE or fatal Pulmonary Embolism, occurred in 2.4% of patients given dabigatran and in 2.1% of those treated with warfarin. Major bleeding occurred in 1.6 and 1.9% of patients given dabigatran and warfarin, respectively. Based on the results of this trial, unmonitored fixed-dose dabigatran appears to be noninferior to warfarin for treatment of patients with VTE. Taken together with the results of the RE-LY trial, these findings suggest that the new oral anticoagulants will gradually replace warfarin.

FIBRINOLYTIC DRUGS

ROLE OF FIBRINOLYTIC THERAPY

Fibrinolytic drugs can be used to degrade thrombi and are administered systemically or can be delivered via catheters directly into the substance of the thrombus. Systemic delivery is used for treatment of acute MI, acute ischemic stroke, and most cases of massive Pulmonary Embolism. The goal of therapy is to produce rapid thrombus dissolution, thereby restoring antegrade blood flow. In the coronary circulation, restoration of blood flow reduces morbidity and mortality rates by limiting myocardial damage, whereas in the cerebral circulation, rapid thrombus dissolution decreases the neuronal death and brain infarction that produce irreversible brain injury. For patients with massive Pulmonary Embolism, the goal of thrombolytic therapy is to restore pulmonary artery perfusion.

Peripheral arterial thrombi and thrombi in the proximal deep veins of the leg are most often treated using catheter-directed thrombolytic therapy. Catheters with multiple side holes can be utilized to enhance drug delivery. In some cases, intravascular devices that fragment and extract the thrombus are used to hasten treatment. These devices can be used alone or in conjunction with fibrinolytic drugs.

MECHANISM OF ACTION

Currently approved fibrinolytic agents include streptokinase; acylated plasminogen streptokinase activator complex (anistreplase); urokinase; recombinant tissue-type plasminogen activator (rtPA), which is also known as alteplase or activase; and two recombinant derivatives of rtPA, tenecteplase and reteplase. All of these agents act by converting the proenzyme, plasminogen, to plasmin, the active enzyme (Fig. 23-7). Plasmin then degrades the fibrin matrix of thrombi and produces soluble fibrin degradation products.

Endogenous fibrinolysis is regulated at two levels. Plasminogen activator inhibitors, particularly the type 1 form (PAI-1), prevent excessive plasminogen activation by regulating the activity of tPA and urokinase-type plasminogen activator. Once plasmin is generated, it is regulated by plasmin inhibitors, the most important of which is α_2-antiplasmin. The plasma concentration of plasminogen is twofold higher than that of α_2-antiplasmin. Consequently, with pharmacologic doses of plasminogen activators, the concentration of plasmin that is generated can exceed that of α_2-antiplasmin. In addition to degrading fibrin, unregulated plasmin can also degrade fibrinogen and other clotting factors.

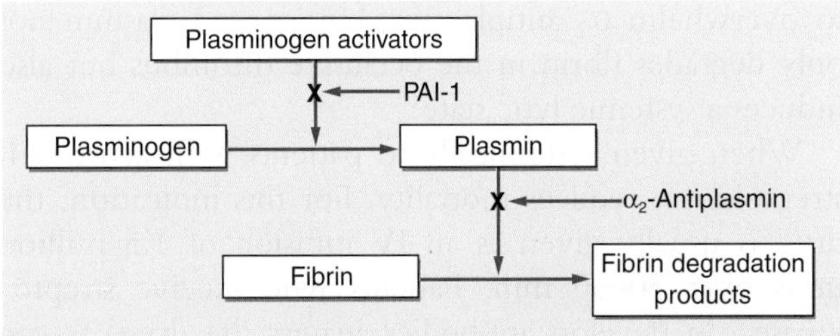

FIGURE 23-7

The fibrinolytic system and its regulation. Plasminogen activators convert plasminogen to plasmin. Plasmin then degrades fibrin into soluble fibrin degradation products. The system is regulated at two levels. Type 1 plasminogen activator inhibitor (PAI-1) regulates the plasminogen activators, whereas α_2-antiplasmin serves as the major inhibitor of plasmin.

This process, which is known as the *systemic lytic state*, reduces the hemostatic potential of the blood and increases the risk of bleeding.

The endogenous fibrinolytic system is geared to localize plasmin generation to the fibrin surface. Both plasminogen and tPA bind to fibrin to form a ternary complex that promotes efficient plasminogen activation. In contrast to free plasmin, plasmin generated on the fibrin surface is relatively protected from inactivation by α_2-antiplasmin, a feature that promotes fibrin dissolution. Furthermore, C-terminal lysine residues, exposed as plasmin degrades fibrin, serve as binding sites for additional plasminogen and tPA molecules. This creates a positive feedback that enhances plasmin generation. When used pharmacologically, the various plasminogen activators capitalize on these mechanisms to a lesser or greater extent.

Plasminogen activators that preferentially activate fibrin-bound plasminogen are considered fibrin-specific. In contrast, nonspecific plasminogen activators do not discriminate between fibrin-bound and circulating plasminogen. Activation of circulating plasminogen results in the generation of unopposed plasmin that can trigger the systemic lytic state. Alteplase and its derivatives are fibrin-specific plasminogen activators, whereas streptokinase, anistreplase, and urokinase are nonspecific agents.

STREPTOKINASE

Unlike other plasminogen activators, streptokinase is not an enzyme and does not directly convert plasminogen to plasmin. Instead, streptokinase forms a 1:1 stoichiometric complex with plasminogen. Formation of this complex induces a conformational change in plasminogen that exposes its active site (Fig. 23-8). This conformationally altered plasminogen then converts additional plasminogen molecules to plasmin.

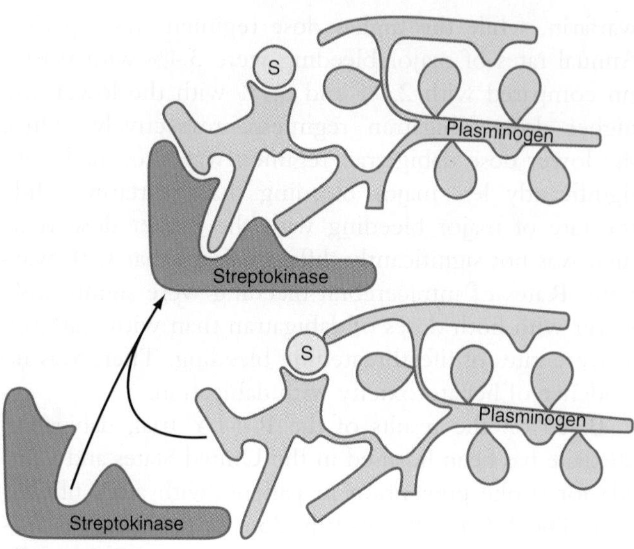

FIGURE 23-8
Mechanism of action of streptokinase. Streptokinase binds to plasminogen and induces a conformational change in plasminogen that exposes its active site (S). The streptokinase–plasmin(ogen) complex then serves as the activator of additional plasminogen molecules.

Streptokinase has no affinity for fibrin, and the streptokinase–plasminogen complex activates both free and fibrin-bound plasminogen. Activation of circulating plasminogen generates sufficient amounts of plasmin to overwhelm α_2-antiplasmin. Unopposed plasmin not only degrades fibrin in the occlusive thrombus but also induces a systemic lytic state.

When given systemically to patients with acute MI, streptokinase reduces mortality. For this indication, the drug is usually given as an IV infusion of 1.5 million units over 30–60 min. Patients who receive streptokinase can develop antibodies against the drug, as can patients with prior streptococcal injection. These antibodies can reduce the effectiveness of streptokinase.

Allergic reactions occur in ~5% of patients treated with streptokinase. These may manifest as a rash, fever, chills, and rigors. Although anaphylactic reactions can occur, these are rare. Transient hypotension is common with streptokinase and has been attributed to plasmin-mediated release of bradykinin from kininogen. The hypotension usually responds to leg elevation and administration of IV fluids and low doses of vasopressors, such as dopamine or norepinephrine.

ANISTREPLASE

To generate this drug, streptokinase is combined with equimolar amounts of Lys-plasminogen, a plasmin-cleaved form of plasminogen with a Lys residue at its N terminus. The active site of Lys-plasminogen that is exposed upon combination with streptokinase is then masked with an anisoyl group. After IV infusion, the anisoyl group is slowly removed by deacylation, giving the complex a half-life of ~100 min. This allows drug administration via a single bolus infusion.

Although it is more convenient to administer, anistreplase offers few mechanistic advantages over streptokinase. Like streptokinase, anistreplase does not distinguish between fibrin-bound and circulating plasminogen. Consequently, it too produces a systemic lytic state. Likewise, allergic reactions and hypotension are just as frequent with anistreplase as they are with streptokinase.

When anistreplase was compared with alteplase in patients with acute MI, reperfusion was obtained more rapidly with alteplase than with anistreplase. Improved reperfusion was associated with a trend toward better clinical outcomes and reduced mortality rate with alteplase. These results and the high cost of anistreplase have dampened the enthusiasm for its use.

UROKINASE

Urokinase is a two-chain serine protease derived from cultured fetal kidney cells with a molecular weight of 34,000. Urokinase converts plasminogen to plasmin directly by cleaving the Arg560-Val561 bond. Unlike streptokinase, urokinase is not immunogenic, and allergic reactions are rare. Urokinase produces a systemic lytic state because it does not discriminate between fibrin-bound and circulating plasminogen.

Despite many years of use, urokinase has never been systemically evaluated for coronary thrombolysis. Instead, urokinase is often employed for catheter-directed lysis of thrombi in the deep veins or the peripheral arteries. Because of production problems, the availability of urokinase is limited.

ALTEPLASE

A recombinant form of single-chain tPA, alteplase has a molecular weight of 68,000. Alteplase is rapidly converted into its two-chain form by plasmin. Although single- and two-chain forms of tPA have equivalent activity in the presence of fibrin, in its absence, single-chain tPA has tenfold lower activity.

Alteplase consists of five discrete domains (Fig. 23-9); the N-terminal A chain of two-chain alteplase contains four of these domains. Residues 4 through 50 make up the finger domain, a region that resembles the finger domain of fibronectin; residues 50 through 87 are homologous with epidermal growth factor, whereas residues 92 through 173 and 180 through 261, which have homology to the kringle domains of plasminogen, are designated as the first and second kringle, respectively. The fifth alteplase domain is the protease domain; it is located on the C-terminal B chain of two-chain alteplase.

The interaction of alteplase with fibrin is mediated by the finger domain and, to a lesser extent, by the second kringle domain. The affinity of alteplase for fibrin is considerably higher than that for fibrinogen. Consequently, the catalytic efficiency of plasminogen activation by alteplase is two to three orders of magnitude higher in the presence of fibrin than in the presence of fibrinogen. This phenomenon helps to localize plasmin generation to the fibrin surface.

Although alteplase preferentially activates plasminogen in the presence of fibrin, alteplase is not as fibrin-selective as was first predicted. Its fibrin specificity is limited because, similar to fibrin, (DD)E, the major soluble degradation product of cross-linked fibrin, binds alteplase and plasminogen with high affinity. Consequently, (DD)E is as potent as fibrin as a stimulator of

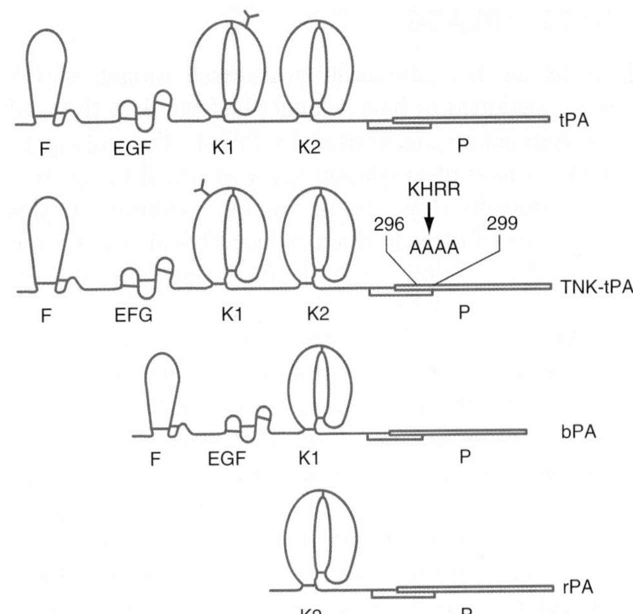

FIGURE 23-9
Domain structures of alteplase (tPA), tenecteplase (TNK-tPA), desmoteplase (bPA), and reteplase (rPA). The finger (F), epidermal growth factor (EGF), first and second kringles (K1 and K2, respectively), and protease (P) domains are illustrated. The glycosylation site (Y) on K1 has been repositioned in tenecteplase to endow it with a longer half-life. In addition, a tetra-alanine substitution in the protease domain renders tenecteplase resistant to type 1 plasminogen activator inhibitor (PAI-1) inhibition. Desmoteplase differs from alteplase and tenecteplase in that it lacks a K2 domain. Reteplase is a truncated variant that lacks the F, EGF, and K1 domains.

plasminogen activation by alteplase. Whereas plasmin generated on the fibrin surface results in thrombolysis, plasmin generated on the surface of circulating (DD)E degrades fibrinogen. Fibrinogenolysis results in the accumulation of fragment X, a high-molecular-weight clottable fibrinogen degradation product. Incorporation of fragment X into hemostatic plugs formed at sites of vascular injury renders them susceptible to lysis. This phenomenon may contribute to alteplase-induced bleeding.

A trial comparing alteplase with streptokinase for treatment of patients with acute MI demonstrated a significantly lower mortality rate with alteplase than with streptokinase, although the absolute difference was small. The greatest benefit was seen in patients age <75 years with anterior MI who presented <6 h after symptom onset.

For treatment of acute MI or acute ischemic stroke, alteplase is given as an IV infusion over 60–90 min. The total dose of alteplase usually ranges from 90 to 100 mg. Allergic reactions and hypotension are rare, and alteplase is not immunogenic.

TENECTEPLASE

Tenecteplase is a genetically engineered variant of tPA and was designed to have a longer half-life than tPA and to be resistant to inactivation by PAI-1. To prolong its half-life, a new glycosylation site was added to the first kringle domain (Fig. 23-9). Because addition of this extra carbohydrate side chain reduced fibrin affinity, the existing glycosylation site on the first kringle domain was removed. To render the molecule resistant to inhibition by PAI-1, a tetra-alanine substitution was introduced at residues 296–299 in the protease domain, the region responsible for the interaction of tPA with PAI-1.

Tenecteplase is more fibrin-specific than tPA. Although both agents bind to fibrin with similar affinity, the affinity of tenecteplase for (DD)E is significantly lower than that of tPA. Consequently, (DD)E does not stimulate systemic plasminogen activation by tenecteplase to the same extent as tPA. As a result, tenecteplase produces less fibrinogenolysis than tPA.

For coronary thrombolysis, tenecteplase is given as a single IV bolus. In a large phase III trial that enrolled >16,000 patients, the 30-day mortality rate with single-bolus tenecteplase was similar to that with accelerated-dose tPA. Although rates of intracranial hemorrhage were also similar with both treatments, patients given tenecteplase had fewer noncerebral bleeds and a reduced need for blood transfusions than those treated with tPA. The improved safety profile of tenecteplase likely reflects its enhanced fibrin specificity.

RETEPLASE

Reteplase is a recombinant tPA derivative and is a single-chain variant that lacks the finger, epidermal growth factor, and first kringle domains (Fig. 23-9). This truncated derivative has a molecular weight of 39,000. Reteplase binds fibrin more weakly than tPA because it lacks the finger domain. Because it is produced in *Escherichia coli*, reteplase is not glycosylated. This endows it with a plasma half-life longer than that of tPA. Consequently, reteplase is given as two IV boluses, which are separated by 30 min. Clinical trials have demonstrated that reteplase is at least as effective as streptokinase for treatment of acute MI, but the agent is not superior to tPA.

NEW FIBRINOLYTIC AGENTS

Several new drugs are under investigation. These include desmoteplase (Fig. 23-9), a recombinant form of the full-length plasminogen activator isolated from the saliva of the vampire bat, and alfimeprase, a truncated form of fibrolase, an enzyme isolated from the venom of the southern copperhead snake. Clinical studies with these agents have been disappointing. Desmoteplase, which is more fibrin-specific than tPA, was investigated for treatment of acute ischemic stroke. Patients presenting 3–9 h after symptom onset were randomized to one of two doses of desmoteplase or to placebo. Overall response rates were low and no different with desmoteplase than with placebo. The mortality rate was higher in the desmoteplase arms.

Alfimeprase is a metalloproteinase that degrades fibrin and fibrinogen in a plasmin-independent fashion. In the circulation, alfimeprase is inhibited by α_2-macroglobulin. Consequently, the drug must be delivered via a catheter directly into the thrombus. Studies of alfimeprase for treatment of peripheral arterial occlusion or for restoration of flow in blocked central venous catheters were stopped due to lack of efficacy. The disappointing results with desmoteplase and alfimeprase highlight the challenges of introducing new fibrinolytic drugs.

CONCLUSIONS AND FUTURE DIRECTIONS

Arterial and venous thromboses reflect a complex interplay among the vessel wall, platelets, the coagulation system, and the fibrinolytic pathways. Activation of coagulation also triggers inflammatory pathways that may contribute to thrombogenesis. A better understanding of the biochemistry of blood coagulation and advances in structure-based drug design have identified new targets and resulted in the development of novel antithrombotic drugs. Well-designed clinical trials have provided detailed information on which drugs to use and when to use them. Despite these advances, however, thromboembolic disorders remain a major cause of morbidity and mortality rates. Therefore, the search for better targets and more potent antiplatelet, anticoagulant, and fibrinolytic drugs continues.

SECTION VII

BIOLOGY OF CANCER

CHAPTER 24

CANCER GENETICS

Pat J. Morin ■ Jeffrey M. Trent ■ Francis S. Collins ■ Bert Vogelstein

CANCER IS A GENETIC DISEASE

Cancer arises through a series of somatic alterations in DNA that result in unrestrained cellular proliferation. Most of these alterations involve actual sequence changes in DNA (i.e., mutations). They may originate as a consequence of random replication errors, exposure to carcinogens (e.g., radiation), or faulty DNA repair processes. While most cancers arise sporadically, familial clustering of cancers occurs in certain families that carry a germline mutation in a cancer gene.

HISTORICAL PERSPECTIVE

The idea that cancer progression is driven by sequential somatic mutations in specific genes has only gained general acceptance in the past 25 years. Before the advent of the microscope, cancer was believed to be composed of aggregates of mucus or other noncellular matter. By the middle of the nineteenth century, it became clear that tumors were masses of cells and that these cells arose from the normal cells of the tissue from which the cancer originated. However, the molecular basis for the uncontrolled proliferation of cancer cells was to remain a mystery for another century. During that time, a number of theories for the origin of cancer were postulated. The great biochemist Otto Warburg proposed the combustion theory of cancer, which stipulated that cancer was due to abnormal oxygen metabolism. In addition, some believed that all cancers were caused by viruses and that cancer was in fact a contagious disease.

In the end, observations of cancer occurring in chimney sweeps, studies of x-rays, and the overwhelming data demonstrating cigarette smoke as a causative agent in lung cancer, together with Ames's work on chemical mutagenesis, provided convincing evidence that cancer originated through changes in DNA. Although the viral theory of cancer did not prove to be generally accurate (with the exception of human papillomaviruses, which can cause cervical cancer in human), the study of retroviruses led to the discovery of the first human *oncogenes* in the late 1970s. Soon after, the study of families with genetic predisposition to cancer was instrumental in the discovery of *tumor-suppressor genes*. The field that studies the type of mutations, as well as the consequence of these mutations in tumor cells, is now known as *cancer genetics*.

THE CLONAL ORIGIN AND MULTISTEP NATURE OF CANCER

Nearly all cancers originate from a single cell; this clonal origin is a critical discriminating feature between neoplasia and hyperplasia. Multiple cumulative mutational events are invariably required for the progression of a tumor from normal to fully malignant phenotype. The process can be seen as Darwinian microevolution in which, at each successive step, the mutated cells gain a growth advantage, resulting in an increased representation relative to their neighbors (Fig. 24-1). Based on observations of cancer frequency increases during aging, as well as recent molecular genetics work, it is believed that 5 to 10 accumulated mutations are necessary for a cell to progress from the normal to the fully malignant phenotype.

We are beginning to understand the precise nature of the genetic alterations responsible for some malignancies and to get a sense of the order in which they occur. The best studied example is colon cancer, in which analyses of DNA from tissues extending from normal colon epithelium through adenoma to carcinoma have identified some of the genes mutated in the process (Fig. 24-2). Other malignancies are believed to progress in a similar step-wise fashion, although the order and identity of genes affected may be different.

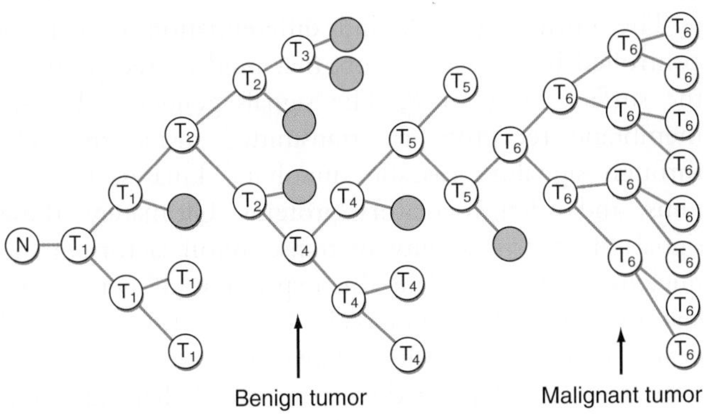

FIGURE 24-1
Multistep clonal development of malignancy. In this diagram, a series of five cumulative mutations (T1, T2, T4, T5, T6), each with a modest growth advantage acting alone, eventually results in a malignant tumor. Note that not all such alterations result in progression; for example, the T3 clone is a dead end. The actual number of cumulative mutations necessary to transform from the normal to the malignant state is unknown in most tumors. *(After P Nowell: The clonal evolution of tumor cell populations. Science 194:23, 1976, with permission.)*

TWO TYPES OF CANCER GENES: ONCOGENES AND TUMOR-SUPPRESSOR GENES

There are two major types of cancer genes. The first type comprises genes that positively influence tumor formation and are known as *oncogenes*. The second type of cancer genes negatively impact tumor growth and have been named *tumor-suppressor genes*. Both oncogenes and tumor-suppressor genes exert their effects on tumor growth through their ability to control cell division (cell birth) or cell death (apoptosis), although the mechanisms can be extremely complex. While tightly regulated in normal cells, oncogenes acquire mutations in cancer cells, and the mutations typically relieve this control and lead to increased activity of the gene products. This mutational event typically occurs in a single allele of the oncogene and acts in a dominant fashion. In contrast, the normal function of tumor-suppressor genes is usually to restrain cell growth, and this function is lost in cancer. Because of the diploid nature of mammalian cells, both alleles must be inactivated for a cell to completely lose the function of a tumor-suppressor gene, leading to a recessive mechanism at the cellular level. From these ideas and studies on the inherited form of retinoblastoma, Knudson and others formulated the *two-hit hypothesis*, which in its modern version states that both copies of a tumor-suppressor gene must be inactivated in cancer.

There is a subset of tumor-suppressor genes, the *caretaker genes*, which do not affect cell growth directly but rather control the ability of the cell to maintain the integrity of its genome. Cells with a deficiency in these genes have an increased rate of mutations throughout their genomes, including in oncogenes and tumor-suppressor genes. This "mutator" phenotype was first hypothesized by Loeb to explain how the multiple mutational events required for tumorigenesis can occur in the lifetime of an individual. A mutator phenotype has now been observed in some forms of cancer, such as those associated with deficiencies in DNA mismatch repair. The great majority of cancers, however, do not harbor repair deficiencies, and their rate of mutation is similar to that observed in normal cells. Many of these cancers, however, appear to harbor a different kind of genetic instability, affecting the loss or gains of whole chromosomes or large parts thereof (as explained in more detail below).

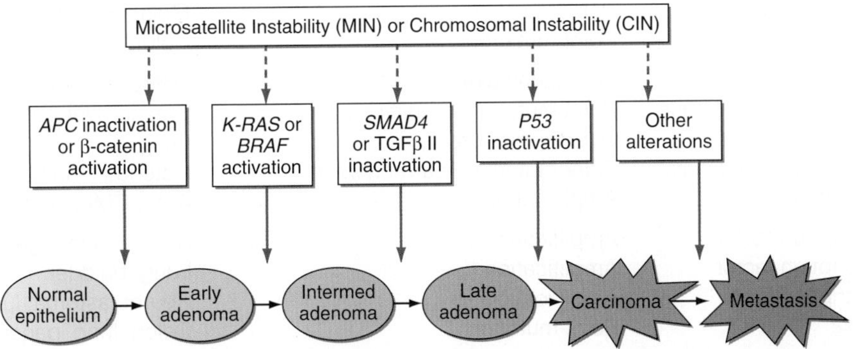

FIGURE 24-2
Progressive somatic mutational steps in the development of colon carcinoma. The accumulation of alterations in a number of different genes results in the progression from normal epithelium through adenoma to full-blown carcinoma. Genetic instability (microsatellite or chromosomal) accelerates the progression by increasing the likelihood of mutation at each step. Patients with familial polyposis are already one step into this pathway, since they inherit a germline alteration of the *APC* gene. TGF, transforming growth factor.

ONCOGENES IN HUMAN CANCER

Work by Peyton Rous in the early 1900s revealed that a chicken sarcoma could be transmitted from animal to animal in cell-free extracts, suggesting that cancer could be induced by an agent acting positively to promote tumor formation. The agent responsible for the transmission of the cancer was a retrovirus (Rous sarcoma virus, RSV) and the oncogene responsible was identified 75 years later as *v-src*. Other oncogenes were also discovered through their presence in the genomes of retroviruses that are capable of causing cancers in chickens, mice, and rats. The cellular homologues of these viral genes are called protooncogenes and are often targets of mutation or aberrant regulation in human cancer. Whereas many oncogenes were discovered because of their presence in retroviruses, other oncogenes, particularly those involved in translocations characteristic of particular leukemias and lymphomas, were isolated through genomic approaches. Investigators cloned the sequences surrounding the chromosomal translocations observed cytogenetically and then deduced the nature of the genes that were the targets of these translocations (see below). Some of these were oncogenes known from retroviruses (e.g., *ABL*, involved in chronic myeloid leukemia [CML]), while others were new (e.g., *BCL2*, involved in B cell lymphoma). In the normal cellular environment, protooncogenes have crucial roles in cell proliferation and differentiation. Table 24-1 is a partial list of oncogenes known to be involved in human cancer.

The normal growth and differentiation of cells is controlled by growth factors that bind to receptors on the surface of the cell. The signals generated by the membrane receptors are transmitted inside the cells through signaling cascades involving kinases, G proteins, and other regulatory proteins. Ultimately, these signals affect the activity of transcription factors in the nucleus, which regulate the expression of genes crucial in cell proliferation, cell differentiation, and cell death. Oncogene products have been found to function at critical steps in these pathways (Chap. 25), and inappropriate activation of these pathways can lead to tumorigenesis.

MECHANISMS OF ONCOGENE ACTIVATION

POINT MUTATION

Point mutation is a common mechanism of oncogene activation. For example, mutations in one of the *RAS* genes (*HRAS*, *KRAS*, or *NRAS*) are present in up to 85% of pancreatic cancers and 45% of colon cancers but are less common in other cancer types, although they can occur at significant frequencies in leukemia, lung, and thyroid cancers. Remarkably—and in contrast to the diversity of mutations found in tumor-suppressor genes (see later discussion)—most of the activated *RAS* genes contain point mutations in codons 12, 13, or 61 (these mutations reduce RAS GTPase activity, leading

TABLE 24-1

COMMON ONCOGENES ALTERED IN HUMAN CANCERS

ONCOGENE	FUNCTION	ALTERATION IN CANCER	NEOPLASM
AKT1	Serine/threonine kinase	Amplification	Stomach
AKT2	Serine/threonine kinase	Amplification	Ovarian, breast, pancreatic
BRAF	Serine/threonine kinase	Point mutation	Melanoma, lung, colorectal
CTNNB1	Signal transduction	Point mutation	Colon, prostate, melanoma, skin, others
FOS	Transcription factor	Overexpression	Osteosarcomas
ERBB2	Receptor tyrosine kinase	Point mutation, amplification	Breast, ovary, stomach, neuroblastoma
JUN	Transcription factor	Overexpression	Lung
MET	Receptor tyrosine kinase	Point mutation, rearrangement	Osteocarcinoma, kidney, glioma
MYB	Transcription factor	Amplification	AML, CML, colorectal, melanoma
C-MYC	Transcription factor	Amplification	Breast, colon, gastric, lung
L-MYC	Transcription factor	Amplification	Lung, bladder
N-MYC	Transcription factor	Amplification	Neuroblastoma, lung
HRAS	GTPase	Point mutation	Colon, lung, pancreas
KRAS	GTPase	Point mutation	Melanoma, colorectal, AML
NRAS	GTPase	Point mutation	Various carcinomas, melanoma
REL	Transcription factor	Rearrangement, amplification	Lymphomas
WNT1	Growth factor	Amplification	Retinoblastoma

Abbreviations: AML, acute myeloid leukemia; CML, chronic myeloid leukemia.

to constitutive activation of the mutant RAS protein). The restricted pattern of mutations observed in oncogenes compared with that of tumor-suppressor genes reflects the fact that gain-of-function mutations are less likely to occur than mutations that simply lead to loss of activity. Indeed, inactivation of a gene can in theory be accomplished through the introduction of a stop codon anywhere in the coding sequence, whereas activations require precise substitutions at residues that can somehow lead to an increase in the activity of the encoded protein. Importantly, the specificity of oncogene mutations provides diagnostic opportunities, as tests that identify mutations at defined positions are easier to design than tests aimed at detecting random changes in a gene.

DNA AMPLIFICATION

The second mechanism for activation of oncogenes is DNA sequence amplification, leading to overexpression of the gene product. This increase in DNA copy number may cause cytologically recognizable chromosome alterations referred to as *homogeneous staining regions* (HSRs) if integrated within chromosomes or *double minutes* (dmins) if extrachromosomal. The recognition of DNA amplification is accomplished through various cytogenetic techniques such as comparative genomic hybridization (CGH) or fluorescence in situ hybridization (FISH), which allow the visualization of chromosomal aberrations using fluorescent dyes. In addition, noncytogenetic, microarray-based approaches are now available for identifying changes in copy number at high resolution. Newer short-tag–based sequencing approaches have been used to evaluate amplifications. When paired with next-generation sequencing instruments, this approach offers the highest degree of resolution and quantification available. With both microarray and sequencing technologies, the entire genome can be surveyed for gains and losses of DNA sequences, thus pinpointing chromosomal regions likely to contain genes important in the development or progression of cancer.

Numerous genes have been reported to be amplified in cancer. Several of these genes, including *NMYC* and *LMYC*, were identified through their presence within the amplified DNA sequences of a tumor and had homology to known oncogenes. Because the region amplified often includes hundreds of thousands of base pairs, multiple oncogenes may be amplified in a single amplicon in some cancers (particularly in sarcomas). Indeed, *MDM2*, *GLI*, *CDK4*, and *SAS* at chromosomal location 12q13-15 have been shown to be simultaneously amplified in several types of sarcomas and other tumors. Amplification of a cellular gene is often a predictor of poor prognosis; for example, *ERBB2/HER2* and *NMYC* are often amplified in aggressive breast cancers and neuroblastoma, respectively.

CHROMOSOMAL REARRANGEMENT

Chromosomal alterations provide important clues to the genetic changes in cancer. The chromosomal alterations in human solid tumors such as carcinomas are heterogeneous and complex and occur as a result of the frequent chromosomal instability (CIN) observed in these tumors (see later discussion). In contrast, the chromosome alterations in myeloid and lymphoid tumors are often simple translocations, i.e., reciprocal transfers of chromosome arms from one chromosome to another. Consequently, many detailed and informative chromosome analyses have been performed on hematopoietic cancers. The breakpoints of recurring chromosome abnormalities usually occur at the site of cellular oncogenes. Table 24-2 lists representative examples of recurring chromosome alterations in malignancy and the associated gene(s) rearranged or deregulated by the chromosomal rearrangement. Translocations are particularly common in lymphoid tumors, probably because these cell types have the capability to rearrange their DNA to generate antigen receptors. Indeed, antigen receptor genes are commonly involved in the translocations, implying that an imperfect regulation of receptor gene rearrangement may be involved in the pathogenesis. An interesting example is Burkitt's lymphoma, a B cell tumor characterized by a reciprocal translocation between chromosomes 8 and 14. Molecular analysis of Burkitt's lymphomas demonstrated that the breakpoints occurred within or near the *MYC* locus on chromosome 8 and within the immunoglobulin heavy chain locus on chromosome 14, resulting in the transcriptional activation of *MYC*. Enhancer activation by translocation, although not universal, appears to play an important role in malignant progression. In addition to transcription factors and signal transduction molecules, translocation may result in the overexpression of cell cycle regulatory proteins or proteins such as cyclins and of proteins that regulate cell death.

The first reproducible chromosome abnormality detected in human malignancy was the Philadelphia chromosome detected in CML. This cytogenetic abnormality is generated by reciprocal translocation involving the *ABL* oncogene on chromosome 9, encoding a tyrosine kinase, being placed in proximity to the *BCR* (breakpoint cluster region) gene on chromosome 22. Figure 24-3 illustrates the generation of the translocation and its protein product. The consequence of expression of the *BCR-ABL* gene product is the activation of signal transduction pathways leading to cell growth independent of normal external signals.

TABLE 24-2

REPRESENTATIVE ONCOGENES AT CHROMOSOMAL TRANSLOCATIONS

GENE (CHROMOSOME)	TRANSLOCATION	MALIGNANCY
ABL (9q34.1)–BCR *(22q11)*	(9;22)(q34;q11)	Chronic myeloid leukemia
ATF1 (12q13)–*EWS* (22q12)	(12;22)(q13;q12)	Malignant melanoma of soft parts
BCL1 (11q13.3)–*IgH* (14q32)	(11;14)(q13;q32)	Mantle cell lymphoma
BCL2 (18q21.3)–*IgH* (14q32)	(14;18)(q32;q21)	Follicular lymphoma
FLI1 (11q24)–*EWS* (22q12)	(11;22)(q24;q12)	Ewing's sarcoma
LCK (1p34)–*TCRB* (7q35)	(1;7)(p34;q35)	T cell acute lymphocytic leukemia
MYC (8q24)–*IgH* (14q32)	(8;14)(q24;q32)	Burkitt's lymphoma, B cell acute lymphocytic leukemia
PAX3 (2q35)–*FKHR/ALV* (13q14)	(2;13)(q35;q14)	Alveolar rhabdomyosarcoma
PAX7 (1p36)–*KHR*/ALV(13q14)	(1;13)(p36;q14)	Alveolar rhabdomyosarcoma
REL (2p13)–*NRG* (2p11.2-14)	Inv(2(p13;p11.2-14)	Non-Hodgkin's lymphoma
RET (10q11.2)–*PKAR1A* (17q23)	(10;17)(q11.2;q23)	Thyroid carcinoma
TAL1(1p32)–*TCTA* (3p21)	(1;3)(p34;p21)	Acute T cell leukemia
TRK (1q23-1q24)–*TPM3* (1q31)	Inv1(q23;q31)	Colon carcinoma
WT1 (11p13)–*EWS* (22q12)	(11;22)(p13;q12)	Desmoplastic small round cell tumor

Source: From R Hesketh: *The Oncogene and Tumour Suppressor Gene Facts Book,* 2nd ed. San Diego, Academic Press, 1997; with permission.

Imatinib (marketed as Gleevec), a drug that specifically blocks the activity of *BCR-ABL*, has shown remarkable efficacy with little toxicity in patients with CML. It is hoped that knowledge of genetic alterations in other cancers will likewise lead to mechanism-based design and development of a new generation of chemotherapeutic agents.

CHROMOSOMAL INSTABILITY IN SOLID TUMORS

Solid tumors are generally highly aneuploid, containing an abnormal number of chromosomes; these chromosomes also exhibit structural alterations such as translocations, deletions, and amplifications. These

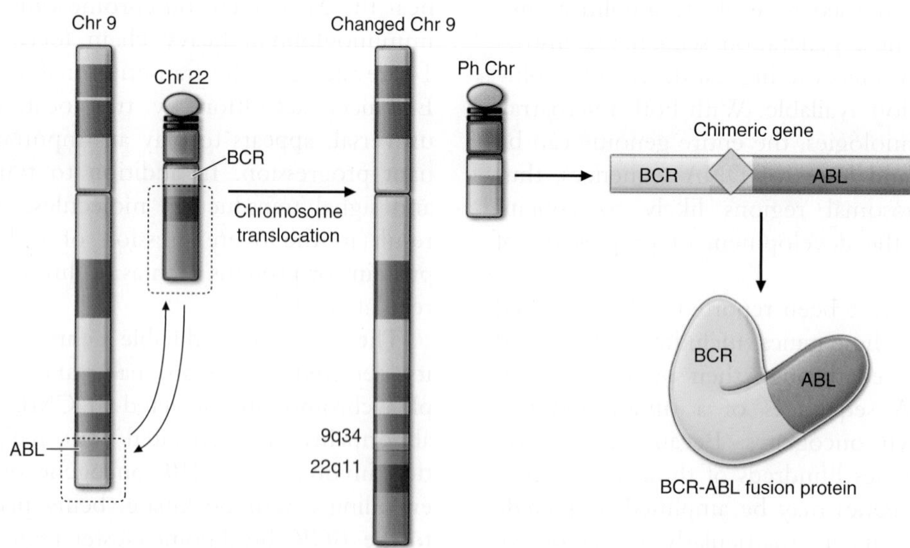

FIGURE 24-3

Specific translocation seen in chronic myeloid leukemia (CML). The Philadelphia chromosome (Ph) is derived from a reciprocal translocation between chromosomes 9 and 22 with the breakpoint joining the sequences of the *ABL* oncogene with the *BCR* gene. The fusion of these DNA sequences allows the generation of an entirely novel fusion protein with modified function.

abnormalities are collectively referred to as CIN. Normal cells possess several cell cycle checkpoints, essentially quality-control requirements that have to be met before subsequent events are allowed to take place. The mitotic checkpoint, which ensures proper chromosome attachment to the mitotic spindle before allowing the sister chromatids to separate, is altered in certain cancers. The molecular basis of CIN remains unclear, although a number of mitotic checkpoint genes are found mutated or abnormally expressed in various tumors. The exact effects of these changes on the mitotic checkpoint are unknown, and both weakening and overactivation of the checkpoint have been proposed. The identification of the cause of CIN in tumors will likely be a formidable task, considering that several hundred genes are thought to control the mitotic checkpoint and other cellular processes ensuring proper chromosome segregation. Regardless of the mechanisms underlying CIN, the measurement of the number of chromosomal alterations present in tumors is now possible with both cytogenetic and molecular techniques, and several studies have shown that this information can be useful for prognostic purposes. In addition, since the mitotic checkpoint is essential for cellular viability, it may become a target for novel therapeutic approaches.

TUMOR-SUPPRESSOR GENE INACTIVATION IN CANCER

The first indication of the existence of tumor-suppressor genes came from experiments showing that fusion of mouse cancer cells with normal mouse fibroblasts led to a nonmalignant phenotype in the fused cells. The normal role of tumor-suppressor genes is to restrain cell growth, and the function of these genes is inactivated in cancer. The two major types of somatic lesions observed in tumor-suppressor genes during tumor development are *point mutations* and *large deletions*. Point mutations in the coding region of tumor-suppressor genes will frequently lead to truncated protein products or otherwise nonfunctional proteins. Similarly, deletions lead to the loss of a functional product and sometimes encompass the entire gene or even the entire chromosome arm, leading to loss of heterozygosity (LOH) in the tumor DNA compared with the corresponding normal tissue DNA (Fig. 24-4). LOH in tumor DNA is considered a hallmark for the presence of a tumor-suppressor gene at a particular chromosomal location, and LOH studies have been useful in the positional cloning of many tumor-suppressor genes.

Gene silencing, an epigenetic change that leads to the loss of gene expression and occurs in conjunction with hypermethylation of the promoter and histone deacetylation, is another mechanism of tumor-suppressor gene inactivation. (An *epigenetic modification* refers to a change in the genome, heritable by cell progeny, that does not involve a change in the DNA sequence. The inactivation of the second X chromosome in female cells is an example of an epigenetic silencing that prevents gene expression from the inactivated chromosome). During embryologic development, regions of chromosomes from one parent are silenced, and gene expression proceeds from the chromosome of the other parent. For most genes, expression occurs from both alleles or randomly from one allele or the other. The preferential expression of a particular gene exclusively from the allele contributed by one parent is called *parental imprinting* and is thought to be regulated by covalent modifications of chromatin protein and DNA (often methylation) of the silenced allele.

The role of epigenetic control mechanisms in the development of human cancer is unclear. However, a general decrease in the level of DNA methylation has been noted as a common change in cancer. In addition, numerous genes, including some tumor-suppressor genes, appear to become hypermethylated and silenced during tumorigenesis. *VHL* and *p16INK4* are well-studied examples of such tumor-suppressor genes. Overall, epigenetic mechanisms may be responsible for reprogramming the expression of a large number of genes in cancer and, together with the mutation of specific genes, are likely to be crucial in the development of human malignancies.

FAMILIAL CANCER SYNDROMES

A small fraction of cancers occur in patients with a genetic predisposition. In these families, the affected individuals have a predisposing loss-of-function mutation in one allele of a tumor-suppressor gene. The tumors in these patients show a loss of the remaining normal allele as a result of somatic events (point mutations or deletions) in agreement with the two-hit hypothesis (Fig. 24-4). Thus, most cells of an individual with an inherited loss-of-function mutation in a tumor-suppressor gene are functionally normal, and only the rare cells that develop a mutation in the remaining normal allele will exhibit uncontrolled regulation.

Roughly 100 syndromes of familial cancer have been reported, although many are rare. The majority are inherited as autosomal dominant traits, although some of those associated with DNA repair abnormalities (xeroderma pigmentosum, Fanconi's anemia, ataxia telangiectasia) are autosomal recessive. Table 24-3 shows a number of cancer predisposition syndromes and the responsible genes. The current paradigm states that the genes mutated in familial syndromes can also be

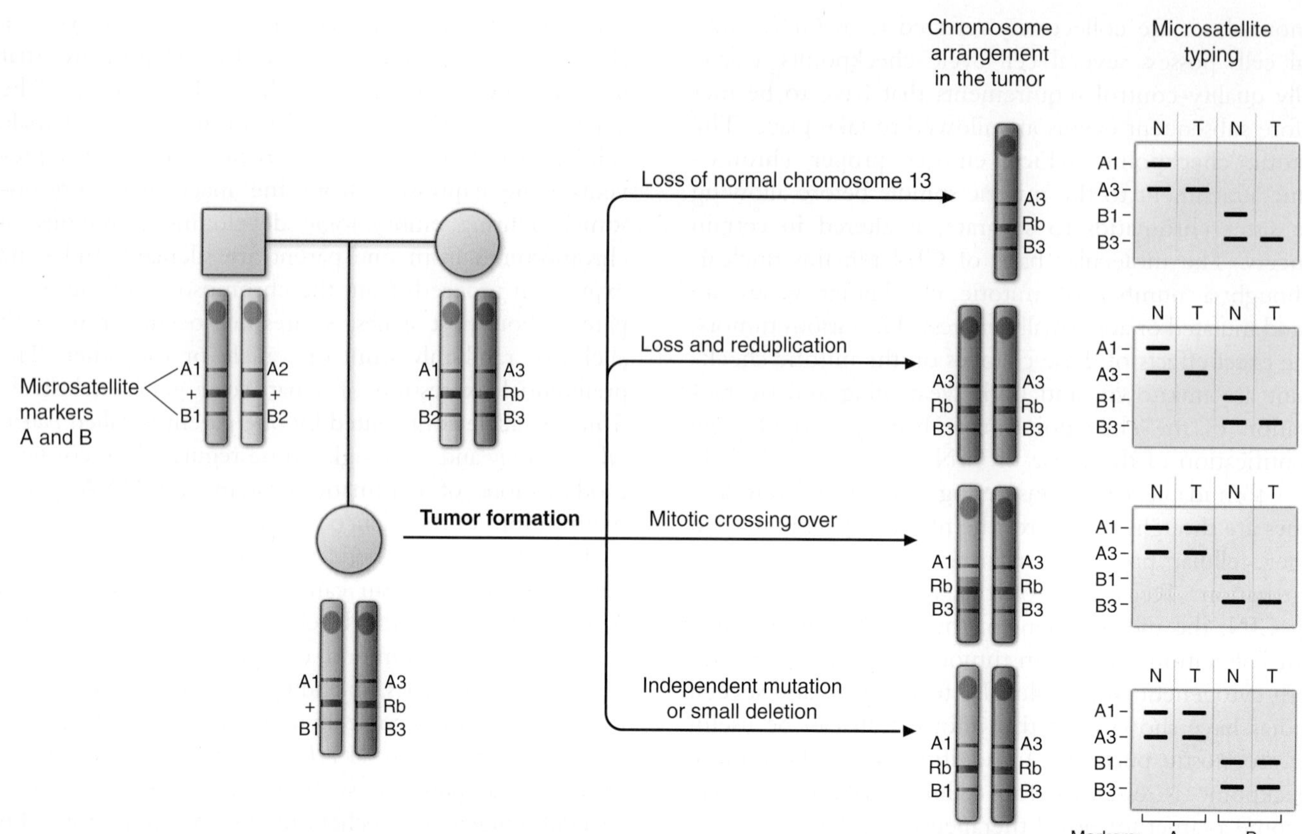

FIGURE 24-4

Diagram of possible mechanisms for tumor formation in an individual with hereditary (familial) retinoblastoma. On the left is shown the pedigree of an affected individual who has inherited the abnormal (Rb) allele from her affected mother. The normal allele is shown as a (+). The four chromosomes of her two parents are drawn to indicate their origin. Flanking the retinoblastoma locus are microsatellite markers (A and B) also analyzed in this family. Markers A3 and B3 are on the chromosome carrying the retinoblastoma disease gene. Tumor formation results when the normal allele, which this patient inherited from her father, is inactivated. On the right are shown four possible ways in which this could occur. In each case, the resulting chromosome 13 arrangement is shown, as well as the results of polymerase chain reaction typing using the microsatellite markers comparing normal tissue (N) with tumor tissue (T). Note that in the first three situations the normal allele (B1) has been lost in the tumor tissue, which is referred to as loss of heterozygosity (LOH) at this locus.

targets for somatic mutations in sporadic (noninherited) tumors. The study of cancer syndromes has thus provided invaluable insights into the mechanisms of progression for many tumor types. This section examines the case of inherited colon cancer in detail, but similar general lessons can be applied to many of the cancer syndromes listed in Table 24-3. In particular, the study of inherited colon cancer will clearly illustrate the difference between two types of tumor-suppressor genes: the *gatekeepers*, which directly regulate the growth of tumors, and the *caretakers*, which, when mutated, lead to genetic instability and therefore act indirectly on tumor growth.

Familial adenomatous polyposis (FAP) is a dominantly inherited colon cancer syndrome due to germline mutations in the adenomatous polyposis coli (*APC*) tumor-suppressor gene on chromosome 5. Patients with this syndrome develop hundreds to thousands of adenomas in the colon. Each of these adenomas has lost the normal remaining allele of *APC* but has not yet accumulated the required additional mutations to generate fully malignant cells (Fig. 24-2). The loss of the second functional *APC* allele in tumors from FAP families often occurs through LOH. However, out of these thousands of benign adenomas, several will invariably acquire further abnormalities, and a subset will even develop into fully malignant cancers. *APC* is thus considered to be a gatekeeper for colon tumorigenesis: in the absence of mutation of this gatekeeper (or a gene acting within the same pathway), a colorectal tumor simply cannot form. Figure 24-5 shows germline and somatic mutations found in the *APC* gene. The function of the APC protein is still not completely understood, but it likely provides differentiation and apoptotic cues to colonic cells as they migrate up the crypts. Defects in this process may lead to abnormal

TABLE 24-3

CANCER PREDISPOSITION SYNDROMES AND ASSOCIATED GENES

SYNDROME	GENE	CHROMOSOME	INHERITANCE	TUMORS
Ataxia telangiectasia	*ATM*	11q22-q23	AR	Breast
Autoimmune lymphoproliferative syndrome	*FAS*	10q24	AD	Lymphomas
	FASL	1q23		
Bloom syndrome	*BLM*	15q26.1	AR	Several types
Cowden syndrome	*PTEN*	10q23	AD	Breast, thyroid
Familial adenomatous polyposis	*APC*	5q21	AD	Intestinal adenoma, colorectal
Familial melanoma	*p16INK4*	9p21	AD	Melanoma, pancreatic
Familial Wilms' tumor	*WT1*	11p13	AD	Kidney (pediatric)
Hereditary breast/ovarian cancer	*BRCA1*	17q21	AD	Breast, ovarian, colon, prostate
	BRCA2	13q12.3		
Hereditary diffuse gastric cancer	*CDH1*	16q22	AD	Stomach
Hereditary multiple exostoses	*EXT1*	8q24	AD	Exostoses, chondrosarcoma
	EXT2	11p11-12		
Hereditary prostate cancer	*HPC1*	1q24-25	AD	Prostate
Hereditary retinoblastoma	*RB1*	13q14.2	AD	Retinoblastoma, osteosarcoma
Hereditary nonpolyposis colon cancer	*MSH2*	2p16	AD	Colon, endometrial, ovarian, stomach, small bowel, ureter carcinoma
	MLH1	3p21.3		
	MSH6	2p16		
	PMS2	7p22		
Hereditary papillary renal carcinoma	*MET*	7q31	AD	Papillary kidney
Juvenile polyposis	*SMAD4*	18q21	AD	Gastrointestinal, pancreatic
Li-Fraumeni	*TP53*	17p13.1	AD	Sarcoma, breast
Multiple endocrine neoplasia type 1	*MEN1*	11q13	AD	Parathyroid, endocrine, pancreas, and pituitary
Multiple endocrine neoplasia type 2a	*RET*	10q11.2		Medullary thyroid carcinoma, pheochromocytoma
Neurofibromatosis type 1	*NF1*	17q11.2	AD	Neurofibroma, neurofibrosarcoma, brain
Neurofibromatosis type 2	*NF2*	22q12.2	AD	Vestibular schwannoma, meningioma, spine
Nevoid basal cell carcinoma syndrome (Gorlin's syndrome)	*PTCH*	9q22.3	AD	Basal cell carcinoma, medulloblastoma, jaw cysts
Tuberous sclerosis	*TSC1*	9q34	AD	Angiofibroma, renal angiomyolipoma
	TSC2	16p13.3		
von Hippel–Lindau	*VHL*	3p25-26	AD	Kidney, cerebellum, pheochromocytoma

Abbreviations: AD, autosomal dominant; AR, autosomal recessive.

accumulation of cells that should normally undergo apoptosis.

In contrast to patients with FAP, patients with hereditary nonpolyposis colon cancer (HNPCC, or Lynch syndrome) do not develop multiple polyposis but instead develop only one or a small number of adenomas that rapidly progress to cancer. Most HNPCC cases are due to mutations in one of four DNA mismatch repair genes (Table 24-3), which are components of a repair system that is normally responsible for correcting errors in freshly replicated DNA. Germline mutations in *MSH2* and *MLH1* account for more than 90% of HNPCC cases, while mutations in *MSH6* and *PMS2* are much less frequent. When a somatic mutation inactivates the remaining wild-type allele of a mismatch repair gene, the cell develops a hypermutable phenotype characterized by profound genomic instability, especially for the short repeated sequences called *microsatellites*. This microsatellite instability (MSI) favors the development of cancer by increasing the rate of mutations in many genes, including oncogenes and tumor-suppressor genes (Fig. 24-2). These genes can thus be considered caretakers. Interestingly, chromosomal instability (CIN) can also be found in colon cancer, but MSI and CIN appear to be mutually exclusive, suggesting that they represent alternative mechanisms for

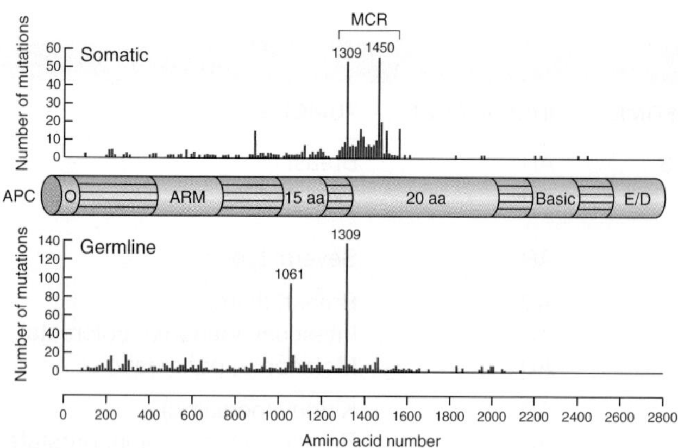

FIGURE 24-5

Germline and somatic mutations in the tumor-suppressor gene *APC*. *APC* encodes a 2843-amino-acid protein with 6 major domains: an oligomerization region (O), armadillo repeats (ARM), 15-amino-acid repeats (15 aa), 20-amino-acid repeats (20 aa), a basic region, and a domain involved in binding EB1 and the *Drosophila* discs large homologue (E/D). Shown are the positions within the *APC* gene of a total of 650 somatic and 826 germline mutations (from the *APC* database at *www.umd.be/APC*). The vast majority of these mutations result in the truncation of the APC protein. Germline mutations are found to be relatively evenly distributed up to codon 1600 except for two mutation hotspots at amino acids 1061 and 1309, which together account for one-third of the mutations found in familial adenomatous polyposis (FAP) families. Somatic *APC* mutations in colon tumors cluster in an area of the gene known as the *mutation cluster region* (MCR). The location of the MCR suggests that the 20-amino-acid domain plays a crucial role in tumor suppression.

the generation of a mutator phenotype in this cancer (Fig. 24-2). Other cancer types rarely exhibit MSI, but most exhibit CIN.

While most autosomal dominant inherited cancer syndromes are due to mutations in tumor-suppressor genes (Table 24-3), there are a few interesting exceptions. Multiple endocrine neoplasia type II, a dominant disorder characterized by pituitary adenomas, medullary carcinoma of the thyroid, and (in some pedigrees) pheochromocytoma, is due to gain-of-function mutations in the protooncogene *RET* on chromosome 10. Similarly, gain-of-function mutations in the tyrosine kinase domain of the *MET* oncogene lead to hereditary papillary renal carcinoma. Interestingly, loss-of-function mutations in the *RET* gene cause a completely different disease, Hirschsprung's disease (aganglionic megacolon [Chap 50]).

Although the Mendelian forms of cancer have taught us much about the mechanisms of growth control, most forms of cancer do not follow simple patterns of inheritance. In many instances (e.g., lung cancer), a strong environmental contribution is at work. Even in such circumstances, however, some individuals may be more genetically susceptible to developing cancer, given the appropriate exposure, due to the presence of modifier alleles.

GENETIC TESTING FOR FAMILIAL CANCER

The discovery of cancer susceptibility genes raises the possibility of DNA testing to predict the risk of cancer in individuals of affected families. An algorithm for cancer risk assessment and decision making in high-risk families using genetic testing is shown in Fig. 24-6. Once a mutation is discovered in a family, subsequent testing of asymptomatic family members can be crucial in patient management. A negative gene test result in these individuals can prevent years of anxiety in the knowledge that their cancer risk is no higher than that

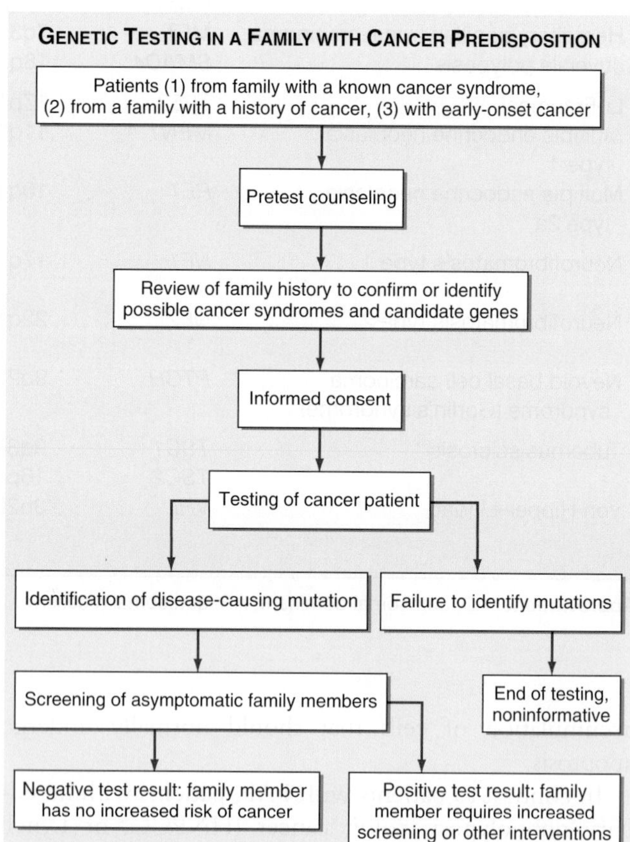

FIGURE 24-6

Algorithm for genetic testing in a family with cancer predisposition. The key step is the identification of a mutation in a cancer patient, which allows testing of asymptomatic family members. Asymptomatic family members who test positive may require increased screening or surgery, whereas others are at no greater risk for cancer than the general population.

of the general population. On the other hand, a positive test result may lead to alteration of clinical management, such as increased frequency of cancer screening and, when feasible and appropriate, prophylactic surgery. Potential negative consequences of a positive test result include psychological distress (anxiety, depression) and discrimination, although the Genetic Information Nondiscrimination Act (GINA) makes it illegal for predictive genetic information to be used to discriminate in health insurance or employment. Testing should therefore not be conducted without counseling before and after disclosure of the test result. In addition, the decision to test should depend on whether effective interventions exist for the particular type of cancer to be tested. Despite these caveats, genetic cancer testing for some cancer syndromes already appears to have greater benefits than risks, and many companies now offer testing for various genes associated with the predisposition to breast cancer (*BRCA1* and *BRCA2*), melanoma (*p16INK4*), and colon cancer (*APC* and the HNPCC genes).

Because of the inherent problems of genetic testing such as cost, specificity, and sensitivity, it is not yet appropriate to offer these tests to the general population. However, testing may be appropriate in some subpopulations with a known increased risk, even without a defined family history. For example, two mutations in the breast cancer susceptibility gene *BRCA1*, 185delAG and 5382insC, exhibit a sufficiently high frequency in the Ashkenazi Jewish population that genetic testing of an individual of this ethnic group may be warranted.

As noted earlier, it is important that genetic test results be communicated to families by trained genetic counselors, especially for high-risk high-penetrance conditions such as the hereditary breast/ovarian cancer syndrome (*BRCA1/BRCA2*). To ensure that the families clearly understand its advantages and disadvantages and the impact it may have on disease management and psyche, genetic testing should never be done before counseling. Significant expertise is needed to communicate the results of genetic testing to families. For example, one common mistake is to misinterpret the result of negative genetic test results. For many cancer predisposition genes, the sensitivity of genetic testing is less than 70% (i.e., of 100 kindreds tested, disease-causing mutations can be identified in 70 at most). Therefore, such testing should in general begin with an affected member of the kindred (the youngest family member still alive who has had the cancer of interest). If a mutation is not identified in this individual, then the test result should be reported as noninformative (Fig. 24-6) rather than negative (because it is possible that, for technical reasons, the mutation in this individual is not detectable by standard genetic assays). On the other hand, if a mutation can be identified in this individual, then testing of other family members can be performed, and the sensitivity of such subsequent tests will be 100% (because the mutation in the family is in this case known to be detectable by the method used).

MICRORNAs AND CANCER

MicroRNAs (miRNAs) are small noncoding RNAs 20–22 nucleotides in length that are involved in posttranscriptional gene regulation. Studies in chronic lymphocytic leukemia first suggested a link between miRNAs and cancer when *miR-15* and *miR-16* were found to be deleted or downregulated in the vast majority of tumors. Various miRNAs have since been found abnormally expressed in several human malignancies. Aberrant expression of miRNAs in cancer has been attributed to several mechanisms, such as chromosomal rearrangements, genomic copy number change, epigenetic modifications, defects in miRNA biogenesis pathway, and regulation by transcriptional factors.

Functionally, miRNAs have been suggested to contribute to tumorigenesis through their ability to regulate oncogenic signaling pathways. For example, *miR-15* and *miR-16* have been shown to target the *BCL2* oncogene, leading to its downregulation in leukemic cells and apoptosis. As another example of miRNAs' involvement in oncogenic pathways, the p53 tumor suppressor can transcriptionally induce *miR-34* following genotoxic stress, and this induction is important in mediating p53 function. The expression of miRNAs is extremely specific, and there is evidence that miRNA expression patterns may be useful in distinguishing lineage and differentiation state, as well as cancer diagnosis and outcome prediction. However, no miRNA gene has ever been observed to be mutated in a cancer, either in the germline or somatically. At present, the only absolutely reliable way to causally implicate a gene in the human neoplastic process is through evidence of its mutant status. Hundreds of other genes, besides miRNAs, are expressed at higher or lower levels in cancers compared with corresponding normal tissues, and the roles of any of these genes in human cancer remain conjectural.

VIRUSES IN HUMAN CANCER

Certain human malignancies are associated with viruses. Examples include Burkitt's lymphoma (Epstein-Barr virus), hepatocellular carcinoma (hepatitis viruses), cervical cancer (human papillomavirus [HPV]), and T cell leukemia (retroviruses). The mechanisms of action of these viruses are varied but always involve activation of growth-promoting pathways or inhibition of tumor-suppressor products in the infected cells. For example,

HPV proteins E6 and E7 bind and inactivate cellular tumor suppressors p53 and pRB, respectively. Viruses are not sufficient for cancer development but constitute one alteration in the multistep process of cancer progression.

GENE EXPRESSION IN CANCER

The tumorigenesis process, driven by alterations in tumor suppressors, oncogenes, and epigenetic regulation, is accompanied by changes in gene expression. The advent of powerful techniques for high-throughput gene expression profiling, based on sequencing or microarrays, has allowed the comprehensive study of gene expression in neoplastic cells. It is indeed possible to identify the expression levels of thousands of genes expressed in normal and cancer tissues. Figure 24-7 shows a typical microarray experiment examining gene expression in cancer. This global knowledge of gene expression allows the identification of differentially expressed genes and, in principle, the understanding of the complex molecular circuitry regulating normal and neoplastic behaviors. Such studies have led to molecular profiling of tumors, which has suggested general methods for distinguishing tumors of various biologic behaviors (molecular classification), elucidating pathways relevant to the development of tumors, and identifying molecular targets for the detection and therapy of cancer. The first practical applications of this technology have suggested that global gene expression profiling can provide prognostic information not evident from other clinical or laboratory tests. The Sanger Cancer Genome Project (*www.sanger.ac.uk/genetics/CGP/*) maintains a database dedicated to collect data on gene expression in normal and malignant tissues and making it available on the Internet. The Gene Expression Omnibus (GEO, *www.ncbi.nlm.nih.gov/geo/*) is another online data repository for expression profiling experiments.

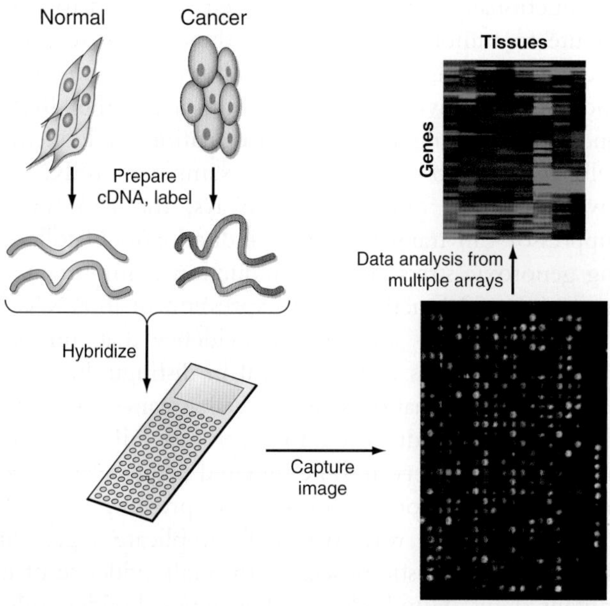

FIGURE 24-7

A microarray experiment. RNA is prepared from cells, reverse transcribed to cDNA, and labeled with fluorescent dyes (typically green for normal cells and red for cancer cells). The fluorescent probes are mixed and hybridized to a cDNA array. Each spot on the array is an oligonucleotide (or cDNA fragment) that represents a different gene. The image is then captured with a fluorescence camera; red spots indicate higher expression in tumor cells compared with reference, while green spots represent the lower expression in tumor cells. Yellow signals indicate equal expression levels in normal and tumor specimens. After clustering analysis of multiple arrays, the results are typically represented graphically using a visualization software, which shows, for each sample, a color-coded representation of gene expression for every gene on the array.

GENOMEWIDE MUTATIONAL PROFILING IN CANCER

With the completion of the Human Genome Project and advances in sequencing technologies, systematic mutational analysis of the cancer genome has become possible. All protein-encoding genes known to be present in the human genome have been sequenced in breast, pancreatic, brain, and colorectal tumors. Interestingly, it was found that there are generally 40 to 100 genetic alterations that affect protein sequence in a typical cancer, although statistical analyses suggested that only 8–15 are functionally involved in tumorigenesis. The picture that emerges from these studies is that most genes found mutated in tumors are actually mutated at relatively low frequencies (<5%), while a small number of genes (such as *p53*, *KRAS*) are mutated in a large proportion of tumors (Fig. 24-8). In the past, the focus of research has been on the frequently mutated genes, but it appears that the large number of genes that are infrequently mutated in cancer are major contributors to the cancer phenotype. Understanding the signaling pathways altered by mutations in these genes, as well as the functional relevance of these different mutations, represents the next challenge in the field. The Cancer Genome Atlas (*http://cancergenome.nih.gov*) is a coordinated effort from the National Cancer Institute and the National Human Genome Research Institute to systematically characterize the entire spectrum of genomic changes involved in human cancers.

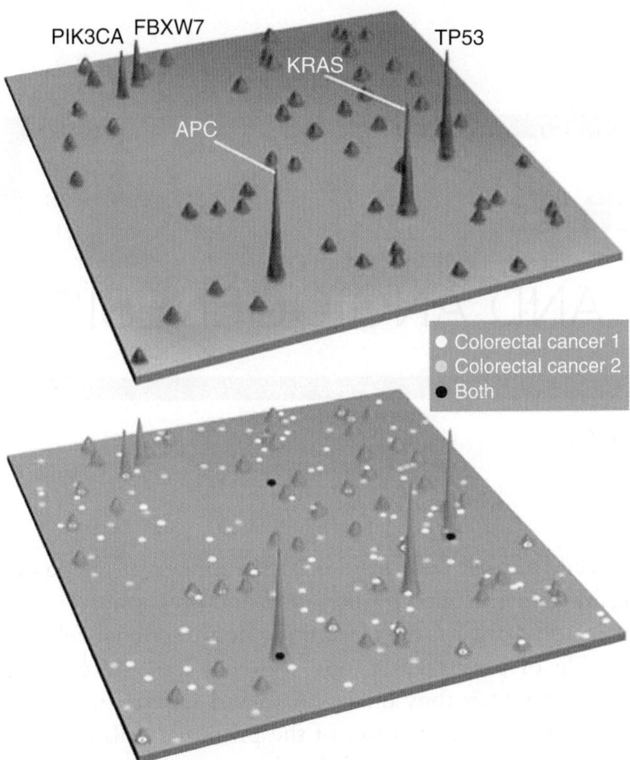

FIGURE 24-8
Two-dimensional maps of genes mutated in colo-rectal cancer. The two-dimensional landscape represent the positions of the RefSeq genes along the chromosomes and the height of the peaks represent the mutation frequency. On the top map, the taller peaks represent the genes that are commonly mutated in colon cancer, while the large number of smaller hills indicates the genes that are mutated at lower frequency. On the lower map, the mutations of two individual tumors are indicated. Note that there is little overlap between the mutated genes of the two colorectal tumors shown. These differences may represent the basis for the heterogeneity in terms of behavior and responsiveness to therapy observed in human cancer. (*From LD Wood et al: The genomic landscapes of human breast and colorectal cancers. Science 318:1108, 2007, with permission.*)

PERSONALIZED CANCER TREATMENT BASED ON MOLECULAR PROFILES

Gene expression profiling and genomewide sequencing approaches have allowed for an unprecedented understanding of cancer at the molecular level. It has been suggested that individualized knowledge of pathways or genes deregulated in a given tumor (personalized genomics) may provide a guide for therapeutic options on this tumor, thus leading to personalized therapy. As tumor behavior is highly heterogeneous, even within a tumor type, personalized information-based medicine may provide a viable alternative to current one-size-fits-all therapy, especially in the case of tumors resistant to conventional therapeutic approaches. The success of this approach will be dependent on accumulated information on cancer behavior and phenotypes. For example, the identification of a particular mutation, such as that in *BRAF*, can indicate whether a certain tumor (such as melanoma) is likely to be susceptible to a specific drug that targets the mutant *BRAF* gene. Similarly, the identification of another mutation, in *KRAS*, can indicate that tumor is unlikely to be sensitive to an antibody targeting EGFR. Gene expression also offers the potential to predict drug sensitivities as well as provide prognostic information. Commercial diagnostic tests, such as Mammaprint and Oncotype DX for breast cancer, are available to help the patients and their physicians make treatment decisions. Personalized medicine is an exciting new avenue for cancer treatment based on molecular profiling, and this approach is in the process of changing our approaches to cancer therapy in fundamental ways.

THE FUTURE

A revolution in cancer genetics has occurred in the past 25 years. Identification of cancer genes has led to a deep understanding of the tumorigenesis process and has had important repercussions on all fields of cancer biology. In particular, the advancement of powerful techniques for genomewide expression profiling and mutation analyses has provided a detailed picture of the molecular defects present in individual tumors. In addition, individualized treatment based on the specific genetic alterations within some tumor types has already become possible. While these advances have not yet translated into overall changes in cancer prevention, prognosis, or treatment, it is expected that breakthroughs in these areas will continue to emerge and be applicable to an ever-increasing number of cancers.

CHAPTER 25

CANCER CELL BIOLOGY AND ANGIOGENESIS

Dan L. Longo

CANCER CELL BIOLOGY

Cancers are characterized by unregulated cell growth, tissue invasion, and metastasis. A neoplasm is *benign* when it grows in an unregulated fashion without tissue invasion. The presence of both features is characteristic of *malignant* neoplasms. Cancers are named based on their origin: those derived from epithelial tissue are called *carcinomas*, those derived from mesenchymal tissues are *sarcomas*, and those derived from hematopoietic tissue are *leukemias* or *lymphomas*.

Cancers nearly always arise as a consequence of genetic alterations. Choriocarcinoma may be an exception to this rule in that experimental insertion of a choriocarcinoma cell into an animal blastocyst can result in the neoplastic cell giving rise to normal body structures under the inductive influence of the developing embryo. Such an occurrence would be unlikely in the setting of irreversible genetic damage.

Occasional cancers appear to be caused by an alteration in a dominant gene that drives uncontrolled cell proliferation. Examples include chronic myeloid leukemia (*abl*) and Burkitt's lymphoma (*c-myc*). The genes that can promote cell growth when altered are often called *oncogenes*. They were first identified as critical elements of viruses that cause animal tumors; later it was found that the viral genes had normal counterparts with important functions in the cell and had been captured and mutated by viruses as they passed from host to host.

However, the vast majority of human cancers are characterized by multiple genetic abnormalities, each of which contributes to the loss of control of cell proliferation and differentiation and the acquisition of capabilities, such as tissue invasion and angiogenesis. Many cancers go through recognizable steps of progressively more abnormal phenotypes: hyperplasia to adenoma to dysplasia to carcinoma in situ to invasive cancer (Table 25-1). These properties are not found in the normal adult cell from which the tumor is derived. Indeed, normal cells have a large number of safeguards against uncontrolled proliferation and invasion.

In most organs, only primitive nonfunctional cells are capable of proliferating, and the cells lose the capacity to proliferate as they differentiate and acquire functional capability. The expansion of the primitive cells is linked to some functional need in the host through receptors that receive signals from the local environment or through hormonal influences delivered by the vascular supply. In the absence of such signals, the cells are at rest. We have a poor understanding of the signals that keep the primitive cells at rest. These signals, too, must be environmental, based on the observations that a regenerating liver stops growing when it has replaced the portion that has been surgically removed and regenerating bone marrow stops growing when the peripheral blood counts return to normal. Cancer cells clearly have lost responsiveness to such controls and do not recognize when they have overgrown the niche normally occupied by the organ from which they are derived. We know very little about this mechanism of growth regulation.

CELL CYCLE CHECKPOINTS

Normal cells have a number of control mechanisms that are targeted by specific genetic alterations in cancer. The progression of a cell through the cell division cycle is regulated at a number of checkpoints by a wide array of genes. In the first phase, G_1, preparations are made to replicate the genetic material. The cell stops before entering the DNA synthesis phase or S phase to take inventory. Are we ready to replicate our DNA? Is the DNA repair machinery in place to fix any mutations that are detected? Are the DNA replicating enzymes available? Is there an adequate supply of nucleotides? Is there sufficient energy? The main brake on the process is the retinoblastoma protein, Rb. When the cell determines that it is prepared to move ahead, sequential

TABLE 25-1

PHENOTYPIC CHARACTERISTICS OF MALIGNANT CELLS

Deregulated cell proliferation: Loss of function of negative growth regulators (suppressor oncogenes, i.e., Rb, p53), and increased action of positive growth regulators (oncogenes, i.e., *Ras, Myc*). Leads to aberrant cell cycle control and includes loss of normal checkpoint responses.

Failure to differentiate: Arrest at a stage before terminal differentiation. May retain stem cell properties. (Frequently observed in leukemias due to transcriptional repression of developmental programs by the gene products of chromosomal translocations.)

Loss of normal apoptosis pathways: Inactivation of p53, increases in Bcl-2 family members. This defect enhances the survival of cells with oncogenic mutations and genetic instability and allows clonal expansion and diversification within the tumor without activation of physiologic cell death pathways.

Genetic instability: Defects in DNA repair pathways leading to either single or oligo-nucleotide mutations (as in microsatellite instability, MIN) or more commonly chromosomal instability (CIN) leading to aneuploidy. Caused by loss of function of p53, BRCA1/2, mismatch repair genes, DNA repair enzymes, and the spindle checkpoint.

Loss of replicative senescence: Normal cells stop dividing in vitro after 25–50 population doublings. Arrest is mediated by the Rb, $p16^{INK4a}$, and p53 pathways. Further replication leads to telomere loss with crisis. Surviving cells often harbor gross chromosomal abnormalities. Relevance to human in vivo cancer remains uncertain. Many human cancers express telomerase.

Increased angiogenesis: Due to increased gene expression of proangiogenic factors (VEGF, FGF, IL-8) by tumor or stromal cells, or loss of negative regulators (endostatin, tumstatin, thrombospondin).

Invasion: Loss of cell-cell contacts (gap junctions, cadherins) and increased production of matrix metalloproteinases (MMPs). Often takes the form of epithelial-to-mesenchymal transition (EMT), with anchored epithelial cells becoming more like motile fibroblasts.

Metastasis: Spread of tumor cells to lymph nodes or distant tissue sites. Limited by the ability of tumor cells to survive in a foreign environment.

Evasion of the immune system: Downregulation of MHC class I and II molecules; induction of T cell tolerance; inhibition of normal dendritic cell and/or T cell function; antigenic loss variants and clonal heterogeneity; increase in regulatory T cells.

Abbreviations: FGF, fibroblast growth factor; IL, interleukin; MHC, major histocompatibility complex; VEGF, vascular endothelial growth factor.

activation of cyclin-dependent kinases (CDKs) results in the inactivation of the brake, Rb, by phosphorylation. Phosphorylated Rb releases the S-phase-regulating transcription factor, E2F/DP1, and genes required for S phase progression are expressed. If the cell determines that it is unready to move ahead with DNA replication, a number of inhibitors are capable of blocking the action of the CDKs, including $p21^{Cip2/Waf1}$, $p16^{Ink4a}$, and $p27^{Kip1}$. *Nearly every cancer has one or more genetic lesions in the G_1 checkpoint that permits progression to S phase.*

At the end of S phase, when the cell has exactly duplicated its DNA content, a second inventory is taken at the S checkpoint. Have all of the chromosomes been fully duplicated? Were any segments of DNA copied more than once? Do we have the right number of chromosomes and the right amount of DNA? If so, the cell proceeds to G_2, in which the cell prepares for division by synthesizing mitotic spindle and other proteins needed to produce two daughter cells. When DNA damage is detected, the p53 pathway is normally activated. Called the guardian of the genome, p53 is a transcription factor that is normally present in the cell in very low levels. Its level is generally regulated through its rapid turnover. Normally, p53 is bound to mdm2, which transports p53 out of the nucleus for degradation in the proteosome. When damage is sensed, the ATM (ataxia-telangiectasia mutated) pathway is activated; ATM phosphorylates mdm2, which no longer binds to p53, and p53 then stops cell cycle progression and directs the synthesis of repair enzymes, or if the damage is too great, initiates apoptosis of the cell to prevent the propagation of a damaged cell (Fig. 25-1).

A second method of activating p53 involves the induction by oncogenes of $p14^{ARF}$ (p19 in mice). ARF competes with p53 for binding to mdm2, allowing p53 to escape the effects of mdm2 and accumulate in the cell. Then p53 stops cell cycle progression by activating CDK inhibitors such as p21 and/or initiating the apoptosis pathway. Mutations in the gene for p53 on chromosome 17p are found in more than 50% of human cancers. Most commonly these mutations are acquired in the malignant tissue in one allele and the second allele is deleted, leaving the cell unprotected from DNA-damaging agents. Some environmental exposures produce signature mutations in p53; for example, aflatoxin exposure leads to mutation of arginine to serine at codon 249 and leads to hepatocellular carcinoma. In rare instances, p53 mutations are in the germ line (Li-Fraumeni syndrome) and produce a familial cancer syndrome. The absence of p53 leads to chromosome instability and the accumulation of DNA damage, including the acquisition of properties that give the abnormal cell a proliferative and survival advantage. *Like Rb dysfunction, most cancers have mutations that disable the p53 pathway.* Indeed, the importance of p53 and Rb in the development of cancer is underscored by the neoplastic transformation mechanism of human papillomavirus. This virus has two main oncogenes, E6 and E7. E6 acts to increase the rapid turnover of p53, and E7 acts to inhibit Rb function; inhibition of these two targets is sufficient to lead to neoplasia.

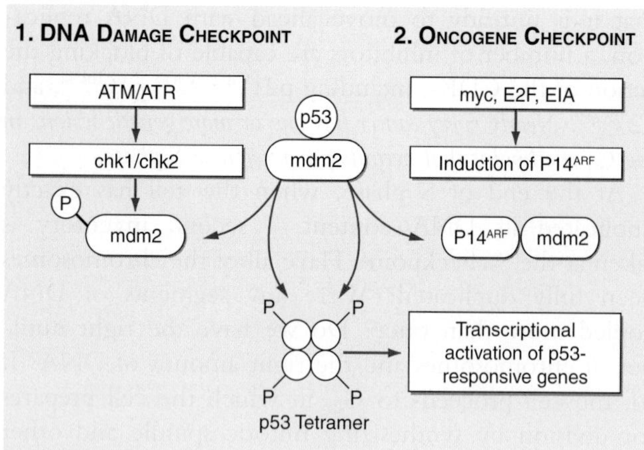

FIGURE 25-1

Induction of p53 by the DNA damage and oncogene checkpoints. In response to noxious stimuli, p53 and mdm2 are phosphorylated by the ataxia-telangiectasia mutated (ATM) and related ATR serine/threonine kinases, as well as the immediate downstream checkpoint kinases, Chk1 and Chk2. This causes dissociation of p53 from mdm2, leading to increased p53 protein levels and transcription of genes leading to cell cycle arrest ($p21^{Cip1/Waf1}$) or apoptosis (e.g., the proapoptotic Bcl-2 family members Noxa and Puma). Inducers of p53 include hypoxemia, DNA damage (caused by ultraviolet radiation, gamma irradiation, or chemotherapy), ribonucleotide depletion, and telomere shortening. A second mechanism of p53 induction is activated by oncogenes such as *Myc*, which promote aberrant G_1/S transition. This pathway is regulated by a second product of the Ink4a locus, $p14^{ARF}$ (p19 in mice), which is encoded by an *a*lternative *r*eading *f*rame of the same stretch of DNA that codes for $p16^{Ink4a}$. Levels of ARF are upregulated by *Myc* and E2F, and ARF binds to mdm2 and rescues p53 from its inhibitory effect. This *oncogene checkpoint* leads to the death or senescence (an irreversible arrest in G_1 of the cell cycle) of renegade cells that attempt to enter S phase without appropriate physiologic signals. Senescent cells have been identified in patients whose premalignant lesions harbor activated oncogenes, for instance, dysplastic nevi that encode an activated form of BRAF (see later discussion), demonstrating that induction of senescence is a protective mechanism that operates in humans to prevent the outgrowth of neoplastic cells.

Another cell cycle checkpoint exists when the cell is undergoing division, the spindle checkpoint. The details of this checkpoint are still being discovered; however, it appears that if the spindle apparatus does not properly align the chromosomes for division, if the chromosome number is abnormal (i.e., > or $<4n$), if the centromeres are not properly paired with their duplicated partners, then the cell initiates a cell death pathway to prevent the production of aneuploid progeny. Abnormalities in the spindle checkpoint facilitate the development of aneuploidy. In some tumors, aneuploidy is a predominant genetic feature. In others, microsatellite instability is the primary genetic lesion. Microsatellite instability arises from defects in DNA mismatch repair genes. In general, tumors either have defects in chromosome number or microsatellite instability but not both. Defects that lead to cancer include abnormal cell cycle checkpoints, inadequate DNA repair, and failure to preserve genome integrity.

Efforts are underway to therapeutically restore the defects in cell cycle regulation that characterize cancer.

CANCER AS AN ORGAN THAT IGNORES ITS NICHE

The fundamental cellular defects that create a malignant neoplasm act at the cellular level. However, that is not the entire story. Cancers behave as organs that have lost their specialized function and stopped responding to signals that normally limit their growth. Human cancers usually become clinically detectable when a primary mass is at least 1 cm in diameter—such a mass consists of about 10^9 cells. More commonly, patients present with tumors that are 10^{10} cells or greater. A lethal tumor burden is about 10^{12} cells. If all tumor cells were dividing at the time of diagnosis, patients would reach a lethal tumor burden in a very short time. However, human tumors grow by Gompertzian kinetics—this means that not every daughter cell produced by a cell division is itself capable of dividing. The growth fraction of a tumor declines exponentially with time. The growth fraction of the first malignant cell is 100%, and by the time a patient presents for medical care, the growth fraction is 2–3% or less. This fraction is similar to the growth fraction of normal bone marrow and normal intestinal epithelium, the most highly proliferative normal tissues in the human body, a fact that may explain the dose-limiting toxicities of agents that target dividing cells.

The implication of these data is that the tumor is slowing its own growth over time. How does it do this? The tumor cells have multiple genetic lesions that tend to promote proliferation, yet by the time the tumor is clinically detectable, its capacity for proliferation has declined. We need to better understand how a tumor stops its own growth. A number of factors can contribute to the failure of tumor cells to proliferate in vivo. Some cells are hypoxemic and have an inadequate supply of nutrients and energy. Some have sustained too much genetic damage to complete the cell cycle and have lost the capacity to undergo apoptosis. However, an important subset is not actively dividing but retains the capacity to divide and starts dividing again when the tumor mass is reduced by treatments. Just as the bone marrow increases its rate of proliferation in response to bone marrow–damaging agents, so too does the tumor seem to sense when the tumor cell numbers have been reduced and responds by increasing its growth rate. However, the marrow stops growing when it has reached its production goals. Tumors do not.

It is not in the long-term interest of a cancer to kill its host. It errs when it overshoots the limits imposed by the organ niche it occupies. Additional tumor cell vulnerabilities are likely to be detected when we learn more about how normal cells respond to "stop" signals from their environment and how tumor cells fail to heed such signals.

IS IN VITRO SENESCENCE RELEVANT TO CARCINOGENESIS?

When normal cells are placed in culture in vitro, most are not capable of sustained growth. Fibroblasts are an exception to this rule. When they are cultured, fibroblasts may divide 30–50 times, and then they undergo what has been termed a "crisis" during which the majority of cells stop dividing (usually due to an increase in p21 expression, a CDK inhibitor), many die, and a small fraction emerge that have acquired genetic changes that permit their uncontrolled growth. The cessation of growth of normal cells in culture has been termed "senescence," and whether this phenomenon is relevant to any physiologic event in vivo is debated.

Among the cellular changes during in vitro propagation is telomere shortening. DNA polymerase is unable to replicate the tips of chromosomes, resulting in the loss of DNA at the specialized ends of chromosomes (called *telomeres*) with each replication cycle. At birth, human telomeres are 15- to 20-kb pairs long and are composed of tandem repeats of a six-nucleotide sequence (TTAGGG) that associates with specialized telomere-binding proteins to form a T-loop structure that protects the ends of chromosomes from being mistakenly recognized as damaged. The loss of telomeric repeats with each cell division cycle causes gradual telomere shortening, leading to growth arrest (called *senescence*) when one or more critically short telomeres trigger a p53-regulated DNA-damage checkpoint response. Cells can bypass this growth arrest if pRb and p53 are nonfunctional, but cell death ensues when the unprotected ends of chromosomes lead to chromosome fusions or other catastrophic DNA rearrangements. *The ability to bypass telomere-based growth limitations is thought to be a critical step in the evolution of most malignancies.* This occurs by the reactivation of telomerase expression in cancer cells. Telomerase is an enzyme that adds TTAGGG repeats onto the 3′ ends of chromosomes. It contains a catalytic subunit with reverse transcriptase activity (hTERT) and an RNA component that provides the template for telomere extension. Most normal somatic cells do not express sufficient telomerase to prevent telomere attrition with each cell division. Exceptions include stem cells (such as those found in hematopoietic tissues, gut and skin epithelium, and germ cells) that require extensive cell division to maintain tissue homeostasis. More than 90% of human cancers express high levels of telomerase that prevent telomere shortening to critical levels and allow indefinite cell proliferation. In vitro experiments indicate that inhibition of telomerase activity leads to tumor cell apoptosis. Major efforts are underway to develop methods to inhibit telomerase activity in cancer cells. The reverse transcriptase activity of telomerase is a prime target for small-molecule pharmaceuticals. In addition, the protein component of telomerase (hTERT) may act as a tumor-associated antigen and be targeted by vaccine approaches.

All of the known functions of telomerase relate to cell division. Thus, it is unclear how short telomeres interfere with the differentiated functions of normal cells. Nevertheless, a major growth industry in medical research has been discovering an association between short telomeres and human diseases ranging from diabetes and coronary artery disease to Alzheimer's disease. The picture is further complicated by the fact that rare genetic defects in the telomerase enzyme seem to cause pulmonary fibrosis but not hematopoietic failure or defects in nutrient absorption in the gut, the sites that might be presumed to be most sensitive to defective cell proliferation. Much remains to be learned about how telomere shortening and telomere maintenance is related to human illness in general and cancer in particular.

SIGNAL TRANSDUCTION PATHWAYS IN CANCER CELLS

Signals that affect cell behavior come from adjacent cells, the stroma in which the cells are located, hormonal signals that originate remotely, and the cells themselves (autocrine signaling). These signals generally exert their influence on the receiving cell through activation of signal transduction pathways that have as their end result the induction of activated transcription factors that mediate a change in cell behavior or function or the acquisition of effector machinery to accomplish a new task. Although signal transduction pathways can lead to a wide variety of outcomes, many such pathways rely on cascades of signals that sequentially activate different proteins or glycoproteins and lipids or glycolipids, and the activation steps often involve the addition or removal of one or more phosphate groups on a downstream target. Other chemical changes can result from signal transduction pathways, but phosphorylation and dephosphorylation play a major role. The protein kinases are generally of two distinct classes; one class acts on tyrosine residues, and the other acts on serine/threonine residues. The tyrosine kinases often play critical roles in signal transduction pathways; they may be receptor tyrosine kinases or may be linked to other cell-surface receptors through associated docking proteins (Fig. 25-2).

Normally, tyrosine kinase activity is short-lived and reversed by protein tyrosine phosphatases (PTPs). However, in many human cancers, tyrosine kinases or components of their downstream pathways are activated by mutation, gene amplification, or chromosomal translocations. Because these pathways regulate proliferation, survival, migration, and angiogenesis, they have been identified as important targets for cancer therapeutics.

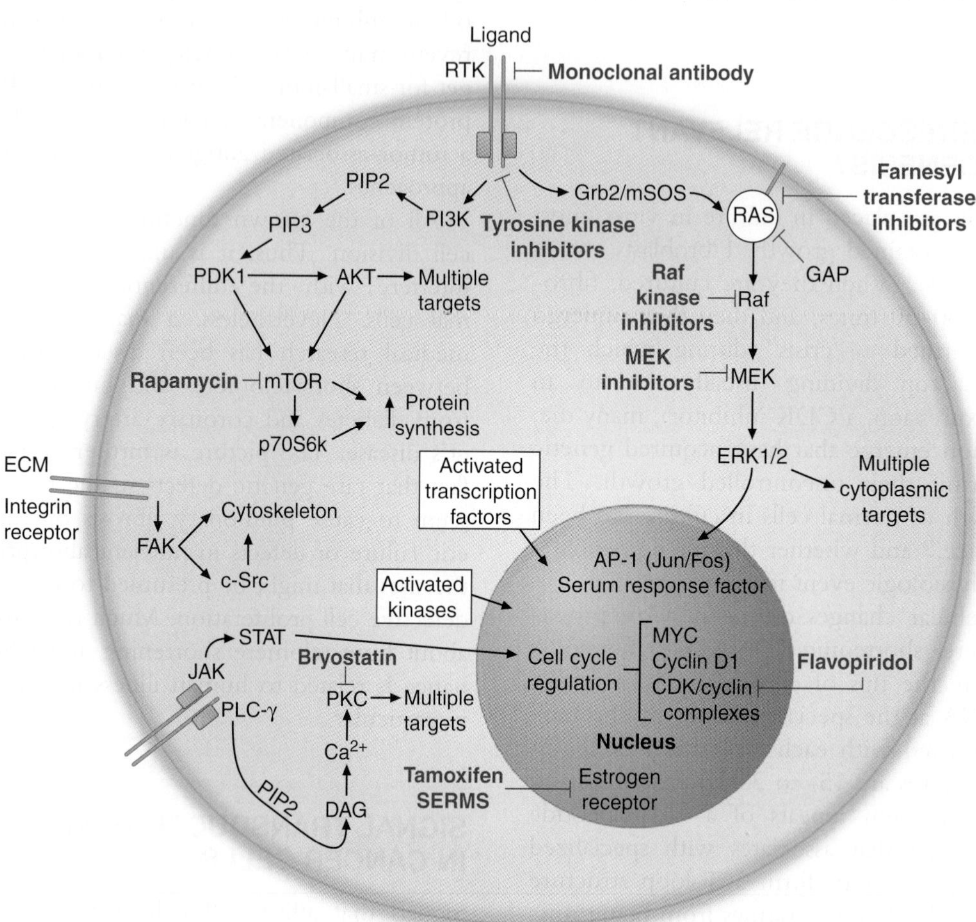

FIGURE 25-2

Therapeutic targeting of signal transduction pathways in cancer cells. Three major signal transduction pathways are activated by receptor tyrosine kinases (RTK). ***1.*** The protooncogene Ras is activated by the Grb2/mSOS guanine nucleotide exchange factor, which induces an association with Raf and activation of downstream kinases (MEK and ERK1/2). ***2.*** Activated PI3K phosphorylates the membrane lipid PIP_2 to generate PIP_3, which acts as a membrane-docking site for a number of cellular proteins including the serine/threonine kinases PDK1 and Akt. PDK1 has numerous cellular targets, including Akt and mTOR. Akt phosphorylates target proteins that promote resistance to apoptosis and enhance cell cycle progression, while mTOR and its target p70S6K upregulate protein synthesis to potentiate cell growth. ***3.*** Activation of PLC-γ leads the formation of diacylglycerol (DAG) and increased intracellular calcium, with activation of multiple isoforms of PKC and other enzymes regulated by the calcium/calmodulin system. Other important signaling pathways involve non-RTKs that are activated by cytokine or integrin receptors. Janus kinases (JAK) phosphorylate STAT (signal transducer and activator of transcription) transcription factors, which translocate to the nucleus and activate target genes. Integrin receptors mediate cellular interactions with the extracellular matrix (ECM), inducing activation of FAK (focal adhesion kinase) and c-Src, which activate multiple downstream pathways, including modulation of the cell cytoskeleton. Many activated kinases and transcription factors migrate into the nucleus, where they regulate gene transcription, thus completing the path from extracellular signals, such as growth factors, to a change in cell phenotype, such as induction of differentiation or cell proliferation. The nuclear targets of these processes include transcription factors (e.g., Myc, AP-1, and serum response factor) and the cell cycle machinery (CDKs and cyclins). Inhibitors of many of these pathways have been developed for the treatment of human cancers. Examples of inhibitors that are currently being evaluated in clinical trials are shown in purple type.

Inhibition of kinase activity is effective in the treatment of a number of neoplasms. Lung cancers with mutations in the epidermal growth factor receptor are highly responsive to erlotinib and gefitinib (Table 25-2). Lung cancers with activation of the anaplastic lymphoma kinase (ALK) respond to crizotinib, an ALK inhibitor. A BRAF inhibitor is highly effective in melanomas and thyroid cancers in which BRAF is overexpressed. Janus kinase inhibitors are active in myeloproliferative syndromes in which JAK2 activation is a pathogenetic event. Imatinib is an effective agent in tumors that overexpress c-Abl (such as chronic myeloid leukemia), c-Kit (gastrointestinal stromal cell tumors), or platelet-derived growth factor receptor (PDGFR; chronic myelomonocytic leukemia); second-generation congeners, dasatinib, and nilotinib are even more effective. Sorafenib and sunitinib, agents that inhibit a large number of kinases, are being widely tested and have shown promising antitumor activity in renal cell cancer and hepatocellular carcinoma. Inhibitors of the mammalian target of rapamycin (mTOR) such as temsirolimus are also active in renal cell cancer. The list of active agents and treatment indications is growing rapidly. These new agents have ushered in a new era

TABLE 25-2

SOME FOOD AND DRUG ADMINSTRATION–APPROVED MOLECULARLY TARGETED AGENTS FOR THE TREATMENT OF CANCER

DRUG	MOLECULAR TARGET	DISEASE	MECHANISM OF ACTION
All-*trans* retinoic acid (ATRA)	PML-RARα oncogene	Acute promyelocytic leukemia M3 AML; t(15;17)	Inhibits transcriptional repression by PML-RARα
Imatinib (Gleevec) Dasatinib (Sprycel) Nilotinib (Tasigna)	Bcr-Abl, c-Abl, c-Kit, PDGFR-α/β	Chronic myeloid leukemia; GIST	Blocks ATP binding to tyrosine kinase active site
Sunitinib (Sutent)	c-Kit, VEGFR-2, PDGFR-β, Flt-3	GIST; renal cell cancer	Inhibits activated c-Kit and PDGFR in GIST; inhibits VEGFR in RCC
Sorafenib (Nexavar)	RAF, VEGFR-2, PDGFR-α/β, Flt-3, c-Kit	RCC; hepatocellular carcinoma	Targets VEGFR pathways in RCC. Possible activity against BRAF in melanoma, colon cancer, and others
Erlotinib (Tarceva)	EGFR	Non–small cell lung cancer; pancreatic cancer	Competitive inhibitor of the ATP-binding site of the EGFR
Gefitinib (Iressa)	EGFR	Non–small cell lung cancer	Inhibitor of EGFR tyrosine kinase
Bortezomib (Velcade)	Proteasome	Multiple myeloma	Inhibits proteolytic degradation of multiple cellular proteins
Monoclonal Antibodies			
Trastuzumab (Herceptin)	HER2/neu (ERBB2)	Breast cancer	Binds HER2 on tumor cell surface and induces receptor internalization
Cetuximab (Erbitux)	EGFR	Colon cancer, squamous cell carcinoma of the head and neck	Binds extracellular domain of EGFR and blocks binding of EGF and TGF-α; induces receptor internalization. Potentiates the efficacy of chemotherapy and radiotherapy
Panitumumab (Vectibix)	EGFR	Colon cancer	Like cetuximab; likely to be very similar in clinical activity
Rituximab (Rituxan)	CD20	B cell lymphomas and leukemias that express CD20	Multiple potential mechanisms, including direct induction of tumor cell apoptosis and immune mechanisms
Alemtuzumab (Campath)	CD52	Chronic lymphocytic leukemia and CD52-expressing lymphoid tumors	Immune mechanisms
Bevacizumab (Avastin)	VEGF	Colon, lung, breast cancers; data pending in other tumors	Inhibits angiogenesis by high-affinity binding to VEGF

Abbreviations: AML, acute myeloid leukemia; ATP, adenosine triphosphate; EGFR, epidermal growth factor receptor; Flt-3, fms-like tyrosine kinase-3; GIST, gastrointestinal stromal tumor; PDGFR, platelet-derived growth factor receptor; PML-RARα, promyelocytic leukemia-retinoic acid receptor-alpha; RCC, renal cell cancer; t(15;17), translocation between chromosomes 15 and 17; TGF-α, transforming growth factor-alpha; VEGFR, vascular endothelial growth factor receptor.

of personalized therapy. It is becoming more routine for resected tumors to be assessed for specific molecular changes that predict response and to have clinical decision-making guided by those results.

However, it must be acknowledged that none of these therapies is curative in any malignancy. The reasons for the failure to cure are not all defined. However, at least some causes of resistance are known. In some tumors, resistance to kinase inhibitors is related to an acquired mutation in the target kinase that inhibits drug binding. Many of these kinase inhibitors act as competitive inhibitors of the adenosine triphosphate (ATP)–binding pocket. ATP is the phosphate donor in these phosphorylation reactions. Mutation in the BCR-ABL kinase in the ATP–binding pocket (such as the tyrosine to isoleucine change at codon 315) can prevent imatinib binding. Other resistance mechanisms include altering other signal transduction pathways to bypass the inhibited pathway. Some kinase inhibitors are less specific for an oncogenic target than was hoped, and toxicities related to off-target kinase inhibition limit the use of the agent at a dose that would inhibit the cancer-relevant kinase. As resistance mechanisms become better defined, rational strategies to overcome resistance will emerge.

Another strategy to enhance the antitumor effects of targeted agents is to use them in rational combinations with each other and in empiric combinations with chemotherapy agents that kill cells in ways distinct from targeted agents. For example, in the c-Kit overexpressing gastrointestinal stromal tumor (GIST), resistance to imatinib develops due to secondary mutations in c-Kit, and many of these tumors are susceptible to treatment with the multitargeted tyrosine kinase (TK) inhibitor sunitinib that has activity against c-Kit as well as the PDGF and vascular endothelial growth factor (VEGF) receptors. Sunitinib is approved by the U.S. Food and Drug Administration (FDA) for treatment of patients with imatinib-resistant GIST or who are intolerant of imatinib (Table 25-2). Interestingly, tumors with mutations in exon 11 of c-Kit's juxtamembrane region are particularly sensitive to imatinib, whereas those with exon 9 mutations (extracellular domain) respond better to sunitinib than imatinib. In the future, primary therapy for GIST may be determined by the specific molecular defect in c-Kit.

While targeted therapies have not yet resulted in cures when used alone, their use in the adjuvant setting and when combined with other effective treatments has substantially increased the fraction of patients cured. For example, the addition of rituximab, an anti-CD20 antibody, to combination chemotherapy in patients with diffuse large B-cell lymphoma improves cure rates by 15–20%. The addition of trastuzumab, antibody to HER2, to combination chemotherapy in the adjuvant treatment of HER2-positive breast cancer reduces relapse rates by 50%.

Targeted therapies are being developed for the ras/mitogen-activated protein (MAP) kinase pathways, the hedgehog pathway, various angiogenesis pathways, and phospholipid signaling pathways such as the phosphatidylinositol-3-kinase (PI3K) and phospholipase C-gamma pathways, which are involved in a large number of cellular processes that are important in cancer development and progression.

One of the strategies for new drug development is to take advantage of so-called oncogene addiction. This situation (Fig. 25-3) is created when a tumor cell develops an activating mutation in an oncogene that becomes a dominant pathway with reduced contributions from auxiliary pathways. This dependency on a single pathway creates a cell that is vulnerable to inhibitors of the oncogene pathway. For example, cells harboring mutations in *BRAF* are very sensitive to MEK inhibitors.

Many transcription factors are activated by phosphorylation, which can be prevented by tyrosine- or serine/threonine kinase inhibitors. The transcription factor NF-κB is a heterodimer composed of p65 and p50 subunits that associate with an inhibitor, IκB, in the cell cytoplasm. In response to growth factor or cytokine signaling, a multi-subunit kinase called IKK (IκB-kinase) phosphorylates IκB and directs its degradation by the ubiquitin/proteasome system. NF-κB, free of its inhibitor, translocates to the nucleus and activates target genes, many of which promote the survival of tumor cells. Novel drugs called *proteasome inhibitors* block the proteolysis of IκB, thereby preventing NF-κB activation. For unexplained reasons, this is selectively toxic to tumor cells. The antitumor effects of proteasome inhibitors are more complicated and involve the inhibition of the degradation of multiple cellular proteins. Proteasome inhibitors (bortezomib [Velcade]) have activity in patients with multiple myeloma, including partial and complete remissions. Inhibitors of IKK are also in development, with the hope of more selectively blocking the degradation of IκB, thus "locking" NF-κB in an inhibitory complex and rendering the cancer cell more susceptible to apoptosis-inducing agents.

Estrogen receptors (ERs) and androgen receptors, members of the steroid hormone family of nuclear receptors, are targets of inhibition by drugs used to treat breast and prostate cancers, respectively. Tamoxifen, a partial agonist and antagonist of ER function, can mediate tumor regression in metastatic breast cancer and can prevent disease recurrence in the adjuvant setting. Tamoxifen binds to the ER and modulates its transcriptional activity, inhibiting activity in the breast but promoting activity in bone and uterine epithelium. Selective estrogen receptor modulators (SERMs) have been developed with the hope of a more beneficial modulation of ER activity, i.e., antiestrogenic activity in the breast, uterus, and ovary, but estrogenic

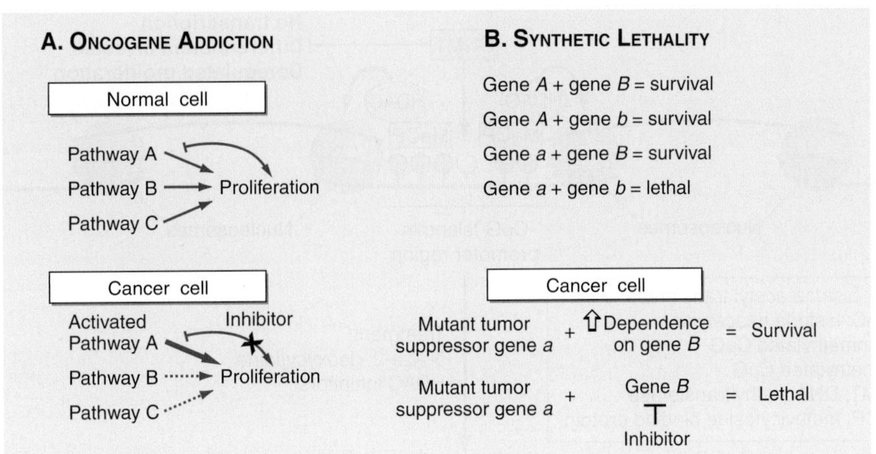

FIGURE 25-3

Oncogene addiction and synthetic lethality: keys to discovery of new anticancer drugs. *A.* Normal cells receive environmental signals that activate signaling pathways (pathways A, B, and C) that together promote G_1 to S phase transition and passage through the cell cycle. Inhibition of one pathway (such as pathway A by a targeted inhibitor) has no significant effect due to redundancy provided by pathways B and C. In cancer cells, oncogenic mutations lead over time to dependency on the activated pathway, with loss of significant input from pathways B and C. The dependency or addiction of the cancer cell to pathway A makes it highly vulnerable to inhibitors that target components of this pathway. Clinically relevant examples include Bcr-Abl (CML), amplified HER2/*neu* (breast cancer), overexpressed or mutated EGF receptors (lung cancer), and mutated *BRAF* (melanoma). ***B.*** Genes are said to have a synthetic lethal relationship when mutation of either gene alone is tolerated by the cell but mutation of both genes leads to lethality. Thus, in the example, mutant *gene a* and *gene b* have a synthetic lethal relationship, implying that the loss of one gene makes the cell dependent on the function of the other gene. In cancer cells, loss of function of a tumor-suppressor gene (wild-type designated *gene A*; mutant designated *gene a*) may render the cancer cells dependent on an alternative pathway of which *gene B* is a component. As shown in the figure, if an inhibitor of *gene B* can be identified, this can cause death of the cancer cell, without harming normal cells (which maintain wild-type function for *gene A*). High-throughput screens can now be performed using isogenic cell line pairs in which one cell line has a defined defect in a tumor-suppressor pathway. Compounds can be identified that selectively kill the mutant cell line; targets of these compounds have a synthetic lethal relationship to the tumor-suppressor pathway and are potentially important targets for future therapeutics. Note that this approach allows discovery of drugs that indirectly target deleted tumor-suppressor genes and hence greatly expands the list of physiologically relevant cancer targets.

for bone, brain, and cardiovascular tissues. Aromatase inhibitors, which block the conversion of androgens to estrogens in breast and subcutaneous fat tissues, have demonstrated improved clinical efficacy compared with tamoxifen and are often used as first-line therapy in patients with ER-positive disease (Chap. 37).

EPIGENETIC INFLUENCES ON CANCER GENE TRANSCRIPTION

Chromatin structure regulates the hierarchical order of sequential gene transcription that governs differentiation and tissue homeostasis. Disruption of chromatin remodeling leads to aberrant gene expression and can induce proliferation of undifferentiated cells. *Epigenetics* is defined as changes that alter the pattern of gene expression that persist across at least one cell division but are not caused by changes in the DNA code. Epigenetic changes include alterations of chromatin structure mediated by methylation of cytosine residues in CpG dinucleotides, modification of histones by acetylation or methylation, or changes in higher-order chromosome structure (Fig. 25-4). The transcriptional regulatory regions of active genes often contain a high frequency of CpG dinucleotides (referred to as *CpG islands*), which are normally unmethylated. Expression of these genes is controlled by transient association with repressor or activator proteins that regulate transcriptional activation. However, hypermethylation of promoter regions is a common mechanism by which tumor-suppressor loci are epigenetically silenced in cancer cells. Thus, one allele may be inactivated by mutation or deletion (as occurs in loss of heterozygosity), while expression of the other allele is epigenetically silenced. The mechanisms that target tumor-suppressor genes for this form of gene silencing are unknown.

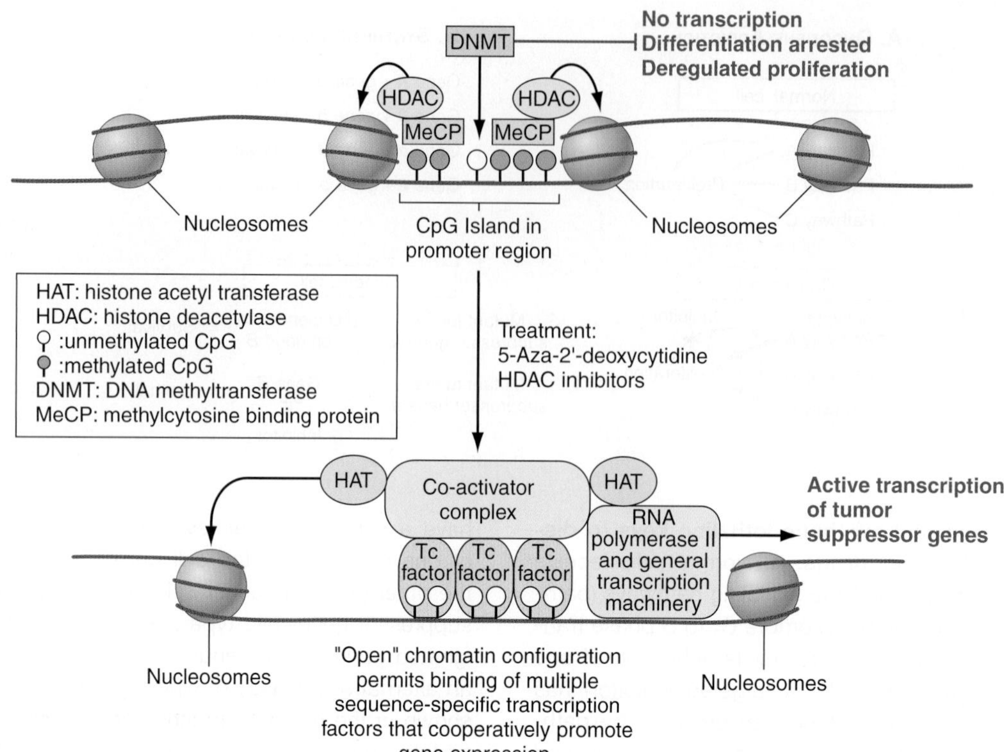

FIGURE 25-4

Epigenetic regulation of gene expression in cancer cells. Tumor-suppressor genes are often epigenetically silenced in cancer cells. In the upper portion, a CpG island within the promoter and enhancer regions of the gene has been methylated, resulting in the recruitment of methyl-cytosine binding proteins (MeCP) and complexes with histone deacetylase (HDAC) activity. Chromatin is in a condensed, nonpermissive conformation that inhibits transcription. Clinical trials are under way utilizing the combination of demethylating agents such as 5-aza-2′-deoxycytidine plus HDAC inhibitors, which together confer an open, permissive chromatin structure (*lower portion*). Transcription factors bind to specific DNA sequences in promoter regions and, through protein–protein interactions, recruit coactivator complexes containing histone acetyl transferase (HAT) activity. This enhances transcription initiation by RNA polymerase II and associated general transcription factors. The expression of the tumor-suppressor gene commences, with phenotypic changes that may include growth arrest, differentiation, or apoptosis.

Acetylation of the amino terminus of the core histones H3 and H4 induces an open chromatin conformation that promotes transcription initiation. Histone acetylases are components of coactivator complexes recruited to promoter/enhancer regions by sequence-specific transcription factors during the activation of genes (Fig. 25-4). Histone deacetylases (HDACs; at least 17 are encoded in the human genome) are recruited to genes by transcriptional repressors and prevent the initiation of gene transcription. Methylated cytosine residues in promoter regions become associated with methyl cytosine–binding proteins that recruit protein complexes with HDAC activity. The balance between permissive and inhibitory chromatin structure is therefore largely determined by the activity of transcription factors in modulating the "histone code" and the methylation status of the genetic regulatory elements of genes.

The pattern of gene transcription is aberrant in all human cancers, and in many cases, epigenetic events are responsible. Unlike genetic events that alter DNA primary structure (e.g., deletions), epigenetic changes are potentially reversible and appear amenable to therapeutic intervention. In certain human cancers, including pancreatic cancer and multiple myeloma, the $p16^{Ink4a}$ promoter is inactivated by methylation, thus permitting the unchecked activity of CDK4/cyclin D and rendering pRb nonfunctional. In sporadic forms of renal, breast, and colon cancer, the von Hippel–Lindau (*VHL*), breast cancer 1 (*BRCA1*), and serine/threonine kinase 11 (*STK11*) genes, respectively, are epigenetically silenced. Other targeted genes include the $p15^{Ink4b}$ CDK inhibitor, glutathione-S-transferase (which detoxifies reactive oxygen species), and the E-cadherin molecule (important for junction formation between epithelial cells). Epigenetic silencing can occur in premalignant lesions and can affect genes involved in DNA repair, thus predisposing to further genetic damage. Examples include MLH1 (mut L homologue) in hereditary nonpolyposis colon cancer (HNPCC, also called Lynch's syndrome), which is critical for repair of mismatched bases that occur during DNA synthesis, and O^6-methylguanine-DNA methyltransferase, which removes alkylated guanine adducts from DNA and is often silenced in colon, lung, and lymphoid tumors.

Human leukemias often have chromosomal translocations that code for novel fusion proteins with enzymatic activities that alter chromatin structure. The promyelocytic leukemia–retinoic acid receptor (PML-RAR) fusion protein, generated by the t(15;17) observed in most cases of acute promyelocytic leukemia (APL), binds to promoters containing retinoic acid response elements and recruits HDAC to these promoters, effectively inhibiting gene expression. This arrests differentiation at the promyelocyte stage and promotes tumor cell proliferation and survival. Treatment with pharmacologic doses of all-*trans* retinoic acid (ATRA), the ligand for RARα, results in the release of HDAC activity and the recruitment of coactivators, which overcome the differentiation block. This induced differentiation of APL cells has improved treatment of these patients but also has led to a novel treatment toxicity when newly differentiated tumor cells infiltrate the lungs. However, ATRA represents a treatment paradigm for the reversal of epigenetic changes in cancer. For other leukemia-associated fusion proteins, such as acute myeloid leukemia (AML)-eight-twenty-one (ETO) and the MLL fusion proteins seen in AML and ALL, no ligand is known. Therefore, efforts are ongoing to determine the structural basis for interactions between translocation fusion proteins and chromatin-remodeling proteins and to use this information to rationally design small molecules that will disrupt specific protein–protein associations. Drugs that block the enzymatic activity of HDAC are being tested. HDAC inhibitors have demonstrated antitumor activity in clinical studies against cutaneous T cell lymphoma (e.g., vorinostat) and some solid tumors. HDAC inhibitors may target cancer cells via a number of mechanisms, including upregulation of death receptors (DR4/5 and FAS and their ligands) and $p21^{Cip1/Waf1}$, as well as inhibition of cell cycle checkpoints.

Efforts are also under way to reverse the hypermethylation of CpG islands that characterizes many solid tumors. Drugs that induce DNA demethylation, such as 5-aza-2′-deoxycytidine, can lead to reexpression of silenced genes in cancer cells with restoration of function. However, 5-aza-2′-deoxycytidine has limited aqueous solubility and is myelosuppressive. Other inhibitors of DNA methyltransferases are in development. In ongoing clinical trials, inhibitors of DNA methylation are being combined with HDAC inhibitors. The hope is that by reversing coexisting epigenetic changes, the deregulated patterns of gene transcription in cancer cells will be at least partially reversed.

Another epigenetic form of gene regulation is microRNAs. These are short (average 22 nucleotides in length) RNA molecules that silence gene expression after transcription by binding and inhibiting the translation or promoting the degradation of mRNA transcripts. It is estimated that more than 1000 microRNAs are encoded in the human genome. Each tissue has a distinctive repertoire of microRNA expression, and this pattern is altered in specific ways in cancers. However, specific correlations between microRNA expression and tumor biology and clinical behavior are just now emerging. Therapies targeting microRNAs are not currently at hand but represent a novel area of treatment development.

APOPTOSIS

Tissue homeostasis requires a balance between the death of aged, terminally differentiated cells and their renewal by proliferation of committed progenitors. Genetic damage to growth-regulating genes of stem cells could lead to catastrophic results for the host as a whole. However, genetic events causing activation of oncogenes or loss of tumor suppressors, which would be predicted to lead to unregulated cell proliferation, may instead activate signal transduction pathways that block aberrant cell proliferation. These pathways can lead to programmed cell death (*apoptosis*) or irreversible growth arrest (*senescence*). Much as a panoply of intra- and extracellular signals impinge upon the core cell cycle machinery to regulate cell division, so too these signals are transmitted to a core enzymatic machinery that regulates cell death and survival.

Apoptosis is induced by two main pathways (Fig. 25-5). The extrinsic pathway of apoptosis is activated by cross-linking members of the tumor necrosis factor (TNF) receptor superfamily, such as CD95 (Fas) and death receptors DR4 and DR5, by their ligands, Fas ligand or TRAIL (TNF-related apoptosis-inducing ligand), respectively. This induces the association of FADD (Fas-associated death domain) and procaspase-8 to death domain motifs of the receptors. Caspase-8 is activated and then cleaves and activates effector caspases-3 and -7, which then target cellular constituents (including caspase-activated DNAse, cytoskeletal proteins, and a number of regulatory proteins), inducing the morphologic appearance characteristic of apoptosis, which pathologists term "karyorrhexis." The intrinsic pathway of apoptosis is initiated by the release of cytochrome c and SMAC (second mitochondrial activator of caspases) from the mitochondrial intermembrane

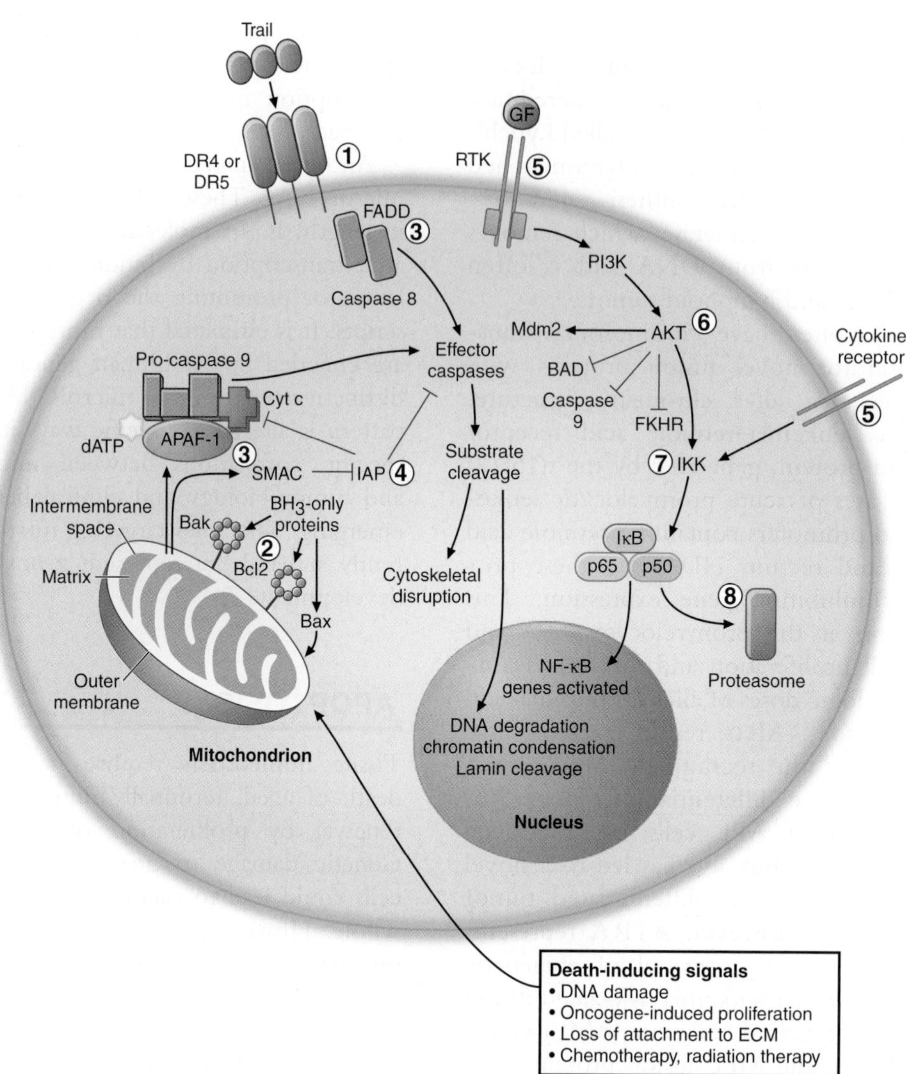

FIGURE 25-5

Therapeutic strategies to overcome aberrant survival pathways in cancer cells. ***1.*** The extrinsic pathway of apoptosis can be selectively induced in cancer cells by TRAIL (the ligand for death receptors 4 and 5) or by agonistic monoclonal antibodies. ***2.*** Inhibition of antiapoptotic Bcl-2 family members with antisense oligonucleotides or inhibitors of the BH_3-binding pocket will promote formation of Bak- or Bax-induced pores in the mitochondrial outer membrane. ***3.*** Epigenetic silencing of APAF-1, caspase-8, and other proteins can be overcome using demethylating agents and inhibitors of histone deacetylases. ***4.*** Inhibitor of apoptosis proteins (IAP) blocks activation of caspases; small-molecule inhibitors of IAP function (mimicking SMAC action) should lower the threshold for apoptosis. ***5.*** Signal transduction pathways originating with activation of receptor tyrosine kinase receptors (RTKs) or cytokine receptors promote survival of cancer cells by a number of mechanisms. Inhibiting receptor function with monoclonal antibodies, such as trastuzumab or cetuximab, or inhibiting kinase activity with small-molecule inhibitors can block the pathway. ***6.*** The Akt kinase phosphorylates many regulators of apoptosis to promote cell survival; inhibitors of Akt may render tumor cells more sensitive to apoptosis-inducing signals; however, the possibility of toxicity to normal cells may limit the therapeutic value of these agents. ***7*** and ***8.*** Activation of the transcription factor NF-κB (composed of p65 and p50 subunits) occurs when its inhibitor, IκB, is phosphorylated by IκB-kinase (IKK), with subsequent degradation of IκB by the proteasome. Inhibition of IKK activity should selectively block the activation of NF-κB target genes, many of which promote cell survival. Inhibitors of proteasome function are approved by the Food and Drug Administration and may work in part by preventing destruction of IκB, thus blocking NF-κB nuclear localization. NF-κB is unlikely to be the only target for proteasome inhibitors. SMAC, small mitochondrial activator of caspases; TRAIL, TNF-related apoptosis-inducing ligand; APAP-1, apoptotic protease activating factor.

space in response to a variety of noxious stimuli, including DNA damage, loss of adherence to the extracellular matrix (ECM), oncogene-induced proliferation, and growth factor deprivation. Upon release into the cytoplasm, cytochrome c associates with dATP, procaspase-9, and the adaptor protein APAF-1, leading to the sequential activation of caspase-9 and effector caspases. SMAC binds to and blocks the function of inhibitor of apoptosis proteins (IAP), negative regulators of caspase activation.

The release of apoptosis-inducing proteins from the mitochondria is regulated by pro- and antiapoptotic members of the Bcl-2 family. Antiapoptotic members (e.g., Bcl-2, Bcl-XL, and Mcl-1) associate with the mitochondrial outer membrane via their carboxyl termini, exposing to the cytoplasm a hydrophobic binding pocket composed of Bcl-2 homology (BH) domains 1, 2, and 3 that is crucial for their activity. Perturbations of normal physiologic processes in specific cellular compartments lead to the activation of BH3-only proapoptotic family members (such as Bad, Bim, Bid, Puma, Noxa, and others) that can alter the conformation of the outer-membrane proteins Bax and Bak, which then oligomerize to form pores in the mitochondrial outer membrane resulting in cytochrome c release. If proteins comprised only by BH3 domains are sequestered by Bcl-2, Bcl-XL, or Mcl-1, pores do not form and apoptosis-inducing proteins are not released from the mitochondria. The ratio of levels of antiapoptotic Bcl-2 family members and the levels of proapoptotic BH3-only proteins at the mitochondrial membrane determines the activation state of the intrinsic pathway. The mitochondrion must therefore be recognized not only as an organelle with vital roles in intermediary metabolism and oxidative phosphorylation but also as a central regulatory structure of the apoptotic process.

The evolution of tumor cells to a more malignant phenotype requires the acquisition of genetic changes that subvert apoptosis pathways and promote cancer cell survival and resistance to anticancer therapies. However, cancer cells may be more vulnerable than normal cells to therapeutic interventions that target the apoptosis pathways that cancer cells depend upon. For instance, overexpression of Bcl-2 as a result of the t(14;18) translocation contributes to follicular lymphoma. Upregulation of Bcl-2 expression is also observed in prostate, breast, and lung cancers and melanoma. Targeting of antiapoptotic Bcl-2 family members has been accomplished by the identification of several low-molecular-weight compounds that bind to the hydrophobic pockets of either Bcl-2 or Bcl-XL and block their ability to associate with death-inducing BH3-only proteins. These compounds inhibit the antiapoptotic activities of Bcl-2 and Bcl-XL at nanomolar concentrations in the laboratory and are entering clinical trials.

Preclinical studies targeting death receptors DR4 and -5 have demonstrated that recombinant, soluble, human TRAIL or humanized monoclonal antibodies with agonist activity against DR4 or -5 can induce apoptosis of tumor cells while sparing normal cells. The mechanisms for this selectivity may include expression of decoy receptors or elevated levels of intracellular inhibitors (such as FLIP, which competes with caspase-8 for FADD) by normal cells but not tumor cells. Synergy has been shown between TRAIL-induced apoptosis and chemotherapeutic agents. For instance, some colon cancers encode mutated Bax protein as the result of mismatch repair (MMR) defects and are resistant to TRAIL. However, upregulation of Bak by chemotherapy restores the ability of TRAIL to activate the mitochondrial pathway of apoptosis. However, clinical studies have not yet shown that clinical activity correlates with activation of the extrinsic pathway of apoptosis.

Many of the signal transduction pathways perturbed in cancer promote tumor cell survival (Fig. 25-5). These include activation of the PI3K/Akt pathway, increased levels of the NF-κB transcription factor, and epigenetic silencing of genes such as APAF-1 and caspase-8. Each of these pathways is a target for therapeutic agents that, in addition to affecting cancer cell proliferation or gene expression, may render cancer cells more susceptible to apoptosis, thus promoting synergy when combined with other chemotherapeutic agents.

Some tumor cells resist drug-induced apoptosis by expression of one or more members of the ABC family of ATP-dependent efflux pumps that mediate the multidrug-resistance (MDR) phenotype. The prototype, P-glycoprotein (PGP), spans the plasma membrane 12 times and has two ATP-binding sites. Hydrophobic drugs (e.g., anthracyclines and vinca alkaloids) are recognized by PGP as they enter the cell and are pumped out. Numerous clinical studies have failed to demonstrate that drug resistance can be overcome using inhibitors of PGP. However, ABC transporters have different substrate specificities, and inhibition of a single family member may not be sufficient to overcome the MDR phenotype. Efforts to reverse PGP-mediated drug resistance continue.

METASTASIS

The three major features of tissue invasion are cell adhesion to the basement membrane, local proteolysis of the membrane, and movement of the cell through the rent in the membrane and the ECM. Malignant cells that gain access to the circulation must then repeat those steps at a remote site, find a hospitable niche in a foreign tissue, avoid detection by host defenses, and induce the growth of new blood vessels. Few drugs directly target the process of metastasis. Metalloproteinase inhibitors (see "Tumor Angiogenesis;" see later discussion) represent an initial attempt to inhibit the migration of tumor cells into blood and lymphatic vessels. The rate-limiting step for metastasis is the ability for tumor cells to survive and expand in the novel microenvironment of the metastatic site, and multiple host–tumor interactions determine the ultimate outcome (Fig. 25-6).

The metastatic phenotype is likely restricted to a small fraction of tumor cells (Fig. 25-6). Some data

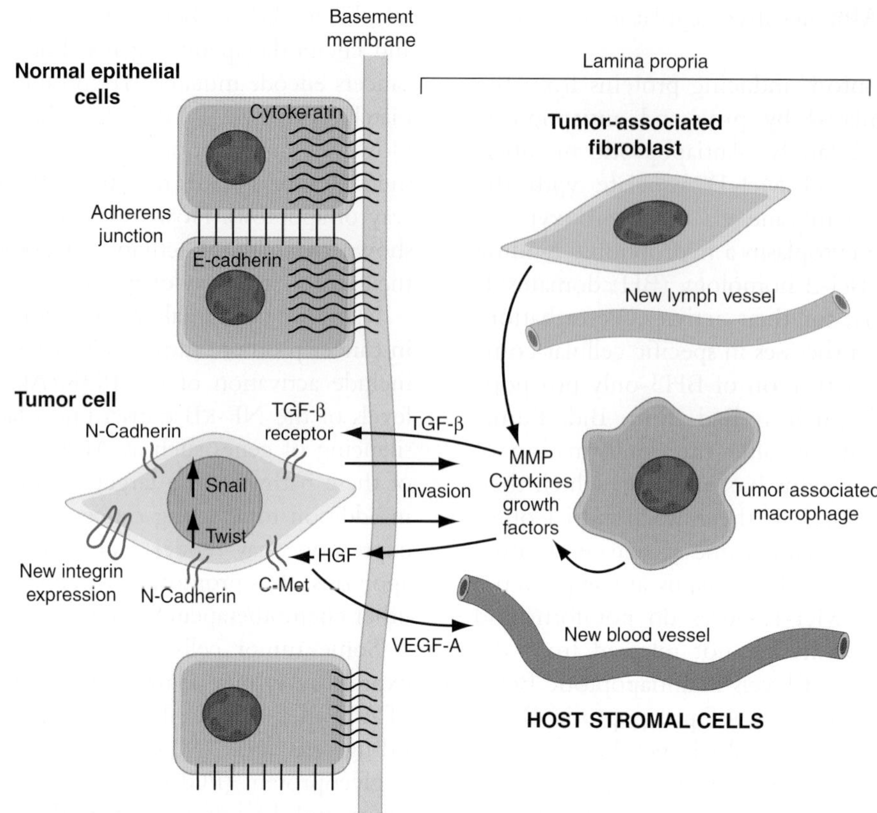

FIGURE 25-6

Oncogene signaling pathways are activated during tumor progression and promote metastatic potential. This figure shows a cancer cell that has undergone epithelial to mesenchymal transition (EMT) under the influence of several environmental signals. Critical components include activated transforming growth factor beta (TGF-β) and the hepatocyte growth factor (HGF)/c-Met pathways, as well as changes in the expression of adhesion molecules that mediate cell–cell and cell–extracellular matrix interactions. Important changes in gene expression are mediated by the Snail and Twist family of transcriptional repressors (whose expression is induced by the oncogenic pathways), leading to reduced expression of E-cadherin, a key component of adherens junctions between epithelial cells. This, in conjunction with upregulation of N-cadherin, a change in the pattern of expression of integrins (which mediate cell–extracellular matrix associations that are important for cell motility), and a switch in intermediate filament expression from cytokeratin to vimentin, results in the phenotypic change from adherent highly organized epithelial cells to motile and invasive cells with a fibroblast or mesenchymal morphology. EMT is thought to be an important step leading to metastasis in some human cancers. Host stromal cells, including tumor-associated fibroblasts and macrophages, play an important role in modulating tumor cell behavior through secretion of growth factors and proangiogenic cytokines, and matrix metalloproteinases that degrade the basement membrane. Vascular endothelial growth factor (VEGF)-A, -C, and -D are produced by tumor cells and stromal cells in response to hypoxemia or oncogenic signals and induce production of new blood vessels and lymphatic channels through which tumor cells metastasize to lymph nodes or tissues.

suggest that cells with the appropriate capability express chemokine receptors. A number of candidate metastasis-suppressor genes have been identified. The loss of function of these genes enhances metastasis, and although the molecular mechanisms are in many cases uncertain, one common theme is enhancing the ability of the metastatic tumor cells to overcome apoptosis signals. Gene expression profiling is being used to study the metastatic process and other properties of tumor cells that may predict susceptibilities.

Bone metastases are extremely painful, cause fractures of weight-bearing bones, can lead to hypercalcemia, and are a major cause of morbidity for cancer patients. Osteoclasts and their monocyte-derived precursors express the surface receptor RANK (receptor activator of NF-κB), which is required for terminal differentiation and activation of osteoclasts. Osteoblasts and other stromal cells express RANK ligand, as both a membrane-bound and soluble cytokine. Osteoprotegerin (OPG), a soluble receptor for RANK ligand produced by stromal cells, acts as a decoy receptor to inhibit RANK activation. The relative balance of RANK ligand and OPG determines the activation state of RANK on osteoclasts. Many tumors increase osteoclast activity by secretion of substances such as parathyroid hormone (PTH), PTH-related peptide, interleukin (IL)-1, or Mip1 that perturb the homeostatic balance of bone remodeling by increasing RANK signaling. One example is multiple myeloma, in which tumor cell–stromal cell interactions activate osteoclasts and inhibit osteoblasts, leading to the development of multiple lytic bone lesions. Inhibition of RANK ligand by an antibody (denosumab) can prevent further bone destruction. Bisphosphonates are also effective inhibitors of osteoclast function that are used in the treatment of cancer patients with bone metastases.

CANCER STEM CELLS

Only a small proportion of the cells within a tumor are capable of initiating colonies in vitro or forming tumors at high efficiency when injected into immunocompromised nonobese diabetic/severe combined immunodeficiency (NOD/SCID) mice. Acute and chronic myeloid leukemias (AML and CML) have a small population of cells (<1%) that have properties of stem cells, such as unlimited self-renewal and the capacity to cause leukemia when serially transplanted in mice. These cells have an undifferentiated phenotype (Thy1 $CD34^+CD38^-$ and do not express other differentiation markers) and resemble normal stem cells in many ways but are no longer under homeostatic control (Fig. 25-7). Solid tumors may also contain a population of stem cells. Cancer stem cells, like their normal counterparts, have unlimited proliferative capacity and paradoxically traverse the cell cycle at a very slow rate; cancer growth occurs largely due to expansion of the stem cell pool, unregulated proliferation of an amplifying population, and failure of apoptosis pathways (Fig. 25-7). Slow cell cycle progression and high levels of expression of antiapoptotic Bcl-2 family members and drug efflux pumps of the MDR family render cancer stem cells less vulnerable to cancer chemotherapy or radiation therapy. Implicit in the cancer stem cell hypothesis is the idea that failure to cure most human cancers is due to the fact that current therapeutic agents do not kill the stem cells. If cancer stem cells can be identified and isolated, then aberrant signaling pathways that distinguish these cells from normal tissue stem cells can be identified and targeted.

ONCOGENE ADDICTION AND SYNTHETIC LETHALITY

The concepts of oncogene addiction and synthetic lethality have spurred new drug development targeting oncogene- and tumor-suppressor pathways. As discussed earlier in this chapter and outlined in Fig. 25-3, cancer cells become dependent upon signaling pathways containing activated oncogenes; this can effect proliferation (i.e., mutated Ras, BRAF, overexpressed Myc, or activated tyrosine kinases), survival (overexpression of Bcl-2 or NF-κB), cell metabolism (as occurs when hypoxemia-inducible factor (HIF)-1α and Akt increase dependence on glycolysis), and perhaps angiogenesis (production of VEGF, e.g., renal cell cancer). In such cases, targeted inhibition of the pathway can lead to specific killing of the cancer cells. However, targeting defects in tumor-suppressor genes has been much more difficult, since the target of the mutation is often deleted. However, identifying genes that have a synthetic lethal relationship to tumor-suppressor pathways may allow targeting of proteins required uniquely by the tumor cells (Fig. 25-3, *B*). Several examples of this have been identified. For instance, the von Hippel–Lindau tumor-suppressor protein is inactivated in 60% of renal cell cancers, leading to overexpression of HIF-1α and the subsequent activation of downstream genes that promote angiogenesis, proliferation, survival, and altered glucose metabolism. HIF-1α mRNA has a complex 5′-terminus that indirectly requires the activity of mTOR (via activation of p70S6K and inhibition of 4E-BP) for efficient protein translation. Inhibitors of mTOR block HIF-1α translation and have significant clinical activity in renal cell cancer. In this case, mTOR is synthetic lethal to VHL loss (Fig. 25-3), and its inhibition results in selective killing of cancer cells. Conceptually, this provides a framework for genetic screens to identify other synthetic lethal combinations involving known tumor-suppressor genes and development of novel therapeutic agents to target dependent pathways.

TUMOR ANGIOGENESIS

The growth of primary and metastatic tumors to larger than a few millimeters requires the recruitment of blood vessels and vascular endothelial cells to support their metabolic requirements. The diffusion limit for oxygen in tissues is ~100 mm. A critical element in the growth of primary tumors and formation of metastatic sites is the *angiogenic switch*: the ability of the tumor to promote the formation of new capillaries from preexisting host vessels. The angiogenic switch is a phase in tumor development when the dynamic balance of pro- and antiangiogenic factors is tipped in favor of vessel formation by the effects of the tumor on its immediate environment. Stimuli for tumor angiogenesis include hypoxemia, inflammation, and genetic lesions in oncogenes or tumor suppressors that alter tumor cell gene expression. Angiogenesis consists of several steps,

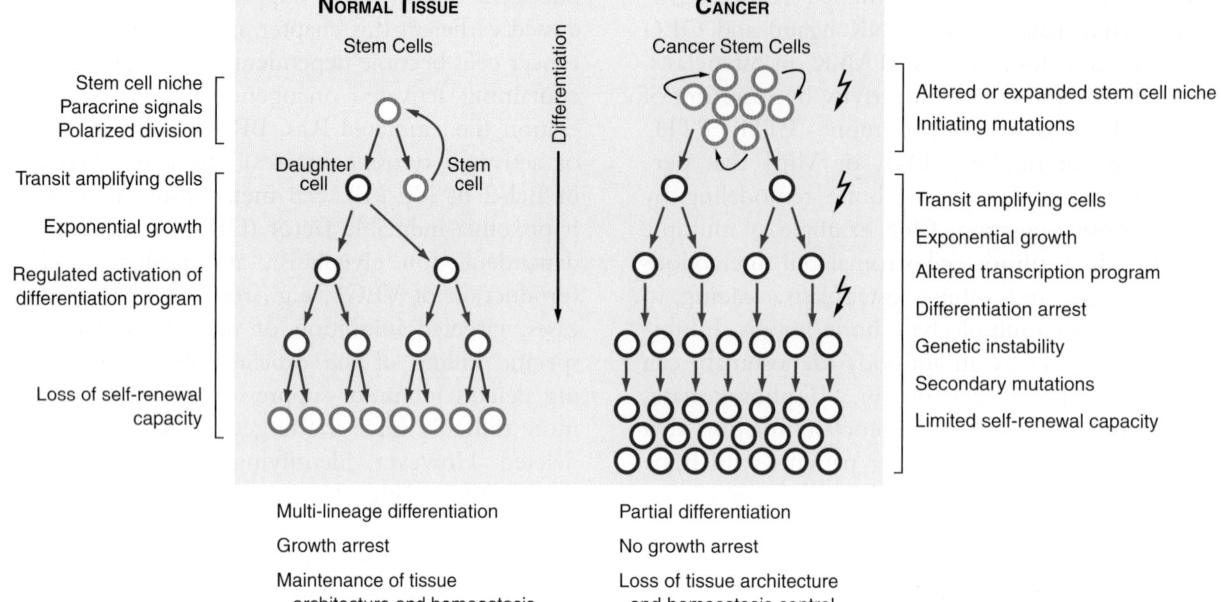

FIGURE 25-7

Cancer stem cells play a critical role in the initiation, progression, and resistance to therapy of malignant neoplasms. In normal tissues (left), homeostasis is maintained by asymmetric division of stem cells, leading to one progeny cell that will differentiate and one cell that will maintain the stem cell pool. This occurs within highly specific niches unique to each tissue, such as in close apposition to osteoblasts in bone marrow, or at the base of crypts in the colon. Here, paracrine signals from stromal cells, such as sonic hedgehog or Notch-ligands, as well as upregulation of β-catenin and telomerase, help to maintain stem cell features of unlimited self-renewal while preventing differentiation or cell death. This occurs in part through upregulation of the transcriptional repressor Bmi-1 and inhibition of the p16^{Ink4a}/Arf and p53 pathways. Daughter cells leave the stem cells niche and enter a proliferative phase (referred to as *transit-amplifying*) for a specified number of cell divisions, during which time a developmental program is activated, eventually giving rise to fully differentiated cells that have lost proliferative potential. Cell renewal equals cell death, and homeostasis is maintained. In this hierarchical system, only stem cells are long-lived. The hypothesis is that cancers harbor stem cells that make up a small fraction (i.e., 0.001–1%) of all cancer cells. These cells share several features with normal stem cells, including an undifferentiated phenotype, unlimited self-renewal potential, a capacity for some degree of differentiation; however, due to initiating mutations (mutations are indicated by lightning bolts), they are no longer regulated by environmental cues. The cancer stem cell pool is expanded, and rapidly proliferating progeny, through additional mutations, may attain stem cell properties, although most of this population is thought to have a limited proliferative capacity. Differentiation programs are dysfunctional due to reprogramming of the pattern of gene transcription by oncogenic signaling pathways. Within the cancer transit-amplifying population, genomic instability generates aneuploidy and clonal heterogeneity as cells attain a fully malignant phenotype with metastatic potential. The cancer stem cell hypothesis has led to the idea that current cancer therapies may be effective at killing the bulk of tumor cells but do not kill tumor stem cells, leading to a regrowth of tumors that is manifested as tumor recurrence or disease progression. Research is in progress to identify unique molecular features of cancer stem cells that can lead to their direct targeting by novel therapeutic agents.

including the stimulation of endothelial cells (ECs) by growth factors, the degradation of the ECM by proteases, proliferation of ECs and migration into the tumor, and the eventual formation of new capillary tubes.

Tumor blood vessels are not normal; they have chaotic architecture and blood flow. Due to an imbalance of angiogenic regulators such as VEGF and angiopoietins (see later discussion), tumor vessels are tortuous and dilated with an uneven diameter, excessive branching, and shunting. Tumor blood flow is variable, with areas of hypoxemia and acidosis leading to the selection of variants that are resistant to hypoxemia-induced apoptosis (often due to the loss of p53 expression). Tumor vessel walls have numerous openings, widened interendothelial junctions, and discontinuous or absent basement membranes; this contributes to the high vascular permeability of these vessels and, together with lack of functional intratumoral lymphatics, causes increased interstitial pressure within the tumor (which also interferes with the delivery of therapeutics to the tumor; Figs. 25-8, 25-9, and 25-10). Tumor blood vessels lack perivascular cells such as pericytes and smooth-muscle cells that normally regulate flow in response to tissue metabolic needs.

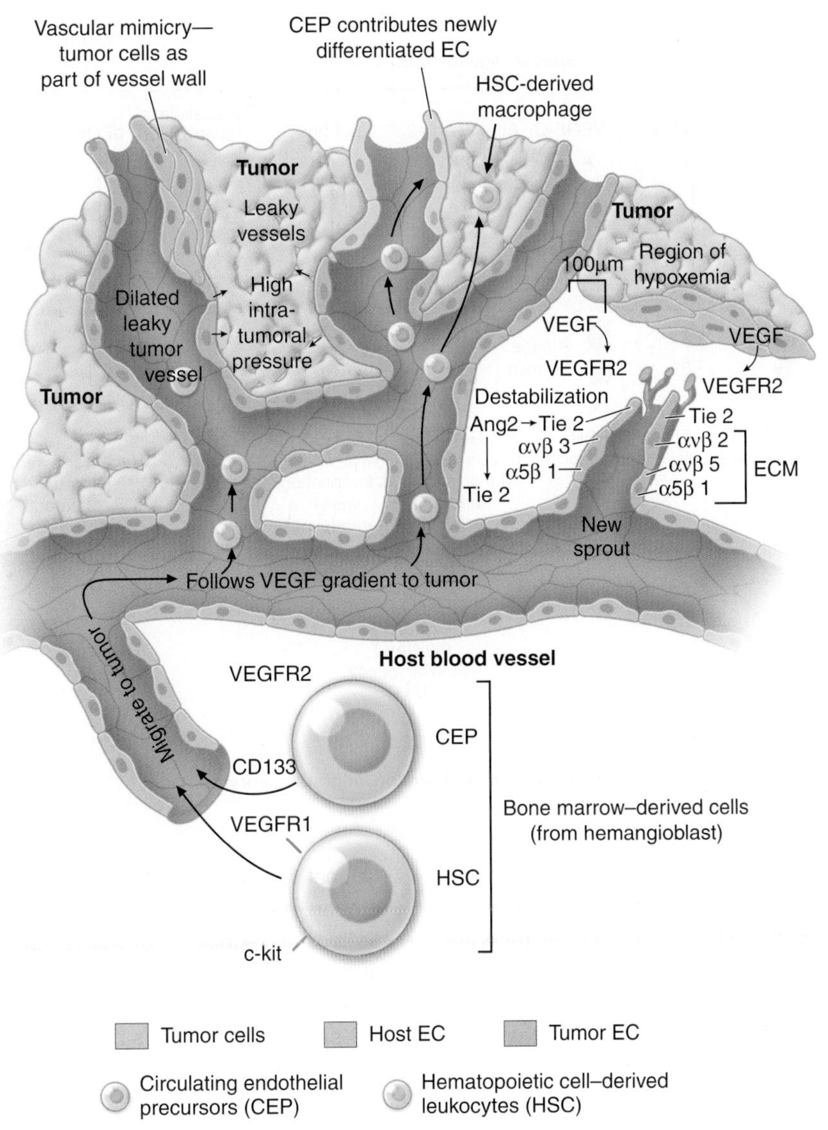

FIGURE 25-8

Tumor angiogenesis is a complex process involving many different cell types that must proliferate, migrate, invade, and differentiate in response to signals from the tumor microenvironment. Endothelial cells (ECs) sprout from host vessels in response to vascular endothelial growth factor (VEGF), basic fibroblast growth factor (bFGF), Ang2, and other proangiogenic stimuli. Sprouting is stimulated by VEGF/VEGFR2, Ang2/Tie-2, and integrin–extracellular matrix (ECM) interactions. Bone marrow–derived circulating endothelial precursors (CEPs) migrate to the tumor in response to VEGF and differentiate into ECs, while hematopoietic stem cells differentiate into leukocytes, including tumor-associated macrophages that secrete angiogenic growth factors and produce matrix metalloproteinases (MMPs) that remodel the ECM and release bound growth factors. Tumor cells themselves may directly form parts of vascular channels within tumors. The pattern of vessel formation is haphazard: vessels are tortuous, dilated, and leaky and branch in random ways. This leads to uneven blood flow within the tumor, with areas of acidosis and hypoxemia (which stimulate release of angiogenic factors) and high intratumoral pressures that inhibit delivery of therapeutic agents.

Unlike normal blood vessels, the vascular lining of tumor vessels is not a homogeneous layer of ECs but often consists of a mosaic of ECs and tumor cells; the concept of cancer cell–derived vascular channels, which may be lined by ECM secreted by the tumor cells, is referred to as *vascular mimicry*. It is unclear whether tumor cells actually form structural elements of vascular channels or represent tumor cells in transit into or out of the vessel. However, the former is supported by evidence that in some human colon cancers, tumor cells can comprise up to 15% of vessel walls. The ECs of angiogenic blood vessels are unlike quiescent ECs found in adult vessels, where only 0.01% of ECs are dividing. During tumor angiogenesis, ECs are highly proliferative and express a number of plasma membrane proteins that are characteristic of activated endothelium, including

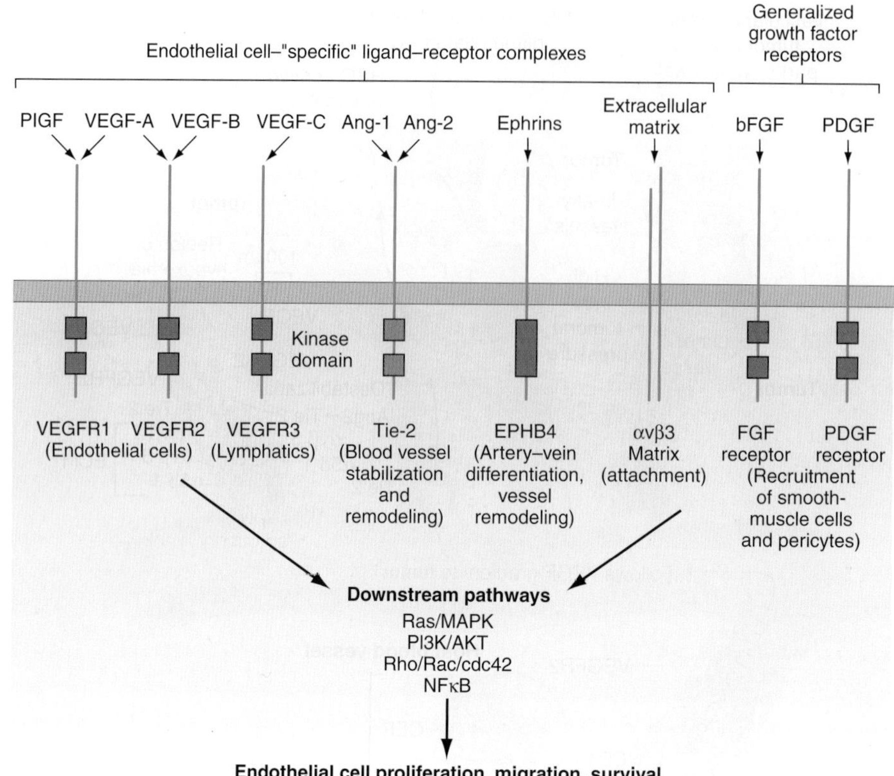

FIGURE 25-9

Critical molecular determinants of endothelial cell biology. Angiogenic endothelium expresses a number of receptors not found on resting endothelium. These include receptor tyrosine kinases (RTKs) and integrins that bind to the extracellular matrix and mediate endothelial cell (EC) adhesion, migration, and invasion. ECs also express RTK (i.e., the fibroblast growth factor [FGF] and platelet-derived growth factor [PDGF] receptors) that are found on many other cell types. Critical functions mediated by activated RTK include proliferation, migration, and enhanced survival of endothelial cells, as well as regulation of the recruitment of perivascular cells and bloodborne circulating endothelial precursors and hematopoietic stem cells to the tumor. Intracellular signaling via EC-specific RTK utilizes molecular pathways that may be targets for future antiangiogenic therapies.

growth factor receptors and adhesion molecules such as integrins.

MECHANISMS OF TUMOR VESSEL FORMATION

Tumors use a number of mechanisms to promote vascularization, subverting normal angiogenic processes for this purpose (Fig. 25-8). Primary or metastatic tumor cells sometimes arise in proximity to host blood vessels and grow around these vessels, parasitizing nutrients by co-opting the local blood supply. However, most tumor blood vessels arise by the process of *sprouting*, in which tumors secrete trophic angiogenic molecules, the most potent being VEGF, that induce the proliferation and migration of host ECs into the tumor. Sprouting in normal and pathogenic angiogenesis is regulated by three families of transmembrane receptor tyrosine kinases (RTKs) expressed on ECs and their ligands (VEGFs, angiopoietins, ephrins; Fig. 25-9), which are produced by tumor cells, inflammatory cells, or stromal cells in the tumor microenvironment.

When tumor cells arise in or metastasize to an avascular area, they grow to a size limited by hypoxemia and nutrient deprivation. Hypoxemia, a key regulator of tumor angiogenesis, causes the transcriptional induction of the gene encoding VEGF by a process that involves stabilization of HIF-1α. Under normoxemic conditions, HIF-1α levels are maintained at a low level by proteasome-mediated destruction regulated by a ubiquitin E3-ligase encoded by the VHL tumor-suppressor locus. However, under hypoxemic conditions, HIF-1α is not hydroxylated and association with VHL does not occur; therefore HIF-1 levels increase, and target genes including VEGF, nitric oxide synthetase (NOS), and Ang2 are induced. Loss of the *VHL* genes, as occurs in familial and sporadic renal cell carcinomas, results in HIF-1α stabilization and induction of VEGF. Most tumors have hypoxemic regions due to poor blood flow, and tumor cells in these areas stain positive for HIF-1α expression;

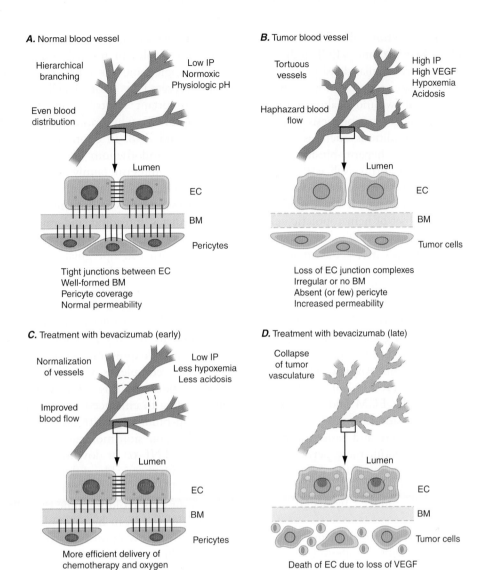

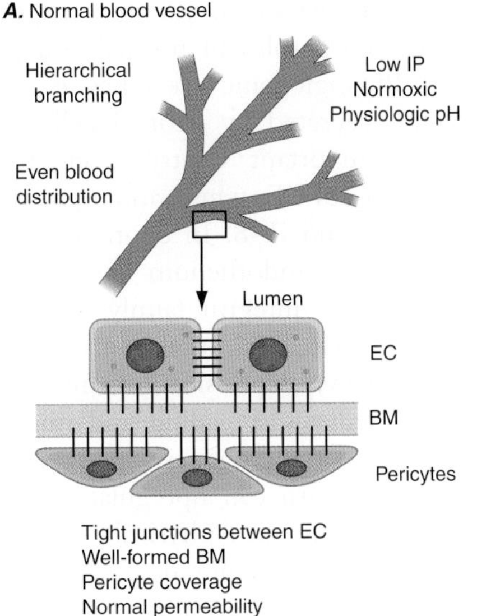

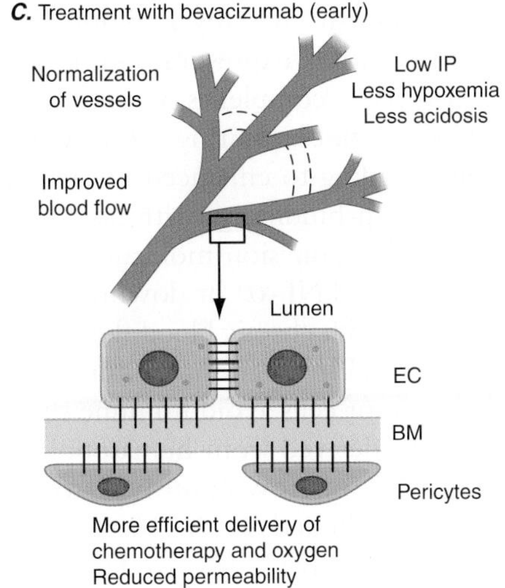

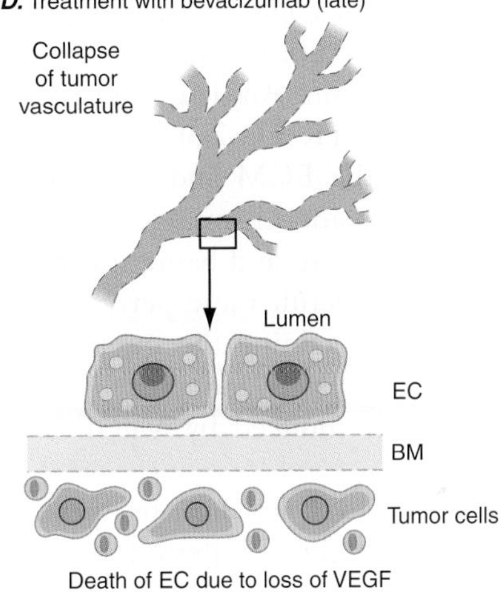

FIGURE 25-10

Normalization of tumor blood vessels due to inhibition of vascular endothelial growth factor (VEGF) signaling. *A.* Blood vessels in normal tissues exhibit a regular hierarchical branching pattern that delivers blood to tissues in a spatially and temporally efficient manner to meet the metabolic needs of the tissue (top). At the microscopic level, tight junctions are maintained between endothelial cells (ECs), which are adherent to a thick and evenly distributed basement membrane (BM). Pericytes form a surrounding layer that provides trophic signals to the EC and helps maintain proper vessel tone. Vascular permeability is regulated, interstitial fluid pressure is low, and oxygen tension and pH are physiologic. ***B.*** Tumors have abnormal vessels with tortuous branching and dilated, irregular interconnecting branches, causing uneven blood flow with areas of hypoxemia and acidosis. This harsh environment selects genetic events that result in resistant tumor variants, such as the loss of p53. High levels of VEGF (secreted by tumor cells) disrupt gap junction communication, tight junctions, and adherens junctions between EC via src-mediated phosphor-ylation of proteins such as connexin 43, zonula occludens-1, VE-cadherin, and α/β-catenins. Tumor vessels have thin, irregular BM, and pericytes are sparse or absent. Together, these molecular abnormalities result in a vasculature that is permeable to serum macromolecules, leading to high tumor interstitial pressure, which can prevent the delivery of drugs to the tumor cells. This is made worse by the binding and activation of platelets at sites of exposed BM, with release of stored VEGF and microvessel clot formation, creating more abnormal blood flow and regions of hypoxemia. ***C.*** In experimental systems, treatment with bevacizumab or blocking antibodies to VEGFR2 leads to changes in the tumor vasculature that has been termed *vessel normalization*. During the first week of treatment, abnormal vessels are eliminated or pruned (dotted lines), leaving a more normal branching pattern. ECs partially regain features such as cell–cell junctions, adherence to a more normal BM, and pericyte coverage. These changes lead to a decrease in vascular permeability, reduced interstitial pressure, and a transient increase in blood flow within the tumor. Note that in murine models, this normalization period lasts only for ~5–6 days. ***D.*** After continued anti-VEGF/VEGFR therapy (which is often combined with chemo- or radiotherapy), ECs die, leading to tumor cell death (either due to direct effects of the chemotherapy or lack of blood flow).

in renal cancers with *VHL* deletion, all of the tumor cells express high levels of HIF-1α, and VEGF-induced angiogenesis leads to high microvascular density.

VEGF and its receptors are required for embryonic *vasculogenesis*, and normal (wound healing, corpus luteum formation) and pathologic angiogenesis (tumor angiogenesis, inflammatory conditions such as rheumatoid arthritis). VEGF-A is a heparin-binding glycoprotein with at least four isoforms (splice variants) that regulates blood vessel formation by binding to the RTKs VEGFR1 and VEGFR2, which are expressed on all ECs in addition to a subset of hematopoietic cells (Fig. 25-8). VEGFR2 regulates EC proliferation, migration, and survival, while VEGFR1 may act as an antagonist of R2 in ECs but is probably also important for angioblast differentiation during embryogenesis. Tumor vessels may be more dependent on VEGFR signaling for growth and survival than normal ECs. While VEGF signaling is a critical initiator of angiogenesis, this is a complex process regulated by additional signaling pathways (Fig. 25-9). The angiopoietin, Ang1, produced by stromal cells, binds to the EC RTK Tie-2 and promotes the interaction of ECs with the ECM and perivascular cells, such as pericytes and smooth-muscle cells, to form tight, nonleaky vessels. PDGF and basic fibroblast growth factor (bFGF) help to recruit these perivascular cells. Ang1 is required for maintaining the quiescence and stability of mature blood vessels and prevents the vascular permeability normally induced by VEGF and inflammatory cytokines.

For tumor cell–derived VEGF to initiate sprouting from host vessels, the stability conferred by the Ang1/Tie2 pathway must be perturbed; this occurs by the secretion of Ang2 by ECs that are undergoing active remodeling. Ang2 binds to Tie2 and is a competitive inhibitor of Ang1 action: under the influence of Ang2, preexisting blood vessels become more responsive to remodeling signals, with less adherence of ECs to stroma and associated perivascular cells and more responsiveness to VEGF. Therefore, Ang2 is required at early stages of tumor angiogenesis for destabilizing the vasculature by making host ECs more sensitive to angiogenic signals. Since tumor ECs are blocked by Ang2, there is no stabilization by the Ang1–Tie2 interaction, and tumor blood vessels are leaky, hemorrhagic, and have poor association of ECs with underlying stroma. Sprouting tumor ECs express high levels of the transmembrane protein ephrin-B2 and its receptor, the RTK EPH, whose signaling appears to work with the angiopoietins during vessel remodeling. During embryogenesis, EPH receptors are expressed on the endothelium of primordial venous vessels while the transmembrane ligand ephrin-B2 is expressed by cells of primordial arteries; the reciprocal expression may regulate differentiation and patterning of the vasculature.

A number of ubiquitously expressed host molecules play critical roles in normal and pathologic angiogenesis. Proangiogenic cytokines, chemokines, and growth factors secreted by stromal cells or inflammatory cells make important contributions to neovascularization, including bFGF, transforming growth factor-α (TGF-α), TNF-α, and IL-8. In contrast to normal endothelium, angiogenic endothelium overexpresses specific members of the integrin family of ECM-binding proteins that mediate EC adhesion, migration, and survival. Specifically, expression of integrins $\alpha_v\beta_3$, $\alpha_v\beta_5$, and $\alpha_5\beta_1$ mediates spreading and migration of ECs and is required for angiogenesis induced by VEGF and bFGF, which in turn can upregulate EC integrin expression. The $\alpha_v\beta_3$ integrin physically associates with VEGFR2 in the plasma membrane and promotes signal transduction from each receptor to promote EC proliferation (via focal adhesion kinase, src, PI3K, and other pathways) and survival (by inhibition of p53 and increasing the Bcl-2/Bax expression ratio). In addition, $\alpha_v\beta_3$ forms cell-surface complexes with matrix metalloproteinases (MMPs), zinc-requiring proteases that cleave ECM proteins, leading to enhanced EC migration and the release of heparin-binding growth factors, including VEGF and bFGF. EC adhesion molecules can be upregulated (i.e., by VEGF, TNF-α) or downregulated (by TGF-β); this, together with chaotic blood flow, explains poor leukocyte-endothelial interactions in tumor blood vessels and may help tumor cells avoid immune surveillance.

Cells derived from hematopoietic progenitors in the host bone marrow contribute to tumor angiogenesis in a process linked to the secretion of VEGF and PlGF (placenta-derived growth factor) by tumor cells and their surrounding stroma. VEGF promotes the mobilization and recruitment of circulating endothelial cell precursors (CEPs) and hematopoietic stem cells (HSCs) to tumors where they co-localize and appear to cooperate in neovessel formation. CEPs express VEGFR2, while HSCs express VEGFR1, a receptor for VEGF and PlGF. Both CEPs and HSCs are derived from a common precursor, the hemangioblast. CEPs are thought to differentiate into ECs, whereas the role of HSC-derived cells (such as tumor-associated macrophages) may be to secrete angiogenic factors required for sprouting and stabilization of ECs (VEGF, bFGF, angiopoietins) and to activate MMPs, resulting in ECM remodeling and growth factor release. In mouse tumor models and in human cancers, increased numbers of CEPs and subsets of VEGFR-expressing HSCs can be detected in the circulation, which may correlate with increased levels of serum VEGF. It is not yet known whether levels of these cells have prognostic value or if changes during treatment correlate with inhibition of tumor angiogenesis. Whether CEPs and VEGFR1-expressing HSCs are required to maintain the long-term integrity of established tumor vessels is also unknown.

Lymphatic vessels also exist within tumors. Development of tumor lymphatics is associated with expression of VEGFR3 and its ligands VEGF-C and VEGF-D. The role of these vessels in tumor cell metastasis to regional lymph nodes remains to be determined, since, as discussed earlier, interstitial pressures within tumors are high and most lymphatic vessels may exit in a collapsed and nonfunctional state. However, VEGF-C levels correlate significantly with metastasis to regional lymph nodes in lung, prostate, and colorectal cancers.

ANTIANGIOGENIC THERAPY

ECs comprising the tumor vasculature are genetically stable and do not share genetic changes with tumor cells; the EC apoptosis pathways are therefore intact. Each EC of a tumor vessel helps provide nourishment to many tumor cells, and although tumor angiogenesis can be driven by a number of exogenous proangiogenic stimuli, experimental data indicate that at least in some tumor types, blockade of a single growth factor (e.g., VEGF) may inhibit tumor-induced vascular growth. Angiogenesis inhibitors function by targeting the critical molecular pathways involved in EC proliferation, migration, and/or survival, many of which are unique to the activated endothelium in tumors. Inhibition of growth factor and adhesion-dependent signaling pathways can induce EC apoptosis with concomitant inhibition of tumor growth. Different types of tumors use distinct molecular mechanisms to activate the angiogenic switch. Therefore, it is doubtful that a single antiangiogenic strategy will suffice for all human cancers; rather, a number of agents will be needed, each responding to distinct programs of angiogenesis used by different human cancers.

Bevacizumab, an antibody to VEGF, appears to potentiate the effects of many different types of active chemotherapeutic regimens used to treat a variety of different tumor types. It lacks single-agent antitumor activity and its strategy, the sopping up of locally produced VEGF after systemic administration, does not seem as likely to be effective as a therapy that interferes with the VEGF receptor on target cells. Bevacizumab appears to augment the antitumor effects of chemotherapy in colon cancer and additional testing in other tumor types is underway.

Bevacizumab is administered IV every 2–3 weeks (its half-life is nearly 20 days) and is generally well tolerated. Hypertension has been noted in most trials that utilize inhibitors of VEGF receptors, but only 10% of patients require treatment with antihypertensive agents and this rarely requires discontinuation of therapy. A mechanism for the hypertension may be a bevacizumab-induced decrease in vessel production of nitric oxide, resulting in vasoconstriction and increased blood pressure. Rare but serious side effects of bevacizumab include an increased risk of arterial thromboembolic events including stroke and myocardial infarction, usually in patients older than age 65 years with a history of cardiovascular disease. An increased risk of hemorrhage was noted in lung cancer patients with a squamous histology and large central tumors near the major mediastinal blood vessels. Cavitation of the tumor with vessel rupture and massive hemoptysis lead to the exclusion of squamous cell cancers from treatment with bevacizumab. This potentially fatal side effect may actually reflect an increased activity of bevacizumab plus chemotherapy in squamous cell cancers. Other serious complications include bowel perforations that have been observed in 1–3% of patients (mainly those with colon and ovarian cancers).

The bevacizumab experience suggests that inhibition of the VEGF pathway will be most efficacious when combined with agents that directly target tumor cells. This also appears to be the case in the development of small-molecule inhibitors (SMIs) that target VEGF receptor tyrosine kinase activity but are also inhibitory to other kinases that are expressed by tumor cells and important for their proliferation and survival. Sunitinib, FDA approved for the treatment of GIST (see earlier discussion and Table 25-2), has activity directed against mutant c-Kit receptors but also targets VEGFR and PDGFR and has shown significant antitumor activity against metastatic renal cell carcinoma (RCC), presumably on the basis of its antiangiogenic activity. Similarly, sorafenib, originally developed as a Raf kinase inhibitor but with potent activity against VEGF and PDGF receptors, increases progression-free survival in RCC. Thus, agents that target both angiogenesis and tumor-specific signaling pathways may have greater efficacy against a broad range of cancers. A caveat is that RCC and GIST are highly dependent upon single signaling pathways (VEGF and c-Kit, respectively), whereas most solid tumors use a panoply of interconnected proliferation and survival pathways that are redundant and likely to be less amenable to single-agent targeting.

The success in targeting tumor angiogenesis has led to enhanced enthusiasm for the development of drugs that target other aspects of the angiogenic process; some of these therapeutic approaches are outlined in Fig. 25-11.

SUMMARY

The explosion of information on tumor cell biology, metastasis, and angiogenesis has ushered in a new era of rational targeted therapy for cancer. Furthermore, it

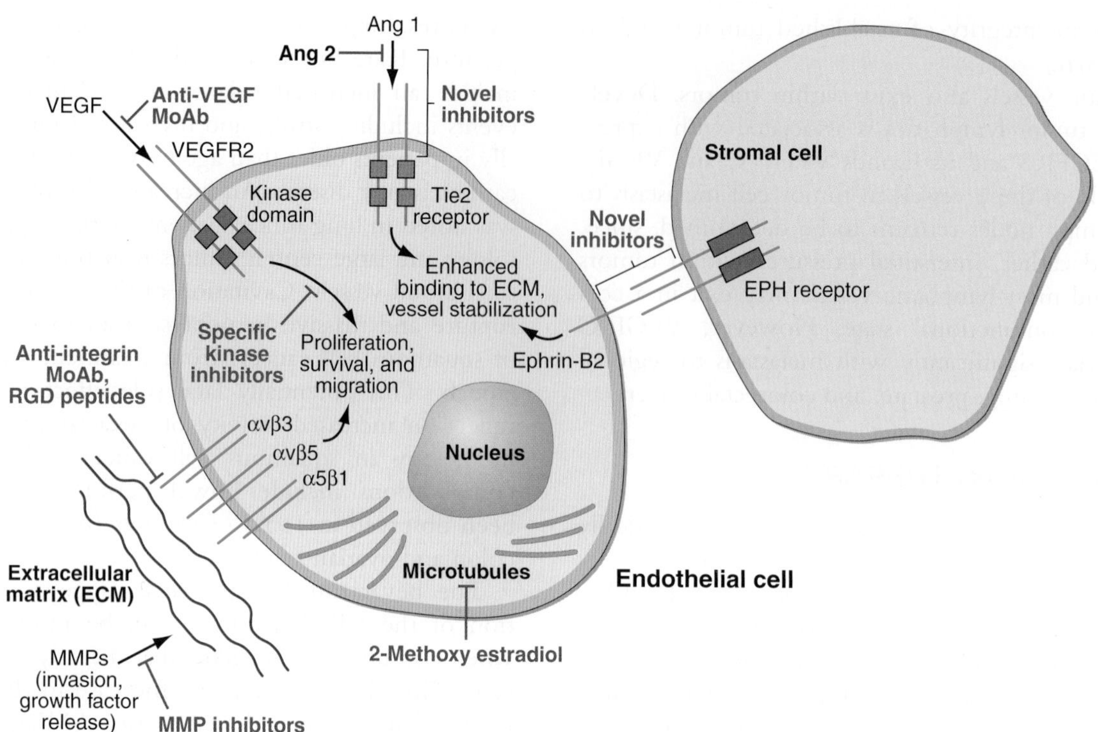

FIGURE 25-11

Knowledge of the molecular events governing tumor angiogenesis has led to a number of therapeutic strategies to block tumor blood vessel formation. The successful therapeutic targeting of vascular endothelial growth factor (VEGF) is described in the text. Other endothelial cell–specific receptor tyrosine kinase pathways (e.g., angiopoietin/Tie2 and ephrin/EPH) are likely targets for the future. Ligation of the $\alpha_v\beta_3$ integrin is required for endothelial cell (EC) survival. Integrins are also required for EC migration and are important regulators of matrix metalloproteinase (MMP) activity, which modulates EC movement through the ECM as well as release of bound growth factors. Targeting of integrins includes development of blocking antibodies, small peptide inhibitors of integrin signaling, and arg-gly-asp–containing peptides that prevent integrin–ECM binding. Peptides derived from normal proteins by proteolytic cleavage, including endostatin and tumstatin, inhibit angiogenesis by mechanisms that include interfering with integrin function. Signal transduction pathways that are dysregulated in tumor cells indirectly regulate EC function. Inhibition of epidermal growth factor (EGF)-family receptors, whose signaling activity is upregulated in a number of human cancers (e.g., breast, colon, and lung cancers), results in downregulation of VEGF and interleukin 8 (IL-8), while increasing expression of the antiangiogenic protein thrombospondin-1. The Ras/MAPK, PI3K/Akt, and Src kinase pathways constitute important antitumor targets that also regulate the proliferation and survival of tumor-derived EC. The discovery that EC from normal tissues express tissue-specific "vascular addressins" on their cell surfaces suggests that targeting specific EC subsets may be possible.

has become clear that specific molecular factors detected in individual tumors (specific gene mutations, gene-expression profiles, microRNA expression) can be used to tailor therapy and maximize antitumor effects.

Acknowledgement

Robert G. Fenton contributed to this chapter in prior editions of Harrison's Principles of Internal Medicine and important material from those prior chapters has been included here.

SECTION VIII

PRINCIPLES OF CANCER PREVENTION AND TREATMENT

CHAPTER 26

APPROACH TO THE PATIENT WITH CANCER

Dan L. Longo

The application of current treatment techniques (surgery, radiation therapy, chemotherapy, and biologic therapy) results in the cure of nearly two of three patients diagnosed with cancer. Nevertheless, patients experience the diagnosis of cancer as one of the most traumatic and revolutionary events that has ever happened to them. Independent of prognosis, the diagnosis brings with it a change in a person's self-image and in his or her role in the home and workplace. The prognosis of a person who has just been found to have pancreatic cancer is the same as the prognosis of a person with aortic stenosis who develops the first symptoms of congestive heart failure (median survival, ~8 months). However, the patient with heart disease may remain functional and maintain a self-image as a fully intact person with just a malfunctioning part, a diseased organ ("a bum ticker"). By contrast, the patient with pancreatic cancer has a completely altered self-image and is viewed differently by family and anyone who knows the diagnosis. He or she is being attacked and invaded by a disease that could be anywhere in the body. Every ache or pain takes on desperate significance. Cancer is an exception to the coordinated interaction among cells and organs. In general, the cells of a multicellular organism are programmed for collaboration. Many diseases occur because the specialized cells fail to perform their assigned task. Cancer takes this malfunction one step further. Not only is there a failure of the cancer cell to maintain its specialized function, but it also strikes out on its own; the cancer cell competes to survive using natural mutability and natural selection to seek advantage over normal cells in a recapitulation of evolution. One consequence of the traitorous behavior of cancer cells is that the patient feels betrayed by his or her body. The cancer patient feels that he or she, and not just a body part, is diseased.

THE MAGNITUDE OF THE PROBLEM

No nationwide cancer registry exists; therefore, the incidence of cancer is estimated on the basis of the National Cancer Institute's Surveillance, Epidemiology, and End Results (SEER) database, which tabulates cancer incidence and death figures from nine sites, accounting for about 10% of the U.S. population, and from population data from the U.S. Census Bureau. In 2010, 1.530 million new cases of invasive cancer (789,620 men, 739,940 women) were diagnosed, and 569,490 persons (299,200 men, 270,290 women) died from cancer. The percent distribution of new cancer cases and cancer deaths by site for men and women are shown in Table 26-1. Cancer incidence has been declining by about 2% each year since 1992.

The most significant risk factor for cancer overall is age; two-thirds of all cases were in those older than age 65 years. Cancer incidence increases as the third, fourth, or fifth power of age in different sites. For the interval between birth and age 39 years, 1 in 70 men and 1 in 48 women will develop cancer; for the interval between ages 40 and 59 years, 1 in 12 men and 1 in 11 women will develop cancer; and for the interval between ages 60 and 79 years, 1 in 3 men and 1 in 5 women will develop cancer. Overall, men have a 44% risk of developing cancer at some time during their lives; women have a 38% lifetime risk.

Cancer is the second leading cause of death behind heart disease. Deaths from heart disease have declined 45% in the United States since 1950 and continue to decline. Cancer has overtaken heart disease as the number one cause of death in persons younger than age 85 years (Fig. 26-1). After a 70-year period of increase, cancer deaths began to decline in 1990–1991

TABLE 26-1

DISTRIBUTION OF CANCER INCIDENCE AND DEATHS FOR 2010

MALE			FEMALE		
SITES	%	NUMBER	SITES	%	NUMBER
Cancer Incidence					
Prostate	28	217,730	Breast	28	207,090
Lung	15	116,750	Lung	14	105,770
Colorectal	9	72,090	Colorectal	10	70,480
Bladder	7	52,760	Endometrial	6	43,470
Melanoma	5	38,870	Thyroid	5	33,930
Lymphoma	4	35,380	Lymphoma	4	30,160
Kidney	4	35,370	Melanoma	4	29,260
Oral cavity	3	25,420	Kidney	3	22,870
Leukemia	3	24,690	Ovary	3	21,880
Pancreas	3	21,370	Pancreas	3	21,770
All others	19	149,190	All others	20	153,260
All sites	100	789,620	All sites	100	739,940
Cancer Deaths					
Lung	29	86,220	Lung	26	71,080
Prostate	11	32,050	Breast	15	39,840
Colorectal	9	26,580	Colorectal	9	24,790
Pancreas	6	18,770	Pancreas	7	18,030
Liver	4	12,720	Ovary	5	13,850
Leukemia	4	12,660	Lymphoma	4	9500
Esophagus	4	11,650	Leukemia	3	9180
Lymphoma	4	10,710	Endometrial	3	7950
Bladder	3	10,410	Liver	2	6190
Kidney	3	8210	CNS	2	5720
All others	23	69,220	All others	21	64,160
All sites	100	299,200	All sites	100	270,290

Abbreviation: CNS, central nervous system.

(Fig. 26-2). Between 1990 and 2006, cancer deaths decreased by 21% among men and 12.3% among women. The five leading causes of cancer deaths are shown for various populations in Table 26-2. The 5-year survival rates for white patients were 39% in 1960–1963 and 69% in 1999–2005. Cancers are more often deadly in blacks; the 5-year survival rate was 59% for the 1999–2005 interval. Incidence and mortality vary among racial and ethnic groups (Table 26-3). The basis for these differences is unclear.

CANCER AROUND THE WORLD

In 2002, 11 million new cancer cases and 7 million cancer deaths were estimated worldwide. When broken down by region of the world, ~45% of cases were in Asia, 26% in Europe, 14.5% in North America, 7.1% in Central/South America, 6% in Africa, and 1% in Australia and New Zealand (Fig. 26-3). Lung cancer is the most common cancer and the most common cause of cancer death in the world. Its incidence is highly variable, affecting only 2 per 100,000 African women but as many as 61 per 100,000 North American men. Breast cancer is the second most common cancer worldwide; however, it ranks fifth as a cause of death behind lung, stomach, liver, and colorectal cancer. Among the eight most common forms of cancer, lung (2-fold), breast (3-fold), prostate (2.5-fold), and colorectal (3-fold) cancers are more common in more developed countries than in less developed countries. By contrast, liver (2-fold), cervical (2-fold), and esophageal (2- to 3-fold) cancers are more common in less developed countries. Stomach cancer incidence is similar in more and less developed countries but is much more common in Asia than North America or Africa. The most common cancers in Africa are cervical, breast, and liver cancers. It has been estimated that nine modifiable risk factors are responsible for more than one-third of cancers worldwide. These include smoking, alcohol consumption, obesity, physical inactivity, low fruit and vegetable consumption, unsafe sex, air pollution, indoor smoke from household fuels, and contaminated injections.

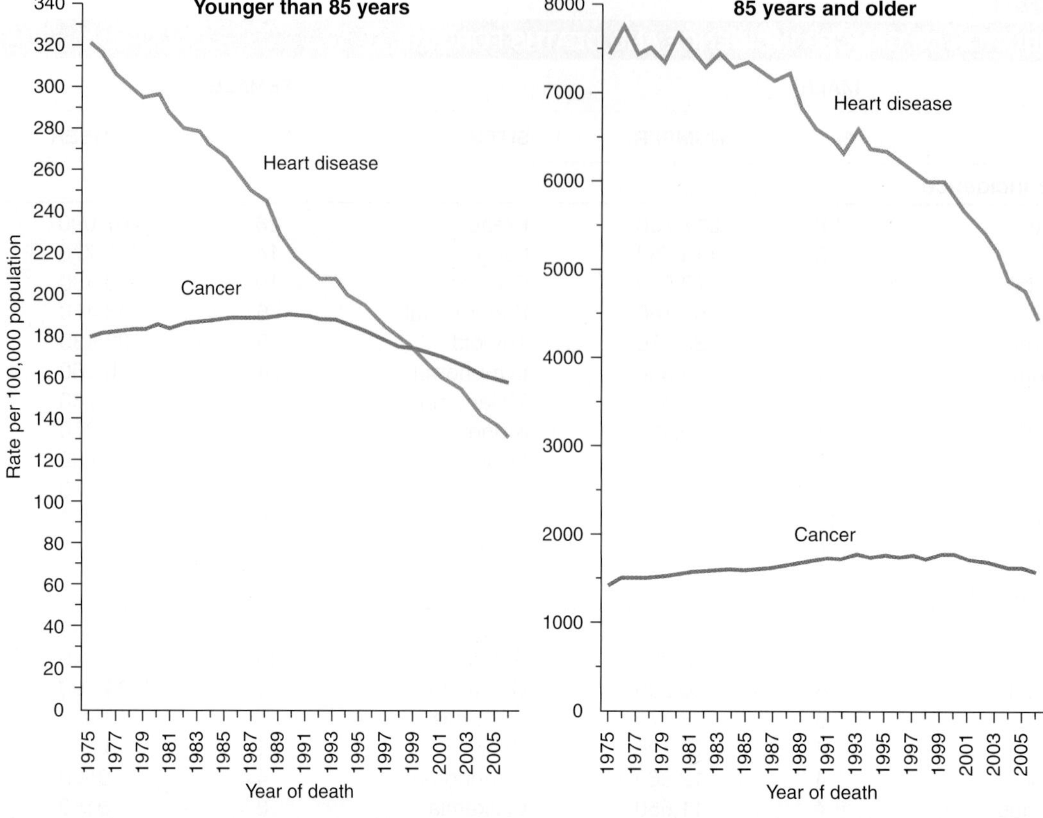

FIGURE 26-1
Death rates for heart disease and cancer among people younger and older than age 85 years. ***A.*** In people younger than age 85 years, cancer has overtaken heart disease as the largest cause of death. ***B.*** In people older than age 85 years, heart disease is by far the major cause of death. *(From A Jemal et al: CA Cancer J Clin 60:277, 2010.)*

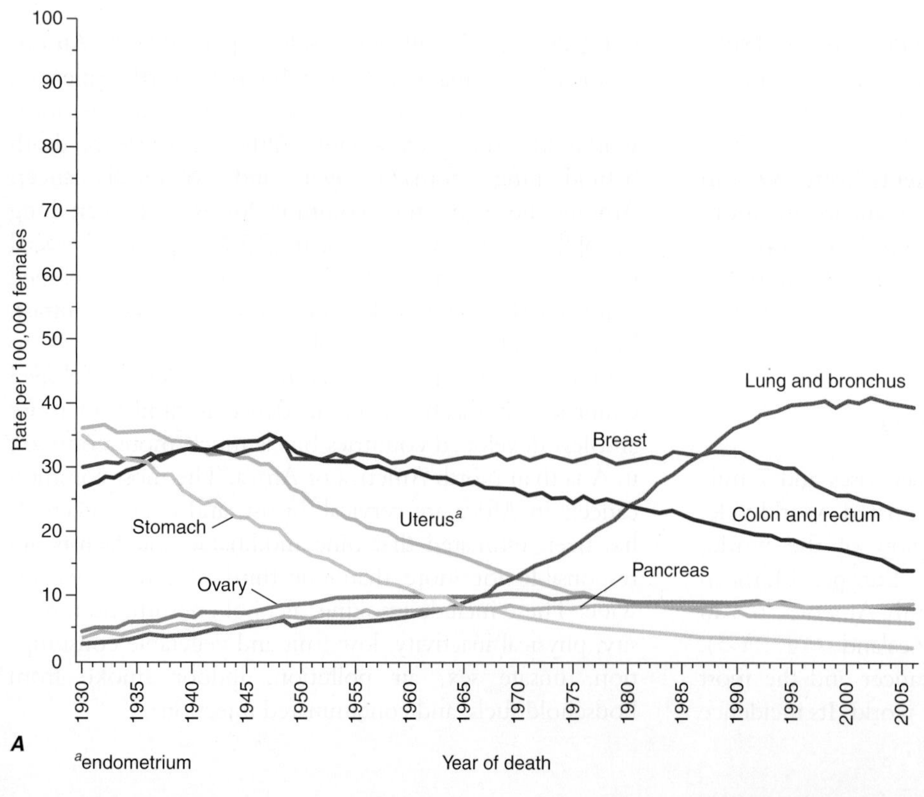

FIGURE 26-2
Sixty-five-year trend in cancer death rates for (***A***) women and (***B***) men by site in the United States, 1930–2006. Rates are per 100,000 age-adjusted to the 2000 U.S. standard population. *(From A Jemal et al: CA Cancer J Clin 60:277, 2010.)*

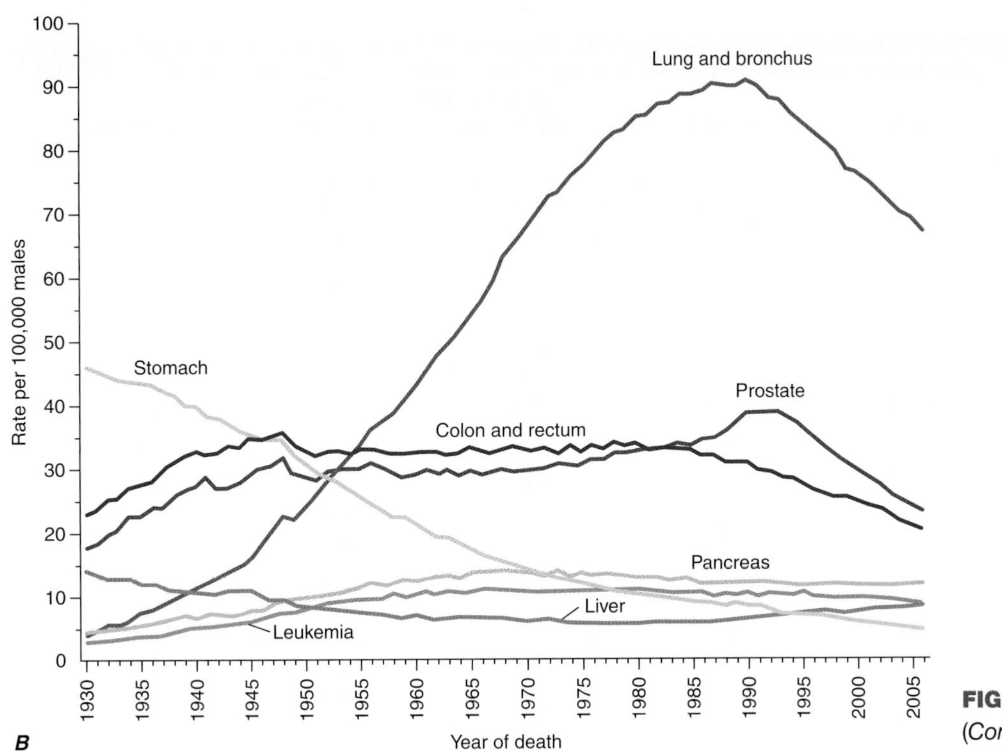

FIGURE 26-2
(Continued)

PATIENT MANAGEMENT

Important information is obtained from every portion of the routine history and physical examination. The duration of symptoms may reveal the chronicity of disease. The past medical history may alert the physician to the presence of underlying diseases that may affect the choice of therapy or the side effects of treatment. The social history may reveal occupational exposure to carcinogens or habits, such as smoking or alcohol consumption, that may influence the course of disease and its treatment. The family history may suggest an underlying familial cancer predisposition and point out the need to begin surveillance or other preventive therapy for unaffected siblings of the patient. The review of systems may suggest early symptoms of metastatic disease or a paraneoplastic syndrome.

DIAGNOSIS

The diagnosis of cancer relies most heavily on invasive tissue biopsy and should never be made without obtaining tissue; no noninvasive diagnostic test is sufficient to define a disease process as cancer. Although in

TABLE 26-2

THE FIVE LEADING PRIMARY TUMOR SITES FOR PATIENTS DYING OF CANCER BASED ON AGE AND SEX IN 2007

			AGE, YEARS				
RANK		**ALL AGES**	**UNDER 20**	**20–39**	**40–59**	**60–79**	**>80**
1	M	Lung	Leukemia	Leukemia	Lung	Lung	Lung
	F	Lung	Leukemia	Breast	Breast	Lung	Lung
2	M	Prostate	CNS	CNS	Colorectal	Colorectal	Prostate
	F	Breast	CNS	Cervix	Lung	Breast	Colorectal
3	M	Colorectal	Bone sarcoma	Colorectal	Liver	Prostate	Colorectal
	F	Colorectal	Endocrine	Leukemia	Colorectal	Colorectal	Breast
4	M	Pancreas	Endocrine	Lymphoma	Pancreas	Pancreas	Bladder
	F	Pancreas	Bone sarcoma	Colorectal	Ovary	Pancreas	Pancreas
5	M	Leukemia	Soft tissue sarcoma	Lung	Esophagus	Esophagus	Pancreas
	F	Ovary	Soft tissue sarcoma	CNS	Pancreas	Ovary	Lymphoma

Abbreviations: CNS, central nervous system. F, female; M, male.

TABLE 26-3

CANCER INCIDENCE AND MORTALITY RATES IN RACIAL AND ETHNIC GROUPS, UNITED STATES, 2002–2006

SITE		WHITE	BLACK	ASIAN/PACIFIC ISLANDER	AMERICAN INDIAN	HISPANIC
Incidence per 100,000 Population						
All	M	550.1	626.8	334.5	318.4	430.3
	F	420.0	389.5	276.3	265.1	326.8
Breast		123.5	113.0	81.6	67.2	90.2
Colorectal	M	58.2	68.4	44.1	38.1	50.0
	F	42.6	51.7	33.1	30.7	35.1
Kidney	M	19.7	20.6	9.0	16.6	18.2
	F	10.3	10.6	4.5	10.6	10.3
Liver	M	8.0	12.5	21.4	8.9	15.9
	F	2.8	3.8	8.1	4.6	6.2
Lung	M	85.9	104.8	50.6	57.9	49.2
	F	57.1	50.7	27.6	41.3	26.5
Prostate		146.3	231.9	82.3	82.7	131.1
Deaths per 100,000 Population						
All	M	226.7	304.2	135.4	183.3	154.8
	F	157.3	183.7	95.1	140.1	103.9
Breast		23.9	33.0	12.5	17.6	15.5
Colorectal	M	21.4	31.4	13.8	20.0	16.2
	F	14.9	21.6	10.0	13.7	10.7
Kidney	M	6.1	6.0	2.4	9.0	5.2
	F	2.8	2.7	1.2	4.2	2.4
Liver	M	6.8	10.8	15.0	10.3	11.2
	F	2.9	3.9	6.6	6.5	5.1
Lung	M	69.9	90.1	36.9	48.0	33.9
	F	41.9	40.0	18.2	33.5	14.4
Prostate		23.6	56.3	10.6	20.0	19.6

Abbreviations: F, female; M, male.

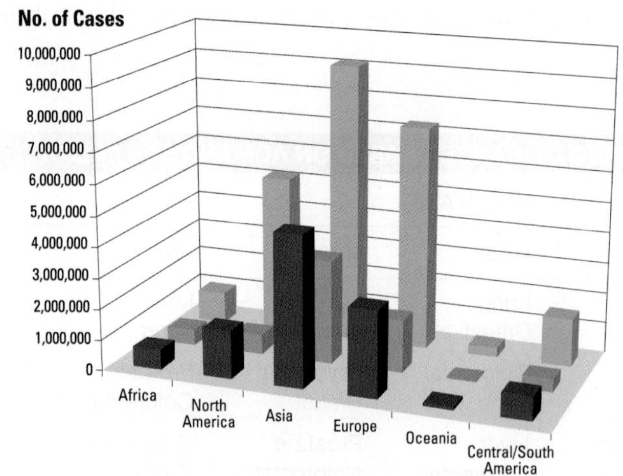

FIGURE 26-3

Worldwide overall annual cancer incidence, mortality and 5-year prevalence for the period of 1993–2001. *(From F Kamangar et al: J Clin Oncol 24:2137, 2006.)*

rare clinical settings (e.g., thyroid nodules) fine-needle aspiration is an acceptable diagnostic procedure, the diagnosis generally depends on obtaining adequate tissue to permit careful evaluation of the histology of the tumor, its grade, and its invasiveness and to yield further molecular diagnostic information, such as the expression of cell-surface markers or intracellular proteins that typify a particular cancer, or the presence of a molecular marker, such as the t(8;14) translocation of Burkitt's lymphoma. Increasing evidence links the expression of certain genes with the prognosis and response to therapy (Chaps. 24 and 25).

Occasionally a patient will present with a metastatic disease process that is defined as cancer on biopsy but has no apparent primary site of disease. Efforts should be made to define the primary site based on age, sex, sites of involvement, histology and tumor markers, and personal and family history. Particular attention should be focused on ruling out the most treatable causes (Chap. 47).

Once the diagnosis of cancer is made, the management of the patient is best undertaken as a multidisciplinary collaboration among the primary care physician, medical oncologists, surgical oncologists, radiation oncologists, oncology nurse specialists, pharmacists, social workers, rehabilitation medicine specialists, and a number of other consulting professionals working closely with each other and with the patient and family.

DEFINING THE EXTENT OF DISEASE AND THE PROGNOSIS

The first priority in patient management after the diagnosis of cancer is established and shared with the patient is to determine the extent of disease. The curability of a tumor usually is inversely proportional to the tumor burden. Ideally, the tumor will be diagnosed before symptoms develop or as a consequence of screening efforts (Chap. 27). A very high proportion of such patients can be cured. However, most patients with cancer present with symptoms related to the cancer caused either by mass effects of the tumor or by alterations associated with the production of cytokines or hormones by the tumor.

For most cancers, the extent of disease is evaluated by a variety of noninvasive and invasive diagnostic tests and procedures. This process is called *staging*. There are two types. *Clinical staging* is based on physical examination, radiographs, isotopic scans, computed tomography scans, and other imaging procedures; *pathologic staging* takes into account information obtained during a surgical procedure, which might include intraoperative palpation, resection of regional lymph nodes or tissue adjacent to the tumor, and inspection and biopsy of organs commonly involved in disease spread. Pathologic staging includes histologic examination of all tissues removed during the surgical procedure. Surgical procedures performed may include a simple lymph node biopsy or more extensive procedures such as thoracotomy, mediastinoscopy, or laparotomy. Surgical staging may occur in a separate procedure or may be done at the time of definitive surgical resection of the primary tumor.

Knowledge of the predilection of particular tumors for spreading to adjacent or distant organs helps direct the staging evaluation.

Information obtained from staging is used to define the extent of disease either as localized, as exhibiting spread outside of the organ of origin to regional but not distant sites, or as metastatic to distant sites. The most widely used system of staging is the TNM (tumor, node, metastasis) system codified by the International Union Against Cancer and the American Joint Committee on Cancer. The TNM classification is an anatomically based system that categorizes the tumor on the basis of the size of the primary tumor lesion (T1–T4, where a higher number indicates a tumor of larger size), the presence of nodal involvement (usually N0 and N1 for the absence and presence, respectively, of involved nodes, although some tumors have more elaborate systems of nodal grading), and the presence of metastatic disease (M0 and M1 for the absence and presence, respectively, of metastases). The various permutations of T, N, and M scores (sometimes including tumor histologic grade, G) are then broken into stages, usually designated by the roman numerals I through IV. Tumor burden increases and curability decreases with increasing stage. Other anatomic staging systems are used for some tumors, e.g., the Dukes classification for colorectal cancers, the International Federation of Gynecologists and Obstetricians classification for gynecologic cancers, and the Ann Arbor classification for Hodgkin's disease.

Certain tumors cannot be grouped on the basis of anatomic considerations. For example, hematopoietic tumors such as leukemia, myeloma, and lymphoma are often disseminated at presentation and do not spread like solid tumors. For these tumors, other prognostic factors have been identified (Chaps. 14, 15, and 17).

In addition to tumor burden, a second major determinant of treatment outcome is the physiologic reserve of the patient. Patients who are bedridden before developing cancer are likely to fare worse, stage for stage, than fully active patients. Physiologic reserve is a determinant of how a patient is likely to cope with the physiologic stresses imposed by the cancer and its treatment. This factor is difficult to assess directly. Instead, surrogate markers for physiologic reserve are used, such as the patient's age or Karnofsky performance status (Table 26-4) or Eastern Cooperative Oncology Group (ECOG) performance status (Table 26-5). Older patients and those with a Karnofsky performance status <70 or ECOG performance status ≥3 have a poor prognosis unless the poor performance is a reversible consequence of the tumor.

Increasingly, biologic features of the tumor are being related to prognosis. The expression of particular oncogenes, drug-resistance genes, apoptosis-related genes, and genes involved in metastasis are being found to influence response to therapy and prognosis. The presence of selected cytogenetic abnormalities may influence survival. Tumors with higher growth fractions, as assessed by expression of proliferation-related markers such as proliferating cell nuclear antigen, behave more aggressively than tumors with lower growth fractions. Information obtained from studying the tumor itself will increasingly be used to influence treatment decisions. Host genes involved in drug metabolism can influence the safety and efficacy of particular treatments.

TABLE 26-4

KARNOFSKY PERFORMANCE INDEX

PERFORMANCE STATUS	FUNCTIONAL CAPABILITY OF THE PATIENT
100	Normal; no complaints; no evidence of disease
90	Able to carry on normal activity; minor signs or symptoms of disease
80	Normal activity with effort; some signs or symptoms of disease
70	Cares for self; unable to carry on normal activity or do active work
60	Requires occasional assistance but is able to care for most needs
50	Requires considerable assistance and frequent medical care
40	Disabled; requires special care and assistance
30	Severely disabled; hospitalization is indicated, although death is not imminent
20	Very sick; hospitalization necessary; active supportive treatment is necessary
10	Moribund; fatal processes progressing rapidly
0	Dead

MAKING A TREATMENT PLAN

From information on the extent of disease and the prognosis and in conjunction with the patient's wishes, it is determined whether the treatment approach should be curative or palliative in intent. Cooperation among the various professionals involved in cancer treatment is of the utmost importance in treatment planning. For some cancers, chemotherapy or chemotherapy plus radiation therapy delivered before the use of definitive surgical treatment (so-called neoadjuvant therapy) may improve the outcome, as seems to be the case for locally advanced breast cancer and head and neck cancers. In certain settings in which combined modality therapy is intended, coordination among the medical oncologist, radiation oncologist, and surgeon is crucial to achieving optimal results. Sometimes the chemotherapy and radiation therapy need to be delivered sequentially and other times concurrently. Surgical procedures may precede or follow other treatment approaches. It is best for the treatment plan either to follow a standard protocol precisely or else to be part of an ongoing clinical research protocol evaluating new treatments. Ad hoc modifications of standard protocols are likely to compromise treatment results.

The choice of treatment approaches was formerly dominated by the local culture in both the university and the practice settings. However, it is now possible to gain access electronically to standard treatment protocols and to every approved clinical research study in North America through a personal computer interface with the Internet.[1]

The skilled physician also has much to offer the patient for whom curative therapy is no longer an option. Often a combination of guilt and frustration over the inability to cure the patient and the pressure of a busy schedule greatly limit the time a physician spends with a patient who is receiving only palliative care. Resist these forces. In addition to the medicines administered to alleviate symptoms (see below), it is important to remember the comfort that is provided by holding the patient's hand, continuing regular examinations, and taking time to talk.

TABLE 26-5

THE EASTERN COOPERATIVE ONCOLOGY GROUP (ECOG) PERFORMANCE SCALE

ECOG Grade 0: Fully active; able to carry on all predisease performance without restriction

ECOG Grade 1: Restricted in physically strenuous activity but ambulatory and able to carry out work of a light or sedentary nature, e.g., light housework, office work

ECOG Grade 2: Ambulatory and capable of all self-care but unable to carry out any work activities. Up and about more than 50% of waking hours

ECOG Grade 3: Capable of only limited self-care; confined to bed or chair more than 50% of waking hours

ECOG Grade 4: Completely disabled. Cannot carry on any self-care. Totally confined to bed or chair

ECOG Grade 5: Dead

Source: From MM Oken et al: Am J Clin Oncol 5:649, 1982.

MANAGEMENT OF DISEASE AND TREATMENT COMPLICATIONS

Because cancer therapies are toxic (Chap. 28), patient management involves addressing complications of both the disease and its treatment as well as the complex

[1]The National Cancer Institute maintains a database called PDQ (Physician Data Query) that is accessible on the Internet under the name CancerNet at *www.cancer.gov/cancertopics/pdq/cancerdatabase*. Information can be obtained through a facsimile machine using CancerFax by dialing 301-402-5874. Patient information is also provided by the National Cancer Institute in at least three formats: on the Internet via CancerNet at *www.cancer.gov*, through the CancerFax number listed above or by calling 800-4-CANCER. The quality control for the information provided through these services is rigorous.

psychosocial problems associated with cancer. In the short term during a course of curative therapy, the patient's functional status may decline. Treatment-induced toxicity is less acceptable if the goal of therapy is palliation. The most common side effects of treatment are nausea and vomiting (see later discussion), febrile neutropenia (Chap. 29), and myelosuppression (Chap. 28). Tools are now available to minimize the acute toxicity of cancer treatment.

New symptoms developing in the course of cancer treatment should always be assumed to be reversible until proven otherwise. The fatalistic attribution of anorexia, weight loss, and jaundice to recurrent or progressive tumor could result in a patient dying from a reversible intercurrent cholecystitis. Intestinal obstruction may be due to reversible adhesions rather than progressive tumor. Systemic infections, sometimes with unusual pathogens, may be a consequence of the immunosuppression associated with cancer therapy. Some drugs used to treat cancer or its complications (e.g., nausea) may produce central nervous system symptoms that look like metastatic disease or may mimic paraneoplastic syndromes such as the syndrome of inappropriate antidiuretic hormone. A definitive diagnosis should be pursued and may even require a repeat biopsy.

A critical component of cancer management is assessing the response to treatment. In addition to a careful physical examination in which all sites of disease are physically measured and recorded in a flow chart by date, response assessment usually requires periodic repeating of imaging test results that were abnormal at the time of staging. If imaging test results have become normal, repeat biopsy of previously involved tissue is performed to document complete response by pathologic criteria. Biopsies are not usually required if there is macroscopic residual disease. A *complete response* is defined as disappearance of all evidence of disease, and a *partial response* as >50% reduction in the sum of the products of the perpendicular diameters of all measurable lesions. The determination of partial response may also be based on a 30% decrease in the sums of the longest diameters of lesions (Response Evaluation Criteria in Solid Tumors, or RECIST, criteria). *Progressive disease* is defined as the appearance of any new lesion or an increase of >25% in the sum of the products of the perpendicular diameters of all measurable lesions (or an increase of 20% in the sums of the longest diameters by RECIST). Tumor shrinkage or growth that does not meet any of these criteria is considered *stable disease*. Some sites of involvement (e.g., bone) or patterns of involvement (e.g., lymphangitic lung or diffuse pulmonary infiltrates) are considered unmeasurable. No response is complete without biopsy documentation of their resolution, but partial responses may exclude their assessment unless clear objective progression has occurred.

Tumor markers may be useful in patient management in certain tumors. Response to therapy may be difficult to gauge with certainty. However, some tumors produce or elicit the production of markers that can be measured in the serum or urine, and in a particular patient, rising and falling levels of the marker are usually associated with increasing or decreasing tumor burden, respectively. Some clinically useful tumor markers are shown in Table 26-6. Tumor markers are not in themselves specific enough to permit a diagnosis of malignancy to be made, but once a malignancy has been diagnosed and shown to be associated with elevated levels of a tumor marker, the marker can be used to assess response to treatment.

The recognition and treatment of depression are important components of management. The incidence of depression in cancer patients is ~25% overall and may be greater in patients with greater debility. This diagnosis is likely in a patient with a depressed mood (dysphoria) or a loss of interest in pleasure (anhedonia) for at least 2 weeks. In addition, three or more of the following symptoms are usually present: appetite change, sleep problems, psychomotor retardation or agitation, fatigue, feelings of guilt or worthlessness, inability to concentrate, and suicidal ideation. Patients with these symptoms should receive therapy. Medical therapy with a serotonin reuptake inhibitor such as fluoxetine (10–20 mg/d), sertraline (50–150 mg/d), or paroxetine (10–20 mg/d) or a tricyclic antidepressant such as amitriptyline (50–100 mg/d) or desipramine (75–150 mg/d) should be tried, allowing 4–6 weeks for response. Effective therapy should be continued at least 6 months after resolution of symptoms. If therapy is unsuccessful, other classes of antidepressants may be used. In addition to medication, psychosocial interventions such as support groups, psychotherapy, and guided imagery may be of benefit.

Many patients opt for unproven or unsound approaches to treatment when it appears that conventional medicine is unlikely to be curative. Those seeking such alternatives are often well educated and may be early in the course of their disease. Unsound approaches are usually hawked on the basis of unsubstantiated anecdotes and not only cannot help the patient but may be harmful. Physicians should strive to keep communications open and nonjudgmental, so that patients are more likely to discuss with the physician what they are actually doing. The appearance of unexpected toxicity may be an indication that a supplemental therapy is being taken.[2]

[2]Information about unsound methods may be obtained from the National Council Against Health Fraud, Box 1276, Loma Linda, CA 92354 or from the Center for Medical Consumers and Health Care Information, 237 Thompson Street, New York, NY 10012.

TABLE 26-6

TUMOR MARKERS

TUMOR MARKERS	CANCER	NONNEOPLASTIC CONDITIONS
Hormones		
Human chorionic gonadotropin	Gestational trophoblastic disease, gonadal germ cell tumor	Pregnancy
Calcitonin	Medullary cancer of the thyroid	
Catecholamines	Pheochromocytoma	
Oncofetal Antigens		
α Fetoprotein	Hepatocellular carcinoma, gonadal germ cell tumor	Cirrhosis, hepatitis
Carcinoembryonic antigen	Adenocarcinomas of the colon, pancreas, lung, breast, ovary	Pancreatitis, hepatitis, inflammatory bowel disease, smoking
Enzymes		
Prostatic acid phosphatase	Prostate cancer	Prostatitis, prostatic hypertrophy
Neuron-specific enolase	Small cell cancer of the lung, neuroblastoma	
Lactate dehydrogenase	Lymphoma, Ewing's sarcoma	Hepatitis, hemolytic anemia, many others
Tumor-Associated Proteins		
Prostate-specific antigen	Prostate cancer	Prostatitis, prostatic hypertrophy
Monoclonal immunoglobulin	Myeloma	Infection, MGUS
CA-125	Ovarian cancer, some lymphomas	Menstruation, peritonitis, pregnancy
CA 19-9	Colon, pancreatic, breast cancer	Pancreatitis, ulcerative colitis
CD30	Hodgkin's disease, anaplastic large cell lymphoma	—
CD25	Hairy cell leukemia, adult T cell leukemia/ lymphoma	—

Abbreviation: MGUS, monoclonal gammopathy of uncertain significance.

LONG-TERM FOLLOW-UP AND LATE COMPLICATIONS

At the completion of treatment, sites originally involved with tumor are reassessed, usually by radiography or imaging techniques, and any persistent abnormality is biopsied. If disease persists, the multidisciplinary team discusses a new salvage treatment plan. If the patient has been rendered disease-free by the original treatment, the patient is followed regularly for disease recurrence. The optimal guidelines for follow-up care are not known. For many years, a routine practice has been to follow the patient monthly for 6–12 months, then every other month for a year, every 3 months for 1 year, every 4 months for 1 year, every 6 months for 1 year, and then annually. At each visit, a battery of laboratory and radiographic and imaging tests were obtained on the assumption that it is best to detect recurrent disease before it becomes symptomatic. However, when follow-up procedures have been examined, this assumption has been found to be untrue. Studies of breast cancer, melanoma, lung cancer, colon cancer, and lymphoma have all failed to support the notion that asymptomatic relapses are more readily cured by salvage therapy than symptomatic relapses. In view of the enormous cost of a full battery of diagnostic tests and their manifest lack of impact on survival, new guidelines are emerging for less frequent follow-up visits, during which the history and physical examination are the major investigations performed.

As time passes, the likelihood of recurrence of the primary cancer diminishes. For many types of cancer, survival for 5 years without recurrence is tantamount to cure. However, important medical problems can occur in patients treated for cancer and must be examined (Chap. 55). Some problems emerge as a consequence of the disease and some as a consequence of the treatment. An understanding of these disease- and treatment-related problems may help in their detection and management.

Despite these concerns, most patients who are cured of cancer return to normal lives.

SUPPORTIVE CARE

In many ways, the success of cancer therapy depends on the success of the supportive care. Failure to control the symptoms of cancer and its treatment may lead patients to abandon curative therapy. Of equal importance, supportive care is a major determinant of quality of life. Even when life cannot be prolonged, the physician must strive to preserve its quality. Quality-of-life measurements have become common endpoints of clinical research studies. Furthermore, palliative care has been shown to be cost-effective when approached in an organized fashion. A credo for oncology could be to cure sometimes, to extend life often, and to comfort always.

Pain

Pain occurs with variable frequency in cancer patients: 25–50% of patients present with pain at diagnosis, 33% have pain associated with treatment, and 75% have pain with progressive disease. The pain may have several causes. In ~70% of cases, pain is caused by the tumor itself—by invasion of bone, nerves, blood vessels, or mucous membranes or obstruction of a hollow viscus or duct. In ~20% of cases, pain is related to a surgical or invasive medical procedure, radiation injury (mucositis, enteritis, or plexus or spinal cord injury), or chemotherapy injury (mucositis, peripheral neuropathy, phlebitis, steroid-induced aseptic necrosis of the femoral head). In 10% of cases, pain is unrelated to cancer or its treatment.

Assessment of pain requires the methodical investigation of the history of the pain, its location, character, temporal features, provocative and palliative factors, and intensity; a review of the oncologic history and past medical history as well as personal and social history; and a thorough physical examination. The patient should be given a 10-division visual analogue scale on which to indicate the severity of the pain. The clinical condition is often dynamic, making it necessary to reassess the patient frequently. Pain therapy should not be withheld while the cause of pain is being sought.

A variety of tools are available with which to address cancer pain. About 85% of patients will have pain relief from pharmacologic intervention. However, other modalities, including antitumor therapy (such as surgical relief of obstruction, radiation therapy, and strontium-89 or samarium-153 treatment for bone pain), neurostimulatory techniques, regional analgesia, or neuroablative procedures, are effective in an additional 12% or so. Thus, very few patients will have inadequate pain relief if appropriate measures are taken. A specific approach to pain relief is detailed in Chap. 32.

Nausea

Emesis in cancer patients is usually caused by chemotherapy (Chap. 28). Its severity can be predicted from the drugs used to treat the cancer. Three forms of emesis are recognized on the basis of their timing with regard to the noxious insult. *Acute emesis*, the most common variety, occurs within 24 h of treatment. *Delayed emesis* occurs 1–7 days after treatment; it is rare, but, when present, usually follows cisplatin administration. *Anticipatory emesis* occurs before administration of chemotherapy and represents a conditioned response to visual and olfactory stimuli previously associated with chemotherapy delivery.

Acute emesis is the best understood form. Stimuli that activate signals in the chemoreceptor trigger zone in the medulla, the cerebral cortex, and peripherally in the intestinal tract lead to stimulation of the vomiting center in the medulla, the motor center responsible for coordinating the secretory and muscle contraction activity that leads to emesis. Diverse receptor types participate in the process, including dopamine, serotonin, histamine, opioid, and acetylcholine receptors. The serotonin receptor antagonists ondansetron and granisetron are the most effective drugs against highly emetogenic agents, but they are expensive.

As with the analgesia ladder, emesis therapy should be tailored to the situation. For mildly and moderately emetogenic agents, prochlorperazine, 5–10 mg orally (PO) or 25 mg per rectume, is effective. Its efficacy may be enhanced by administering the drug before the chemotherapy is delivered. Dexamethasone, 10–20 mg intravenously (IV), is also effective and may enhance the efficacy of prochlorperazine. For highly emetogenic agents such as cisplatin, mechlorethamine, dacarbazine, and streptozocin, combinations of agents work best, and administration should begin 6–24 h before treatment. Ondansetron, 8 mg PO every 6 h the day before therapy and IV on the day of therapy, plus dexamethasone, 20 mg IV before treatment, is an effective regimen. Addition of oral aprepitant (a substance P/neurokinin 1 receptor antagonist) to this regimen (125 mg on day 1, 80 mg on days 2 and 3) further decreases the risk of both acute and delayed vomiting. Like pain, emesis is easier to prevent than to alleviate.

Delayed emesis may be related to bowel inflammation from the therapy and can be controlled with oral dexamethasone and oral metoclopramide, a dopamine receptor antagonist that also blocks serotonin receptors at high dosages. The best strategy for preventing anticipatory emesis is to control emesis in the early cycles of therapy to prevent the conditioning from taking place. If this is unsuccessful, prophylactic antiemetics the day before treatment may help. Experimental studies are evaluating behavior modification.

Effusions

Fluid may accumulate abnormally in the pleural cavity, pericardium, or peritoneum. Asymptomatic malignant effusions may not require treatment. Symptomatic effusions occurring in tumors responsive to systemic therapy usually do not require local treatment but respond to the treatment for the underlying tumor. Symptomatic effusions occurring in tumors unresponsive to systemic therapy may require local treatment in patients with a life expectancy of at least 6 months.

Pleural effusions due to tumors may or may not contain malignant cells. Lung cancer, breast cancer, and lymphomas account for ~75% of malignant pleural effusions. Their exudative nature is usually gauged by an effusion/serum protein ratio of ≥0.5 or an effusion/serum lactate dehydrogenase ratio of ≥0.6. When the condition is symptomatic, thoracentesis is usually performed first. In most cases, symptomatic improvement occurs for <1 month. Chest tube drainage is required if symptoms recur within 2 weeks. Fluid is aspirated until the flow rate is <100 mL in 24 h. Then 60 units of bleomycin or 1 g of doxycycline is infused into the chest tube in 50 mL of 5% dextrose in water; the tube is clamped; the patient is rotated on four sides, spending 15 min in each position; and, after 1–2 h, the tube is again attached to suction for another 24 h. The tube is then disconnected from suction and allowed to drain by gravity. If <100 mL drains over the next 24 h, the chest tube is pulled, and a radiograph is taken 24 h later. If the chest tube continues to drain fluid at an unacceptably high rate, sclerosis can be repeated. Bleomycin may be somewhat more effective than doxycycline but is very expensive. Doxycycline is usually the drug of first choice. If neither doxycycline nor bleomycin is effective, talc can be used.

Symptomatic pericardial effusions are usually treated by creating a pericardial window or by stripping the pericardium. If the patient's condition does not permit a surgical procedure, sclerosis can be attempted with doxycycline and/or bleomycin.

Malignant ascites is usually treated with repeated paracentesis of small volumes of fluid. If the underlying malignancy is unresponsive to systemic therapy, peritoneovenous shunts may be inserted. Despite the fear of disseminating tumor cells into the circulation, widespread metastases are an unusual complication. The major complications are occlusion, leakage, and fluid overload. Patients with severe liver disease may develop disseminated intravascular coagulation.

Nutrition

Cancer and its treatment may lead to a decrease in nutrient intake of sufficient magnitude to cause weight loss and alteration of intermediary metabolism. The prevalence of this problem is difficult to estimate because of variations in the definition of cancer cachexia, but most patients with advanced cancer experience weight loss and decreased appetite. A variety of both tumor-derived factors (e.g., bombesin, adrenocorticotropic hormone) and host-derived factors (e.g., tumor necrosis factor, interleukins 1 and 6, growth hormone) contribute to the altered metabolism, and a vicious cycle is established in which protein catabolism, glucose intolerance, and lipolysis cannot be reversed by the provision of calories.

It remains controversial how to assess nutritional status and when and how to intervene. Efforts to make the assessment objective have included the use of a prognostic nutritional index based on albumin levels, triceps skinfold thickness, transferrin levels, and delayed-type hypersensitivity skin testing. However, a simpler approach has been to define the threshold for nutritional intervention as >10% unexplained body weight loss, serum transferrin level <1500 mg/L (150 mg/dL), and serum albumin <34 g/L (3.4 g/dL).

The decision is important because it appears that cancer therapy is substantially more toxic and less effective in the face of malnutrition. Nevertheless, it remains unclear whether nutritional intervention can alter the natural history. Unless some pathology is affecting the absorptive function of the gastrointestinal tract, enteral nutrition provided orally or by tube feeding is preferred over parenteral supplementation. However, the risks associated with the tube may outweigh the benefits. Megestrol acetate, a progestational agent, has been advocated as a pharmacologic intervention to improve nutritional status. Research in this area may provide more tools in the future as cytokine-mediated mechanisms are further elucidated.

Psychosocial support

The psychosocial needs of patients vary with their situation. Patients undergoing treatment experience fear, anxiety, and depression. Self-image is often seriously compromised by deforming surgery and loss of hair. Women who receive cosmetic advice that enables them to look better also feel better. Loss of control over how one spends time can contribute to the sense of vulnerability. Juggling the demands of work and family with the demands of treatment may create enormous stresses. Sexual dysfunction is highly prevalent and needs to be discussed openly with the patient. An empathetic health care team is sensitive to the individual patient's needs and permits negotiation when such flexibility will not adversely affect the course of treatment.

Cancer survivors have other sets of difficulties. Patients may have fears associated with the termination of a treatment they associate with their continued survival. Adjustments are required to physical losses and disabilities, real and perceived. Patients may be preoccupied with minor physical problems. They perceive a decline in their job mobility and view themselves as less desirable workers. They may be victims of job or insurance discrimination. Patients may experience difficulty reentering their normal past lives. They may feel guilty for having survived and may carry a sense of vulnerability to colds and other illnesses. Perhaps the most pervasive and threatening concern is the ever-present fear of relapse (the Damocles syndrome).

Patients in whom therapy has been unsuccessful have other problems related to the end of life.

Death and dying

The most common causes of death in patients with cancer are infection (leading to circulatory failure), respiratory failure, hepatic failure, and renal failure. Intestinal blockage may lead to inanition and starvation. Central nervous system disease may lead to seizures, coma, and central hypoventilation. About 70% of patients develop dyspnea preterminally. However, many months usually pass between the diagnosis of cancer and the occurrence of these complications, and during this period, the patient is severely affected by the possibility of death. The path of unsuccessful cancer treatment usually occurs in three phases. First, there is optimism at the hope of cure; when the tumor recurs, there is the acknowledgment of an incurable disease, and the goal of palliative therapy is embraced in the hope of being able to live with disease; finally, at the disclosure of imminent death, another adjustment in outlook takes place. The patient imagines the worst in preparation for the end of life and may go through stages of adjustment to the diagnosis. These stages include denial, isolation, anger, bargaining, depression, acceptance, and hope. Of course, patients do not all progress through all the stages or proceed through them in the same order or at the same rate. Nevertheless, developing an understanding of how the patient has been affected by the diagnosis and is coping with it is an important goal of patient management.

It is best to speak frankly with the patient and the family regarding the likely course of disease. These discussions can be difficult for the physician as well as for the patient and family. The critical features of the interaction are to reassure the patient and family that everything that can be done to provide comfort will be done. They will not be abandoned. Many patients prefer to be cared for in their homes or in a hospice setting rather than a hospital. The American College of Physicians has published a book called *Home Care Guide for Cancer: How to Care for Family and Friends at Home* that teaches an approach to successful problem-solving in home care. With appropriate planning, it should be possible to provide the patient with the necessary medical care as well as the psychological and spiritual support that will prevent the isolation and depersonalization that can attend in-hospital death.

The care of dying patients may take a toll on the physician. A "burnout" syndrome has been described that is characterized by fatigue, disengagement from patients and colleagues, and a loss of self-fulfillment. Efforts at stress reduction, maintenance of a balanced life, and setting realistic goals may combat this disorder.

End-of-life decisions

Unfortunately, a smooth transition in treatment goals from curative to palliative may not be possible in all cases because of the occurrence of serious treatment-related complications or rapid disease progression. Vigorous and invasive medical support for a reversible disease or treatment complication is assumed to be justified. However, if the reversibility of the condition is in doubt, the patient's wishes determine the level of medical care. These wishes should be elicited before the terminal phase of illness and reviewed periodically. Information about advance directives can be obtained from the American Association of Retired Persons, 601 E Street, NW, Washington, DC 20049, 202-434-2277 or Choice in Dying, 250 West 57th Street, New York, NY 10107, 212-366-5540. A full discussion of end-of-life management is in Chap. 32.

CHAPTER 27

PREVENTION AND EARLY DETECTION OF CANCER

Jennifer M. Croswell ■ Otis W. Brawley ■ Barnett S. Kramer

Improved understanding of carcinogenesis has allowed cancer prevention and early detection (also known as cancer control) to expand beyond the identification and avoidance of carcinogens. Specific interventions to prevent cancer in those at risk and effective screening for early detection of cancer are the goals.

Carcinogenesis is not simply an event but a process, a continuum of discrete tissue and cellular changes over time, resulting in more autonomous cellular processes. Prevention concerns the identification and manipulation of the biologic, environmental, and genetic factors in the causal pathway of cancer.

EDUCATION AND HEALTHFUL HABITS

Public education on the avoidance of identified risk factors for cancer and encouraging healthy habits contribute to cancer prevention and control. The clinician is a powerful messenger in this process. The patient-provider encounter provides an opportunity to teach patients about the hazards of smoking, the features of a healthy lifestyle, use of proven cancer screening methods, and sun avoidance.

SMOKING CESSATION

Tobacco smoking is a strong, modifiable risk factor for cardiovascular disease, pulmonary disease, and cancer. Smokers have an approximately one in three lifetime risk of dying prematurely from a tobacco-related cancer or cardiovascular or pulmonary disease. Tobacco use causes more deaths from cardiovascular disease than from cancer. Lung cancer and cancers of the larynx, oropharynx, esophagus, kidney, bladder, pancreas, and stomach are all tobacco-related.

The number of cigarettes smoked per day and the level of inhalation of cigarette smoke are correlated with risk of lung cancer mortality. Light- and low-tar cigarettes are not safer because smokers tend to inhale them more frequently and deeply.

Those who stop smoking have a 30–50% lower 10-year lung cancer mortality rate compared with those who continue smoking, despite the fact that some carcinogen-induced gene mutations persist for years after smoking cessation. Smoking cessation and avoidance have the potential to save more lives than any other public health activity.

The risk of tobacco smoke is not limited to the smoker. Environmental tobacco smoke, known as secondhand or passive smoke, causes lung cancer and other cardiopulmonary diseases in nonsmokers.

Tobacco prevention is a pediatric issue. More than 80% of adult American smokers began smoking before the age of 18 years. Approximately 20% of Americans in grades 9 through 12 have smoked a cigarette in the past month. Counseling of adolescents and young adults is critical to prevent smoking. A clinician's simple advice to not start smoking or to quit smoking can be of benefit. Providers should query patients on tobacco use and offer smokers assistance in quitting.

Current approaches to smoking cessation recognize that smoking is an addiction. A smoker who is quitting goes through a process with identifiable stages that include contemplation of quitting, an action phase in which the smoker quits, and a maintenance phase. Smokers who quit completely are more likely to be successful than those who gradually reduce the number of cigarettes smoked or change to lower-tar or lower-nicotine cigarettes. More than 90% of the Americans who have successfully quit smoking did so on their own, without participation in an organized cessation program, but cessation programs are helpful for some smokers. The Community Intervention Trial for Smoking Cessation (COMMIT) was a 4-year program showing that light smokers (<25 cigarettes per day) were more likely to benefit from simple cessation messages and cessation programs than those who did not receive an intervention. Quit rates were 30.6% in the intervention group and 27.5% in the control group. The COMMIT interventions were not successful in heavy smokers (>25 cigarettes per day). Heavy smokers may need an intensive broad-based cessation program that includes counseling, behavioral strategies, and pharmacologic adjuncts, such as nicotine replacement (gum, patches, sprays, lozenges, and inhalers), bupropion, and/or varenicline.

The health risks of cigars are similar to those of cigarettes. Smoking one or two cigars daily doubles the risk for oral and esophageal cancers; three or four cigars daily increases the risk of oral cancers more than eightfold and esophageal cancer fourfold. The risks of occasional use are unknown.

Smokeless tobacco also represents a substantial health risk. Chewing tobacco is a carcinogen linked to dental caries, gingivitis, oral leukoplakia, and oral cancer. The systemic effects of smokeless tobacco (including snuff) may increase risks for other cancers. Esophageal cancer is linked to carcinogens in tobacco dissolved in saliva and swallowed.

PHYSICAL ACTIVITY

Physical activity is associated with a decreased risk of colon and breast cancer. A variety of mechanisms have been proposed. However, such studies are prone to confounding factors such as recall bias, association of exercise with other health-related practices, and effects of preclinical cancers on exercise habits (reverse causality).

DIET MODIFICATION

International epidemiologic studies suggest that diets high in fat are associated with an increased risk for cancers of the breast, colon, prostate, and endometrium. These cancers have their highest incidence and mortalities in western cultures, where fat comprises an average of one-third of the total calories consumed.

Despite correlations, dietary fat has not been proven to cause cancer. Case-control and cohort epidemiologic studies give conflicting results. In addition, diet is a highly complex exposure to many nutrients and chemicals. Low-fat diets are associated with many dietary changes beyond simple subtraction of fat. Other lifestyle changes are also associated with adherence to a low-fat diet.

In observational studies, dietary fiber is associated with a reduced risk of colonic polyps and invasive cancer of the colon. However, cancer-protective effects of increasing fiber and lowering dietary fat have not been proven in the context of a prospective clinical trial. The putative protective mechanisms are complex and speculative. Fiber binds oxidized bile acids and generates soluble fiber products, such as butyrate, that may have differentiating properties. Fiber does not increase bowel transit times. High-fiber diets could lower the risk of breast and prostate cancer by absorbing and inactivating dietary estrogenic and androgenic cancer promoters. However, two large prospective cohort studies of >100,000 health professionals showed no association between fruit and vegetable intake and risk of cancer.

The Polyp Prevention Trial randomly assigned 2000 elderly persons, who had polyps removed, to a low-fat, high-fiber diet versus routine diet for 4 years. No differences were noted in polyp formation.

The U.S. National Institutes of Health Women's Health Initiative, launched in 1994, was a long-term clinical trial enrolling >100,000 women aged 45–69 years. It placed women in 22 intervention groups. Participants received calcium/vitamin D supplementation; hormone-replacement therapy; and counseling to increase exercise, eat a low-fat diet with increased consumption of fruits, vegetables, and fiber, and cease smoking. The study showed that while dietary fat intake was lower in the diet intervention group, invasive breast cancers were not reduced over an 8-year follow-up period compared with the control group. No reduction was seen in the incidence of colorectal cancer in the dietary intervention arm. The difference in dietary fat averaged ~10% between the two groups. Evidence does not currently establish the anti-carcinogenic value of vitamin, mineral, or nutritional supplements in amounts greater than those provided by a balanced diet.

ENERGY BALANCE

The risk of cancer appears to increase as body mass index increases to more than 25 kg/m^2. Obesity is associated with increased risk for cancers of the colon, breast (female postmenopausal), endometrium, kidney (renal cell), and esophagus, although causality has not been established.

In observational studies, relative risks of colon cancer are increased in obesity by 1.5–2 for men and 1.2–1.5 for women. Obese postmenopausal women have a 30–50% increased risk of breast cancer. A hypothesis for the association is that adipose tissue serves as a depot for aromatase that facilitates estrogen production.

SUN AVOIDANCE

Nonmelanoma skin cancers (basal cell and squamous cell) are induced by cumulative exposure to ultraviolet radiation. Intermittent acute sun exposure and sun damage have been linked to melanoma, but the evidence is inconsistent. Sunburns, especially in childhood and adolescence, may be associated with an increased risk of melanoma in adulthood. Reduction of sun exposure through use of protective clothing and changing patterns of outdoor activities can reduce the skin cancer risk. Sunscreens decrease the risk of actinic keratoses, the precursor to squamous cell skin cancer, but melanoma risk may not be reduced. Sunscreens prevent burning, but they may encourage more prolonged exposure to the sun and may not filter out wavelengths of energy that cause melanoma.

Educational interventions to help individuals accurately assess their risk of developing skin cancer have some impact. Self-examination for skin pigment characteristics associated with skin cancer, such as freckling, may be useful in identifying people at high risk. Those who recognize themselves as being at risk tend to be more compliant with sun-avoidance recommendations. Risk factors for melanoma include a propensity to sunburn, a large number of benign melanocytic nevi, and atypical nevi.

CANCER CHEMOPREVENTION

Chemoprevention involves the use of specific natural or synthetic chemical agents to reverse, suppress, or prevent carcinogenesis before the development of invasive malignancy.

Cancer develops through an accumulation of tissue abnormalities associated with genetic and epigenetic changes that are potential points of intervention to prevent cancer. The initial changes are termed *initiation*. The alteration can be inherited or acquired through the action of physical, infectious, or chemical carcinogens. Like most human diseases, cancer arises from an interaction between genetics and environmental exposures (Table 27-1). Influences that cause the initiated cell to progress through the carcinogenic process and change phenotypically are termed *promoters*. Promoters include hormones such as androgens, linked to prostate cancer, and estrogen, linked to breast and endometrial cancer. The distinction between an initiator and promoter is sometimes arbitrary; some components of cigarette smoke are "complete carcinogens," acting as both initiators and promoters. Cancer can be prevented or controlled through interference with the factors that cause cancer initiation, promotion, or progression. Compounds of interest in chemoprevention often have antimutagenic, hormone modulation, anti-inflammatory, antiproliferative, or pro-apoptotic activity (or a combination).

TABLE 27-1

SUSPECTED CARCINOGENS

CARCINOGENS[a]	ASSOCIATED CANCER OR NEOPLASM
Alkylating agents	Acute myeloid leukemia, bladder cancer
Androgens	Prostate cancer
Aromatic amines (dyes)	Bladder cancer
Arsenic	Cancer of the lung, skin
Asbestos	Cancer of the lung, pleura, peritoneum
Benzene	Acute myelocytic leukemia
Chromium	Lung cancer
Diethylstilbestrol (prenatal)	Vaginal cancer (clear cell)
Epstein-Barr virus	Burkitt's lymphoma, nasal T cell lymphoma
Estrogens	Cancer of the endometrium, liver, breast
Ethyl alcohol	Cancer of the liver, esophagus, head and neck
Helicobacter pylori	Gastric cancer, gastric MALT lymphoma
Hepatitis B or C virus	Liver cancer
Human immunodeficiency virus	Non-Hodgkin's lymphoma, Kaposi's sarcoma, squamous cell carcinomas (especially of the urogenital tract)
Human papilloma virus	Cervix cancer, head and neck cancer
Human T cell lymphotropic virus type I (HTLV-I)	Adult T cell leukemia/ lymphoma
Immunosuppressive agents (azathioprine, cyclosporine, glucocorticoids)	Non-Hodgkin's lymphoma
Ionizing radiation (therapeutic or diagnostic)	Breast, bladder, thyroid, soft tissue, bone, hematopoietic, and many more
Nitrogen mustard gas	Cancer of the lung, head and neck, nasal sinuses
Nickel dust	Cancer of the lung, nasal sinuses
Phenacetin	Cancer of the renal pelvis and bladder
Polycyclic hydrocarbons	Cancer of the lung, skin (especially squamous cell carcinoma of scrotal skin)
Schistosomiasis	Bladder cancer (squamous cell)
Sunlight (ultraviolet)	Skin cancer (squamous cell and melanoma)
Tobacco (including smokeless)	Cancer of the upper aerodigestive tract, bladder
Vinyl chloride	Liver cancer (angiosarcoma)

[a]Agents that are thought to act as cancer initiators and/or promoters.

CHEMOPREVENTION OF CANCERS OF THE UPPER AERODIGESTIVE TRACT

Smoking causes diffuse epithelial injury in the oral cavity, neck, esophagus, and lung. Patients cured of squamous cell cancers of the lung, esophagus, oral cavity, and neck are at risk (as high as 5% per year) of developing second cancers of the upper aerodigestive tract. Cessation of cigarette smoking does not markedly decrease the cured cancer patient's risk of second malignancy even though it does lower the cancer risk in those who have never developed a malignancy. Smoking cessation may halt the early stages of the carcinogenic process (such as metaplasia), but it may have no effect on late stages of carcinogenesis. This "field carcinogenesis" hypothesis for upper aerodigestive tract cancer has made "cured" patients an important population for chemoprevention of second malignancies.

Oral human papilloma virus (HPV) infection, particularly HPV-16, increases the risk for cancers of the oropharynx. This association exists even in the absence of other risk factors such as smoking or alcohol use (although the magnitude of increased risk appears greater than additive when HPV infection and smoking are both present). Oral HPV infection is believed to be largely sexually acquired. The introduction of the HPV vaccine might eventually reduce oropharyngeal cancer rates.

Oral leukoplakia, a premalignant lesion commonly found in smokers, has been used as an intermediate marker allowing demonstration of chemopreventive activity in smaller shorter-duration, randomized, placebo-controlled trials. Response was associated with upregulation of retinoic acid receptor-β (RAR-β). Therapy with high, relatively toxic doses of isotretinoin (13-*cis*-retinoic acid) causes regression of oral leukoplakia. However, the lesions recur when the therapy is withdrawn, suggesting the need for long-term administration. More tolerable doses of isotretinoin have not proven beneficial in the prevention of head and neck cancer. Isotretinoin also failed to prevent second malignancies in patients cured of early-stage non-small cell lung cancer; mortality rates were actually increased in current smokers.

Several large-scale trials have assessed agents in the chemoprevention of lung cancer in patients at high risk. In the α-tocopherol/β-carotene (ATBC) Lung Cancer Prevention Trial, participants were male smokers, ages 50–69 years at entry. Participants had smoked an average of one pack of cigarettes per day for 35.9 years. Participants received α-tocopherol, β-carotene, and/or placebo in a randomized, two-by-two factorial design. After a median follow-up of 6.1 years, lung cancer incidence and mortality were statistically significantly increased in those receiving β-carotene. α-Tocopherol had no effect on lung cancer mortality, and no evidence suggested interaction between the two drugs. Patients receiving α-tocopherol had a higher incidence of hemorrhagic stroke.

The β-Carotene and Retinol Efficacy Trial (CARET) involved 17,000 American smokers and workers with asbestos exposure. Entrants were randomly assigned to one of four arms and received β-carotene, retinol, and/or placebo in a two-by-two factorial design. This trial also demonstrated harm from β-carotene: a lung cancer rate of 5 per 1000 subjects per year for those taking placebo and of 6 per 1000 subjects per year for those taking β-carotene.

The ATBC and CARET results demonstrate the importance of testing chemoprevention hypotheses thoroughly before their widespread implementation as the results contradict a number of observational studies. The Physicians' Health Trial showed no change in the risk of lung cancer for those taking β-carotene; however, fewer of its participants were smokers than those in the ATBC and CARET studies.

CHEMOPREVENTION OF COLON CANCER

Many colon cancer prevention trials are based on the premise that most colorectal cancers develop from adenomatous polyps. These trials use adenoma recurrence or disappearance as a surrogate endpoint (not yet validated) for colon cancer prevention. Early clinical trial results suggest that nonsteroidal anti-inflammatory drugs (NSAIDs), such as piroxicam, sulindac, and aspirin, may prevent adenoma formation or cause regression of adenomatous polyps. The mechanism of action of NSAIDs is unknown, but they are presumed to work through the cyclooxygenase (COX) pathway. Pooled findings from observational cohort studies demonstrate a relative reduction in colorectal cancer incidence of approximately 22% and a relative reduction in colorectal adenoma incidence of about 28% with regular aspirin use; however, in two randomized controlled trials (the Physicians' Health Study and the Women's Health Study), aspirin had no effect on colon cancer or adenoma incidence in persons with no previous history of colonic lesions, at up to 10 years of therapy. The randomized controlled trials did show an approximately 18% relative risk reduction for colonic adenoma incidence in persons with a previous history of adenomas after 1 year's therapy.

COX-2 inhibitors have also been considered for colorectal cancer and polyp prevention. Trials with COX-2 inhibitors were initiated, but an increased risk of cardiovascular events in those taking the COX-2 inhibitors was noted, suggesting that these agents are not suitable for chemoprevention in the general population.

Epidemiologic studies suggest that diets high in calcium lower colon cancer risk. Calcium binds bile and fatty acids, which cause proliferation of colonic epithelium. It is hypothesized that calcium reduces intraluminal exposure to these compounds. The randomized controlled Calcium Polyp Prevention Study found that calcium supplementation decreased the absolute risk of adenomatous polyp recurrence by 7% at 4 years; extended observational follow-up demonstrated a 12% absolute risk reduction 5 years after cessation of treatment. However, in the Women's Health Initiative, combined use of calcium carbonate and vitamin D twice daily did not reduce the incidence of invasive colorectal cancer compared with placebo after 7 years.

The Women's Health Initiative demonstrated that postmenopausal women taking estrogen plus progestin have a 44% lower risk of colorectal cancer compared with women taking placebo. Of >16,600 women randomized and followed for a median of 5.6 years, 43 invasive colorectal cancers occurred in the hormone group and 72 in the placebo group. The positive effect on colon cancer is mitigated by the modest increase in cardiovascular and breast cancer risks associated with combined estrogen plus progestin therapy.

A case-control study suggested that statins decrease the incidence of colorectal cancer; however, several subsequent case-control and cohort studies have not demonstrated an association between regular statin use and a reduced risk of colorectal cancer. No randomized controlled trials have addressed this hypothesis. A meta-analysis of statin use showed no protective effect of statins on overall cancer incidence or death.

CHEMOPREVENTION OF BREAST CANCER

Tamoxifen is an antiestrogen with partial estrogen agonistic activity in some tissues, such as endometrium and bone. One of its actions is to upregulate transforming growth factor β, which decreases breast cell proliferation. In randomized placebo-controlled trials to assess tamoxifen as adjuvant therapy for breast cancer, tamoxifen reduced the number of new breast cancers in the opposite breast by more than one-third. In a randomized placebo-controlled prevention trial involving >13,000 women at high risk, tamoxifen decreased the risk of developing breast cancer by 49% (from 43.4 to 22 per 1000 women) after a median follow-up of nearly 6 years. Tamoxifen also reduced bone fractures; a small increase in risk of endometrial cancer, stroke, pulmonary emboli, and deep-vein thrombosis was noted. The International Breast Cancer Intervention Study (IBIS-I) and the Italian Randomized Tamoxifen Prevention Trial also demonstrated a reduction in breast cancer incidence with tamoxifen use. Tamoxifen has been approved by the U.S. Food and Drug Administration for reduction of breast cancer in women at high risk for the disease (1.66% risk at 5 years based on the Gail risk model: *www.nci.nih.gov/cancertopics/pdq/genetics/breast-and-ovarian/healthprofessional#Section_66*).

A trial comparing tamoxifen with another selective estrogen receptor modulator, raloxifene, showed that raloxifene is comparable to tamoxifen in cancer prevention. This trial only included postmenopausal women. Raloxifene was associated with more noninvasive breast cancer than tamoxifen; the drugs are similar in risks of other cancers, fractures, ischemic heart disease, and stroke. Because the aromatase inhibitors are even more effective than tamoxifen in adjuvant breast cancer therapy, it is hoped that they would be more effective in breast cancer prevention. However, no data are yet available on this point.

CHEMOPREVENTION OF PROSTATE CANCER

Finasteride is a 5-α-reductase inhibitor. It inhibits conversion of testosterone to dihydrotestosterone (DHT), a potent stimulator of prostate cell proliferation. The Prostate Cancer Prevention Trial (PCPT) randomly assigned men aged 55 years or older at average risk of prostate cancer to finasteride or placebo. All men in the trial were being regularly screened with prostate-specific antigen (PSA) and digital rectal examination (DRE). After 7 years of therapy, the incidence of prostate cancer was 18.4% in the finasteride arm and 24.8% in the placebo arm, a statistically significant difference. However, the finasteride group had more patients with tumors of Gleason score 7 and higher compared with the placebo arm (6.4 vs 5.1%). The clinical significance of this finding, if any, is unknown. The observed increase in high-grade tumors was spurious and likely due to an increased sensitivity of PSA and DRE for high-grade tumors in men receiving finasteride.

Another 5-α-reductase inhibitor, dutasteride, has also been evaluated as a preventive agent for prostate cancer. The Reduction by Dutasteride of Prostate Cancer Events (REDUCE) trial was a randomized double-blind trial in which approximately 8200 men with an elevated PSA (2.5–10 ng/mL for men aged 50–60 years and 3–10 ng/mL for men aged 60 years or older) and negative prostate biopsy results on enrollment received 0.5 mg/d of dutasteride or placebo. A preliminary report from this trial noted a statistically significant 23% relative risk reduction in the incidence of biopsy-detected prostate cancer in the dutasteride arm at 4 years of treatment (659 cases vs 857 cases, respectively). Unlike the PCPT, no difference was observed in the rates of high-grade prostate cancer. Since all men in both the PCPT and REDUCE trials were being screened and since screening approximately doubles the rate of prostate cancer, it is not known if finasteride or dutasteride decrease the risk of prostate cancer in men who are not being screened.

Several favorable laboratory and observational studies led to the formal evaluation of selenium and α-tocopherol (vitamin E) as potential prostate cancer preventives. The Selenium and Vitamin E Cancer Prevention Trial (SELECT) assigned 35,533 men to receive 200 μg/d selenium, 400 IU/d α-tocopherol, selenium plus vitamin E, or placebo. After a median follow-up of 5.5 years, no significant difference in the prostate cancer incidence rate was observed for any group. In fact, compared with placebo, a trend toward an increased risk of developing prostate cancer was observed for those men taking vitamin E alone (hazard ratio, 1.13; 95% confidence interval [CI], 0.99–1.29)

VACCINES AND CANCER PREVENTION

A number of infectious agents cause cancer. Hepatitis B and C are linked to liver cancer, some HPV strains are linked to cervical and head and neck cancer, and *Helicobacter pylori* is associated with gastric adenocarcinoma and gastric lymphoma. Vaccines to protect against these agents may reduce the risk of their associated cancers.

The hepatitis B vaccine is effective in preventing hepatitis and hepatomas due to chronic hepatitis B infection. Public health officials are encouraging widespread administration of the hepatitis B vaccine, especially in Asia, where the disease is epidemic.

A quadrivalent HPV vaccine (covering HPV strains 6, 11, 16, and 18) and a bivalent vaccine (covering HPV strains 16 and 18) are available for use in the United States. HPV types 16 and 18 cause cervical cancer, and types 6 and 11 cause genital papillomas. For females not previously infected with these HPV strains, the vaccines demonstrate high efficacy in preventing persistent strain-specific HPV infections. Trials that evaluated the vaccines' ability to prevent cervical cancer relied on surrogate outcome measures (cervical intraepithelial neoplasia [CIN] I, II, and III), and no cases of cervical cancer were observed in either the vaccine or control arms. The vaccines do not appear to impact preexisting infections; efficacy was markedly lower for populations that had previously been exposed to vaccine-specific HPV strains. The vaccine is recommended for girls and women ages 9–26 years. Reduction in these HPV types could prevent >70% of cervical cancers worldwide.

SURGICAL PREVENTION OF CANCER

Some organs in some individuals are at such high risk of developing cancer that surgical removal of the organ at risk may be considered. Women with severe cervical dysplasia are treated with conization and occasionally even hysterectomy. Colectomy is used to prevent colon cancer in patients with familial polyposis or ulcerative colitis.

Prophylactic bilateral mastectomy may be chosen for breast cancer prevention among women with genetic predisposition to breast cancer. In a prospective series of 139 women with *BRCA1* and *BRCA2* mutations, 76 chose to undergo prophylactic mastectomy, and 63 chose close surveillance. At 3 years, no cases of breast cancer had been diagnosed in those opting for surgery, but 8 in the surveillance group had developed breast cancer. A larger (n = 639) retrospective cohort study reported that 3 patients developed breast cancer after prophylactic mastectomy compared with an expected incidence of 30–53 cases, a 90–94% reduction in breast cancer risk. The effect of the procedure on mortality is unknown.

Prophylactic oophorectomy may also be employed for the prevention of ovarian and breast cancers among high-risk women. A case-control study of women with *BRCA1* or *BRCA2* mutations found that 6 (2.8%) of 259 women who underwent bilateral prophylactic oophorectomy had stage I ovarian cancer at the time of surgery, and 2 (0.8%) developed papillary serous peritoneal carcinoma over 9 years. By comparison, 58 (19.9%) of 292 women in the matched control group developed ovarian cancer: this corresponds to a 96% relative risk reduction for ovarian cancer with the use of prophylactic surgery. Studies of prophylactic oophorectomy for prevention of breast cancer in women with genetic mutations have shown relative risk reductions of approximately 50%.

At present, all of the evidence concerning the use of prophylactic mastectomy and oophorectomy for prevention of breast and ovarian cancer in high-risk women has been observational in nature; such studies are prone to a variety of biases, including case selection bias, family relationships between patients and control participants, and inadequate information about hormone use. Thus, they may give an overestimate of the magnitude of benefit.

Orchiectomy is an effective method of androgen deprivation in prostate cancer.

CANCER SCREENING

Screening is a means of detecting disease early in asymptomatic individuals, with the goal of decreasing morbidity and mortality. While screening can potentially reduce disease-specific deaths and has been shown to do so in cervical, colon, and breast cancer, it is also subject to a number of biases that can suggest a benefit when actually there is none. Biases can even mask net harm. Early detection does not in itself confer benefit. To be of value, screening must detect disease earlier, and treatment of earlier disease must yield a better outcome than treatment at the onset of symptoms. Cause-specific mortality, rather than survival after diagnosis, is the preferred endpoint (see later discussion).

Because screening is done on asymptomatic, healthy persons, it should offer a substantial likelihood of benefit that outweighs harm. Screening tests and their appropriate use should be carefully evaluated before their use is widely encouraged in screening programs as a matter of public policy.

A large and increasing number of genetic mutations and nucleotide polymorphisms have been associated with an increased risk of cancer. Testing for these genetic mutations could in theory define a high-risk population. However, most of the identified mutations have very low penetrance and individually provide minimal predictive accuracy. The ability to predict the development of a particular cancer may some day present therapeutic options as well as ethical dilemmas. It may eventually allow for early intervention to prevent a cancer or limit its severity. People at high risk may be ideal candidates for chemoprevention and screening; however, the efficacy of these interventions in the high-risk population should be investigated. Currently, persons at high risk for a particular cancer can engage in intensive screening. While this course is clinically reasonable, it is not known if it saves lives in these populations.

The accuracy of screening

A screening test's accuracy or ability to discriminate disease is described by four indices: sensitivity, specificity, positive predictive value, and negative predictive value (Table 27-2). *Sensitivity*, also called the true positive rate, is the proportion of persons with the disease who test positive in the screen (i.e., the ability of the test to detect disease when it is present). *Specificity*, or 1 minus the false-positive rate, is the proportion of persons who do not have the disease and test negative in the screening test (i.e., the ability of a test to correctly identify that the disease is not present). The *positive predictive value* is the proportion of persons who test positive and actually have the disease. Similarly, *negative predictive value* is the proportion testing negative who do not have the disease. The sensitivity and specificity of a test are independent of the underlying prevalence (or risk) of the disease in the population screened, but the predictive values depend strongly on the prevalence of the disease.

Screening is most beneficial, efficient, and economical when the target disease is common in the population being screened. To be valuable, the screening test should have a high specificity; sensitivity need not be very high.

TABLE 27-2

ASSESSMENT OF THE VALUE OF A DIAGNOSTIC TEST[a]

	CONDITION PRESENT	CONDITION ABSENT
Positive test result	*a*	*b*
Negative test result	*c*	*d*

a = true positive
b = false positive
c = false negative
d = true negative

Sensitivity	The proportion of persons with the condition who test positive: $a/(a + c)$
Specificity	The proportion of persons without the condition who test negative: $d/(b + d)$
Positive predictive value (PPV)	The proportion of persons with a positive test who have the condition: $a/(a + b)$
Negative predictive value	The proportion of persons with a negative test who do not have the condition: $d/(c + d)$

Prevalence, sensitivity, and specificity determine PPV

$$\text{PPV} = \frac{\text{prevalence} \times \text{sensitivity}}{(\text{prevalence} \times \text{sensitivity}) + (1 - \text{prevalence})(1 - \text{specificity})}$$

[a]For diseases of low prevalence, such as cancer, poor specificity has a dramatic adverse effect on PPV such that only a small fraction of positive test results are true positives.

Potential biases of screening tests

Common biases of screening are lead time, length-biased sampling, and selection. These biases can make a screening test seem beneficial when actually it is not (or even causes net harm). Whether beneficial or not, screening can create the false impression of an epidemic by increasing the number of cancers diagnosed. It can also produce a shift in the proportion of patients diagnosed at an early stage and inflated survival statistics without reducing mortality (i.e., the number of deaths from a given cancer relative to the number of those at risk for the cancer). In such a case, the *apparent* duration of survival (measured from the date of diagnosis) increases without lives being saved or life expectancy changed.

Lead-time bias occurs when a test does not influence the natural history of the disease; the patient is merely diagnosed at an earlier date. When lead-time bias occurs, survival *appears* increased, but life is not really prolonged. The screening test only prolongs the time the subject is aware of the disease and spends as a patient.

Length-biased sampling occurs because screening tests generally can more easily detect slow-growing, less aggressive cancers than fast-growing cancers. Cancers diagnosed due to the onset of symptoms between scheduled screenings are on average more aggressive, and treatment outcomes are not as favorable. An extreme form of length bias sampling is termed *overdiagnosis*, the detection of "pseudo disease." The reservoir of some undetected slow-growing tumors is large. Many of these tumors fulfill the histologic criteria of cancer but will never become clinically significant or cause death. This problem is compounded by the fact that the most common cancers appear most frequently at ages when competing causes of death are more frequent.

Selection bias must be considered in assessing the results of any screening effort. The population most likely to seek screening may differ from the general population to which the screening test might be applied. In general, volunteers for studies are more health conscious and likely to have a better prognosis or lower mortality rate, irrespective of the screening result. This is termed the *healthy volunteer effect*.

Potential drawbacks of screening

Risks associated with screening include harm caused by the screening intervention itself, harm due to the further investigation of persons with positive tests (both true and false positives), and harm from the treatment of persons with a true-positive result, even if life is extended by treatment. The diagnosis and treatment of cancers that would never have caused medical problems can lead to the harm of unnecessary treatment and give patients the anxiety of a cancer diagnosis. The psychosocial impact of cancer screening can also be substantial when applied to the entire population.

Assessment of screening tests

Good clinical trial design can offset some biases of screening and demonstrate the relative risks and benefits of a screening test. A randomized controlled screening trial with cause-specific mortality as the endpoint provides the strongest support for a screening intervention. Overall mortality should also be reported to detect an adverse effect of screening and treatment on other disease outcomes (e.g., cardiovascular disease). In a randomized trial, two like populations are randomly established. One is given the usual standard of care (which may be no screening at all), and the other receives the screening intervention being assessed. The two populations are compared over time. Efficacy for the population studied is established when the group receiving the screening test has a better cause-specific mortality rate than the control group. Studies showing a reduction in the incidence of advanced-stage disease, an improved survival, or a stage shift are weaker (and possibly misleading) evidence of benefit. These latter criteria are necessary but not sufficient to establish the value of a screening test.

Although a randomized, controlled screening trial provides the strongest evidence to support a screening test, it is not perfect. Unless the trial is population-based, it does not remove the question of generalizability to the target population. Screening trials generally involve thousands of persons and last for years. Less definitive study designs are therefore often used to estimate the effectiveness of screening practices. However, every non-randomized study design is subject to strong confounders. In descending order of strength, evidence may also be derived from the findings of internally controlled trials using intervention allocation methods other than randomization (e.g., allocation by birth date, date of clinic visit), the findings of cohort or case-control analytic observational studies, or the results of multiple time series studies with or without the intervention.

Screening for specific cancers

Widespread screening for cervical, colon, and breast cancer is beneficial for certain age groups. A number of organizations have considered whether or not to endorse routine use of certain screening tests. Because these groups have not used the same criteria to judge whether a screening test should be endorsed, they have arrived at different recommendations. The American Cancer Society (ACS) and the U.S. Preventive Services Task Force (USPSTF) publish screening guidelines (Table 27-3); the American College of Physicians (ACP) and the American Academy of Family Practitioners (AAFP) generally follow or endorse the USPSTF recommendations. Special surveillance of those at high risk for a specific cancer because of a family history or a genetic risk factor may be prudent, but few studies have assessed the influence on mortality.

Breast cancer

Breast self-examination, clinical breast examination by a caregiver, mammography, and magnetic resonance imaging (MRI) have all been variably advocated as useful screening tools.

A number of trials have suggested that annual or biennial screening with mammography or mammography plus clinical breast examination in normal-risk women older than age 50 years decreases the breast cancer mortality rate. Each trial has been criticized for design flaws. In most trials, the breast cancer mortality rate is decreased by 15–30%. Experts disagree on whether average-risk women aged 40–49 years should receive regular screening (Table 27-3). The U.K. Age Trial, the only randomized trial of breast cancer screening to specifically evaluate the impact of mammography in women aged 40–49 years, found no statistically significant difference in breast cancer mortality rate for screened women versus controls after about 11 years of follow-up (relative risk [RR], 0.83; 95% CI, 0.66–1.04); however, fewer than 70% of women received screening in the intervention arm, potentially diluting the observed effect. A meta-analysis of eight large randomized trials showed a 15% relative reduction in mortality (RR, 0.85; 95% CI, 0.75–0.96) from

TABLE 27-3

SCREENING RECOMMENDATIONS FOR ASYMPTOMATIC NORMAL-RISK SUBJECTS[a]

TEST OR PROCEDURE	USPSTF	ACS
Sigmoidoscopy	Adults 50–75 years: every 5 years ("A")[b] Adults 76–85 years: "C" Adults ≥85 years: "D"	Adults ≥50 years: Screen every 5 years
Fecal occult blood testing (FOBT)	Adults 50–75 years: Annually ("A") Adults 76–85 years: "C" Adults ≥85 years: "D"	Adults ≥50 years: Screen every year
Colonoscopy	Adults 50–75 years: every 10 years ("A") Adults 76–85 years: "C" Adults ≥85 years: "D"	Adults ≥50 years: Screen every 10 years
Fecal DNA testing	"I"	Adults ≥50 years: Screen, but interval uncertain
Fecal immunochemical testing (FIT)	"I"	Adults ≥50 years: Screen every year
CT colonography	"I"	Adults ≥50 years: Screen every 5 years
Digital rectal examination (DRE)	No recommendation	Men ≥50 years with a 10-year life expectancy; men ≥45 years, if African American, or men with a first-degree relative diagnosed with prostate cancer <65 years; ≥40, if has several relatives with prostate cancer <65 years: Discuss and offer (with PSA testing) annually
Prostate-specific antigen (PSA)	Men <75 years: "I" Men ≥75 years: "D"	As for DRE
Pap test	Women <65 years: Beginning 3 years after first intercourse or by age 21 years, screen at least every 3 years ("A") Women ≥65 years, with adequate, normal recent Pap screenings: "D" Women after total hysterectomy for noncancerous causes: "D"	Women <30 years: Beginning 3 years after first intercourse or by age 21. Yearly for standard Pap; every 2 years with liquid test. Women 30–70 years: Every 2–3 years if last 3 tests normal Women ≥70 years: May stop screening if no abnormal Pap in past 10 years Women after total hysterectomy for noncancerous causes: Do not screen
Breast self-examination	"D"	Women ≥20 years: Breast self-exam is an option
Breast clinical examination	Women ≥40 years: "I" (as a stand-alone without mammography)	Women 20–40 years: Perform every 3 years Women ≥40 years: Perform annually
Mammography	Women 40–49 years: The decision should be an individual one and take patient context into account ("C") Women 50–74 years: every 2 years ("B") Women ≥75 years: ("I")	Women ≥40 years: Screen annually
Magnetic resonance imaging (MRI)	"I"	Women >20% lifetime risk of breast cancer: Screen with MRI plus mammography annually Women 15–20% lifetime risk of breast cancer: Discuss option of MRI plus mammography annually Women <15% lifetime risk of breast cancer: Do not screen annually with MRI
Complete skin examination	"I"	Self-examination monthly; clinical exam as part of routine cancer-related checkup

[a]Summary of the screening procedures recommended for the general population by the U.S. Preventive Services Task Force (USPSTF) and the American Cancer Society (ACS). These recommendations refer to asymptomatic persons who have no risk factors, other than age or gender, for the targeted condition.

[b]USPSTF lettered recommendations are defined as follows: "A": The USPSTF strongly recommends that clinicians provide (the service) to eligible patients; "B": The USPSTF recommends that clinicians provide (this service) to eligible patients; "C": The USPSTF makes no recommendation for or against routine provision of (the service); "D": The USPSTF recommends against routinely providing [the service] to asymptomatic patients; "I": The USPSTF concludes that the evidence is insufficient to recommend for or against routinely providing (the service).

mammography screening for women aged 39–49 years after 11–20 years of follow-up. This is equivalent to a number needed to invite to screening of 1904 over 10 years to prevent one breast cancer death. At the same time, nearly half of women aged 40–49 years screened annually will have false-positive mammograms necessitating further evaluation, often including biopsy. Estimates of overdiagnosis range from 10 to 40% of diagnosed invasive cancers.

No study of breast self-examination has shown it to decrease the mortality rate. A randomized controlled trial of approximately 266,000 women in China demonstrated no difference in the mortality rate between a group that received intensive breast self-exam instruction and reinforcement and reminders and control participants at 10 years of follow-up. However, more benign breast lesions were discovered, and more breast biopsies were performed in the self-examination arm.

Genetic screening for *BRCA1* and *BRCA2* mutations and other markers of breast cancer risk has identified a group of women at high risk for breast cancer. Unfortunately, when to begin and the optimal frequency of screening have not been defined. Mammography is less sensitive at detecting breast cancers in women carrying *BRCA1* and *-2* mutations, possibly because such cancers occur in younger women, in whom mammography is known to be less sensitive. MRI screening may be more sensitive than mammography in women at high risk due to genetic predisposition or in women with very dense breast tissue, but specificity may be lower. An increase in overdiagnosis may accompany the higher sensitivity. The impact of MRI on breast cancer mortality with or without concomitant use of mammography has not been evaluated in a randomized controlled trial.

Cervical cancer

Screening with Papanicolaou smears decreases cervical cancer mortality rates. The cervical cancer mortality rate has fallen substantially since the widespread use of the Pap smear. Screening guidelines recommend regular Pap testing for all women who have reached the age of 21 years; some organizations advocate beginning earlier depending on sexual history. With the onset of sexual activity comes the risk of sexual transmission of HPV, the most common etiologic factor for cervical cancer. The recommended interval for Pap screening varies from 1 to 3 years. At age 30 years, women who have had three normal test results in a row may get screened every 2–3 years. An upper age limit at which screening ceases to be effective is not known, but women aged 65–70 years with no abnormal results in the previous 10 years may choose to stop screening. Screening should be discontinued in women who have undergone a hysterectomy for non cancerous reasons.

Although the efficacy of the Papanicolaou smear in reducing cervical cancer mortality rates has never been directly confirmed in a randomized, controlled setting, a clustered randomized trial in India evaluated the impact of one-time cervical visual inspection and immediate colposcopy, biopsy, and/or cryotherapy (when indicated) versus counseling on cervical cancer deaths in women aged 30–59 years. After 7 years of follow-up, the age-standardized rate of death due to cervical cancer was 39.6 per 100,000 person-years in the intervention group versus 56.7 per 100,000 person-years in control participants.

Colorectal cancer

Fecal occult blood testing (FOBT), DRE rigid and flexible sigmoidoscopy, colonoscopy, and computed tomography (CT) colonography have been considered for colorectal cancer screening. Annual FOBT could reduce colorectal cancer mortality by one-third. The sensitivity for fecal occult blood is increased if specimens are rehydrated before testing but at the cost of lower specificity. The false-positive rate for rehydrated FOBT is high; 1–5% of persons tested have a positive test result. Only 2–10% of those with occult blood in the stool have cancer, and 20–30% have adenomas. The high false-positive rate of FOBT dramatically increases the number of colonoscopies performed.

Fecal immunochemical tests appear to have higher sensitivity for colorectal cancer than nonrehydrated FOBT tests. Fecal DNA testing is an emerging testing modality; it appears to have increased sensitivity and comparable specificity to FOBT and could potentially reduce harms associated with follow-up of false-positive test results. The body of evidence on the operating characteristics and effectiveness of fecal DNA tests in reducing colorectal cancer mortality rates is limited.

Two case-control studies suggest that regular screening of those older than age 50 years with sigmoidoscopy decreases mortality rates. This type of study is prone to selection biases. One-quarter to one-third of polyps can be discovered with the rigid sigmoidoscope; half are found with a 35-cm flexible scope, and two-thirds to three-quarters are found with a 60-cm scope. Diagnosis of adenomatous polyps by sigmoidoscopy should lead to evaluation of the entire colon with colonoscopy. The most efficient interval for screening sigmoidoscopy is unknown, but 5 years is often recommended. Case-control studies suggest that intervals of up to 15 years may confer benefit.

One-time colonoscopy detects ~25% more advanced lesions (polyps >10 mm, villous adenomas, adenomatous polyps with high-grade dysplasia, invasive cancer) than one-time FOBT with sigmoidoscopy. Perforation rates are about 3/1000 for colonoscopy and 1/1000 for sigmoidoscopy. Debate continues on whether colonoscopy is too expensive and invasive for widespread use as a screening tool in standard-risk populations. Two observational studies suggest that efficacy of colonoscopy to decrease colorectal cancer mortality rates is restricted to the left side of the colon. CT colonography, if done at expert centers, appears to have a sensitivity for polyps ≥6 mm comparable to colonoscopy. However, the rate of extracolonic findings of abnormalities of uncertain significance that must nevertheless be worked up is high (~15–30%); the long-term cumulative radiation risk of repeated colonography screenings is also a concern.

Lung cancer

Chest radiography and sputum cytology have been evaluated in randomized lung cancer screening trials. No reduction in lung cancer mortality has been seen, although all controlled trials have had low statistical power. Preliminary (unpublished) findings from the National Lung Screening Trial, a randomized controlled trial of screening for lung cancer in ~53,000 persons aged 55-74 years with a 30+ pack-year smoking history, have shown a statistically significant 20% reduction in lung cancer mortality in the spiral CT arm (354 deaths) compared with the chest radiography arm (442 deaths). However, the mortality benefits must be weighed against the disadvantages of spiral CT for a given population. These include the potential radiation risks associated with multiple scans, the discovery of incidental findings of unclear significance, and a high rate of false-positive test results. Both incidental findings and false-positive test results can lead to invasive diagnostic procedures associated with anxiety, expense, and complications (e.g., pneumo- or hemothorax after lung biopsy).

Ovarian cancer

Adnexal palpation, transvaginal ultrasound, and serum CA-125 assay have been considered for ovarian cancer screening. These tests alone and in combination do not have sufficiently high sensitivity or specificity to be recommended for routine screening of ovarian cancer. The risks and costs associated with the high number of false-positive results is an impediment to routine use of these modalities for screening. A large randomized controlled trial has shown that of female participants receiving at least one false-positive serum CA-125 test result, 14% underwent a major surgical procedure (e.g., laparotomy with oophorectomy) for benign disease. For transvaginal ultrasound, the rate was close to 40%.

Prostate cancer

The most common prostate cancer screening modalities are DRE and serum PSA assay. Newer serum tests, such as measurement of bound to free serum PSA, have yet to be fully evaluated. An emphasis on PSA screening has caused prostate cancer to become the most common non-skin cancer diagnosed in American males. This disease is prone to lead-time bias, length bias, and overdiagnosis, and substantial debate rages among experts as to whether it is effective. Prostate cancer screening clearly detects many asymptomatic cancers, but the ability to distinguish tumors that are lethal but still curable from those that pose little or no threat to health is limited. Men older than age 50 years have a high prevalence of indolent, clinically insignificant prostate cancers.

Two randomized controlled trials of the impact of PSA screening on prostate cancer mortality have been published. The Prostate, Lung, Colorectal, and Ovarian (PLCO) Cancer Screening Trial was a multicenter U.S. trial that randomized almost 77,000 men ages 55–74 years to receive annual PSA testing for 6 years or usual care. At 7 years of follow-up, no statistically significant difference in the number of prostate cancer deaths was noted between the arms (rate ratio, 1.13; 95% CI, 0.75–1.90). The data at 10 years (67% complete) showed similar results. Approximately 44% of men in the control arm received at least one PSA test during the trial, which may have potentially diluted an observed effect.

The European Randomized Study of Screening for Prostate Cancer (ERSPC) was a multinational study that randomized approximately 162,000 men between ages 50 and 74 years (with a predefined "core" screening group of men ages 55–69 years) to receive PSA testing every 4 years or no screening. Recruitment and randomization procedures and actual frequency of PSA testing varied by country. After a median follow-up of 9 years, a 20% relative reduction in the risk of prostate cancer death in the screened arm was noted in the "core" screening group (no difference in mortality was observed in the overall study population). The trial also found that 1140 men would need to be screened and 48 additional cases treated to avert 1 death from prostate cancer.

The effectiveness of treatments for low-stage prostate cancer is under study. However, both surgery and radiation therapy may cause significant morbidity, such as impotence and urinary incontinence. Comparison of radical prostatectomy with "watchful waiting" in clinically diagnosed (not screen-detected) prostate cancers showed a small decrease in prostate cancer death rate in the surgery arm, but no statistically significant decrease in overall mortality was seen after 11 years of follow-up. Benefits were restricted to men younger than age 65 years. Urinary incontinence and sexual impotence were more common in the surgery arm. A man should have a life expectancy of at least 10 years to be eligible for screening. The USPSTF has found insufficient evidence to recommend prostate cancer screening for men younger than age 75 years; it recommends against screening for prostate cancer in men age 75 years or older ("D" recommendation) (Table 27-3).

Endometrial cancer

Transvaginal ultrasound and endometrial sampling have been advocated as screening tests for endometrial cancer. Benefit from routine screening has not been shown. Transvaginal ultrasound and endometrial sampling are indicated for workup of vaginal bleeding in postmenopausal women but are not considered as screening tests in symptomatic women.

Skin cancer

Visual examination of all skin surfaces by the patient or by a health care provider is used in screening for basal and squamous cell cancers and melanoma. No prospective randomized study has been performed to look for a mortality decrease. Unfortunately, screening is associated with a substantial rate of overdiagnosis.

CHAPTER 28

PRINCIPLES OF CANCER TREATMENT

Edward A. Sausville ■ Dan L. Longo

The goal of cancer treatment is first to eradicate the cancer. If this primary goal cannot be accomplished, the goal of cancer treatment shifts to palliation, the amelioration of symptoms, and preservation of quality of life while striving to extend life. The dictum *primum non nocere* may not always be the guiding principle of cancer therapy. When cure of cancer is possible, cancer treatments may be undertaken despite the certainty of severe and perhaps life-threatening toxicities. Every cancer treatment has the potential to cause harm, and treatment may be given that produces toxicity with no benefit. The therapeutic index of many interventions is quite narrow, and most treatments are given to the point of toxicity. Conversely, when the clinical goal is palliation, careful attention to minimizing the toxicity of potentially toxic treatments becomes a significant goal. Irrespective of the clinical scenario, the guiding principle of cancer treatment should be *primum succerrere*, "first hasten to help." Radical surgical procedures, large-field hyperfractionated radiation therapy, high-dose chemotherapy, and maximum tolerable doses of cytokines such as interleukin (IL) 2 are all used in certain settings where 100% of the patients will experience toxicity and side effects from the intervention and only a fraction of the patients will experience benefit. One of the challenges of cancer treatment is to use the various treatment modalities alone and together in a fashion that maximizes the chances for patient benefit.

Cancer treatments are divided into four main types: surgery, radiation therapy (including photodynamic therapy), chemotherapy (including hormonal therapy and molecularly targeted therapy), and biologic therapy (including immunotherapy and gene therapy). The modalities are often used in combination, and agents in one category can act by several mechanisms. For example, cancer chemotherapy agents can induce differentiation, and antibodies (a form of immunotherapy) can be used to deliver radiation therapy. Surgery and radiation therapy are considered local treatments, though their effects can influence the behavior of tumor at remote sites. Chemotherapy and biologic therapy are usually systemic treatments. *Oncology*, the study of tumors, including treatment approaches, is a multidisciplinary effort with surgical-, radiotherapy-, and internal medicine–related areas of expertise. Treatments for patients with hematologic malignancies are often shared by hematologists and medical oncologists.

In many ways, cancer mimics an organ attempting to regulate its own growth. However, cancers have not set an appropriate limit on how much growth should be permitted. Normal organs and cancers share the properties of having (1) a population of cells in cycle and actively renewing and (2) a population of cells not in cycle. In cancers, cells that are not dividing are heterogeneous; some have sustained too much genetic damage to replicate but have defects in their death pathways that permit their survival, some are starving for nutrients and oxygen, and some are out of cycle but poised to be recruited back into cycle and expand if needed (i.e., reversibly growth-arrested). Severely damaged and starving cells are unlikely to kill the patient. The problem is that the cells that are reversibly not in cycle are capable of replenishing tumor cells physically removed or damaged by radiation and chemotherapy. These include *cancer stem cells*, whose properties are being elucidated. The stem cell fraction may define new targets for therapies that will retard their ability to reenter the cell cycle.

Tumors follow a Gompertzian growth curve (Fig. 28-1); the growth fraction of a neoplasm starts at 100% with the first transformed cell and declines exponentially over time until at the time of diagnosis, with a tumor burden of $1–5 \times 10^9$ tumor cells, the growth fraction is usually 1–4%. Thus, the peak growth rate occurs before the tumor is detectable. A key feature of a successful tumor is the ability to stimulate the development of a new supporting

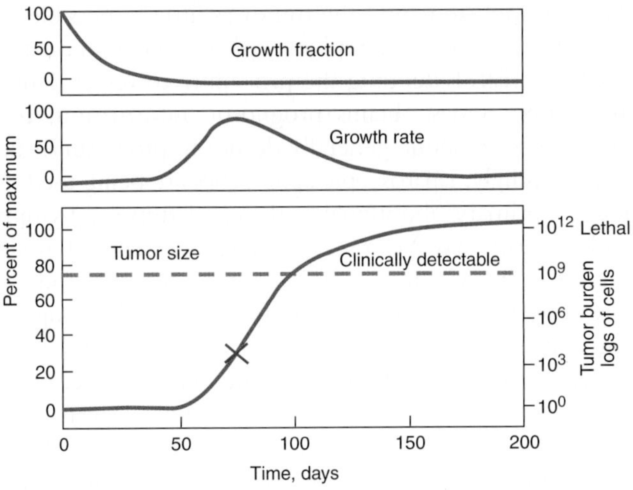

FIGURE 28-1

Gompertzian tumor growth. The growth fraction of a tumor declines exponentially over time *(top)*. The growth rate of a tumor peaks before it is clinically detectable *(middle)*. Tumor size increases slowly, goes through an exponential phase, and slows again as the tumor reaches the size at which limitation of nutrients or auto- or host regulatory influences can occur. The maximum growth rate occurs at 1/e, the point at which the tumor is about 37% of its maximum size *(marked with an X)*. Tumor becomes detectable at a burden of about 10^9 (1 cm^3) cells and kills the patient at a tumor cell burden of about 10^{12} (1 kg). Efforts to treat the tumor and reduce its size can result in an increase in the growth fraction and an increase in growth rate.

stroma through angiogenesis and production of proteases to allow invasion through basement membranes and normal tissue barriers (Chap. 25). Specific cellular mechanisms promote entry or withdrawal of tumor cells from the cell cycle. For example, when a tumor recurs after surgery or chemotherapy, frequently its growth is accelerated, and the growth fraction of the tumor is increased. This pattern is similar to that seen in regenerating organs. Partial resection of the liver results in the recruitment of cells into the cell cycle, and the resected liver volume is replaced. Similarly, chemotherapy-damaged bone marrow increases its growth to replace cells killed by chemotherapy. However, cancers do not recognize a limit on their expansion. Monoclonal gammopathy of uncertain significance may be an example of a clonal neoplasm with intrinsic features that stop its growth before a lethal tumor burden is reached. A fraction of patients with this disorder go on to develop fatal multiple myeloma, but probably this occurs because of the accumulation of additional genetic lesions. Elucidation of the mechanisms that regulate this "organ-like" behavior of tumors may provide additional clues to cancer control and treatment.

PRINCIPLES OF CANCER SURGERY

Surgery is used in cancer prevention, diagnosis, staging, treatment (for both localized and metastatic disease), palliation, and rehabilitation.

PROPHYLAXIS

Cancer can be prevented by surgery in people who have premalignant lesions resected (e.g., premalignant lesions of skin, colon, cervix) and in those who are at increased risk of cancer from an underlying disease (colectomy in those with pancolonic involvement with ulcerative colitis), the presence of genetic lesions (colectomy for familial polyposis, thyroidectomy for multiple endocrine neoplasia type 2, bilateral mastectomy or oophorectomy for familial breast or ovarian cancer syndromes), or a developmental anomaly (orchiectomy in those with an undescended testis). In some cases, prophylactic surgery is more radical than the surgical procedures used to treat the cancer after it develops. The assessment of risk involves many factors and should be undertaken with care before advising a patient to undergo such a major procedure. For breast cancer prevention, many experts use a 20% risk of developing breast cancer over the next 5 years as a threshold. However, patient fears play a major role in defining candidates for cancer prevention surgery. Counseling and education may not be enough to allay the fears of someone who has lost close family members to a malignancy.

DIAGNOSIS

The underlying principle in cancer diagnosis is to obtain as much tissue as safely possible. Owing to tumor heterogeneity, pathologists are better able to make the diagnosis when they have more tissue to examine. In addition to light-microscopic inspection of a tumor for pattern of growth, degree of cellular atypia, invasiveness, and morphologic features that aid in the differential diagnosis, sufficient tissue is of value in searching for genetic abnormalities and protein expression patterns, such as hormone receptor expression in breast cancers, that may aid in differential diagnosis or provide information about prognosis or likely response to treatment. Efforts to define "personalized" information from the biology of each patient's tumor and pertinent to each patient's treatment plan are becoming increasingly important in selecting treatment options. Histologically similar tumors may have very different gene expression patterns when assessed by such techniques as microarray analysis using gene chips, with important differences in response to treatment. Such testing requires that the tissue be handled properly (e.g., immunologic detection of proteins is more effective in fresh-frozen tissue rather than in formalin-fixed tissue). Coordination among the surgeon, pathologist, and primary care physician is essential to ensure that the amount of information learned from the biopsy material is maximized.

These goals are best met by an *excisional biopsy* in which the entire tumor mass is removed with a small margin of normal tissue surrounding it. If an excisional biopsy cannot be performed, *incisional biopsy* is the procedure of second choice. A wedge of tissue is removed, and an effort is made to include the majority of the cross-sectional diameter of the tumor in the biopsy to minimize sampling error. The biopsy techniques that involve cutting into tumor carry with them a risk of facilitating the spread of the tumor. *Core-needle biopsy* usually obtains considerably less tissue, but this procedure often provides enough information to plan a definitive surgical procedure. *Fine-needle aspiration* generally obtains only a suspension of cells from within a mass. This procedure is minimally invasive, and if positive for cancer, it may allow inception of systemic treatment when metastatic disease is evident, or it can provide a basis for planning a more meticulous and extensive surgical procedure.

STAGING

As noted in Chap. 26 an important component of patient management is defining the extent of disease. Radiographic and other imaging tests can be helpful in defining the clinical stage; however, pathologic staging requires defining the extent of involvement by documenting the histologic presence of tumor in tissue biopsies obtained through a surgical procedure. Axillary lymph node sampling in breast cancer and lymph node sampling at laparotomy for testicular, colon, and other intraabdominal cancers may provide crucial information for treatment planning and may determine the extent and nature of primary cancer treatment.

TREATMENT

Surgery is the most effective means of treating cancer. Today about 40% of cancer patients are cured by surgery. Unfortunately, a large fraction of patients with solid tumors (perhaps 60%) have metastatic disease that is not accessible for removal. However, even when the disease is not curable by surgery alone, the removal of tumor can obtain important benefits, including local control of tumor, preservation of organ function, debulking that permits subsequent therapy to work better, and staging information on extent of involvement. Cancer surgery aiming for cure is usually planned to excise the tumor completely with an adequate margin of normal tissue (the margin varies with the tumor and the anatomy), touching the tumor as little as possible to prevent vascular and lymphatic spread, and minimizing operative risk. Extending the procedure to resect draining lymph nodes obtains prognostic information, but such resections alone generally do not improve survival.

Increasingly, laparoscopic approaches are being used to address primary abdominal and pelvic tumors. Lymph node spread may be assessed using the sentinel node approach in which the first draining lymph node a spreading tumor would encounter is defined by injecting a dye into the tumor site at operation and then resecting the first node to turn blue. The sentinel node assessment is continuing to undergo clinical evaluation but appears to provide reliable information without the risks (lymphedema, lymphangiosarcoma) associated with resection of all the regional nodes. Advances in adjuvant chemotherapy and radiation therapy following surgery have permitted a substantial decrease in the extent of primary surgery necessary to obtain the best outcomes. Thus, lumpectomy with radiation therapy is as effective as modified radical mastectomy for breast cancer, and limb-sparing surgery followed by adjuvant radiation therapy and chemotherapy has replaced radical primary surgical procedures involving amputation and disarticulation for childhood rhabdomyosarcomas. More limited surgery is also being employed to spare organ function, as in larynx and bladder cancer. The magnitude of operations necessary to optimally control and cure cancer has also been diminished by technical advances; for example, the circular anastomotic stapler has allowed narrower (<2-cm) margins in colon cancer without compromise of local control rates, and many patients who would have had colostomies are able to maintain normal anatomy.

In some settings—e.g., bulky testicular cancer or stage III breast cancer—surgery is not the first treatment modality employed. After an initial diagnostic biopsy, chemotherapy and/or radiation therapy is delivered to reduce the size of the tumor and clinically control undetected metastatic disease. Such therapy is followed by a surgical procedure to remove residual masses; this is called *neoadjuvant therapy*. Because the sequence of treatment is critical to success and is different from the standard surgery-first approach, coordination among the surgical oncologist, radiation oncologist, and medical oncologist is crucial.

Surgery may be curative in a subset of patients with metastatic disease. Patients with lung metastases from osteosarcoma may be cured by resection of the lung lesions. In patients with colon cancer who have fewer than five liver metastases restricted to one lobe and no extrahepatic metastases, hepatic lobectomy may produce long-term disease-free survival in 25% of selected patients. Surgery can also be associated with systemic antitumor effects. In the setting of hormonally responsive tumors, oophorectomy and/or adrenalectomy may control estrogen production, and orchiectomy may reduce androgen production; both have effects on metastatic tumor growth. If resection of the primary lesion takes place in the presence of metastases, acceleration of metastatic growth may occur, perhaps based on the removal of a source of angiogenesis inhibitors and mass-related growth regulators in the tumor.

In selecting a surgeon or center for primary cancer treatment, consideration must be given to the volume of cancer surgeries undertaken by the site. Studies in a variety of cancers have shown that increased annual procedure volume appears to correlate with outcome. In addition, facilities with extensive support systems—e.g., for joint thoracic and abdominal surgical teams with cardiopulmonary bypass, if needed—may allow resection of certain tumors that would otherwise not be possible.

PALLIATION

Surgery is employed in a number of ways for supportive care, including insertion of central venous catheters, control of pleural and pericardial effusions and ascites, caval interruption for recurrent pulmonary emboli, stabilization of cancer-weakened weight-bearing bones, and control of hemorrhage, among others. Surgical bypass of gastrointestinal, urinary tract, or biliary tree obstruction can alleviate symptoms and prolong survival. Surgical procedures may provide relief of otherwise intractable pain or reverse neurologic dysfunction (cord decompression). Splenectomy may relieve symptoms and reverse hypersplenism. Intrathecal or intrahepatic therapy relies on surgical placement of appropriate infusion portals. Surgery may correct other treatment-related toxicities such as adhesions or strictures.

REHABILITATION

Surgical procedures are also valuable in restoring a cancer patient to full health. Orthopedic procedures may be necessary to ensure proper ambulation. Breast reconstruction can make an enormous impact on the patient's perception of successful therapy. Plastic and reconstructive surgery can correct the effects of disfiguring primary treatment.

PRINCIPLES OF RADIATION THERAPY

PHYSICAL PROPERTIES AND BIOLOGIC EFFECTS

Radiation is a physical form of treatment that damages any tissue in its path; its selectivity for cancer cells may be due to defects in a cancer cell's ability to repair sublethal DNA and other damage. Radiation causes breaks in DNA and generates free radicals from cell water that may damage cell membranes, proteins, and organelles. Radiation damage is augmented dependent on only oxygen; hypoxemic cells are more resistant. Augmentation of oxygen is the basis for radiation sensitization. Sulfhydryl compounds interfere with free radical generation and may act as radiation protectors.

Most radiation-induced cell damage is due to the formation of hydroxyl radicals:

$$\text{Ionizing radiation} + H_2O \rightarrow H_2O^+ + e^-$$

$$H_2O^+ + H_2O \rightarrow H_3O^+ + OH^\bullet$$

$$OH^\bullet \rightarrow \text{cell damage}$$

The dose-response curve for cells has both linear and exponential components. The linear component is from double-strand DNA breaks produced by single hits. The exponential component represents breaks produced by multiple hits. Plotting the fraction of surviving cells against doses of x-rays or gamma radiation, the curve has a shoulder that reflects the cell's repair of sublethal damage followed by a linear portion reflecting greater cell kill with larger doses. The features that make a particular cell more sensitive or more resistant to the biologic effects of radiation are not completely defined.

Therapeutic radiation is delivered in three ways: (1) *teletherapy*, with beams of radiation generated at a distance and aimed at the tumor within the patient; (2) *brachytherapy*, with encapsulated sources of radiation implanted directly into or adjacent to tumor tissues; and (3) *systemic therapy*, with radionuclides targeted in some fashion to a site of tumor. Teletherapy is the most commonly used form of radiation therapy.

X-rays and gamma rays are the forms of radiation most commonly used to treat cancer. They are both electromagnetic, nonparticulate waves that cause the ejection of an orbital electron when absorbed. This orbital electron ejection is called *ionization*. X-rays are generated by linear accelerators; gamma rays are generated from decay of atomic nuclei in radioisotopes such as cobalt and radium. These waves behave biologically as packets of energy, called *photons*. Particulate forms of radiation are also used in certain circumstances. Electron beams have a very low tissue penetrance and are used to treat skin conditions such as mycosis fungoides. Proton beams are becoming more widely available and may be more able to delimit dose to tumor in certain anatomic locations. However, aside from these specialized uses, particulate forms of radiation such as neutrons, protons, and negative mesons, which should do more tissue damage because of their higher linear energy transfer and lesser dependence on oxygen, are in most applications not superior to X- or gamma rays in clinical studies reported thus far.

A number of parameters influence the damage done to tissue by radiation. Hypoxemic cells are relatively resistant. Nondividing cells are more resistant than dividing cells. In addition to these biologic parameters, physical parameters of the radiation are also crucial. The energy of the radiation determines its ability to penetrate tissue. Low-energy orthovoltage beams (150–400 kV) scatter when they strike the body, much like light diffuses when it strikes particles in the air. Such beams result in more damage to adjacent normal tissues and less radiation delivered to the tumor. Megavoltage radiation (>1 MeV) has very low lateral scatter; this produces a skin-sparing effect, more homogeneous distribution of the radiation energy, and greater deposit of the energy in the tumor, or *target volume*. The tissues that the beam passes through to get to the tumor are called the *transit volume*. The maximum dose in the target volume is often the cause of complications to tissues in the transit volume, and the minimum dose in the target volume influences the likelihood of tumor recurrence. Dose homogeneity in the target volume is the goal. Computational approaches and delivery of many beams to converge on a target lesion are the basis for "gamma knife" and related approaches to deliver high dose to small volumes of tumor, sparing normal tissue.

Radiation is quantitated on the basis of the amount of radiation absorbed in the patient; it is not based on the amount of radiation generated by the machine. The *rad* (*r*adiation *a*bsorbed *d*ose) is defined as 100 ergs of energy per gram of tissue. The International System (SI) unit for rad is the Gray (Gy); 1 Gy = 100 rad. Radiation dose is measured by placing detectors at the body surface or calculating the dose based on radiating phantoms that resemble human form and substance. Radiation dose has three determinants: total absorbed dose, number of fractions, and time. A frequent error is to omit the number of fractions and the duration of treatment. This is analogous to saying that a runner completed a race in 20 s; without knowing how far he or she ran, the result is difficult to interpret. The time could be very good for a 200-m race or very poor for a 100-m race. Thus, a typical course of radiation therapy should be described as 4500 cGy delivered to a particular target (e.g., mediastinum) over 5 weeks in 180-cGy fractions. Most curative radiation treatment programs are delivered once a day, 5 days a week in 150- to 200-cGy fractions.

Certain drugs used in cancer treatment may also act as radiation sensitizers. For example, compounds that incorporate into DNA and alter its stereochemistry (e.g., halogenated pyrimidines, cisplatin) augment radiation effects, as does hydroxyurea, another DNA synthesis inhibitor.

APPLICATION TO PATIENTS

Teletherapy

Radiation therapy can be used alone or together with chemotherapy to produce cure of localized tumors and control of the primary site of disease in tumors that have disseminated. Therapy is planned based on the use of a simulator with the treatment field or fields designed to accommodate an individual patient's anatomic features. Individualized treatment planning employs lead shielding tailored to shape the field and limit the radiation exposure of normal tissue. Often the radiation is delivered from two or three different positions. Conformal three-dimensional treatment planning permits the delivery of higher doses of radiation to the target volume without increasing complications in the transit volume.

Radiation therapy is a component of curative therapy for a number of diseases, including breast cancer, Hodgkin's disease, head and neck cancer, prostate cancer, and gynecologic cancers. Radiation therapy can also palliate disease symptoms in a variety of settings, including relief of bone pain from metastatic disease, control of brain metastases, reversal of spinal cord compression and superior vena caval obstruction, shrinkage of painful masses, and opening of threatened airways. In high-risk settings, radiation therapy can prevent the development of leptomeningeal disease and brain metastases in acute leukemia and lung cancer.

Brachytherapy

Brachytherapy involves placing a sealed source of radiation into or adjacent to the tumor and withdrawing the radiation source after a period of time precisely calculated to deliver a chosen dose of radiation to the tumor. This approach is often used to treat prostate tumors and cervical cancer. The difficulty with brachytherapy is the short range of radiation effects (the inverse square law) and the inability to shape the radiation to fit the target volume. Normal tissue may receive toxic exposure to the radiation, with attendant radiation enteritis or cystitis in cervix cancer or brain injury in brain tumors.

Radionuclides and radioimmunotherapy

Nuclear medicine physicians and radiation oncologists may administer radionuclides with therapeutic effects. Iodine 131 is used to treat thyroid cancer since iodine is naturally taken up preferentially by the thyroid; it emits gamma rays that destroy the normal thyroid as well as the tumor. Strontium 89 and samarium 153 are two radionuclides that are preferentially taken up in bone, particularly sites of new bone formation. Both are capable of controlling bone metastases and the pain associated with them, but the dose-limiting toxicity is myelosuppression.

Monoclonal antibodies and other ligands can be attached to radioisotopes by conjugation (for nonmetal isotopes) or by chelation (for metal isotopes), and the targeting moiety can result in the accumulation of the radionuclide preferentially in tumor. Iodine 131–labeled anti-CD20 and yttrium 90–labeled anti-CD20 are active in B cell lymphoma, and other labeled antibodies are being evaluated. Thyroid uptake of labeled iodine is blocked by cold iodine. Dose-limiting toxicity is myelosuppression.

Photodynamic therapy

Some chemical structures (porphyrins, phthalocyanines) are selectively taken up by cancer cells by mechanisms not fully defined. When light, usually delivered by a laser, is shone on cells containing these compounds, free radicals are generated, and the cells die. Hematoporphyrins and light are being used with increasing frequency to treat skin cancer; ovarian cancer; and cancers of the lung, colon, rectum, and esophagus. Palliation of recurrent locally advanced disease can sometimes be dramatic and last many months.

TOXICITY

Though radiation therapy is most often administered to a local region, systemic effects, including fatigue, anorexia, nausea, and vomiting, may develop that are related in part to the volume of tissue irradiated, dose fractionation, radiation fields, and individual susceptibility. Bone is among the most radioresistant organs, radiation effects being manifested mainly in children through premature fusion of the epiphyseal growth plate. By contrast, the male testis, female ovary, and bone marrow are the most sensitive organs. Any bone marrow in a radiation field will be eradicated by therapeutic irradiation. Organs with less need for cell renewal, such as heart, skeletal muscle, and nerves, are more resistant to radiation effects. In radiation-resistant organs, the vascular endothelium is the most sensitive component. Organs with more self-renewal as a part of normal homeostasis, such as the hematopoietic system and mucosal lining of the intestinal tract, are more sensitive. Acute toxicities include mucositis, skin erythema (ulceration in severe cases), and bone marrow toxicity. Often these can be alleviated by interruption of treatment.

Chronic toxicities are more serious. Radiation of the head and neck region often produces thyroid failure. Cataracts and retinal damage can lead to blindness. Salivary glands stop making saliva, which leads to dental caries and poor dentition. Taste and smell can be affected. Mediastinal irradiation leads to a threefold increased risk of fatal myocardial infarction. Other late vascular effects include chronic constrictive pericarditis, lung fibrosis, viscus stricture, spinal cord transection, and radiation enteritis. A serious late toxicity is the development of second solid tumors in or adjacent to the radiation fields. Such tumors can develop in any organ or tissue and occur at a rate of about 1% per year beginning in the second decade after treatment. Some organs vary in susceptibility to radiation carcinogenesis. A woman who receives mantle field radiation therapy for Hodgkin's disease at age 25 years has a 30% risk of developing breast cancer by age 55 years. This is comparable in magnitude to genetic breast cancer syndromes. Women treated after age 30 years have little or no increased risk of breast cancer. No data suggest that a threshold dose of therapeutic radiation exists below which the incidence of second cancers is decreased. High rates of second tumors occur in people who receive as little as 1000 cGy.

PRINCIPLES OF CHEMOTHERAPY

Medical oncology is the subspecialty of internal medicine that cares for and designs treatment approaches to patients with cancer in conjunction with surgical and radiation oncologists. The core skills of the medical oncologist include the use of drugs that may have a beneficial effect on the natural history of the patient's illness or favorably influence the patient's quality of life.

ENDPOINTS OF DRUG ACTION

The concept that systemically administered drugs may have a useful effect on cancers was historically derived from three sets of observations. Paul Ehrlich in the nineteenth century observed that different dyes reacted with different cell and tissue components. He hypothesized the existence of compounds that would be "magic bullets" that might bind to tumors, owing to the affinity of the agent for the tumor. A second observation was the toxic effects of certain mustard gas derivatives on the bone marrow during World War I, leading to the idea that smaller doses of these agents might be used to treat tumors of marrow-derived cells. Finally, the observation that certain tumors from hormone-responsive tissues, e.g. breast tumors, could shrink after oophorectomy led to the idea that endogenous substances promoting the growth of a tumor might be antagonized. Chemicals achieving each of the goals are actually or intellectually the forbearers of the currently used cancer chemotherapy agents.

Chemotherapy agents may be used for the treatment of active, clinically apparent cancer. Table 28-1, *A* lists tumors considered curable by conventionally available chemotherapeutic agents when used to address disseminated or metastatic cancers. If a tumor is localized to a single site, serious consideration of surgery or primary radiation therapy should be given, as these treatment modalities may be curative as local treatments. Chemotherapy may be employed after the failure of these modalities to eradicate a local tumor or as part of multimodality approaches to offer primary treatment to

TABLE 28-1

CURABILITY OF CANCERS WITH CHEMOTHERAPY

A. Advanced Cancers with Possible Cure	**D. Cancers Possibly Cured with "High-Dose" Chemotherapy With Stem Cell Support**
Acute lymphoid and acute myeloid leukemia (pediatric/adult)	Relapsed leukemias, lymphoid and myeloid
Hodgkin's disease (pediatric/adult)	Relapsed lymphomas, Hodgkin's and non-Hodgkin's
Lymphomas—certain types (pediatric/adult)	Chronic myeloid leukemia
Germ cell neoplasms	Multiple myeloma
Embryonal carcinoma	**E. Cancers Responsive With Useful Palliation, But Not Cure, by Chemotherapy**
Teratocarcinoma	Bladder carcinoma
Seminoma or dysgerminoma	Chronic myeloid leukemia
Choriocarcinoma	Hairy cell leukemia
Gestational trophoblastic neoplasia	Chronic lymphocytic leukemia
Pediatric neoplasms	Lymphoma—certain types
Wilms' tumor	Multiple myeloma
Embryonal rhabdomyosarcoma	Gastric carcinoma
Ewing's sarcoma	Cervix carcinoma
Peripheral neuroepithelioma	Endometrial carcinoma
Neuroblastoma	Soft tissue sarcoma
Small cell lung carcinoma	Head and neck cancer
Ovarian carcinoma	Adrenocortical carcinoma
B. Advanced Cancers Possibly Cured by Chemotherapy and Radiation	Islet-cell neoplasms
Squamous carcinoma (head and neck)	Breast carcinoma
Squamous carcinoma (anus)	Colorectal carcinoma
Breast carcinoma	Renal carcinoma
Carcinoma of the uterine cervix	**F. Tumor Poorly Responsive in Advanced Stages to Chemotherapy**
Non-small cell lung carcinoma (stage III)	Pancreatic carcinoma
Small cell lung carcinoma	Biliary tract neoplasms
C. Cancers Possibly Cured With Chemotherapy as Adjuvant to Surgery	Thyroid carcinoma
Breast carcinoma	Carcinoma of the vulva
Colorectal carcinoma[a]	Non-small cell lung carcinoma
Osteogenic sarcoma	Prostate carcinoma
Soft tissue sarcoma	Melanoma
	Hepatocellular carcinoma
	Salivary gland cancer

[a]Rectum also receives radiation therapy.

a clinically localized tumor. In this event, it can allow organ preservation when given with radiation, as in the larynx or other upper airway sites, or sensitize tumors to radiation when given, e.g., to patients concurrently receiving radiation for lung or cervix cancer (Table 28-1, *B*). Chemotherapy can be administered as an adjuvant, i.e., in addition to surgery (Table 28-1, *C*) or radiation after all clinically apparent disease has been removed. This use of chemotherapy may have curative potential in breast and colorectal neoplasms, as it attempts to eliminate clinically unapparent tumor that may have already disseminated. As noted earlier, small tumors frequently have high growth fractions and therefore may be intrinsically more susceptible to the action of antiproliferative agents. Chemotherapy is routinely used in "conventional" dose regimens. In general, these doses produce reversible acute side effects, primarily consisting of transient myelosuppression with or without gastrointestinal toxicity (usually nausea), which are readily managed. High-dose chemotherapy regimens are predicated on the observation that the dose-response curve for many anticancer agents is rather steep, and increased doses can produce markedly increased therapeutic effect, although at the cost of potentially life-threatening complications that require intensive support, usually in the form of hematopoietic stem cell support from the patient (*autologous*) or from donors matched for histocompatibility loci (*allogeneic*). High-dose regimens have definite curative potential in defined clinical settings (Table 28-1, *D*).

Karnofsky was among the first to champion the evaluation of a chemotherapeutic agent's benefit by carefully quantitating its effect on tumor size and using these measurements to objectively decide the basis for further treatment of a particular patient or further clinical evaluation of a drug's potential. A partial response (PR) is defined conventionally as a decrease by at least 50% in a tumor's bidimensional area, a complete response (CR) connotes disappearance of all tumor, progression of disease signifies an increase in size of existing lesions by >25% from baseline or best response or development of new lesions, and "stable" disease fits into none of the above categories. Newer evaluation systems such as RECIST (Response Evaluation Criteria In Solid Tumors) utilize unidimensional measurement, but the intent is similar in rigorously defining evidence for the activity of the agent in assessing its value to the patient.

If cure is not possible, chemotherapy may be undertaken with the goal of palliating some aspect of the tumor's effect on the host. Common tumors that may be meaningfully addressed with palliative intent are listed in Table 28-1, *E*. Usually, tumor-related symptoms may manifest as pain, weight loss, or some local symptom related to the tumor's effect on normal structures. Patients treated with palliative intent should be aware of their diagnosis and the limitations of the proposed treatments, have access to supportive care, and have suitable "performance status," according to assessment algorithms such as the one developed by Karnofsky or by the Eastern Cooperative Oncology Group (ECOG).

ECOG performance status 0 (PS0) patients are without symptoms, PS1 patients are ambulatory but restricted in strenuous physical activity, PS2 patients are ambulatory but unable to work and are up and about 50% or more of the time, PS3 patients are capable of limited self-care and are up <50% of the time, and PS4 patients are totally confined to bed or chair and incapable of self-care. Only PS0, PS1, and PS2 patients are generally considered suitable for palliative (noncurative) treatment. If there is curative potential, even poor–performance status patients may be treated, but their prognosis is usually inferior to that of good–performance status patients treated with similar regimens.

An important perspective the primary care provider may bring to patients and their families facing incurable cancer is that, given the limited value of chemotherapeutic approaches at some point in the natural history, *palliative care* or *hospice-based* approaches, with meticulous and ongoing attention to symptom relief and with family, psychological, and spiritual support, should receive prominent attention as a valuable therapeutic plan. (Chap. 32). Optimizing the quality of life rather than attempting to extend it becomes a valued intervention. Patients facing the impending progression of disease in a life-threatening way frequently choose to undertake toxic treatments of little to no potential value, and support provided by the primary caregiver in accessing palliative and hospice-based options in contrast to receiving toxic and ineffective regimen can be critical in providing a basis for patients to make sensible choices.

CANCER DRUGS: OVERVIEW AND PRINCIPLES FOR USE

Cancer drug treatments are of four broad types. *Conventional chemotherapy agents* were historically derived by the empirical observation that these "small molecules" (generally with molecular mass <1500 Da) could cause major regression of experimental tumors growing in animals. These agents mainly target DNA structure or segregation of DNA as chromosomes in mitosis. *Targeted agents* refer to small molecules or "biologicals" (generally macromolecules such as antibodies or cytokines) designed and developed to interact with a defined molecular target important in either maintaining the malignant state or selectively expressed by the tumor cells. As described in Chap. 25, successful tumors have activated biochemical pathways that lead to uncontrolled proliferation through the action of, e.g., oncogene products, loss of cell cycle inhibitors, or loss of cell death regulation, and have acquired the capacity to replicate chromosomes indefinitely, invade, metastasize, and evade the immune system. Targeted therapies seek to capitalize on the biology behind the aberrant cellular behavior as a basis for therapeutic effects. *Hormonal therapies* (the first form of targeted therapy) capitalize on the biochemical pathways underlying estrogen and androgen function and action as a therapeutic basis for approaching patients with tumors of breast, prostate, uterus, and ovarian origin. *Biologic therapies* are often macromolecules that have a particular target (e.g., anti-growth factor or cytokine antibodies) or may have the capacity to regulate growth of tumor cells or induce a host immune response to kill tumor cells. Thus, biologic therapies include not only antibodies but cytokines and gene therapies.

The usefulness of any drug is governed by the extent to which a given dose causes a useful result (therapeutic effect; in the case of anticancer agents, toxicity to tumor cells) as opposed to a toxic effect to the host. The *therapeutic index* is the degree of separation between toxic and therapeutic doses. Really useful drugs have large therapeutic indices, and this usually occurs when the drug target is expressed in the disease-causing compartment as opposed to the normal compartment. Classically, selective toxicity of an agent for an organ is governed by the expression of an agent's target or by differential accumulation into or elimination from compartments where toxicity is experienced or ameliorated, respectively. Currently used chemotherapeutic agents have the unfortunate property that their targets are present in both normal and tumor tissues. Therefore, they have relatively narrow therapeutic indices.

Figure 28-2 illustrates steps in cancer drug discovery and development. Following demonstration of antitumor activity in animal models, potentially useful anticancer agents are further evaluated to define an optimal schedule of administration and arrive at a drug formulation designed for a given route and schedule. Safety testing in two species on an analogous schedule of administration defines the starting dose for a phase I trial in humans. This is established as a fraction, usually one-sixth to one-tenth, of the dose just causing easily reversible toxicity in the more sensitive animal species. Escalating doses of the drug are then given during the human phase I trial until reversible toxicity is observed. Dose-limiting toxicity (DLT) defines a dose that conveys greater toxicity than would be acceptable in routine practice, allowing definition of a lower maximal tolerated dose (MTD). The occurrence of toxicity is, if possible, correlated with plasma drug concentrations. The MTD or a dose just lower than the MTD is usually the dose suitable for phase II trials, in which a fixed dose is administered to a relatively homogeneous set of patients with a particular tumor type in an effort to define whether the drug causes regression of tumors. An "active" agent conventionally has PR rates of at least 20–25% with reversible non-life-threatening side effects, and it may then be suitable for study in phase III trials to assess efficacy compared with standard or no therapy.

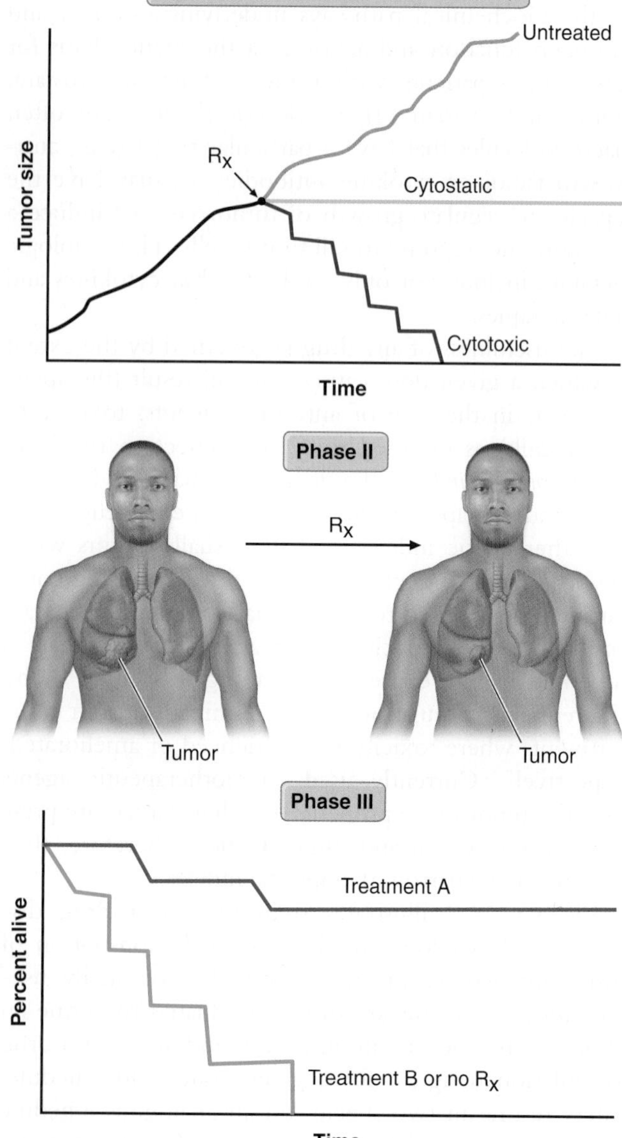

FIGURE 28-2

Steps in cancer drug discovery and development. Preclinical activity *(top)* in animal models of cancers may be used as evidence to support the entry of the drug candidate into phase I trials in humans to define a correct dose and observe any clinical antitumor effect that may occur. The drug may then be advanced to phase II trials directed against specific cancer types, with rigorous quantitation of antitumor effects *(middle)*. Phase III trials then may reveal activity superior to standard or no treatment *(lowest panel)*.

Response, defined as tumor shrinkage, is but the most immediate indicator of drug effect. To be clinically valuable, responses must translate into clinical benefit. This is conventionally established by a beneficial effect on overall survival, or at least an increased time to further progression of disease. Active efforts are being made to quantitate effects of anticancer agents on quality of life. Cancer drug clinical trials conventionally use a toxicity grading scale in which grade I toxicities do not require treatment, grade II often require symptomatic treatment but are not life-threatening, grade III toxicities are potentially life-threatening if untreated, grade IV toxicities are actually life-threatening, and grade V toxicities are those that result in the patient's death.

Development of "targeted agents" may proceed quite differently. While phase I–III trials are still conducted, molecular analysis of human tumors may allow the precise definition of target expression in a patient's tumor that is necessary for or relevant to the drug's action. This information might then allow selection of patients expressing the drug target for participation in all trial phases. These patients may then have a greater chance of developing a useful response to the drug by virtue of expressing the target in the tumor. Clinical trials may be designed to incorporate an assessment of the behavior of the target in relation to the drug (pharmacodynamic studies). Ideally, the plasma concentration that affects the drug target is known, so escalation to MTD may not be necessary. Rather, the correlation of host toxicity while achieving an "optimal biologic dose" becomes a more relevant endpoint for phase I and early phase II trials with targeted agents.

Useful cancer drug treatment strategies using conventional chemotherapy agents, targeted agents, hormonal treatments, or biologicals have one of two valuable outcomes. They can induce cancer cell death, resulting in tumor shrinkage with corresponding improvement in patient survival or increase the time until the disease progresses. Another potential outcome is to induce cancer cell *differentiation* or dormancy with loss of tumor cell replicative potential and reacquisition of phenotypic properties resembling normal cells. Blocking tumor cell differentiation may be a key feature in the pathogenesis of certain leukemias.

Cell death is a closely regulated process. *Necrosis* refers to cell death induced, for example, by physical damage with the hallmarks of cell swelling and membrane disruption. *Apoptosis*, or programmed cell death, refers to a highly ordered process whereby cells respond to defined stimuli by dying, and it recapitulates the necessary cell death observed during the ontogeny of the organism. *Anoikis* refers to the death of epithelial cells after removal from the normal milieu of substrate, particularly from cell-to-cell contact. Cancer chemotherapeutic agents can cause both necrosis and apoptosis. Apoptosis is characterized by chromatin condensation (giving rise to "apoptotic bodies"); cell shrinkage; and, in living animals, phagocytosis by surrounding stromal cells without evidence of inflammation. This process is regulated either by signal transduction systems that promote a cell's demise after a certain level of insult is achieved or in response to specific cell-surface receptors that mediate cell death signals. Modulation of apoptosis by manipulation of signal transduction pathways has emerged as a basis for understanding the actions of drugs and designing new strategies to improve their use. *Autophagy* is a cellular response to injury in which the cell does not initially die but catabolizes itself in a way that can lead to loss of replicative potential.

A general view of how cancer treatments work is that the interaction of a chemotherapeutic drug with its target induces a "cascade" of further signaling steps. These signals ultimately lead to cell death by triggering an "execution phase" in which proteases, nucleases, and endogenous regulators of the cell death pathway are activated (Fig. 28-3).

Targeted agents differ from chemotherapy agents in that they do not indiscriminately cause macromolecular lesions but regulate the action of particular pathways. For example, the p210[bcr-abl] fusion protein tyrosine kinase drives chronic myeloid leukemia (CML), and HER-2/neu stimulates the proliferation of certain breast cancers. The tumor has been described as "addicted" to the function of these molecules in the sense that without the pathway's continued action, the tumor cell cannot survive. In this way, targeted agents may alter the "threshold" tumors have for undergoing apoptosis

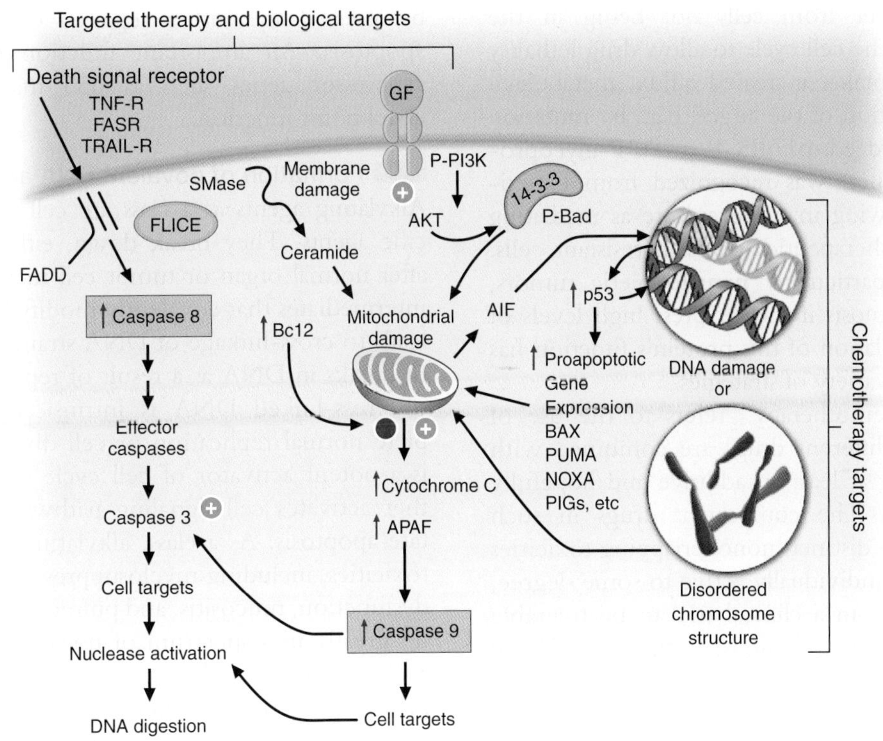

FIGURE 28-3

Integration of cell death responses. Cell death through an apoptotic mechanism requires active participation of the cell. In response to interruption of growth factor (GF) or propagation of certain cytokine death signals (e.g., tumor necrosis factor receptor, TNF-R), there is activation of "upstream" cysteine aspartyl proteases (caspases), which then directly digest cytoplasmic and nuclear proteins, resulting in activation of "downstream" caspases; these cause activation of nucleases, resulting in the characteristic DNA fragmentation that is a hallmark of apoptosis. Chemotherapy agents that create lesions in DNA or alter mitotic spindle function seem to activate aspects of this process by damage ultimately conveyed to the mitochondria, perhaps by activating the transcription of genes whose products can produce or modulate the toxicity of free radicals. In addition, membrane damage with activation of sphingomyelinases results in the production of ceramides that can have a direct action at mitochondria. The antiapoptotic protein bcl2 attenuates mitochondrial toxicity, while proapoptotic gene products such as bax antagonize the action of bcl2. Damaged mitochondria release cytochrome C and apoptosis-activating factor (APAF), which can directly activate caspase 9, resulting in propagation of a direct signal to other downstream caspases through protease activation. Apoptosis-inducing factor (AIF) is also released from the mitochondrion and then can translocate to the nucleus, bind to DNA, and generate free radicals to further damage DNA. An additional proapoptotic stimulus is the bad protein, which can heterodimerize with *bcl2* gene family members to antagonize apoptosis. Importantly, though, bad protein function can be retarded by its sequestration as phospho-bad through the 14-3-3 adapter proteins. The phosphorylation of bad is mediated by the action of the AKT kinase in a way that defines how growth factors that activate this kinase can retard apoptosis and promote cell survival.

without actually creating any molecular lesions such as direct DNA strand breakage or altered membrane function.

While apoptotic mechanisms are important in regulating cellular proliferation and the behavior of tumor cells in vitro, in vivo it is unclear whether all of the actions of chemotherapeutic agents to cause cell death can be attributed to apoptotic mechanisms. However, changes in molecules that regulate apoptosis are correlated with clinical outcomes (e.g., *bcl2* overexpression in certain lymphomas conveys poor prognosis; proapoptotic bax expression is associated with a better outcome after chemotherapy for ovarian carcinoma). A better understanding of the relationship of cell death and cell survival mechanisms is needed.

Resistance to chemotherapy drugs has been postulated to arise either from cells not being in the appropriate phase of the cell cycle to allow drug lethality or from decreased uptake, increased efflux, metabolism of the drug, or alteration of the target, e.g., by mutation or overexpression. Indeed, p170PGP (p170 P-glycoprotein; *mdr* gene product) was recognized from experiments with cells growing in tissue culture as mediating the efflux of chemotherapeutic agents in resistant cells. Certain neoplasms, particularly hematopoietic tumors, have an adverse prognosis if they express high levels of p170PGP, and modulation of this protein's function has been attempted by a variety of strategies.

"Combination chemotherapy" refers to the use of regimens in which different drugs are combined with the goal of achieving at least an additive and hopefully supra-additive effect. The component drugs in such regimens ideally have distinct, nonoverlapping toxicities to the host, are each individually active to some degree, and have been shown in a clinical trial to be tolerable and convey clinical value in contrast to the use of single agents.

CHEMOTHERAPEUTIC AGENTS USED FOR CANCER TREATMENT

Table 28-2 lists commonly used cancer chemotherapy agents and pertinent clinical aspects of their use. The drugs and schedules listed are examples that have proved tolerable and useful; the specific doses that may be used in a particular patient may vary somewhat with the particular protocol, or plan, of treatment. Significant variation from these dose ranges should be carefully verified to avoid or anticipate toxicity. Not included in Table 28-2 are hormone receptor–directed agents, as the side effects are generally those expected from the interruption or augmentation of hormonal effect, and doses used in most cases are those that adequately saturate the intended hormone receptor. The drugs listed may be usefully grouped into three general categories: those affecting DNA, those affecting microtubules, and molecularly targeted agents.

Direct DNA-interactive agents

DNA replication occurs during the synthesis or S-phase of the cell cycle, with chromosome segregation of the replicated DNA occurring in the M, or mitosis, phase. The G_1 and G_2 "gap phases" precede S and M, respectively. Historically, chemotherapeutic agents have been divided into "phase-nonspecific" agents, which can act in any phase of the cell cycle, and "phase-specific" agents, which require the cell to be at a particular cell cycle phase to cause greatest effect. Once the agent has acted, cells may progress to "checkpoints" in the cell cycle in which the drug-related damage may be assessed and either repaired or allowed to initiate apoptosis. An important function of certain tumor-suppressor genes such as p53 may be to modulate checkpoint function.

Formation of covalent DNA adducts

Alkylating agents as a class are cell cycle phase–nonspecific agents. They break down, either spontaneously or after normal organ or tumor cell metabolism, to reactive intermediates that covalently modify bases in DNA. This leads to cross-linkage of DNA strands or the appearance of breaks in DNA as a result of repair efforts. "Broken" or cross-linked DNA is intrinsically unable to complete normal replication or cell division; in addition, it is a potent activator of cell cycle checkpoints and further activates cell-signaling pathways that can precipitate apoptosis. As a class, alkylating agents share similar toxicities, including myelosuppression, alopecia, gonadal dysfunction, mucositis, and pulmonary fibrosis. They differ greatly in a spectrum of normal organ toxicities. As a class they share the capacity to cause "second" neoplasms, particularly leukemia, many years after use, particularly when used in low doses for protracted periods.

Cyclophosphamide is inactive unless metabolized by the liver to 4-hydroxy-cyclophosphamide, which decomposes into an alkylating species, as well as to chloroacetaldehyde and acrolein. The latter causes chemical cystitis; therefore, excellent hydration must be maintained while using cyclophosphamide. If severe, the cystitis may be effectively treated by mesna (2-*me*rcapto*e*thane*s*ulfo*na*te). Liver disease impairs drug activation. Sporadic interstitial pneumonitis leading to pulmonary fibrosis can accompany the use of cyclophosphamide, and high doses used in conditioning regimens for bone marrow transplant can cause cardiac dysfunction. Ifosfamide is a cyclophosphamide analogue also activated in the liver, but more slowly, and it requires coadministration of mesna to prevent bladder injury. Central nervous system (CNS) effects, including somnolence, confusion, and psychosis, can follow

TABLE 28-2

COMMONLY USED CANCER CHEMOTHERAPY AGENTS

DRUG	EXAMPLES OF USUAL DOSES	TOXICITY	INTERACTIONS, ISSUES
Direct DNA-Interacting Agents			
Alkylators			
Cyclophosphamide	400–2000 mg/m^2 IV 100 mg/m^2 PO qd	Marrow (relative platelet sparing) Cystitis Common alkylator[a] Cardiac (high dose)	Liver metabolism required to activate to phosphoramide mustard + acrolein Mesna protects against "high-dose" bladder damage
Mechlorethamine	6 mg/m^2 IV day 1 and day 8	Marrow Vesicant Nausea	Topical use in cutaneous lymphoma
Chlorambucil	1–3 mg/m^2 qd PO	Marrow Common alkylator[a]	
Melphalan	8 mg/m^2 qd × 5, PO	Marrow (delayed nadir) GI (high dose)	Decreased renal function delays clearance
Carmustine (BCNU)	200 mg/m^2 IV 150 mg/m^2 PO	Marrow (delayed nadir) GI, liver (high dose) Renal	
Lomustine (CCNU)	100–300 mg/m^2 PO	Marrow (delayed nadir)	
Ifosfamide	1.2 g/m^2 per day qd × 5 + mesna	Myelosuppressive Bladder Neurologic Metabolic acidosis Neuropathy	Isomeric analogue of cyclophosphamide More lipid soluble Greater activity vs testicular neoplasms and sarcomas Must use mesna
Procarbazine	100 mg/m^2 per day qd × 14	Marrow Nausea Neurologic Common alkylator[a]	Liver and tissue metabolism required Disulfiram-like effect with ethanol Acts as MAOI HBP after tyrosinase-rich foods
Dacarbazine (DTIC)	375 mg/m^2 IV day 1 and day 15	Marrow Nausea Flulike	Metabolic activation
Temozolomide	150–200 mg/m^2 qd × 5 q28d *or* 75 mg/m^2 qd × 6–7 weeks	Nausea/vomiting Headache/fatigue Constipation	Infrequent myelosuppression
Altretamine (formerly hexamethylmelamine)	260 mg/m^2 per day qd × 14–21 as 4 divided oral doses	Nausea Neurologic (mood swing) Neuropathy Marrow (less)	Liver activation Barbiturates enhance/cimetidine diminishes
Cisplatin	20 mg/m^2 qd × 5 IV 1 q3–4 weeks or 100–200 mg/m^2 per dose IV q3–4 weeks	Nausea Neuropathy Auditory Marrow platelets > WBCs Renal Mg^{2+}, Ca^{2+}	Maintain high urine flow; osmotic diuresis, monitor intake/output K^+, Mg^{2+} Emetogenic—prophylaxis needed Full dose if CrCl > 60 mL/min and tolerate fluid push
Carboplatin	365 mg/m^2 IV q3–4 weeks as adjusted for CrCl	Marrow platelets > WBCs Nausea Renal (high dose)	Reduce dose according to CrCl: to AUC of 5–7 mg/mL per min [AUC = dose/(CrCl + 25)]
Oxaliplatin	130 mg/m^2 q3 weeks over 2 h *or* 85 mg/m^2 q2 weeks	Nausea Anemia	Acute reversible neurotoxicity; chronic sensory neurotoxicity cumulative with dose; reversible laryngopharyngeal spasm
Antitumor Antibiotics and Topoisomerase Poisons			
Bleomycin	15–25 mg/d qd × 5 IV bolus *or* continuous IV	Pulmonary Skin effects Raynaud's phenomenon Hypersensitivity	Inactivate by bleomycin hydrolase (decreased in lung/skin) O_2 enhances pulmonary toxicity Cisplatin-induced decrease in CrCl may increase skin/lung toxicity Reduce dose if CrCl < 60 mL/min

(continued)

TABLE 28-2

COMMONLY USED CANCER CHEMOTHERAPY AGENTS (*CONTINUED*)

DRUG	EXAMPLES OF USUAL DOSES	TOXICITY	INTERACTIONS, ISSUES
Actinomycin D	10–15 μg/kg per day qd × 5 IV bolus	Marrow Nausea Mucositis Vesicant Alopecia	Radiation recall
Etoposide (VP16-213)	100–150 mg/m² IV qd × 3–5d *or* 50 mg/m² PO qd × 21 d *or* up to 1500 mg/m² per dose (high dose with stem cell support)	Marrow (WBCs > platelet) Alopecia Hypotension Hypersensitivity (rapid IV) Nausea Mucositis (high dose)	Hepatic metabolism—renal 30% Reduce doses with renal failure Schedule-dependent (5 day better than 1 day) Late leukemogenic Accentuate antimetabolite action
Topotecan	20 mg/m² IV q3–4 weeks over 30 min *or* 1.5–3 mg/m² q3–4 weeks over 24 h *or* 0.5 mg/m² per day over 21 days	Marrow Mucositis Nausea Mild alopecia	Reduce dose with renal failure No liver toxicity
Irinotecan (CPT II)	100–150 mg/m² IV over 90 min q3–4 weeks *or* 30 mg/m² per day over 120 h	Diarrhea: "early onset" with cramping, flushing, vomiting; "late onset" after several doses Marrow Alopecia Nausea Vomiting Pulmonary	Prodrug requires enzymatic clearance to active drug "SN 38" Early diarrhea likely due to biliary excretion Late diarrhea, use "high-dose" loperamide (2 mg q2–4 h)
Doxorubicin and daunorubicin	45–60 mg/m² dose q3–4 weeks *or* 10–30 mg/m² dose q week *or* continuous-infusion regimen	Marrow Mucositis Alopecia Cardiovascular acute/ chronic Vesicant	Heparin aggregate; coadministration increases clearance Acetaminophen, BCNU increase liver toxicity Radiation recall
Idarubicin	10–15 mg/m² IV q 3 weeks *or* 10 mg/m² IV qd × 3	Marrow Cardiac (less than doxorubicin)	None established
Epirubicin	150 mg/m² IV q3 weeks	Marrow Cardiac	None established
Mitoxantrone	12 mg/m² qd × 3 *or* 12–14 mg/m² q3 weeks	Marrow Cardiac (less than doxorubicin) Vesicant (mild) Blue urine, sclerae, nails	Interacts with heparin Less alopecia, nausea than doxorubicin Radiation recall
Indirect DNA-Interacting Agents			
Antimetabolites			
Deoxycoformycin	4 mg/m² IV every other week	Nausea Immunosuppression Neurologic Renal	Excretes in urine Reduce dose for renal failure Inhibits adenosine deaminase
6-Mercaptopurine	75 mg/m² PO *or* up to 500 mg/m² PO (high dose)	Marrow Liver Nausea	Variable bioavailability Metabolize by xanthine oxidase Decrease dose with allopurinol Increased toxicity with thiopurine methyltransferase deficiency
6-Thioguanine	2–3 mg/kg per day for up to 3–4 weeks	Marrow Liver Nausea	Variable bioavailability Increased toxicity with thiopurine methyltransferase deficiency

(*continued*)

TABLE 28-2

COMMONLY USED CANCER CHEMOTHERAPY AGENTS (*CONTINUED*)

DRUG	EXAMPLES OF USUAL DOSES	TOXICITY	INTERACTIONS, ISSUES
Azathioprine	1–5 mg/kg per day	Marrow Nausea Liver	Metabolizes to 6MP; therefore, reduce dose with allopurinol Increased toxicity with thiopurine methyltransferase deficiency
2-Chlorodeoxy-adenosine	0.09 mg/kg per day qd × 7 as continuous infusion	Marrow Renal Fever	Notable use in hairy cell leukemia
Hydroxyurea	20–50 mg/kg (lean body weight) PO qd *or* 1–3 g/d	Marrow Nausea Mucositis Skin changes Rare renal, liver, lung, CNS	Decrease dose with renal failure Augments antimetabolite effect
Methotrexate	15–30 mg PO or IM qd × 3–5 *or* 30 mg IV days 1 and 8 *or* 1.5–12g/m^2 per day (with leucovorin)	Marrow Liver/lung Renal tubular Mucositis	Rescue with leucovorin Excreted in urine Decrease dose in renal failure NSAIDs increase renal toxicity
5-Fluorouracil (5FU)	375 mg/m^2 IV qd × 5 *or* 600 mg/m^2 IV days 1 and 8	Marrow Mucositis Neurologic Skin changes	Toxicity enhanced by leucovorin Dihydropyrimidine dehydrogenase deficiency increases toxicity Metabolizes in tissues
Capecitabine	665 mg/m^2 bid continuous; 1250 mg/m^2 bid 2 weeks on / 1 off; 829 mg/m^2 bid 2 weeks on / 1 off + 60 mg/d leucovorin	Diarrhea Hand–foot syndrome	Prodrug of 5FU due to intratumoral metabolism
Cytosine arabinoside	100 mg/m^2 per day qd × 7 by continuous infusion *or* 1–3 g/m^2 dose IV bolus	Marrow Mucositis Neurologic (high dose) Conjunctivitis (high dose) Noncardiogenic pulmonary edema	Enhances activity of alkylating agents Metabolizes in tissues by deamination
Azacytidine	750 mg/m^2 per week or 75–200 mg/m^2 per day × 5–10 (bolus) or (continuous IV or subcutaneous)	Marrow Nausea Liver Neurologic Myalgia	Use limited to leukemia Altered methylation of DNA alters gene expression
Gemcitabine	1000 mg/m^2 IV weekly × 7	Marrow Nausea Hepatic Fever/"flu syndrome"	
Fludarabine phosphate	25 mg/m^2 IV qd × 5	Marrow Neurologic Lung	Dose reduction with renal failure Metabolized to F-ara converted to F-ara ATP in cells by deoxycytidine kinase
Asparaginase	25,000 IU/m^2 q3–4 weeks *or* 6000 IU/m^2 per day qod for 3–4 weeks *or* 1000–2000 IU/m^2 for 10–20 days	Protein synthesis Clotting factors Glucose Albumin Hypersensitivity CNS Pancreatitis Hepatic	Blocks methotrexate action
Pemetrexed	200 mg/m^2 q3 weeks	Anemia Neutropenia Thrombocytopenia	Supplement folate/B_{12} Caution in renal failure

(*continued*)

TABLE 28-2

COMMONLY USED CANCER CHEMOTHERAPY AGENTS (*CONTINUED*)

DRUG	EXAMPLES OF USUAL DOSES	TOXICITY	INTERACTIONS, ISSUES
Antimitotic Agents			
Vincristine	1–1.4 mg/m^2 per week (frequently cap at 2 mg total dose)	Vesicant Marrow Neurologic GI: ileus/constipation; bladder hypotoxicity; SIADH Cardiovascular	Hepatic clearance Dose reduction for bilirubin >1.5 mg/dL Prophylactic bowel regimen
Vinblastine	6–8 mg/m^2 per week	Vesicant Marrow Neurologic (less common but similar spectrum to other vincas) Hypertension Raynaud's phenomenon	Hepatic clearance Dose reduction as with vincristine
Vinorelbine	15–30 mg/m^2 per week	Vesicant Marrow Allergic/bronchospasm (immediate) Dyspnea/cough (subacute) Neurologic (less prominent but similar spectrum to other vincas)	Hepatic clearance
Paclitaxel	135–175 mg/m^2 per 24-h infusion *or* 175 mg/m^2 per 3-h infusion *or* 140 mg/m^2 per 96-h infusion *or* 250 mg/m^2 per 24-h infusion plus G-CSF	Hypersensitivity Marrow Mucositis Alopecia Sensory neuropathy CV conduction disturbance Nausea—infrequent	Premedicate with steroids, H_1 and H_2 blockers Hepatic clearance Dose reduction as with vincas
Docetaxel	100 mg/m^2 per 1-h infusion q3 weeks	Hypersensitivity Fluid retention syndrome Marrow Dermatologic Sensory neuropathy Nausea infrequent Some stomatitis	Premedicate with steroids, H_1 and H_2 blockers
Estramustine phosphate	14 mg/kg per day in 3–4 divided doses with water >2 h after meals Avoid Ca^{2+}-rich foods	Nausea Vomiting Diarrhea CHF Thrombosis Gynecomastia	
Nab-paclitaxel (protein bound)	260 mg/m^2 q3 weeks	Neuropathy Anemia Neutropenia Thrombocytopenia	Caution in hepatic insufficiency
Ixabepilone	40 mg/m^2 q3 weeks	Myelosuppression Neuropathy	
Molecularly Targeted Agents			
Retinoids			
Tretinoin	45 mg/m^2 per day until complete response + anthracycline-based regimen in APL	Teratogenic Cutaneous	APL differentiation syndrome: pulmonary dysfunction/infiltrate, pleural/pericardial effusion, fever
Bexarotene	300–400 mg/m^2 per day, continuous	Hypercholesterolemia Hypertriglyceridemia Cutaneous Teratogenic	Central hypothyroidism

(*continued*)

TABLE 28-2

COMMONLY USED CANCER CHEMOTHERAPY AGENTS (*CONTINUED*)

DRUG	EXAMPLES OF USUAL DOSES	TOXICITY	INTERACTIONS, ISSUES
Targeted Toxins			
Denileukin diftitox	9–18 μg/kg per day × 5 d q3 weeks	Nausea/vomiting Chills/fever Asthenia Hepatic	Acute hypersensitivity: hypotension, vasodilation, rash, chest tightness Vascular leak: hypotension, edema, hypoalbuminemia, thrombotic events (MI, DVT, CVA)
Tyrosine Kinase Inhibitors			
Imatinib	400 mg/d, continuous	Nausea Periorbital edema	Myelosuppression not frequent in solid tumor indications
Gefitinib	250 mg PO per day	Rash Diarrhea	In U.S., only with prior documented benefit
Erlotinib	150 mg PO per day	Rash Diarrhea	1 h before, 2 h after meals
Dasatinib	70 mg PO bid; 100 mg PO per day	Liver changes Rash Neutropenia Thrombocytopenia	
Sorafenib	400 mg PO bid	Diarrhea Hand–foot syndrome Other rash	
Sunitinib	50 mg PO qd for 4 of 6 weeks	Fatigue Diarrhea Neutropenia	
Proteosome Inhibitors			
Bortezomib	1.3 mg/m² day 1,4	Neuropathy Thrombocytopenia	
Histone Deacetylase Inhibitors			
Vorinostat	400 mg/day	Fatigue Diarrhea Thrombocytopenia Embolism	
Romidepsin	14 mg/m² day 1, 8, 15	Nausea Vomiting Cytopenias Cardiac conduction	
mTOR Inhibitors			
Temsirolimus	25 mg weekly	Stomatitis Thrombocytopenia Nausea Anorexia, fatigue Metabolic (glucose, lipid)	
Everolimus	10 mg daily	Stomatitis Fatigue	
Miscellaneous			
Arsenic trioxide	0.16 mg/kg per day up to 50 days in APL	↑ QT_c Peripheral neuropathy Musculoskeletal pain Hyperglycemia	APL differentiation syndrome (see under tretinoin)

[a]Common alkylator: alopecia, pulmonary, infertility, plus teratogenesis.

Abbreviations: APL, acute promyelocytic leukemia; ATP, adenosine triphosphate; AUC, area under the curve; bid, twice a day; CHF, congestive heart failure; CNS, central nervous system; CrCl, creatinine clearance; CV, cardiovascular; CVA, cerebrovascular accident; DVT, deep-vein thrombosis; G-CSF, granulocyte colony-stimulating factor; GI, gastrointestinal; HBP, high blood pressure; IV, intravenous; MAOI, monoamine oxidase inhibitors; MI, myocardial infarction; 6MP, 6-mercaptopurine; mTOR, mammalian target of rapamycin; NSAID, nonsteroidal anti-inflammatory drug; PO, oral; qd, every day; SIADH, syndrome of inappropriate antidiuretic hormone; WBC, white blood cell.

ifosfamide use; the incidence appears related to low body surface area or decreased creatinine clearance.

Several alkylating agents are less commonly used. Nitrogen mustard (mechlorethamine) is the prototypic agent of this class, decomposing rapidly in aqueous solution to potentially yield a bifunctional carbonium ion. It must be administered shortly after preparation into a rapidly flowing intravenous line. It is a powerful vesicant, and infiltration may be symptomatically ameliorated by infiltration of the affected site with 1/6 *M* thiosulfate. Even without infiltration, aseptic thrombophlebitis is frequent. It can be used topically as a dilute solution in cutaneous lymphomas, with a notable incidence of hypersensitivity reactions. It causes moderate nausea after intravenous administration. Bendamustine is a nitrogen mustard derivative with evidence of activity in chronic lymphocytic leukemia and certain lymphomas.

Chlorambucil causes predictable myelosuppression, azoospermia, nausea, and pulmonary side effects. Busulfan can cause profound myelosuppression, alopecia, and pulmonary toxicity but is relatively "lymphocyte sparing." Its routine use in treatment of CML has been curtailed in favor of imatinib (Gleevec) or dasatinib, but it is still employed in transplant preparation regimens. Melphalan shows variable oral bioavailability and undergoes extensive binding to albumin and α_1-acidic glycoprotein. Mucositis appears more prominently; however, it has prominent activity in multiple myeloma.

Nitrosoureas break down to carbamylating species that not only cause a distinct pattern of DNA base pair–directed toxicity but also can covalently modify proteins. They share the feature of causing relatively delayed bone marrow toxicity, which can be cumulative and long-lasting. Methyl CCNU (lomustine) causes direct glomerular as well as tubular damage, cumulatively related to dose and time of exposure.

Procarbazine is metabolized in the liver and possibly in tumor cells to yield a variety of free radical and alkylating species. In addition to myelosuppression, it causes hypnotic and other CNS effects, including vivid nightmares. It can cause a disulfiram-like syndrome on ingestion of ethanol. Altretamine (formerly hexamethylmelamine) and thiotepa can chemically give rise to alkylating species, although the nature of the DNA damage has not been well characterized in either case. Dacarbazine (DTIC) is activated in the liver to yield the highly reactive methyl diazonium cation. It causes only modest myelosuppression 21–25 days after a dose but causes prominent nausea on day 1. Temozolomide is structurally related to dacarbazine but was designed to be activated by nonenzymatic hydrolysis in tumors and is bioavailable orally.

Cisplatin was discovered fortuitously by observing that bacteria present in electrolysis solutions could not divide. Only the *cis* diamine configuration is active as an antitumor agent. It is hypothesized that in the intracellular environment, a chloride is lost from each position, being replaced by a water molecule. The resulting positively charged species is an efficient bifunctional interactor with DNA, forming Pt-based cross-links. Cisplatin requires administration with adequate hydration, including forced diuresis with mannitol to prevent kidney damage; even with the use of hydration, a gradual decrease in kidney function is common, along with noteworthy anemia. Hypomagnesemia frequently attends cisplatin use and can lead to hypocalcemia and tetany. Other common toxicities include neurotoxocity with stocking-and-glove sensorimotor neuropathy. Hearing loss occurs in 50% of patients treated with conventional doses. Cisplatin is intensely emetogenic, requiring prophylactic antiemetics. Myelosuppression is less evident than with other alkylating agents. Chronic vascular toxicity (Raynaud's phenomenon, coronary artery disease) is a more unusual toxicity. Carboplatin displays less nephro-, oto-, and neurotoxicity. However, myelosuppression is more frequent, and as the drug is exclusively cleared through the kidneys, adjustment of dose for creatinine clearance must be accomplished through use of various dosing nomograms. Oxaliplatin is a platinum analogue with noteworthy activity in colon cancers refractory to other treatments. It is prominently neurotoxic.

Antitumor antibiotics and topoisomerase poisons

Antitumor antibiotics are substances produced by bacteria that in nature appear to provide a chemical defense against other hostile microorganisms. As a class they bind to DNA directly and can frequently undergo electron transfer reactions to generate free radicals in close proximity to DNA, leading to DNA damage in the form of single-strand breaks or cross-links. Topoisomerase poisons include natural products or semisynthetic species derived ultimately from plants, and they modify enzymes that regulate the capacity of DNA to unwind to allow normal replication or transcription. These include topoisomerase I, which creates single-strand breaks that then rejoin following the passage of the other DNA strand through the break. Topoisomerase II creates double-strand breaks through which another segment of DNA duplex passes before rejoining. DNA damage from these agents can occur in any cell cycle phase, but cells tend to arrest in S-phase or G_2 of the cell cycle in cells with p53 and Rb pathway lesions as the result of defective checkpoint mechanisms in cancer cells. Owing to the role of topoisomerase I in the procession of the replication fork, topoisomerase I poisons cause lethality if the topoisomerase I–induced lesions are made in S-phase.

Doxorubicin can intercalate into DNA, thereby altering DNA structure, replication, and topoisomerase II function. It can also undergo reduction reactions by accepting electrons into its quinone ring system, with the capacity to undergo reoxidation to form reactive oxygen radicals after reoxidation. It causes predictable myelosuppression, alopecia, nausea, and mucositis. In addition, it causes acute cardiotoxicity in the form of atrial and ventricular dysrhythmias, but these are rarely of clinical significance. In contrast, cumulative doses >550 mg/m^2 are associated with a 10% incidence of chronic cardiomyopathy. The incidence of cardiomyopathy appears to be related to schedule (peak serum concentration), with low-dose, frequent treatment or continuous infusions better tolerated than intermittent higher-dose exposures. Cardiotoxicity has been related to iron-catalyzed oxidation and reduction of doxorubicin, and not to topoisomerase action. Cardiotoxicity is related to peak plasma dose; thus, lower doses and continuous infusions are less likely to cause heart damage. Doxorubicin's cardiotoxicity is increased when given together with trastuzumab (Herceptin), the anti-HER2/neu antibody. Radiation recall or interaction with concomitantly administered radiation to cause local site complications is frequent. The drug is a powerful vesicant, with necrosis of tissue apparent 4–7 days after an extravasation; therefore, it should be administered into a rapidly flowing intravenous line. Dexrazoxane is an antidote to doxorubicin-induced extravasation. Doxorubicin is metabolized by the liver, so doses must be reduced by 50–75% in the presence of liver dysfunction. Daunorubicin is closely related to doxorubicin and was actually introduced first into leukemia treatment, where it remains part of curative regimens and has been shown preferable to doxorubicin owing to less mucositis and colonic damage. Idarubicin is also used in acute myeloid leukemia treatment and may be preferable to daunorubicin in activity. Encapsulation of daunorubicin into a liposomal formulation has attenuated cardiac toxicity and antitumor activity in Kaposi's sarcoma and ovarian cancer.

Bleomycin refers to a mixture of glycopeptides that have the unique feature of forming complexes with Fe^{2+} while also bound to DNA. It remains an important component of curative regimens for Hodgkin's disease and germ cell neoplasms. Oxidation of Fe^{2+} gives rise to superoxide and hydroxyl radicals. The drug causes little, if any, myelosuppression. The drug is cleared rapidly, but augmented skin and pulmonary toxicity in the presence of renal failure have led to the recommendation that doses be reduced by 50–75% in the face of a creatinine clearance <25 mL/min. Bleomycin is not a vesicant and can be administered intravenously, intramuscularly, or subcutaneously. Common side effects include fever and chills, facial flush, and Raynaud's phenomenon. Hypertension can follow rapid intravenous administration, and the incidence of anaphylaxis with early preparations of the drug has led to the practice of administering a test dose of 0.5–1 unit before the rest of the dose. The most feared complication of bleomycin treatment is pulmonary fibrosis, which increases in incidence at >300 cumulative units administered and is minimally responsive to treatment (e.g., glucocorticoids). The earliest indicator of an adverse effect is a decline in the carbon monoxide diffusing capacity (DL_{CO}), although cessation of drug immediately upon documentation of a decrease in DL_{CO} may not prevent further decline in pulmonary function. Bleomycin is inactivated by a bleomycin hydrolase, whose concentration is diminished in skin and lung. Because bleomycin-dependent electron transport is dependent on O_2, bleomycin toxicity may become apparent after exposure to transient very high PI_{O2}. Thus, during surgical procedures, patients with prior exposure to bleomycin should be maintained on the lowest PI_{O2} consistent with maintaining adequate tissue oxygenation.

Mitoxantrone is a synthetic compound that was designed to recapitulate features of doxorubicin but with less cardiotoxicity. It is quantitatively less cardiotoxic (comparing the ratio of cardiotoxic with therapeutically effective doses) but is still associated with a 10% incidence of cardiotoxicity at cumulative doses of >150 mg/m^2. It also causes alopecia. Cases of acute promyelocytic leukemia (APL) have arisen shortly after exposure of patients to mitoxantrone, particularly in the adjuvant treatment of breast cancer. While chemotherapy-associated leukemia is generally of the acute myeloid type, APL arising in the setting of prior mitoxantrone treatment had the typical t(15;17) chromosome translocation associated with APL, but the breakpoints of the translocation appeared to be at topoisomerase II sites that would be preferred sites of mitoxantrone action, clearly linking the action of the drug to the generation of the leukemia.

Etoposide was synthetically derived from the plant product podophyllotoxin; it binds directly to topoisomerase II and DNA in a reversible ternary complex. It stabilizes the covalent intermediate in the enzyme's action where the enzyme is covalently linked to DNA. This "alkali-labile" DNA bond was historically a first hint that an enzyme such as a topoisomerase might exist. The drug therefore causes a prominent G_2 arrest, reflecting the action of a DNA damage checkpoint. Prominent clinical effects include myelosuppression, nausea, and transient hypotension related to the speed of administration of the agent. Etoposide is a mild vesicant but is relatively free from other large-organ toxicities. When given at high doses or very frequently, topoisomerase II inhibitors may cause acute leukemia associated with chromosome 11q23 abnormalities in up to 1% of exposed patients.

Camptothecin was isolated from extracts of a Chinese tree and had notable antileukemia activity in preclinical mouse models. Early human clinical studies with the sodium salt of the hydrolyzed camptothecin lactone showed evidence of toxicity with little antitumor activity. Identification of topoisomerase I as the target of camptothecins and the need to preserve lactone structure allowed additional efforts to identify active members of this series. Topoisomerase I is responsible for unwinding the DNA strand by introducing single-strand breaks and allowing rotation of one strand about the other. In S-phase, topoisomerase I–induced breaks that are not promptly resealed lead to progress of the replication fork off the end of a DNA strand. The DNA damage is a potent signal for induction of apoptosis. Camptothecins promote the stabilization of the DNA linked to the enzyme in a so-called cleavable complex, analogous to the action of etoposide with topoisomerase II. Topotecan is a camptothecin derivative approved for use in gynecologic tumors and small cell lung cancer. Toxicity is limited to myelosuppression and mucositis. CPT-11, or irinotecan, is a camptothecin with evidence of activity in colon carcinoma. In addition to myelosuppression, it causes a secretory diarrhea related to the toxicity of a metabolite called SN-38. The diarrhea can be treated effectively with loperamide or octreotide.

Indirect effectors of DNA function: antimetabolites

A broad definition of antimetabolites would include compounds with structural similarity to precursors of purines or pyrimidines, or compounds that interfere with purine or pyrimidine synthesis. Antimetabolites can cause DNA damage indirectly, through misincorporation into DNA, abnormal timing or progression through DNA synthesis, or altered function of pyrimidine and purine biosynthetic enzymes. They tend to convey greatest toxicity to cells in S-phase, and the degree of toxicity increases with duration of exposure. Common toxic manifestations include stomatitis, diarrhea, and myelosuppression. Second malignancies are not associated with their use.

Methotrexate inhibits dihydrofolate reductase, which regenerates reduced folates from the oxidized folates produced when thymidine monophosphate is formed from deoxyuridine monophosphate. Without reduced folates, cells die a "thymine-less" death. *N*5-tetrahydrofolate or *N*5-formyltetrahydrofolate (leucovorin) can bypass this block and rescue cells from methotrexate, which is maintained in cells by polyglutamylation. The drug and other reduced folates are transported into cells by the folate carrier, and high concentrations of drug can bypass this carrier and allow diffusion of drug directly into cells. These properties have suggested the design of "high-dose" methotrexate regimens with leucovorin rescue of normal marrow and mucosa as part of curative approaches to osteosarcoma in the adjuvant setting and hematopoietic neoplasms of children and adults. Methotrexate is cleared by the kidney via both glomerular filtration and tubular secretion, and toxicity is augmented by renal dysfunction and drugs such as salicylates, probenecid, and nonsteroidal anti-inflammatory drugs (NSAIDs) that undergo tubular secretion. With normal renal function, 15 mg/m^2 of leucovorin will rescue 10^{-8} to 10^{-6} M methotrexate in three to four doses. However, with decreased creatinine clearance, doses of 50–100 mg/m^2 are continued until methotrexate levels are $<5 \times 10^{-8}$ M. In addition to bone marrow suppression and mucosal irritation, methotrexate can cause renal failure itself at high doses owing to crystallization in renal tubules; therefore, high-dose regimens require alkalinization of urine with increased flow by hydration. Methotrexate can be sequestered in third-space collections and leach back into the general circulation, causing prolonged myelosuppression. Less frequent adverse effects include reversible increases in transaminases and hypersensitivity-like pulmonary syndrome. Chronic low-dose methotrexate can cause hepatic fibrosis. When administered to the intrathecal space, methotrexate can cause chemical arachnoiditis and CNS dysfunction.

Pemetrexed is a novel folate-directed antimetabolite. It is "multitargeted" in that it inhibits the activity of several enzymes, including thymidylate synthetase, dihydrofolate reductase, and glycinamide ribonucleotide formyltransferase, thereby affecting the synthesis of both purine and pyrimidine nucleic acid precursors. To avoid significant toxicity to the normal tissues, patients receiving pemetrexed should also receive low-dose folate and vitamin B_{12} supplementation. Pemetrexed has notable activity against certain lung cancers and, in combination with cisplatin, also against mesotheliomas. Palatrexate is an antifolate approved for use in T cell lymphoma that is very efficiently transported into cancer cells.

5-Fluorouracil (5FU) represents an early example of "rational" drug design in that it originated from the observation that tumor cells incorporate radiolabeled uracil more efficiently into DNA than normal cells, especially gut. 5FU is metabolized in cells to 5′FdUMP, which inhibits thymidylate synthetase (TS). In addition, misincorporation can lead to single-strand breaks, and RNA can aberrantly incorporate FUMP. 5FU is metabolized by dihydropyrimidine dehydrogenase, and deficiency of this enzyme can lead to excessive toxicity from 5FU. Oral bioavailability varies unreliably, but orally administered analogues of 5FU such as capecitabine have been developed that allow at least equivalent activity to many parenteral 5FU-based approaches. Intravenous administration of 5FU leads to bone marrow suppression after short infusions but to stomatitis after prolonged infusions. Leucovorin augments the activity of 5FU by promoting formation of the ternary covalent complex of 5FU, the reduced folate, and TS. Less frequent toxicities include CNS dysfunction, with prominent cerebellar signs, and endothelial toxicity manifested by thrombosis, including pulmonary embolus and myocardial infarction.

Cytosine arabinoside (ara-C) is incorporated into DNA after formation of ara-CTP, resulting in S-phase–related toxicity. Continuous infusion schedules allow maximal efficiency, with uptake maximal at 5–7 μ*M*. Ara-C can be administered intrathecally. Adverse effects include nausea, diarrhea, stomatitis, chemical conjunctivitis, and cerebellar ataxia. Gemcitabine is a cytosine derivative that is similar to ara-C in that it is incorporated into DNA after anabolism to the triphosphate, rendering DNA susceptible to breakage and repair synthesis, which differs from that in ara-C in that gemcitabine-induced lesions are very inefficiently removed. In contrast to ara-C, gemcitabine appears to have useful activity in a variety of solid tumors, with limited nonmyelosuppressive toxicities. 6-Thioguanine and 6-mercaptopurine (6MP) are used in the treatment of acute lymphoid leukemia. Although administered orally, they display variable bioavailability. 6MP is metabolized by xanthine oxidase and therefore requires dose reduction when used with allopurinol.

Fludarabine phosphate is a prodrug of F-adenine arabinoside (F-ara-A), which in turn was designed to diminish the susceptibility of ara-A to adenosine deaminase. F-ara-A is incorporated into DNA and can cause delayed cytotoxicity even in cells with low growth fraction, including chronic lymphocytic leukemia and follicular B cell lymphoma. CNS and peripheral nerve dysfunction and T cell depletion leading to opportunistic infections can occur in addition to myelosuppression. 2-Chlorodeoxyadenosine is a similar compound with activity in hairy cell leukemia. 2-Deoxycoformycin inhibits adenosine deaminase, with resulting increase in dATP levels. This causes inhibition of ribonucleotide reductase as well as augmented susceptibility to apoptosis, particularly in T cells. Renal failure and CNS dysfunction are notable toxicities in addition to immunosuppression. Hydroxyurea inhibits ribonucleotide reductase, resulting in S-phase block. It is orally bioavailable and useful for the acute management of myeloproliferative states.

Asparaginase is a bacterial enzyme that causes breakdown of extracellular asparagine required for protein synthesis in certain leukemic cells. This effectively stops tumor cell DNA synthesis, as DNA synthesis requires concurrent protein synthesis. The outcome of asparaginase action is therefore very similar to the result of the small-molecule antimetabolites. As asparaginase is a foreign protein, hypersensitivity reactions are common, as are effects on organs such as pancreas and liver that normally require continuing protein synthesis. This may result in decreased insulin secretion with hyperglycemia, with or without hyperamylasemia and clotting function abnormalities. Close monitoring of clotting functions should accompany use of asparaginase. Paradoxically, owing to depletion of rapidly turning over anticoagulant factors, thromboses particularly affecting the CNS may also be seen with asparaginase.

Mitotic spindle inhibitors

Microtubules are cellular structures that form the mitotic spindle, and in interphase cells they are responsible for the cellular "scaffolding" along which various motile and secretory processes occur. Microtubules are composed of repeating noncovalent multimers of a heterodimer of α and β isoform of the protein tubulin. Vincristine binds to the tubulin dimer with the result that microtubules are disaggregated. This results in the block of growing cells in M-phase; however, toxic effects in G_1 and S-phase are also evident, reflecting effects on normal cellular activities of microtubules. Vincristine is metabolized by the liver, and dose adjustment in the presence of hepatic dysfunction is required. It is a powerful vesicant, and infiltration can be treated by local heat and infiltration of hyaluronidase. At clinically used intravenous doses, neurotoxicity in the form of glove-and-stocking neuropathy is frequent. Acute neuropathic effects include jaw pain, paralytic ileus, urinary retention, and the syndrome of inappropriate antidiuretic hormone secretion. Myelosuppression is not seen. Vinblastine is similar to vincristine, except that it tends to be more myelotoxic, with more frequent thrombocytopenia and also mucositis and stomatitis. Vinorelbine is a vinca alkaloid that appears to have differences in resistance patterns in comparison to vincristine and vinblastine; it may be administered orally.

The taxanes include paclitaxel and docetaxel. These agents differ from the vinca alkaloids in that the taxanes stabilize microtubules against depolymerization. The "stabilized" microtubules function abnormally and are not able to undergo the normal dynamic changes of microtubule structure and function necessary for cell cycle completion. Taxanes are among the most broadly active antineoplastic agents for use in solid tumors, with evidence of activity in ovarian cancer, breast cancer, Kaposi's sarcoma, and lung tumors. They are administered intravenously, and paclitaxel requires use of a Cremophor-containing vehicle that can cause hypersensitivity reactions. Premedication with dexamethasone (8–16 mg orally or intravenously 12 and 6 h before treatment) and diphenhydramine (50 mg) and cimetidine (300 mg), both 30 min before treatment, decreases but does not eliminate the risk of hypersensitivity reactions to the paclitaxel vehicle. Docetaxel uses a polysorbate 80 formulation, which can cause fluid retention in addition to hypersensitivity reactions, and dexamethasone premedication with or without antihistamines is frequently used. A protein-bound formulation of paclitaxel (called *nab-paclitaxel*) has at least equivalent antineoplastic activity and decreased risk of hypersensitivity reactions. Paclitaxel may also cause hypersensitivity reactions, myelosuppression, neurotoxicity in the form of glove-and-stocking numbness, and paresthesia. Cardiac rhythm disturbances were observed in phase I and II trials, most commonly asymptomatic bradycardia but also, much more rarely, varying degrees of heart block. These have not emerged as clinically significant in the majority of patients. Docetaxel causes comparable degrees of myelosuppression and neuropathy. Hypersensitivity reactions, including bronchospasm, dyspnea, and hypotension, are less frequent but occur to some degree in up to 25% of patients. Fluid retention appears to result from a vascular leak syndrome that can aggravate preexisting effusions. Rash can complicate docetaxel administration, appearing prominently as a pruritic maculopapular rash affecting the forearms, but it has also been associated with fingernail ridging, breakdown, and skin discoloration. Stomatitis appears to be somewhat more frequent than with paclitaxel.

Resistance to taxanes has been related to the emergence of efficient efflux of taxanes from tumor cells through the p170 P-glycoprotein (*mdr* gene product) or the presence of variant or mutant forms of tubulin. Epothilones represent a class of novel microtubule-stabilizing agents that have been conscientiously optimized for activity in taxane-resistant tumors. Ixabepilone has clear evidence of activity in breast cancers resistant to taxanes and anthracyclines such as doxorubicin. It retains acceptable expected side effects, including myelosuppression, and can also cause peripheral sensory neuropathy.

Estramustine was originally synthesized as a mustard derivative that might be useful in neoplasms that possessed estrogen receptors. However, no evidence of interaction with DNA was observed. Surprisingly, the drug caused metaphase arrest, and subsequent study revealed that it binds to microtubule-associated proteins, resulting in abnormal microtubule function. Estramustine binds to estramustine-binding proteins (EMBPs), which are notably present in prostate tumor tissue. The drug is used in patients with prostate cancer. Gastrointestinal and cardiovascular adverse effects related to the estrogen moiety occur in up to 10% of patients, including worsened heart failure and thromboembolic phenomena. Gynecomastia and nipple tenderness can also occur.

Hormonal agents

Steroid hormone receptor–related molecules have emerged as prominent targets for small molecules useful in cancer treatment. When bound to their cognate ligands, these receptors can alter gene transcription and, in certain tissues, induce apoptosis. The pharmacologic effect is a mirror or parody of the normal effects of the agents acting on nontransformed normal tissues, although the effects on tumors are mediated by indirect effects in some cases.

Glucocorticoids are generally given in "pulsed" high doses in leukemias and lymphomas, where they induce apoptosis in tumor cells. Cushing's syndrome or inadvertent adrenal suppression on withdrawal from high-dose glucocorticoids can be significant complications, along with infections common in immunosuppressed patients, in particular *Pneumocystis* pneumonia, which classically appears a few days after completing a course of high-dose glucocorticoids.

Tamoxifen is a partial estrogen receptor antagonist; it has a tenfold greater antitumor activity in breast cancer patients whose tumors express estrogen receptors than in those who have low or no levels of expression. It might be considered the prototypic "molecularly targeted" agent. Owing to its agonistic activities in vascular and uterine tissue, side effects include a somewhat increased risk of cardiovascular complications, such as thromboembolic phenomena, and a small increased incidence of endometrial carcinoma, which appears after chronic use (usually >5 years). Progestational agents—including medroxyprogesterone acetate, androgens including fluoxymesterone (Halotestin), and, paradoxically, estrogens—have approximately the same degree of activity in primary hormonal treatment of breast cancers that have elevated expression of estrogen receptor protein. Estrogen itself is not used often owing to prominent cardiovascular and uterotropic activity.

Aromatase refers to a family of enzymes that catalyze the formation of estrogen in various tissues, including the ovary and peripheral adipose tissue and some tumor cells. Aromatase inhibitors are of two types, the irreversible steroid analogues such as exemestane and the reversible inhibitors such as anastrozole or letrozole. Anastrozole is superior to tamoxifen in the adjuvant treatment of breast cancer in postmenopausal patients with estrogen receptor–positive tumors. Letrozole treatment affords benefit following tamoxifen treatment. Adverse effects of aromatase inhibitors may include an increased risk of osteoporosis.

Prostate cancer is classically treated by androgen deprivation. Diethylstilbestrol (DES) acting as an estrogen at the level of the hypothalamus to downregulate hypothalamic luteinizing hormone (LH) production results in decreased elaboration of testosterone by the testicle. For this reason, orchiectomy is equally as effective as moderate-dose DES, inducing responses in 80% of previously untreated patients with prostate cancer but without the prominent cardiovascular side effects of DES, including thrombosis and exacerbation of coronary artery disease. In the event that orchiectomy is not accepted by the patient, testicular androgen suppression can also be effected by luteinizing hormone–releasing hormone (LHRH) agonists such as leuprolide and goserelin. These agents cause tonic stimulation of the LHRH receptor, with the loss of its normal pulsatile activation resulting in decreased output of LH by the anterior pituitary.

Therefore, as primary hormonal manipulation in prostate cancer, one can choose orchiectomy or leuprolide but not both. The addition of androgen receptor blockers, including flutamide or bicalutamide, is of uncertain additional benefit in extending overall response duration; the combined use of orchiectomy or leuprolide plus flutamide is referred to as *total androgen blockade*.

Tumors that respond to a primary hormonal manipulation may frequently respond to second and third hormonal manipulations. Thus, breast tumors that had previously responded to tamoxifen have, on relapse, notable response rates to withdrawal of tamoxifen itself or to subsequent addition of an aromatase inhibitor or progestin. Likewise, initial treatment of prostate cancers with leuprolide plus flutamide may be followed after disease progression by response to withdrawal of flutamide. These responses may result from the removal of antagonists from mutant steroid hormone receptors that have come to depend on the presence of the antagonist as a growth-promoting influence.

Additional strategies to treat refractory breast and prostate cancers that possess steroid hormone receptors may also address adrenal capacity to produce androgens and estrogens, even after orchiectomy or oophorectomy, respectively. Thus, aminoglutethimide or ketoconazole can be used to block adrenal synthesis by interfering with the enzymes of steroid hormone metabolism. Administration of these agents requires concomitant hydrocortisone replacement and additional glucocorticoid doses administered in the event of physiologic stress.

Humoral mechanisms can also result in complications from an underlying malignancy producing the hormone. Adrenocortical carcinomas can cause Cushing's syndrome as well as syndromes of androgen or estrogen excess. Mitotane can counteract these by decreasing synthesis of steroid hormones. Islet cell neoplasms can cause debilitating diarrhea, treated with the somatostatin analogue octreotide. Prolactin-secreting tumors can be effectively managed by the dopaminergic agonist bromocriptine.

TARGETED THERAPIES

A better understanding of cancer cell biology has suggested many new targets for cancer drug discovery and development. These include the products of oncogenes and tumor-suppressor genes, regulators of cell death pathways, mediators of cellular immortality such as telomerase, and molecules responsible for microenvironmental molding such as proteases or angiogenic factors. The essential difference in the development of agents that would target these processes is that the basis for discovery of the candidate drug is the a priori importance of the target in the biology of the tumor, rather than the initial detection of drug candidates based on the phenomenon of tumor cell regression in tissue culture or in animals. The following examples reflect the rapidly evolving clinical research activity in this area. Figure 28-4 summarizes how Food and Drug Administration (FDA)–approved targeted agents act.

Hematopoietic neoplasms

Imatinib targets the adenosine triphosphate (ATP) binding site of the $p210^{bcr\text{-}abl}$ protein tyrosine kinase that is formed as the result of the chromosome 9,22 translocation producing the Philadelphia chromosome in CML. Imatinib is superior to interferon plus chemotherapy in the initial treatment of the chronic phase of this disorder. It has lesser activity in the blast phase of CML, where the cells may have acquired additional mutations in $p210^{bcr\text{-}abl}$ itself or other genetic lesions. Its side effects are relatively tolerable in most patients and include hepatic dysfunction, diarrhea, and fluid retention. Rarely, patients receiving imatinib have decreased cardiac function, which may persist after discontinuation of the drug. The quality of response to imatinib enters into the decision about when to refer patients with CML for consideration of transplant approaches. Nilotinib is a tyrosine protein kinase inhibitor with a similar spectrum of activity to imatinib but with increased potency and perhaps better tolerance by certain patients. Dasatinib, another inhibitor of the $p210^{bcr\text{-}abl}$ oncoproteins, is active in certain mutant variants of $p210^{bcr\text{-}abl}$ that are refractory to imatinib and arise during therapy with imatinib or are present de novo. Dasatinib also has inhibitory action against kinases belonging to the src tyrosine protein kinase family; this activity may contribute to its effects in hematopoietic tumors and suggest a role in solid tumors where src kinases are active. Only the T315I mutant is resistant to dasatinib; a new class of inhibitors called aurora kinase inhibitors is in development to address this problem.

All-*trans*-retinoic acid (ATRA) targets the PML-retinoic acid receptor (RAR) α fusion protein, which is the result of the chromosome 15,17 translocation pathogenic for most forms of APL. Administered orally, it causes differentiation of the neoplastic promyelocytes to mature granulocytes and attenuates the rate of hemorrhagic complications. Adverse effects include headache with or without pseudotumor cerebri and gastrointestinal and cutaneous toxicities. Another active retinoid is the synthetic retinoid X receptor ligand bexarotene, which has activity in cutaneous T cell lymphoma.

Bortezomib is an inhibitor of the proteasome, the multisubunit assembly of protease activities responsible for the selective degradation of proteins important in regulating activation of transcription factors, including NF-κB and proteins regulating cell cycle progression.

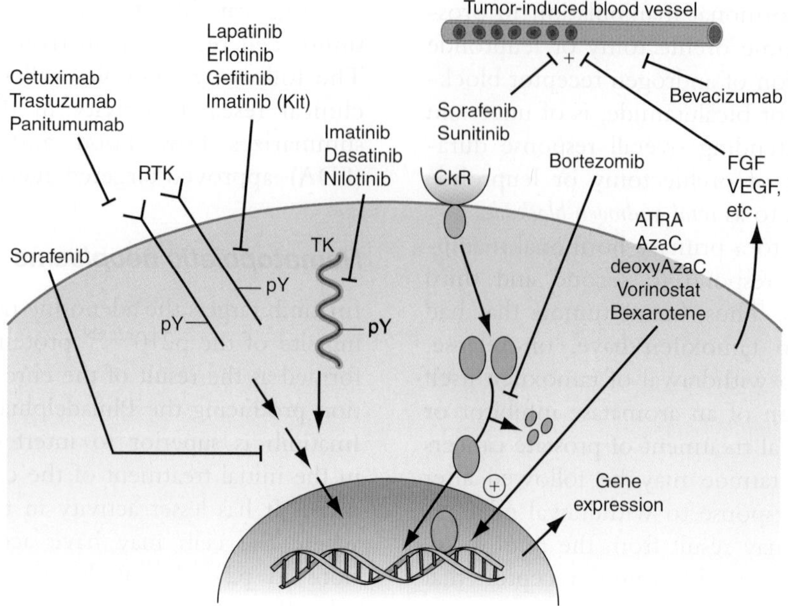

FIGURE 28-4

Site of action of targeted agents. Signals proceeding from growth factor–related receptor tyrosine kinases (RTKs) such as epidermal growth factor receptor (EGF-R), erbB2, or c-kit can be interrupted by lapatinib, erlotinib, gefitinib, and imatinib, acting at the adenosine triphosphate (ATP) binding site; or by cetuximab, trastuzumab, or panitumumab acting at the receptor. Tyrosine kinases (TKs) that are not directly stimulated by growth factors such as p210 bcr-abl or src can be inhibited by imatinib, dasatinib, or nilotinib. Signals projected downstream from growth factor receptors can be affected by the multitargeted kinase inhibitor sorafenib, acting on c-raf, and, upon arrival at the nucleus, affect gene expression, which can be affected by the targeted transcriptional modulators vorinostat (targeting histone deacetylase), azacytidine derivatives (targeting DNA methyltransferase), or retinoid receptor modulators all-*trans*-retinoic acid (ATRA) or bexarotene. Cytokine receptors (CkRs) are one stimulus for degradation of the inhibitory subunit of the NFκB transcription factor by the proteosome. Bortezomib inhibits this process and can prevent activation of NFκB-dependent genes, among other growth-related effects. Sorafenib and sunitinib, acting as inhibitors of vascular endothelial growth factor (VEGF) receptors, can modulate tumor blood vessel function through their action on endothelial cells, while bevacizumab targets the same process by combining with VEGF itself.

It has activity in multiple myeloma and certain lymphomas. Adverse effects include neuropathy, orthostatic hypotension with or without hyponatremia, and reversible thrombocytopenia.

Vorinostat is an inhibitor of histone deacetylases, responsible for maintaining the proper orientation of histones on DNA, with resulting capacity for transcriptional readiness. Acetylated histones allow entry of transcription factors and therefore increased expression of genes that are selectively repressed in tumors. The result can be differentiation with the emergence of a more normal cellular phenotype or cell-cycle arrest with expression of endogenous regulators of cell cycle progression. Vorinostat is approved for clinical use in cutaneous T cell lymphoma, with dramatic skin clearing and very few side effects. Romidepsin is a distinct molecular class of histone deacetylase inhibitor also active in cutaneous T cell lymphoma.

DNA methyltransferase inhibitors, including 5-aza-cytidine and 2′-deoxy-5-azacytidine (decitabine), can also increase transcription of genes "silenced" during the pathogenesis of a tumor by causing demethylation of the methylated cytosines that are acquired as an "epigenetic" (i.e., after the DNA is replicated) modification of DNA. These drugs were originally considered antimetabolites but have clinical value in myelodysplastic syndromes and certain leukemias when administered at low doses. Combinations of DNA methyltransferase inhibitors and histone deacetylase inhibitors may offer new approaches to regulate chromatin function.

Targeted toxins utilize macromolecules such as antibodies or cytokines with high affinity for defined tumor cell-surface molecules, such as a leukemia differentiation antigen, to which a therapeutic antibody can deliver a covalently linked potent cytotoxin or a growth factor such as IL-2 to deliver a toxin (in the form of diphtheria toxin in denileukin diftitox) to cells bearing the IL-2 receptor. The value of such targeted approaches is that in addition to maximizing the therapeutic index by differential expression of the target in tumor (as opposed to nonrenewable normal cells), selection of patients for clinical use can capitalize on assessing the target in the tumor.

Solid tumors

Small-molecule epidermal growth factor (EGF) antagonists act at the ATP binding site of the EGF receptor tyrosine kinase. In early clinical trials, gefitinib showed evidence of responses in a small fraction of patients with non-small cell lung cancer (NSCLC). Side effects were generally acceptable, consisting mostly of rash and diarrhea. Subsequent analysis of responding patients revealed a high frequency of activating mutations in the EGF receptor. Often patients who developed resistance to gefitinib have acquired additional mutations in the enzyme, similar to what was seen in imatinib-resistant CML. Erlotinib is another EGF receptor tyrosine kinase antagonist with somewhat superior outcome in clinical trials in NSCLC. Even patients with wild-type EGF receptors may benefit from erlotinib treatment. Lapatinib is a combined EGF receptor and erbB2 tyrosine kinase antagonist with activity in breast cancers refractory to anti-erbB2 antibodies.

In addition to the $p210^{bcr\text{-}abl}$ kinase, imatinib also has activity against the c-kit tyrosine kinase, activated in gastrointestinal stromal sarcoma, and the platelet-derived growth factor receptor (PDGF-R), activated by translocation in certain sarcomas. Imatinib has found clinical utility in these neoplasms previously refractory to chemotherapeutic approaches.

"Multitargeted" kinase antagonists are small-molecule ATP site-directed antagonists that inhibit more than one protein kinase. Drugs of this type with prominent activity against the vascular endothelial growth factor receptor (VEGF-R) tyrosine kinase have activity in renal cell carcinoma. Sorafenib is a VEGF-R antagonist with activity against the *raf* serine-threonine protein kinase as well. Sunitinib has anti-VEGF-R as well as anti-PDGF-R and anti-c-kit activity. It causes prominent responses as well as stabilization of disease in renal cell cancers and gastrointestinal stromal tumors. Side effects for both agents are mostly acceptable, with fatigue and diarrhea encountered with both agents. The "hand–foot syndrome" with erythema and desquamation of the distal extremities, in some cases requiring dose modification, may be seen with sorafenib. Temsirolimus and everolimus are mammalian target of rapamycin (mTOR) inhibitors with activity in renal cancers. They produce stomatitis, fatigue, and some hyperlipidemia (10%), myelosuppression (10%), and rare lung toxicity.

Personalized cancer treatment

The recognition that targeted therapies may benefit subsets of patients with an identical histologic diagnosis, but whose tumor is dependent for viability on the target's function, has spurred research to define molecular diagnostic approaches to define potentially responding patients. In addition, a patient's germ-line DNA may contain indicators of differential capacity to metabolize cancer chemotherapy agents and thus be susceptible to drug-induced toxicity. While efforts in this area are still a focus of both clinical and basic research, the following conclusions can be drawn and are applicable to patients being initially managed in the primary care setting.

All patients undergoing initial diagnostic evaluation for breast cancer should have their tumors tested for the expression of the estrogen receptor (ER), progesterone receptor (PR), and the c-erbB2 (HER2; HER2/neu) oncoprotein by immunohistochemistry or fluorescence in situ hybridization (FISH). Patients expressing the ER and/or PR are candidates for adjuvant hormone receptor–directed therapies. Patients with evidence of abundant HER2 expression or HER2 gene amplification will likely derive benefit from trastuzumab. In addition, Oncotype Dx is a 21-gene expression test that has been approved by the FDA for defining patients without lymph node involvement but with ER+ tumors who may have the greatest chance of benefiting from adjuvant chemotherapy added to adjuvant estrogen therapy. The MammaPrint test is similar in intent for node-negative patients but without reference to ER expression status.

The value of characterizing the mutational status of the EGF receptor pathway in patients with lung cancer is also a matter of current clinical investigations. While the tyrosine kinase inhibitor erlotinib is approved for use in all patients with NSCLC who have had progression of disease despite treatment with platinum-based chemotherapy, subsets of patients, such as female Asian nonsmokers, have a high evidence of EGF-R mutations, resulting in marked sensitivity to erlotinib. And it is possible that in the larger population of patients with NSCLC, such testing may allow selection of patients in whom initial use of erlotinib may also be considered. Conversely, a mutated K-ras oncogene in patients with lung adenocarcinoma is associated with no benefit from erlotinib treatment.

In patients with colon cancer, a mutated K-ras oncogene is clearly associated with no benefit to the use of the EGF-R–directed antibody cetuximab, and characterization of K-ras mutational status should be undertaken as part of the routine diagnostic evaluation of patients with newly diagnosed metastatic or newly recurrent colon cancer. Patients undergoing diagnostic evaluation for initial treatment of metastatic colon cancer might usefully undergo evaluation of their germ-line uridine diphosphate glucuronosyl transferase (UGT) 1A1 allele status, as the expression of variant alleles at that locus influences susceptibility to irinotecan-induced hematologic toxicity. Patients with known Gilbert's disease should receive irinotecan very cautiously or perhaps not at all.

ACUTE COMPLICATIONS OF CANCER CHEMOTHERAPY

Myelosuppression

The common cytotoxic chemotherapeutic agents almost invariably affect bone marrow function. Titration of this effect determines the MTD of the agent on a given schedule. The normal kinetics of blood cell turnover influences the sequence and sensitivity of each of the formed elements. Polymorphonuclear leukocytes (PMNs; $t_{1/2}$ = 6–8 h), platelets ($t_{1/2}$ = 5–7 days), and red blood cells (RBCs; $t_{1/2}$ = 120 days), respectively, have most, less, and least susceptibility to usually administered cytotoxic agents. The nadir count of each cell type in response to classes of agents is characteristic. Maximal neutropenia occurs 6–14 days after conventional doses of anthracyclines, antifolates, and antimetabolites. Alkylating agents differ from each other in the timing of cytopenias. Nitrosoureas, DTIC, and procarbazine can display delayed marrow toxicity, first appearing 6 weeks after dosing.

Complications of myelosuppression result from the predictable sequelae of the missing cells' function. *Febrile neutropenia* refers to the clinical presentation of fever (one temperature ≥38.5°C or three readings ≥38°C but ≤38.5°C per 24 h) in a neutropenic patient with an uncontrolled neoplasm involving the bone marrow or, more usually, in a patient undergoing treatment with cytotoxic agents. Mortality from uncontrolled infection varies inversely with the neutrophil count. If the nadir neutrophil count is >1000/μL, there is little risk; if <500/μL, risk of death is markedly increased. Management of febrile neutropenia has conventionally included empirical coverage with antibiotics for the duration of neutropenia (Chap. 29). Selection of antibiotics is governed by the expected association of infections with certain underlying neoplasms; careful physical examination (with scrutiny of catheter sites, dentition, mucosal surfaces, and perirectal and genital orifices by gentle palpation); chest radiography; and Gram stain and culture of blood, urine, and sputum (if any) to define a putative site of infection. In the absence of any originating site, a broadly acting β-lactam with anti-*Pseudomonas* activity, such as ceftazidime, is begun empirically. The addition of vancomycin to cover potential cutaneous sites of origin (until these are ruled out or shown to originate from methicillin-sensitive organisms) or metronidazole or imipenem for abdominal or other sites favoring anaerobes reflects modifications tailored to individual patient presentations. The coexistence of pulmonary compromise raises a distinct set of potential pathogens, including *Legionella*, *Pneumocystis*, and fungal agents that may require further diagnostic evaluations, such as bronchoscopy with bronchoalveolar lavage. Febrile neutropenic patients can be stratified broadly into two prognostic groups. The first, with expected short duration of neutropenia and no evidence of hypotension or abdominal or other localizing symptoms, may be expected to do well even with oral regimens, e.g., ciprofloxacin or moxifloxacin, or amoxicillin plus clavulanic acid. A less favorable prognostic group is patients with expected prolonged neutropenia, evidence of sepsis, and end-organ compromise, particularly pneumonia. These patients require tailoring of their antibiotic regimen to their underlying presentation, with frequent empirical addition of antifungal agents if fever persists for 7 days without identification of an adequately treated organism or site.

Transfusion of granulocytes has no role in the management of febrile neutropenia, owing to their exceedingly short half-life, mechanical fragility, and clinical syndromes of pulmonary compromise with leukostasis after their use. Instead, colony-stimulating factors (CSFs) are used to augment bone marrow production of PMNs. Early-acting factors such as IL-1, IL-3, and stem cell factor have not been as useful clinically as late-acting, lineage-specific factors such as G-CSF (granulocyte colony-stimulating factor) or GM-CSF (granulocyte-macrophage colony-stimulating factor), erythropoietin (EPO), thrombopoietin, IL-6, and IL-11. CSFs may easily become overused in oncology practice. The settings in which their use has been proved effective are limited. G-CSF, GM-CSF, EPO, and IL-11 are currently approved for use. The American Society of Clinical Oncology has developed practice guidelines for the use of G-CSF and GM-CSF (Table 28-3).

Primary prophylaxis (i.e., shortly after completing chemotherapy to reduce the nadir) administers G-CSF to patients receiving cytotoxic regimens associated with a 20% incidence of febrile neutropenia. "Dose-dense" regimens, in which cycling of chemotherapy is intended to be completed without delay of administered doses, may also benefit, but such patients should be on a clinical trial. Administration of G-CSF in these circumstances has reduced the incidence of febrile neutropenia in several studies by about 50%. Most patients, however, receive regimens that do not have such a high risk of expected febrile neutropenia, and therefore most patients initially should not receive G-CSF or GM-CSF. Special circumstances—such as a documented history of febrile neutropenia with the regimen in a particular patient or categories of patients at increased risk, such as patients older than age 65 years with aggressive lymphoma treated with curative chemotherapy regimens; extensive compromise of marrow by prior radiation or chemotherapy; or active, open wounds or deep-seated infection may support primary treatment with G-CSF or GM-CSF. Administration of G-CSF or GM-CSF to afebrile neutropenic patients or to patients with low-risk febrile neutropenia is not recommended, and patients receiving concomitant chemoradiation treatment, particularly those with thoracic neoplasms,

TABLE 28-3

INDICATIONS FOR THE CLINICAL USE OF G-CSF OR GM-CSF

Preventive Uses
With the first cycle of chemotherapy (so-called primary CSF administration)
Not needed on a routine basis
Use if the probability of febrile neutropenia is ≥20%
Use if patient has preexisting neutropenia or active infection
Age >65 years treated for lymphoma with curative intent or other tumor treated by similar regimens
Poor performance status
Extensive prior chemotherapy
Dose-dense regimens in a clinical trial or with strong evidence of benefit
With subsequent cycles if febrile neutropenia has previously occurred (so-called secondary CSF administration)
Not needed after short-duration neutropenia without fever
Use if patient had febrile neutropenia in previous cycle
Use if prolonged neutropenia (even without fever) delays therapy
Therapeutic Uses
Afebrile neutropenic patients
No evidence of benefit
Febrile neutropenic patients
No evidence of benefit
May feel compelled to use in the face of clinical deterioration from sepsis, pneumonia, or fungal infection, but benefit unclear
In bone marrow or peripheral blood stem cell transplantation
Use to mobilize stem cells from marrow
Use to hasten myeloid recovery
In acute myeloid leukemia
G-CSF of minor or no benefit
GM-CSF of no benefit and may be harmful
In myelodysplastic syndromes
Not routinely beneficial
Use intermittently in subset with neutropenia and recurrent infection
What Dose and Schedule Should Be Used?
G-CSF: 5 mg/kg per day subcutaneously
GM-CSF: 250 mg/m^2 per day subcutaneously
Peg-filgrastim: one dose of 6 mg 24 h after chemotherapy
When Should Therapy Begin and End?
When indicated, start 24–72 h after chemotherapy
Continue until absolute neutrophil count is 10,000/µL
Do not use concurrently with chemotherapy or radiation therapy

Abbreviations: G-CSF, granulocyte colony-stimulating factor; GM-CSF, granulocyte-macrophage colony-stimulating factor.

Source: From the American Society of Clinical Oncology: J Clin Oncol 24:3187, 2006.

likewise are not generally recommended for treatment. In contrast, administration of G-CSF to high-risk patients with febrile neutropenia and evidence of organ compromise, including sepsis syndrome, invasive fungal infection, concurrent hospitalization at the time fever develops, pneumonia, profound neutropenia (<0.1 × 10^9/L), or age >65 years, is reasonable.

Secondary prophylaxis refers to the administration of CSFs in patients who have experienced a neutropenic complication from a prior cycle of chemotherapy; dose reduction or delay may be a reasonably considered alternative. G-CSF or GM-CSF is conventionally started 24–72 h after completion of chemotherapy and continued until a PMN count of 10,000/µL is achieved unless a "depot" preparation of G-CSF such as pegfilgrastim is used, in which one dose is administered at least 14 days before the next scheduled administration of chemotherapy. Also, patients with myeloid leukemias undergoing induction therapy may have a slight reduction in the duration of neutropenia if G-CSF is commenced after completion of therapy and may be of particular value in elderly patients, but the influence on long-term outcome has not been defined. GM-CSF probably has a more restricted utility than G-CSF, with its use currently limited to patients after autologous bone marrow transplants, although proper head-to-head comparisons with G-CSF have not been conducted in most instances. GM-CSF may be associated with more systemic side effects.

Dangerous degrees of thrombocytopenia do not frequently complicate the management of patients with solid tumors receiving cytotoxic chemotherapy (with the possible exception of certain carboplatin-containing regimens), but they are frequent in patients with certain hematologic neoplasms in whom marrow is infiltrated with tumor. Severe bleeding related to thrombocytopenia occurs with increased frequency at platelet counts <20,000/µL and is very prevalent at counts <5000/µL.

The precise "trigger" point at which to transfuse patients is being evaluated in a randomized study. This issue is important not only because of the costs of frequent transfusion, but unnecessary platelet transfusions expose the patient to the risks of allosensitization and loss of value from subsequent transfusion owing to rapid platelet clearance, as well as the infectious and hypersensitivity risks inherent in any transfusion. Prophylactic transfusions to keep platelets >20,000/µL are reasonable in patients with leukemia who are stressed by fever or concomitant medical conditions (the threshold for transfusion is 10,000/µL in patients with solid tumors and no other bleeding diathesis or physiologic stressors such as fever or hypotension, a level that might also be reasonably considered for leukemia patients who are thrombocytopenic but not stressed or bleeding). In contrast, patients with myeloproliferative states may have functionally altered platelets despite normal platelet counts, and transfusion with normal donor platelets should be considered for evidence of bleeding in these patients. Careful review of medication lists to prevent exposure to NSAIDs and maintenance of clotting factor levels adequate to support near-normal prothrombin and partial thromboplastin time test results are important in minimizing the risk of bleeding in the thrombocytopenic patient.

Certain cytokines in clinical investigation have shown an ability to increase platelets (e.g., IL-6, IL-1, thrombopoietin), but clinical benefit and safety are not yet proven. IL-11 (oprelvekin) is approved for use in the setting of expected thrombocytopenia, but its effects on platelet counts are small, and it is associated with side effects such as headache, fever, malaise, syncope, cardiac arrhythmias, and fluid retention.

Anemia associated with chemotherapy can be managed by transfusion of packed RBCs. Transfusion is not undertaken until the hemoglobin falls to <80 g/L (8 g/dL) or if compromise of end-organ function occurs, or an underlying condition (e.g., coronary artery disease) calls for maintenance of hemoglobin >90 g/L (9 g/dL). Patients who are to receive therapy for >2 months on a "stable" regimen and who are likely to require continuing transfusions are also candidates for EPO. Randomized trials in certain tumors have raised the possibility that EPO use may promote tumor-related adverse events. This information should be considered in the care of individual patients. In the event EPO treatment is undertaken, maintenance of hemoglobin of 90–100 g/L (9–10 g/dL) should be the target. In the setting of adequate iron stores and serum EPO levels <100 ng/mL, EPO, 150 U three times a week, can produce a slow increase in hemoglobin over about 2 months of administration. Depot formulations can be administered less frequently. It is unclear whether higher hemoglobin levels, up to 110–120 g/L (11–12 g/dL), are associated with improved quality of life to a degree that justifies the more intensive EPO use. Efforts to achieve levels at or above 120 g/L (12 g/dL) have been associated with increased thromboses and mortality rates. EPO may rescue hypoxemic cells from death and contribute to tumor radioresistance.

Nausea and vomiting

The most common side effect of chemotherapy administration is nausea, with or without vomiting. Nausea may be acute (within 24 h of chemotherapy), delayed (>24 h), or anticipatory of the receipt of chemotherapy. Patients may be likewise stratified for their risk of susceptibility to nausea and vomiting, with increased risk in young, female, heavily pretreated patients without a history of alcohol or drug use but with a history of motion or morning sickness. Antineoplastic agents vary in their capacity to cause nausea and vomiting. Highly emetogenic drugs (>90%) include mechlorethamine, streptozotocin, DTIC, cyclophosphamide at >1500 mg/m^2, and cisplatin; moderately emetogenic drugs (30–90% risk) include carboplatin, cytosine arabinoside (>1 mg/m^2), ifosfamide, conventional-dose cyclophosphamide, and anthracyclines; low-risk (10–30%) agents include fluorouracil, taxanes, etoposide, and bortezomib, with minimal risk (<10%) afforded by treatment with antibodies, bleomycin, busulfan, fludarabine, and vinca alkaloids. *Emesis* is a reflex caused by stimulation of the vomiting center in the medulla. Input to the vomiting center comes from the chemoreceptor trigger zone (CTZ) and afferents from the peripheral gastrointestinal tract, cerebral cortex, and heart. The different emesis "syndromes" require distinct management approaches. In addition, a conditioned reflex may contribute to anticipatory nausea arising after repeated cycles of chemotherapy. Accordingly, antiemetic agents differ in their locus and timing of action. Combining agents from different classes or the sequential use of different classes of agent is the cornerstone of successful management of chemotherapy-induced nausea and vomiting. Of great importance are the prophylactic administration of agents and such psychological techniques as the maintenance of a supportive milieu, counseling, and relaxation to augment the action of antiemetic agents.

Serotonin antagonists (5-HT3) and neurokine (NK1) receptor antagonists are useful in "high-risk" chemotherapy regimens. The combination acts at both peripheral gastrointestinal as well as CNS sites that control nausea and vomiting. For example, the 5-HT3 blocker dolasetron (Anzamet), 100 mg intravenously or orally; dexamethasone, 12 mg; and the NK1 antagonist aprepitant, 125 mg orally, are combined on the day of administration of severely emetogenic regimens, with repetition of dexamethasone (8 mg) and aprepitant (80 mg) on days 2 and 3 for delayed nausea. Alternate 5-HT3 antagonists include ondansetron (Zofran), given as 0.15 mg/kg intravenously for three doses just before and at 4 and 8 h after chemotherapy; palonosetron (Aloxi) at 0.25 mg over 30 s, 30 min prechemotherapy; and granisetron (Kytril), given as a single dose of 0.01 mg/kg just before chemotherapy. Emesis from moderately emetic chemotherapy regimens may be prevented with a 5-HT3 antagonist and dexamethasone alone for patients not receiving doxorubicin and cyclophosphamide combinations; the latter combination requires the 5-HT3/dexamethasone/aprepitant on day 1 but aprepitant alone on days 2 and 3. Emesis from low-emetic-risk regimens may be prevented with 8 mg of dexamethasone alone, or with non-5-HT3, non-NK1 antagonist approaches including the following.

Antidopaminergic phenothiazines act directly at the CTZ and include prochlorperazine (Compazine), 10 mg intramuscularly or intravenously, 10–25 mg orally or 25 mg per rectum every 4–6 h for up to four doses, and thiethylperazine (Torecan), 10 mg by potentially all the above routes every 6 h. Haloperidol (Haldol) is a butyrophenone dopamine antagonist given at 1.0 to 1 mg intramuscularly or orally every 8 h. Antihistamines such as diphenhydramine (Benadryl) have little intrinsic antiemetic capacity but are frequently given to prevent or treat dystonic reactions that can complicate use of the antidopaminergic agents. Lorazepam (Ativan) is a short-acting benzodiazepine that provides an anxiolytic effect to augment the effectiveness of a variety of agents when used at 1–2 mg intramuscularly, intravenously, or orally every 4–6 h. Metoclopramide (Reglan) acts on peripheral dopamine receptors to augment gastric emptying and is used in high doses for highly emetogenic regimens (1–2 mg/kg intravenously 30 min before chemotherapy and every 2 h for up to three additional doses as needed); intravenous doses of 10–20 mg every 4–6 h as needed or 50 mg orally 4 h before and 8 and 12 h after chemotherapy are used for moderately emetogenic regimens. 5-9-Tetrahydrocannabinol (Marinol) is a rather weak antiemetic compared with other available agents, but it may be useful for persisting nausea and is used orally at 10 mg every 3–4 h as needed.

Diarrhea

Regimens that include fluorouracil infusions and/or irinotecan may produce severe diarrhea. Similar to the vomiting syndromes, chemotherapy-induced diarrhea may be immediate or can occur in a delayed fashion up to 48–72 h after the drugs. Careful attention to maintained hydration and electrolyte repletion, intravenously if necessary, along with antimotility treatments such as "high-dose" loperamide, commenced with 4 mg at the first occurrence of diarrhea, with 2 mg repeated every 2 h until 12 h without loose stools, not to exceed a total daily dose of 16 mg. Octreotide (100–150 μg), a somatostatin analogue, or opiate-based preparations may be considered for patients not responding to loperamide.

Mucositis

Irritation and inflammation of the mucous membranes particularly afflicting the oral and anal mucosa, but potentially involving the gastrointestinal tract, may accompany cytotoxic chemotherapy. Mucositis is due to damage to the proliferating cells at the base of the mucosal squamous epithelia or in the intestinal crypts. Topical therapies, including anesthetics and barrier-creating preparations, may provide symptomatic relief in mild cases. Palifermin or keratinocyte growth factor, a member of the fibroblast growth factor family, is effective in preventing severe mucositis in the setting of high-dose chemotherapy with stem cell transplantation for hematologic malignancies. It may also prevent or ameliorate mucositis from radiation.

Alopecia

Chemotherapeutic agents vary widely in causing alopecia, with anthracyclines, alkylating agents, and topoisomerase inhibitors reliably causing near-total alopecia when given at therapeutic doses. Antimetabolites are more variably associated with alopecia. Psychological support and the use of cosmetic resources are to be encouraged, and "chemo caps" that reduce scalp temperature to decrease the degree of alopecia should be discouraged, particularly during treatment with curative intent of neoplasms, such as leukemia or lymphoma, or in adjuvant breast cancer therapy. The richly vascularized scalp can certainly harbor micrometastatic or disseminated disease.

Gonadal dysfunction and pregnancy

Cessation of ovulation and azoospermia reliably result from alkylating agent– and topoisomerase poison–containing regimens. The duration of these effects varies with age and sex. Males treated for Hodgkin's disease with mechlorethamine- and procarbazine-containing regimens are effectively sterile, whereas fertility usually returns after regimens that include cisplatin, vinblastine, or etoposide and after bleomycin for testicular cancer. Sperm banking before treatment may be considered to support patients likely to be sterilized by treatment. Females experience amenorrhea with anovulation after alkylating agent therapy; they are likely to recover normal menses if treatment is completed before age 30 years but unlikely to recover menses after age 35 years. Even those who regain menses usually experience premature menopause. As the magnitude and extent of decreased fertility can be difficult to predict, patients should be counseled to maintain effective contraception, preferably by barrier means, during and after therapy. Resumption of efforts to conceive should be considered in the context of the patient's likely prognosis. Hormone replacement therapy should be undertaken in women who do not have a hormonally responsive tumor. For patients who have had a hormone-sensitive tumor primarily treated by a local modality, conventional practice would counsel against hormone replacement, but this issue is under investigation.

Chemotherapy agents have variable effects on the success of pregnancy. All agents tend to have increased risk of adverse outcomes when administered during the first trimester, and strategies to delay chemotherapy, if possible, until after this milestone should be considered if the pregnancy is to continue to term. Patients in their second or third trimester can be treated with most regimens for the common neoplasms affecting women in their childbearing years, with the exception of antimetabolites, particularly antifolates, which have notable teratogenic or fetotoxic effects throughout pregnancy. The need for anticancer chemotherapy per se is infrequently a clear basis to recommend termination of a concurrent pregnancy, although each treatment strategy in this circumstance must be tailored to the individual needs of the patient. Chronic effects of cancer treatment are reviewed in Chap. 55.

BIOLOGIC THERAPY

The goal of biologic therapy is to manipulate the host–tumor interaction in favor of the host, potentially at an optimum biologic dose that might be different than an MTD. As a class, biologic therapies may be distinguished from molecularly targeted agents in that many biologic therapies require an active response (e.g., reexpression of silenced genes, or antigen expression) on the part of the tumor cell or on the part of the host (e.g., immunologic effects) to allow therapeutic effect. This may be contrasted with the more narrowly defined antiproliferative or apoptotic response that is the ultimate goal of molecularly targeted agents discussed above. However, there is much commonality in the strategies to evaluate and use molecularly targeted and biologic therapies.

IMMUNE MEDIATORS OF ANTITUMOR EFFECTS

Tumors have a variety of means of avoiding the immune system: (1) they are often only subtly different from their normal counterparts; (2) they are capable of downregulating their major histocompatibility complex antigens, effectively masking them from recognition by T cells; (3) they are inefficient at presenting antigens to the immune system; (4) they can cloak themselves in a protective shell of fibrin to minimize contact with surveillance mechanisms; and (5) they can produce a range of soluble molecules, including potential immune targets, that can distract the immune system from recognizing the tumor cell or can kill the immune effector cells. Some of the cell products initially polarize the immune response away from cellular immunity (shifting from T_H1 to T_H2 responses) and ultimately lead to defects in T cells that prevent their activation and cytotoxic activity. Cancer treatment further suppresses host immunity. A variety of strategies are being tested to overcome these barriers.

Cell-mediated immunity

The strongest evidence that the immune system can exert clinically meaningful antitumor effects comes from allogeneic bone marrow transplantation. Adoptively transferred T cells from the donor expand in the tumor-bearing host, recognize the tumor as being foreign, and can mediate impressive antitumor effects (graft-versus-tumor effects). Three types of experimental interventions are being developed to take advantage of the ability of T cells to kill tumor cells.

1. Allogeneic T cells are transferred to cancer-bearing hosts in three major settings: in the form of allogeneic bone marrow transplantation, as pure lymphocyte transfusions following bone marrow recovery after allogeneic bone marrow transplantation, and as pure lymphocyte transfusions following immunosuppressive (but not myeloablative) therapy (so-called mini-transplants). In each of these settings, the effector cells are donor T cells that recognize the tumor as being foreign, probably through minor histocompatibility differences. The main risk of such therapy is the development of graft-versus-host disease because of the minimal difference between the cancer and the normal host cells. This approach has been highly effective in certain hematologic cancers.
2. Autologous T cells are removed from the tumor-bearing host, manipulated in several ways in vitro, and given back to the patient. The two major classes of autologous T cell manipulation are (a) to develop tumor antigen–specific T cells and expand them to large numbers over many weeks ex vivo before administration and (b) to activate the cells with polyclonal stimulators such as anti-CD3 and anti-CD28 after a short period ex vivo and try to expand them in the host after adoptive transfer with stimulation by IL-2, for example. Short periods removed from the patient permit the cells to overcome the tumor-induced T cell defects, and such cells traffic and home to sites of disease better than cells that have been in culture for many weeks.
3. Tumor vaccines are aimed at boosting T cell immunity. The finding that mutant oncogenes that are expressed only intracellularly can be recognized as targets of T cell killing greatly expanded the possibilities for tumor vaccine development. No longer is it difficult to find something different about tumor cells. However, major difficulties remain in getting the tumor-specific peptides presented in a fashion to prime the T cells. Tumors themselves are very poor at presenting their own antigens to T cells at the first antigen exposure (*priming*). Priming is best accomplished by professional antigen-presenting cells (dendritic cells). Thus, a number of experimental strategies are aimed at priming host T cells against tumor-associated peptides. Vaccine adjuvants such as GM-CSF appear capable of attracting antigen-presenting cells to a skin site containing a tumor antigen. Such an approach has been documented to eradicate microscopic residual disease in follicular lymphoma and give rise to tumor-specific T cells. Purified antigen-presenting cells can be pulsed with tumor, its membranes, or particular tumor antigens and delivered as a vaccine. One such vaccine, Sipuleucel-T, is approved for use in patients with hormone-independent prostate cancer. In this approach, the patient undergoes leukapheresis, wherein mononuclear cells (that include antigen-presenting cells) are removed from

the patient's blood. The cells are pulsed in a laboratory with an antigenic fusion protein comprising a protein frequently expressed by prostate cancer cells, prostate acid phosphatase, fused to GM-CSF, and matured to increase their capacity to present the antigen to immune effector cells. The cells are then returned to the patient, in a well-tolerated treatment. While no objective tumor response was documented, median survival was increased about 4 months. Tumor cells can also be transfected with genes that attract antigen-presenting cells. Vaccines against viruses that cause cancers are safe and effective. Hepatitis B vaccine prevents hepatocellular carcinoma, and a tetravalent human papilloma virus vaccine prevents infection by virus types currently accounting for 70% of cervical cancer. These vaccines are ineffective at treating patients who have developed a virus-induced cancer.

Antibodies

In general, antibodies are not very effective at killing cancer cells. Because the tumor seems to influence the host toward making antibodies rather than generating cellular immunity, it is inferred that antibodies are easier for the tumor to fend off. Many patients can be shown to have serum antibodies directed at their tumors, but these do not appear to influence disease progression. However, the ability to grow very large quantities of high-affinity antibody directed at a tumor by the hybridoma technique has led to the application of antibodies to the treatment of cancer.

Clinical antitumor efficacy has been obtained using antibodies in which the antigen-combining regions are grafted onto human immunoglobulin gene products (chimerized or humanized) or derive de novo from mice bearing human immunoglobulin gene loci. Such humanized antibodies against the CD20 molecule expressed on B cell lymphomas (rituximab) and against the HER-2/neu receptor overexpressed on epithelial cancers, especially breast cancer (trastuzumab), have become reliable tools in the oncologist's armamentarium. Each used alone can cause tumor regression (rituximab more than trastuzumab), and both appear to potentiate the effects of combination chemotherapy given just after antibody administration. Antibodies to CD52 are active in chronic lymphoid leukemia and T cell malignancies. EGF-R–directed antibodies (such as cetuximab and panitumumab) have activity in colorectal cancer refractory to chemotherapy, particularly when utilized to augment the activity of an additional chemotherapy program, and in the primary treatment of head and neck cancers treated with radiation therapy. The mechanism of action is unclear. Direct effects on the tumor may mediate an antiproliferative effect as well as stimulate the participation of host mechanisms involving immune cell or complement-mediated response to tumor cell–bound antibody. Alternatively, the antibody may alter the release of paracrine factors promoting tumor cell survival.

The anti-VEGF antibody bevacizumab shows little evidence of antitumor effect when used alone, but when combined with chemotherapeutic agents it improves the magnitude of tumor shrinkage and time to disease progression in colorectal, lung, and breast cancer. The mechanism for the effect is unclear and may relate to the capacity of the antibody to alter delivery and tumor uptake of the active chemotherapeutic agent.

Side effects include infusion-related hypersensitivity reactions, usually limited to the first infusion, which can be managed with glucocorticoid and/or antihistamine prophylaxis. In addition, distinct syndromes have emerged with different antibodies. Anti-EGF-R antibodies produce an acneiform rash that poorly responds to steroid cream treatment. Trastuzumab (anti-HER2) can inhibit cardiac function, particularly in those patients with prior exposure to anthracyclines. Bevacizumab has a number of side effects of medical significance, including hypertension, thrombosis, proteinuria, hemorrhage, and gastrointestinal perforations with or without prior surgeries.

Conjugation of antibodies to drugs and toxins is discussed above; conjugates of antibodies with isotopes, photodynamic agents, and other killing moieties may also be effective. Radioconjugates targeting CD20 on lymphomas have been approved for use [ibritumomab tiuxetan (Zevalin), using yttrium-90 or ^{131}I-tositumomab]. Other conjugates are associated with problems that have not yet been solved (e.g., antigenicity, instability, poor tumor penetration).

Cytokines

There are >70 separate proteins and glycoproteins with biologic effects in humans: interferon (IFN) α, β, γ; IL-1 through -29 (so far); the tumor necrosis factor (TNF) family (including lymphotoxin, TNF-related apoptosis-inducing ligand [TRAIL], CD40 ligand, and others); and the chemokine family. Only a fraction of these has been tested against cancer; only IFN-α and IL-2 are in routine clinical use.

About 20 different genes encode IFN-α, and their biologic effects are indistinguishable. Interferon induces the expression of many genes, inhibits protein synthesis, and exerts a number of different effects on diverse cellular processes. The two recombinant forms that are commercially available are IFN-α2a and -α2b. Interferon is not curative for any tumor but can induce partial responses in follicular lymphoma, hairy cell leukemia,

CML, melanoma, and Kaposi's sarcoma. It has been used in the adjuvant setting in stage II melanoma, multiple myeloma, and follicular lymphoma, with uncertain effects on survival. It produces fever, fatigue, a flulike syndrome, malaise, myelosuppression, and depression and can induce clinically significant autoimmune disease.

IL-2 must exert its antitumor effects indirectly through augmentation of immune function. Its biologic activity is to promote the growth and activity of T cells and natural killer cells. High doses of IL-2 can produce tumor regression in certain patients with metastatic melanoma and renal cell cancer. About 2–5% of patients may experience complete remissions that are durable, unlike any other treatment for these tumors. IL-2 is associated with myriad clinical side effects, including intravascular volume depletion, capillary leak syndrome, adult respiratory distress syndrome, hypotension, fever, chills, skin rash, and impaired renal and liver function. Patients may require blood pressure support and intensive care to manage the toxicity. However, when the agent is stopped, most of the toxicities reverse completely within 3–6 days.

GENE THERAPIES

No gene therapy has been approved for routine clinical use. Several strategies are under evaluation, including the use of viruses that cannot replicate to express genes that can allow the action of drugs or directly inhibit cancer cell growth, viruses that can actually replicate but only in the context of the tumor cell, or viruses that can express antigens in the context of the tumor and therefore provoke a host-mediated immune response. Key issues in the success of these approaches will be in defining safe viral vector systems that escape host immune function and effectively target the tumor or tumor cell milieu. Other gene therapy strategies would utilize therapeutic oligonucleotides to target the expression of genes important in the maintenance of tumor cell viability.

Acknowledgments

Stephen M. Hahn, MD, and Eli Glatstein, MD, contributed a chapter on radiation therapy in a prior edition of Harrison's Principles of Internal Medicine, and some of their material has been incorporated into this chapter.

CHAPTER 29

INFECTIONS IN PATIENTS WITH CANCER

Robert Finberg

Infections are a common cause of death and an even more common cause of morbidity in patients with a wide variety of neoplasms. Autopsy studies show that most deaths from acute leukemia and half of deaths from lymphoma are caused directly by infection. With more intensive chemotherapy, patients with solid tumors have also become more likely to die of infection. Fortunately, an evolving approach to prevention and treatment of infectious complications of cancer has decreased infection-associated mortality rates and will probably continue to do so. This accomplishment has resulted from three major steps:

1. The concept of "early empirical" antibiotics reduced mortality rates among patients with leukemia and bacteremia from 84% in 1965 to 44% in 1972. This dramatic improvement is attributed to early intervention with appropriate antimicrobial therapy.
2. "Empirical" antifungal therapy has lowered the incidence of disseminated fungal infection; in trial settings, mortality rates now range from 7% to 21%. An antifungal agent is administered—on the basis of likely fungal infection—to neutropenic patients who, after 4–7 days of antibiotic therapy, remain febrile but have no positive cultures. In one study, the 7-day survival rate was ~85% among patients who had fever and neutropenia as a result of cancer chemotherapy and who required antifungal therapy.
3. Use of antibiotics for afebrile neutropenic patients as broad-spectrum prophylaxis against infections has decreased both mortality and morbidity even further. The current approach to treatment of severely neutropenic patients (e.g., those receiving high-dose chemotherapy for leukemia or high-grade lymphomas) is based on initial prophylactic therapy at the onset of neutropenia, with subsequent "empirical" antibacterial therapy targeting the organisms whose involvement is likely in light of physical findings (most often fever alone), and finally "empirical" antifungal therapy based on the known likelihood that fungal infection will become a serious issue after 4–7 days of broad-spectrum antibacterial therapy.

A physical predisposition to infection in patients with cancer (Table 29-1) can be a result of the neoplasm's production of a break in the skin. For example, a squamous cell carcinoma may cause local invasion of the epidermis, which allows bacteria to gain access to the subcutaneous tissue and permits the development of cellulitis. The artificial closing of a normally patent orifice can also predispose to infection; for example, obstruction of a ureter by a tumor can cause urinary tract infection, and obstruction of the bile duct can cause cholangitis. Part of the host's normal defense against infection depends on the continuous emptying of a viscus; without emptying, a few bacteria that are present as a result of bacteremia or local transit can multiply and cause disease.

A similar problem can affect patients whose lymph node integrity has been disrupted by radical surgery, particularly patients who have had radical node dissections. A common clinical problem following radical mastectomy is the development of cellulitis (usually caused by streptococci or staphylococci) because of lymphedema and/or inadequate lymph drainage. In most cases, this problem can be addressed by local measures designed to prevent fluid accumulation and breaks in the skin, but antibiotic prophylaxis has been necessary in refractory cases.

A life-threatening problem common to many cancer patients is the loss of the reticuloendothelial capacity to clear microorganisms after splenectomy, which may be performed as part of the management of hairy cell leukemia, chronic lymphocytic leukemia (CLL), and chronic myelocytic leukemia (CML) and in Hodgkin's disease. Even after curative therapy for the underlying disease, the lack of a spleen predisposes such patients to rapidly fatal infections. The loss of the spleen through

TABLE 29-1

DISRUPTION OF NORMAL BARRIERS THAT MAY PREDISPOSE TO INFECTIONS IN PATIENTS WITH CANCER

TYPE OF DEFENSE	SPECIFIC LESION	CELLS INVOLVED	ORGANISM	CANCER ASSOCIATION	DISEASE
Physical barrier	Breaks in skin	Skin epithelial cells	Staphylococci, streptococci	Head and neck, squamous cell carcinoma	Cellulitis, extensive skin infection
Emptying of fluid collections	Occlusion of orifices: ureters, bile duct, colon	Luminal epithelial cells	Gram-negative bacilli	Renal, ovarian, biliary tree, metastatic diseases of many cancers	Rapid, overwhelming bacteremia; urinary tract infection
Lymphatic function	Node dissection	Lymph nodes	Staphylococci, streptococci	Breast cancer surgery	Cellulitis
Splenic clearance of microorganisms	Splenectomy	Splenic reticuloendothelial cells	*Streptococcus pneumoniae, Haemophilus influenzae, Neisseria meningitidis, Babesia, Capnocytophaga canimorsus*	Hodgkin's disease, leukemia, idiopathic thrombocytopenic purpura	Rapid, overwhelming sepsis
Phagocytosis	Lack of granulocytes	Granulocytes (neutrophils)	Staphylococci, streptococci, enteric organisms, fungi	Hairy cell, acute myelocytic, and acute lymphocytic leukemias	Bacteremia
Humoral immunity	Lack of antibody	B cells	*S. pneumoniae, H. influenzae, N. meningitidis*	Chronic lymphocytic leukemia, multiple myeloma	Infections with encapsulated organisms, sinusitis, pneumonia
Cellular immunity	Lack of T cells	T cells and macrophages	*Mycobacterium tuberculosis, Listeria,* herpesviruses, fungi, intracellular parasites	Hodgkin's disease, leukemia, T cell lymphoma	Infections with intracellular bacteria, fungi, parasites

trauma similarly predisposes the normal host to overwhelming infection throughout life. The splenectomized patient should be counseled about the risks of infection with certain organisms, such as the protozoan *Babesia* spp. and *Capnocytophaga canimorsus*, a bacterium carried in the mouths of animals. Since encapsulated bacteria (*Streptococcus pneumoniae*, *Haemophilus influenzae*, and *Neisseria meningitidis*) are the organisms most commonly associated with postsplenectomy sepsis, splenectomized persons should be vaccinated (and revaccinated; Table 29-2) against the capsular polysaccharides of these organisms. Many clinicians recommend giving splenectomized patients a small supply of antibiotics effective against *S. pneumoniae*, *N. meningitidis*, and *H. influenzae* to avert rapid, overwhelming sepsis in the event that they cannot present for medical attention immediately after the onset of fever or other signs or symptoms of bacterial infection. A few amoxicillin/clavulanic acid tablets are a reasonable choice for this purpose.

The level of suspicion of infections with certain organisms should depend on the type of cancer diagnosed (Table 29-3). Diagnosis of multiple myeloma or CLL should alert the clinician to the possibility of hypogammaglobulinemia. While immunoglobulin replacement therapy can be effective, in most cases, prophylactic antibiotics are a cheaper, more convenient method of eliminating bacterial infections in CLL patients with hypogammaglobulinemia. Patients with acute lymphocytic leukemia (ALL), patients with non-Hodgkin's lymphoma, and all cancer patients treated with high-dose glucocorticoids (or glucocorticoid-containing chemotherapy regimens) should receive antibiotic prophylaxis for *Pneumocystis* infection (Table 29-3) for the duration of their chemotherapy. In addition to exhibiting susceptibility to certain infectious organisms, patients with cancer are likely to manifest their infections in characteristic ways. For example, fever—generally a sign of infection in normal hosts—continues to be a reliable indicator in neutropenic patients. In contrast, patients receiving glucocorticoids and agents that impair T cell function and cytokine secretion may have serious infections in the absence of fever. Similarly, neutropenic patients commonly present with cellulitis without

TABLE 29-2

VACCINATION OF CANCER PATIENTS RECEIVING CHEMOTHERAPY[a]

	USE IN INDICATED PATIENTS		
VACCINE	**INTENSIVE CHEMOTHERAPY**	**HODGKIN'S DISEASE**	**HEMATOPOIETIC STEM CELL TRANSPLANTATION**
Diphtheria–tetanus[b]	Primary series and boosters as necessary	No special recommendation	3 doses given 6–12 months after transplantation
Poliomyelitis[c]	Complete primary series and boosters	No special recommendation	3 doses given 6–12 months after transplantation
Haemophilus influenzae type b conjugate	Primary series and booster for children	Immunization before treatment and booster 3 months afterward	3 doses given 6–12 months after transplantation
Human papillomavirus	3 doses for girls and women through 26 years of age	3 doses for girls and women through 26 years of age	3 doses for girls and women through 26 years of age
Hepatitis A	As indicated for normal hosts based on occupation and lifestyle	As indicated for normal hosts based on occupation and lifestyle	As indicated for normal hosts based on occupation and lifestyle
Hepatitis B	Same as for normal hosts	As indicated for normal hosts based on occupation and lifestyle	3 doses given 6–12 months after transplantation
23-Valent pneumococcal polysaccharide[d]	Every 5 years	Immunization before treatment and booster 3 months afterward	1 or 2 doses given 6–12 months after transplantation
4-Valent meningococcal vaccine[e]	Should be administered to splenectomized patients and patients living in endemic areas, including college students in dormitories	Should be administered to splenectomized patients and patients living in endemic areas, including college students in dormitories	Should be administered to splenectomized patients and patients living in endemic areas, including college students in dormitories
Influenza	Seasonal immunization	Seasonal immunization	Seasonal immunization
Measles–mumps–rubella	Contraindicated	Contraindicated during chemotherapy	After 24 months in patients without graft-vs-host disease
Varicella-zoster virus[f]	Contraindicated[g]	Contraindicated	Contraindicated

[a]The latest recommendations by the Advisory Committee on Immunization Practices and the Centers for Disease Control and Prevention guidelines can be found at *http://www.cdc.gov/vaccines.*

[b]The Td (tetanus–diphtheria) combination was recommended for adults. Pertussis vaccine was not recommended for people >6 years of age in the past. However, recent data indicate that the Tdap (tetanus–diphtheria–acellular pertussis) product is both safe and efficacious in adults. A single Tdap booster is now recommended for adults.

[c]Live-virus vaccine is contraindicated; inactivated vaccine should be used.

[d]The 7- and 13-valent pneumococcal conjugate vaccines are currently recommended for children.

[e]Meningococcal conjugate vaccine (MCV4) is recommended for adults ≤55 years old and meningococcal polysaccharide vaccine (MPSV4) for those ≥56 years old.

[f]Includes both varicella vaccine for children and zoster vaccine for adults.

[g]Contact the manufacturer for more information on use in children with acute lymphocytic leukemia.

purulence and with pneumonia without sputum or even radiographic findings (see later discussion).

The use of monoclonal antibodies that target B and T cells as well as drugs that interfere with lymphocyte signal transduction events is associated with reactivation of latent infections. The use of rituximab, the antibody to CD20 (a B–cell surface protein), is associated with the development of reactivation tuberculosis as well as hepatitis B, cytomegalovirus (CMV) infection, and other latent infections. Like organ transplant recipients, patients with positive purified protein derivative test results and underlying viral infection should be carefully monitored for reactivation disease.

SYSTEM-SPECIFIC SYNDROMES

SKIN-SPECIFIC SYNDROMES

Skin lesions are common in cancer patients, and the appearance of these lesions may permit the diagnosis of systemic bacterial or fungal infection. While cellulitis

TABLE 29-3

INFECTIONS ASSOCIATED WITH SPECIFIC TYPES OF CANCER

CANCER	UNDERLYING IMMUNE ABNORMALITY	ORGANISMS CAUSING INFECTION
Multiple myeloma	Hypogammaglobulinemia	*Streptococcus pneumoniae, Haemophilus influenzae, Neisseria meningitidis*
Chronic lymphocytic leukemia	Hypogammaglobulinemia	*S. pneumoniae, H. influenzae, N. meningitidis*
Acute myelocytic or lymphocytic leukemia	Granulocytopenia, skin and mucous membrane lesions	Extracellular gram-positive and gram-negative bacteria, fungi
Hodgkin's disease	Abnormal T cell function	Intracellular pathogens *(Mycobacterium tuberculosis, Listeria, Salmonella, Cryptococcus, Mycobacterium avium)*
Non-Hodgkin's lymphoma and acute lymphocytic leukemia	Glucocorticoid chemotherapy, T and B cell dysfunction	*Pneumocystis*
Colon and rectal tumors	Local abnormalities[a]	*Streptococcus bovis* (bacteremia)
Hairy cell leukemia	Abnormal T cell function	Intracellular pathogens (*M. tuberculosis, Listeria, Cryptococcus, M. avium*)

[a]The reason for this association is not well defined.

caused by skin organisms such as *Streptococcus* or *Staphylococcus* is common, neutropenic patients i.e., those with <500 functional polymorphonuclear leukocytes (PMNs)/μL—and patients with impaired blood or lymphatic drainage may develop infections with unusual organisms. Innocent-looking macules or papules may be the first sign of bacterial or fungal sepsis in immunocompromised patients (Fig. 29-1). In a neutropenic host, a macule progresses rapidly to ecthyma gangrenosum (Fig. e7-35), a usually painless, round, necrotic lesion consisting of a central black or gray-black eschar with surrounding erythema. Ecthyma gangrenosum, which is located in nonpressure areas (as distinguished from necrotic lesions associated with lack of circulation), is often associated with *Pseudomonas aeruginosa* bacteremia but may be caused by other bacteria.

Candidemia is also associated with a variety of skin conditions and commonly presents as a maculopapular rash. Punch biopsy of the skin may be the best method for diagnosis.

Cellulitis, an acute spreading inflammation of the skin, is most often caused by infection with group A *Streptococcus* or *Staphylococcus aureus*, virulent organisms normally found on the skin. Although cellulitis tends to

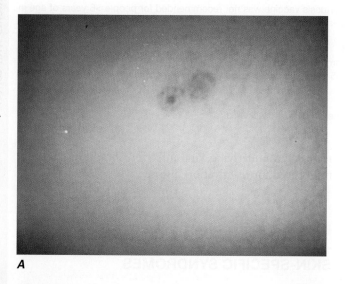

A

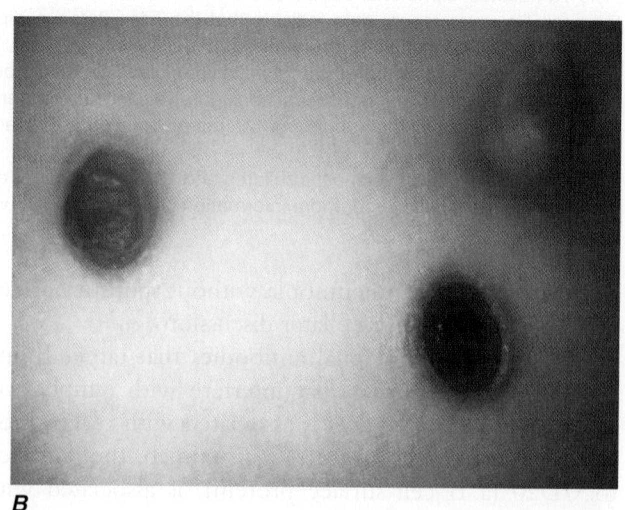

B

FIGURE 29-1

A.* Papules related to *Escherichia coli* bacteremia** in a neutropenic patient with acute lymphocytic leukemia. ***B. The same lesion the following day.

TABLE 29-4

ORGANISMS LIKELY TO CAUSE INFECTIONS IN GRANULOCYTOPENIC PATIENTS

Gram-positive cocci	*Enterobacter* spp.
Staphylococcus epidermidis	*Serratia* spp.
Staphylococcus aureus	*Acinetobacter* spp.[a]
Viridans *Streptococcus*	*Citrobacter* spp.
Enterococcus faecalis	Gram-positive bacilli
Streptococcus pneumoniae	Diphtheroids
Gram-negative bacilli	JK bacillus[a]
Escherichia coli	Fungi
Klebsiella spp.	*Candida* spp.
Pseudomonas aeruginosa	*Aspergillus* spp.
Non-*aeruginosa Pseudomonas* spp.[a]	

[a]Often associated with intravenous catheters.

be circumscribed in normal hosts, it may spread rapidly in neutropenic patients. A tiny break in the skin may lead to spreading cellulitis, which is characterized by pain and erythema; in affected patients, signs of infection (e.g., purulence) are often lacking. What might be a furuncle in a normal host may require amputation because of uncontrolled infection in a patient presenting with leukemia. A dramatic response to an infection that might be trivial in a normal host can mark the first sign of leukemia. Fortunately, granulocytopenic patients are likely to be infected with certain types of organisms (Table 29-4); thus the selection of an antibiotic regimen is somewhat easier than it might otherwise be (see "Antibacterial Therapy" later in this chapter). It is essential to recognize cellulitis early and to treat it aggressively. Patients who are neutropenic or have previously received antibiotics for other reasons may develop cellulitis with unusual organisms (e.g., *Escherichia coli*, *Pseudomonas* spp., or fungi). Early treatment, even of innocent-looking lesions, is essential to prevent necrosis and loss of tissue. Debridement to prevent spread may sometimes be necessary early in the course of disease, but it can often be performed after chemotherapy, when the PMN count increases.

Sweet's syndrome, or *febrile neutrophilic dermatosis*, was originally described in women with elevated white blood cell (WBC) counts. The disease is characterized by the presence of leukocytes in the lower dermis, with edema of the papillary body. Ironically, this disease now is usually seen in neutropenic patients with cancer, most often in association with acute leukemia but also in association with a variety of other malignancies. Sweet's syndrome usually presents as red or bluish-red papules or nodules that may coalesce and form sharply bordered plaques (Fig. e7-41). The edema may suggest vesicles, but on palpation, the lesions are solid, and vesicles probably never arise in this disease. The lesions are most common on the face, neck, and arms. On the legs, they may be confused with erythema nodosum. The development of lesions is often accompanied by high fevers and an elevated erythrocyte sedimentation rate. Both the lesions and the temperature elevation respond dramatically to glucocorticoid administration. Treatment begins with high doses of glucocorticoids (60 mg/d of prednisone) followed by tapered doses over the next 2–3 weeks.

Data indicate that *erythema multiforme* with mucous membrane involvement is often associated with herpes simplex virus (HSV) infection and is distinct from Stevens-Johnson syndrome, which is associated with drugs and tends to have a more widespread distribution. Since cancer patients are both immunosuppressed (and therefore susceptible to herpes infections) and heavily treated with drugs and therefore subject to Stevens-Johnson syndrome, both of these conditions are common in this population.

Cytokines, which are used as adjuvants or primary treatments for cancer, can themselves cause characteristic rashes, further complicating the differential diagnosis. This phenomenon is a particular problem in bone marrow transplant recipients, who, in addition to having the usual chemotherapy-, antibiotic-, and cytokine-induced rashes, are plagued by graft-versus-host disease.

CATHETER-RELATED INFECTIONS

Because intravenous (IV) catheters are commonly used in cancer chemotherapy and are prone to infection, they pose a major problem in the care of patients with cancer. Some catheter-associated infections can be treated with antibiotics, while in others, the catheter must be removed (Table 29-5). If the patient has a "tunneled" catheter (which consists of an entrance site, a subcutaneous tunnel, and an exit site), a red streak over the subcutaneous part of the line (the tunnel) is grounds for immediate device removal. Failure to remove catheters under these circumstances may result in extensive cellulitis and tissue necrosis.

More common than tunnel infections are exit-site infections, often with erythema around the area where the line penetrates the skin. Most authorities recommend treatment (usually with vancomycin) for an exit-site infection caused by coagulase-negative *Staphylococcus*. Treatment of coagulase-positive staphylococcal infection is associated with a poorer outcome, and it is advisable to remove the catheter if possible. Similarly, many clinicians remove catheters associated with infections due to *P. aeruginosa* and *Candida* spp. since such infections are difficult to treat and bloodstream infections with these organisms are likely to be deadly. Catheter infections caused by *Burkholderia*

TABLE 29-5

APPROACH TO CATHETER INFECTIONS IN IMMUNOCOMPROMISED PATIENTS

CLINICAL PRESENTATION	CATHETER REMOVAL	ANTIBIOTICS	COMMENTS
Evidence of Infection, Negative Blood Cultures			
Exit-site erythema	Not necessary if infection responds to treatment	Usually begin treatment for gram-positive cocci.	Coagulase-negative staphylococci are most common.
Tunnel-site erythema	Required	Treat for gram-positive cocci pending culture results.	Failure to remove the catheter may lead to complications.
Blood Culture–Positive Infections			
Coagulase-negative staphylococci	Line removal optimal but may be unnecessary if patient is clinically stable and responds to antibiotics	Usually start with vancomycin. (Linezolid, quinupristin/dalfopristin, and daptomycin are all appropriate.)	If there are no contraindications to line removal, this course of action is optimal. If the line is removed, antibiotics may not be necessary.
Other gram-positive cocci (e.g., *Staphylococcus aureus, Enterococcus*); gram-positive rods (*Bacillus, Corynebacterium* spp.)	Recommended	Treat with antibiotics to which the organism is sensitive, with duration based on the clinical setting.	The incidence of metastatic infections following *S. aureus* infection and the difficulty of treating enterococcal infection make line removal the recommended course of action. In addition, gram-positive rods do not respond readily to antibiotics alone.
Gram-negative bacteria	Recommended	Use an agent to which the organism is shown to be sensitive.	Organisms like *Stenotrophomonas, Pseudomonas*, and *Burkholderia* are notoriously hard to treat.
Fungi	Recommended	—	Fungal infections of catheters are extremely difficult to treat.

cepacia, Stenotrophomonas spp., *Agrobacterium* spp., and *Acinetobacter baumannii* as well as *Pseudomonas* spp. other than *aeruginosa* are likely to be very difficult to eradicate with antibiotics alone. Similarly, isolation of *Bacillus, Corynebacterium*, and *Mycobacterium* spp. should prompt removal of the catheter.

GASTROINTESTINAL TRACT–SPECIFIC SYNDROMES

Upper gastrointestinal tract disease

Infections of the mouth

The oral cavity is rich in aerobic and anaerobic bacteria that normally live in a commensal relationship with the host. The antimetabolic effects of chemotherapy cause a breakdown of host defenses, leading to ulceration of the mouth and the potential for invasion by resident bacteria. Mouth ulcerations affect most patients receiving cytotoxic chemotherapy and have been associated with viridans streptococcal bacteremia. *Candida* infections of the mouth are very common. Fluconazole is clearly effective in the treatment of both local infections (thrush) and systemic infections (esophagitis) due to *Candida albicans*. Other azoles (e.g., voriconazole) as well as echinocandins offer similar efficacy as well as activity against the fluconazole-resistant organisms that are associated with extensive fluconazole treatment.

Noma (*cancrum oris*), commonly seen in malnourished children, is a penetrating disease of the soft and hard tissues of the mouth and adjacent sites, with resulting necrosis and gangrene. It has a counterpart in immunocompromised patients and is thought to be due to invasion of the tissues by *Bacteroides, Fusobacterium*, and other normal inhabitants of the mouth. Noma is associated with debility, poor oral hygiene, and immunosuppression.

Viruses, particularly HSV, are a prominent cause of morbidity in immunocompromised patients, in whom they are associated with severe mucositis. The use of acyclovir, either prophylactically or therapeutically, is of value.

Esophageal infections

The differential diagnosis of esophagitis (usually presenting as substernal chest pain upon swallowing) includes HSV and candidiasis, both of which are readily treatable.

Lower gastrointestinal tract disease

Hepatic candidiasis (Chap. 203) results from seeding of the liver (usually from a gastrointestinal source) in neutropenic patients. It is most common among patients being treated for acute leukemia and usually presents symptomatically around the time the neutropenia resolves. The characteristic picture is that of persistent fever unresponsive to antibiotics, abdominal pain and tenderness or nausea, and elevated serum levels of alkaline phosphatase in a patient with hematologic malignancy who has recently recovered from neutropenia. The diagnosis of this disease (which may present in an indolent manner and persist for several months) is based on the finding of yeasts or pseudohyphae in granulomatous lesions. Hepatic ultrasound or CT may reveal bull's-eye lesions. In some cases, MRI reveals small lesions not visible by other imaging modalities. The pathology (a granulomatous response) and the timing (with resolution of neutropenia and an elevation in granulocyte count) suggest that the host response to *Candida* is an important component of the manifestations of disease. In many cases, although organisms are visible, cultures of biopsied material may be negative. The designation *hepatosplenic candidiasis* or *hepatic candidiasis* is a misnomer because the disease often involves the kidneys and other tissues; the term *chronic disseminated candidiasis* may be more appropriate. Because of the risk of bleeding with liver biopsy, diagnosis is often based on imaging studies (MRI, CT). Treatment should be directed to the causative agent (usually *C. albicans* but sometimes *C. tropicalis* or other less common *Candida* spp).

Typhlitis

Typhlitis (also referred to as necrotizing colitis, neutropenic colitis, necrotizing enteropathy, ileocecal syndrome, and cecitis) is a clinical syndrome of fever and right-lower-quadrant tenderness in an immunosuppressed host. This syndrome is classically seen in neutropenic patients after chemotherapy with cytotoxic drugs. It may be more common among children than among adults and appears to be much more common among patients with acute myelocytic leukemia (AML) or ALL than among those with other types of cancer; a similar syndrome has been reported in patients infected with HIV type 1. Physical examination reveals right-lower-quadrant tenderness, with or without rebound tenderness. Associated diarrhea (often bloody) is common, and the diagnosis can be confirmed by the finding of a thickened cecal wall on CT, MRI, or ultrasonography. Plain films may reveal a right-lower-quadrant mass, but CT with contrast or MRI is a much more sensitive means of diagnosis. Although surgery is sometimes attempted to avoid perforation from ischemia, most cases resolve with medical therapy alone. The disease is sometimes associated with positive blood cultures (which usually yield aerobic gram-negative bacilli), and therapy is recommended for a broad spectrum of bacteria (particularly gram-negative bacilli, which are likely to be found in the bowel flora). Surgery is indicated in the case of perforation.

Clostridium difficile–induced diarrhea

Patients with cancer are predisposed to the development of *C. difficile* diarrhea (Chap. 129) as a consequence of chemotherapy alone. Thus, they may have positive toxin tests before receiving antibiotics. Obviously, such patients are also subject to *C. difficile*–induced diarrhea as a result of antibiotic pressure. *C. difficile* should always be considered as a possible cause of diarrhea in cancer patients who have received antibiotics.

CENTRAL NERVOUS SYSTEM–SPECIFIC SYNDROMES

Meningitis

The presentation of meningitis in patients with lymphoma or CLL, patients receiving chemotherapy (particularly with glucocorticoids) for solid tumors, and patients who have received bone marrow transplants suggests a diagnosis of cryptococcal or listerial infection. As noted previously, splenectomized patients are susceptible to rapid, overwhelming infection with encapsulated bacteria (including *S. pneumoniae*, *H. influenzae*, and *N. meningitidis*). Similarly, patients who are antibody-deficient (e.g., those with CLL, those who have received intensive chemotherapy, or those who have undergone bone marrow transplantation) are likely to have infections caused by these bacteria. Other cancer patients, however, because of their defective cellular immunity, are likely to be infected with other pathogens (Table 29-3).

Encephalitis

The spectrum of disease resulting from viral encephalitis is expanded in immunocompromised patients. A predisposition to infections with intracellular organisms similar to those encountered in patients with AIDS (Chap. 189) is seen in cancer patients receiving (1) high-dose cytotoxic chemotherapy, (2) chemotherapy affecting T cell function (e.g., fludarabine), or (3) antibodies that eliminate T cells (e.g., anti-CD3, alemtuzumab, anti-CD52) or cytokine activity (anti-tumor necrosis factor agents or interleukin 1 receptor antagonists). Infection with varicella-zoster virus (VZV)

TABLE 29-6

DIFFERENTIAL DIAGNOSIS OF CENTRAL NERVOUS SYSTEM INFECTIONS IN PATIENTS WITH CANCER

	UNDERLYING PREDISPOSITION	
FINDINGS ON CT OR MRI	PROLONGED NEUTROPENIA	DEFECTS IN CELLULAR IMMUNITY[a]
Mass lesions	*Aspergillus, Nocardia,* or *Cryptococcus* brain abscess	Toxoplasmosis EBV-LPD
Diffuse encephalitis	PML (JC virus)	Infection with VZV, CMV, HSV, HHV-6, JC virus (PML), *Listeria*

[a]High-dose glucocorticoid therapy, cytotoxic chemotherapy.

Abbreviations: CMV, cytomegalovirus; CT, computed tomography; EBV-LPD, Epstein-Barr virus lymphoproliferative disease; HHV-6, human herpesvirus type 6; HSV, herpes simplex virus; MRI, magnetic resonance imaging; PML, progressive multifocal leukoencephalopathy; VZV, varicella-zoster virus.

TABLE 29-7

DIFFERENTIAL DIAGNOSIS OF CHEST INFILTRATES IN IMMUNOCOMPROMISED PATIENTS

	CAUSE OF PNEUMONIA	
INFILTRATE	INFECTIOUS	NONINFECTIOUS
Localized	Bacteria (including *Legionella,* mycobacteria)	Local hemorrhage or embolism, tumor
Nodular	Fungi (e.g., *Aspergillus* or *Mucor*), *Nocardia*	Recurrent tumor
Diffuse	Viruses (especially CMV), *Chlamydia, Pneumocystis, Toxoplasma gondii,* mycobacteria	Congestive heart failure, radiation pneumonitis, drug-induced lung injury, diffuse alveolar hemorrhage (described after BMT)

Abbreviations: BMT, bone marrow transplantation; CMV, cytomegalovirus.

has been associated with encephalitis that may be caused by VZV-related vasculitis. Chronic viral infections may also be associated with dementia and encephalitic presentations, and a diagnosis of progressive multifocal leukoencephalopathy should be considered when a patient who has received chemotherapy presents with dementia (Table 29-6). Other abnormalities of the central nervous system (CNS) that may be confused with infection include normal-pressure hydrocephalus and vasculitis resulting from CNS irradiation. It may be possible to differentiate these conditions by MRI.

Brain masses

Mass lesions of the brain most often present as headache with or without fever or neurologic abnormalities. Infections associated with mass lesions may be caused by bacteria (particularly *Nocardia*), fungi (particularly *Cryptococcus* or *Aspergillus*), or parasites (*Toxoplasma*). Epstein-Barr virus (EBV)–associated lymphoproliferative disease may also present as single or multiple mass lesions of the brain. A biopsy may be required for a definitive diagnosis.

PULMONARY INFECTIONS

Pneumonia in immunocompromised patients may be difficult to diagnose because conventional methods of diagnosis depend on the presence of neutrophils. Bacterial pneumonia in neutropenic patients may present without purulent sputum—or, in fact, without any sputum at all—and may not produce physical findings suggestive of chest consolidation (rales or egophony).

In granulocytopenic patients with persistent or recurrent fever, the chest x-ray pattern may help to localize an infection and thus to determine which investigative tests and procedures should be undertaken and which therapeutic options should be considered (Table 29-7). In this setting, a simple chest x-ray is a screening tool; because the impaired host response results in less evidence of consolidation or infiltration, high-resolution CT is recommended for the diagnosis of pulmonary infections. The difficulties encountered in the management of pulmonary infiltrates relate in part to the difficulties of performing diagnostic procedures on the patients involved. When platelet counts can be increased to adequate levels by transfusion, microscopic and microbiologic evaluation of the fluid obtained by endoscopic bronchial lavage is often diagnostic. Lavage fluid should be cultured for *Mycoplasma, Chlamydia, Legionella, Nocardia,* more common bacterial pathogens, and fungi. In addition, the possibility of *Pneumocystis* pneumonia should be considered, especially in patients with ALL or lymphoma who have not received prophylactic trimethoprim-sulfamethoxazole (TMP-SMX). The characteristics of the infiltrate may be helpful in decisions about further diagnostic and therapeutic maneuvers. Nodular infiltrates suggest fungal pneumonia (e.g., that caused by *Aspergillus* or *Mucor*). Such lesions may best be approached by visualized biopsy procedures.

Aspergillus species can colonize the skin and respiratory tract or cause fatal systemic illness. Although this fungus may cause aspergillomas in a previously existing cavity or may produce allergic bronchopulmonary disease, the major problem posed by this genus in neutropenic patients is invasive disease due to *A. fumigatus* or *A. flavus*. The organisms enter the host following colonization of the respiratory tract, with subsequent invasion of blood vessels. The disease is likely to present as a thrombotic or embolic event because of this ability of the fungi to invade blood vessels. The risk of infection with *Aspergillus* correlates directly with the duration of neutropenia. In prolonged neutropenia, positive surveillance cultures for nasopharyngeal colonization with *Aspergillus* may predict the development of disease.

Patients with *Aspergillus* infection often present with pleuritic chest pain and fever, which are sometimes accompanied by cough. Hemoptysis may be an ominous sign. Chest x-rays may reveal new focal infiltrates or nodules. Chest CT may reveal a characteristic halo consisting of a mass-like infiltrate surrounded by an area of low attenuation. The presence of a "crescent sign" on chest x-ray or chest CT, in which the mass progresses to central cavitation, is characteristic of invasive *Aspergillus* infection but may develop as the lesions are resolving.

In addition to causing pulmonary disease, *Aspergillus* may invade through the nose or palate, with deep sinus penetration. The appearance of a discolored area in the nasal passages or on the hard palate should prompt a search for invasive *Aspergillus*. This situation is likely to require surgical debridement. Catheter infections with *Aspergillus* usually require both removal of the catheter and antifungal therapy.

Diffuse interstitial infiltrates suggest viral, parasitic, or *Pneumocystis* pneumonia. If the patient has a diffuse interstitial pattern on chest x-ray, it may be reasonable, while considering invasive diagnostic procedures, to institute empirical treatment for *Pneumocystis* with TMP-SMX and for *Chlamydia*, *Mycoplasma*, and *Legionella* with a quinolone or an erythromycin derivative (e.g., azithromycin). Noninvasive procedures, such as staining of sputum smears for *Pneumocystis*, serum cryptococcal antigen tests, and urine testing for *Legionella* antigen, may be helpful. Serum galactomannan and β-d-glucan tests may be helpful in diagnosing *Aspergillus* infection, but their utility is limited by their lack of sensitivity. In transplant recipients who are seropositive for CMV, a determination of CMV load in the serum should be considered. Viral load studies (which allow physicians to quantitate viruses) have superseded simple measurement of serum IgG, which merely documents prior exposure to virus. Infections with viruses that cause only upper respiratory symptoms in immunocompetent hosts, such as respiratory syncytial virus (RSV), influenza viruses, and parainfluenza viruses, may be associated with fatal pneumonitis in immunocompromised hosts. Polymerase chain reaction testing now allows rapid diagnosis of viral pneumonia, which can lead to treatment in some cases (e.g., influenza).

Bleomycin is the most common cause of chemotherapy-induced lung disease. Other causes include alkylating agents (such as cyclophosphamide, chlorambucil, and melphalan), nitrosoureas (carmustine [BCNU], lomustine [CCNU], and methyl-CCNU), busulfan, procarbazine, methotrexate, and hydroxyurea. Both infectious and noninfectious (drug- or radiation-induced) pneumonitis can cause fever and abnormalities on chest radiographs; thus, the differential diagnosis of an infiltrate in a patient receiving chemotherapy encompasses a broad range of conditions (Table 29-7). The treatment of radiation pneumonitis (which may respond dramatically to glucocorticoids) or drug-induced pneumonitis is different from that of infectious pneumonia, and a biopsy may be important in the diagnosis. Unfortunately, no definitive diagnosis can be made in ~30% of cases, even after bronchoscopy.

Open-lung biopsy is the gold standard of diagnostic techniques. Biopsy via a visualized thoracostomy can replace an open procedure in many cases. When a biopsy cannot be performed, empirical treatment can be undertaken; a quinolone or an erythromycin derivative (azithromycin) and TMP-SMX are used in the case of diffuse infiltrates, and an antifungal agent is administered in the case of nodular infiltrates. The risks should be weighed carefully in these cases. If inappropriate drugs are administered, empirical treatment may prove toxic or ineffective; either of these outcomes may be riskier than biopsy.

CARDIOVASCULAR INFECTIONS

Patients with Hodgkin's disease are prone to persistent infections by *Salmonella*, sometimes (and particularly often in elderly patients) affecting a vascular site. The use of IV catheters deliberately lodged in the right atrium is associated with a high incidence of bacterial endocarditis, presumably related to valve damage followed by bacteremia. Nonbacterial thrombotic endocarditis has been described in association with a variety of malignancies (most often solid tumors) and may follow bone marrow transplantation as well. The presentation of an embolic event with a new cardiac murmur suggests this diagnosis. Blood cultures are negative in this disease of unknown pathogenesis.

ENDOCRINE SYNDROMES

Infections of the endocrine system have been described in immunocompromised patients. *Candida* infection of the thyroid may be difficult to diagnose during the neutropenic period. It can be defined by indium-labeled WBC scans or gallium scans after neutrophil counts increase. CMV infection can cause adrenalitis with or without resulting adrenal insufficiency. The presentation of a sudden endocrine anomaly in an immunocompromised patient may be a sign of infection in the involved end organ.

MUSCULOSKELETAL INFECTIONS

Infection that is a consequence of vascular compromise, resulting in gangrene, can occur when a tumor restricts the blood supply to muscles, bones, or joints. The process of diagnosis and treatment of such infection is similar to that in normal hosts, with the following caveats:

1. *In terms of diagnosis*, a lack of physical findings resulting from a lack of granulocytes in a granulocytopenic patient should make the clinician more aggressive in obtaining tissue rather than relying on physical signs.
2. *In terms of therapy*, aggressive debridement of infected tissues may be required, but it is usually difficult to operate on patients who have recently received chemotherapy, both because of a lack of platelets (which results in bleeding complications) and because of a lack of WBCs (which may lead to secondary infection). A blood culture positive for *Clostridium perfringens*—an organism commonly associated with gas gangrene—can have a number of meanings. Bloodstream infections with intestinal organisms such as *Streptococcus bovis* and *C. perfringens* may arise spontaneously from lower gastrointestinal lesions (tumor or polyps); alternatively, these lesions may be harbingers of invasive disease. The clinical setting must be considered in order to define the appropriate treatment for each case.

RENAL AND URETERAL INFECTIONS

Infections of the urinary tract are common among patients whose ureteral excretion is compromised (Table 29-1). *Candida*, which has a predilection for the kidney, can invade either from the bloodstream or in a retrograde manner (via the ureters or bladder) in immunocompromised patients. The presence of "fungus balls" or persistent candiduria suggests invasive disease. Persistent funguria (with *Aspergillus* as well as *Candida*) should prompt a search for a nidus of infection in the kidney.

Certain viruses are typically seen only in immunosuppressed patients. BK virus (polyomavirus hominis 1) has been documented in the urine of bone marrow transplant recipients and, like adenovirus, may be associated with hemorrhagic cystitis. BK-induced cystitis usually remits with decreasing immunosuppression. Anecdotal reports have described the treatment of infections due to adenovirus and BK virus with cidofovir.

ABNORMALITIES THAT PREDISPOSE TO INFECTION

See Table 29-1.

THE LYMPHOID SYSTEM

It is beyond the scope of this chapter to detail how all the immunologic abnormalities that result from cancer or from chemotherapy for cancer lead to infections. Disorders of the immune system are discussed in other sections of this book. As has been noted, patients with antibody deficiency are predisposed to overwhelming infection with encapsulated bacteria (including *S. pneumoniae*, *H. influenzae*, and *N. meningitidis*). It is worth mentioning, however, that patients undergoing intensive chemotherapy for any form of cancer will have not only defects due to granulocytopenia but also lymphocyte dysfunction, which may be profound. Thus, these patients—especially those receiving glucocorticoid-containing regimens or drugs that inhibit either T cell activation (calcineurin inhibitors or drugs like fludarabine, which affect lymphocyte function) or cytokine induction—should be given prophylaxis for *Pneumocystis* pneumonia.

THE HEMATOPOIETIC SYSTEM

Initial studies in the 1960s revealed a dramatic increase in the incidence of infections (fatal and nonfatal) among cancer patients with granulocyte counts of <500/μL. The use of prophylactic antibacterial agents has reduced the number of bacterial infections, but 35–78% of febrile neutropenic patients being treated for hematologic malignancies develop infections at some time during chemotherapy. Aerobic pathogens (both gram-positive and gram-negative) predominate in all series, but the exact organisms isolated vary from center to center. Infections with anaerobic organisms are uncommon. Geographic patterns affect the types of fungi isolated. Tuberculosis and malaria are common causes of fever in the developing world and may present in this setting as well.

Neutropenic patients are unusually susceptible to infection with a wide variety of bacteria; thus, antibiotic therapy should be initiated promptly to cover likely pathogens if infection is suspected. Indeed, early initiation of antibacterial agents is mandatory to prevent deaths. Like most immunocompromised patients,

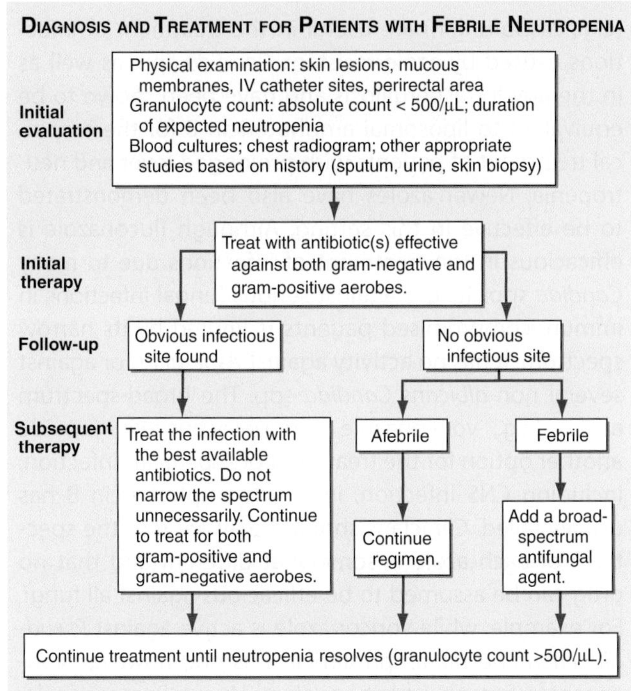

FIGURE 29-2

Algorithm for the diagnosis and treatment of febrile neutropenic patients.

neutropenic patients are threatened by their own microbial flora, including gram-positive and gram-negative organisms found commonly on the skin and in the bowel (Table 29-4). Because treatment with narrow-spectrum agents leads to infection with organisms not covered by the antibiotics used, the initial regimen should target all pathogens likely to be initial causes of bacterial infection in neutropenic hosts. As noted in the algorithm shown in Fig. 29-2, administration of antimicrobial agents is routinely continued until neutropenia resolves—i.e., the granulocyte count is sustained above 500/μL for at least 2 days. In some cases, patients remain febrile after resolution of neutropenia. In these instances, the risk of sudden death from overwhelming bacteremia is greatly reduced, and the following diagnoses should be seriously considered: (1) fungal infection, (2) bacterial abscesses or undrained foci of infection, and (3) drug fever (including reactions to antimicrobial agents as well as to chemotherapy or cytokines). In the proper setting, viral infection or graft-versus-host disease should be considered. In clinical practice, antibacterial therapy is usually discontinued when the patient is no longer neutropenic and all evidence of bacterial disease has been eliminated. Antifungal agents are then discontinued if there is no evidence of fungal disease. If the patient remains febrile, a search for viral diseases or unusual pathogens is conducted while unnecessary cytokines and other drugs are systematically eliminated from the regimen.

TREATMENT Infections in Cancer Patients

ANTIBACTERIAL THERAPY Hundreds of antibacterial regimens have been tested for use in patients with cancer. The major risk of infection is related to the degree of neutropenia seen as a consequence of either the disease or the therapy. Many of the relevant studies have involved small populations in which the outcomes have generally been good, and most have lacked the statistical power to detect differences among the regimens studied. Each febrile neutropenic patient should be approached as a unique problem, with particular attention given to previous infections and recent antibiotic exposures. Several general guidelines are useful in the initial treatment of neutropenic patients with fever (Fig. 29-2):

1. In the initial regimen, it is necessary to use antibiotics active against both gram-negative and gram-positive bacteria (Table 29-4).
2. Monotherapy with an aminoglycoside or an antibiotic without good activity against gram-positive organisms (e.g., ciprofloxacin or aztreonam) is not adequate in this setting.
3. The agents used should reflect both the epidemiology and the antibiotic resistance pattern of the hospital.
4. If the pattern of resistance justifies its use, a single third-generation cephalosporin constitutes an appropriate initial regimen in many hospitals.
5. Most standard regimens are designed for patients who have not previously received prophylactic antibiotics. The development of fever in a patient who has received antibiotics affects the choice of subsequent therapy, which should target resistant organisms and organisms known to cause infections in patients being treated with the antibiotics already administered.
6. Randomized trials have indicated the safety of oral antibiotic regimens in the treatment of "low-risk" patients with fever and neutropenia. Outpatients who are expected to remain neutropenic for <10 days and who have no concurrent medical problems (such as hypotension, pulmonary compromise, or abdominal pain) can be classified as low risk and treated with a broad-spectrum oral regimen.
7. Several large-scale studies indicate that prophylaxis with a fluoroquinolone (ciprofloxacin or levofloxacin) decreases morbidity and mortality rates among afebrile patients who are anticipated to have neutropenia of long duration.

The initial antibacterial regimen should be refined on the basis of culture results (Fig. 29-2). Blood cultures are the most relevant on which to base therapy; surface cultures of skin and mucous membranes may be misleading. In the case of gram-positive bacteremia or another gram-positive infection, it is important that the antibiotic be optimal for the organism isolated. Although it is not desirable to leave the patient unprotected, the addition of more and more antibacterial agents to the regimen is not appropriate unless there is a clinical or microbiologic reason to do so. Planned progressive therapy (the serial, empirical addition of one drug after another without culture data) is not efficacious in most settings and may have unfortunate consequences. Simply adding another antibiotic for fear that a gram-negative infection is present is a dubious practice. The synergy exhibited by β-lactams and aminoglycosides against certain gram-negative organisms (especially *P. aeruginosa*) provides the rationale for using two antibiotics in this setting, but recent analyses suggest that efficacy is not enhanced by the addition of aminoglycosides, while toxicity may be increased. Mere "double coverage," with the addition of a quinolone or another antibiotic that is not likely to exhibit synergy, has not been shown to be of benefit and may cause additional toxicities and side effects. Cephalosporins can cause bone marrow suppression, and vancomycin is associated with neutropenia in some healthy individuals. Furthermore, the addition of multiple cephalosporins may induce β-lactamase production by some organisms; cephalosporins and double β-lactam combinations should probably be avoided altogether in *Enterobacter* infections.

ANTIFUNGAL THERAPY Fungal infections in cancer patients are most often associated with neutropenia. Neutropenic patients are predisposed to the development of invasive fungal infections, most commonly those due to *Candida* and *Aspergillus* spp. and occasionally those caused by *Fusarium*, *Trichosporon*, and *Bipolaris* spp. Cryptococcal infection, which is common among patients taking immunosuppressive agents, is uncommon among neutropenic patients receiving chemotherapy for AML. Invasive candidal disease is usually caused by *C. albicans* or *C. tropicalis* but can be caused by *C. krusei*, *C. parapsilosis*, and *C. glabrata*.

For decades, it has been common clinical practice to add amphotericin B to antibacterial regimens if a neutropenic patient remains febrile despite 4–7 days of treatment with antibacterial agents. The rationale for this empirical addition is that it is difficult to culture fungi before they cause disseminated disease and that mortality rates from disseminated fungal infections in granulocytopenic patients are high. Before the introduction of newer azoles into clinical practice, amphotericin B was the mainstay of antifungal therapy. The insolubility of amphotericin B has resulted in the marketing of several lipid formulations that are less toxic than the amphotericin B deoxycholate complex. Echinocandins (e.g., caspofungin) are useful in the treatment of infections caused by azole-resistant *Candida* spp. as well as in therapy for aspergillosis and have been shown to be equivalent to liposomal amphotericin B for the empirical treatment of patients with prolonged fever and neutropenia. Newer azoles have also been demonstrated to be effective in this setting. Although fluconazole is efficacious in the treatment of infections due to many *Candida* spp., its use against serious fungal infections in immunocompromised patients is limited by its narrow spectrum: it has no activity against *Aspergillus* or against several non-*albicans Candida* spp. The broad-spectrum azoles (e.g., voriconazole and posaconazole) provide another option for the treatment of *Aspergillus* infection, including CNS infection, in which amphotericin B has usually failed. Clinicians should be aware that the spectrum of each azole is somewhat different and that no drug can be assumed to be efficacious against all fungi. For example, while voriconazole is active against *Pseudallescheria boydii*, amphotericin B is not; however, voriconazole has no activity against *Mucor*. Posaconazole, which is administered orally, is useful as a prophylactic agent in patients with prolonged neutropenia. Studies in progress are assessing the use of these agents in combinations.

ANTIVIRAL THERAPY The availability of a variety of agents active against herpes-group viruses, including some new agents with a broader spectrum of activity, has heightened focus on the treatment of viral infections, which pose a major problem in cancer patients. Viral diseases caused by the herpes group are prominent. Serious (and sometimes fatal) infections due to HSV and CMV are well documented, and VZV infections may be fatal to patients receiving chemotherapy. The roles of human herpesvirus (HHV)-6, HHV-7, and HHV-8 (Kaposi's sarcoma–associated herpesvirus) in cancer patients are still being defined. While clinical experience is most extensive with acyclovir, which can be used therapeutically or prophylactically, a number of derivative drugs offer advantages over this agent (Table 29-8).

In addition to the herpes group, several respiratory viruses (especially RSV) may cause serious disease in cancer patients. While influenza vaccination is recommended (see later discussion), it may be ineffective in this patient population. The availability of antiviral drugs with activity against influenza viruses gives the clinician additional options for the treatment of these patients (Table 29-9).

OTHER THERAPEUTIC MODALITIES Another way to address the problems of the febrile neutropenic patient is to replenish the neutrophil population. Although granulocyte transfusions are effective in the treatment of refractory gram-negative bacteremia, they

TABLE 29-8

ANTIVIRAL AGENTS ACTIVE AGAINST HERPESVIRUSES

AGENT	DESCRIPTION	SPECTRUM	TOXICITY	OTHER ISSUES
Acyclovir	Inhibits HSV polymerase	HSV, VZV (± CMV, EBV)	Rarely has side effects; crystalluria can occur at high doses	Long history of safety; original antiviral agent
Famciclovir	Prodrug of penciclovir (a guanosine analogue)	HSV, VZV (± CMV)	Associated with cancerin rats	Longer effective half-life than acyclovir
Valacyclovir	Prodrug of acyclovir; better absorption	HSV, VZV (± CMV)	Associated with thrombotic microangiopathy in one study of immunocompromised patients	Better oral absorption and longer effective half-life than acyclovir; can be given as a single daily dose for prophylaxis
Ganciclovir	More potent polymerase inhibitor; more toxic than acyclovir	HSV, VZV, CMV, HHV-6	Bone marrow suppression	Neutropenia may respond to G-CSF or GM-CSF
Valganciclovir	Prodrug of ganciclovir; better absorption	HSV, VZV, CMV, HHV-6	Bone marrow suppression	—
Cidofovir	Nucleotide analogue of cytosine	HSV, VZV, CMV; good in vitro activity against adenovirus and others	Nephrotoxic marrow suppression	Given IV once a week
Foscarnet	Phosphonoformic acid; inhibits viral DNA polymerase	HSV, VZV, CMV, HHV-6	Nephrotoxic; electrolyte abnormalities common	IV only

Abbreviations: ±, agent has some activity but not enough for the treatment of infections; CMV, cytomegalovirus; EBV, Epstein-Barr virus; G-CSF, granulocyte colony-stimulating factor; GM-CSF, granulocyte-macrophage colony-stimulating factor; HHV, human herpesvirus; HSV, herpes simplex virus; IV, intravenous; VZV, varicella-zoster virus.

TABLE 29-9

OTHER ANTIVIRAL AGENTS USEFUL IN THE TREATMENT OF INFECTIONS IN CANCER PATIENTS

AGENT	DESCRIPTION	SPECTRUM	TOXICITY	OTHER ISSUES
Amantadine, rimantadine	Interfere with uncoating	Influenza A only	5–10% fewer CNS effects with rimantadine	May be given prophylactically
Zanamivir	Neuraminidase inhibitor	Influenza A and B	Usually well tolerated	Inhalation only
Oseltamivir	Neuraminidase inhibitor	Influenza A and B	Usually well tolerated	PO dosing
Pleconaril	Blocks enterovirus binding and uncoating	90% of enteroviruses, 80% of rhinoviruses	Generally well tolerated	Decreases duration of meningitis; available for compassionate use only
Interferons	Cytokines with broad spectrum of activity	Used locally for warts, systemically for hepatitis	Fever, myalgias, bone marrow suppression	Not shown to be helpful in CMV infection; use limited by toxicity
Ribavirin	Purine analogue (precise mechanism of action unknown)	Broad theoretical spectrum; documented use against RSV, Lassa fever virus, and hepatitis viruses (with interferon)	IV form causes anemia	Given by aerosol for RSV infection (efficacy in doubt); approved for use in children with heart/lung disease; given with interferon for hepatitis C

Abbreviations: CMV, cytomegalovirus; CNS, central nervous system; IV, intravenous; RSV, respiratory syncytial virus.

do not have a documented role in prophylaxis. Because of the expense, the risk of leukoagglutinin reactions (which has probably been decreased by improved cell-separation procedures), and the risk of transmission of CMV from unscreened donors (which has been reduced by the use of filters), granulocyte transfusion is reserved for patients unresponsive to antibiotics. This modality is efficacious for documented gram-negative bacteremia refractory to antibiotics, particularly when granulocyte numbers will be depressed for only a short period. The demonstrated usefulness of granulocyte colony-stimulating factor (G-CSF) in mobilizing neutrophils and advances in preservation techniques may make this option more useful than in the past.

A variety of cytokines, including G-CSF and granulocyte-macrophage colony-stimulating factor (GM-CSF), enhance granulocyte recovery after chemotherapy and consequently shorten the period of maximal vulnerability to fatal infections. Interferon γ has been demonstrated to be effective in some infections caused by intracellular organisms, presumably because of its ability to activate macrophages. The role of these cytokines in routine practice is still a matter of some debate. Most authorities recommend their use only when neutropenia is both severe and prolonged. The cytokines themselves may have adverse effects, including fever, hypoxemia, and pleural effusions or serositis in other areas.

Once neutropenia has resolved, the risk of infection decreases dramatically. However, depending on what drugs they receive, patients who continue on chemotherapeutic protocols remain at high risk for certain diseases. Any patient receiving more than a maintenance dose of glucocorticoids (including many treatment regimens for diffuse lymphoma) should also receive prophylactic TMP-SMX because of the risk of *Pneumocystis* infection; those with ALL should receive such prophylaxis for the duration of chemotherapy.

PREVENTION OF INFECTION IN CANCER PATIENTS

EFFECT OF THE ENVIRONMENT

Outbreaks of fatal *Aspergillus* infection have been associated with construction projects and materials in several hospitals. The association between spore counts and risk of infection suggests the need for a high-efficiency air-handling system in hospitals that care for large numbers of neutropenic patients. The use of laminar-flow rooms and prophylactic antibiotics has decreased the number of infectious episodes in severely neutropenic patients. However, because of the expense of such a program and the failure to show that it dramatically affects mortality rates, most centers do not routinely use laminar flow to care for neutropenic patients. Some centers use "reverse isolation," in which health care providers and visitors to a patient who is neutropenic wear gowns and gloves. Since most of the infections these patients develop are due to organisms that colonize the patients' own skin and bowel, the validity of such schemes is dubious, and limited clinical data do not support their use. Hand washing by all staff caring for neutropenic patients should be required to prevent the spread of resistant organisms.

The presence of large numbers of bacteria (particularly *P. aeruginosa*) in certain foods, especially fresh vegetables, has led some authorities to recommend a special "low-bacteria" diet. A diet consisting of cooked and canned food is satisfactory to most neutropenic patients and does not involve elaborate disinfection or sterilization protocols. However, there are no studies to support even this type of dietary restriction. Counseling of patients to avoid leftovers, deli foods, and unpasteurized dairy products is recommended.

PHYSICAL MEASURES

Although few studies address this issue, patients with cancer are predisposed to infections resulting from anatomic compromise (e.g., lymphedema resulting from node dissections after radical mastectomy). Surgeons who specialize in cancer surgery can provide specific guidelines for the care of such patients, and patients benefit from commonsense advice about how to prevent infections in vulnerable areas.

IMMUNOGLOBULIN REPLACEMENT

Many patients with multiple myeloma or CLL have immunoglobulin deficiencies as a result of their disease, and all allogeneic bone marrow transplant recipients are hypogammaglobulinemic for a period after transplantation. However, current recommendations reserve intravenous immunoglobulin replacement therapy for patients with severe (<400 mg/dL), prolonged hypogammaglobulinemia. Antibiotic prophylaxis has been shown to be cheaper and is efficacious in preventing infections in most CLL patients with hypogammaglobulinemia. Routine use of immunoglobulin replacement is not recommended.

SEXUAL PRACTICES

The use of condoms is recommended for severely immunocompromised patients. Any sexual practice that results in oral exposure to feces is not recommended. Neutropenic patients should be advised to avoid any practice that results in trauma, as even microscopic cuts may result in bacterial invasion and fatal sepsis.

ANTIBIOTIC PROPHYLAXIS

Several studies indicate that the use of oral fluoroquinolones prevents infection and decreases mortality rates among severely neutropenic patients. Fluconazole prevents *Candida* infections when given prophylactically to patients receiving bone marrow transplants. The use of broader-spectrum antifungal agents (e.g., posaconazole) appears to be more efficacious. Prophylaxis for *Pneumocystis* is mandatory for patients with ALL and for all cancer patients receiving glucocorticoid-containing chemotherapy regimens.

VACCINATION OF CANCER PATIENTS

In general, patients undergoing chemotherapy respond less well to vaccines than do normal hosts. Their greater need for vaccines thus leads to a dilemma in their management. Purified proteins and inactivated vaccines are almost never contraindicated and should be given to patients even during chemotherapy. For example, all adults should receive diphtheria–tetanus toxoid boosters at the indicated times as well as seasonal influenza vaccine. However, if possible, vaccination should not be undertaken concurrent with cytotoxic chemotherapy. If patients are expected to be receiving chemotherapy for several months and vaccination is indicated (e.g., influenza vaccination in the fall), the vaccine should be given midcycle—as far apart in time as possible from the antimetabolic agents that will prevent an immune response. The meningococcal and pneumococcal polysaccharide vaccines should be given to patients before splenectomy, if possible. The *H. influenzae* type b conjugate vaccine should be administered to all splenectomized patients.

In general, live virus (or live bacterial) vaccines should not be given to patients during intensive chemotherapy because of the risk of disseminated infection. Recommendations on vaccination are summarized in Table 29-2.

CHAPTER 30
HEMATOPOIETIC CELL TRANSPLANTATION

Frederick R. Appelbaum

Bone marrow transplantation was the original term used to describe the collection and transplantation of hematopoietic stem cells, but with the demonstration that the peripheral blood and umbilical cord blood are also useful sources of stem cells, *hematopoietic cell transplantation* has become the preferred generic term for this process. The procedure is usually carried out for one of two purposes: (1) to replace an abnormal but nonmalignant lymphohematopoietic system with one from a normal donor or (2) to treat malignancy by allowing the administration of higher doses of myelosuppressive therapy than would otherwise be possible. The use of hematopoietic cell transplantation has been increasing, both because of its efficacy in selected diseases and because of increasing availability of donors. The Center for International Blood and Marrow Transplant Research (*www.cibmtr.org*) estimates that about 65,000 transplants are performed each year.

THE HEMATOPOIETIC STEM CELL

Several features of the hematopoietic stem cell make transplantation clinically feasible, including its remarkable regenerative capacity, its ability to home to the marrow space following intravenous injection, and the ability of the stem cell to be cryopreserved (Chap. 1). Transplantation of a single stem cell can replace the entire lymphohematopoietic system of an adult mouse. In humans, transplantation of a few percent of a donor's bone marrow volume regularly results in complete and sustained replacement of the recipient's entire lymphohematopoietic system, including all red cells, granulocytes, B and T lymphocytes, and platelets, as well as cells comprising the fixed macrophage population, including Kupffer cells of the liver, pulmonary alveolar macrophages, osteoclasts, Langerhans cells of the skin, and brain microglial cells. The ability of the hematopoietic stem cell to home to the marrow following intravenous injection is mediated, in part, by an interaction between stromal cell–derived factor 1 (SDF1) produced by marrow stromal cells and the alpha-chemokine receptor CXCR4 found on stem cells. Homing is also influenced by the interaction of cell-surface molecules, termed *selectins*, on bone marrow endothelial cells with ligands, termed *integrins*, on early hematopoietic cells. Human hematopoietic stem cells can survive freezing and thawing with little, if any, damage, making it possible to remove and store a portion of the patient's own bone marrow for later reinfusion following treatment of the patient with high-dose myelotoxic therapy.

CATEGORIES OF HEMATOPOIETIC CELL TRANSPLANTATION

Hematopoietic cell transplantation can be described according to the relationship between the patient and the donor and by the anatomic source of stem cells. In ~1% of cases, patients have identical twins who can serve as donors. With the use of syngeneic donors, there is no risk of graft-versus-host disease (GVHD), which often complicates allogeneic transplantation, and unlike the use of autologous marrow, there is no risk that the stem cells are contaminated with tumor cells.

Allogeneic transplantation involves a donor and a recipient who are not genetically identical. Following allogeneic transplantation, immune cells transplanted with the stem cells or developing from them can react against the patient, causing GVHD. Alternatively, if the immunosuppressive preparative regimen used to treat the patient before transplant is inadequate, immunocompetent cells of the patient can cause graft rejection. The risks of these complications are greatly influenced by the degree of matching between donor and recipient for antigens encoded by genes of the major histocompatibility complex.

The human leukocyte antigen (HLA) molecules are responsible for binding antigenic proteins and presenting them to T cells. The antigens presented by HLA molecules may derive from exogenous sources (e.g., during active infections) or may be endogenous proteins. If individuals are not HLA-matched, T cells from one individual will react strongly to the mismatched HLA, or "major antigens," of the second. Even if the individuals are HLA-matched, the T cells of the donor may react to differing endogenous or "minor antigens" presented by the HLA of the recipient. Reactions to minor antigens tend to be less vigorous. The genes of major relevance to transplantation include HLA-A, -B, -C, and -D; they are closely linked and therefore tend to be inherited as haplotypes, with only rare crossovers between them. Thus, the odds that any one full sibling will match a patient are one in four, and the probability that the patient has an HLA-identical sibling is $1 - (0.75)^n$, where n equals the number of siblings.

With current techniques, the risk of graft rejection is 1–3%, and the risk of severe, life-threatening acute GVHD is ~15% following transplantation between HLA-identical siblings. The incidence of graft rejection and GVHD increases progressively with the use of family member donors mismatched for one, two, or three antigens. While survival following a one-antigen mismatched transplant is not markedly altered, survival following two- or three-antigen mismatched transplants is significantly reduced, and such transplants should be performed only as part of clinical trials.

Since the formation of the National Marrow Donor Program and other registries, it has become possible to identify HLA-matched unrelated donors for many patients. The genes encoding HLA antigens are highly polymorphic, and thus the odds of any two unrelated individuals being HLA-identical are extremely low, somewhat less than 1 in 10,000. However, by identifying and typing >14 million volunteer donors, HLA-matched donors can now be found for ~50% of patients for whom a search is initiated. It takes, on average, 3–4 months to complete a search and schedule and initiate an unrelated donor transplant. With improvements in HLA- typing and supportive care measures, survival following matched unrelated donor transplantation is essentially the same as that seen with HLA-matched siblings.

Autologous transplantation involves the removal and storage of the patient's own stem cells with subsequent reinfusion after the patient receives high-dose myeloablative therapy. Unlike allogeneic transplantation, there is no risk of GVHD or graft rejection with autologous transplantation. On the other hand, autologous transplantation lacks a graft-versus-tumor (GVT) effect, and the autologous stem cell product can be contaminated with tumor cells, which could lead to relapse. A variety of techniques have been developed to "purge" autologous products of tumor cells. Some use antibodies directed at tumor-associated antigens plus complement, antibodies linked to toxins, or antibodies conjugated to immunomagnetic beads. In vitro incubation with certain chemotherapeutic agents such as 4-hydroperoxycyclophosphamide and long-term culture of bone marrow have also been shown to diminish tumor cell numbers in stem cell products. Another technique is positive selection of stem cells using antibodies to CD34, with subsequent column adherence or flow techniques to select normal stem cells while leaving tumor cells behind. All these approaches can reduce the number of tumor cells from 1000- to 10,000-fold and are clinically feasible; however, no prospective randomized trials have yet shown that any of these approaches results in a decrease in relapse rates or improvements in disease-free or overall survival.

Bone marrow aspirated from the posterior and anterior iliac crests has traditionally been the source of hematopoietic stem cells for transplantation. Typically, anywhere from 1.5 to 5×10^8 nucleated marrow cells per kilogram are collected for allogeneic transplantation. Several studies have found improved survival in the settings of both matched sibling and unrelated transplantation by transplanting higher numbers of bone marrow cells.

Hematopoietic stem cells circulate in the peripheral blood but in very low concentrations. Following the administration of certain hematopoietic growth factors, including granulocyte colony-stimulating factor (G-CSF) or granulocyte-macrophage colony-stimulating factor (GM-CSF), and during recovery from intensive chemotherapy, the concentration of hematopoietic progenitor cells in blood, as measured either by colony-forming units or expression of the CD34 antigen, increases markedly. This has made it possible to harvest adequate numbers of stem cells from the peripheral blood for transplantation. Donors are typically treated with 4 or 5 days of hematopoietic growth factor, following which stem cells are collected in one or two 4-h pheresis sessions. In the autologous setting, transplantation of $>2.5 \times 10^6$ CD34 cells per kilogram, a number that can be collected in most circumstances, leads to rapid and sustained engraftment in virtually all cases. In the 10–20% of patients who fail to mobilize sufficient CD34+ cells with growth factor alone, the addition of plerixafor, an antagonist of CXCR4, may be useful. Compared with the use of autologous marrow, use of peripheral blood stem cells results in more rapid hematopoietic recovery, with granulocytes recovering to 500/μL by day 12 and platelets recovering to 20,000/μL by day 14. While this more rapid recovery diminishes the morbidity rate of transplantation, no studies show improved survival.

Hesitation in studying the use of peripheral blood stem cells for allogeneic transplantation was because peripheral blood stem cell products contain as much as 1 log more T cells than are contained in the typical marrow harvest; in animal models, the incidence of GVHD is related to the number of T cells transplanted. Nonetheless, clinical trials have shown that the use of growth factor–mobilized peripheral blood stem cells from HLA-matched family members leads to faster engraftment without an increase in acute GVHD. Chronic GVHD may be increased with peripheral blood stem cells, but in trials conducted so far, this has been more than balanced by reductions in relapse rates and nonrelapse mortality rates, with the use of peripheral blood stem cells resulting in improved overall survival. Randomized trials are now evaluating the use of peripheral blood versus bone marrow for matched unrelated donor transplantation.

Umbilical cord blood contains a high concentration of hematopoietic progenitor cells, allowing for its use as a source of stem cells for transplantation. Cord blood transplantation from family members has been explored when the immediate need for transplantation precludes waiting the 9 or so months generally required for the baby to mature to the point of donating marrow. Use of cord blood results in slower engraftment and peripheral count recovery than seen with marrow but a low incidence of GVHD, perhaps reflecting the low number of T cells in cord blood. Several banks have been developed to harvest and store cord blood for possible transplantation to unrelated patients from material that would otherwise be discarded. A summary of the first 562 unrelated cord blood transplants, facilitated by the New York Blood Center, reported engraftment in ~85% of patients but at a slower pace than seen with marrow. Severe GVHD was seen in 23% of patients. The risk of graft failure and transplant-related mortality were related to the dose of cord blood cells per kilogram, thus limiting the application of single cord blood transplantation for the treatment of larger adolescent and adult patients. Subsequent trials suggest that the use of double cord transplants diminishes the risk of graft failure and early mortality even though only one of the donors ultimately engrafts.

THE TRANSPLANT PREPARATIVE REGIMEN

The treatment regimen administered to patients immediately preceding transplantation is designed to eradicate the patient's underlying disease and, in the setting of allogeneic transplantation, immunosuppress the patient adequately to prevent rejection of the transplanted marrow. The appropriate regimen therefore depends on the disease setting and source of marrow. For example, when transplantation is performed to treat severe combined immunodeficiency and the donor is a histocompatible sibling, no treatment is needed because no host cells require eradication and the patient is already too immunoincompetent to reject the transplanted marrow. For aplastic anemia, there is no large population of cells to eradicate, and high-dose cyclophosphamide plus antithymocyte globulin are sufficient to immunosuppress the patient adequately to accept the marrow graft. In the setting of thalassemia and sickle cell anemia, high-dose busulfan is frequently added to cyclophosphamide in order to eradicate hyperplastic host hematopoiesis. A variety of different regimens have been developed to treat malignant diseases. Most of these regimens include agents that have high activity against the tumor in question at conventional doses and have myelosuppression as their predominant dose-limiting toxicity. Therefore, these regimens commonly include busulfan, cyclophosphamide, melphalan, thiotepa, carmustine, etoposide, and total-body irradiation in various combinations.

Although high-dose treatment regimens have typically been used in transplantation, the understanding that much of the antitumor effect of transplantation derives from an immunologically mediated GVT response has led investigators to ask if reduced-intensity conditioning regimens might be effective and more tolerable. Evidence for a GVT effect comes from studies showing that posttransplant relapse rates are lowest in patients who develop acute and chronic GVHD, higher in those without GVHD, and higher still in recipients of T cell–depleted allogeneic or syngeneic marrow. The demonstration that complete remissions can be obtained in many patients who have relapsed posttransplant by simply administering viable lymphocytes from the original donor further strengthens the argument for a potent GVT effect. Accordingly, a variety of less-intensive nonmyeloablative regimens have been studied, ranging in intensity from the very minimum required to achieve engraftment (e.g., fludarabine plus 200 cGy total-body irradiation) to regimens of more immediate intensity (e.g., fludarabine plus melphalan). Studies to date document that engraftment can be readily achieved with less toxicity than seen with conventional transplantation. Furthermore, the severity of acute GVHD appears to be decreased because less tissue damage is done by the lower doses of drugs in the preparative regimen. Complete sustained responses have been documented in many patients, particularly those with more indolent hematologic malignancies. The role of reduced-intensity conditioning in any disease, however, has not been fully defined.

THE TRANSPLANT PROCEDURE

Marrow is usually collected from the donor's posterior and sometimes anterior iliac crests, with the donor under general or spinal anesthesia. Typically, 10–15 mL/kg of marrow is aspirated, placed in heparinized media, and filtered through 0.3- and 0.2-mm screens to remove fat and bony spicules. The collected marrow may undergo further processing depending on the clinical situation, such as the removal of red cells to prevent hemolysis in ABO-incompatible transplants, the removal of donor T cells to prevent GVHD, or attempts to remove possible contaminating tumor cells in autologous transplantation. Marrow donation is safe, with only very rare complications reported.

Peripheral blood stem cells are collected by leukapheresis after the donor has been treated with hematopoietic growth factors or, in the setting of autologous transplantation, sometimes after treatment with a combination of chemotherapy and growth factors. Stem cells for transplantation are generally infused through a large-bore central venous catheter. Such infusions are usually well tolerated, although occasionally patients develop fever, cough, or shortness of breath. These symptoms usually resolve with slowing of the infusion. When the stem cell product has been cryopreserved using dimethyl sulfoxide, patients more often experience short-lived nausea or vomiting due to the odor and taste of the cryoprotectant.

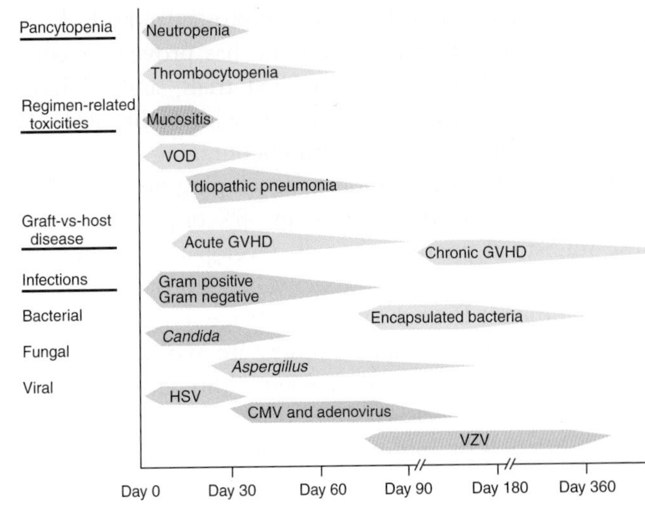

FIGURE 30-1

Major syndromes complicating marrow transplantation. The size of the shaded area roughly reflects the risk of the complication. CMV, cytomegalovirus; GVHD, graft-versus-host disease; HSV, herpes simplex virus; VOD, venoocclusive disease; VZV, varicella-zoster virus.

ENGRAFTMENT

Peripheral blood counts usually reach their nadir several days to a week posttransplant as a consequence of the preparative regimen; then cells produced by the transplanted stem cells begin to appear in the peripheral blood. The rate of recovery depends on the source of stem cells, the use of posttransplant growth factors, and the form of GVHD prophylaxis employed. If marrow is the source of stem cells, recovery to 100 granulocytes/μL occurs by day 16 and to 500/μL by day 22. Use of G-CSF–mobilized peripheral blood stem cells speeds the rate of recovery by ~1 week with marrow, whereas engraftment following cord blood transplantation is typically delayed by ~1 week compared with marrow. Use of a myeloid growth factor (G-CSF or GM-CSF) posttransplant can accelerate recovery by 3–5 days, while use of methotrexate to prevent GVHD delays engraftment by a similar period. Following allogeneic transplantation, engraftment can be documented using fluorescence in situ hybridization of sex chromosomes if donor and recipient are sex-mismatched, HLA-typing if HLA-mismatched, or restriction fragment length polymorphism analysis if sex- and HLA-matched.

COMPLICATIONS FOLLOWING HEMATOPOIETIC CELL TRANSPLANT

Early direct chemoradiotoxicities

The transplant preparative regimen may cause a spectrum of acute toxicities that vary according to intensity of the regimen and the specific agents used but frequently results in nausea, vomiting, and mild skin erythema (Fig. 30-1). Regimens that include high-dose cyclophosphamide can result in hemorrhagic cystitis, which can usually be prevented by bladder irrigation or with the sulfhydryl compound mercaptoethanesulfonate (MESNA); rarely, acute hemorrhagic carditis is seen. Most high-dose preparative regimens will result in oral mucositis, which typically develops 5–7 days posttransplant and often requires narcotic analgesia. Use of a patient-controlled analgesic pump provides the greatest patient satisfaction and results in a lower cumulative dose of narcotic. Keratinocyte growth factor (palifermin) can shorten the duration of mucositis by several days following autologous transplantation. Patients begin losing their hair 5–6 days posttransplant and by 1 week are usually profoundly pancytopenic.

Depending on the intensity of the conditioning regimen, 3–10% of patients will develop sinusoidal obstruction syndrome of the liver, a syndrome that results from direct cytotoxic injury to hepatic-venular and sinusoidal endothelium, with subsequent deposition of fibrin and the development of a local hypercoagulable state. This chain of events leads to the clinical symptoms of tender hepatomegaly, ascites, jaundice, and fluid retention. These symptoms can develop any time during the first month posttransplant, with the peak incidence at day 16. Predisposing factors include prior exposure to intensive chemotherapy, pretransplant hepatitis of any cause, and use of more intense conditioning regimens. The mortality rate of sinusoidal obstruction syndrome is ~30%, with progressive hepatic failure culminating in a terminal hepatorenal syndrome. Both thrombolytic and antithrombotic agents, such as tissue plasminogen activator, heparin, and prostaglandin E, have been studied as therapy, but none has proven of consistent major benefit in controlled trials, and all have significant toxicity. Early studies with defibrotide, a polydeoxyribonucleotide, seem encouraging.

Although most pneumonias developing posttransplant are caused by infectious agents, in ~5% of patients, a diffuse interstitial pneumonia will develop that is thought to be the result of direct toxicity of high-dose preparative regimens. Bronchoalveolar lavage typically shows alveolar hemorrhage, and biopsies are typically characterized by diffuse alveolar damage, although some cases may have a more clearly interstitial pattern. High-dose glucocorticoids or antitumor necrosis factor therapies are sometimes used as treatment, although randomized trials testing their utility have not been reported.

Late direct chemoradiotoxicities

Late complications of the preparative regimen include decreased growth velocity in children and delayed development of secondary sex characteristics. These complications can be partly ameliorated with the use of appropriate growth and sex hormone replacement. Most men become azoospermic, and most postpubertal women will develop ovarian failure, which should be treated. Thyroid dysfunction, usually well compensated, is sometimes seen. Cataracts develop in 10–20% of patients and are most common in patients treated with total-body irradiation and those who receive glucocorticoid therapy posttransplant for treatment of GVHD. Aseptic necrosis of the femoral head is seen in 10% of patients and is particularly frequent in those receiving chronic glucocorticoid therapy. Both acute and late chemoradiotoxicities (except those due to glucocorticoids) are considerably less frequent in recipients of reduced- compared with high-dose preparative regimens.

Graft-versus-host disease

GVHD is the result of allogeneic T cells that are transferred with the donor's stem cell inoculum reacting with antigenic targets on host cells. GVHD developing within the first 3 months posttransplant is termed *acute GVHD*, while GVHD developing or persisting beyond 3 months posttransplant is termed *chronic GVHD*. Acute GVHD most often first becomes apparent 2–4 weeks posttransplant and is characterized by an erythematous maculopapular rash; persistent anorexia or diarrhea or both; and liver disease with increased serum levels of bilirubin, alanine and aspartate aminotransferase, and alkaline phosphatase. Since many conditions can mimic acute GVHD, diagnosis usually requires skin, liver, or endoscopic biopsy for confirmation. In all these organs, endothelial damage and lymphocytic infiltrates are seen. In skin, the epidermis and hair follicles are damaged; in liver, the small bile ducts show segmental disruption; and in intestines, destruction of the crypts and mucosal ulceration may be noted. A commonly used rating system for acute GVHD is shown in Table 30-1. Grade I acute GVHD is of little clinical significance, does not affect the likelihood of survival, and does not require treatment. In contrast, grades II to IV GVHD are associated with significant symptoms and a poorer probability of survival, and they require aggressive therapy. The incidence of acute GVHD is higher in recipients of stem cells from mismatched or unrelated donors, in older patients, and in patients unable to receive full doses of drugs used to prevent the disease.

One general approach to the prevention of GVHD is the administration of immunosuppressive drugs early after transplant. Combinations of methotrexate and either cyclosporine or tacrolimus are among the most effective and widely used regimens. Prednisone, anti–T cell antibodies, mycophenolate mofetil, and other

TABLE 30-1

CLINICAL STAGING AND GRADING OF ACUTE GRAFT-VERSUS-HOST DISEASE

CLINICAL STAGE	SKIN	LIVER—BILIRUBIN, μmol/L (mg/dL)	GUT
1	Rash <25% body surface	34–51 (2–3)	Diarrhea 500–1000 mL/d
2	Rash 25–50% body surface	51–103 (3–6)	Diarrhea 1000–1500 mL/d
3	Generalized erythroderma	103–257 (6–15)	Diarrhea >1500 mL/d
4	Desquamation and bullae	>257 (>15)	Ileus
OVERALL CLINICAL GRADE	**SKIN STAGE**	**LIVER STAGE**	**GUT STAGE**
I	1–2	0	0
II	1–3	1	1
III	1–3	2–3	2–3
IV	2–4	2–4	2–4

immunosuppressive agents have also been or are being studied in various combinations. A second general approach to GVHD prevention is removal of T cells from the stem cell inoculum. While effective in preventing GVHD, T cell depletion is associated with an increased incidence of graft failure and of tumor recurrence post-transplant; as yet, little evidence suggests that T-cell depletion improves cure rates in any specific setting.

Despite prophylaxis, significant acute GVHD will develop in ~30% of recipients of stem cells from matched siblings and in as many as 60% of those receiving stem cells from unrelated donors. The disease is usually treated with glucocorticoids, additional immunosuppressants, or monoclonal antibodies targeted against T cells or T cell subsets.

Between 20 and 50% of patients surviving >6 months after allogeneic transplantation will develop chronic GVHD. The disease is more common in older patients, in recipients of mismatched or unrelated stem cells, and in those with a preceding episode of acute GVHD. The disease resembles an autoimmune disorder with malar rash, sicca syndrome, arthritis, obliterative bronchiolitis, and bile duct degeneration, and cholestasis. Single-agent prednisone or cyclosporine is standard treatment at present, although trials of other agents are under way. In most patients, chronic GVHD resolves, but it may require 1–3 years of immunosuppressive treatment before these agents can be withdrawn without the disease recurring. Because patients with chronic GVHD are susceptible to significant infection, they should receive prophylactic trimethoprim-sulfamethoxazole (TMP-SMX), and all suspected infections should be investigated and treated aggressively.

Graft failure

While complete and sustained engraftment is usually seen posttransplant, occasionally marrow function either does not return or, after a brief period of engraftment, is lost. Graft failure after autologous transplantation can be the result of inadequate numbers of stem cells being transplanted, damage during ex vivo treatment or storage, or exposure of the patient to myelotoxic agents posttransplant. Infections with cytomegalovirus (CMV) or human herpesvirus type 6 have also been associated with loss of marrow function. Graft failure after allogeneic transplantation can also be due to immunologic rejection of the graft by immunocompetent host cells. Immunologically based graft rejection is more common following use of less-immunosuppressive preparative regimens, in recipients of T cell–depleted stem cell products, and in patients receiving grafts from HLA-mismatched donors or cord blood.

Treatment of graft failure usually involves removing all potentially myelotoxic agents from the patient's regimen and attempting a short trial of a myeloid growth factor. Persistence of lymphocytes of host origin in allogeneic transplant recipients with graft failure indicates immunologic rejection. Reinfusion of donor stem cells in such patients is usually unsuccessful unless preceded by a second immunosuppressive preparative regimen. Standard high-dose preparative regimens are generally tolerated poorly if administered within 100 days of a first transplant because of cumulative toxicities. However, use of regimens combining, for example, anti-CD3 antibodies with high-dose glucocorticoids, fludarabine plus low-dose total-body irradiation, or cyclophosphamide plus antithymocyte globulin, has been effective in some cases.

Infection

Posttransplant patients, particularly recipients of allogeneic transplantation, require unique approaches to the problem of infection. Early after transplantation, patients are profoundly neutropenic, and because the risk of bacterial infection is so great, most centers initiate antibiotic treatment once the granulocyte count falls to <500/μL. Fluconazole prophylaxis at a dose of 200–400 mg/kg per day reduces the risk of candidal infections. Patients seropositive for herpes simplex should receive acyclovir prophylaxis. One approach to infection prophylaxis is shown in Table 30-2. Despite these prophylactic measures, most patients will develop fever and signs of infection posttransplant. The management of patients who become febrile despite bacterial and fungal prophylaxis is a difficult challenge and is guided by individual aspects of the patient and by the institution's experience.

Once patients engraft, the incidence of bacterial infection diminishes; however, patients, particularly allogeneic transplant recipients, remain at significant risk of infection. During the period from engraftment until about 3 months posttransplant, the most common causes of infection are gram-positive bacteria; fungi (particularly *Aspergillus*); and viruses, including CMV. CMV infection, which in the past was frequently seen and often fatal, can be prevented in seronegative patients transplanted from seronegative donors by the use of either seronegative blood products or products from which the white blood cells have been removed. In seropositive patients or patients transplanted from seropositive donors, the use of ganciclovir, either as prophylaxis beginning at the time of engraftment or initiated when CMV first reactivates as evidenced by development of antigenemia or viremia, can significantly reduce the risk of CMV disease. Foscarnet is effective for some patients who develop CMV antigenemia or infection despite the use of ganciclovir or who cannot tolerate the drug.

Pneumocystis jiroveci pneumonia, once seen in 5–10% of patients, can be prevented by treating patients with

TABLE 30-2

APPROACH TO INFECTION PROPHYLAXIS IN ALLOGENEIC TRANSPLANT RECIPIENTS

ORGANISM		APPROACH
Bacterial	Levofloxacin	750 mg PO or IV daily
Fungal	Fluconazole	400 mg PO qd to day 75 posttransplant
Pneumocystis carinii	Trimethoprim-sulfamethoxazole	1 double-strength tablet PO bid 2 days/week until day 180 or off immunosuppression
Viral		
Herpes simplex	Acyclovir	800 mg PO bid to day 30
Varicella-zoster	Acyclovir	800 mg PO bid to day 365
Cytomegalovirus	Ganciclovir	5 mg/kg IV bid for 7 days, then 5 (mg/kg)/d 5 days/ week to day 100

Abbreviations: bid, twice a day; IV, intravenous; PO, oral; qd, every day.

oral TMP-SMX for 1 week pretransplant and resuming the treatment once patients have engrafted.

The risk of infection diminishes considerably beyond 3 months after transplant unless chronic GVHD develops, requiring continuous immunosuppression. Most transplant centers recommend continuing TMP-SMX prophylaxis while patients are receiving any immunosuppressive drugs and also recommend careful monitoring for late CMV reactivation. In addition, many centers recommend prophylaxis against varicella-zoster, using acyclovir for 1 year posttransplant. Patients should be revaccinated against tetanus, diphtheria, haemophilus influenza, polio, and pneumococcal pneumonia starting at 12 months posttransplant and against measles, mumps, and rubella at 24 months.

TREATMENT OF SPECIFIC DISEASES USING HEMATOPOIETIC CELL TRANSPLANTATION

TREATMENT Nonmalignant Diseases

IMMUNODEFICIENCY DISORDERS By replacing abnormal stem cells with cells from a normal donor, hematopoietic cell transplantation can cure patients of a variety of immunodeficiency disorders, including severe combined immunodeficiency, Wiskott-Aldrich syndrome, and Chédiak-Higashi syndrome. The widest experience has been with severe combined immunodeficiency disease, in which cure rates of 90% can be expected with HLA-identical donors and success rates of 50–70% have been reported using haplotype-mismatched parents as donors (Table 30-3).

APLASTIC ANEMIA Transplantation from matched siblings after a preparative regimen of high-dose cyclophosphamide and antithymocyte globulin can cure up to 90% of patients age <40 years with severe aplastic anemia. Results in older patients and in recipients of mismatched family member or unrelated marrow are less favorable; therefore, a trial of immunosuppressive therapy is generally recommended for such patients before considering transplantation. Transplantation is effective in all forms of aplastic anemia, including, for example, the syndromes associated with paroxysmal nocturnal hemoglobinuria and Fanconi's anemia. Patients with Fanconi's anemia are abnormally sensitive to the toxic effects of alkylating agents, so less intensive preparative regimens must be used in their treatment (Chap. 11).

HEMOGLOBINOPATHIES Marrow transplantation from an HLA-identical sibling following a preparative regimen of busulfan and cyclophosphamide can cure 70–90% of patients with thalassemia major. The best outcomes can be expected if patients are transplanted before they develop hepatomegaly or portal fibrosis and if they have been given adequate iron chelation therapy. Among such patients, the probabilities of 5-year survival and disease-free survival are 95 and 90%, respectively. Although prolonged survival can be achieved with aggressive chelation therapy, transplantation is the only curative treatment for thalassemia. Transplantation is being studied as a curative approach to patients with sickle cell anemia. Two-year survival and disease-free survival rates of 90 and 80%, respectively, have been reported following matched sibling transplantation. Decisions about patient selection and the timing of transplantation remain difficult, but transplantation represents a reasonable option for younger patients who have repeated crises or other significant complications and who have not responded to other interventions (Chap. 8).

TABLE 30-3

ESTIMATED 5-YEAR SURVIVAL RATES FOLLOWING TRANSPLANTATION[a]

DISEASE	ALLOGENEIC, %	AUTOLOGOUS, %
Severe combined immunodeficiency	90	N/A
Aplastic anemia	90	N/A
Thalassemia	90	N/A
Acute myeloid leukemia		
First remission	55–60	50
Second remission	40	30
Acute lymphocytic leukemia		
First remission	50	40
Second remission	40	30
Chronic myeloid leukemia		
Chronic phase	70	ID
Accelerated phase	40	ID
Blast crisis	15	ID
Chronic lymphocytic leukemia	50	ID
Myelodysplasia	45	ID
Multiple myeloma	30	35
Non-Hodgkin's lymphoma		
First relapse/ second remission	40	40
Hodgkin's disease		
First relapse/ second remission	40	50
Breast cancer		
High-risk stage II	N/A	70
Stage IV	N/A	15

[a]These estimates are generally based on data reported by the International Bone Marrow Transplant Registry. The analysis has not been reviewed by their Advisory Committee.

Abbreviations: ID, insufficient data; N/A, not applicable

OTHER NONMALIGNANT DISEASES Theoretically, hematopoietic cell transplantation should be able to cure any disease that results from an inborn error of the lymphohematopoietic system. Transplantation has been used successfully to treat congenital disorders of white blood cells such as Kostmann's syndrome, chronic granulomatous disease, and leukocyte adhesion deficiency. Congenital anemias such as Blackfan-Diamond anemia can also be cured with transplantation. Infantile malignant osteopetrosis is due to an inability of the osteoclast to resorb bone, and since osteoclasts derive from the marrow, transplantation can cure this rare inherited disorder.

Hematopoietic cell transplantation has been used as treatment for a number of storage diseases caused by enzymatic deficiencies, such as Gaucher's disease, Hurler's syndrome, Hunter's syndrome, and infantile metachromatic leukodystrophy. Transplantation for these diseases has not been uniformly successful, but treatment early in the course of these diseases, before irreversible damage to extramedullary organs has occurred, increases the chance for success.

Transplantation is being explored as a treatment for severe acquired autoimmune disorders. These trials are based on studies demonstrating that transplantation can reverse autoimmune disorders in animal models and on the observation that occasional patients with coexisting autoimmune disorders and hematologic malignancies have been cured of both with transplantation.

TREATMENT Malignant Diseases

ACUTE LEUKEMIA Allogeneic hematopoietic cell transplantation cures 15–20% of patients who do not achieve complete response from induction chemotherapy for acute myeloid leukemia (AML) and is the only form of therapy that can cure such patients. Cure rates of 30–35% are seen when patients are transplanted in second remission or in first relapse. The best results with allogeneic transplantation are achieved when applied during first remission, with disease-free survival rates averaging 55–60%. Meta analyses of studies comparing matched related donor transplantation to chemotherapy for adult AML patients age <60 years show a survival advantage with transplantation. This advantage is greatest for those with unfavorable-risk AML and lost in those with favorable-risk disease. The role of autologous transplantation in the treatment of AML is less well defined. The rates of disease recurrence with autologous transplantation are higher than those seen after allogeneic transplantation, and cure rates are somewhat less.

Similar to patients with AML, adults with acute lymphocytic leukemia who do not achieve a complete response to induction chemotherapy can be cured in 15–20% of cases with immediate transplantation. Cure rates improve to 30–50% in second remission; therefore, transplantation can be recommended for adults who have persistent disease after induction chemotherapy or who have subsequently relapsed. Transplantation in first remission results in cure rates about 55%. Transplantation appears to offer a clear advantage over chemotherapy for patients with high-risk disease, such as those with Philadelphia chromosome–positive disease. Debate continues about whether adults with standard-risk disease should be transplanted in first remission or whether transplantation should be reserved until relapse. Autologous transplantation is associated with a higher relapse rate but a somewhat lower risk of nonrelapse mortality compared with allogeneic transplantation.

There is no obvious role of autologous transplantation for ALL in first remission, and for second-remission patients, most experts recommend use of allogeneic stem cells if an appropriate donor is available.

CHRONIC LEUKEMIA Allogeneic hematopoietic cell transplantation is the only therapy shown to cure a substantial portion of patients with chronic myeloid leukemia (CML). Five-year disease-free survival rates are 15–20% for patients transplanted for blast crisis, 25–50% for accelerated-phase patients, and 60–70% for chronic-phase patients, with cure rates as high as 80% at selected centers. However, with the availability of imatinib mesylate, a remarkably effective, relatively nontoxic oral agent, most physicians favor reserving transplantation for those who fail to achieve a complete cytogenetic response with imatinib, relapse after an initial response, or are intolerant of the drug (Chap. 14).

Allogeneic transplantation using high-dose preparative regimen was rarely used for chronic lymphocytic leukemia (CLL), in large part because of the chronic nature of the disease and because of the age profile of patients. In cases where when it was studied, complete remissions were achieved in the majority of patients, with disease-free survival rates of ~50% at 3 years, despite the advanced stage of the disease at the time of transplant. The marked antitumor effects have resulted in the increased use and study of allogeneic transplantation using reduced-intensity conditioning for the treatment of CLL.

MYELODYSPLASIA Between 40 and 50% of patients with myelodysplasia appear to be cured with allogeneic transplantation. Results are better among younger patients and those with less advanced disease. However, some patients with myelodysplasia can live for extended periods without intervention, so transplantation is generally recommended only for patients with disease categorized as intermediate risk I or greater according to the International Prognostic Scoring System (Chap. 11).

LYMPHOMA Patients with disseminated intermediate- or high-grade non-Hodgkin's lymphoma who have not been cured by first-line chemotherapy and are transplanted in first relapse or second remission can still be cured in 40–50% of cases. This represents a clear advantage over results obtained with conventional-dose salvage chemotherapy. It is unsettled whether patients with high-risk disease benefit from transplantation in first remission. Most experts favor the use of autologous rather than allogeneic transplantation for patients with intermediate- or high-grade non-Hodgkin's lymphoma because fewer complications occur with this approach, and survival appears equivalent. For patients with recurrent disseminated indolent non-Hodgkin's lymphoma, autologous transplantation results in high response rates and improved progression-free survival compared with salvage chemotherapy. However, late relapses are seen after transplantation. The role of autologous transplantation in the initial treatment of patients is under study. Reduced-intensity conditioning regimens followed by allogeneic transplantation result in high response rates in patients with indolent lymphomas, but the exact role of this approach remains to be defined.

The role of transplantation in Hodgkin's disease is similar to that in intermediate- and high-grade non-Hodgkin's lymphoma. With transplantation, 5-year disease-free survival is 20–30% in patients who never achieve a first remission with standard chemotherapy and up to 70% for those transplanted in second remission. Transplantation has no defined role in first remission in Hodgkin's disease.

MYELOMA Patients with myeloma who have progressed on first-line therapy can sometimes benefit from allogeneic or autologous transplantation. Autologous transplantation has been studied as part of the initial therapy of patients, and both disease-free survival and overall survival were improved with this approach in randomized trials. The use of autologous transplantation followed by nonmyeloablative allogeneic transplantation is the subject of ongoing research.

SOLID TUMORS Among women with metastatic breast cancer, 15–20% disease-free survival rates at 3 years have been reported, with better results seen in younger patients who have responded completely to standard-dose therapy before undergoing transplantation. Randomized trials have not shown superior survival for patients treated for metastatic disease with high-dose chemotherapy plus stem cell support. Randomized trials evaluating transplantation as treatment for primary breast cancer have yielded mixed results. No role for autologous transplantation has been established in the treatment of breast cancer.

Patients with testicular cancer who have failed first-line chemotherapy have been treated with autologous transplantation; ~10–20% of such patients apparently have been cured with this approach.

The use of high-dose chemotherapy with autologous stem cell support is being studied for several other solid tumors, including neuroblastoma and pediatric sarcomas. As in most other settings, the best results have been obtained in patients with limited amounts of disease and when the remaining tumor remains sensitive to conventional-dose chemotherapy. Few randomized trials of transplantation in these diseases have been completed.

Partial and complete responses have been reported following nonmyeloablative allogeneic transplantation for some solid tumors, most notably renal cell cancers. The GVT effect, well documented in the treatment of hematologic malignancies, may apply to selected solid tumors under certain circumstances.

POSTTRANSPLANT RELAPSE Patients who relapse following autologous transplantation sometimes respond to further chemotherapy and may be candidates for possible allogeneic transplantation, particularly if the remission following the initial autologous transplant was long. Several options are available for patients who relapse following allogeneic transplantation. Of particular interest are the response rates seen with infusion of unirradiated donor lymphocytes. Complete responses in as many as 75% of patients with chronic myeloid leukemia, 40% in myelodysplasia, 25% in AML, and 15% in myeloma have been reported. Major complications of donor lymphocyte infusions include transient myelosuppression and the development of GVHD. These complications depend on the number of donor lymphocytes given and the schedule of infusions, with less GVHD seen with lower dose, fractionated schedules.

CHAPTER 31

NEOPLASIA DURING PREGNANCY

Dan L. Longo

Cancer develops during ~1 in every 1000 pregnancies. Of all the cancers that occur in women, fewer than 1% occur in pregnant women. The four cancers most commonly developing during pregnancy are cervical cancer, breast cancer, melanoma, and lymphomas (particularly Hodgkin's lymphoma); however, virtually every form of cancer has been reported in pregnant women (Table 31-1). In addition to cancers developing in other organs of the mother, gestational trophoblastic tumors can arise from the placenta. The problem of cancer in a pregnant woman is complex. One must take into account the possible influence of the pregnancy on the natural history of the cancer, the effects of the diagnostic and staging procedures, and the treatments of the cancer on both the mother and the developing fetus. These issues may lead to dilemmas: what is best for the mother may be harmful to the fetus, and what is best for the fetus may be harmful to the mother.

TABLE 31-1

INCIDENCE OF MALIGNANT TUMORS DURING GESTATION

TUMOR TYPE	INCIDENCE PER 10,000 PREGNANCIES[a]	% OF CASES[b]
Breast cancer	1–3	25
Cervical cancer	1.2–4.5	25
Thyroid cancer	1.2	15
Hodgkin's disease	1.6	10
Melanoma	1–2.6	8
Ovarian cancer	0.8	2
All sites	10	100

[a]These are estimates based on extrapolations from a review of more than 3 million pregnancies (Smith LH, Dalrymple JL, Leiserowitz GS, et al: Obstetrical deliveries associated with maternal malignancy in California, 1992 through 1997. *Am J Obstet Gynecol* 2001;184(7): 1504–1512; discussion 1512–1513).

[b]Based on accumulating case reports from the literature; the precision of these data is not high.

Another complicating issue in women who develop cancer during pregnancy is that many of the early symptoms of cancer are ignored in pregnant women. The many changes in a woman's body during pregnancy dull one's senses to changes that may be related to an underlying disease rather than the pregnancy. Thus, many cancers that occur in pregnancy present in advanced stages.

As a general rule, one should assume that no diagnostic or therapeutic intervention is safe in the first trimester of pregnancy other than surgery. If the mother develops life-threatening complications during the first trimester that require radiation therapy or systemic chemotherapy and these interventions cannot be safely delayed, a recommendation should be made for an abortion. Indeed, radiation, even in the form of diagnostic radiography, should be avoided throughout pregnancy. No exposure to radiation is safe, and efforts to shield the fetus with barriers placed on the abdomen cannot block internal scatter radiation. It is safest to omit radiation exposure of any kind. Fortunately, its use is seldom an essential component of treatment before delivery.

Chemotherapy exposure is also to be avoided, if at all possible. It should never be given in the first trimester; a variety of single agents and combinations have been given in the second and third trimesters without a high frequency of catastrophic effects to the pregnancy or the fetus, but data on safety are sparse. Maternal factors that may influence the pharmacology of chemotherapeutic agents include the 50% increase in plasma volume, altered absorption and protein binding, increased glomerular filtration rate, increased hepatic mixed function oxidase activity, and third space created by amniotic fluid. The fetus is protected from some agents by placental expression of drug efflux pumps, but decreased fetal hepatic mixed function oxidase and glucuronidation activity may prolong the half-life of agents that do cross the placenta. A database on the risks associated with individual chemotherapy agents is available on the Internet (*www.motherisk.org*).

The optimal management strategies have not been developed based on prospective clinical trials. Instead, a guiding principle has been to delay therapeutic interventions until as late as possible during the pregnancy. Delivery is recommended at 32 weeks. By and large, this approach minimizes exposure of the child to noxious cancer treatments, spares the mother complications of pregnancy, and is generally accomplished without an adverse impact on treatment outcome. Pregnancy appears to have little or no impact on the natural history of malignancies despite the hormonal influences. Spread of the mother's cancer to the fetus (so-called vertical transmission) is exceedingly rare.

CERVICAL CANCER DURING PREGNANCY

The incidence of cervical cancer in pregnant women is roughly comparable to that of age-matched control participants who are not pregnant. Invasive cervical cancer develops at a rate of about 0.45 in 1000 live births, and carcinoma in situ is seen in 1 in 750 pregnancies. About 1% of women diagnosed with cervical cancer are pregnant at the time of diagnosis. Early signs of cervical cancer include vaginal spotting or discharge, pain, and postcoital bleeding, which are also common features of pregnancy. Early visual changes in the cervix related to invasive cancer can be mistaken for cervical decidualization or ectropion (columnar epithelium on the cervix) due to pregnancy. Women diagnosed with cervical cancer during pregnancy report having had symptoms for 4.5 months on average.

Human papillomavirus (HPV) types 16 and 18 account for about 70% of cervical cancer. The rate of carriage of these serotypes can be reduced with the use of vaccination before exposure. Screening is recommended at the first prenatal visit and 6 weeks postpartum. The rate of cytologic abnormalities on Pap smear in pregnant women is about 5–8% and is not much different than the rate in nonpregnant women of the same age. Consensus guidelines dictate that specific tests are indicated based on the level of atypia seen on Pap smear. Atypical squamous cells of unknown significance (ASCUS) generally trigger HPV testing with colposcopy reserved for the subset of women with a high-risk HPV-type infection. By contrast, the presence of dysplasia is considered an indication for colposcopy regardless of HPV type. Women with either low- or high-grade squamous intraepithelial lesions (LSIL or HSIL) and HIV-infected women with ASCUS are recommended for colposcopy.

At colposcopy, any areas suspicious for invasive disease are biopsied. However, endocervical curettage is contraindicated in pregnant patients. The only indication for therapy of cervical neoplasia in pregnant women is the documentation of invasive cancer. Accordingly, some physicians defer colposcopy in pregnant women until 6 weeks postpartum unless they are at high risk for invasive disease. Cervical intraepithelial neoplasia has a low risk of progression to invasive cancer during pregnancy (~0.4%), and many such lesions (36–70%) regress spontaneously postpartum. If invasive disease is suspected at colposcopy and the pregnancy is between 16 and 20 weeks, a cone biopsy may be performed to make the diagnosis; however, the procedure is associated with bleeding because of the increased vasculature in the gravid cervix and increases the risk of premature rupture of membranes and preterm labor two- to threefold. Cone biopsy should not be done within 4 weeks of delivery.

Management of invasive disease is guided by the stage of disease, the gestational age of the fetus, and the desire of the mother to have the baby. If the disease is in early stage and the pregnancy is desired, it is safe to delay treatment regardless of gestational age until fetal maturity allows for safe delivery. If the disease is in advanced stage and the pregnancy is desired, the safety of delaying therapy is unproven. Abortion followed by definitive therapy is recommended for women with advanced cancer in the first or second trimester (see Chap. 44). In women in the third trimester with advanced disease, the baby should be delivered at the earliest possible time and followed immediately by stage-appropriate therapy. Most women with invasive cancer have early-stage disease. If the disease is microinvasive, vaginal delivery can take place and be followed by definitive treatment, usually conization. If a lesion is visible on the cervix, delivery is best done by cesarean section and followed by radical hysterectomy.

BREAST CANCER DURING PREGNANCY

Breast cancer occurs once in 3000 to 10,000 live births. About 5% of all breast cancers occur in women 40 years of age or younger. Among all premenopausal women with breast cancer, 25–30% were pregnant at the time of diagnosis. While early pregnancy is a protective factor against breast cancer in women as a whole, the breast cancers diagnosed during pregnancy are often diagnosed at a later stage of disease and so have a poorer outcome. The late diagnosis has at least two contributions. One is the more aggressive behavior of the cancer possibly related to the hormonal milieu (estrogen increases 100-fold; progesterone increases 1000-fold) of the pregnancy. However, about 70% of the breast cancers found in pregnancy are estrogen receptor–negative. Another factor is that early physical signs of the disease are often attributed to the changes that occur in the breast normally as a part of pregnancy. However, a breast mass in a pregnant woman is never normal. Younger women with breast cancer have a higher likelihood of having mutations in *BRCA1* or *BRCA2*. Pregnancy retains its protective effects in carriers of *BRCA1* mutations; such women with four or more children had a 38% reduction in breast cancer risk compared with nulliparous carriers. However, pregnancy seems to increase the risk of breast cancer among carriers of *BRCA2* mutations, particularly in the first 2 years after pregnancy. About 28–58% of the tumors express HER-2.

Primary tumors in pregnant women are 3.5 cm on average compared with <2 cm in nonpregnant women. A dominant mass and a nipple discharge are the most common presenting signs, and they should prompt ultrasonography and breast magnetic resonance imaging (MRI) (if available) followed by lumpectomy if the mass is solid and aspiration if the mass is cystic. Mammography is less reliable in pregnancy due to the increased breast density. Needle aspirates of breast masses in pregnant women are often nondiagnostic or falsely positive. Even in pregnancy, most breast masses are benign (~80% are adenoma, lobular hyperplasia, milk retention cyst, fibrocystic disease, fibroadenoma, and other rarer entities).

Differences between pregnancy-associated breast cancer (often defined as cancer detected during pregnancy and up to 1 year after delivery) are shown in Table 31-2. About 20% of breast cancers are detected in the first trimester, 45% in the second trimester, and 35% in the third trimester. Some argue that stage for stage, the outcome is the same for breast cancer diagnosed in pregnant and nonpregnant women.

Staging the axillary lymph nodes is currently somewhat controversial. Sentinel lymph node sampling is not straightforward in pregnant women. Blue dye has been carcinogenic in rats, and shielding the fetus from administered radionuclides is of unproven efficacy. For this reason, many surgeons favor axillary node dissection to stage the nodes. Largely due to the typical delay in diagnosis, axillary nodes are more often positive in pregnant than in nonpregnant women.

As with other types of cancer in pregnant women, diagnosis in the first trimester often triggers a recommendation for an abortion to allow definitive therapeutic intervention at the earliest possible time. While definitive local surgery is applicable in the first trimester, radiation therapy and chemotherapy are considerably more risky. Delay in administration of systemic therapy can increase the risk of axillary spread. In the second and third trimesters, chemotherapy (particularly anthracycline-based combinations) is both safe and effective (see Chap. 37). Lumpectomy followed by adjuvant chemotherapy is frequently used; fluorouracil and cyclophosphamide with either doxorubicin or epirubicin have been given without major risk to the fetus. Taxanes and gemcitabine are also beginning to be used; however, safety data are sparse. Methotrexate and other folate antagonists are to be avoided because of effects on the fetal nervous system. Myelotoxic therapy is generally not administered after the 33rd or 34th week of gestation to allow 3 weeks off therapy before delivery for recovery of blood counts. Endocrine therapy and trastuzumab are unsafe during pregnancy. Experience with lapatinib is anecdotal, but no fetal malformations have been reported. Antiemetics and colony-stimulating factors are also considered safe. Women being treated into the postpartum period should not nurse their babies because of excretion of cancer chemotherapy agents, particularly alkylating agents, in milk.

Subsequent pregnancies following gestational breast cancer do not appear to influence relapse rate or overall survival. Indeed, a meta-analysis has suggested that pregnancy in breast cancer survivors may reduce the risk of dying from breast cancer by as much as 42%.

TABLE 31-2

DIFFERENCES IN BREAST CANCERS IN PREGNANT AND NONPREGNANT WOMEN

	PREGNANT	NONPREGNANT
Tumor size	3.5 cm	2 cm
Estrogen receptor +	30%[a]	67%
HER-2 +	≤58%	10–25%
Stage II, III	65–90%	45–66%
Lymph node +	56–89%	38–54%

[a]Lower measured levels could be in part artifactual due to the increased levels of estrogen in the milieu

MELANOMA DURING PREGNANCY

Speculation about melanoma occurring during pregnancy based largely on anecdotal evidence and small case series concluded that it occurred with increased frequency, was more aggressive in its natural history, and was caused in part by the hormonal changes that also produced hyperpigmentation (so-called melasma) during pregnancy. However, more complete epidemiologic data suggest that melanoma is no more frequent in pregnant women than in nonpregnant women in the same age group, melanoma is not more aggressive during pregnancy, and hormones seem to have little or nothing to do with the etiology. Pregnant and nonpregnant women do not differ in the location of primary tumor, depth of primary tumor, tumor ulceration, or vascular invasion.

Suspicious lesions should be looked for and managed definitively with excisional biopsy during pregnancy.

Wide excision with sampling of regional lymph nodes is warranted. If lymph nodes are involved, the course of action is less clear. Several agents have demonstrated some activity in melanoma, but none have been used during pregnancy. Adjuvant interferon-alfa is toxic, and its safety in pregnancy has not been documented. Agents active in advanced disease include dacarbazine, interleukin 2, and ipilumimab (antibody to CTLA-4) and in those with BRAF mutation V600E, a BRAF kinase inhibitor. In the setting of metastatic disease, abortion may be indicated so that systemic therapy can be initiated as soon as possible (see Chap. 33).

Pregnancy subsequent to the diagnosis and treatment of melanoma is also not associated with an increased risk of melanoma recurrence.

HODGKIN'S DISEASE AND NON-HODGKIN'S LYMPHOMADURING PREGNANCY

(See Chap. 15.) Hodgkin's disease occurs mainly in the age range of people who are of child-bearing age. However, Hodgkin's disease is not more common in pregnant than nonpregnant women. Hodgkin's disease is diagnosed in approximately 1 in 6,000 pregnancies. It generally presents as a nontender lymph node swelling, most often in the left supraclavicular region. It may be accompanied by B symptoms (fever, night sweats, unexplained weight loss). Excisional biopsy is the preferred diagnostic procedure as fine-needle aspiration cannot reveal the architectural framework that is an essential component of Hodgkin's disease diagnosis. The stage at presentation appears to be unaffected by pregnancy. Women diagnosed in the second and third trimester can be treated safely with combination chemotherapy, usually doxorubicin, bleomycin, vinblastine, and dacarbazine (ABVD). In general, the patient in the first trimester is asymptomatic, and a woman with a desired pregnancy can be followed until the second or third trimester when definitive multiagent chemotherapy can be safely given. Radiation therapy is not given during pregnancy. If symptoms requiring treatment appear during the first trimester, anecdotal evidence suggests that Hodgkin's disease symptoms can be controlled with weekly low-dose vinblastine. Such an approach has been safely used to avoid termination of pregnancy. Pregnancy does not have an adverse effect on treatment outcome.

Non-Hodgkin's lymphomas are more unusual in pregnancy (~0.8 per 100,000 pregnancies) but are usually tumors with an aggressive natural history like diffuse large B-cell lymphoma, Burkitt's lymphoma, or peripheral T-cell lymphoma. Diagnosis relies on an excisional biopsy of a tumor mass, not fine-needle aspiration. Staging evaluation is generally limited to ultrasound or MRI examinations. Diagnosis in the first trimester should prompt termination of the pregnancy followed by definitive treatment with combination chemotherapy, as aggressive lymphomas are not likely to be held at bay with single-agent chemotherapy. Women diagnosed in the second or third trimesters can be treated with standard chemotherapy, such as with cyclophosphamide, doxorubicin, vincristine, and prednisone (CHOP). The experience with rituximab in this setting is anecdotal. However, infants born to mothers who have received rituximab may have transient delay in B cell development that typically normalizes by 6 months. The treatment outcome is similar in lymphomas diagnosed in pregnant and nonpregnant women of the same clinical stage.

THYROID CANCER DURING PREGNANCY

(See Chap. 48.) Thyroid cancer along with melanomas, brain tumors, and lymphomas are cancers that are increasing in incidence in the general population. Thyroid cancers are rising faster among women in North America than the other increasing tumor types. The Endocrine Society has developed practice guidelines to inform the management of patients with thyroid disease during pregnancy (*www.endo-society.org/guidelines/final/upload/Clinical-Guideline-Executive-Summary-Management-of-Thyroid-Dysfunction-during-Pregnancy-Postpartum.pdf*). Thyroid nodules 1 cm or larger are approached by fine-needle aspiration. If a malignancy is diagnosed, surgery is generally recommended in the second and third trimesters. However, surgical complications appear to be twice as common when the patient is pregnant. Because the growth of thyroid tumors is often indolent, surgery is not recommended in the first trimester. Patients with follicular cancer or early papillary cancer can be observed until the postpartum period. Radioactive iodine can be safely administered after delivery. Patients with a history of thyroid cancer who become pregnant should be maintained on thyroid hormone replacement during pregnancy because of the adverse impact of maternal hypothyroidism on the fetus. Women who are breastfeeding should not be treated with radioactive iodine, and women treated with radioactive iodine should not become pregnant for 6–12 months after treatment.

The assessment of thyroid function during pregnancy is challenging because of the physiologic changes that occur during pregnancy. Women who have previously been treated for thyroid cancer are at risk of hypothyroidism. The demand for thyroid hormone increases during pregnancy and doses to maintain normal function may increase by 30–50%. Total T4 levels are higher during pregnancy, but target therapeutic levels

TABLE 31-3

THYROID FUNCTION TEST DURING PREGNANCY (MEAN LEVELS)

	NONPREGNANT	FIRST TRIMESTER	SECOND TRIMESTER	THIRD TRIMESTER
TSH (mIU/L)	1.38	0.91	1.03	1.32
Total thyroxine (μg/dL)	7.35	10.98	11.88	11.08

Abbreviation: TSH, thyroid-stimulating hormone.
Source: Based on the National Health and Nutrition Examination Survey III (NHANES III) (OP Soldin et al: Gestation-specific thyroxine and thyroid stimulating hormone levels in the United States and worldwide. Ther Drug Monit 2007;29(5):553–559).

also increase (Table 31-3). It is recommended that the upper and lower limits of the laboratory range be multiplied by 1.5 in the second and third trimester to establish a pregnancy-specific normal range. The target TSH level is lower than 2.5 mIU/L.

GESTATIONAL TROPHOBLASTIC DISEASE

(See Chap. 44.) Gestational trophoblastic disease encompasses hydatidiform mole, choriocarcinoma, placental site trophoblastic tumor, and assorted miscellaneous and unclassifiable trophoblastic tumors. Moles are the most common, occurring in 1 in 1500 pregnancies in the United States. The incidence is higher in Asia. In general, if the serum level of beta-human chorionic gonadotropin (HCG) returns to normal after surgical removal (evacuation) of the mole, the illness is considered gestational trophoblastic disease. By contrast, if the HCG level remains elevated after mole evacuation, the patient is considered to have gestational trophoblastic neoplasia. Choriocarcinoma occurs in 1 in 25,000 pregnancies. Maternal age >45 years and history of molar pregnancy are risk factors. A previous molar pregnancy makes choriocarcinoma about 1000 times more likely to occur (incidence, 1–2%).

Hydatidiform moles are characterized by clusters of villi with hydropic changes, trophoblastic hyperplasia, and absence of fetal blood vessels. Invasive moles are distinguished by invasion of the myometrium. Placental site trophoblastic tumors are composed mainly of cytotrophoblast cells arising at the site of placental origin. Choriocarcinomas contain anaplastic trophoblastic tissue with both cytotrophoblast and syncytiotrophoblast features and no identifiable villi.

Moles can be partial or complete. Partial moles have a distinct molecular origin and usually are smaller tumors with less hydropic villi. Partial moles result from fertilization of an egg by two sperm, resulting in diandric triploidy. Complete moles usually have a 46,XX genotype; 95% develop by a single male sperm fertilizing an empty egg and undergoing gene duplication (diandric diploidy), and 5% develop from dispermic fertilization of an empty egg (diandric dispermy).

Women with gestational trophoblastic disease often present with first-trimester bleeding and unusually large uterine size. Ultrasound shows absence of fetal parts or heart sounds. Patients are monitored by chest radiography, pelvic examination, and weekly measurement of HCG levels.

Patients with molar pregnancies require suction curettage with postoperative HCG monitoring. In 80% of cases, HCG declines within 8–10 days. Patients should not become pregnant for at least 12 months. Women with invasive moles generally undergo hysterectomy followed by chemotherapy. About half of choriocarcinomas develop after a molar pregnancy and half develop after ectopic pregnancy or rarely, after a normal full-term pregnancy. Disease is classified as stage I if it is confined to the uterus; stage II if disease is limited to genital structures (~30% have vaginal involvement); stage III if disease has spread to the lungs but no other organs; and stage IV if disease has spread to liver, brain, or other organs.

Specific criteria have been developed to aid the decision about when disease becomes neoplasia:

1. Four consecutive increased HCG levels over the 3 weeks after evacuation surgery
2. A rise in HCG of 10% or more on three consecutive values over 2 or more weeks
3. The presence of choriocarcinoma
4. Persistent HCG elevations 6 months after evacuation

Patients without widely metastatic disease are generally managed with single-agent methotrexate (either 30 mg/m^2 intramuscularly [IM] weekly until HCG normalizes or 1 mg/kg IM every other day for 4 doses followed by leukovorin 0.1 mg/kg IV 24 hours after methotrexate), which cures >90% of patients. Patients with very high HCG levels, presenting >4 months after a pregnancy, with brain or liver metastases, or failing to be cured by single agent methotrexate are treated with combination chemotherapy. Etoposide, methotrexate, and dactinomycin alternating with cyclophosphamide and vincristine (EMA-CO) is the most commonly used regimen producing long-term survival in >80% of patients. Brain metastases can usually be controlled with brain radiation therapy. Women cured of trophoblastic disease who have not undergone hysterectomy do not appear to have increased risk of fetal abnormalities or maternal complications with subsequent pregnancies.

CHAPTER 32

PALLIATIVE AND END-OF-LIFE CARE

Ezekiel J. Emanuel

EPIDEMIOLOGY

In 2007, 2,423,712 individuals died in the United States (Table 32-1). Approximately 72% of all deaths occur in those >65 years of age. The epidemiology of mortality is similar in most developed countries; cardiovascular diseases and cancer are the predominant causes of death, a marked change since 1900, when heart disease caused ~8% of all deaths and cancer accounted for <4% of all deaths. In 2006, the year with the most recent available data, AIDS accounted for <1% of all U.S. deaths, although among those age 35–44 years, it remained one of the top five causes.

It is estimated that in developed countries, ~70% of all deaths are preceded by a disease or condition, making it reasonable to plan for dying in the foreseeable future. Cancer has served as the paradigm for terminal care, but it is not the only type of illness with a recognizable and predictable terminal phase. Since heart failure, chronic obstructive pulmonary disease (COPD), chronic liver failure, dementia, and many other conditions have recognizable terminal phases, a systematic approach to end-of-life care should be part of all medical specialties. Many patients with illness-related suffering also can benefit from palliative care regardless of

TABLE 32-1

TEN LEADING CAUSES OF DEATH IN THE UNITED STATES AND BRITAIN

	UNITED STATES			BRITAIN	
CAUSE OF DEATH	NUMBER OF DEATHS	PERCENT OF TOTAL	NUMBER OF DEATHS AMONG PEOPLE ≥65 YEARS OF AGE	NUMBER OF DEATHS	PERCENT OF TOTAL
All deaths	2,423,712	100	1,759,423	538,254	100
Heart disease	616,067	25.4	510,542	129,009	24
Malignant neoplasms	562,875	23.2	387,515	135,955	25.3
Cerebrovascular diseases	135,952	5.6	117,010	57,808	10.7
Chronic lower respiratory diseases	127,924	5.1	106,845	27,905	5.2
Accidents	123,706	5.1	36,689	10,979	2
Alzheimer's disease	74,632	2.2	71,660	6316	1.2
Diabetes mellitus	71,382	2.9	52,351	34,477	6.4
Influenza and pneumonia	52,717	2.2	49,346	5055	0.9
Nephritis, nephritic syndrome, nephrosis	46,448	1.9	37,377	3287	0.6
Septicemia	34,828	1.4	26,201	2206	0.4

Source: National Center for Health Statistics (data for all age groups from 2007; for age >65 years, from 2006), *http://www.cdc.gov/nchs*; National Statistics (Great Britain, 2003), *http://www.statistics.gov.uk*.

prognosis. Ideally, palliative care should be considered part of comprehensive care for all patients. Reviews of the recent literature have found strong evidence that palliative care can be improved by coordination among caregivers, doctors, and patients for advance care planning, as well as dedicated teams of physicians, nurses, and other providers.

The rapid increases in life expectancy in the United States over the past century have been accompanied by new difficulties facing individuals, families, and society as a whole in addressing the needs of an aging population. These challenges include both more complicated conditions and technologies to address them at the end of life. The development of technologies that can prolong life without restoring full health has led many Americans to seek out alternative end-of-life care settings and approaches that relieve suffering for those with terminal diseases. Over the past few decades in the United States, a significant change in the site of death has occurred that coincides with patient and family preferences. Nearly 60% of Americans died as inpatients in hospitals in 1980. By 2000, the trend was reversing, with ~40% of Americans dying as hospital inpatients (Fig. 32-1). This shift has been most dramatic for those dying from cancer and COPD and for younger and very old individuals. In the past decade, it has been associated with the increased use of hospice care; in 2008, approximately 39% of all decedents in the United States received such care. Cancer patients currently constitute ~38.3% of hospice users. About 79% of patients receiving hospice care die out of the hospital, and around 41% of those receiving hospice care die in a private residence. In addition, in 2008, for the first time, the American Board of Medical Specialties (ABMS) offered certification in hospice and palliative medicine. With shortening of hospital stays, many serious conditions are being treated at home or on an outpatient basis. Consequently, providing optimal palliative and end-of-life care requires ensuring that appropriate services are available in a variety of settings, including noninstitutional settings.

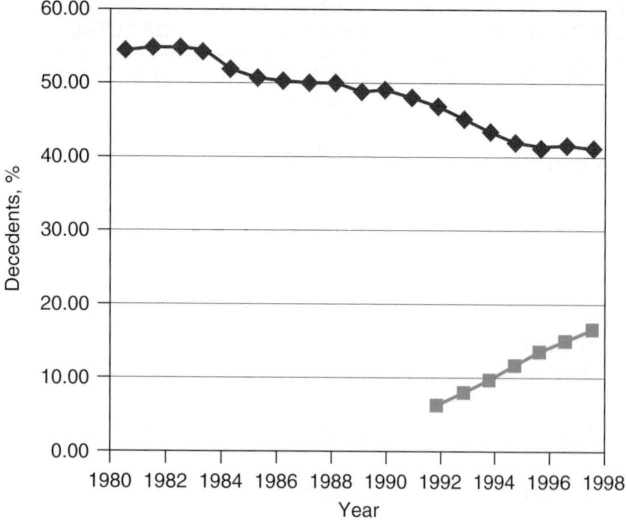

FIGURE 32-1
Graph showing trends in the site of death in the past two decades. ◆, percentage of hospital inpatient deaths; ■, percentage of decedents enrolled in a hospice.

HOSPICE AND THE PALLIATIVE CARE FRAMEWORK

Central to this type of care is an interdisciplinary team approach that typically encompasses pain and symptom management, spiritual and psychological care for the patient, and support for family caregivers during the patients illness and the bereavement period.

Terminally ill patients have a wide variety of advanced diseases, often with multiple symptoms that demand relief, and require noninvasive therapeutic regimens to be delivered in flexible care settings. Fundamental to ensuring quality palliative and end-of-life care is a focus on four broad domains: (1) physical symptoms; (2) psychological symptoms; (3) social needs that include interpersonal relationships, caregiving, and economic concerns; and (4) existential or spiritual needs.

A comprehensive assessment screens for and evaluates needs in each of these four domains. Goals for care are established in discussions with the patient and/or family, based on the assessment in each of the domains. Interventions then are aimed at improving or managing symptoms and needs. Although physicians are responsible for certain interventions, especially technical ones, and for coordinating the interventions, they cannot be responsible for providing all of them. Since failing to address any one of the domains is likely to preclude a good death, a well-coordinated, effectively communicating interdisciplinary team takes on special importance in end-of-life care. Depending on the setting, critical members of the interdisciplinary team will include physicians, nurses, social workers, chaplains, nurses aides, physical therapists, bereavement counselors, and volunteers.

ASSESSMENT AND CARE PLANNING

Comprehensive assessment

Standardized methods for conducting a comprehensive assessment focus on evaluating the patients condition in all four domains affected by illness: physical, psychological, social, and spiritual. The assessment of physical and mental symptoms should follow a modified version of the traditional medical history and physical examination that emphasizes symptoms. Questions should aim at elucidating symptoms and discerning sources of suffering and gauging how much those symptoms interfere with the patients quality of life. Standardized assessment is critical. Currently, there are 21 symptom assessment instruments for cancer alone. Further research on and validation of these assessment tools, especially taking into account patient perspectives, could improve their effectiveness. Instruments with good psychometric properties that assess a wide range of symptoms include the Memorial Symptom Assessment Scale (MSAS), the Rotterdam Symptom Checklist, the Worthing Chemotherapy Questionnaire, and the Computerized Symptom Assessment Instrument. These instruments are long and may be useful for initial clinical or for research assessments. Shorter instruments are useful for patients whose performance status does not permit comprehensive assessments. Suitable shorter instruments include the Condensed Memorial Symptom Assessment Scale, the Edmonton Symptom Assessment System, the M.D. Anderson Symptom Assessment Inventory, and the Symptom Distress Scale. Using such instruments ensures that the assessment is comprehensive and does not focus only on pain and a few other physical symptoms. Invasive tests are best avoided in end-of-life care, and even minimally invasive tests should be evaluated carefully for their benefit-to-burden ratio for the patient. Aspects of the physical examination that are uncomfortable and unlikely to yield useful information can be omitted.

Regarding social needs, health care providers should assess the status of important relationships, financial burdens, caregiving needs, and access to medical care. Relevant questions will include the following: *How often is there someone to feel close to? How has this illness been for your family? How has it affected your relationships? How much help do you need with things like getting meals and getting around? How much trouble do you have getting the medical care you need?* In the area of existential needs, providers should assess distress and the patient's sense of being emotionally and existentially settled and of finding purpose or meaning. Helpful assessment questions can include the following: *How much are you able to find meaning since your illness began? What things are most important to you at this stage?* In addition, it can be helpful to ask how the patient perceives his or her care: *How much do you feel your doctors and nurses respect you? How clear is the information from us about what to expect regarding your illness? How much do you feel that the medical care you are getting fits with your goals?* If concern is detected in any of these areas, deeper evaluative questions are warranted.

Communication

Especially when an illness is life-threatening, there are many emotionally charged and potentially conflict-creating moments, collectively called "bad news" situations, in which empathic and effective communication skills are essential. These moments include communicating with the patient and/or family about a terminal diagnosis, the patients prognosis, any treatment failures, deemphasizing efforts to cure and prolong life while focusing more on symptom management and palliation, advance care planning, and the patient's death. Although these conversations can be difficult and lead to tension, research indicates that end-of-life discussions can lead to earlier hospice referrals rather than overly aggressive treatment, benefiting quality of life for patients and improving the bereavement process for families.

Just as surgeons plan and prepare for major operations and investigators rehearse a presentation of research results, physicians and health care providers caring for patients with significant or advanced illness can develop a practiced approach to sharing important information and planning interventions. In addition, families identify as important both how well the physician was prepared to deliver bad news and the setting in which it was delivered. For instance, 27% of families making critical decisions for patients in an intensive care unit (ICU) desired better and more private physical space to communicate with physicians, and 48% found having clergy present reassuring.

An organized and effective seven-step procedure for communicating bad news goes by the acronym P-SPIKES: (1) ***p***repare for the discussion, (2) ***s***et up a suitable environment, (3) begin the discussion by finding out what the ***p***atient and/or family understand, (4) determine how they will comprehend new ***i***nformation best and how much they want to know, (5) provide needed new ***k***nowledge accordingly, (6) allow for ***e***motional responses, and (7) ***s***hare plans for the next steps in care. Table 32-2 provides a summary of these steps along with suggested phrases and underlying rationales for each one. Additional research that further considers the response of patients to systematic methods of delivering bad news could build the evidence base for even more effective communication procedures.

Continuous goal assessment

Major barriers to ensuring quality palliative and end-of-life care include difficulty providing an accurate prognosis and emotional resistance of patients and their families to accepting the implications of a poor prognosis. A practical solution to these barriers is to integrate palliative care with curative care regardless of prognosis. With this approach, palliative care no longer conveys the message of failure, having no more treatments, or "giving up hope." Fundamental to integrating palliative care with curative therapy is to include continuous goal assessment as part of the routine patient reassessment that occurs at most patient–physician encounters.

Goals for care are numerous, ranging from cure of a specific disease, to prolonging life, to relief of a

TABLE 32-2

ELEMENTS OF COMMUNICATING BAD NEWS—THE P-SPIKES APPROACH

ACRONYM	STEPS	AIM OF THE INTERACTION	PREPARATIONS, QUESTIONS, OR PHRASES
P	Preparation	Mentally prepare for the interaction with the patient and/or family.	Review what information needs to be communicated. Plan how you will provide emotional support. Rehearse key steps and phrases in the interaction.
S	Setting of the interaction	Ensure the appropriate setting for a serious and potentially emotionally charged discussion.	Ensure that patient, family, and appropriate social supports are present. Devote sufficient time. Ensure privacy and prevent interruptions by people or beeper. Bring a box of tissues.
P	Patient's perception and preparation	Begin the discussion by establishing the baseline and whether the patient and family can grasp the information. Ease tension by having the patient and family contribute.	Start with open-ended questions to encourage participation. Possible phrases to use: *What do you understand about your illness?* *When you first had symptom X, what did you think it might be?* *What did Dr. X tell you when he or she sent you here?* *What do you think is going to happen?*
I	Invitation and information needs	Discover what information needs the patient and/or family have and what limits they want regarding the bad information.	Possible phrases to use: *If this condition turns out to be something serious, do you want to know?* *Would you like me to tell you all the details of your condition? If not, who would you like me to talk to?*
K	Knowledge of the condition	Provide the bad news or other information to the patient and/or family sensitively.	Do not just dump the information on the patient and family. Check for patient and family understanding. Possible phrases to use: *I feel badly to have to tell you this, but. . .* *Unfortunately, the tests showed. . .* *I'm afraid the news is not good. . .*
E	Empathy and exploration	Identify the cause of the emotions—e.g., poor prognosis. Empathize with the patient and/or family's feelings. Explore by asking open-ended questions.	Strong feelings in reaction to bad news are normal. Acknowledge what the patient and family are feeling. Remind them such feelings are normal, even if frightening. Give them time to respond. Remind patient and family you wont abandon them. Possible phrases to use: *I imagine this is very hard for you to hear.* *You look very upset. Tell me how you are feeling.* *I wish the news were different.* *We'll do whatever we can to help you.*
S	Summary and planning	Delineate for the patient and the family the next steps, including additional tests or interventions.	It is the unknown and uncertain that can increase anxiety. Recommend a schedule with goals and landmarks. Provide your rationale for the patient and/or family to accept (or reject). If the patient and/or family is not ready to discuss the next steps, schedule a follow-up visit.

Source: Adapted from R Buckman: *How to Break Bad News: A Guide for Health Care Professionals.* Baltimore, Johns Hopkins University Press, 1992.

symptom, to delaying the course of an incurable disease, to adapting to progressive disability without disrupting the family, to finding peace of mind or personal meaning, to dying in a manner that leaves loved ones with positive memories. Discernment of goals for care can be approached through a seven-step protocol: (1) ensure that medical and other information is as complete as reasonably possible and is understood by all relevant parties (see earlier discussion); (2) explore what the patient and/or family are hoping for while identifying relevant and realistic goals; (3) share all the options with the patient and family; (4) respond with empathy as they adjust to changing expectations; (5) make a plan, emphasizing what can be done toward achieving the realistic goals; (6) follow through with the plan; and (7) review and revise the plan periodically, considering at every encounter whether the goals of care should be reviewed with the patient and/or family. Each of these steps need not be followed in rote order, but together they provide a helpful framework for interactions with patients and their families about goals for care. It can be especially challenging if a patient or family member has difficulty letting go of an unrealistic goal. One strategy is to help them refocus on more realistic goals and suggest that while hoping for the best, it is still prudent to plan for other outcomes as well.

Advance care planning

Practices

Advance care planning is a process of planning for future medical care in case the patient becomes incapable of making medical decisions. A 2010 study of adults 60 years of age or older who died between 2000 and 2006 found that 42% required decision-making about treatment in the final days of life but 70% lacked decision-making capacity. Among those lacking decision-making capacity, around one-third did not have advance planning directives. Ideally, such planning would occur before a health care crisis or the terminal phase of an illness. Unfortunately, diverse barriers prevent this. Although 80% of Americans endorse advance care planning and completing living wills, only 47% have actually done so. Most patients expect physicians to initiate advance care planning and wait for physicians to broach the subject. Patients also wish to discuss advance care planning with their families. Yet patients with unrealistic expectations are significantly more likely to prefer aggressive treatments. Fewer than one-third of health care providers have completed advance care planning for themselves. Hence, a good first step is for health care providers to complete their own advance care planning. This makes providers aware of the critical choices in the process and the issues that are especially charged and allows them to tell their patients truthfully that they personally have done advance planning.

Steps in effective advance care planning center on (1) introducing the topic, (2) structuring a discussion, (3) reviewing plans that have been discussed by the patient and family, (4) documenting the plans, (5) updating them periodically, and (6) implementing the advance care directives (Table 32-3). Two of the main barriers to advance care planning are problems in raising the topic and difficulty in structuring a succinct discussion. Raising the topic can be done efficiently as a routine matter, noting that it is recommended for all patients, analogous to purchasing insurance or estate planning. Many of the most difficult cases have involved unexpected, acute episodes of brain damage in young individuals.

Structuring a focused discussion is a central communication skill. Identify the health care proxy and recommend his or her involvement in the process of advance care planning. Select a worksheet, preferably one that has been evaluated and demonstrated to produce reliable and valid expressions of patient preferences, and orient the patient and proxy to it. Such worksheets exist for both general and disease-specific situations. Discuss with the patient and proxy one scenario as an example to demonstrate how to think about the issues. It is often helpful to begin with a scenario in which the patient is likely to have settled preferences for care, such as being in a persistent vegetative state. Once the patient's preferences for interventions in this scenario are determined, suggest that the patient and proxy discuss and complete the worksheet for the others. If appropriate, suggest that the patient involve other family members in the discussion. On a return visit, go over the patient's preferences, checking and resolving any inconsistencies. After having the patient and proxy sign the document, place it in the medical chart and be sure that copies are provided to relevant family members and care sites. Since patients preferences can change, these documents have to be reviewed periodically.

Types of documents

Advance care planning documents are of two broad types. The first includes living wills or instructional directives; these are advisory documents that describe the types of decisions that should direct care. Some are more specific, delineating different scenarios and interventions for the patient to choose from. Among these, some are for general use, and others are designed for use by patients with a specific type of disease, such as cancer or HIV. Less specific directives can be general statements of not wanting life-sustaining interventions or forms that describe the values that should guide specific discussions about terminal care. The second type of advance directive allows the designation of a health care proxy (sometimes also referred to as a durable attorney for health care), who is an individual selected by the patient to make decisions. The choice is not either/or; a combined directive that includes a living will and designates a proxy is often used, and the directive should indicate clearly whether the specified patient's preferences or the proxy's choice takes precedence if they conflict. Some states have begun to put into practice a "Physician Orders for Life-Sustaining Treatment (POLST)" paradigm, which builds on communication between providers and patients to include guidance for end-of-life care in a color-coordinated form that follows the patient across treatment settings.

TABLE 32-3
STEPS IN ADVANCE CARE PLANNING

STEP	GOALS TO BE ACHIEVED AND MEASURES TO COVER	USEFUL PHRASES OR POINTS TO MAKE
Introducing advance care planning	Ask the patient what he or she knows about advance care planning and if he or she has already completed an advance care directive. Indicate that you as a physician have completed advance care planning. Indicate that you try to perform advance care planning with all patients regardless of prognosis. Explain the goals of the process as empowering the patient and ensuring that you and the proxy understand the patients preferences. Provide the patient relevant literature, including the advance care directive that you prefer to use. Recommend the patient identify a proxy decision-maker who should attend the next meeting.	*I'd like to talk with you about something I try to discuss with all my patients. It's called advance care planning. In fact, I feel that this is such an important topic that I have done this myself. Are you familiar with advance care planning or living wills?* *Have you thought about the type of care you would want if you ever became too sick to speak for yourself? That is the purpose of advance care planning.* *There is no change in health that we have not discussed. I am bringing this up now because it is sensible for everyone, no matter how well or ill, old or young.* I have many copies of advance care directives available, including in the waiting room, for patients and families. Know resources for state-specific forms (available at *www.nhpco.org*).
Structured discussion of scenarios and patient	Affirm that the goal of the process is to follow the patient's wishes if the patient loses decision-making capacity. Elicit the patient's overall goals related to health care. Elicit the patient's preferences for specific interventions in a few salient and common scenarios. Help the patient define the threshold for withdrawing and withholding interventions. Define the patient's preference for the role of the proxy.	Use a structured worksheet with typical scenarios. Begin the discussion with persistent vegetative state and consider other scenarios, such as recovery from an acute event with serious disability, asking the patient about his or her preferences regarding specific interventions, such as ventilators, artificial nutrition, and CPR, and then proceeding to less invasive interventions, such as blood transfusions and antibiotics.
Review the patients preferences	After the patient has made choices of interventions, review them to ensure they are consistent and the proxy is aware of them.	
Document the patients preferences	Formally complete the advance care directive and have a witness sign it. Provide a copy for the patient and the proxy. Insert a copy into the patient's medical record and summarize in a progress note.	
Update the directive	Periodically, and with major changes in health status, review the directive with the patient and make any modifications.	
Apply the directive	The directive goes into effect only when the patient becomes unable to make medical decisions for himself or herself. Reread the directive to be sure about its content. Discuss your proposed actions based on the directive with the proxy.	

Abbreviation: CPR, cardiopulmonary resuscitation.

The procedures for completing advance care planning documents vary according to state law.

A potentially misleading distinction relates to statutory as opposed to advisory documents. Statutory documents are drafted to fulfill relevant state laws. Advisory documents are drafted to reflect the patient's wishes. Both are legal, the first under state law and the latter under common or constitutional law.

Legal aspects

As of 2006, 48 states and the District of Columbia had enacted living will legislation. Many states have their own statutory forms. Massachusetts and Michigan do not have living will laws, although both have health care proxy laws. In 25 states, the laws state that the living will is not valid if a woman is pregnant. However, like all other states except Alaska, these states have enacted durable power of attorney for health care laws that permit patients to designate a proxy decision-maker with authority to terminate life-sustaining treatments. Only in Alaska does the law prohibit proxies from terminating life-sustaining treatments. The health reform legislation, the Affordable Care Act of 2010, raised substantial controversy when early versions of the law included Medicare reimbursement for advance care planning consultations. These provisions were withdrawn over accusations that they would lead to the rationing of care for the elderly.

The U.S. Supreme Court has ruled that patients have a constitutional right to decide about refusing and terminating medical interventions, including life-sustaining interventions, and that mentally incompetent patients can exercise this right by providing "clear and convincing evidence" of their preferences. Since advance care directives permit patients to provide such evidence, commentators agree that they are constitutionally protected. Most commentators believe that a state is required to honor any clear advance care directive whether or not it is written on an "official" form. Many states have enacted laws explicitly to honor out-of-state directives. If a patient is not using a statutory form, it may be advisable to attach a statutory form to the advance care directive being used. State-specific forms are readily available free of charge for health care providers and patients and families through the website of the National Hospice and Palliative Care Organization (*www.nhpco.org*).

INTERVENTIONS

PHYSICAL SYMPTOMS AND THEIR MANAGEMENT

Great emphasis has been placed on addressing dying patients pain. Some institutions have made pain assessment a fifth vital sign to emphasize its importance. This also has been advocated by large health care systems such as the Veterans Administration and accrediting bodies such as The Joint Commission. Although this embrace of pain as the fifth vital sign has been symbolically important, no data document that it has improved pain management practices. Although good palliative care requires good pain management, it also requires more. The frequency of symptoms varies by disease and other factors. The most common physical and psychological symptoms among all terminally ill patients include pain, fatigue, insomnia, anorexia, dyspnea, depression, anxiety, and nausea and vomiting. In the last days of life, terminal delirium is also common. Assessments of patients with advanced cancer have shown that patients experienced an average of 11.5 different physical and psychological symptoms (Table 32-4).

TABLE 32-4

COMMON PHYSICAL AND PSYCHOLOGICAL SYMPTOMS OF TERMINALLY ILL PATIENTS

PHYSICAL SYMPTOMS	PSYCHOLOGICAL SYMPTOMS
Pain	Anxiety
Fatigue and weakness	Depression
Dyspnea	Hopelessness
Insomnia	Meaninglessness
Dry mouth	Irritability
Anorexia	Impaired concentration
Nausea and vomiting	Confusion
Constipation	Delirium
Cough	Loss of libido
Swelling of arms or legs	
Itching	
Diarrhea	
Dysphagia	
Dizziness	
Fecal and urinary incontinence	
Numbness or tingling in the hands or feet	

Evaluations to determine the etiology of these symptoms usually can be limited to the history and physical examination. In some cases, radiologic or other diagnostic examinations will provide sufficient benefit in directing optimal palliative care to warrant the risks, potential discomfort, and inconvenience, especially to a seriously ill patient. Only a few of the common symptoms that present difficult management issues will be addressed in this chapter. Additional information on the management of other symptoms, such as nausea and vomiting can be found in Chap. 26.

Pain

Frequency

The frequency of pain among terminally ill patients varies widely. Substantial pain occurs in 36–90% of patients with advanced cancer. In the SUPPORT study of hospitalized patients with diverse conditions and an estimated survival ≤6 months, 22% reported moderate to severe pain, and caregivers of those patients noted that 50% had similar levels of pain during the last few days of life. A meta-analysis found pain prevalence of 58–69% in studies that included patients characterized as having advanced, metastatic, or terminal cancer; 44–73% in studies that included patients characterized as undergoing cancer treatment; and 21–46% in studies that included posttreatment individuals.

Etiology

Nociceptive pain is the result of direct mechanical or chemical stimulation of nociceptors and normal neural signaling to the brain. It tends to be localized, aching, throbbing, and cramping. The classic example is bone metastases. *Visceral pain* is caused by nociceptors in gastrointestinal (GI), respiratory, and other organ systems. It is a deep or colicky type of pain classically associated with pancreatitis, myocardial infarction, or tumor invasion of viscera. *Neuropathic pain* arises from disordered nerve signals. It is described by patients as burning, electrical, or shocklike pain. Classic examples are post-stroke pain, tumor invasion of the brachial plexus, and herpetic neuralgia.

Assessment

Pain is a subjective experience. Depending on the patient's circumstances, perspective, and physiologic condition, the same physical lesion or disease state can produce different levels of reported pain and need for pain relief. Systematic assessment includes eliciting the following: (1) type: throbbing, cramping, burning, etc.; (2) periodicity: continuous, with or without exacerbations, or incident; (3) location; (4) intensity; (5) modifying factors; (6) effects of treatments; (7) functional impact; and (8) impact on patient. Several validated pain assessment measures may be used, such as the Visual Analogue Scale, the Brief Pain Inventory, and the pain component of one of the more comprehensive symptom assessment instruments. Frequent reassessments are essential to assess the effects of interventions.

Interventions

Interventions for pain must be tailored to each individual, with the goal of preempting chronic pain and relieving breakthrough pain. At the end of life, there is rarely reason to doubt a patient's report of pain. Pain medications are the cornerstone of management. If they are failing and nonpharmacologic interventions—including radiotherapy and anesthetic or neurosurgical procedures such as peripheral nerve blocks or epidural medications—are required, a pain consultation is appropriate.

Pharmacologic interventions follow the World Health Organization three-step approach involving nonopioid analgesics, mild opioids, and strong opioids, with or without adjuvants. Nonopioid analgesics, especially nonsteroidal anti-inflammatory drugs (NSAIDs), are the initial treatments for mild pain. They work primarily by inhibiting peripheral prostaglandins and reducing inflammation but also may have central nervous system (CNS) effects. They have a ceiling effect. Ibuprofen, up to 1600 mg/d qid, has a minimal risk of causing bleeding and renal impairment and is a good initial choice. In patients with a history of severe GI or other bleeding, it should be avoided. In patients with a history of mild gastritis or gastroesophageal reflux disease (GERD), acid-lowering therapy such as a proton pump inhibitor should be used. Acetaminophen is an alternative in patients with a history of GI bleeding and can be used safely at up to 4 g/d qid. In patients with liver dysfunction due to metastases or other causes and in patients with heavy alcohol use, doses should be reduced.

If nonopioid analgesics are insufficient, opioids should be introduced. They work by interacting with mu opioid receptors in the CNS to activate pain-inhibitory neurons; most are receptor antagonists. The mixed agonist/antagonist opioids useful for post-acute pain should not be used for the chronic pain in end-of-life care. Weak opioids such as codeine can be used initially. However, if they are escalated and fail to relieve pain, strong opioids such as morphine, 5–10 mg every 4 h, should be used. Nonopioid analgesics should be combined with opioids because they potentiate the effect of opioids.

For continuous pain, opioids should be administered on a regular, around-the-clock basis consistent with their duration of analgesia. They should not be provided only when the patient experiences pain; the goal is to prevent patients from experiencing pain. Patients also should be provided rescue medication, such as liquid morphine, for breakthrough pain, generally at 20% of the baseline dose. Patients should be informed that using the rescue medication does not obviate the need to take the next standard dose of pain medication. If after 24 h the patient's pain remains uncontrolled and recurs before the next dose, requiring the patient to utilize the rescue medication, the daily opioid dose can be increased by the total dose of rescue medications used by the patient or by 50% for moderate pain and 100% for severe pain of the standing opioid daily dose.

It is inappropriate to start with extended-release preparations. Instead, an initial focus on using short-acting preparations to determine how much is required in the first 24–48 h will allow clinicians to determine opioid needs. Once pain relief is obtained with short-acting preparations, one should switch to extended-release preparations. Even with a stable extended-release preparation regimen, the patient may have incident pain, such as during movement or dressing changes. Short-acting preparations should be taken before such predictable episodes. Although less common, patients may have "end-of-dose failure" with long-acting opioids, meaning that they develop pain after 8 h in the case of an every-12-h medication. In these cases, a trial of giving an every-12-h medication every 8 h is appropriate.

Because of differences in opioid receptors, cross-tolerance among opioids is incomplete, and patients may experience different side effects with different opioids. Therefore, if a patient is not experiencing pain relief or is experiencing too many side effects, a change to another opioid preparation is appropriate. When switching, one should begin with 50–75% of the published equianalgesic dose of the new opioid.

Unlike NSAIDs, opioids have no ceiling effect; therefore, there is no maximum dose no matter how many milligrams the patient is receiving. The appropriate dose is the dose needed to achieve pain relief. This is an important point for clinicians to explain to patients and families. Addiction or excessive respiratory depression is extremely unlikely in terminally ill individuals; fear of these side effects should neither prevent escalating opioid medications when the patient is experiencing insufficient pain relief nor justify using opioid antagonists.

Opioid side effects should be anticipated and treated preemptively. Nearly all patients experience constipation that can be debilitating (see later discussion). Failure to prevent constipation often results in noncompliance with opioid therapy. Methylnaltrexone is a drug that targets opioid-induced constipation by blocking peripheral opioid receptors but not central receptors for analgesia. In placebo-controlled trials, it has been shown to cause laxation within 24 h of administration. As with the use of opioids, about one-third of patients using methylnaltrexone experience nausea and vomiting, but unlike constipation, tolerance develops, usually within 1 week. Therefore, when one is beginning opioids, an antiemetic such as metoclopramide or a serotonin antagonist often is prescribed prophylactically and stopped after 1 week. Olanzapine also has been shown to have antinausea properties and can be effective in countering delirium or anxiety, with the advantage of some weight gain.

Drowsiness, a common side effect of opioids, also usually abates within 1 week. During this period, drowsiness can be treated with psychostimulants such as dextroamphetamine, methylphenidate, and modafinil. Modafinil has the advantage of everyday dosing. Pilot reports suggest that donepezil may also be helpful for opiate-induced drowsiness as well as relieving fatigue and anxiety. Metabolites of morphine and most opioids are cleared renally; doses may have to be adjusted for patients with renal failure.

Seriously ill patients who require chronic pain relief rarely if ever become addicted. Suspicion of addiction should not be a reason to withhold pain medications from terminally ill patients. Patients and families may withhold prescribed opioids for fear of addiction or dependence. Physicians and health care providers should reassure patients and families that the patient will not become addicted to opioids if they are used as prescribed for pain relief; this fear should not prevent the patient from taking the medications around the clock. However, diversion of drugs for use by other family members or illicit sale may occur. It may be necessary to advise the patient and caregiver about secure storage of opioids. Contract writing with the patient and family can help. If that fails, transfer to a safe facility may be necessary.

Tolerance is the need to increase medication dosage for the same pain relief without a change in disease. In the case of patients with advanced disease, the need for increasing opioid dosage for pain relief usually is caused by disease progression rather than tolerance. Physical dependence is indicated by symptoms from the abrupt withdrawal of opioids and should not be confused with addiction.

Adjuvant analgesic medications are nonopioids that potentiate the analgesic effects of opioids. They are especially important in the management of neuropathic pain. Gabapentin, an anticonvulsant initially studied in the setting of herpetic neuralgia, is now the first-line treatment for neuropathic pain from a variety of causes. It is begun at 100–300 mg bid or tid, with 50–100% dose increments every 3 days. Usually 900–3600 mg/d in two or three doses is effective. The combination of gabapentin and nortriptyline may be more effective than gabapentin alone. One potential side effect of gabapentin to be aware of is confusion and drowsiness, especially in the elderly. Other effective adjuvant medications include pregabalin, which has the same mechanism of action as gabapentin but is absorbed more efficiently from the GI tract. Lamotrigine is a novel agent whose mechanism of action is unknown, but it has shown effectiveness. It is recommended to begin at 25–50 mg/d, increasing to 100 mg/d. Carbamazepine, a first-generation agent, has been proved effective in randomized trials for neuropathic pain. Other potentially effective anticonvulsant adjuvants include topiramate (25–50 mg qd or bid, rising to 100–300 mg/d) and oxcarbazepine (75–300 mg bid, rising to 1200 mg bid). Glucocorticoids, preferably dexamethasone given once a day, can be useful in reducing inflammation that causes pain while elevating mood, energy, and appetite. Its main side effects include confusion, sleep difficulties, and fluid retention. Glucocorticoids are especially effective for bone pain and abdominal pain from distention of the GI tract or liver. Other drugs, including clonidine and baclofen, can be effective in pain relief. These drugs are adjuvants and generally should be used in conjunction with—not instead of—opioids. Methadone, carefully dosed because of its unpredictable half-life in many patients, has activity at the *N*-methyl-D-aspartamate (NMDA) receptor and is useful for complex pain syndromes and neuropathic pain. It generally is reserved for cases in which first-line opioids (morphine, oxycodone, hydromorphone) are either ineffective or unavailable.

Radiation therapy can treat bone pain from single metastatic lesions. Bone pain from multiple metastases can be amenable to radiopharmaceuticals such as strontium 89 and samarium 153. Bisphosphonates (such as pamidronate [90 mg every 4 weeks]) and calcitonin

(200 IU intranasally once or twice a day) also provide relief from bone pain but have onset of action of days.

Constipation

Frequency

Constipation is reported in up to 87% of patients requiring palliative care.

Etiology

Although hypercalcemia and other factors can cause constipation, it is most frequently a predictable consequence of the use of opioids for the relief of pain and dyspnea and of tricyclic antidepressants, from their anticholinergic effects, as well as of the inactivity and poor diet that are common among seriously ill patients. If untreated, constipation can cause substantial pain and vomiting and also is associated with confusion and delirium. Whenever opioids and other medications known to cause constipation are used, preemptive treatment for constipation should be instituted.

Assessment

The physician should establish the patient's previous bowel habits, including the frequency, consistency, and volume. Abdominal and rectal examinations should be performed to exclude impaction or acute abdomen. A number of constipation assessment scales are available, although guidelines issued in the *Journal of Palliative Medicine* did not recommend them for routine practice. Four commonly used assessment scales are the Bristol Stool Form Scale, the Constipation Assessment Scale, the Constipation Visual Analogue Scale, and the Eton Scale Risk Assessment for Constipation. Radiographic assessments beyond a simple flat plate of the abdomen in cases in which obstruction is suspected are rarely necessary.

Intervention

Intervention to reestablish comfortable bowel habits and relieve pain and discomfort should be the goals of any measures to address constipation during end-of-life care. Although physical activity, adequate hydration, and dietary treatments with fiber can be helpful, each is limited in its effectiveness for most seriously ill patients, and fiber may exacerbate problems in the setting of dehydration and if impaired motility is the etiology. Fiber is contraindicated in the presence of opioid use. Stimulant and osmotic laxatives, stool softeners, fluids, and enemas are the mainstays of therapy (Table 32-5). In preventing constipation from opioids and other medications, a combination of a laxative and a stool softener (such as senna and docusate) should be used. If after several days of treatment a bowel movement has not occurred, a rectal examination to remove impacted stool and place a suppository is necessary. For patients with impending bowel obstruction or gastric stasis, octreotide to reduce secretions can be helpful. For patients in whom the suspected mechanism is dysmotility, metoclopramide can be helpful.

Nausea

Frequency

Up to 70% of patients with advanced cancer have nausea, defined as the subjective sensation of wanting to vomit.

Etiology

Nausea and vomiting are both caused by stimulation at one of four sites: the GI tract, the vestibular system, the chemoreceptor trigger zone (CTZ), and the cerebral cortex. Medical treatments for nausea are aimed at receptors at each of these sites: The GI tract contains

TABLE 32-5

MEDICATIONS FOR THE MANAGEMENT OF CONSTIPATION

INTERVENTION	DOSE	COMMENT
Stimulant laxatives		These agents directly stimulate peristalsis and may reduce colonic absorption of water.
Prune juice	120–240 mL/d	
Senna (Senokot)	2–8 tablets PO bid	Works in 6–12 h.
Bisacodyl	5–15 mg/d PO, PR	
Osmotic laxatives		These agents are not absorbed. They attract and retain water in the gastrointestinal tract.
Lactulose	15–30 mL PO q4–8h	
Magnesium hydroxide (Milk of Magnesia)	15–30 mL/d PO	Lactulose may cause flatulence and bloating.
Magnesium citrate	125–250 mL/d PO	Lactulose works in 1 day, magnesium products in 6 h.
Stool softeners		These agents work by increasing water secretion and as detergents, increasing water penetration into the stool.
Sodium docusate (Colace)	300–600 mg/d PO	
Calcium docusate	300–600 mg/d PO	Work in 1–3 days.
Suppositories and enemas		
Bisacodyl	10–15 PR qd	
Sodium phosphate enema	PR qd	Fixed dose, 4.5 oz, Fleets.

Abbreviations: bid, twice a day; PO, oral; PR, per rectum; qd, every day.

mechanoreceptors, chemoreceptors, and 5-hydroxytryptamine type 3 (5-HT3) receptors; the vestibular system probably contains histamine and acetylcholine receptors; and the CTZ contains chemoreceptors, dopamine type 2 receptors, and 5-HT3 receptors. An example of nausea that most likely is mediated by the cortex is anticipatory nausea before a dose of chemotherapy or other noxious stimuli.

Specific causes of nausea include metabolic changes (liver failure, uremia from renal failure, hypercalcemia), bowel obstruction, constipation, infection, GERD, vestibular disease, brain metastases, medications (including antibiotics, NSAIDs, proton pump inhibitors, opioids, and chemotherapy), and radiation therapy. Anxiety can also contribute to nausea.

Intervention

Medical treatment of nausea is directed at the anatomic and receptor-mediated cause that a careful history and physical examination reveals. When a single specific cause is not found, many advocate beginning treatment with a dopamine antagonist such as haloperidol or prochlorperazine. Prochlorperazine is usually more sedating than haloperidol. When decreased motility is suspected, metoclopramide can be an effective treatment. When inflammation of the GI tract is suspected, glucocorticoids such as dexamethasone are an appropriate treatment. For nausea that follows chemotherapy and radiation therapy, one of the 5-HT3 receptor antagonists (ondansetron, granisetron, dolasetron) is recommended. Clinicians should attempt prevention of postchemotherapy nausea rather than provide treatment after the fact. Current clinical guidelines recommend tailoring the strength of treatments to the specific emetic risk posed by a specific chemotherapy drug. When a vestibular cause (such as "motion sickness" or labyrinthitis) is suspected, antihistamines such as meclizine (whose primary side effect is drowsiness) or anticholinergics such as scopolamine can be effective. In anticipatory nausea, a benzodiazepine such as lorazepam is indicated. As with antihistamines, drowsiness and confusion are the main side effects.

Dyspnea

Frequency

Dyspnea is a subjective experience of being short of breath. Nearly 75% of dying patients experience dyspnea at some point in their illness. Dyspnea is among the most distressing physical symptoms and can be even more distressing than pain.

Assessment

As with pain, dyspnea is a subjective experience that may not correlate with objective measures of P_{O_2}, P_{CO_2}, or respiratory rate. Consequently, measurements of oxygen saturation through pulse oximetry or blood gases are rarely helpful in guiding therapy. Despite the limitations of existing assessment methods, physicians should regularly assess and document patients' experience of dyspnea and its intensity. Guidelines recommend visual or analogue dyspnea scales to assess the severity of symptoms and the effects of treatment. Potentially reversible or treatable causes of dyspnea include infection, pleural effusions, pulmonary emboli, pulmonary edema, asthma, and tumor encroachment on the airway. However, the risk-versus-benefit ratio of the diagnostic and therapeutic interventions for patients with little time left to live must be considered carefully before one undertakes diagnostic steps. Frequently, the specific etiology cannot be identified, and dyspnea is the consequence of progression of the underlying disease that cannot be treated. The anxiety caused by dyspnea and the choking sensation can significantly exacerbate the underlying dyspnea in a negatively reinforcing cycle.

Interventions

When reversible or treatable etiologies are diagnosed, they should be treated as long as the side effects of treatment, such as repeated drainage of effusions or anticoagulants, are less burdensome than the dyspnea itself. More aggressive treatments such as stenting a bronchial lesion may be warranted if it is clear that the dyspnea is due to tumor invasion at that site and if the patient and family understand the risks of such a procedure. Usually, treatment will be symptomatic (Table 32-6). A dyspnea scale and careful monitoring should guide dose adjustment. Low-dose opioids reduce the sensitivity of the central respiratory center and the sensation of dyspnea. If patients are not receiving opioids, weak opioids can be initiated; if patients are already receiving opioids, morphine or other strong opioids should be used. Controlled trials do not support the use of nebulized opioids for dyspnea at the end of life. Phenothiazines and chlorpromazine may be helpful when combined with opioids. Benzodiazepines can be helpful if anxiety is present but should be neither used as first-line therapy nor used alone in the treatment of dyspnea. If the patient has a history of COPD or asthma, inhaled bronchodilators and glucocorticoids may be helpful. If the patient has pulmonary edema due to heart failure, diuresis with a medication such as furosemide is indicated. Excess secretions can be dried with scopolamine, transdermally or intravenously. Oxygen can be used, although it may only be an expensive placebo. For some families and patients, oxygen is distressing; for others, it is reassuring. More general interventions that medical staff can do include sitting the patient upright, removing smoke or other irritants such as perfume, ensuring a supply of fresh air with sufficient humidity, and minimizing other factors that can increase anxiety.

TABLE 32-6

MEDICATIONS FOR THE MANAGEMENT OF DYSPNEA

INTERVENTION	DOSE	COMMENTS
Weak opioids		For patients with mild dyspnea
Codeine (or codeine with 325 mg acetaminophen)	30 mg PO q4h	For opioid-naïve patients
Hydrocodone	5 mg PO q4h	
Strong opioids		For opioid-naïve patients with moderate to severe dyspnea
Morphine	5–10 mg PO q4h	
	30–50% of baseline opioid dose q4h	For patients already taking opioids for pain or other symptoms
Oxycodone	5–10 mg PO q4h	
Hydromorphone	1–2 mg PO q4h	
Anxiolytics		Give a dose every hour until the patient is relaxed; then provide a dose for maintenance
Lorazepam	0.5–2.0 mg PO/SL/IV qh then q4–6h	
Clonazepam	0.25–2.0 mg PO q12h	
Midazolam	0.5 mg IV q15min	

Abbreviations: IV, intravenous; PO, oral; SL, sublingual.

Fatigue

Frequency

More than 90% of terminally ill patients experience fatigue and/or weakness. Fatigue is one of the most commonly reported symptoms of cancer treatment as well as in the palliative care of multiple sclerosis, COPD, heart failure, and HIV. Fatigue frequently is cited as among the most distressing symptoms.

Etiology

The multiple causes of fatigue in terminally ill individuals can be categorized as resulting from the underlying disease; from disease-induced factors such as tumor necrosis factor and other cytokines; and from secondary factors such as dehydration, anemia, infection, hypothyroidism, and drug side effects. Apart from low caloric intake, loss of muscle mass and changes in muscle enzymes may play important roles in fatigue of terminal illness. The importance of changes in the CNS, especially the reticular activating system, have been hypothesized based on reports of fatigue in patients receiving cranial radiation, experiencing depression, or having chronic pain in the absence of cachexia or other physiologic changes. Finally, depression and other causes of psychological distress can contribute to fatigue.

Assessment

Fatigue is subjective; objective changes, even in body mass, may be absent. Consequently, assessment must rely on patient self-reporting. Scales used to measure fatigue, such as the Edmonton Functional Assessment Tool, the Fatigue Self-Report Scales, and the Rhoten Fatigue Scale, are usually appropriate for research rather than clinical purposes. In clinical practice, a simple performance assessment such as the Karnofsky Performance Status or the Eastern Cooperative Oncology Group's question: "How much of the day does the patient spend in bed?" may be the best measure. In this 0–4 performance status assessment, 0 = normal activity; 1 = symptomatic without being bedridden; 2 = requiring some but <50%, bed time; 3 = bedbound more than half the day; and 4 = bedbound all the time. Such a scale allows for assessment over time and correlates with overall disease severity and prognosis. A 2008 review by the European Association of Palliative Care also described several longer assessment tools with 9–20 items, including the Piper Fatigue Inventory, the Multidimensional Fatigue Inventory, and the Brief Fatigue Inventory (BFI).

Interventions

At the end of life, fatigue will not be "cured." The goal is to ameliorate it and help patients and families adjust expectations. Behavioral interventions should be utilized to avoid blaming the patient for inactivity and to educate both the family and the patient that the underlying disease causes physiologic changes that produce low energy levels. Understanding that the problem is physiologic and not psychological can help alter expectations regarding the patient's level of physical activity. Practically, this may mean reducing routine activities such as housework and cooking or social events outside the house and making it acceptable to receive guests lying on a couch. At the same time, institution of exercise regimens and physical therapy can raise endorphins, reduce muscle wasting, and reduce the risk of depression. In addition, ensuring good hydration without worsening edema may help reduce fatigue. Discontinuing medications that worsen fatigue may help, including cardiac medications, benzodiazepines, certain antidepressants, or opioids if pain is well-controlled. As end-of-life care proceeds into its final stages, fatigue may protect patients from further suffering, and continued treatment could be detrimental.

Only a few pharmacologic interventions target fatigue and weakness. Glucocorticoids can increase energy and enhance mood. Dexamethasone is preferred for its once-a-day dosing and minimal mineralocorticoid activity. Benefit, if any, usually is seen within the first month. Psychostimulants such as dextroamphetamine (5–10 mg orally [PO]) and methylphenidate (2.5–5 mg PO) may also enhance energy levels, although a randomized trial did not show methylphenidate beneficial compared with placebo in cancer fatigue. Doses should be given in the morning and at noon to minimize the risk of counterproductive insomnia. Modafinil, developed for narcolepsy, has shown some promise in the treatment of fatigue and has the advantage of once-daily dosing. Its precise role in fatigue at the end of life has not been determined. Anecdotal evidence suggests that l-carnitine may improve fatigue, depression, and sleep disruption.

PSYCHOLOGICAL SYMPTOMS AND THEIR MANAGEMENT

Depression

Frequency

Depression at the end of life presents an apparently paradoxical situation. Many people believe that depression is normal among seriously ill patients because they are dying. People frequently say, "Wouldnt you be depressed?" However, depression is not a necessary part of terminal illness and can contribute to needless suffering. Although sadness, anxiety, anger, and irritability are normal responses to a serious condition, they are typically of modest intensity and transient. Persistent sadness and anxiety and the physically disabling symptoms that they can lead to are abnormal and suggestive of major depression. Although as many as 75% of terminally ill patients experience depressive symptoms, <25% of terminally ill patients have major depression.

Etiology

Previous history of depression, family history of depression or bipolar disorder, and prior suicide attempts are associated with increased risk for depression among terminally ill patients. Other symptoms, such as pain and fatigue, are associated with higher rates of depression; uncontrolled pain can exacerbate depression, and depression can cause patients to be more distressed by pain. Many medications used in the terminal stages, including glucocorticoids, and some anticancer agents, such as tamoxifen, interleukin 2, interferon α, and vincristine, also are associated with depression. Some terminal conditions, such as pancreatic cancer, certain strokes, and heart failure, have been reported to be associated with higher rates of depression, although this is controversial. Finally, depression may be attributable to grief over the loss of a role or function, social isolation, or loneliness.

Assessment

Diagnosing depression among seriously ill patients is complicated because many of the vegetative symptoms in the DSM-IV (*Diagnostic and Statistical Manual of Mental Disorders*) criteria for clinical depression—insomnia, anorexia and weight loss, fatigue, decreased libido, and difficulty concentrating—are associated with the dying process itself. The assessment of depression in seriously ill patients therefore should focus on the dysphoric mood, helplessness, hopelessness, and lack of interest and enjoyment and concentration in normal activities. The single questions: "How often do you feel downhearted and blue?" (more than a good bit of the time or similar responses) and "Do you feel depressed most of the time?" are appropriate for screening.

Certain conditions may be confused with depression. Endocrinopathies such as hypothyroidism and Cushing's syndrome; electrolyte abnormalities such as hypercalcemia; and akathisia, especially from dopamine-blocking antiemetics such as metoclopramide and prochlorperazine, can mimic depression and should be excluded.

Interventions

Physicians must treat any physical symptom, such as pain, that may be causing or exacerbating depression. Fostering adaptation to the many losses that the patient is experiencing can also be helpful. Nonpharmacologic interventions, including group or individual psychological counseling, and behavioral therapies such as relaxation and imagery can be helpful, especially in combination with drug therapy.

Pharmacologic interventions remain the core of therapy. The same medications are used to treat depression in terminally ill as in non–terminally ill patients. Psychostimulants may be preferred for patients with a poor prognosis or for those with fatigue or opioid-induced somnolence. Psychostimulants are comparatively fast acting, working within a few days instead of the weeks required for selective serotonin reuptake inhibitors (SSRIs). Dextroamphetamine or methylphenidate should be started at 2.5–5.0 mg in the morning and at noon, the same starting doses used for treating fatigue. The dose can be escalated up to 15 mg bid. Modafinil is started at 100 mg qd and can be increased to 200 mg if there is no effect at the lower dose. Pemoline is a nonamphetamine psychostimulant with minimal abuse potential. It is also effective as an antidepressant beginning at 18.75 mg in the morning and at noon. Because it can be absorbed through the buccal mucosa, it is preferred for patients with intestinal obstruction or dysphagia. If it is used for prolonged periods, liver function must be monitored. The psychostimulants can also be combined with more traditional antidepressants while waiting for the antidepressants to become effective and then tapered after a few weeks if necessary. Psychostimulants have side effects, particularly initial anxiety, insomnia, and rarely paranoia, which may necessitate lowering the dose or discontinuing treatment.

Mirtazapine, an antagonist at the postsynaptic serotonin receptors, is a promising psychostimulant. It should be started at 7.5 mg before bed. It has sedating, antiemetic, and anxiolytic properties with few drug interactions. Its side effect of weight gain may be beneficial for seriously ill patients; it is available in orally disintegrating tablets.

For patients with a prognosis of several months or longer, SSRIs, including fluoxetine, sertraline, paroxetine and citalopram, and serotonin–noradrenaline reuptake inhibitors such as venlafaxine, are the preferred treatment because of their efficacy and comparatively few side effects. Because low doses of these medications may be effective for seriously ill patients, one should use half the usual starting dose for healthy adults. The starting dose for fluoxetine is 10 mg once a day. In most cases, once-a-day dosing is possible. The choice of which SSRI to use should be driven by (1) the patient's past success or failure with the specific medication and (2) the most favorable side-effect profile for that specific agent. For instance, for a patient in whom fatigue is a major symptom, a more activating SSRI (fluoxetine) would be appropriate. For a patient in whom anxiety and sleeplessness are major symptoms, a more sedating SSRI (paroxetine) would be appropriate.

Atypical antidepressants are recommended only in selected circumstances, usually with the assistance of a specialty consultation. Trazodone can be an effective antidepressant but is sedating and can cause orthostatic hypotension and, rarely, priapism. Therefore, it should be used only when a sedating effect is desired and is often used for patients with insomnia, at a dose starting at 25 mg. In addition to its antidepressant effects, bupropion is energizing, making it useful for depressed patients who experience fatigue. However, it can cause seizures, preventing its use for patients with a risk of CNS neoplasms or terminal delirium. Finally, alprazolam, a benzodiazepine, starting at 0.25–1.0 mg tid, can be effective in seriously ill patients who have a combination of anxiety and depression. Although it is potent and works quickly, it has many drug interactions and may cause delirium, especially among very ill patients, because of its strong binding to the benzodiazepine–γ-aminobutyric acid (GABA) receptor complex.

Unless used as adjuvants for the treatment of pain, tricyclic antidepressants are not recommended. Similarly, monoamine oxidase (MAO) inhibitors are not recommended because of their side effects and dangerous drug interactions.

Delirium

Frequency

In the weeks or months before death, delirium is uncommon, although it may be significantly underdiagnosed. However, delirium becomes relatively common in the hours and days immediately before death. Up to 85% of patients dying from cancer may experience terminal delirium.

Etiology

Delirium is a global cerebral dysfunction characterized by alterations in cognition and consciousness. It frequently is preceded by anxiety, changes in sleep patterns (especially reversal of day and night), and decreased attention. In contrast to dementia, delirium has an acute onset; is characterized by fluctuating consciousness and inattention; and is reversible, although reversibility may be more theoretical than real for patients near death. Delirium may occur in a patient with dementia; indeed, patients with dementia are more vulnerable to delirium.

Causes of delirium include metabolic encephalopathy arising from liver or renal failure, hypoxemia, or infection; electrolyte imbalances such as hypercalcemia; paraneoplastic syndromes; dehydration; and primary brain tumors, brain metastases, or leptomeningeal spread of tumor. Commonly, among dying patients, delirium can be caused by side effects of treatments, including radiation for brain metastases, and medications, including opioids, glucocorticoids, anticholinergic drugs, antihistamines, antiemetics, benzodiazepines, and chemotherapeutic agents. The etiology may be multifactorial; e.g., dehydration may exacerbate opioid-induced delirium.

Assessment

Delirium should be recognized in any terminally ill patient with a new onset of disorientation, impaired cognition, somnolence, fluctuating levels of consciousness, or delusions with or without agitation. Delirium must be distinguished from acute anxiety and depression as well as dementia. The central distinguishing feature is altered consciousness, which usually is not noted in anxiety, depression, and dementia. Although "hyperactive" delirium characterized by overt confusion and agitation is probably more common, patients also should be assessed for "hypoactive" delirium characterized by sleep–wake reversal and decreased alertness.

In some cases, use of formal assessment tools such as the Mini-Mental Status Examination (which does not distinguish delirium from dementia) and the Delirium Rating Scale (which does distinguish delirium from dementia) may be helpful in distinguishing delirium from other processes. The patients list of medications must be evaluated carefully. Nonetheless, a reversible etiologic factor for delirium is found in fewer than half of terminally ill patients. Because most terminally ill patients experiencing delirium will be very close to death and may be at home, extensive diagnostic evaluations such as lumbar punctures and neuroradiologic examinations are usually inappropriate.

Interventions

One of the most important objectives of terminal care is to provide terminally ill patients the lucidity to say goodbye to the people they love. Delirium, especially with agitation during the final days, is distressing to family and caregivers. A strong determinant of bereavement difficulties is witnessing a difficult death. Thus, terminal delirium should be treated aggressively.

At the first sign of delirium, such as day–night reversal with slight changes in mentation, the physician should let the family members know that it is time to be sure that everything they want to say has been said. The family should be informed that delirium is common just before death.

If medications are suspected of being a cause of the delirium, unnecessary agents should be discontinued. Other potentially reversible causes, such as constipation, urinary retention, and metabolic abnormalities, should be treated. Supportive measures aimed at providing a familiar environment should be instituted, including restricting visits only to individuals with whom the patient is familiar and eliminating new experiences; orienting the patient, if possible, by providing a clock and calendar; and gently correcting the patient's hallucinations or cognitive mistakes.

Pharmacologic management focuses on the use of neuroleptics and, in the extreme, anesthetics (Table 32-7). Haloperidol remains first-line therapy. Usually, patients can be controlled with a low dose (1–3 mg/d), usually given every 6 h, although some may require as much as 20 mg/d. It can be administered PO, subcutaneously, or intravenously (IV), Intramuscular injections should not be used, except when this is the only way to get a patient under control. Olanzapine, an atypical neuroleptic, has shown significant effectiveness in completely resolving delirium in cancer patients. It has other beneficial effects for terminally ill patients, including antinausea, antianxiety, and weight gain. It is useful for patients with longer anticipated life expectancies because it is less likely to cause dysphoria and has a lower risk of dystonic reactions. Also, because it is metabolized through multiple pathways, it can be used in patients with hepatic and renal dysfunction. Olanzapine has the disadvantage that it is available only orally and that it takes 1 week to reach steady state. The usual dose is 2.5–5 mg PO twice a day. Chlorpromazine (10–25 mg every 4–6 h) can be useful if sedation is desired and can be administered IV or per rectum in addition to PO. Dystonic reactions resulting from dopamine blockade are a side effect of neuroleptics, although they are reported to be rare when these drugs are used to treat terminal delirium. If patients develop dystonic reactions, benztropine should be administered. Neuroleptics may be combined with lorazepam to reduce agitation when the delirium is the result of alcohol or sedative withdrawal.

If no response to first-line therapy is seen, a specialty consultation should be obtained with a change to a different medication. If patients fail to improve after a second neuroleptic, sedation with an anesthetic such as propofol or continuous-infusion midazolam may be necessary. By some estimates, at the very end of life, as many as 25% of patients experiencing delirium, especially restless delirium with myoclonus or convulsions, may require sedation.

Physical restraints should be used with great reluctance only when the patient's violence is threatening to him- or herself or others. If they are used, their appropriateness should be reevaluated frequently.

TABLE 32-7

MEDICATIONS FOR THE MANAGEMENT OF DELIRIUM

INTERVENTIONS	DOSE
Neuroleptics	
Haloperidol	0.5–5 mg q2–12h, PO/IV/SC/IM
Thioridazine	10–75 mg q4–8h, PO
Chlorpromazine	12.5–50 mg q4–12h, PO/IV/IM
Atypical neuroleptics	
Olanzapine	2.5–5 mg qd or bid, PO
Risperidone	1–3 mg q12h, PO
Anxiolytics	
Lorazepam	0.5–2 mg q1–4h, PO/IV/IM
Midazolam	1–5 mg/h continuous infusion, IV/SC
Anesthetics	
Propofol	0.3–2.0 mg/h continuous infusion, IV

Abbreviations: IM, intramuscular; IV, intravenous; PO, oral; SC, subcutaneous.

Insomnia

Frequency

Sleep disorders, defined as difficulty initiating sleep or maintaining sleep, sleep difficulty at least 3 nights a week, or sleep difficulty that causes impairment of daytime functioning, occurs in 19–63% of patients with advanced cancer. Some 30–74% of patients with other end-stage conditions, including AIDS, heart disease, COPD, and renal disease, experience insomnia.

Etiology

Patients with cancer may have changes in sleep efficiency such as an increase in stage I sleep. Other etiologies of insomnia are coexisting physical illness such as thyroid disease and coexisting psychological illnesses such as depression and anxiety. Medications, including antidepressants, psychostimulants, steroids, and β agonists, are significant contributors to sleep disorders, as are caffeine and alcohol. Multiple over-the-counter medications contain caffeine and antihistamines, which can contribute to sleep disorders.

Assessment

Assessment should include specific questions concerning sleep onset, sleep maintenance, and early-morning wakening as these will provide clues to the causative agents and to management. Patients should be asked about previous sleep problems, screened for depression and anxiety, and asked about symptoms of thyroid disease. Caffeine and alcohol are prominent causes of sleep problems, and a careful history of the use of these substances should be obtained. Both excessive use and withdrawal from alcohol can be causes of sleep problems.

Interventions

The mainstays of intervention include improvement of sleep hygiene (encouragement of regular time for sleep, decreased nighttime distractions, elimination of caffeine and other stimulants and alcohol), intervention to treat anxiety and depression, and treatment for the insomnia itself. For patients with depression who have insomnia and anxiety, a sedating antidepressant such as mirtazapine can be helpful. In the elderly, trazodone, beginning at 25 mg at nighttime is an effective sleep aid at doses lower than those which cause its antidepressant effect. Zolpidem may have a decreased incidence of delirium in patients compared with traditional benzodiazepines, but this has not been clearly established. When benzodiazepines are prescribed, short-acting ones (such as lorazepam) are favored over longer-acting (such as diazepam). Patients who receive these medications should be observed for signs of increased confusion and delirium.

SOCIAL NEEDS AND THEIR MANAGEMENT

Financial burdens

Frequency

Dying can impose substantial economic strains on patients and families, causing distress. In the United States, with one of the least comprehensive health insurance systems among the developed countries, ~20% of terminally ill patients and their families spend >10% of family income on health care costs over and above health insurance premiums. Between 10 and 30% of families sell assets, use savings, or take out a mortgage to pay for the patient's health care costs. Nearly 40% of terminally ill patients in the United States report that the cost of their illness is a moderate or great economic hardship for their family.

The patient is likely to reduce and eventually stop working. In 20% of cases, a family member of the terminally ill patient also stops working to provide care. The major underlying causes of economic burden are related to poor physical functioning and care needs, such as the need for housekeeping, nursing, and personal care. More debilitated patients and poor patients experience greater economic burdens.

Intervention

This economic burden should not be ignored as a private matter. It has been associated with a number of adverse health outcomes, including preferring comfort care over life-prolonging care as well as consideration of euthanasia or physician-assisted suicide. Economic burdens increase the psychological distress of families and caregivers of terminally ill patients, and poverty is associated with many adverse health outcomes. Importantly, recent studies found that "patients with advanced cancer who reported having end-of-life conversations with physicians had significantly lower health care costs in their final week of life. Higher costs were associated with worse quality of death." Assistance from a social worker, early on if possible, to ensure access to all available benefits may be helpful. Many patients, families, and health care providers are unaware of options for long term care insurance, respite care, the Family Medical Leave Act (FMLA), and other sources of assistance. Some of these options (such as respite care) may be part of a formal hospice program, but others (such as the FMLA) do not require enrollment in a hospice program.

Relationships

Frequency

Settling personal issues and closing the narrative of lived relationships are universal needs. When asked if sudden death or death after an illness is preferable, respondents often initially select the former but soon change to the latter as they reflect on the importance of saying goodbye. Bereaved family members who have not had the chance to say goodbye often have a more difficult grief process.

Interventions

Care of seriously ill patients requires efforts to facilitate the types of encounters and time spent with family and friends that are necessary to meet those needs. Family and close friends may need to be accommodated with unrestricted visiting hours, which may include sleeping near the patient even in otherwise regimented institutional settings. Physicians and other health care providers may be able to facilitate and resolve strained interactions between the patient and other family members. Assistance for patients and family members who are unsure about how to create or help preserve memories, whether by providing materials such as a scrapbook or memory box or by offering them suggestions and informational resources, can be deeply appreciated. Taking photographs and creating videos can be especially helpful to terminally ill patients who have younger children or grandchildren.

Family caregivers

Frequency

Caring for seriously ill patients places a heavy burden on families. Families frequently are required to provide transportation and homemaking as well as other services. Typically, paid professionals such as home health nurses and hospice workers supplement family care; only about a quarter of all caregiving consists of exclusively paid professional assistance. The trend toward more out-of-hospital deaths will increase reliance on families for end-of-life care. Increasingly, family members are being called upon to provide physical care (such as moving and bathing patients) and medical care (such as assessing symptoms and giving medications) in addition to emotional care and support.

Three-quarters of family caregivers of terminally ill patients are women—wives, daughters, sisters, and even daughters-in-law. Since many are widowed, women tend to be able to rely less on family for caregiving assistance and may need more paid assistance. About 20% of terminally ill patients report substantial unmet needs for nursing and personal care. The impact of caregiving on family caregivers is substantial: both bereaved and current caregivers have a higher mortality rate than that of non-caregiving control participants.

Interventions

It is imperative to inquire about unmet needs and to try to ensure that those needs are met either through the family or by paid professional services when possible. Community assistance through houses of worship or other community groups often can be mobilized by telephone calls from the medical team to someone the patient or family identifies. Sources of support specifically for family caregivers should be identified through local sources or nationally through groups such as the National Family Caregivers Association (*www.nfcacares.org*), the American Cancer Society (*www.cancer.org*), and the Alzheimer's Association (*www.alz.org*).

EXISTENTIAL NEEDS AND THEIR MANAGEMENT

Frequency

Religion and spirituality are often important to dying patients. Nearly 70% of patients report becoming more religious or spiritual when they became terminally ill, and many find comfort in religious or spiritual practices such as prayer. However, ~20% of terminally ill patients become less religious, frequently feeling cheated or betrayed by becoming terminally ill. For other patients, the need is for existential meaning and purpose that is distinct from and may even be antithetical to religion or spirituality. When asked, patients and family caregivers frequently report wanting their professional caregivers to be more attentive to religion and spirituality.

Assessment

Health care providers are often hesitant about involving themselves in the religious, spiritual, and existential experiences of their patients because it may seem private or not relevant to the current illness. But physicians and other members of the care team should be able at least to detect spiritual and existential needs. Screening questions have been developed for a physicians' spiritual history taking. Spiritual distress can amplify other types of suffering and even masquerade as intractable physical pain, anxiety, or depression. The screening questions in the comprehensive assessment are usually sufficient. Deeper evaluation and intervention are rarely appropriate for the physician unless no other member of a care team is available or suitable. Pastoral care providers may be helpful, whether from the medical institution or from the patient's own community.

Interventions

Precisely how religious practices, spirituality, and existential explorations can be facilitated and improve end-of-life care is not well established. What is clear is that for physicians, one main intervention is to inquire about the role and importance of spirituality and religion in a patient's life. This will help a patient feel heard and help physicians identify specific needs. In one study, only 36% of respondents indicated that a clergy member would be comforting. Nevertheless, the increase in religious and spiritual interest among a substantial fraction of dying patients suggests inquiring of individual patients how this need can be addressed. Some evidence supports specific methods of addressing existential needs in patients, ranging from establishing a supportive group environment for terminal patients to individual treatments emphasizing a patient's dignity and sources of meaning.

MANAGING THE LAST STAGES

WITHDRAWING AND WITHHOLDING LIFE-SUSTAINING TREATMENT

Legal aspects

For centuries, it has been deemed ethical to withhold or withdraw life-sustaining interventions. The current legal consensus in the United States and most developed countries is that patients have a moral as well as constitutional or common law right to refuse medical interventions. American courts also have held that incompetent patients have a right to refuse medical interventions. For patients who are incompetent and terminally ill and who have not completed an advance care directive, next of kin can exercise that right, although this may be restricted in some states, depending how clear and convincing the evidence is of the patients preferences. Courts have limited families' ability to terminate life-sustaining treatments in patients who are conscious and incompetent but not terminally ill.

In theory, patients' right to refuse medical therapy can be limited by four countervailing interests: (1) preservation of life, (2) prevention of suicide, (3) protection of third parties such as children, and (4) preservation of the integrity of the medical profession. In practice, these interests almost never override the right of competent patients and incompetent patients who have left explicit and advance care directives.

For incompetent patients who either appointed a proxy without specific indications of their wishes or never completed an advance care directive, three criteria have been suggested to guide the decision to terminate medical interventions. First, some commentators suggest that ordinary care should be administered but extraordinary care could be terminated. Because the ordinary/extraordinary distinction is too vague, courts and commentators widely agree that it should not be used to justify decisions about stopping treatment. Second, many courts have advocated the use of the substituted-judgment criterion, which holds that the proxy decision-makers should try to imagine what the incompetent patient would do if he or she were competent. However, multiple studies indicate that many proxies, even close family members, cannot accurately predict what the patient would have wanted. Therefore, substituted judgment becomes more of a guessing game than a way of fulfilling the patients wishes. Finally, the best-interests criterion holds that proxies should evaluate treatments by balancing their benefits and risks and select those treatments in which the benefits maximally outweigh the burdens of treatment. Clinicians have a clear and crucial role in this by carefully and dispassionately explaining the known benefits and burdens of specific treatments. Yet even when that information is as clear as possible, different individuals can have very different views of what is in the patient's best interests, and families may have disagreements or even overt conflicts. This criterion has been criticized because there is no single way to determine the balance between benefits and burdens; it depends on a patient's personal values. For instance, for some people, being alive even if mentally incapacitated is a benefit, but for others it may be the worst possible existence. As a matter of practice, physicians rely on family members to make decisions that they feel are best and object only if those decisions seem to demand treatments that the physicians consider not beneficial.

Practices

Withholding and withdrawing acutely life-sustaining medical interventions from terminally ill patients are now standard practice. More than 90% of American patients die without cardiopulmonary resuscitation (CPR), and just as many forgo other potentially life-sustaining interventions. For instance, in intensive care units (ICUs) in the period 1987–1988, CPR was performed 49% of the time, but it was performed only 10% of the time in 1992–1993. On average, 3.8 interventions, such as vasopressors and transfusions, were stopped for each dying ICU patient. However, up to 19% of decedents in hospitals received interventions such as extubation, ventilation, and surgery in the 48 h preceding death. However, practices vary widely among hospitals and ICUs, suggesting an important element of physician preferences rather than objective data.

Mechanical ventilation may be the most challenging intervention to withdraw. The two approaches are *terminal extubation*, which is the removal of the endotracheal tube, and *terminal weaning*, which is the gradual reduction of the $\mathrm{FI}_{\mathrm{O}_2}$ or ventilator rate. One-third of ICU physicians prefer to use the terminal weaning technique, and 13% extubate; the majority of physicians utilize both techniques. The American Thoracic Society's 2008 clinical policy guidelines note that there is no single correct process of ventilator withdrawal and that physicians use and should be proficient in both methods but that the chosen approach should carefully balance benefits and burdens as well as patient and caregiver preferences. Physicians' assessment of patients likelihood of survival, their prediction of possible cognitive damage, and patients' preferences about the use of life support are primary factors in determining the likelihood of withdrawal of mechanical ventilation. Some recommend terminal weaning because patients do not develop upper airway obstruction and the distress caused by secretions or stridor; however, terminal weaning can prolong the dying process and not allow a patients family to be with him or her unencumbered by an endotracheal tube. To ensure comfort for conscious or semiconscious patients before withdrawal of the ventilator, neuromuscular blocking agents should be terminated and sedatives and analgesics administered. Removing the neuromuscular blocking agents permits patients to show discomfort, facilitating the titration of sedatives and analgesics; it also permits interactions between patients and their families. A common practice is to inject a bolus of midazolam (2–4 mg) or lorazepam (2–4 mg) before withdrawal followed by 5–10 mg of morphine and continuous infusion of morphine (50% of the bolus dose per hour) during weaning. In patients who have significant upper airway secretions, IV scopolamine at a rate of 100 μg/h can be administered. Additional boluses of morphine or increases in the infusion rate should be administered for respiratory distress or signs of pain. Higher doses will be needed for patients already receiving sedatives and opioids. Families need to be reassured about treatments for common symptoms after withdrawal of ventilatory support, such as dyspnea and agitation, and warned about the uncertainty of length of survival after withdrawal of ventilatory support: up to 10% of patients unexpectedly survive for 1 day or more after mechanical ventilation is stopped.

FUTILE CARE

Beginning in the late 1980s, some commentators argued that physicians could terminate futile treatments demanded by the families of terminally ill patients. Although no objective definition or standard of futility exists, several categories have been proposed. Physiologic futility means that an intervention will have no physiologic effect. Some have defined qualitative futility as applying to procedures that "fail to end a patient's total dependence on intensive medical care." Quantitative futility occurs "when physicians conclude (through personal experience, experiences shared with colleagues, or consideration of reported empiric data) that in the last 100 cases, a medical treatment has been useless." The term conceals subjective value judgments about when a treatment is "not beneficial." Deciding whether a treatment that obtains an additional 6 weeks of life or a 1% survival advantage confers benefit depends on patients' preferences and goals. Furthermore, physicians' predictions of when treatments were futile deviated markedly from the quantitative definition. When residents thought CPR was quantitatively futile, more than one in five patients had a >10% chance of survival to hospital discharge. Most studies that purport to guide determinations of futility are based on insufficient data to provide statistical confidence for clinical decision-making. Quantitative futility rarely applies in ICU settings. Many commentators reject using futility as a criterion for withdrawing care, preferring instead to consider futility situations as ones that represent conflict that calls for careful negotiation between families and health care providers.

In the wake of a lack of consensus over quantitative measures of futility, many hospitals adopted process-based approaches to resolve disputes over futility and enhance communication with patients and surrogates, including focusing on interests and alternatives rather than opposing positions and generating a wide range of options. Some hospitals have enacted "unilateral do not resuscitate (DNR)" policies to allow clinicians to provide a DNR order in cases in which consensus cannot be reached with families and medical opinion is that resuscitation would be futile if attempted. This type of a policy is not a replacement for careful and patient communication and negotiation but recognizes that agreement cannot always be reached. Over the past 15 years, many states, such as Texas, Virginia, Maryland, and California, have enacted so-called medical futility laws that provide physicians a "safe harbor" from liability if they refuse a patient or family's request for life-sustaining interventions. For instance, in Texas, when a disagreement about terminating interventions between the medical team and the family has not been resolved by an ethics consultation, the hospital is supposed to try to facilitate transfer of the patient to an institution willing to provide treatment. If this fails after 10 days, the hospital and physician may unilaterally withdraw treatments determined to be futile. The family may appeal to a state court. Early data suggest that the law increases futility consultations for the ethics committee and that although most families concur with withdrawal, about 10–15% of families refuse to withdraw treatment. Approximately 12 cases have gone to court in Texas in the 7 years since the adoption of the law. As of 2007, there had been 974 ethics committee consultations on medical futility cases and 65 in which committees ruled against families and gave notice that treatment would be terminated. Treatment was withdrawn for 27 of those patients, and the remainder transferred to other facilities or died while awaiting transfer.

EUTHANASIA AND PHYSICIAN-ASSISTED SUICIDE

Euthanasia and physician-assisted suicide are defined in Table 32-8. Terminating life-sustaining care and providing opioid medications to manage symptoms have long been considered ethical by the medical profession and legal by courts and should not be confused with euthanasia or physician-assisted suicide.

Legal aspects

Euthanasia is legal in the Netherlands, Belgium, and Luxembourg. It was legalized in the Northern Territory of Australia in 1995, but that legislation was repealed in 1997. Euthanasia is not legal in any state in the United States. With certain conditions, in Switzerland, a layperson can legally assist suicide. In the United States, physician-assisted suicide is legal in Oregon and Washington State if multiple criteria are met and then only after a process that includes a 15-day waiting period. In 2009, the state supreme court of Montana ruled that state law permits physician-assisted suicide for terminally ill patients. In all other countries and all other states in the United States, physician-assisted suicide and euthanasia are illegal explicitly or by common law.

Practices

Fewer than 10–20% of terminally ill patients actually consider euthanasia and/or physician-assisted suicide for themselves. In the Netherlands and Oregon, >70% of patients utilizing these interventions are dying of cancer; <10% of deaths by euthanasia or physician-assisted suicide involve patients with AIDS or amyotrophic lateral sclerosis. In the Netherlands, the share of deaths attributable to euthanasia or physician-assisted suicide declined from around 2.8% of all deaths in 2001 to around 1.8% in 2005. In 2009, the last year with complete data, around 60 patients in Oregon (~0.2% of all deaths) died by physician-assisted

TABLE 32-8

DEFINITIONS OF ASSISTED SUICIDE AND EUTHANASIA

TERM	DEFINITION	LEGAL STATUS
Voluntary active euthanasia	Intentionally administering medications or other interventions to cause a patient's death with the patient's informed consent	Netherlands Belgium
Involuntary active euthanasia	Intentionally administering medications or other interventions to cause a patient's death when the patient was competent to consent but did not—e.g., the patient may not have been asked	Nowhere
Passive euthanasia	Withholding or withdrawing life-sustaining medical treatments from a patient to let him or her die (terminating life-sustaining treatments)	Everywhere
Physician-assisted suicide	A physician provides medications or other interventions to a patient with the understanding that the patient can use them to commit suicide	Oregon Netherlands Belgium Switzerland

suicide, although this may be an underestimate. In Washington state, between March 2009 (when the law allowing physician-assisted suicide went into force) and December 2009, 36 individuals died from prescribed lethal doses.

Pain is not a primary motivator for patients' requests for or interest in euthanasia and/or physician-assisted suicide. Among the first patients to receive physician-assisted suicide in Oregon, only 1 patient of 15 had inadequate pain control compared with 15 of 43 patients in a control group experiencing inadequate pain relief. Depression; hopelessness; and, more profoundly, concerns about loss of dignity or autonomy or being a burden on family members appear to be primary factors motivating a desire for euthanasia or physician-assisted suicide. In Oregon, fewer than 25% of patients cite pain as the reason for desiring physician-assisted suicide. Most cite losing autonomy, dignity, or enjoyable activities. Over one-third note being a burden on family. A study from the Netherlands showed that depressed terminally ill cancer patients were four times more likely to request euthanasia and confirmed that uncontrolled pain was not associated with greater interest in euthanasia.

Euthanasia and physician-assisted suicide are no guarantee of a painless, quick death. Data from the Netherlands indicate that in as many as 20% of cases, technical and other problems arose, including patients waking from coma, not becoming comatose, regurgitating medications, and experiencing a prolonged time to death. Data from Oregon indicate that between 1997 and 2009, 20 patients (around 5%) regurgitated after taking prescribed medication, 1 patient awaked, and none experienced seizures. Problems were significantly more common in physician-assisted suicide, sometimes requiring the physician to intervene and provide euthanasia.

Whether practicing in a setting where euthanasia is legal or not, over a career, 12–54% of physicians receive a request for euthanasia or physician-assisted suicide from a patient. Competency in dealing with such a request is crucial. Although challenging, the request can also provide a chance to address intense suffering. After receiving a request for euthanasia and/or physician-assisted suicide, health care providers should carefully clarify the request with empathic, open-ended questions to help elucidate the underlying cause for the request, such as: "What makes you want to consider this option?" Endorsing either moral opposition or moral support for the act tends to be counterproductive, giving an impression of being judgmental or of endorsing the idea that the patient's life is worthless. Health care providers must reassure the patient of continued care and commitment. The patient should be educated about alternative, less controversial options, such as symptom management and withdrawing any unwanted treatments and the reality of euthanasia and/or physician-assisted suicide, since the patient may have misconceptions about their effectiveness as well as the legal implications of the choice. Depression, hopelessness, and other symptoms of psychological distress as well as physical suffering and economic burdens are likely factors motivating the request, and such factors should be assessed and treated aggressively. After these interventions and clarification of options, most patients proceed with another approach, declining life-sustaining interventions, possibly including refusal of nutrition and hydration.

CARE DURING THE LAST HOURS

Most laypersons have limited experiences with the actual dying process and death. They frequently do not know what to expect of the final hours and afterward. The family and other caregivers must be prepared, especially if the plan is for the patient to die at home.

Patients in the last days of life typically experience extreme weakness and fatigue and become bedbound;

this can lead to pressure sores. The issue of turning patients who are near the end of life, however, must be balanced against the potential discomfort that movement may cause. Patients stop eating and drinking with drying of mucosal membranes and dysphagia. Careful attention to oral swabbing, lubricants for the lips, and use of artificial tears can provide forms of care to substitute for attempts at feeding the patient. With loss of the gag reflex and dysphagia, patients may also experience accumulation of oral secretions, producing noises during respiration sometimes called "the death rattle." Scopolamine can reduce the secretions. Patients also experience changes in respiration with periods of apnea or Cheyne-Stokes breathing. Decreased intravascular volume and cardiac output cause tachycardia, hypotension, peripheral coolness, and livedo reticularis (skin mottling). Patients can have urinary and, less frequently, fecal incontinence. Changes in consciousness and neurologic function generally lead to two different paths to death (Fig. 32-2).

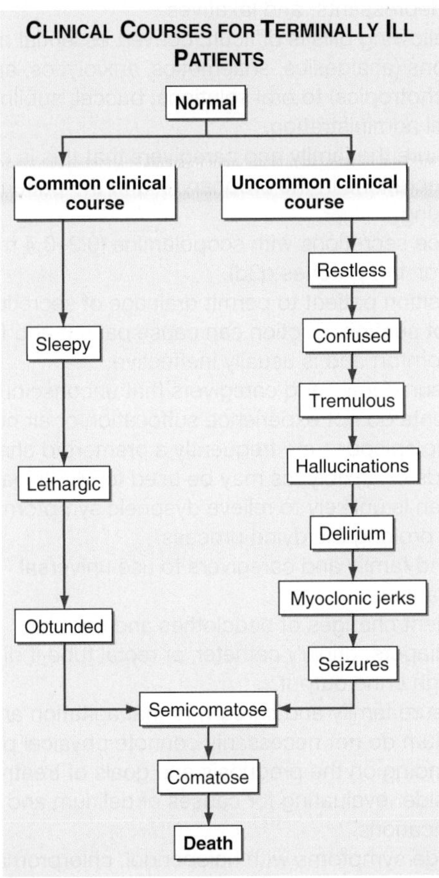

FIGURE 32-2

Common and uncommon clinical courses in the last days of terminally ill patients. *(Adapted from Ferris FD, et al: Module 4: Palliative care, in Comprehensive Guide for the Care of Persons with HIV Disease. Toronto: Mt. Sinai Hospital and Casey Hospice, 1995, http://www.cpsonline.info/content/resources/hivmodule/module4complete.pdf.)*

Each of these terminal changes can cause patients and families distress, requiring reassurance and targeted interventions (Table 32-9). Informing families that these changes might occur and providing them with an information sheet can help preempt problems and minimize distress. Understanding that patients stop eating because they are dying, not dying because they have stopped eating, can reduce family and caregiver anxiety. Similarly, informing the family and caregivers that the "death rattle" may occur and that it is not indicative of suffocation, choking, or pain can reduce their worry regarding the breathing sounds.

Families and caregivers may also feel guilty about stopping treatments, fearing that they are "killing" the patient. This may lead to demands for interventions, such as feeding tubes, that may be ineffective. In such cases, the physician should remind the family and caregivers about the inevitability of events and the palliative goals. Interventions may prolong the dying process and cause discomfort. Physicians also should emphasize that withholding treatments is both legal and ethical and that the family members are not the cause of the patient's death. This reassurance may have to be provided multiple times.

Hearing and touch are said to be the last senses to stop functioning. Whether this is the case or not, families and caregivers can be encouraged to communicate with the dying patient. Encouraging them to talk directly to the patient, even if he or she is unconscious, and hold the patient's hand or demonstrate affection in other ways can be an effective way to channel their urge "to do something" for the patient.

When the plan is for the patient to die at home, the physician must inform the family and caregivers how to determine that the patient has died. The cardinal signs are cessation of cardiac function and respiration; the pupils become fixed; the body becomes cool; muscles relax; and incontinence may occur. Remind the family and caregivers that the eyes may remain open even after the patient has died because the retroorbital fat pad may be depleted, permitting the orbit to fall posteriorly, which makes it difficult for the eyelids to cover the eyeball.

The physician should establish a plan for who the family or caregivers will contact when the patient is dying or has died. Without a plan, they may panic and call 911, unleashing a cascade of unwanted events, from arrival of emergency personnel and resuscitation to hospital admission. The family and caregivers should be instructed to contact the hospice (if one is involved), the covering physician, or the on-call member of the palliative care team. They should also be told that the medical examiner need not be called unless the state requires it for all deaths. Unless foul play is suspected, the health care team need not contact the medical examiner either.

TABLE 32-9

MANAGING CHANGES IN THE PATIENT'S CONDITION DURING THE FINAL DAYS AND HOURS

CHANGES IN THE PATIENT'S CONDITION	POTENTIAL COMPLICATION	FAMILY'S POSSIBLE REACTION AND CONCERN	ADVICE AND INTERVENTION
Profound fatigue	Bedbound with development of pressure ulcers that are prone to infection, malodor, and pain, and joint pain	Patient is lazy and giving up.	Reassure family and caregivers that terminal fatigue will not respond to interventions and should not be resisted. Use an air mattress if necessary.
Anorexia	None	Patient is giving up; patient will suffer from hunger and will starve to death.	Reassure family and caregivers that the patient is not eating because he or she is dying; not eating at the end of life does not cause suffering or death. Forced feeding, whether oral, parenteral, or enteral, does not reduce symptoms or prolong life.
Dehydration	Dry mucosal membranes (see below)	Patient will suffer from thirst and die of dehydration.	Reassure family and caregivers that dehydration at the end of life does not cause suffering because patients lose consciousness before any symptom distress. Intravenous hydration can worsen symptoms of dyspnea by pulmonary edema and peripheral edema as well as prolong dying process.
Dysphagia	Inability to swallow oral medications needed for palliative care		Do not force oral intake. Discontinue unnecessary medications that may have been continued, including antibiotics, diuretics, antidepressants, and laxatives. If swallowing pills is difficult, convert essential medications (analgesics, antiemetics, anxiolytics, and psychotropics) to oral solutions, buccal, sublingual, or rectal administration.
"Death rattle"—noisy breathing		Patient is choking and suffocating.	Reassure the family and caregivers that this is caused by secretions in the oropharynx and the patient is not choking. Reduce secretions with scopolamine (0.2–0.4 mg SC q4h or 1–3 patches q3d). Reposition patient to permit drainage of secretions. Do not suction. Suction can cause patient and family discomfort and is usually ineffective.
Apnea, Cheyne-Stokes respirations, dyspnea		Patient is suffocating.	Reassure family and caregivers that unconscious patients do not experience suffocation or air hunger. Apneic episodes are frequently a premorbid change. Opioids or anxiolytics may be used for dyspnea. Oxygen is unlikely to relieve dyspneic symptoms and may prolong the dying process.
Urinary or fecal incontinence	Skin breakdown if days until death Potential transmission of infectious agents to caregivers	Patient is dirty, malodorous, and physically repellent.	Remind family and caregivers to use universal precautions. Frequent changes of bedclothes and bedding. Use diapers, urinary catheter, or rectal tube if diarrhea or high urine output.
Agitation or delirium	Day–night reversal Hurt self or caregivers	Patient is in horrible pain and going to have a horrible death.	Reassure family and caregivers that agitation and delirium do not necessarily connote physical pain. Depending on the prognosis and goals of treatment, consider evaluating for causes of delirium and modify medications. Manage symptoms with haloperidol, chlorpromazine, diazepam, or midazolam.
Dry mucosal membranes	Cracked lips, mouth sores, and candidiasis can also cause pain. Odor	Patient may be malodorous and physically repellent.	Use baking soda mouthwash or saliva preparation q15–30min. Use topical nystatin for candidiasis. Coat lips and nasal mucosa with petroleum jelly q60–90min. Use ophthalmic lubricants q4h or artificial tears q30min.

Abbreviation: SC, subcuataneous.

Just after the patient dies, even the best-prepared family may experience shock and loss and be emotionally distraught. They need time to assimilate the event and be comforted. Health care providers are likely to find it meaningful to write a bereavement card or letter to the family. The purpose is to communicate about the patient, perhaps emphasizing the patient's virtues and the honor it was to care for the patient and to express concern for the family's hardship. Some physicians attend the funerals of their patients. Although this is beyond any medical obligation, the presence of the physician can be a source of support to the grieving family and provides an opportunity for closure for the physician.

Death of a spouse is a strong predictor of poor health, and even mortality, for the surviving spouse. It may be important to alert the spouse's physician about the death so that he or she is aware of symptoms that might require professional attention.

PALLIATIVE CARE SERVICES: HOW AND WHERE

Determining the best approach to providing palliative care to patients will depend on patient preferences, the availability of caregivers and specialized services in close proximity, institutional resources, and reimbursement. Hospice is a leading, but not the only, model of palliative care services. In the United States, a plurality—40.7%—of hospice care is provided in residential homes. In 2008, just over 20% of hospice care was provided in nursing homes. In the United States, Medicare pays for hospice services under Part A, the hospital insurance part of reimbursement. Two physicians must certify that the patient has a prognosis of ≤6 months if the disease runs its usual course. Prognoses are probabilistic by their nature; patients are not required to die within 6 months but rather to have a condition from which half of individuals with it would not be alive within 6 months. Patients sign a hospice enrollment form that states their intent to forgo curative services related to their terminal illness, but they can still receive medical services for other comorbid conditions. Patients also can withdraw enrollment and reenroll later; the hospice Medicare benefit can be revoked later to secure traditional Medicare benefits. Payments to the hospice are per diem (or capitated), not fee-for-service. Payments are intended to cover physician services for the medical direction of the care team; regular home care visits by registered nurses and licensed practical nurses; home health aid and homemaker services; chaplain services; social work services; bereavement counseling; and medical equipment, supplies, and medications. No specific therapy is excluded, and the goal is for each therapy to be considered for its symptomatic (as opposed to disease-modifying) effect. Additional clinical care, including services of the primary physician, is covered by Medicare Part B even while the hospice Medicare benefit is in place. The health reform legislation signed into law in March 2010—the Affordable Care Act—directs the Secretary of Health and Human Services to gather data on Medicare hospice reimbursement with the goal of reforming payment rates to account for resource use over an entire episode of care. The legislation also requires additional evaluations and reviews of eligibility for hospice care by hospice physicians or nurses. Finally, the legislation establishes a demonstration project for concurrent hospice care in Medicare, which would test and evaluate allowing patients to remain eligible for regular Medicare during hospice care.

By 2008, the mean length of enrollment in a hospice was around 70 days, with the median being 21 days. Such short stays create barriers to establishing high-quality palliative services in patients' homes and also place financial strains on hospice providers since the initial assessments are resource intensive. Physicians should initiate early referrals to the hospice to allow more time for patients to receive palliative care.

Hospice care has been the main method for securing palliative services for terminally ill patients. However, efforts are being made to ensure continuity of palliative care across settings and through time. Palliative care services are becoming available as consultative services and more rarely as palliative care units in hospitals, in day care and other outpatient settings, and in nursing homes. Palliative care consultations for non-hospice patients can be billed as for other consultations under Medicare Part B, the physician reimbursement part. Many believe palliative care should be offered to patients regardless of their prognosis. A patient, his or her family, and physicians should not have to make a "curative versus palliative care" decision because it is rarely possible to make such a decisive switch to embracing mortality.

FUTURE DIRECTIONS

OUTCOME MEASURES

Care near the end of life cannot be measured by most of the available validated outcome measures since palliative care does not consider death a bad outcome. Similarly, the family and patients receiving end-of-life care may not desire the elements elicited in current quality-of-life measurements. Symptom control, enhanced family relationships, and quality of bereavement are difficult to measure and are rarely the primary focus of carefully developed or widely used outcome measures. Nevertheless, outcomes are as important in end-of-life care as in any other field of medical care. Specific end-of-life care instruments are being developed both for assessment, such as The Brief Hospice Inventory and NEST (*n*eeds near the *e*nd of life *s*creening *t*ool), and for outcome measures, such as the Palliative Care Outcomes Scale, as well as for prognosis, such as the Palliative Prognostic Index. The field of end-of-life care is entering an era of evidence-based practice and continuous improvement through clinical trials.

SECTION IX

NEOPLASTIC DISORDERS

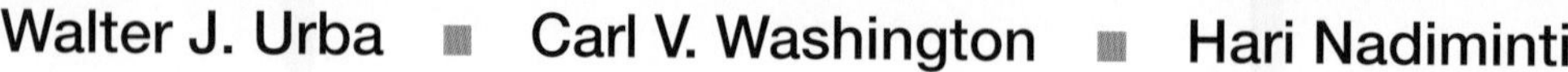

CHAPTER 33

CANCER OF THE SKIN

Walter J. Urba ■ Carl V. Washington ■ Hari Nadiminti

MELANOMA

Pigmented lesions are among the most common findings on skin examination. The challenge is to distinguish cutaneous melanomas, which account for the overwhelming majority of deaths resulting from skin cancer, from the remainder, which with rare exceptions are benign. Cutaneous melanoma can occur in adults of all ages, even young individuals, and people of all colors; it is located on the skin, where it is visible; and it has distinct clinical features that make it detectable at a time when complete surgical excision is possible. Examples of malignant and benign pigmented lesions are shown in Fig. 33-1.

EPIDEMIOLOGY

Melanoma is an aggressive malignancy of melanocytes: pigment-producing cells that originate from the neural crest and migrate to the skin, meninges, mucous membranes, upper esophagus, and eyes. Melanocytes in each of these locations have the potential for malignant transformation. In the United States, nearly 69,000 individuals were expected to develop melanoma and approximately 9000 were expected to die in 2010. Although the overall incidence and mortality have increased over the past decades, the mortality rates for younger patients have flattened, but those rates for individuals older than age 65 years have continued to increase. It is predominantly a malignancy of white-skinned people (98% of cases), and the incidence correlates with latitude of residence, providing strong evidence for the role of sun exposure. Men are affected slightly more than women (1.3:1), and the median age at diagnosis is the late fifties. Dark-skinned populations (such as those of India and Puerto Rico), blacks, and East Asians also develop melanoma, albeit at rates 10–20 times lower than those in whites. Cutaneous melanomas in these populations are diagnosed more often at a higher stage, and patients tend to have worse outcomes. Furthermore, in nonwhite populations, there is a much higher frequency of acral (subungual, plantar, palmar) and mucosal melanomas.

RISK FACTORS

The strongest risk factors for melanoma are the presence of multiple benign or atypical nevi and a family or personal history of melanoma (Table 33-1). The presence of melanocytic nevi, common or dysplastic, is a marker for an increased risk of melanoma. Nevi have been referred to as precursor lesions because they can transform into melanomas; however, the actual risk for any specific nevus is exceedingly low. About one-quarter of melanomas are histologically associated with nevi, but the majority arise de novo. Table 33-2 lists the characteristic features of clinically atypical moles and the features that differentiate them from benign acquired nevi. The number of clinically atypical moles may vary from one to several hundred, and they usually differ from one another in appearance. The borders are often hazy and indistinct, and the pigment pattern is more highly varied than that in benign acquired nevi. Individuals with clinically atypical moles and a strong family history of melanoma have been reported to have a >50% lifetime risk for developing melanoma and warrant close follow-up with a dermatologist. Of the 90% of melanoma patients whose disease is regarded as sporadic (i.e., who lack a family history of melanoma), ~40% have clinically atypical moles compared with an estimated 5–10% of the population at large.

Congenital melanocytic nevi, which are classified as small (≤1.5 cm), medium (1.5–20 cm), and giant (>20 cm), can be precursors for melanoma. The risk is highest for the giant melanocytic nevus, also called the bathing trunk nevus, which is a rare malformation that affects 1 in 30,000–100,000 individuals, with a lifetime risk of melanoma development estimated to be as

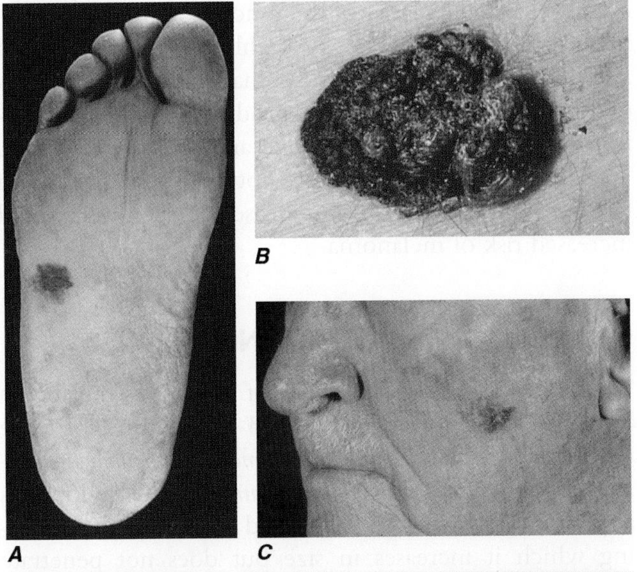

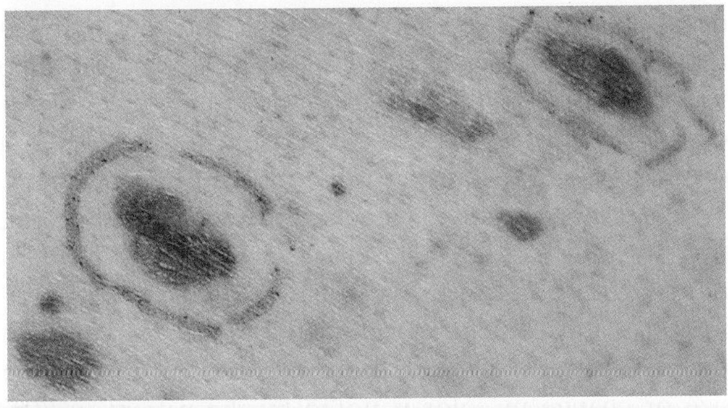

FIGURE 33-1

Atypical and malignant pigmented lesions. The most common melanoma is superficial spreading melanoma (not pictured). ***A.*** Acral lentiginous melanoma is the most common melanoma in blacks, Asians, and Hispanics and occurs as an enlarging hyperpigmented macule or plaque on the palms and soles. Lateral pigment diffusion is present. ***B.*** Nodular melanoma most commonly manifests as a rapidly growing, often ulcerated or crusted black nodule. ***C.*** Lentigo maligna melanoma occurs on sun-exposed skin as a large, hyperpigmented macule or plaque with irregular borders and variable pigmentation. ***D.*** Dysplastic nevi are irregularly pigmented and shaped nevomelanocytic lesions that may be associated with familial melanoma.

high as 6%. At present, there are no uniform management guidelines for giant congenital nevi, but because of the potential for malignancy, prophylactic excision early in life is prudent. This usually requires staged removal with coverage by split-thickness skin grafts. Surgery cannot remove all at-risk nevus cells, as some may penetrate into the muscles or central nervous system (CNS) below the nevus. Small- to medium-size congenital melanocytic nevi affect approximately 1% of persons; the risk of melanoma developing in these lesions is not known but appears to be relatively low. The management of small- to medium-size congenital melanocytic nevi remains controversial.

TABLE 33-1

FACTORS ASSOCIATED WITH INCREASED RISK OF MELANOMA
Total body nevi (higher number = higher risk)
Family or personal history
Dysplastic nevi
Light skin, hair, or eye color
Poor tanning ability
Freckling
Ultraviolet exposure, sunburns, or tanning booths
CDKN2A mutation
MC1R variants

Personal and family history

Perhaps the single greatest risk factor for melanoma is a personal history of melanoma. Once diagnosed, patients with melanoma require a lifetime of surveillance because their risk is 10 times that of the general population. First-degree relatives have a higher risk of developing melanoma than do individuals without a family history, but only 5–10% of all melanomas are truly familial. In familial melanoma, patients tend to be younger at first diagnosis, lesions are thinner, survival is improved, and multiple primary melanomas are common.

Genetic susceptibility

Approximately 20–40% of cases of hereditary melanoma (0.2–2% of all melanomas) are due to germ-line mutations in the cell cycle regulatory gene cyclin-dependent kinase inhibitor 2A (*CDKN2A*). In fact, 70% of all cutaneous melanomas have somatic mutations or deletions affecting the CDKN2A locus on chromosome 9p21. This locus encodes two distinct tumor suppressor proteins from alternate reading frames: p16 and ARF ($p14^{ARF}$). The p16 protein inhibits CDK4/6-mediated phosphorylation and inactivation of the retinoblastoma (RB) protein, whereas ARF inhibits MDM2 ubiquitin-mediated degradation of p53. The end result of the loss of *CDKN2A* is inactivation of two critical tumor suppressor pathways, RB and p53, which control entry of cells into the cell cycle. Several studies have shown an increased risk of pancreatic cancer among melanoma-prone families with *CDKN2A* mutations.

The melanocortin-1 receptor (*MC1R*) gene is also an inherited melanoma susceptibility factor. Solar radiation stimulates the production of melanocortin (α-melanocyte-stimulating hormone [α-MSH]), the ligand for MC1R, which is a G-protein–coupled receptor that signals via

TABLE 33-2

PIGMENTED LESIONS THAT MUST BE DISTINGUISHED FROM CUTANEOUS MELANOMA AND ITS PRECURSORS

Blue nevus	Gunmetal or cerulean blue, blue-gray. Stable over time. One-half occur on dorsa of hands and feet. Lesions are usually single, small, 3 mm–<1 cm. Must be distinguished from nodular melanoma.
Compound nevus	Round or oval shape, well demarcated, smooth-bordered. May be dome-shaped or papillomatous; colors range from flesh-colored to very dark brown, with individual nevi being relatively homogeneous in color.
Hemangioma	Dome-shaped reddish, purple, blue nodule. Compression with a glass microscope slide may result in blanching. Must be distinguished from nodular melanoma.
Junctional nevus	Flat to barely raised brown lesion. Sharp border. Fine pigmentary stippling visible, especially upon magnification.
Lentigo	
Juvenile	Flat, uniformly medium or dark brown lesion with sharp border.
Solar	Solar lentigines are acquired lesions on sites of chronic solar exposure (face and backs of hands). Lesions are 2 mm–≥1 cm. Solar lentigines have reticulate pigmentation upon magnification.
Pigmented basal cell carcinoma	Papular border. May have central ulceration. Usually on a sun-exposed surface in an older patient. Patient usually has dark brown eyes and dark brown or black hair.
Pigmented dermatofibroma	Lesion is not well-demarcated visually, is firm, and dimples downward when compressed laterally. Usually on extremities. Usually <6 mm.
Seborrheic keratosis	Rough, sharp-bordered lesions that feel waxy and "stuck on"; range in color from flesh to tan to dark brown. Presence of keratin plugs in surface is helpful for discriminating especially dark lesions from melanoma.
Subungual hematoma	Maroon (red-brown) coloration. As lesion grows out from nail fold, a curving clear area is seen.
Tattoo (medical or traumatic)	In medical tattoos, lesions are small pigmentary dots, often blue or green, which make a regular pattern (rectangle). Traumatic tattoos are irregular, and pigmentation may appear black.

cyclic AMP and regulates the amount and type of pigment produced. *MC1R* is highly polymorphic, and among its 80 variants are those that result in partial loss of signaling and lead to the production of pheomelanin, which is not sun-protective and produces red hair. This red hair color (RHC) phenotype is associated with fair skin, red hair, freckles, increased sun sensitivity, and increased risk of melanoma.

CLINICAL CLASSIFICATION

Traditionally, four major types of cutaneous melanoma have been recognized (Table 33-3). In three of these types—*superficial spreading melanoma*, *lentigo maligna melanoma*, and *acral lentiginous melanoma*—the lesion has a period of superficial (so-called radial) growth during which it increases in size but does not penetrate deeply. It is during this period that the melanoma is most capable of being cured by surgical excision. The fourth type—*nodular melanoma*—does not have a recognizable radial growth phase and usually presents as a deeply invasive lesion that is capable of early metastasis. When tumors begin to penetrate deeply into the skin, they are in the so-called vertical growth phase. Melanomas with a radial growth phase are characterized by irregular and sometimes notched borders, variation in pigment pattern, and variation in color. An increase in size or change in color is noted by the patient in 70% of early lesions. Bleeding, ulceration, and pain are late signs and are of little help in early recognition. Superficial spreading melanoma is the most common variant observed in the white population. The back is the most common site for melanoma in men. In women, the back and the lower leg (from knee to ankle) are common sites. Nodular melanomas are dark brown-black to blue-black nodules. Lentigo maligna melanoma usually is confined to chronically sun-damaged, sun-exposed sites (face, neck, back of hands) in older individuals. Acral lentiginous melanoma occurs on the palms, soles, nail beds, and mucous membranes. Although this type occurs in whites, it occurs most frequently (along with nodular melanoma) in blacks and East Asians. A fifth type of melanoma, *desmoplastic melanoma*, is associated with a fibrotic response, neural invasion, and a greater tendency for local recurrence. Occasionally, melanomas appear clinically to be amelanotic, in which case the diagnosis is established histologically after biopsy of a new or a changing skin nodule or because of suspicion of a basal cell carcinoma.

Although melanoma subtypes are clinically and histopathologically distinct, this classification does not have independent prognostic value and has fallen out of favor. Histologic subtype is not part of American Joint Committee on Cancer (AJCC) staging and often is not identified in current pathology reports. Future

TABLE 33-3

CLASSIFICATION OF MALIGNANT MELANOMA

TYPE	SITE	AVERAGE AGE AT DIAGNOSIS, YEARS	DURATION OF KNOWN EXISTENCE, YEARS	COLOR
Lentigo maligna melanoma	Sun-exposed surfaces, particularly malar region of cheek and temple	70	5–20 or longer[a]	In flat portions, shades of brown and tan predominate, but whitish gray occasionally present; in nodules, shades of reddish brown, bluish gray, bluish black
Superficial spreading melanoma	Any site (more common on upper back and, in women, lower legs)	40–50	1–7	Shades of brown mixed with bluish red (violaceous), bluish black, reddish brown, and often whitish pink, and the border of lesion is at least in part visibly and/or palpably elevated
Nodular melanoma	Any	40–50	Months–<5 years	Reddish blue (purple) or bluish black; either uniform in color or mixed with brown or black
Acral lentiginous melanoma	Palm, sole, nail bed, mucous membranes	60	1–10	In flat portions, dark brown predominantly; in raised lesions (plaques), brown-black or blue-black predominantly

[a]During much of this time, the precursor stage, lentigo maligna, is confined to the epidermis.
Source: Adapted from AJ Sober, in NA Soter, HP Baden (eds): *Pathophysiology of Dermatologic Diseases*. New York, McGraw-Hill, 1984.

classification schemes will be based on molecular features of each melanoma (see later discussion). The molecular analysis of individual melanomas will provide a basis for distinguishing benign nevi from melanomas, identify distinct subclasses of melanoma on the basis of the anatomic site, indicate the extent of ultraviolet (UV) exposure, and determine the mutational status of the tumor, which will help elucidate the molecular mechanisms of tumorigenesis and identify targets that will serve as a basis for selection of therapy.

PATHOGENESIS AND MOLECULAR CLASSIFICATION

Considerable evidence from epidemiologic and molecular studies suggests that cutaneous melanomas arise via multiple pathways. There are both environmental and genetic components. Uv solar radiation causes genetic changes in the skin, impairs cutaneous immune function, increases the production of growth factors, and induces the formation of DNA-damaging reactive oxygen species that affect keratinocytes and melanocytes. A comprehensive catalog of somatic mutations from a human melanoma revealed more than 33,000 base mutations with damage to almost 300 protein-coding segments compared with normal cells from the same patient. The dominant mutational signature reflected DNA damage due to UV light exposure. The melanoma also contained previously described driver mutations (i.e., mutations that confer selective clonal growth advantage and are implicated in oncogenesis). These driver mutations affect pathways that promote cell proliferation and inhibit normal pathways of apoptosis in response to DNA repair (see later discussion). The altered melanocytes accumulate DNA damage, and selection occurs for all the attributes that constitute the malignant phenotype: invasion, metastasis, and angiogenesis.

An understanding of the molecular changes that occur during the transformation of normal melanocytes into malignant melanoma not only would help classify patients in similar prognostic groups but also would contribute to the understanding of etiology and help identify new therapeutic options. A genomewide assessment of melanomas classified into four groups based on their location and degree of exposure to the sun has confirmed that there are distinct genetic pathways in the development of melanoma. The four groups were melanomas on skin without chronic sun-induced damage, melanomas on skin with chronic sun-induced damage, mucosal melanomas, and acral melanomas. Remarkably, distinct patterns of DNA alterations were noted that varied with the site of origin and were independent of the histologic subtype of the tumor. What that work and research done by others have shown is that the overall pattern of mutation, amplification, and loss of cancer genes indicate that although the genetic changes are diverse, they have convergent effects on key biochemical pathways involved in

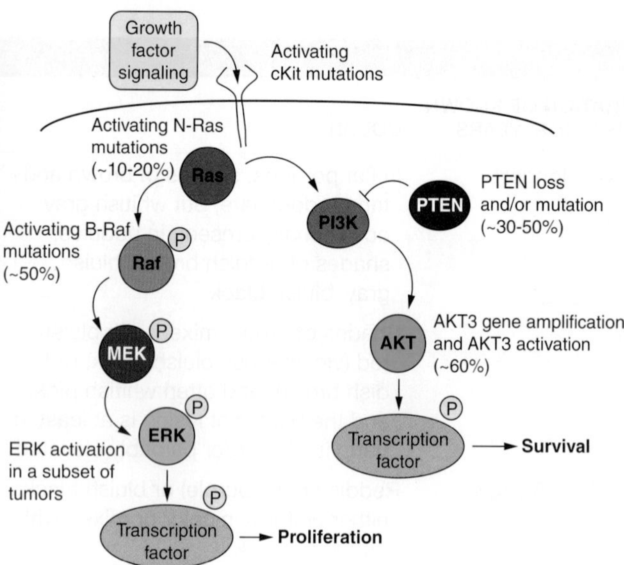

FIGURE 33-2

Major pathways involved in melanoma. The MAP kinase and AKT pathways, which promote proliferation and inhibit apoptosis, respectively, are subject to mutations in melanoma. ERK, extracellular signal-regulated kinase; MEK, MAP kinase kinase; PTEN, phosphatase and tensin homolog.

proliferation, senescence, and apoptosis. The p16 mutation that leads to cell cycle arrest and the ARF mutation that results in defective apoptotic responses to genotoxic damage were described earlier. The proliferative pathways affected were the mitogen-activated protein (MAP) kinase and phosphatidylinositol 3′ kinase/AKT pathways (Fig. 33-2).

The RAS family and BRAF, members of the MAP kinase pathway, which classically mediates the transcription of genes involved in cell proliferation and survival, undergo somatic mutation in melanoma. N-RAS is mutated in approximately 20% of melanomas, and somatic activating BRAF mutations are found in most benign nevi and 40–60% of melanomas. Neither mutation by itself appears to be sufficient to cause melanoma; they often are accompanied by other mutations, (e.g., *CDKN2A*) or phosphatidylinositol 3′ kinase pathway (e.g., loss of PTEN). The BRAF mutation is almost always a point mutation (T→A nucleotide change) that results in a valine-to-glutamate amino acid substitution (V600E). V600E BRAF mutations do not have the standard UV signature mutation (pyrimidine dimer) but are present in most melanomas that arise on sites with intermittent sun exposure and are absent in melanomas from chronically sun-damaged skin.

Melanomas also contain mutations in AKT (primarily in AKT3) and PTEN (phosphatase and tensin homolog). AKT can be amplified, and PTEN may be deleted or undergo epigenetic silencing that leads to constitutive activation of the PI3K/AKT pathway and enhanced cell survival by antagonizing the intrinsic pathway of apoptosis. Loss of PTEN, which dysregulates AKT activity, and mutation of AKT3 prolong survival through inactivation of BAD, Bc12-antagonist of cell death, and activation of the forkhead transcription factor FOXO1, which leads to synthesis of prosurvival genes. In melanoma, these two signaling pathways enhance tumorigenesis, chemoresistance, migration, and cell cycle dysregulation. Targeted agents are being employed that inhibit each pathway, but it is likely that effective antimelanoma therapy will require simultaneous inhibition of both MAPK and PI3K.

DIAGNOSIS

The main goal is to diagnose melanoma early in its natural history, before tumor invasion and life-threatening metastases have occurred. Early detection of melanoma may be facilitated by applying the ABCDEs: asymmetry (benign lesions are usually symmetric), border irregularity (most nevi have clear-cut borders), color variegation (benign lesions usually have uniform light or dark pigment), diameter >6 mm (the size of a pencil eraser); evolving (any change in size, shape, color, or elevation or new symptoms such as bleeding, itching, and crusting). The aim of differential diagnosis is to distinguish benign pigmented lesions from melanoma and its precursor. If melanoma is a consideration, biopsy is appropriate. Some benign look-alikes may be removed in the process of trying to detect melanoma. Several factors may help distinguish benign nevi from atypical moles:

1. Size: Benign nevi usually are <6 mm in diameter; atypical moles usually are >6 mm in diameter.
2. Shape: Benign nevi usually are round with distinct borders and may be flat or elevated; atypical moles usually have irregular borders with pigment fading off at the edge.
3. Color: Benign nevi usually are uniformly brown or tan; atypical moles usually have variable mixtures of brown, tan, black, and reddish pigment and differ from one another.
4. Location: Benign nevi usually appear on sun-exposed skin above the waist, rarely involving the scalp, breasts, or buttocks; atypical moles usually appear on sun-exposed skin, most often on the back, but can involve the scalp, breasts, or buttocks.
5. Number: Benign nevi are present in 85% of adults, with 10–40 moles scattered over the body; atypical nevi can be present in the hundreds.

The entire cutaneous surface, including the scalp and mucous membranes, as well as the nails should be examined in each patient. Bright room illumination is important, and a hand lens is helpful for evaluating variation in pigment pattern. Any suspicious lesions should be biopsied, evaluated by a specialist, or recorded by chart and/or photography for follow-up. A focused method for examining individual lesions, dermoscopy, employs low-level magnification of the epidermis and may allow a more precise visualization of patterns of pigmentation than is possible with the naked eye. Complete physical examination with attention to the regional lymph nodes is part of the initial evaluation in a patient with suspected melanoma. The patient should be advised to have other family members screened if either melanoma or clinically atypical moles (dysplastic nevi) are present. Patients who fit into high-risk groups should be instructed to perform monthly self-examinations.

Biopsy

Any pigmented cutaneous lesion that has changed in size or shape or has other features suggestive of malignant melanoma is a candidate for biopsy. The recommended technique is an excisional biopsy, which facilitates pathologic assessment of the lesion, permits accurate measurement of thickness if the lesion is melanoma, and constitutes treatment if the lesion is benign. For large lesions or lesions on anatomic sites where excisional biopsy may not be feasible (such as the face, hands, and feet), an incisional biopsy through the most nodular or darkest area of the lesion is acceptable; this should include the vertical growth phase of the primary tumor, if present. Incisional biopsy does not appear to facilitate the spread of melanoma. For suspicious lesions, every attempt should be made to preserve the ability to assess the deep and peripheral margins and to perform immunohistochemistry. Shave biopsies and cauterization should be avoided. The biopsy should be read by a pathologist experienced in pigmented lesions, and the minimal elements of the report should include Breslow thickness, mitoses per square millimeter for lesions ≤1 mm, presence or absence of ulceration, and peripheral and deep margin status. Breslow thickness is the greatest thickness of a primary cutaneous melanoma measured on the slide from the top of the epidermal granular layer, or from the ulcer base, to the bottom of the tumor. To distinguish melanomas from benign nevi in cases with challenging histology, fluorescence in situ hybridization (FISH) with multiple probes can be helpful.

PROGNOSTIC FACTORS

The prognostic factors of greatest importance to a newly diagnosed patient are included in the staging classification (Table 33-4). The best predictor of metastatic risk is the lesion's Breslow thickness. The Clark level, which defines melanomas on the basis of the layer of skin to which a melanoma has invaded, does not add significant prognostic information and no longer is used. Other important factors recognized via the staging classification include the presence of ulceration, evidence of nodal involvement, serum lactate dehydrogenase (LDH) level, and presence and site of distant metastases. The effects of these important prognostic factors on survival can be seen in Fig. 33-3, where survival is depicted according to stage (Table 33-4). Another determinant is anatomic site; favorable sites are the forearm and leg (excluding the feet), and unfavorable sites include the scalp, hands, feet, and mucous membranes. In general, women with stage I or II disease have better survival than men, perhaps in part because of earlier diagnosis; women frequently have melanomas on the lower leg, where self-recognition is more likely and the prognosis is better. The impact of age is not straightforward. Older individuals, especially men older than age 60 years, have worse prognoses, a finding that has been explained in part by a tendency toward later diagnosis (and thus thicker tumors) and in part by a higher proportion of acral melanomas in men. However, there is a greater risk of lymph node metastasis in young patients.

STAGING

Once the diagnosis of melanoma has been made, the tumor must be staged to determine the prognosis and treatment. The 2009 AJCC revised melanoma staging and classification are depicted in Table 33-4. The clinical stage of the patient is determined after the pathologic evaluation of the melanoma skin lesion and any clinical or radiologic assessment for metastatic disease. Pathologic staging also includes the pathologic evaluation of the regional lymph nodes obtained at sentinel lymph node biopsy or complete lymphadenectomy. All patients with melanoma should have a complete history and physical examination with attention to symptoms that may represent metastatic disease such as malaise, weight loss, headaches, visual difficulty, and pain. The physical examination should be directed to the site of the primary melanoma, looking for persistent disease or for dermal or subcutaneous nodules that could represent satellite or in-transit metastases. Physical examination also should include the regional draining lymph nodes, CNS, liver, and lungs. A complete blood count (CBC), complete metabolic panel, and LDH level should be performed. Although these are low-yield tests for uncovering metastatic disease, a microcytic anemia would raise the possibility of bowel metastases, particularly in the small bowel, and an unexplained elevated LDH should prompt a more extensive evaluation, including CT scan or possibly a positron emission tomography (PET) (or CT and PET combined) scan. If signs or symptoms of metastatic disease are uncovered, appropriate diagnostic imaging should be performed. At initial presentation, more than 80% of patients will have disease confined to the skin and a negative history and physical examination, in which case imaging generally is not indicated.

TABLE 33-4

STAGING CRITERIA FOR MELANOMA

PATHOLOGIC AND TNM STAGE	THICKNESS, mm	ULCERATION	NO. INVOLVED LYMPH NODES	NODAL INVOLVEMENT
0				
Tis	In situ	No	0	None
IA				
T1a	<1	No; mitosis <1/mm	0	None
IB				
T1b	<1	Yes or mitosis >1/mm	0	None
T2a	1.01–2	No	0	None
IIA				
T2b	1.01–2	Yes	0	None
T3a	2.01–4	No	0	None
IIB				
T3b	2.01–4	Yes	0	None
T4a	>4	No	0	None
IIC				
T4b	>4	Yes	0	None
IIIA				
N1a	T1-4a	No	1	Microscopic
N2a	T1-4a	No	2 or 3	Microscopic
IIIB				
N1a	Any	Yes	1	Microscopic
N2a	Any	Yes	2 or 3	Microscopic
N1b	Any	Yes or no	1	Macroscopic
N2b	Any	Yes or no	2 or 3	Macroscopic
N2c	Any	Yes or no	In-transit metastases or satellites; no nodal involvement	
IIIC				
N1b	Any	Yes or no	1	Macroscopic
N2b	Any	Yes or no	2 or 3	Macroscopic
N2c	Any	Yes or no	In-transit metastases or satellites, no nodal involvement	
N3	Any	Yes or no	4+ metastatic nodes, matted nodes, or in-transit metastases or satellites with metastatic nodes	
IV				
M1a		Distant metastasis		
M1b		Skin, subcutaneous		
M1c		Lung		
		Other visceral site		
		Elevated lactate dehydrogenase		

Abbreviation: TNM, tumor, node, metastasis.

Source: 2009 AJCC staging criteria and modified after H Tsao et al: N Engl J Med 351:998, 2004.

TREATMENT Melanoma

MANAGEMENT OF CLINICALLY LOCALIZED MELANOMA (STAGE I, II) For a newly diagnosed cutaneous melanoma, wide surgical excision of the lesion with a margin of normal skin is necessary to remove all malignant cells and minimize possible local recurrence. The following margins are recommended for primary melanoma: in situ, 0.5 cm; invasive up to 1 mm thick, 1 cm; >1.01–2 mm, 1–2 cm; and >2 mm, 2 cm. For lesions on the face, hands, and feet, strict adherence to these margins must give way to individual considerations about the constraints of surgery and minimization of morbidity. In all instances, however, inclusion of subcutaneous fat in the surgical specimen facilitates adequate thickness measurement and assessment of

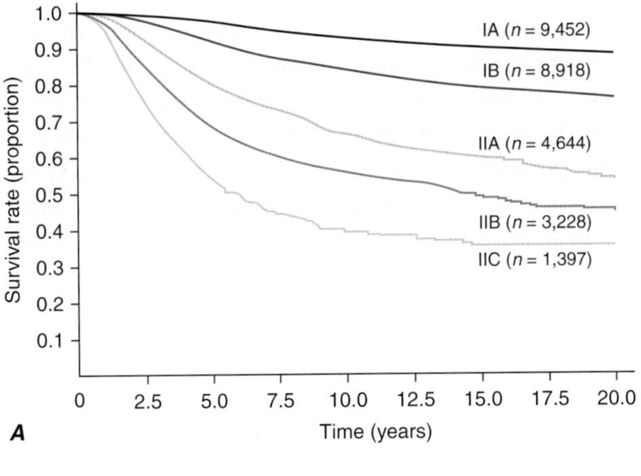

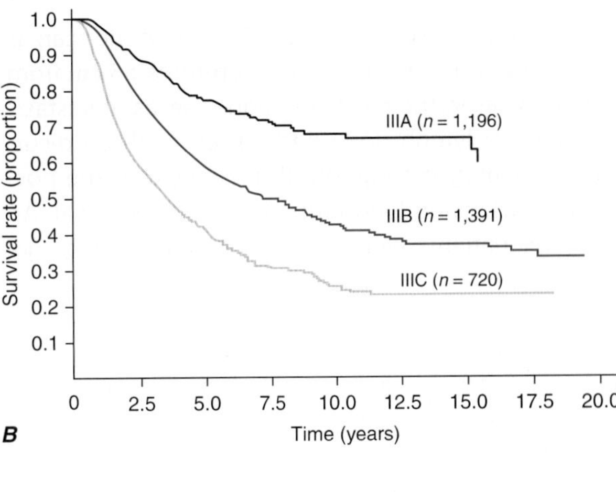

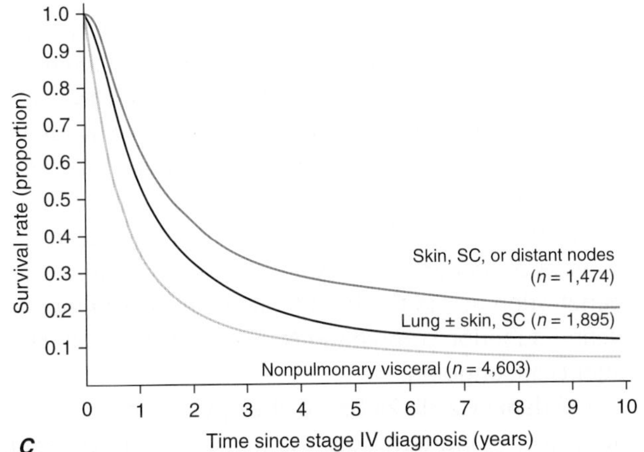

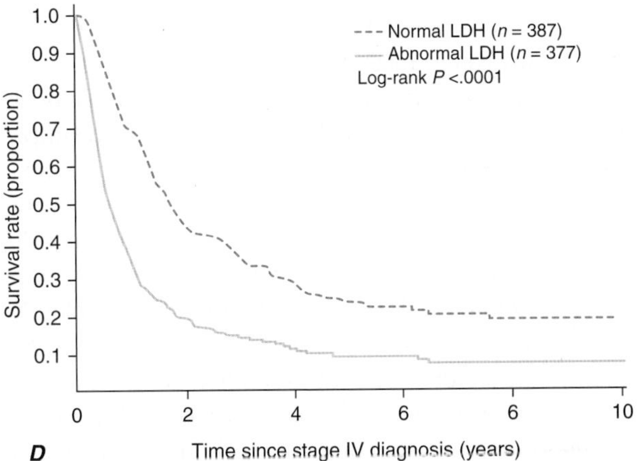

FIGURE 33-3

Survival curves for patients with melanoma. *A.* stage I and II disease; ***B.*** stage III disease; ***C.*** stage IV by site of metastatic disease; ***D.*** stage IV according to lactate dehydrogenase (LDH) level. SC, subcutaneous. (*From CM Balch et al: J Clin Oncol 27:199, 2009, with permission.*)

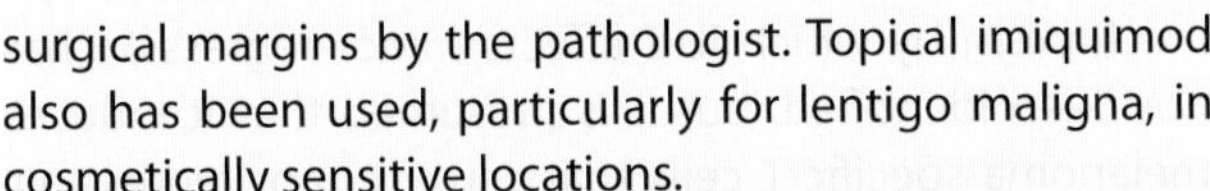

surgical margins by the pathologist. Topical imiquimod also has been used, particularly for lentigo maligna, in cosmetically sensitive locations.

Sentinel lymph node biopsy (SLNB) is a valuable staging tool that has replaced elective regional nodal dissection for the evaluation of regional nodal status. SLNB provides prognostic information and helps identify patients at high risk for relapse who may be candidates for adjuvant therapy. The initial (sentinel) draining node(s) from the primary site is (are) identified by injecting a blue dye and a radioisotope around the primary site. The sentinel node(s) then is (are) identified by inspection of the nodal basin for the blue-stained node and/or the node with high uptake of the radioisotope. The identified nodes are removed and subjected to careful histopathologic processing with serial section with hematoxylin and eosin stains as well as immunohistochemical stains to identify melanocytes (e.g., S100, HMB45, and MelanA).

Not every patient is a candidate for an SLNB. Patients whose melanomas are ≤1 mm thick and have <1 mitotic figure/mm^2 have an excellent prognosis and generally do not need an SLNB unless they have high-risk features such as young age, an ulcerated primary, and positive deep margins. They usually can be referred for wide excision as definitive therapy. Most other patients with clinically negative lymph nodes should undergo an SLNB. Patients whose SLNB findings are negative are spared a complete node dissection and its attendant morbidities. They can simply be followed or considered for adjuvant therapy or a clinical trial as appropriate for the primary lesion. The current standard of care for all patients with a positive SLN result is to perform a complete lymphadenectomy; however, ongoing clinical studies are attempting to determine whether patients with small-volume metastases in the sentinel node can be managed safely without additional surgery. Patients with microscopically positive lymph nodes should be considered for adjuvant therapy with interferon (IFN) or enrolled in a clinical trial.

MANAGEMENT OF REGIONALLY METASTATIC MELANOMA (STAGE III) Regional metastases may occur as a local recurrence at the edge of the scar or graft; as satellite metastases, which are separate from the scar but within 2–5 cm of the scar; as in-transit metastases, which are recurrences >5 cm from the scar; or, as in the most common case, as metastasis to a draining lymph node basin. Each of these recurrences is managed surgically, if possible, with the possibility of achieving long-term disease-free survival. An option for patients with extensive cutaneous regional recurrences in an extremity is isolated limb perfusion or infusion with melphalan and hyperthermia. High complete response rates have been reported, and responses are associated with significant palliation of symptoms.

After surgery, patients with regional metastases who are rendered free of disease may be at high risk for a local or distant recurrence. Therefore, some patients should be considered for adjuvant therapy. Adjuvant radiotherapy can reduce the risk of local recurrence after lymphadenectomy but does not affect overall survival. Patients with large (>3–4 cm) or multiple involved lymph nodes or extranodal spread on microscopic examination should be considered for radiation. Systemic adjuvant therapy is indicated primarily for patients with stage III disease, but high-risk, node-negative patients (>4 mm thick or ulcerated lesions) and patients with completely resected stage IV disease also may benefit. IFN-α2b, which is given for 1 year at 20 million units/m^2 intravenously 5 days a week for 4 weeks followed by 10 million units/m^2 subcutaneously three times a week for 11 months, is the only U.S. Food and Drug Administration (FDA)–approved agent for adjuvant therapy. High-dose IFN is associated with significant toxicity, including a flulike illness, decline in performance status, and the development of depression in a large fraction of patients. The toxicity can be managed in most patients by appropriate therapy for symptoms, dose reduction; treatment interruption; and, for one-third of patients, early discontinuation of IFN. Adjuvant treatment with high-dose IFN has been associated with improved disease-free survival, but its impact on overall survival is unclear. Enrollment in a clinical trial is appropriate for these patients, many of whom will otherwise be observed without treatment either because they are poor candidates for IFN or because a patient (or his or her oncologist) does not believe the beneficial effects of IFN outweigh the toxicity.

TREATMENT Metastatic Disease

When a patient with a history of melanoma develops signs or symptoms of recurrent disease, he or she should undergo restaging. This typically includes an MRI of the brain and total-body PET/CT or CT scans of the chest, abdomen, and pelvis. Distant metastases (stage IV), which may involve any organ, commonly include skin and lymph node metastases as well as visceral, bone, or brain metastases. Metastatic melanoma is generally incurable, and the median survival time ranges from 6 to 15 months, depending on the organ involved (Fig. 33-3*C*, *D*). The prognosis is better for skin and subcutaneous metastases (Mla) than for lung (M1b) or other visceral metastases (Mlc). An elevated serum LDH in a patient with metastatic disease is a poor prognostic factor and puts the patient in stage Mlc regardless of the site of the metastases.

The only FDA-approved chemotherapy for melanoma is dacarbazine (DTIC). Other agents with modest activity include temozolomide (TMZ), cisplatin and carboplatin, the taxanes, paclitaxel and docetaxel alone or albumin-bound, and carmustine (BCNU), which have reported response rates of 12–20%. Although limited in efficacy, single-agent DTIC is still considered the standard treatment because drug combinations have never been shown to improve survival. Although not FDA-approved for melanoma, TMZ, which shares an active metabolite with DTIC, has been used widely because of its ease of oral administration, excellent tolerance, and penetration across the blood–brain barrier. Attempts to define superior combinations and identify new active agents are ongoing.

Interleukin 2 (IL-2)–based therapy has been associated with long-term disease-free survival (probable cures) in 5% of treated patients. Treatment usually consists of high-dose IL-2 alone, but some centers combine IL-2 with IFN-α and chemotherapy (biochemotherapy). IL-2 therapy generally is reserved for patients with a good performance status and administered at centers with experience managing IL-2–related toxicity. The mechanism by which IL-2 effects tumor regression has not been identified, but it is presumed that it induces melanoma-specific T cells that cause tumor regression. Based on this assumption, Rosenberg and his colleagues in the National Cancer Institute (NCI) Surgery Branch have used adoptive immunotherapy with in vitro-expanded tumor-infiltrating lymphocytes with high-dose IL-2. A series of studies of adoptive T cell therapy in patients who have been treated with non-myeloablative chemotherapy (sometimes combined with total-body irradiation) have reported tumor regression in more than 50% of patients with IL-2–refractory melanoma. Multiple investigators have attempted to develop vaccination strategies against melanoma using purified tumor proteins, peptides, DNA vectors, dendritic cells, and unmodified or genetically altered tumor cells as immunogens to elicit melanoma-specific T cell responses, but none of these approaches has met with much clinical success.

A promising new approach is CTLA-4 blockade with a monoclonal antibody. CTLA-4 antibodies block the inhibitory signal produced when CTLA-4 is engaged on activated T cells, enhance T cell function, and cause tumor regression in animal models. Administration of anti–CTLA-4 (ipilimumab) to patients with previously treated metastatic melanoma in a randomized study was shown to improve overall survival compared with patients receiving a peptide vaccine. A novel spectrum of side effects that implies development of autoimmunity, so-called immune-related adverse events, has been noted. Patients who develop skin rashes, diarrhea and colitis, and hypophysitis, all of which can be managed, appear to have higher rates of tumor regression.

Targeted therapies are an exciting approach for patients with metastatic melanoma. The most promising available agents are those that target activating mutations in BRAF and c-kit, which result in constitutive activation of the MAP kinase pathway. V600E BRAF is the most common kinase mutation in melanoma. A highly selective oral BRAF inhibitor, PLX4032, has been developed, and tumor regression rates up to 70% have been reported in early clinical trials; to date, most remissions appear to be partial and of limited duration. Activating mutations in the c-kit receptor tyrosine kinase are also found in melanoma but primarily in mucosal, acral lentiginous, and lentigo maligna melanoma. Since these tumors are found in only 5% of the patients with metastatic melanoma, the number of patients with c-kit mutations is exceedingly small. Nevertheless, if present, they are largely identical to mutations found in gastrointestinal stromal tumors (GISTs), and melanomas with activating c-kit mutations can have rather dramatic responses to imatinib. The availability of targeted therapies will require that selected patients have their tumors sent for molecular typing to determine their suitability for treatment with available agents or their eligibility for clinical trials of newly developed agents. Some patients with stage IV disease will experience long-term disease-free survival after surgical resection of their metastases (metastatectomy). Surgery often is performed in patients with metastatic disease involving a small number of sites, either before or after systemic therapy. These patients may have a solitary lung or brain metastasis, but surgery increasingly is being employed in patients with metastases at more than one site. After surgery, patients with no evidence of disease can be considered for INF therapy or a clinical trial because their risk of developing additional metastases is very high.

Current therapy for the overwhelming majority of patients is palliative, so enrollment in a clinical trial is always an appropriate option, even for previously untreated patients. However, because most stage IV disease is incurable, a major focus of care, particularly for patients with poor performance status, should be the timely integration of palliative care and hospice.

FOLLOW-UP

Skin examination and surveillance at least once a year is recommended for all patients with melanoma. The National Cancer Comprehensive Network (NCCN) guidelines for patients with stage IB–IV melanoma recommend a comprehensive history and physical examination every 3–6 months for 2 years, then every 3–12 months for 3 years, and annually thereafter, as clinically indicated. Particular attention should be paid to the draining lymph nodes in stage I–III patients as resection of lymph node recurrences may still be curative. A CBC, LDH, and chest radiography are recommended at the physician's discretion. Routine imaging for metastatic disease is not recommended at this time because there is no discernible survival benefit to the early detection of metastatic disease.

PREVENTION

Primary melanoma prevention is based on protection from the sun, which includes wearing protective clothing, avoiding intense midday UV exposure and tanning booths, and routine application of a broad-spectrum ultraviolet-A/ultraviolet-B (UV-A/UV-B) sunblock with sun protection factor ≥15. This includes use of protective clothing and avoidance of intense midday UV exposure. Secondary prevention consists of education and screening. Patients should be educated in the clinical features of melanoma (ABCDEs) and advised to report any growth or other change in a pigmented lesion. Brochures are available from the American Cancer Society, the American Academy of Dermatology, the National Cancer Institute, and the Skin Cancer Foundation. Self-examination at 6- to 8-week intervals may enhance the likelihood of detecting change. Although the U.S. Preventive Services Task Force states that evidence is insufficient to recommend for or against skin cancer screening, a full-body skin cancer screening seems to be a simple, practical way to approach reducing the mortality rate for skin cancer. This is particularly true for patients with clinically atypical moles (dysplastic nevi) and those with a personal history of melanoma. Individuals with three or more primary melanomas and families with at least one invasive melanoma and two or more cases of melanoma and/or pancreatic cancer among first- or second-degree relatives on the same side of the family may benefit from genetic testing.

NONMELANOMA SKIN CANCER

Nonmelanoma skin cancer (NMSC) is the most common cancer in the United States, with an estimated annual incidence of 1.5–2 million cases. Basal cell carcinomas (BCCs) account for 70–80% of NMSCs. Squamous cell carcinomas (SCCs), though representing only

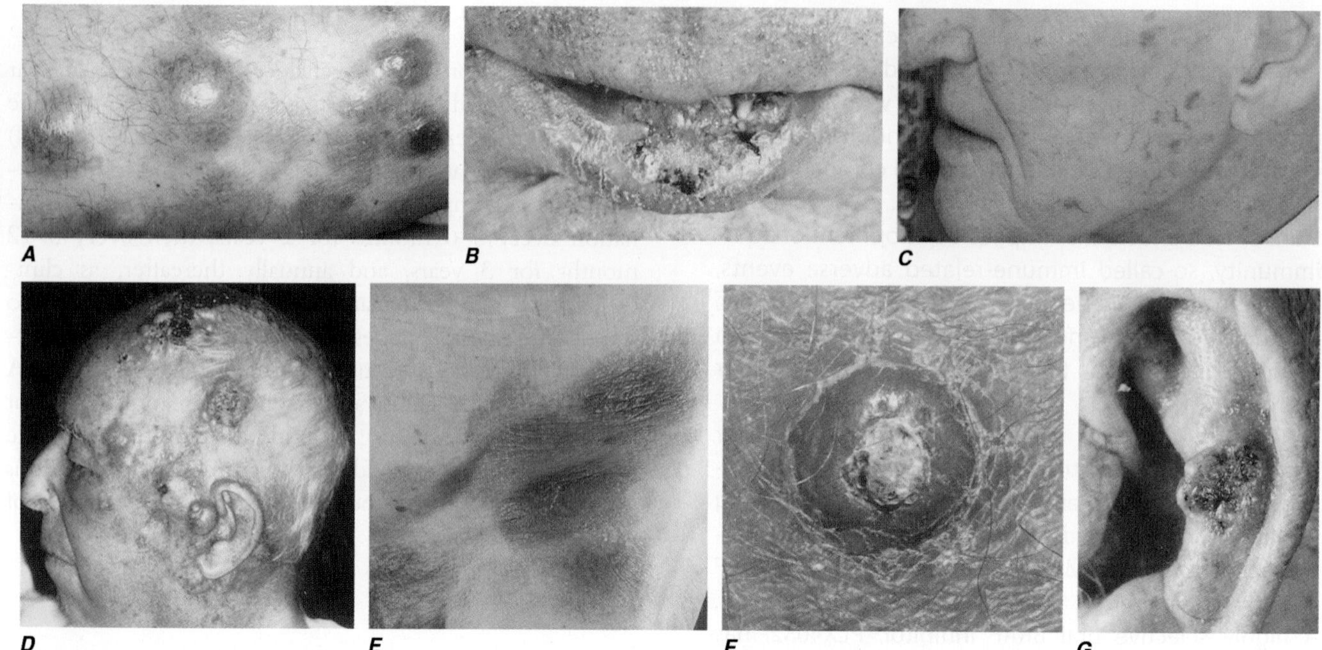

FIGURE 33-4

Cutaneous neoplasms. *A.* Non-Hodgkin's lymphoma involves the skin with typical violaceous, "plum-colored" nodules. ***B.*** Squamous cell carcinoma is seen here as a hyperkeratotic crusted and somewhat eroded plaque on the lower lip. Sun-exposed skin in areas such as the head, neck, hands, and arms represent other typical sites of involvement. ***C.*** Actinic keratoses consist of hyperkeratotic erythematous papules and patches on sun-exposed skin. They arise in middle-aged to older adults and have some potential for malignant transformation. ***D.*** Metastatic carcinoma to the skin is characterized by inflammatory, often ulcerated dermal nodules. ***E.*** Mycosis fungoides is a cutaneous T cell lymphoma, and plaque-stage lesions are seen in this patient. ***F.*** Keratoacanthoma is a low-grade squamous cell carcinoma that presents as an exophytic nodule with central keratinous debris. ***G.*** This basal cell carcinoma shows central ulceration and a pearly, rolled telangiectatic tumor border.

~20% of NMSCs, are more significant because of their ability to metastasize (Fig. 33-4). They account for most of the 2400 deaths annually. Incidence rates have risen dramatically over the past decade.

ETIOLOGY

The causes of BCC and SCC are multifactorial. Cumulative exposure to sunlight, principally the UV-B spectrum, is the most significant factor. Other factors associated with a higher incidence of skin cancer are male sex, older age, Celtic descent, a fair complexion, blond or red hair, blue or green eyes, a tendency to sunburn easily, and an outdoor occupation. The incidence of these tumors increases with decreasing latitude. Most tumors develop on sun-exposed areas of the head and neck. Tumors are more common on the left side of the body in the United States but on the right side in England, presumably owing to asymmetric exposure during driving. As the earth's protective ozone shield continues to thin, further increases in the incidence of skin cancer can be anticipated. In certain geographic areas, exposure to arsenic in well water or from industrial sources may increase the risk of BCC and SCC significantly. Skin cancer in affected individuals may be seen with or without other cutaneous markers of chronic arsenism (e.g., arsenical keratoses). Less common is exposure to the cyclic aromatic hydrocarbons in tar, soot, or shale. The risk of lip or oral SCC is increased with cigarette smoking. Human papillomaviruses and UV radiation may act as cocarcinogens.

Host factors associated with a higher risk of skin cancer include immunosuppression induced by disease or drugs. Solid-organ transplant recipients on chronic immunosuppressive therapy have a dramatically higher incidence of NMSCs. SCCs are most common, with a 65-fold increase in incidence, whereas BCCs have a tenfold increase in incidence. The frequency of skin cancer is proportional to the level and duration of immunosuppression as well as the extent of sun exposure both before and after transplantation. SCCs in this population also demonstrate more aggressive behavior with higher rates of local recurrence, metastasis, and mortality.

Skin cancer is not uncommon in patients infected with HIV, and tumors may be more aggressive in this setting. Other factors include ionizing radiation, thermal burn scars, and chronic ulcerations. Several heritable conditions are associated with skin cancer (e.g., albinism, xeroderma pigmentosum, Rombo's syndrome, Bazex-Dupré-Christol syndrome, and basal cell nevus syndrome). Background mutations in hedgehog pathway genes, primarily genes encoding patched homolog 1 (*PTCH1*) and smoothened homolog (*SMO*), occur in BCC. In fact, an oral hedgehog inhibitor has shown promise in clinical trials treating advanced inoperable or metastatic BCC.

CLINICAL PRESENTATION

NMSCs are often asymptomatic, but nonhealing ulceration, bleeding, or pain can occur in advanced lesions.

Basal cell carcinoma

BCC is a malignancy arising from epidermal basal cells. The least invasive of BCC subtypes, *superficial BCC*, classically consists of truncal erythematous scaling plaques that slowly enlarge. This BCC subtype may be confused with benign inflammatory dermatoses, especially nummular eczema and psoriasis. BCC also can present as a small, slowly growing pearly nodule, often with small telangiectatic vessels on its surface (*nodular BCC*). The occasional presence of melanin in this variant of nodular BCC (*pigmented BCC*) may lead to confusion clinically with melanoma. *Morpheaform (fibrosing) and micronodular BCC*, the most invasive subtypes, manifest as solitary, flat or slightly depressed, indurated whitish or yellowish plaques. Borders are typically indistinct, a feature associated with a greater potential for extensive subclinical spread.

Squamous cell carcinoma

Primary *cutaneous SCC* is a malignant neoplasm of keratinizing epidermal cells. SCC can grow rapidly and metastasize. The clinical features of SCC vary widely. Commonly, SCC appears as an ulcerated erythematous nodule or superficial erosion on the skin or lower lip, but it may present as a verrucous papule or plaque. Overlying telangiectasias are uncommon. The margins of this tumor may be ill defined, and fixation to underlying structures may occur. Cutaneous SCC may develop anywhere on the body but usually arises on sun-damaged skin. A related neoplasm, keratoacanthoma, typically appears as a dome-shaped papule with a central keratotic crater, expands rapidly, and commonly regresses without therapy. This lesion can be difficult to differentiate from SCC.

Actinic keratoses and *cheilitis*, both premalignant forms of SCC, present as hyperkeratotic papules on sun-exposed areas. The potential for malignant degeneration in untreated lesions ranges from 0.25 to 20%. *Bowen's disease*, the in situ form of SCC, presents as a scaling, erythematous plaque. Treatment of premalignant and in situ lesions reduces the subsequent risk of invasive disease.

NATURAL HISTORY

Basal cell carcinoma

The natural history of BCC is that of a slowly enlarging, locally invasive neoplasm. The degree of local destruction and risk of recurrence vary with the size, duration, location, and histologic subtype of the tumor; presence of recurrent disease; and various patient characteristics. Location on the central face, ears, or scalp may portend a higher risk. Small nodular, pigmented, cystic, or superficial BCCs respond well to most treatments. Large lesions and micronodular and morpheaform subtypes may be more aggressive. The metastatic potential of BCC has been estimated to be 0.0028–0.1%. Persons with either BCC or SCC have an increased risk of developing subsequent skin cancers that is estimated to be up to 40% in 5 years.

Squamous cell carcinoma

The natural history of SCC depends on both tumor and host characteristics. Tumors arising on sun-damaged skin have a lower metastatic potential than do those on protected surfaces. Cutaneous SCC metastasizes in 0.3–5.2% of individuals, most frequently to regional draining lymph nodes. Tumors occurring on the lower lip and ear have metastatic potentials approaching 13 and 11%, respectively. The metastatic potential of SCC arising in scars, chronic ulcerations, and genital or mucosal surfaces is higher. The overall metastatic rate for recurrent tumors may approach 30%. Large, poorly differentiated, deep tumors with perineural or lymphatic invasion often behave aggressively. Multiple tumors with rapid growth and aggressive behavior can be a therapeutic challenge in immunosuppressed patients.

TREATMENT Basal Cell Carcinoma

The most frequently employed treatment modalities for BCC include electrodesiccation and curettage (ED&C), excision, cryosurgery, radiation therapy, laser therapy, Mohs micrographic surgery (MMS), topical 5-fluorouracil, photodynamic therapy, and topical immunomodulators. The mode of therapy chosen depends on tumor characteristics, patient age, medical status, preferences of the patient, and other factors. ED&C remains the method most commonly employed by dermatologists. This method is selected for low-risk tumors (e.g., a small primary tumor of a less aggressive subtype in a favorable location). Excision that offers the advantage of histologic control, usually is selected for more aggressive tumors or those in high-risk locations or, in many instances, for aesthetic reasons. Cryosurgery using liquid nitrogen may be used in certain low-risk tumors but requires specialized equipment (cryoprobes) to be employed effectively.

Radiation therapy, although not used as often as a primary modality, offers an excellent chance for cure in many cases of BCC. It is useful in patients not considered surgical candidates and as a surgical adjunct in high-risk tumors. Younger patients may not be good candidates for radiation therapy because of the risks of long-term carcinogenesis and radiodermatitis. Despite rapidly advancing technology in laser development, its long-term efficacy in treating infiltrative or recurrent lesions is unknown. In contrast, MMS, a specialized type of surgical excision that permits the best histologic control and preservation of uninvolved tissue, is associated with cure rates >98%. It is the preferred modality for lesions that are recurrent, in a high-risk location, or are large and ill defined and in which maximal tissue conservation is critical (e.g., the eyelids). Topical 5-fluorouracil therapy should be limited to superficial BCC. Topical immunomodulators (e.g., imiquimod) show promise in treating superficial and even smaller nodular BCCs. Intralesional chemotherapy (5-fluorouracil and IFN) and photodynamic therapy (which employs selective activation of a photoactive drug by visible light) have been used successfully in patients with numerous tumors. A topical endonuclease (T4N5 liposome lotion) has been shown to repair DNA and may decrease the rate of NMSC in xeroderma pigmentosum.

SQUAMOUS CELL CARCINOMA Therapy for cutaneous SCC should be based on an analysis of risk factors influencing the biologic behavior of the tumor. These factors include the size, location, and degree of histologic differentiation of the tumor as well as the age and physical condition of the patient. Surgical excision, MMS, and radiation therapy are standard methods of treatment. Cryosurgery and ED&C have been used successfully for premalignant lesions and small primary tumors. Metastases are treated with lymph node dissection, irradiation, or both. 13-*cis*-Retinoic acid (1 mg/kg PO qd) plus IFN-α (3 million U SC or IM qd) may produce a partial response in most patients. Systemic chemotherapy combinations that include cisplatin may also be palliative in some patients. An oral inhibitor of the hedgehog pathway, vismodegib, produces meaningful responses in advanced disease.

PREVENTION

As the vast majority of skin cancers are related to chronic UV radiation exposure, patient and physician education could reduce their incidence dramatically. Emphasis should be placed on preventive measures that begin early in life. Patients must understand that damage from UV-B begins early despite the fact that cancers develop years later. Regular use of sunscreens and protective clothing should be encouraged. Avoidance of tanning salons and midday (10 A.M. to 2 P.M.) sun exposure is recommended. Precancerous and in situ lesions should be treated early. Early detection of small tumors allows the use of simpler treatment modalities with higher cure rates and lower morbidity rates. In patients with a history of skin cancer, long-term follow-up for the detection of recurrence, metastasis, and new skin cancers should be emphasized. Chemoprophylaxis using synthetic retinoids as well as immunosuppression reduction in transplant patients may be useful in controlling new lesions in those with multiple tumors.

OTHER NONMELANOMA CUTANEOUS MALIGNANCIES

Neoplasms of cutaneous adnexa and sarcomas of fibrous, mesenchymal, fatty, and vascular tissues make up the remaining 1–2% of NMSCs (Table 33-1) *Merkel cell carcinoma* is a neural crest–derived (cytokeratin-20-positive), highly aggressive malignancy that exhibits mortality rates of about 33% at 3 years. Recent studies have implicated a novel oncogenic Merkel cell polyomavirus that is present in 80% of tumors. Prognosis largely depends on extent of disease: 90% survival with local disease, 52% with nodal involvement, and 10% with distant disease at 3 years. Incidence tripled from 1986 to 2001 with a current estimate of 1200 cases per year in the United States. It typically presents as an asymptomatic rapidly expanding red/pink tumor on sun-exposed skin of older white patients. Treatment is surgical excision with or without sentinel lymph node biopsy, often followed by adjuvant radiation.

Extramammary Paget's disease is an uncommon apocrine malignancy arising from stem cells of the epidermis that are characterized histologically by the presence of Paget cells. These tumors present as moist erythematous patches on anogenital or, less commonly, axillary skin of the elderly. Treatment may be challenging as these tumors characteristically extend far beyond clinical margins; surgical excision with MMS has the highest cure rates. Similarly, MMS is the treatment of choice in other rare cutaneous tumors with extensive subclinical extension such as *dermatofibromasarcoma protuberans*.

Kaposi's sarcoma (KS) is a soft tissue sarcoma of vascular origin that is induced by the human herpes virus 8. The incidence of KS was rare before the AIDS epidemic. AIDS-associated KS has decreased 10-fold with the institution of highly active antiretroviral therapy.

Acknowledgment

Hensin Tsao, MD, and Arthur J. Sober, MD, contributed to this chapter in the 17th edition of Harrison's Principles of Internal Medicine, and material from that chapter is included here.

CHAPTER 34

HEAD AND NECK CANCER

Everett E. Vokes

Epithelial carcinomas of the head and neck arise from the mucosal surfaces in the head and neck area and typically are squamous cell in origin. This category includes tumors of the paranasal sinuses; the oral cavity; and the nasopharynx, oropharynx, hypopharynx, and larynx. Tumors of the salivary glands differ from the more common carcinomas of the head and neck in etiology, histopathology, clinical presentation, and therapy. Thyroid malignancies are described in Chap. 48.

INCIDENCE AND EPIDEMIOLOGY

The number of new cases of head and neck cancers in the United States was 36,540 in 2010, accounting for about 3% of adult malignancies; 7880 people died from the disease. The worldwide incidence exceeds half a million cases annually. In North America and Europe, the tumors usually arise from the oral cavity, oropharynx, or larynx, whereas nasopharyngeal cancer is more commonly seen in the Mediterranean countries and in the Far East.

ETIOLOGY AND GENETICS

Alcohol and tobacco use are the most significant risk factors for head and neck cancer in the United States. Smokeless tobacco is an etiologic agent for oral cancers. Other potential carcinogens include marijuana and occupational exposures such as nickel refining, exposure to textile fibers, and woodworking.

Dietary factors may contribute. The incidence of head and neck cancer is higher in people with the lowest consumption of fruits and vegetables. Certain vitamins, including carotenoids, may be protective if included in a balanced diet. Supplements of retinoids such as *cis*-retinoic acid have not been shown to prevent head and neck cancers (or lung cancer) and may increase the risk in active smokers.

Some head and neck cancers have a viral etiology. Epstein-Barr virus (EBV) infection is frequently associated with nasopharyngeal cancer. Nasopharyngeal cancer occurs endemically in some countries of the Mediterranean and Far East, where EBV antibody titers can be measured to screen high-risk populations. Nasopharyngeal cancer has also been associated with consumption of salted fish.

In Western countries, the human papilloma virus (HPV) is associated with approximately 50% of tumors arising from the oropharynx, i.e., the tonsillar bed and base of tongue. Similar to cervical cancer, HPV 16 and 18 are the commonly associated viral subtypes. The incidence of oropharyngeal cancers is increasing in Western counties. Epidemiologically, HPV-related oropharyngeal cancer occurs in a younger patient population and is associated with increased numbers of sexual partners and oral sexual practices.

No specific risk factors or environmental carcinogens have been identified for salivary gland tumors.

HISTOPATHOLOGY, CARCINOGENESIS, AND MOLECULAR BIOLOGY

Squamous cell head and neck cancers can be divided into well-differentiated, moderately well-differentiated, and poorly differentiated categories. Poorly differentiated tumors have a worse prognosis than well-differentiated tumors. For nasopharyngeal cancers, the less common differentiated squamous cell carcinoma is distinguished from nonkeratinizing and undifferentiated carcinoma (lymphoepithelioma) that contains infiltrating lymphocytes and is commonly associated with EBV.

Salivary gland tumors can arise from the major (parotid, submandibular, sublingual) or minor salivary glands (located in the submucosa of the upper aerodigestive tract). Most parotid tumors are benign, but half of submandibular and sublingual gland tumors and most minor salivary gland tumors are malignant. Malignant tumors include mucoepidermoid and adenoid cystic carcinomas and adenocarcinomas.

The mucosal surface of the entire pharynx is exposed to alcohol- and tobacco-related carcinogens and is at risk for the development of a premalignant or malignant lesion. Erythroplakia (a red patch) or leukoplakia (a white patch) can be histopathologically hyperplasia, dysplasia, carcinoma in situ, or carcinoma. However, most head and neck cancers do not present with a history of premalignant lesions. Multiple synchronous or metachronous cancers can also be observed. In fact, over time patients with early-stage head and neck cancer are at greater risk of dying from a second malignancy than from a recurrence of the primary disease.

Second head and neck malignancies are usually not therapy-induced; they reflect the exposure of the upper aerodigestive mucosa to the same carcinogens that caused the first cancer. These second primaries develop in the head and neck area, the lung, or the esophagus. Rarely, patients can develop a radiation therapy–induced sarcoma after having undergone radiotherapy for a head and neck cancer.

The molecular carcinogenesis of head and neck cancer is a developing story. Activation of oncogenes and inactivation of tumor suppressor genes (frequently of p53) have been described. Overexpression of the epidermal growth factor receptor (EGF-R) is common and of prognostic importance.

Resected tumor specimens with histopathologically negative margins ("complete resection") can have residual tumor cells with persistent p53 mutations at the margins. Thus, a tumor-specific p53 mutation can be detected in some phenotypically "normal" surgical margins, indicating residual disease. Patients with such submicroscopic marginal involvement may have a worse prognosis than patients with truly negative margins.

CLINICAL PRESENTATION AND DIFFERENTIAL DIAGNOSIS

Most head and neck cancers occur in patients older than age 50 years. HPV-related malignancies are frequently diagnosed in patients in their 40s, while EBV-related nasopharyngeal cancer can occur in all ages, including teenagers. The manifestations vary according to the stage and primary site of the tumor. Patients with nonspecific signs and symptoms in the head and neck area should be evaluated with a thorough otolaryngologic exam, particularly if symptoms persist longer than 2–4 weeks.

Cancer of the nasopharynx typically does not cause early symptoms. However, on occasion it may cause unilateral serous otitis media due to obstruction of the eustachian tube, unilateral or bilateral nasal obstruction, or epistaxis. Advanced nasopharyngeal carcinoma causes neuropathies of the cranial nerves due to skull base involvement.

Carcinomas of the oral cavity present as nonhealing ulcers, changes in the fit of dentures, or painful lesions. Tumors of the tongue base or oropharynx can cause decreased tongue mobility and alterations in speech. Cancers of the oropharynx or hypopharynx rarely cause early symptoms, but they may cause sore throat and/or otalgia.

Hoarseness may be an early symptom of laryngeal cancer, and persistent hoarseness requires referral to a specialist for indirect laryngoscopy and/or radiographic studies. If a head and neck lesion treated initially with antibiotics does not resolve in a short period, further workup is indicated; to simply continue the antibiotic treatment may be to lose the chance of early diagnosis of a malignancy.

Advanced head and neck cancers in any location can cause severe pain, otalgia, airway obstruction, cranial neuropathies, trismus, odynophagia, dysphagia, decreased tongue mobility, fistulas, skin involvement, and massive cervical lymphadenopathy, which may be unilateral or bilateral. Some patients have enlarged lymph nodes even though no primary lesion can be detected by endoscopy or biopsy; these patients are considered to have carcinoma of unknown primary (Fig. 34-1). If the enlarged nodes are located in the upper neck and the tumor cells are of squamous cell histology, the malignancy probably arose from

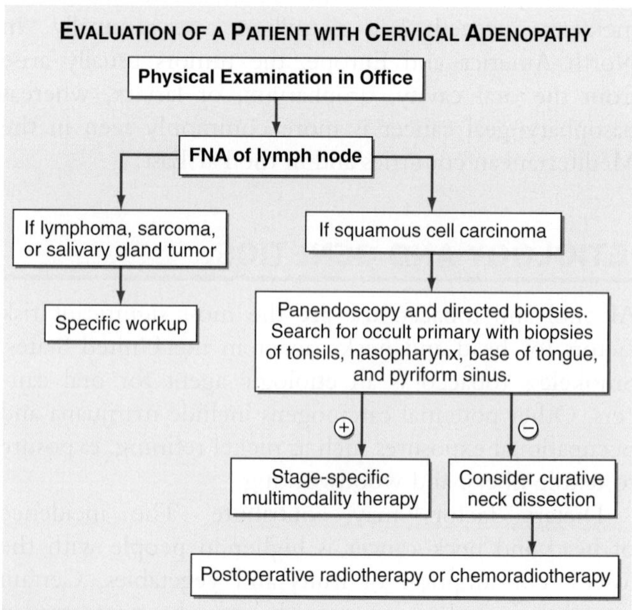

FIGURE 34-1

Evaluation of a patient with cervical adenopathy without a primary mucosal lesion; a diagnostic workup. FNA, fine-needle aspiration.

a mucosal surface in the head or neck. Tumor cells in supraclavicular lymph nodes may also arise from a primary site in the chest or abdomen.

The physical examination should include inspection of all visible mucosal surfaces and palpation of the floor of mouth and tongue and of the neck. In addition to tumors themselves, leukoplakia (a white mucosal patch) or erythroplakia (a red mucosal patch) may be observed; these "premalignant" lesions can represent hyperplasia, dysplasia, or carcinoma in situ and require biopsy. Further examination should be performed by a specialist. Additional staging procedures include CT of the head and neck to identify the extent of the disease. Patients with lymph node involvement should have chest radiography and a bone scan to screen for distant metastases. A positron emission tomographic scan may also be administered and can help to identify or exclude distant metastases. The definitive staging procedure is an endoscopic examination under anesthesia, which may include laryngoscopy, esophagoscopy, and bronchoscopy; during this procedure, multiple biopsy samples are obtained to establish a primary diagnosis, define the extent of primary disease, and identify any additional premalignant lesions or second primaries.

Head and neck tumors are classified according to the TNM (tumor, node, metastasis) system of the American Joint Committee on Cancer. This classification varies according to the specific anatomic subsite (Tables 34-1 and 34-2). Distant metastases are found in <10% of patients at initial diagnosis and are more common in patients with advanced lymph nodal stage; microscopic involvement of the lungs, bones, or liver is more common, particularly in patients with advanced neck lymph node disease. Modern imaging techniques may increase the number of patients with clinically detectable distant metastases in the future.

In patients with lymph node involvement and no visible primary, the diagnosis should be made by lymph node excision. If the results indicate squamous cell carcinoma, a panendoscopy should be performed, with biopsy of all suspicious-appearing areas and directed biopsies of common primary sites, such as the nasopharynx, tonsil, tongue base, and pyriform sinus.

TABLE 34-1

TUMOR, NODE, METASTASIS CLASSIFICATION FOR HEAD AND NECK CANCER

	PRIMARY TUMOR SITE (EXAMPLE)	
T GRADE	**OROPHARYNX**	**HYPOPHARYNX**
T1	0–2 cm	0–2 cm
T2	2.1–4 cm	>1 site, 2.1–4 cm
T3	>4 cm	>4 cm or fixation of hemilarynx
T4a	Invasion of larynx, muscle of tongue, medial pterygoid, hard palate, mandible	Invasion of thyroid/cricoid cartilage, hyoid bone, thyroid gland, esophagus, or central compartment soft tissue invasion
T4b	Invasion of lateral pterygoid muscle, pterygoid plates, lateral nasopharynx, or skull base or encases carotid artery	Invasion of prevertebral fascia, encases carotid artery, or involvement of mediastinal structures

Regional Lymph Nodes (N)

NX	Regional lymph nodes cannot be assessed
N0	No regional lymph node metastasis
N1	Unilateral metastasis in lymph node(s), ≤3 cm in greatest dimension
N2	Single ipsilateral lymph node >3.1, ≤6 cm, or multiple ipsilateral, or contralateral lymph nodes ≤6 cm. Bilateral metastasis in lymph node(s), ≤6 cm in greatest dimension, above the supraclavicular fossa
N3	Lymph node >6 cm in greatest dimension

Stage Grouping

Stage 0	Tis	N0	M0
Stage I	T1	N0	M0
Stage II	T2	N0	M0
Stage III	T3	N0	M0
	T1-T3	N1	M0
Stage IVA	T4a	N0	M0
	T4a	N1	M0
	T1-T4a	N2	M0
Stage IVB	T4b	Any N	M0
	Any T	N3	M0
Stage IVC	Any T	Any N	M1

TREATMENT Head and Neck Cancer

Patients with head and neck cancer can be grossly categorized into three clinical groups: those with localized disease, those with locally or regionally advanced disease, and those with recurrent and/or metastatic disease. Comorbidities associated with tobacco and alcohol abuse can affect treatment outcome and define long-term risks for patients who are cured of their disease.

LOCALIZED DISEASE Nearly one-third of patients have localized disease, that is, T1 or T2 (stage I or stage II) lesions without detectable lymph node involvement or distant metastases. These lesions are treated with curative intent by either surgery or radiation therapy. The choice of modality differs according to anatomic location and institutional expertise. Radiation therapy is often preferred for laryngeal cancer to preserve voice

TABLE 34-2

DEFINITION OF TUMOR, NODE, METASTASIS–NASOPHARYNX

PRIMARY TUMOR (T)	STAGE GROUPING
Tis	Carcinoma in situ
T1	Tumor confined to the nasopharynx
T2	Tumor extends to parapharyngeal soft tissues
T3	Tumor involves bony structures of skull base and/or paranasal sinuses
T4	Tumor with intracranial extension and/or involvement of cranial nerves, infratemporal fossa, hypopharynx, orbit, or masticator space
Regional Lymph Nodes (N)	
	The distribution and the prognostic impact of regional lymph node spread from nasopharynx cancer, particularly of the undifferentiated type, are different from those of other head and neck mucosal cancers and justify the use of a different N classification scheme
N0	No regional lymph node metastasis
N1	Unilateral metastasis in lymph node(s), ≤6 cm in greatest dimension, above the supraclavicular fossa
N2	Bilateral metastasis in lymph node(s), ≤6 cm in greatest dimension, above the supraclavicular fossa
N3	Metastasis in lymph node(s), >6 cm and/or to supraclavicular fossa
N3a	Greater than 6 cm in dimension
N3b	Extension to the supraclavicular fossa

ANATOMIC STAGE/PROGNOSTIC GROUPS

Nasopharynx			
Stage 0	Tis	N0	M0
Stage I	T1	N0	M0
Stage II	T1	N1	M0
	T2	N0–N1	M0
Stage III	T1	N2	M0
	T2	N2	M0
	T3	N0–N2	M0
Stage IVA	T4	N0–N2	M0
Stage IVB	Any T	N3	M0
Stage IVC	Any T	Any N	M1

function, and surgery is preferred for small lesions in the oral cavity to avoid the long-term complications of radiation, such as xerostomia and dental decay. Overall 5-year survival is 60–90%. Most recurrences occur within the first 2 years following diagnosis and are usually local.

LOCALLY OR REGIONALLY ADVANCED DISEASE Locally or regionally advanced disease—disease with a large primary tumor and/or lymph node metastases—is the stage of presentation for >50% of patients. Such patients can also be treated with curative intent but not with surgery or radiation therapy alone. Combined modality therapy including surgery, radiation therapy, and chemotherapy is most successful. It can be administered as induction chemotherapy (chemotherapy before surgery and/or radiotherapy) or as concomitant (simultaneous) chemotherapy and radiation therapy. The latter is currently most commonly used and best evidence–supported. In patients with intermediate stage (stage III and early stage IV), concomitant chemoradiotherapy is given postoperatively. It can be administered either as a primary treatment for patients with unresectable disease, to pursue an organ-preserving approach, or in the postoperative setting for intermediate-stage resectable tumors.

Induction chemotherapy In this strategy, patients receive chemotherapy (current standard is a three-drug regimen of docetaxel, cisplatin, and fluorouracil [5-FU]) before surgery and radiation therapy. Most patients who receive three cycles show tumor reduction, and the response is clinically "complete" in up to half. This "sequential" multimodality therapy allows for organ preservation (omission of surgery) in patients with laryngeal and hypopharyngeal cancer, and it has been shown to result in higher cure rates compared with radiotherapy alone.

Concomitant chemoradiotherapy With the concomitant strategy, chemotherapy and radiation therapy are given simultaneously rather than in sequence. Tumor recurrences from head and neck cancer develop most commonly locoregionally (in the head and neck area of the primary and draining lymph nodes). The concomitant approach is aimed at enhancing tumor cell killing by radiation therapy in the presence of chemotherapy (radiation enhancement). Toxicity (especially mucositis, grade 3 or 4 in 70–80%) is increased with concomitant chemoradiotherapy. However, meta-analyses of randomized trials document an improvement in 5-year survival of 8% with concomitant chemotherapy and radiation therapy. Results seem more favorable in recent trials as more active drugs or more intensive radiotherapy schedules are used. The 5-year survival rate is 34–50%. In addition, concomitant chemoradiotherapy produces better laryngectomy-free survival (organ preservation) than radiation therapy alone in patients with advanced larynx cancer. The use of radiation therapy together with cisplatin has also produced improved survival in patients with advanced nasopharyngeal cancer. The outcome of HPV-related cancers seems to be especially favorable following cisplatin-based chemoradiotherapy.

The success of concomitant chemoradiotherapy in patients with unresectable disease has led to the testing of a similar approach in patients with resected intermediate-stage disease as a postoperative therapy. Concomitant chemoradiotherapy produces a significant improvement over postoperative radiation therapy alone for patients whose tumors demonstrate higher risk features, such as extracapsular spread beyond involved lymph nodes, involvement of multiple lymph nodes, or positive margins at the primary site following surgery.

A monoclonal antibody to the EGF-R (cetuximab) increases survival rates when administered during radiotherapy. EGF-R blockade results in radiation sensitization and has milder systemic side effects than traditional chemotherapy agents, although an acneiform skin rash is commonly observed. The integration of cetuximab into current standard chemoradiotherapy regimens is under investigation.

RECURRENT OR METASTATIC DISEASE Ten percent of patients present with metastatic disease, and more than half of patients with locoregionally advanced disease have recurrence, frequently outside the head and neck region. Patients with recurrent and/or metastatic disease are, with few exceptions, treated with palliative intent. Some patients may require local or regional radiation therapy for pain control, but most are given chemotherapy. Response rates to chemotherapy average only 30–50%; the duration of response averages only 3 months, and the median survival time is 6–8 months. Therefore, chemotherapy provides transient symptomatic benefit. Drugs with single-agent activity in this setting include methotrexate, 5-FU, cisplatin, paclitaxel, and docetaxel. Combinations of cisplatin with 5-FU, carboplatin with 5-FU, and cisplatin or carboplatin with paclitaxel or docetaxel are frequently used.

EGF-R–directed therapies, including monoclonal antibodies (e.g., cetuximab) and tyrosine kinase inhibitors (TKIs) of the EGF-R signaling pathway (e.g., erlotinib or gefitinib) have single-agent activity of approximately 10%. Side effects are usually limited to an acneiform rash and diarrhea (for the TKIs). The addition of cetuximab to standard combination chemotherapy with cis- or carboplatin and 5-FU was shown to result in a significant increase in median survival.

COMPLICATIONS Complications from treatment of head and neck cancer are usually correlated to the extent of surgery and exposure of normal tissue structures to radiation. Currently, the extent of surgery has been limited or completely replaced by chemotherapy and radiation therapy as the primary approach. Acute complications of radiation include mucositis and dysphagia. Long-term complications include xerostomia, loss of taste, decreased tongue mobility, second malignancies, dysphagia, and neck fibrosis. The complications of chemotherapy vary with the regimen used but usually include myelosuppression, mucositis, nausea and vomiting, and nephrotoxicity (with cisplatin).

The mucosal side effects of therapy can lead to malnutrition and dehydration. Many centers address issues of dentition before starting treatment, and some place feeding tubes to ensure control of hydration and nutrition intake. About 50% of patients develop hypothyroidism from the treatment; thus, thyroid function should be monitored.

SALIVARY GLAND TUMORS

Most benign salivary gland tumors are treated with surgical excision, and patients with invasive salivary gland tumors are treated with surgery and radiation therapy. These tumors may recur regionally; adenoid cystic carcinoma has a tendency to recur along the nerve tracks. Distant metastases may occur as late as 10–20 years after the initial diagnosis. For metastatic disease, therapy is given with palliative intent, usually chemotherapy with doxorubicin and/or cisplatin. Identification of novel agents with activity in these tumors is a high priority.

CHAPTER 35

NEOPLASMS OF THE LUNG

Leora Horn ■ William Pao ■ David H. Johnson

Lung cancer is largely a disease of modern humans and was considered quite rare before 1900, with fewer than 400 cases described in the medical literature. However, by the mid-twentieth century, lung cancer had become epidemic and firmly established as the leading cause of cancer-related death in North America and Europe, killing more than three times as many men as prostate cancer and nearly twice as many women as breast cancer. This fact is particularly distressing since lung cancer is one of the most preventable of all of the common malignancies. Tobacco consumption is the primary cause of lung cancer, a fact firmly established in the mid-twentieth century and codified with the release of the U.S. Surgeon General's 1964 report on the health effects of tobacco smoking. Following the report, cigarette use started to decline in North America and parts of Europe and with it so did the incidence of lung cancer. To date, the decline in lung cancer is seen most clearly in men; only recently has the decline become apparent among women in the United States. Unfortunately, in many parts of the world, especially in countries with developing economies, cigarette use continues to increase, and along with it, the incidence of lung cancers is also rising. While tobacco smoking remains the primary cause of lung cancer worldwide, more than 60% of new lung cancers occur in never smokers (smoked <100 cigarettes per lifetime) or former smokers (smoked ≥100 cigarettes per lifetime, quit ≥1 year), many of whom quit decades ago. Moreover, 1 in 5 women and 1 in 12 men diagnosed with lung cancer have never smoked. Given the magnitude of the problem, it is incumbent that every internist has a broad knowledge of lung cancer and its management.

EPIDEMIOLOGY

Lung cancer is the most common cause of cancer death among American men and women. It was predicted that more than 220,000 individuals would be diagnosed with lung cancer in the United States in 2010. The incidence of lung cancer peaked among men in the late 1980s and has plateaued in women. Lung cancer is rare before age 40 years, with rates increasing until age 80 years, after which the rate tapers off. The projected lifetime probability of developing lung cancer is estimated to be approximately 8% among males and approximately 6% among females. The incidence of lung cancer varies by racial and ethnic group, with the highest age-adjusted incidence rates among African Americans. The excess in age-adjusted rates among African Americans occurs only among men, but age-specific rates show that before age 50 years, mortality from lung cancer is more than 25% higher among African American than white women. Incidence and mortality rates among Hispanic and Native and Asian Americans are approximately 40–50% those of whites.

RISK FACTORS

While the large majority (80–90%) of lung cancers is caused by cigarette smoking, several other factors have been implicated, although none to the extent of tobacco. Cigarette smokers have a 10-fold or greater increase in risk of this cancer compared with those who have never smoked. A deep sequencing study suggested that one genetic mutation is induced for every 15 cigarettes smoked. The risk of lung cancer is lower among persons who quit smoking than among those who continue smoking; former smokers have a ninefold increased risk of developing lung cancer compared with men who have never smoked versus the 20-fold excess in those who continue to smoke. The size of the risk reduction increases with the length of time the person has quit smoking, although generally even long-term former smokers have higher risks of lung cancer than those who never smoked. Cigarette smoking increases the risk of all the major lung cancer cell types. Environmental tobacco smoke (ETS) or second-hand smoke is also an established cause of lung cancer. The risk from ETS is less than from active smoking, with a 20–30% increase in lung cancer observed among never smokers married for many years to smokers compared with the 2000% increase among continuing active smokers.

While cigarette smoking is the dominant cause of lung cancer, several other risk factors have been identified, including occupational exposures to asbestos, arsenic, bischloromethyl ether, hexavalent chromium, mustard gas, nickel (as in certain nickel-refining processes), and polycyclic aromatic hydrocarbons. Occupational studies also have provided insight into possible mechanisms of lung cancer induction. For example, the risk of lung cancer among asbestos-exposed workers is increased primarily among those with underlying asbestosis, raising the possibility that the scarring and inflammation produced by this fibrotic nonmalignant lung disease may in many cases (though likely not in all) be the trigger for asbestos-induced lung cancer. Several other occupational exposures have been associated with increased rates of lung cancer, but the causal nature of the association is not as clear.

The risk of lung cancer appears higher among individuals with low fruit and vegetable intake during adulthood. This observation led to hypotheses that specific nutrients, in particular retinoids and carotenoids, might have chemopreventive effects for lung cancer. However, randomized trials failed to validate this hypothesis. In fact, studies found the incidence of lung cancer was increased among smokers with supplementation. Ionizing radiation is also an established lung carcinogen, most convincingly demonstrated from studies showing increased rates of lung cancer among survivors of the atom bombs dropped on Hiroshima and Nagasaki and large excesses among workers exposed to alpha irradiation from radon in underground uranium mining. Prolonged exposure to low-level radon in homes might impart a risk of lung cancer equal or greater than that of ETS. Prior lung diseases such as chronic bronchitis, emphysema, and tuberculosis have been linked to increased risks of lung cancer as well.

Smoking cessation

Given the undeniable link between cigarette smoking and lung cancer (not even addressing other tobacco-related illnesses), physicians must promote tobacco abstinence. Physicians also must help their patients who smoke to stop smoking. Smoking cessation, even well into middle age, can minimize an individual's subsequent risk of lung cancer. Stopping tobacco use before middle age avoids more than 90% of the lung cancer risk attributable to tobacco. However, little health benefit is derived from just "cutting back." Importantly, smoking cessation can even be beneficial in individuals with an established diagnosis of lung cancer, as it is associated with improved survival, fewer side effects from therapy, and an overall improvement in quality of life. Moreover, smoking can alter the metabolism of many chemotherapy drugs, potentially adversely altering the toxicities and therapeutic benefits of the agents. Consequently, it is important to promote smoking cessation even *after* the diagnosis of lung cancer is established.

Physicians need to understand the essential elements of smoking cessation therapy. The individual must want to stop smoking and must be willing to work hard to achieve the goal of smoking abstinence. Self-help strategies alone only marginally affect quit rates, whereas individual and combined pharmacotherapies in combination with counseling can significantly increase rates of cessation. Therapy with an antidepressant (e.g., bupropion) or nicotine replacement therapy (varenicline, an $\alpha_4\beta_2$ nicotinic acetylcholine receptor partial agonist), are approved by the U.S. Food and Drug Administration (FDA) as first-line treatments for nicotine dependence. However, both drugs have been reported to increase suicidal ideation and must be used with caution. In a randomized trial, varenicline was more efficacious than bupropion or placebo. Prolonged use of varenicline beyond the initial induction phase proved useful in maintaining smoking abstinence. Clonidine and nortriptyline are recommended as second-line treatments.

Inherited predisposition to lung cancer

Exposure to environmental carcinogens, such as those found in tobacco smoke, induce or facilitate the transformation from bronchoepithelial cells to the malignant phenotype. The contribution of carcinogens on transformation is modulated by polymorphic variations in genes that affect aspects of carcinogen metabolism. Certain genetic polymorphisms of the P450 enzyme system, specifically CYP1A1, or chromosome fragility are associated with the development of lung cancer. These genetic variations occur at relatively high frequency in the population, but their contribution to an individual's lung cancer risk is generally low. However, because of their population frequency, the overall impact on lung cancer risk could be high. In addition, environmental factors, as modified by inherited modulators, likely affect specific genes by deregulating important pathways to enable the cancer phenotype.

First-degree relatives of lung cancer probands have a two- to threefold excess risk of lung cancer and other cancers, many of which are not smoking-related. These data suggest that specific genes and/or genetic variants may contribute to susceptibility to lung cancer. However, very few such genes have yet been identified.

Individuals with inherited mutations in *RB* (patients with retinoblastoma living to adulthood) and *p53* (Li-Fraumeni syndrome) genes may develop lung cancer. Three genetic loci for lung cancer risk have been identified by genomewide association studies, including 5p15 (TERT-CLPTM1L), 15q25(CHRNA5-CHRNA-3 nicotinic acetylcholine receptor subunits), and 6p21 (BAT3-MSH5). A rare germline mutation (T790M) involving the epidermal growth factor receptor (EGF-R) maybe be linked to lung cancer susceptibility in never smokers. Currently, however, no molecular criteria are used to select patients for more intense screening regimens or for specific chemopreventive strategies.

PATHOLOGY

The term *lung cancer* is used for tumors arising from the respiratory epithelium (bronchi, bronchioles, and alveoli). Mesotheliomas, lymphomas, and stromal tumors (sarcomas) are distinct from epithelial lung cancers. According to the World Health Organization classification, epithelial lung cancers consist of four major cell types: small cell lung cancer (SCLC) and the so-called non–small cell lung cancer (NSCLC) histologies including adenocarcinoma, squamous cell carcinoma, and large cell carcinoma (Fig. 35-1). These four histologies account for approximately 90% of all epithelial lung cancers. The remainder include undifferentiated carcinomas, carcinoids, bronchial gland tumors (including adenoid cystic carcinomas and mucoepidermoid tumors), and rarer tumor types. Tumors may occur as single or mixed-type histology.

All histologic types of lung cancer can be found in current and former smokers. Historically, the histologies associated with heavy tobacco use are squamous and small cell carcinomas. Squamous carcinoma was the most commonly diagnosed form of NSCLC; however, with the steady decline in cigarette consumption over the past four decades and changes in cigarette manufacturing (including use of different types of filters), adenocarcinoma has replaced squamous cell carcinoma as the most frequent histologic subtype in North America. The incidence of small cell carcinoma is also on the decline. In lifetime never smokers, all histologic forms of lung cancer can be found, although adenocarcinoma tends to predominate. Among women and young adults (<60 years), adenocarcinoma tends also to be the most common form of lung cancer.

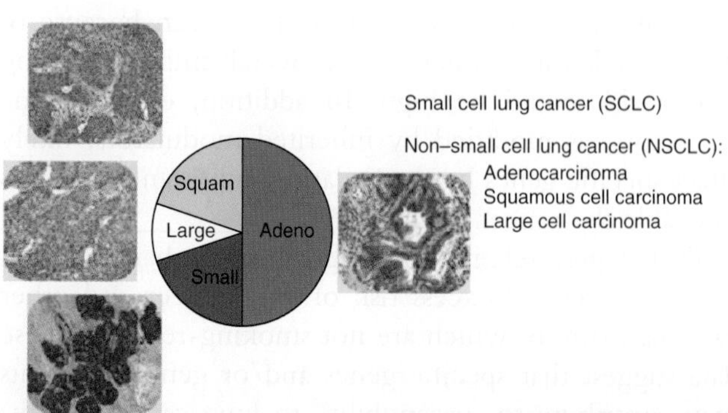

FIGURE 35-1
Traditional view of lung cancer.

Small cell carcinoma is a poorly differentiated neuroendocrine tumor that tends to occur as a central mass with endobronchial growth and is strongly associated with smoking. Small cell carcinoma cells have scant cytoplasm, small hyperchromatic nuclei with a fine ("salt and pepper") chromatin pattern, and prominent nucleoli. Tumors might be arranged in diffuse sheets of cells or may show neuroendocrine patterns such as rosettes, trabeculae, or peripheral palisading of cells at the periphery of nests. There is often widespread cellular necrosis. Small cell carcinomas, more often than non–small cell carcinomas, may produce specific peptide hormones such as adrenocorticotrophic hormone (ACTH), arginine vasopressin (AVP), atrial natriuretic factor (ANF), and gastrin-releasing peptide (GRP). These hormones may be associated with distinctive paraneoplastic syndromes that prompt workup and eventual diagnosis (Chap. 52).

Squamous cell carcinomas of the lung are morphologically identical to extrapulmonary (i.e., head and neck) squamous cell carcinomas and require clinical correlation to differentiate. These tumors tend to occur centrally and are classically associated with a history of smoking. Histologically, the most common pattern is that of an infiltrating nest of tumor cells that lack intercellular bridges. Keratin can usually be seen when present.

Adenocarcinomas often occur in more peripheral lung locations and may be associated with a history of smoking. However, adenocarcinomas are the most common type of lung cancer occurring in never smokers. Histologically, the tissue may contain the presence of glands, papillary structure, bronchioloalveolar pattern, cellular mucin, or solid pattern if poorly differentiated. Variants of adenocarcinomas include signet-ring, clear cell, and mucinous and fetal adenocarcinomas. Bronchioloalveolar carcinoma (BAC) is a subtype of adenocarcinoma that grows along the alveoli without invasion and can present radiographically as a single mass, as a diffuse multinodular lesion, as a fluffy infiltrate, and on screening computed tomography (CT) scans as a "ground-glass" opacity (GGO). Pure BAC is relatively rare. More common is adenocarcinoma with BAC features. BAC may present in a mucinous form, which tends to be multicentric, and a nonmucinous form, which tends to be solitary.

Large cell carcinomas tend to occur peripherally and are defined as poorly differentiated carcinomas of the lung composed of larger malignant cells without evidence of squamous, glandular differentiation, or features of small cell carcinoma by light microscopy. These tumors usually consist of sheets of large malignant cells, often with associated necrosis. Cytologically, the tumor is also arranged in syncytial groups and single cells. Variants of large cell, carcinoma include basaloid carcinoma, which may present as an endobronchial lesion and may resemble a high-grade neuroendocrine tumor, and lymphoepithelioma-like carcinoma, which is similar to the same-named tumor of other sites and is Epstein-Barr virus–related.

Historically, for treatment and prognostication purposes, the major distinction has been between SCLC and NSCLC, as these tumors have quite different natural histories and therapeutic approaches. SCLC is typically widely disseminated at diagnosis. Even if localized, it is rarely curable by surgery. By contrast, NSCLC can be potentially cured by resection in up to 30% of cases. Small cell cancers tend to respond more favorably to traditional cytotoxic chemotherapy agents. Intrinsic drug resistance is the norm for both SCLC and NSCLC. As knowledge of tumor biology improves, more sophisticated classification schemas are under development, including ones based in part on the presence of specific mutations and molecular alterations (Fig. 35-2). Recognition of these molecular distinctions may help guide therapy in the future.

IMMUNOHISTOCHEMISTRY

The diagnosis of lung cancer most often rests on the morphologic or cytologic features correlated with clinical and radiographic findings. Immunohistochemistry may be used to verify neuroendocrine differentiation within a tumor, with markers such as neuron-specific enolase (NSE), CD56 or neural cell adhesion molecule (NCAM), synaptophysin, chromogranin, and Leu7 (Table 35-1). Immunohistochemistry is also helpful in differentiating primary from metastatic adenocarcinomas. Thyroid transcription factor 1 (TTF-1), identified in tumors of thyroid and pulmonary origin, is positive in more than 70% of pulmonary adenocarcinomas and is a reliable indicator of primary lung cancer, provided a thyroid primary has been excluded. A negative TTF-1

TABLE 35-1

COMMON IMMUNOHISTOCHEMICAL MARKERS USED IN THE DIAGNOSIS OF LUNG TUMORS

HISTOLOGY	POSITIVE IMMUNOHISTOCHEMICAL MARKERS
Squamous cell carcinoma	Cytokeratin (CK) cocktail (e.g., AE1/AE3) CK5/6 CK7 rare
Adenocarcinoma	Cytokeratin cocktail (e.g., AE1/AE3) CK7 TTF-1 Neuroendocrine markers rare (e.g., CD56, NSE)
Large cell carcinoma	Cytokeratin TTF-1 rare Neuroendocrine markers rare (e.g., CD56, NSE)
Large cell neuroendocrine carcinoma	Cytokeratin cocktail (e.g., AE1/AE3) TTF-1 CD56 Chromogranin Synaptophysin
Small cell carcinoma	Cytokeratin cocktail (tends to be patchy) TTF-1 CD56 Chromogranin Synaptophysin

Abbreviations: NCAM, neural cell adhesion molecule; NSE, neuron-specific enolase; TTF-1, thyroid transcription factor 1; WT-1, Wilms' tumor gene 1.

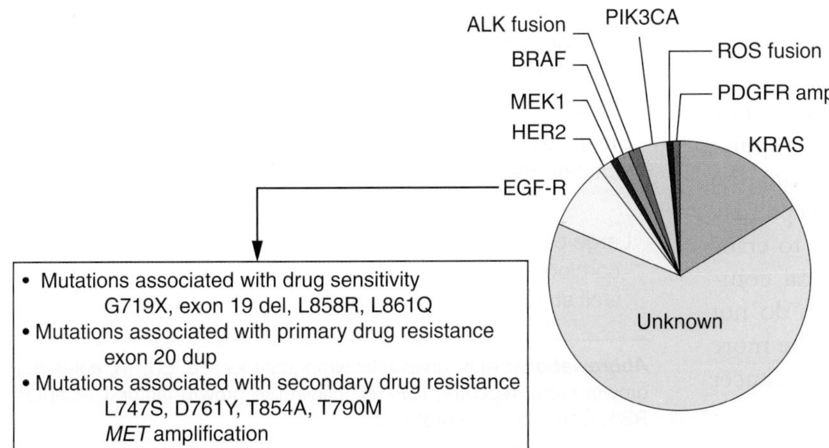

FIGURE 35-2

2010: Lung adenocarcinoma—multiple molecular subsets.

result, however, does not exclude the possibility of a lung primary. TTF-1 is also positive in neuroendocrine tumors of pulmonary and extrapulmonary origin. Cytokeratins 7 and 20 used in combination can help narrow the differential diagnosis; nonsquamous NSCLC, SCLC, and mesothelioma may stain positive for CK7 and negative for CK20, while squamous cell lung cancer will be both CK7 and CK20 negative. Mesothelioma can be easily identified ultrastructurally, but it has historically been difficult to differentiate from adenocarcinoma through morphology and immunohistochemical staining. Several markers in the past few years have proven to be more helpful, including CK5/6, calretinin, and Wilms' tumor gene 1 (WT-1), all of which show positivity in mesothelioma.

MOLECULAR PATHOGENESIS

Cancer is a disease involving dynamic changes in the genome. As proposed by Hanahan and Weinberg, virtually all cancer cells acquire six hallmark capabilities: self-sufficiency in growth signals, insensitivity to antigrowth signals, evading apoptosis, limitless replicative potential, sustained angiogenesis, and tissue invasion and metastasis. The order in which these hallmark capabilities are acquired appears quite variable and can differ from tumor to tumor. Events leading to acquisition of these hallmarks can vary widely, although broadly, cancers arise as a result of accumulations of gain-of-function mutations in oncogenes and loss-of-function mutations in tumor suppressor genes. Further complicating the study of lung cancer, the sequence of events that lead to disease is clearly different for the various histopathologic entities.

The exact cell of origin for lung cancers is not known. Whether one cell of origin leads to all histologic forms of lung cancer is unclear. However, at least for lung adenocarcinoma, type II epithelial cells (or alveolar epithelial cells) have the capacity to give rise to tumors. For SCLC, cells of neuroendocrine origin have been implicated as precursors.

For cancers in general, one theory holds that a small subset of the cells within a tumor (i.e., "stem cells") are responsible for the full malignant behavior of the tumor. As part of this concept, the large bulk of the cells in a cancer are "offspring" of these cancer stem cells. While clonally related to the cancer stem cell subpopulation, most cells by themselves cannot regenerate the full malignant phenotype. The stem cell concept may explain the failure of standard medical therapies to eradicate lung cancers, even when there is a clinical complete response. Disease recurs because therapies do not eliminate the stem cell component, which may be more resistant to chemotherapy. Precise human lung cancer stem cells have yet to be identified.

Lung cancer cells harbor multiple chromosomal abnormalities, including mutations, amplifications, insertions, deletions, and translocations. One of the earliest set of oncogenes found to be aberrant was the MYC family of transcription factors (*MYC, MYCN*, and *MYCL*). *MYC* is most frequently activated via gene amplification or transcriptional dysregulation in both SCLC and NSCLC, whereas abnormalities of *MYCN* and *MYCL* generally occur in SCLC. Currently, there are no MYC-specific drugs.

To date, among lung cancer histologies, adenocarcinomas have been the most extensively catalogued for recurrent genomic gains and losses as well as for somatic mutations. While multiple different kinds of aberrations have been found, a major class involves "driver mutations"—mutations that occur in genes encoding signaling proteins that when aberrant, drive initiation and maintenance of tumor cells (Table 35-2). Importantly, driver mutations can serve as Achilles' heels for tumors if their gene products can be targeted appropriately. For example, one set of mutations involves EGF-R, which belongs to the ERBB (HER) family of protooncogenes, including *EGF-R* (ERBB1), *Her2/neu* (ERBB2), *HER3* (ERBB3), and *HER4* (ERBB4). These genes encode cell-surface receptors consisting of an extracellular ligand-binding domain, a transmembrane structure, and an intracellular tyrosine kinase (TK) domain. The binding of ligand to receptor activates receptor dimerization and TK autophosphorylation, initiating a cascade of intracellular events, leading to increased cell proliferation, angiogenesis, metastasis, and a decrease in apoptosis. Lung adenocarcinomas can

TABLE 35-2

LIST OF SOME GENES SOMATICALLY ALTERED IN DIFFERENT HISTOLOGIC SUBTYPES OF LUNG CANCER

HISTOLOGY	ONCOGENE	TUMOR-SUPPRESSOR GENES
Adenocarcinoma	EGF-R KRAS ALK	TP53 CDKN2A/B (p16, p14) LKB1 (STK11)
Squamous cell carcinoma	EGF-R PIK3CA IGF-1R	TP53 TP63
Small cell carcinoma	MYC BCL-2	TP53 RB1 FHIT
Large cell carcinoma (not well studied)		

Abbreviations: ALK, anaplastic lymphoma kinase; EGF-R, epidermal growth factor receptor; IGF-1R, insulin-like growth factor 1 receptor; RB1, retinoblastoma protein 1.

arise when tumors express mutant *EGF-R*. These same tumors display high sensitivity to small molecule EGF-R TK inhibitors. Additional examples of driver mutations in lung adenocarcinoma include those involving the signaling molecules downstream of EGF-R, e.g., the TK *HER2*; the GTPase, *KRAS*; the serine–threonine kinase, *BRAF*; and the lipid kinase, *PIK3CA*. In 2007, other subsets of lung adenocarcinoma were found to be defined by the presence of specific translocations fusing tyrosine kinases such as ALK and ROS to aberrant upstream partners. Notably, at least *EGF-R*, *KRAS*, and *EML4-ALK* mutations are mutually exclusive, suggesting that acquisition of one of these driver mutations is sufficient to promote tumorigenesis. Thus far, potentially targetable driver mutations have mostly been identified in lung adenocarcinomas as opposed to lung cancers displaying other types of histologies.

A large number of tumor-suppressor genes (recessive oncogenes) have also been identified that are inactivated during the pathogenesis of lung cancer (Table 35-2). Such genes include *TP53*, *RB1*, *RASSF1A*, *CDKN2A/B*, *LKB1* (*STK11*), and *FHIT*. Nearly 90% of SCLCs harbor mutations in *TP53* and *RB1*. Several tumor-suppressor genes on chromosome 3p appear to be involved in nearly all lung cancers. Allelic loss for this region occurs very early in lung cancer pathogenesis, including in histologically normal smoking-damaged lung epithelium.

EARLY DETECTION AND SCREENING

The clinical outcome for lung cancer is related to the stage at diagnosis. Accordingly, it is presumed that early detection of occult tumors will lead to improved survival. Early detection is a process that involves screening tests, surveillance, diagnosis, and early treatment. By contrast, screening is defined as a systematic testing of asymptomatic individuals for preclinical disease. The majority of patients with lung cancer present with advanced disease, raising the question as to whether screening could detect lung tumors at earlier stages when they are theoretically more curable. In order for a screening program to be successful, the burden of disease within the population must be high, effective treatment must be available that can reduce mortality rate, and the test must be accessible, cost-effective, and both sensitive and specific. With any screening procedure, one must keep in mind the possible influence of lead-time bias (i.e., detecting the cancer earlier without an effect on survival), length time bias (i.e., indolent cancers are detected on screening and may actually not affect survival, while aggressive cancers are likely to cause symptoms earlier in patients and are less likely to be detected), and overdiagnosis (i.e., diagnosing cancers so slow growing that they are unlikely to cause the death of the patient) (Chap. 27).

Randomized controlled trials from the 1960s to the 1980s reported no impact on lung cancer–specific mortality rate using screening chest radiographs with or without sputum cytology in high-risk patients (age >50 years or history of smoking). Although these studies have been criticized for their design, statistical analyses, and outdated imaging modalities, they resulted in the current recommendations not to use these tools to screen for lung cancer. The more recent Prostate, Lung, Colorectal and Ovarian (PLCO) Cancer Screening Trial has completed accrual. This study involved more than 150,000 patients randomized to standard care or a baseline single-view posterior-anterior chest radiograph. A total of 5991 (8.9%) baseline chest radiographs were reported as suspicious for lung cancer, highest in current and former smokers. A total of 206 patients had a biopsy, of which 126 (61%) were positive for lung cancer. Among those with positive biopsies, 52% were stage I, 12% were stage II, and 22% were stage III. Long-term follow-up is required to determine the effect on mortality rate, if any.

Low-dose, noncontrast, thin-slice helical or spiral chest CT has emerged as a possible new tool for lung cancer screening. In a spiral chest CT scan, only the pulmonary parenchyma is examined, thus negating the use of intravenous contrast and the necessity of a physician being present at the exam. The scan can usually be done quickly (within a breath) and involves low doses of radiation. However, the benefits of screening with such technology remain to be determined. The International Early Lung Cancer Action Project (I-ECLAP) screened 31,567 asymptomatic patients at high risk for lung cancer (age ≥60 years with history of at least a 10-pack-year smoking history) using low-dose baseline CT and annual screening in 27,456 study participants. Suspicious lesions requiring biopsies were indicated in 535 participants. Lung cancer was diagnosed in 484 participants–405 at baseline, 74 on subsequent screening, and 5 participants due to symptoms between annual visits. Of the 484 participants who received a diagnosis of lung cancer, 412 (85%) were clinical stage I with an estimated 10-year survival rate of 88% regardless of treatment and 92% among the 302 participants who underwent resection within 1 month after diagnosis. A second trial randomized 1276 patients to low-dose CT screening and 1196 to baseline chest radiography followed by yearly medical examination. At 3-year follow-up, this study found a trend toward more patients being diagnosed with stage I lung cancer in the low-dose CT arm, with no difference in the number of patients diagnosed with advanced lung cancer or lung cancer deaths. More mature data from all trials are required to determine whether screening reduces lung cancer mortality rates.

A major challenge confronting advocates of CT screening is the high false-positive rate; on initial screening of at-risk populations, false-positive rates range between 10 and 20% but can be as high as 50%, depending on the geographical region. Positive predictive values range from 2.8 to 11.6%. False-positive results can have a substantial impact on patients through the expense and risk of unneeded further evaluation and emotional stress. False-positive rates and positive predictive values are somewhat improved in annual follow-up CT scans, but there is still significant room for improvement. Based on extant data, it appears that nodules <0.5 mm are unlikely to be cancerous and those 5–10 mm in diameter (25–40% of noncalcified nodules detected) are of uncertain significance. The management of these patients usually consists of serial CT scans over time to see if the nodules grow, attempted fine-needle aspirates, or surgical resection (Fig. 35-3).

Two additional screening studies are ongoing, the National Lung Cancer Screening Trial (NLST), a prospective comparison of spiral CT and standard chest radiographs in 50,000 current or ex-smokers and a similar study in Europe comparing CT scanning with standard of care in subjects with a history of heavy smoking. Until these data and more mature data from the above-mentioned trials become available, routine CT screening for lung cancer cannot be recommended for any risk group. For patients who want to be screened, physicians need to discuss the possible benefits and risks of screening. While lung cancers may be found, patients are at risk for more radiation exposure and false-positive results. The latter can result in multiple follow-up CTs and possible invasive procedures, with potential added costs, anxiety, and morbidity and mortality rates. There are no data on screening never smokers for lung cancer.

CLINICAL MANIFESTATIONS

More than half of all patients diagnosed with lung cancer present with advanced disease at the time of diagnosis. The majority of patients present with signs, symptoms, or laboratory abnormalities that can be attributed to the primary lesion, local tumor growth, invasion or obstruction of adjacent structures, growth

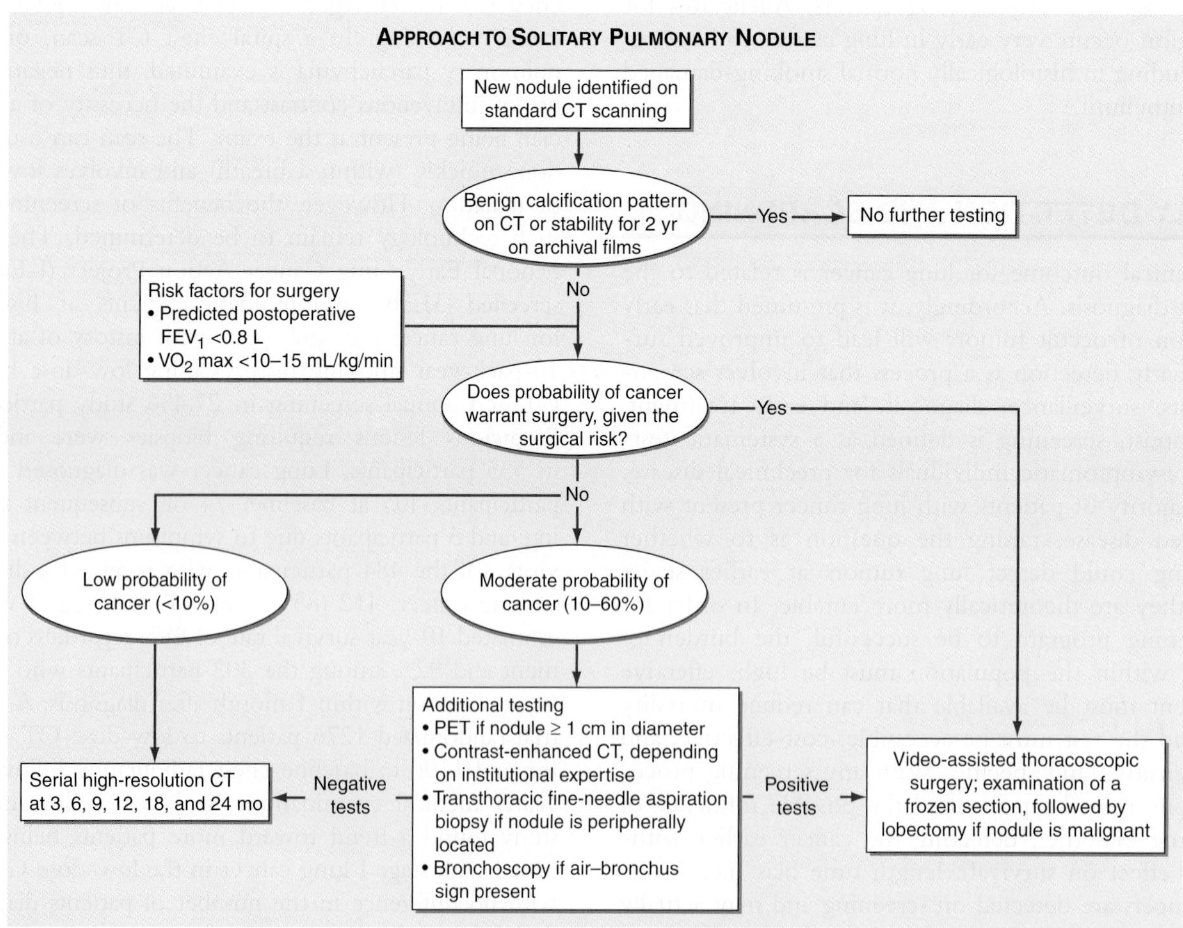

FIGURE 35-3

Approach to solitary pulmonary nodule. CT, computed tomography; FEV1, forced expiratory volume in 1 second; PET, positron emission tomography.

TABLE 35-3

PRESENTING SIGNS AND SYMPTOMS OF LUNG CANCER

SYMPTOM AND SIGNS	RANGE OF FREQUENCY, %
Cough	8–75
Weight loss	0–68
Dyspnea	3–60
Chest pain	20–49
Hemoptysis	6–35
Bone pain	6–25
Clubbing	0–20
Fever	0–20
Weakness	0–10
SVCO	0–4
Dysphagia	0–2
Wheezing and stridor	0–2

Abbreviation: SVCO, superior vena cava obstruction.
Source: Reproduced with permission from MA Beckles et al: Chest 123:97, 2003.

at distant metastatic sites, or a paraneoplastic syndrome (**Tables 35-3 and 35-4**). The prototypical lung cancer patient is a current or former smoker of either sex, usually in the seventh decade of life. A history of chronic cough with or without hemoptysis in a current or former smoker with chronic obstructive pulmonary disease (COPD) age 40 years or older should prompt a thorough investigation for lung cancer even in the face of normal chest radiography findings. A persistent pneumonia without constitutional symptoms and unresponsive to repeated courses of antibiotics also should prompt an evaluation for the underlying cause.

TABLE 35-4

CLINICAL FINDINGS SUGGESTIVE OF METASTATIC DISEASE

Symptoms elicited in history	• Constitutional: weight loss >10 lb • Musculoskeletal: focal skeletal pain • Neurologic: headaches, syncope, seizures, extremity weakness, recent change in mental status
Signs found on physical examination	• Lymphadenopathy (>1 cm) • Hoarseness, superior vena cava syndrome • Bone tenderness • Hepatomegaly (>13 cm span) • Focal neurologic signs, papilledema • Soft-tissue mass
Routine laboratory tests	• Hematocrit: <40% in men, <35% in women • Elevated alkaline phosphatase, GGT, SGOT, and calcium levels

Abbreviations: GGT, gamma-glutamyltransferase; SGOT, serum glutamic-oxaloacetic transaminase.
Source: Reproduced with permission from GA Silvestri et al: Chest 123(1 Suppl):147S, 2003.

Lung cancer arising in a lifetime never smoker is more common in women and East Asians. Such patients also tend to be younger than their smoking counterparts at the time of diagnosis. The clinical presentation of lung cancer in never smokers tends to mirror that of current and former smokers.

Patients with central or endobronchial growth of the primary tumor may present with cough, hemoptysis, wheeze, stridor, dyspnea, or postobstructive pneumonitis. Peripheral growth of the primary tumor may cause pain from pleural or chest wall involvement, dyspnea on a restrictive basis, and symptoms of a lung abscess resulting from tumor cavitation. Regional spread of tumor in the thorax (by contiguous growth or by metastasis to regional lymph nodes) may cause tracheal obstruction, esophageal compression with dysphagia, recurrent laryngeal paralysis with hoarseness, phrenic nerve palsy with elevation of the hemidiaphragm and dyspnea, and sympathetic nerve paralysis with Horner's syndrome (enophthalmos, ptosis, miosis, and anhidrosis). Malignant pleural effusions can cause pain or dyspnea. Pancoast (or superior sulcus tumor) syndromes result from local extension of a tumor growing in the apex of the lung with involvement of the eighth cervical and first and second thoracic nerves, with shoulder pain that characteristically radiates in the ulnar distribution of the arm, often with radiologic destruction of the first and second ribs. Often Horner's syndrome and Pancoast syndrome coexist. Other problems of regional spread include superior vena cava syndrome from vascular obstruction; pericardial and cardiac extension with resultant tamponade, arrhythmia, or cardiac failure; lymphatic obstruction with resultant pleural effusion; and lymphangitic spread through the lungs with hypoxemia and dyspnea. In addition, lung cancer can spread transbronchially, producing tumor growth along multiple alveolar surfaces with impairment of gas exchange, respiratory insufficiency, dyspnea, hypoxemia, and sputum production. Constitutional symptoms may include anorexia, weight loss, weakness, fever, and night sweats. Apart from the brevity of symptom duration, these parameters fail to clearly distinguish SCLC from NSCLC or even from neoplasms metastatic to lungs.

Extrathoracic metastatic disease is found at autopsy in >50% of patients with squamous carcinoma, 80% of patients with adenocarcinoma and large cell carcinoma, and >95% of patients with SCLC. Approximately one-third of patients present with symptoms as a result of distant metastases. Lung cancer metastases may occur in virtually every organ system, and the site of metastatic involvement largely determines other symptoms.

Patients with brain metastases may present with headache, nausea and vomiting, or neurologic deficits. Patients with bone metastases may present with pain, pathologic fractures, or cord compression. The latter may also occur with epidural metastases. Individuals with bone marrow invasion may present with cytopenias or leukoerythroblastosis. Those with liver metastases may present with hepatomegaly, right upper quadrant pain, anorexia, and weight loss. Liver dysfunction or biliary obstructions are rare. Adrenal metastases are common but rarely cause pain or adrenal insufficiency unless they are large.

Paraneoplastic syndromes are common in patients with lung cancer, especially those with SCLC, and may be the presenting finding or the first sign of recurrence. In addition, paraneoplastic syndromes may mimic metastatic disease and, unless detected, lead to inappropriate palliative rather than curative treatment. Often the paraneoplastic syndrome may be relieved with successful treatment of the tumor. In some cases, the pathophysiology of the paraneoplastic syndrome is known, particularly when a hormone with biologic activity is secreted by a tumor. However, in many cases, the pathophysiology is not known. Systemic symptoms of anorexia, cachexia, weight loss (seen in 30% of patients), fever, and suppressed immunity are paraneoplastic syndromes of unknown etiology or at least not well defined. Weight loss greater than 10% of total body weight is considered a bad prognostic sign. Endocrine syndromes are seen in 12% of patients; hypercalcemia resulting from ectopic production of parathyroid hormone (PTH), or more commonly, PTH-related peptide, is the most common life-threatening metabolic complication of malignancy, primarily occurring with squamous cell carcinomas of the lung. Clinical symptoms include nausea, vomiting, abdominal pain, constipation, polyuria, thirst, and altered mental status.

Hyponatremia may be caused by the syndrome of inappropriate secretion of antidiuretic hormone (SIADH) or possibly atrial natriuretic peptide (ANP). SIADH resolves within 1–4 weeks of initiating chemotherapy in the vast majority of cases. During this period, serum sodium can usually be managed and maintained above 128 meq/L via fluid restriction. Demeclocycline can be a useful adjunctive measure when fluid restriction alone is insufficient. Of note, patients with ectopic ANP may have worsening hyponatremia if sodium intake is not concomitantly increased. Accordingly, if hyponatremia fails to improve or worsens after 3–4 days of adequate fluid restriction, plasma levels of ANP should be measured to determine the causative syndrome.

Ectopic secretion of ACTH by SCLC and pulmonary carcinoids usually results in additional electrolyte disturbances, especially hypokalemia, rather than the changes in body habitus that occur in Cushing's syndrome from a pituitary adenoma. Treatment with standard medications, such as metyrapone and ketoconazole, is largely ineffective due to extremely high cortisol levels. The most effective strategy for management of Cushing's syndrome is effective treatment of the underlying SCLC. Bilateral adrenalectomy may be considered in extreme cases.

Skeletal–connective tissue syndromes include clubbing in 30% of cases (usually NSCLCs) and hypertrophic primary osteoarthropathy in 1–10% of cases (usually adenocarcinomas). Patients may develop periostitis, causing pain, tenderness, and swelling over the affected bones and a positive bone scan. Neurologic–myopathic syndromes are seen in only 1% of patients but are dramatic and include the myasthenic Eaton-Lambert syndrome and retinal blindness with SCLC, while peripheral neuropathies, subacute cerebellar degeneration, cortical degeneration, and polymyositis are seen with all lung cancer types. Many of these are caused by autoimmune responses such as the development of anti–voltage-gated calcium channel antibodies in Eaton-Lambert syndrome. Patients with this disorder present with proximal muscle weakness, usually in the lower extremities, occasional autonomic dysfunction, and rarely with cranial nerve symptoms or involvement of the bulbar or respiratory muscles. Depressed deep tendon reflexes are frequently present. In contrast to patients with myasthenia gravis, strength improves with serial effort. Some patients who respond to chemotherapy will have resolution of the neurologic abnormalities. Thus, chemotherapy is the initial treatment of choice. Paraneoplastic encephalomyelitis and sensory neuropathies, cerebellar degeneration, limbic encephalitis, and brainstem encephalitis occur in SCLC in association with a variety of antineuronal antibodies such as anti-Hu, anti-CRMP5, and ANNA-3. Paraneoplastic cerebellar degeneration may be associated with anti-Hu, anti-Yo, or P/Q calcium channel autoantibodies. Coagulation, thrombotic, or other hematologic manifestations occur in 1–8% of patients and include migratory venous thrombophlebitis (Trousseau's syndrome); nonbacterial thrombotic (marantic) endocarditis with arterial emboli; and disseminated intravascular coagulation with hemorrhage, anemia, granulocytosis, and leukoerythroblastosis. Thrombotic disease complicating cancer is usually a poor prognostic sign. Cutaneous manifestations such as dermatomyositis and acanthosis nigricans are uncommon (1%), as are the renal manifestations of nephrotic syndrome and glomerulonephritis (≤1%).

DIAGNOSING LUNG CANCER

Tissue sampling is required to confirm a diagnosis in all patients with suspected lung cancer. Tumor tissue may be obtained via minimally invasive techniques such as bronchial or transbronchial biopsy during fiberoptic bronchoscopy, by fine-needle aspiration (FNA) or percutaneous biopsy using image guidance, or via endobronchial ultrasound (EBUS)–guided biopsy. Depending on the location, lymph node sampling may occur via transesophageal endoscopic ultrasound guide biopsy (EUS), EBUS, or blind biopsy. In patients with clinically palpable lymph nodes, an FNA may be obtained. In patients with suspected metastatic disease, a diagnosis may be confirmed by percutaneous biopsy of a soft tissue mass, lytic bone lesion, bone marrow, pleural, or liver lesion or an adequate cell block obtained from a malignant pleural effusion. In patients with a suspected malignant pleural effusion, if the initial thoracentesis findings are negative, a repeat thoracentesis is recommended. While the majority of pleural effusions are due to malignant disease, particularly if they are exudative or bloody, some may be parapneumonic. In this case, patients should be considered for possible curative treatment.

The diagnostic yield of any biopsy depends on several factors, including location (accessibility) of the tumor, tumor size, tumor type, and technical aspects of the diagnostic procedure including the experience level of the bronchoscopist and pathologist. In general, central lesions, such as squamous cell carcinomas, small cell carcinomas, or endobronchial lesions, such as carcinoid tumors, are more readily diagnosed by bronchoscopic examination, while peripheral lesions such as adenocarcinomas and large cell carcinomas are more amenable to transthoracic FNA. Diagnostic accuracy for SCLC versus NSCLC for most specimens is excellent, with lesser accuracy for subtypes of NSCLC.

Bronchoscopic specimens include bronchial brush, bronchial wash, bronchioloalveolar lavage, and transbronchial FNA. Of these, transbronchial FNA consistently demonstrates the highest sensitivity, surpassed only by the use of a combination of bronchoscopic specimens. Overall sensitivity for combined use of bronchoscopic methods is approximately 80%, and together with tissue biopsy, the yield increases to 85–90%. Like transbronchial FNA specimens, transthoracic FNA specimens are also very good, yielding diagnostic material in 70–95% of cases. Sensitivity is highest for larger lesions and peripheral tumors. In general, FNA specimens, whether transbronchial, transthoracic, or endoscopic ultrasound-guided, are superior to other specimen types. This is primarily due to the higher percentage of tumor cells with fewer confounding factors, such as obscuring inflammation and reactive nonneoplastic cells. For more accurate histologic classification, mutation analysis, or for investigational purposes, reasonable efforts (e.g., a core-needle biopsy) should be made to obtain more tissue than what is contained in a routine cytology specimen obtained by FNA.

Sputum cytology is inexpensive and noninvasive but has a lower yield than other specimen types due to poor preservation of the cells and more variability in acquiring a good-quality specimen. The yield for sputum cytology is highest for larger and centrally located tumors such as squamous cell carcinoma and small cell carcinoma histology. The specificity for sputum cytology averages close to 100%, although sensitivity is generally less than 70%. The accuracy of sputum cytology improves with increased numbers of specimens analyzed. Consequently, analysis of at least three sputum specimens is recommended.

STAGING LUNG CANCER

Lung cancer staging consists of two parts: first, a determination of the location of the tumor and possible metastatic sites (anatomic staging), and second, an assessment of a patient's ability to withstand various antitumor treatments (physiologic staging). All patients with lung cancer should have a complete history and physical examination, with evaluation of all other medical problems, determination of performance status, and history of weight loss. The most significant dividing line is between patients who are candidates for surgical resection and those who are inoperable but will benefit from chemotherapy, radiation therapy, or both. Staging with regard to a patient's potential for surgical resection is principally applicable to NSCLC.

ANATOMIC STAGING OF PATIENTS WITH LUNG CANCER

The accurate staging of patients with NSCLC is essential for determining the appropriate treatment in patients with resectable disease and avoiding unnecessary surgical procedures in patients with advanced disease (Fig. 35-4). All patients with NSCLC should undergo initial radiographic imaging with CT scan, positron emission tomography (PET), or preferably CT-PET. PET scanning attempts to identify sites of malignancy based on glucose metabolism by measuring the uptake of fluorodeoxyglucose F18. Rapidly dividing cells, presumably in the lung tumors, will preferentially take up ^{18}F-FDG and appear as a "hot spot." To date, PET has been mostly used for staging and detection of metastases in lung cancer and in the detection of nodules >15 mm in diameter. Combined ^{18}F-FDG PET-CT imaging has been shown to improve the accuracy of staging in NSCLC compared to visual correlation of PET and CT or either study alone. CT-PET has been found to be superior in identifying pathologically enlarged mediastinal lymph nodes and extrathoracic metastases. A standardized uptake value (SUV) of >2.5 on PET is highly suspicious for malignancy. False-negative results can be seen in diabetes, in lesions <8 mm, in slow-growing tumors, and in concurrent infections such as tuberculosis. False-positive results can be seen in

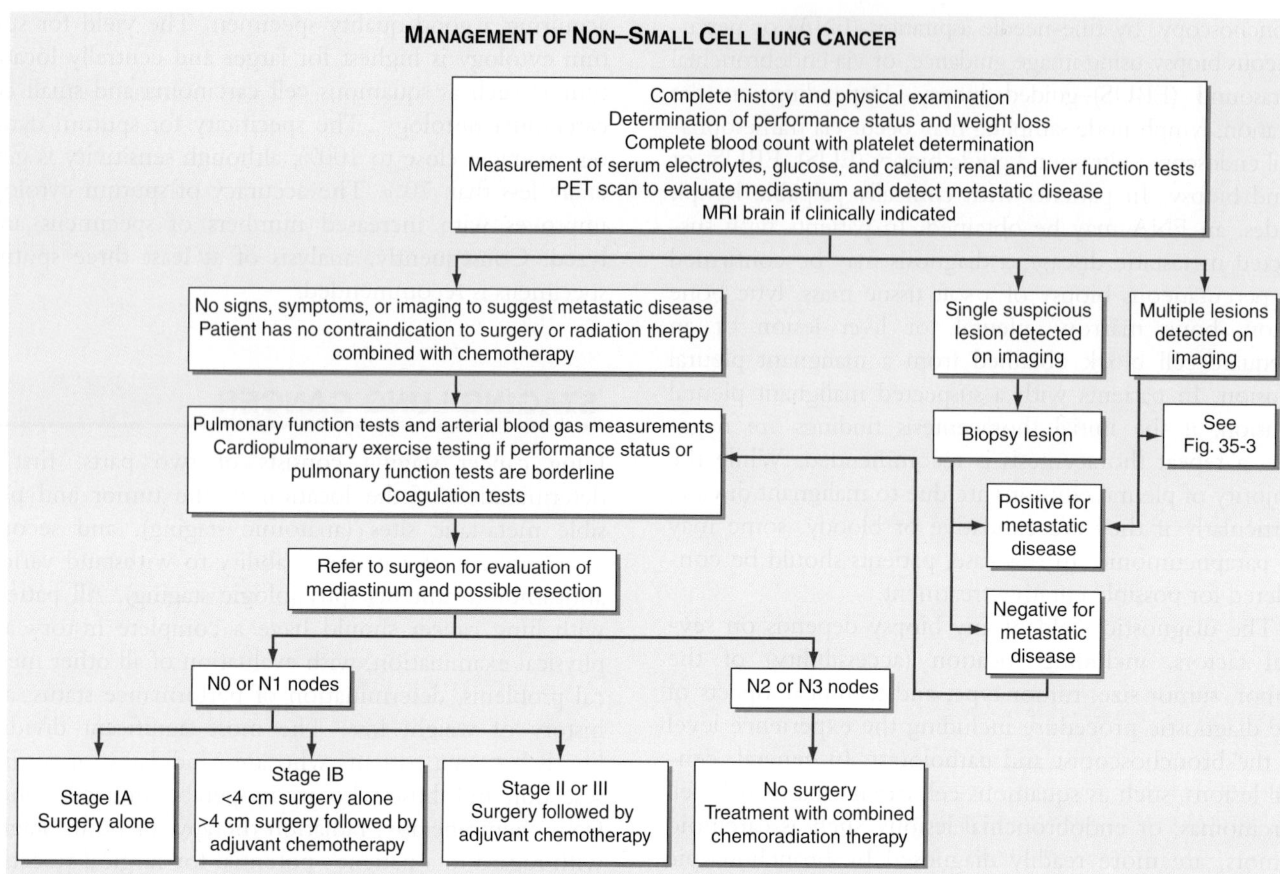

FIGURE 35-4

Algorithm for management of non-small cell lung cancer. MRI, magnetic resonance imaging; PET, positron emission tomography.

infections and granulomatous disease. Thus, PET should never be used alone to diagnose lung cancer, mediastinal involvement, or metastases. Confirmation with tissue biopsy is required. For brain metastases, MRI is the most effective method. MRI can also be useful in selected circumstances, such as for superior sulcus tumors, to rule out brachial plexus involvement but in general does not play a major role in NSCLC staging.

In patients with NSCLC, the following are major contraindications to potential curative resection: extrathoracic metastases; superior vena cava syndrome; vocal cord and, in most cases, phrenic nerve paralysis; malignant pleural effusion; cardiac tamponade; tumor within 2 cm of the carina (potentially curable with combined chemoradiotherapy); metastasis to the contralateral lung; metastases to supraclavicular lymph nodes; contralateral mediastinal node metastases (potentially curable with combined chemoradiotherapy); and involvement of the main pulmonary artery. When it will make a difference in treatment, abnormal scan findings require tissue confirmation of malignancy so that patients are not precluded from having potentially curative surgery.

The best predictor of metastatic disease remains a careful history and physical examination. If signs, symptoms, or findings from physical examination suggest the presence of malignancy, then sequential imaging starting with the most appropriate study should be performed. If the findings from the clinical evaluation are negative, then imaging studies beyond CT-PET are unnecessary, and the search for metastatic disease is complete. More controversial is how one should assess patients with known stage III disease. Because these patients are more likely to have asymptomatic occult metastatic disease, current guidelines recommend a more extensive imaging evaluation, including imaging of the brain with either CT scan or MRI. In patients in whom distant metastatic disease has been ruled out, lymph node status needs to be assessed via a combination of radiographic imaging and/or minimally invasive techniques such as those mentioned earlier and/or invasive techniques such as mediastinoscopy, mediastinotomy, thoracoscopy, and thoracotomy. About one-quarter to half of patients diagnosed with NSCLC have mediastinal lymph node metastases at the time of diagnosis. Lymph node sampling is recommended in all patients with enlarged nodes detected by CT or PET scan and in patients with large tumors or tumors occupying the inner third of the lung. The extent of mediastinal lymph node involvement is important in determining the appropriate treatment strategy: surgical resection followed by adjuvant chemotherapy versus combined chemoradiotherapy alone (see later discussion). A standard nomenclature for referring to the location of lymph nodes involved with lung cancer has evolved (Fig. 35-5).

There are limited data on the use of CT-PET in the staging of patients with SCLC (Fig. 35-6). Current staging recommendations include a CT scan of the chest and abdomen (because of the high frequency of hepatic and adrenal involvement), MRI of the brain (positive in 10% of asymptomatic patients), and radionuclide (bone) scan if symptoms or signs suggest disease involvement in these areas. Bone marrow biopsies and aspirations are rarely performed given the low incidence of isolated bone marrow metastases. Confirmation of metastatic disease, ipsilateral or contralateral lung nodules, or metastases beyond the mediastinum may be achieved by the same modalities recommended above for patients with NSCLC.

If a patient has signs or symptoms of spinal cord compression (pain, weakness, paralysis, urinary retention), a spinal CT or MRI scan and examination of the cerebrospinal fluid cytology should be performed. If metastases are evident on imaging, a neurosurgeon should be consulted for possible palliative surgical resection and/or a radiation oncologist should be consulted for palliative radiotherapy to the site of compression. If signs of symptoms of leptomeningitis develop at any time in a patient with lung cancer, an MRI of the brain and spinal cord should be performed as well as a spinal tap for detection of malignant cells. If the spinal tap findings are negative, a repeat spinal tap should be considered. There is currently no approved therapy for the treatment of leptomeningeal disease.

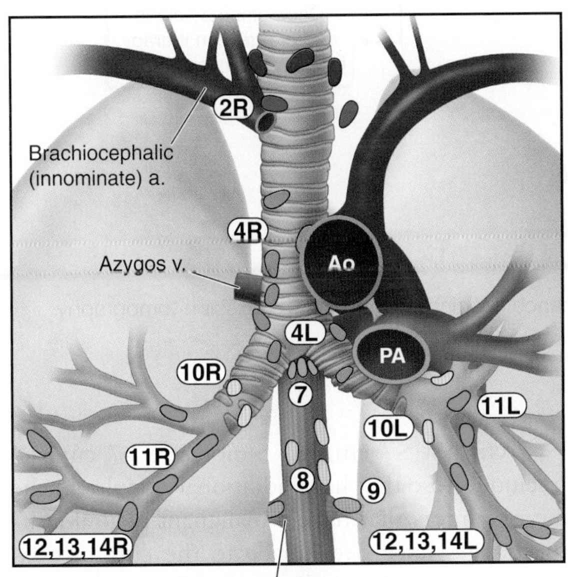

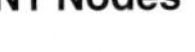

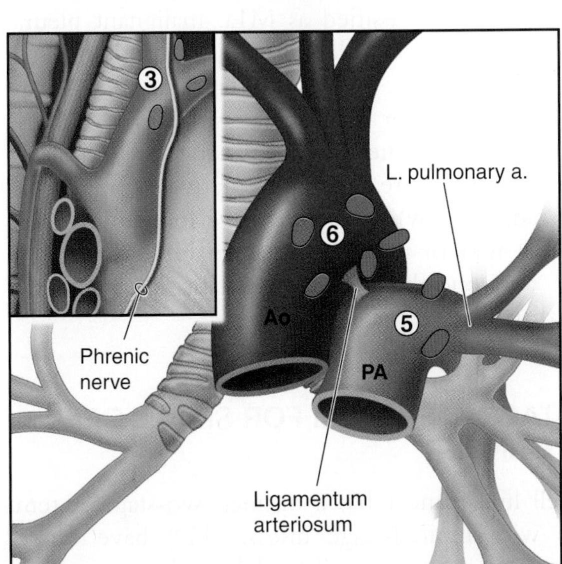

Superior Mediastinal Nodes

- 1. Highest mediastinal
- 2. Upper paratracheal
- 3. Prevascular and retrotracheal
- 4. Lower paratracheal (including azygos nodes)

N2 = single digit, ipsilateral
N3 = single digit, contralateral or supraclavicular

Aortic Nodes

- 5. Subaortic (A-P window)
- 6. Para-aortic (ascending aorta or phrenic)

Inferior Mediastinal Nodes

- 7. Subcarinal
- 8. Paraesophageal (below carina)
- 9. Pulmonary ligament

N1 Nodes

- 10. Hilar
- 11. Interlobar
- 12. Lobar
- 13. Segmental
- 14. Subsegmental

FIGURE 35-5
Lymph node stations in staging non-small cell lung cancer.

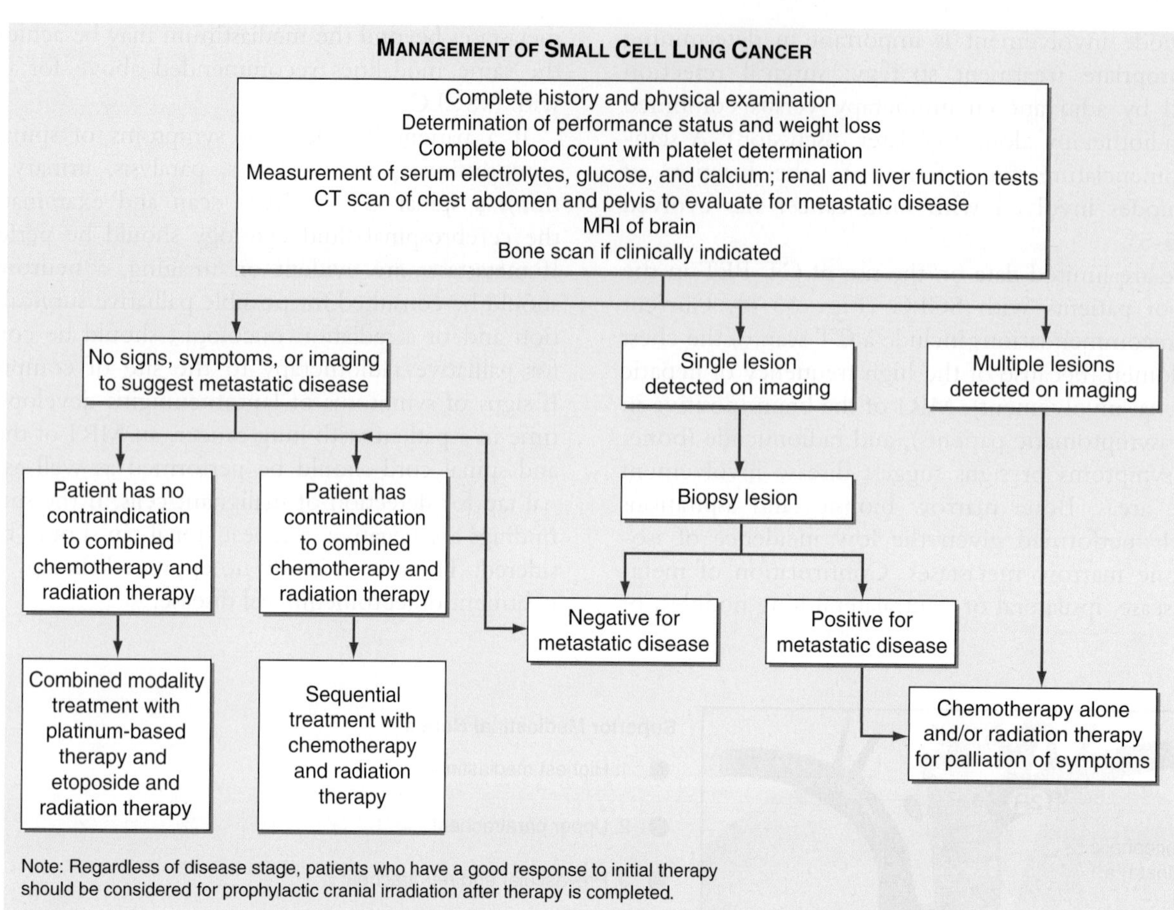

FIGURE 35-6
Algorithm for management of small cell lung cancer. MRI, magnetic resonance imaging; PET, positron emission tomography.

THE STAGING SYSTEM FOR NON–SMALL CELL LUNG CANCER

The TNM International Staging System provides useful prognostic information and is used to stage all patients with NSCLC. The various T (tumor size), N (regional node involvement), and M (presence or absence of distant metastasis) are combined to form different stage groups (Table 35-5). The former TNM staging system for lung cancer (sixth edition) was developed based on a relatively small database of patients from a single institution. In 1999, the International Association for the Study of Lung Cancer established the lung cancer staging project and collected data on more than 68,000 cases from 46 sources in more than 19 countries to develop the new TNM (seventh edition) staging system, which came into use in 2010. As seen in Tables 35-5 and 35-6, the major distinction between the sixth and seventh edition staging system is within the T classification; T1 tumors are divided into tumors ≤2 cm in size, as these patients were found to have a better prognosis compared with tumors >2 cm but ≤3 cm. T2 tumors are divided into those that are >3 cm but ≤5 cm and those that are >5 cm but ≤7 cm. T3 tumors are >7 cm. T4 tumors include those that have additional nodules in the same lobe or tumors that have a malignant pleural effusion. No changes have been made to the current classification of lymph node involvement (N). Patients with metastasis may be classified as M1a, malignant pleural or pericardial effusion, pleural nodules or nodules in the contralateral lung, or M1b distant metastasis (e.g., bone, liver, adrenal, or brain metastasis). Based on these data, approximately one-third of patients have localized disease that can be treated with curative attempt (surgery or radiotherapy), one-third have local or regional disease that may or may not be amenable to a curative attempt, and one-third have metastatic disease at the time of diagnosis.

THE STAGING SYSTEM FOR SMALL CELL LUNG CANCER

Small cell lung cancer has a distinct two-stage system. Patients with limited-stage disease (LD) have cancer that is confined to the ipsilateral hemithorax and can

TABLE 35-5

COMPARISON OF THE SIXTH AND SEVENTH EDITION TUMOR, NODE, METASTASIS STAGING SYSTEMS FOR NON-SMALL CELL LUNG CANCER

	SIXTH EDITION	SEVENTH EDITION
Tumor (T)		
T1	Tumor ≤3 cm diameter without invasion more proximal than lobar bronchus	Tumor ≤3 cm diameter, surrounded by lung or visceral pleura, without invasion more proximal than lobar bronchus
T1a		Tumor ≤2 cm in diameter
T1b		Tumor >2 cm but ≤3 cm in diameter
T2	Tumor >3 cm diameter *or* tumor of any size with any of the following: Visceral pleural invasion Atelectasis of less than entire lung Proximal extent at least 2 cm from carina	Tumor >3 cm but ≤7 cm with any of the following: Involves main bronchus, ≥2 cm distal to carina, invades visceral pleura Associated with atelectasis or obstructive pneumonitis extending to hilar region but not involving the entire lung
T2a		Tumor >3 cm but ≤5 cm in diameter
T2b		Tumor >5 cm but ≤7 cm in diameter
T3	Tumor of any size that invades any of the following: chest wall, diaphragm, mediastinal pleura, parietal pericardium Tumor <2 cm distal to carina	Tumor >7 cm or directly invades any of the following: chest wall (including superior sulcus tumors), phrenic nerve, mediastinal pleura, parietal pericardium Tumor <2 cm distal to carina but without involvement of carina Tumor with associated atelectasis or obstructive pneumonitis of entire lung Separate tumor nodule(s) in same lobe
T4	Tumor of any size that invades any of the following: mediastinum, heart or great vessels, trachea, esophagus, vertebral body, carina Tumor with malignant pleural or pericardial effusion Separate tumor nodules in same lobe	Tumor of any size that invades any of the following: mediastinum, heart or great vessels, trachea, recurrent laryngeal nerve, esophagus, vertebral body, carina Separate tumor nodule(s) in a different ipsilateral lobe
Nodes (N)		
N0	No regional lymph node metastasis	No regional lymph node metastasis
N1	Metastasis in ipsilateral peribronchial and/or hilar lymph node(s)	Metastasis in ipsilateral peribronchial and/or hilar lymph node(s) and intrapulmonary node(s), including involvement by direct extensions
N2	Metastasis in ipsilateral mediastinal and/or subcarinal lymph node(s)	Metastasis in ipsilateral mediastinal and/or subcarinal lymph node(s)
N3	Metastasis in contralateral mediastinal, contralateral hilar, ipsilateral or contralateral scalene or supraclavicular lymph node(s)	Metastasis in contralateral mediastinal, hilar, ipsilateral or contralateral scalene or supraclavicular lymph node(s)
Metastasis (M)		
M0	No distant metastasis	No distant metastasis
M1	Distant metastasis (includes tumor nodules in different lobe from primary)	Distant metastasis
M1a		Separate tumor nodules in a contralateral lobe Tumor with pleural nodules or malignant pleural or pericardial effusion
M1b		Distant metastasis

Source: Reproduced with permission from P Goldstraw et al: J Thorac Oncol 2:706, 2007.

TABLE 35-6

COMPARISON OF SURVIVAL BY STAGE IN TUMOR, NODE, METASTASIS SIXTH AND SEVENTH EDITIONS

STAGE	TNM SIXTH EDITION	TNM SEVENTH EDITION	5-YEAR SURVIVAL (%)[a]
IA	T1N0M0	T1a-T1bN0M0	73
IB	T2N0M0	T2aN0M0	58
IIA	T1N1M0	T1a-T2aN1M0 or T2bN0M0	46
IIB	T2N1M0 or T3N0M0	T2bN1M0 or T3N0M0	36
IIIA	T3N1M0 or T1-3N2M0	T1a-T3N2M0 or T3N1M0 or T4N0-1M0	24
IIIB	Any T N3M0 T4 Any N M0	T4N2M0 or T1a-T4N3M0	9
IV	Any T Any N M1	Any T Any N M1a or M1b	13

[a]Survival according to the seventh edition.

be encompassed within a tolerable radiation port. Thus, contralateral supraclavicular nodes, recurrent laryngeal nerve involvement, and superior vena caval obstruction can all be part of limited-stage disease. Patients with extensive-stage disease (ED) have overt metastatic disease by imaging or physical examination. Cardiac tamponade, malignant pleural effusion, and bilateral pulmonary parenchymal involvement generally qualify disease as extensive-stage because the involved organs cannot be encompassed safely or effectively within a single radiation therapy port. Sixty to 70% of patients are diagnosed with extensive disease at presentation.

PHYSIOLOGIC STAGING

Patients with lung cancer often have other comorbid conditions related to smoking, including cardiovascular disease and COPD. To improve their preoperative condition, correctable problems (e.g., anemia, electrolyte and fluid disorders, infections, cardiac disease, and arrhythmias) should be addressed, appropriate chest physical therapy instituted, and patients should be encouraged to stop smoking. Since it is not always possible to predict whether a lobectomy or pneumonectomy will be required until the time of operation, a conservative approach is to restrict surgical resection to patients who could potentially tolerate a pneumonectomy. Patients with an FEV_1 (forced expiratory volume in 1 s) of greater than 2 L or greater than 80% of predicted can tolerate a pneumonectomy, and those with an FEV_1 greater than 1.5 L have adequate reserve for a lobectomy. In patients with borderline lung function but a resectable tumor, cardiopulmonary exercise testing could be performed as part of the physiologic evaluation. This test allows an estimate of the maximal oxygen consumption (Vo_2max). A Vo_2max <15 mL/(kg·min) predicts for a higher risk of postoperative complications. Patients deemed unable to tolerate lobectomy or pneumonectomy from a pulmonary functional standpoint may be candidates for more limited resections, such as wedge or anatomic segmental resection, although such procedures are associated with significantly higher rates of local recurrence and a trend toward decreased overall survival. All patients should be assessed for cardiovascular risk using American College of Cardiology and American Heart Association guidelines. A myocardial infarction within the past 3 months is a contraindication to thoracic surgery because 20% of patients will die of reinfarction. An infarction in the past 6 months is a relative contraindication. Other major contraindications include uncontrolled arrhythmias, an FEV_1 of less than 1 L, CO_2 retention (resting PCO_2 >45 mm Hg), DL_{CO} (carbon monoxide diffusing capacity) <40%, and severe pulmonary hypertension.

TREATMENT Non–Small Cell Lung Cancer

The overall treatment approach to patients with NSCLC is shown in Fig. 35-4.

MANAGEMENT OF OCCULT AND STAGE 0 CARCINOMAS Patients with severe atypia on sputum cytology have an increased risk of developing lung cancer compared with those without atypia. In the uncommon circumstance where malignant cells are identified in a sputum or bronchial washing specimen but the chest imaging appears normal (TX tumor stage), the lesion must be localized. More than 90% of tumors can be localized by meticulous examination of the bronchial tree with a fiberoptic bronchoscope under general anesthesia and collection of a series of differential brushings and biopsies. Surgical resection following bronchoscopic localization improves survival compared with no treatment. Close follow-up of these patients is indicated because of the high incidence of second primary lung cancers (5% per patient per year).

SOLITARY PULMONARY NODULE AND "GROUND-GLASS" OPACITIES A solitary pulmonary nodule is defined as an x-ray density completely surrounded by normal aerated lung with circumscribed margins, of any shape, usually 1–6 cm at greatest diameter. The approach to a patient with a solitary pulmonary nodule is based on an estimate of the probability of cancer, determined according to the patient's smoking history, age, and characteristics on

TABLE 35-7

ASSESSMENT OF RISK OF CANCER IN PATIENTS WITH SOLITARY PULMONARY NODULES

	RISK		
VARIABLE	**LOW**	**INTERMEDIATE**	**HIGH**
Diameter (cm)	<1.5	1.5–2.2	≥2.3
Age (years)	<45	45–60	>60
Smoking status	Never smoker	Current smoker (<20 cigarettes/d)	Current smoker (>20 cigarettes/d)
Smoking cessation status	Quit ≥7 years ago or quit	Quit <7 years ago	Never quit
Characteristics of nodule margins	Smooth	Scalloped	Corona radiata or spiculated

Source: Reproduced with permission from D Ost et al: N Engl J Med 348:2535, 2003.

imaging (Table 35-7). Prior chest radiographs and CT scans should be obtained if available for comparison. A PET scan may be useful if the lesion is greater than 7–8 mm in diameter. If no diagnosis is apparent, Mayo Clinic investigators reported that clinical characteristics (age, cigarette smoking status, and prior cancer diagnosis) and three radiologic characteristics (nodule diameter, spiculation, and upper lobe location) were independent predictors of malignancy. At present, only two radiographic criteria are thought to predict the benign nature of a solitary pulmonary nodule: lack of growth over a period >2 years and certain characteristic patterns of calcification. Calcification alone, however, does not exclude malignancy; a dense central nidus, multiple punctate foci, and "bull's-eye" (granuloma) and "popcorn ball" (hamartoma) calcifications are highly suggestive of a benign lesion. In contrast, a relatively large lesion, lack of or asymmetric calcification, chest symptoms, associated atelectasis, pneumonitis, or growth of the lesion revealed by comparison with an old radiograph or CT scan or a positive PET scan are suggestive of a malignant process and warrant further attempts to establish a histologic diagnosis. An algorithm for assessing these lesions is shown in Fig. 35-3.

Since the advent of screening CTs, small GGOs have often been observed, particularly as the increased sensitivity of CTs enables detection of smaller lesions. Many of these GGOs, when biopsied, are found to be BAC. Some of the GGOs are semiopaque and referred to as "partial" GGOs. These are often more slow-growing and harbor atypical adenomatous hyperplasia histology and are thought to be precursors to adenocarcinoma. By contrast, "solid" GGOs have faster growth rates and are usually typical adenocarcinoma histologically.

MANAGEMENT OF STAGES I AND II NSCLC

Surgical Resection for Stages I and II NSCLC Surgical resection by an experienced surgeon is the treatment of choice for patients with clinical stage I or II NSCLC who are able to tolerate the procedure. A retrospective review indicated that operative mortality rates for patients whose tumors were resected by noncardiothoracic or cardiothoracic surgeons were lower compared with general surgeons (5.8% vs 5.6% vs 7.6%; $P = .001$). The extent of resection is a matter of surgical judgment based on findings at exploration. A clinical trial in patients with stage IA NSCLC found that lobectomy was superior to wedge resection in reducing the rate of local recurrence, with a trend toward improvement in overall survival. A retrospective review of the Surveillance, Epidemiology, and End Results (SEER) database also reported a survival benefit for lobectomy compared with wedge resection. A limited resection, wedge resection, and segmentectomy (potentially by video-assisted thoracic surgery [VATS]) may be more appropriate in patients with comorbidities, including compromised pulmonary reserve and small peripheral lesions. Pneumonectomy is reserved for patients with very central tumors and should only be performed in patients with excellent pulmonary reserve. The 5-year survival rates are 60–80% for patients with stage I NSCLC and 40–50% for patients with stage II NSCLC.

Accurate pathologic staging requires adequate segmental, hilar, and mediastinal lymph node sampling. Mediastinal lymph node dissection provides for a significantly larger amount of material, which can refine pathologic (nodal) stage. On the right side, mediastinal stations 2R, 4R, 7, 8R, and 9R should be dissected; on the left side, stations 5, 6, 7, 8L, and 9L should be dissected (Fig. 35-5). Hilar lymph nodes are typically resected and sent with the specimen, although it is helpful to specifically dissect and label level 10 lymph nodes when possible. On the left side, level 2 and sometimes level 4 lymph nodes are generally obscured by the aorta. Although the therapeutic benefit of nodal dissection versus nodal sampling remains controversial, in a recent pooled analysis of three trials, 4-year survival was superior in patients undergoing resection with stages I–IIIA NSCLC who had complete mediastinal lymph node dissection compared with lymph node sampling. Moreover, a complete mediastinal lymphadenectomy adds little morbidity to a pulmonary resection for lung cancer. Thus, the recommendation at this time is that patients should have a complete mediastinal node dissection.

Radiation Therapy in Stages I and II NSCLC

There is currently no role for adjuvant radiation therapy in patients following resection of stage I or II NSCLC. Patients with stage I or II disease who refuse or are not candidates for pulmonary resection should be considered for radiation therapy with curative intent. The decision to administer high-dose radiotherapy is based on the extent of disease and the volume of the chest that requires radiation. A systematic review reported 5-year survival rates of 13–39% in patients with stage I or II NSCLC treated with radical radiotherapy. Stereotactic radiation therapy and cryoablation are relatively new techniques that are being used in the treatment of patients with isolated pulmonary nodules who are not candidates for or refuse surgical resection, but their use may be limited by tumor size: ≤5 cm for stereotactic radiotherapy and ≤3 cm for cryoablation therapy.

Chemotherapy in Stages I and II NSCLC

A multitude of trials have evaluated the role of adjuvant chemotherapy in patients with resected stage IA–IIIA NSCLC with conflicting results (Table 35-8). A meta-analysis, the Lung Adjuvant Cisplatin Evaluation Study (LACE), reported a 5.4% improvement in 5-year survival for adjuvant chemotherapy compared with surgery alone in patients with stage I–IIIA NSCLC. The effect of cisplatin plus vinorelbine appeared marginally better than other cisplatin-based doublet regimens. The analysis, however, reported a harmful effect for chemotherapy in patients with stage IA disease, with questionable benefit in patients with stage IB disease. Chemotherapy also appeared to be detrimental in patients with poor performance status (ECOG PS2). The results of these studies have led to the recommendation for adjuvant chemotherapy only in patients with stage II or III NSCLC. Chemotherapy should start 6 to 8 weeks after surgery, if the patient has recovered, and should be administered for four cycles. All patients should be treated with a cisplatin-based regimen. Carboplatin is a reasonable consideration in patients who are unlikely to tolerate cisplatin for reasons such as reduced renal function, presence of neuropathy, or hearing impairment.

The treatment of patients with stage IB NSCLC remains controversial. Retrospective subset analyses of randomized phase III trials have reported no benefit for adjuvant chemotherapy in patients with stage IB disease. The only trial to evaluate adjuvant chemotherapy in patients with stage IB NSCLC reported no improvement in overall survival; however, a retrospective analysis of the trial reported a benefit in patients with tumors that were ≥4 cm. At this time, the risks and benefits of chemotherapy should be considered on an individual patient basis.

Four trials have evaluated neoadjuvant chemotherapy (chemotherapy before surgery) in patients with stage I–III NSCLC, of which three reported a trend toward improvement in progression-free and overall survival. However, at this time, no data support the use of neoadjuvant chemotherapy in NSCLC patients.

All patients with resected NSCLC are at high risk of recurrence or developing a second primary lung cancer. Thus, it is reasonable to follow these patients with regular imaging. The most appropriate modality and frequency has not been defined. Given that the majority of patients recur within the first 2 years after therapy, one guideline suggests CT scans of the chest with contrast every 6 months for the first 2 years after surgery, followed by yearly CT scans of the chest without contrast thereafter.

TABLE 35-8

ADJUVANT CHEMOTHERAPY TRIALS IN NON–SMALL CELL LUNG CANCER

TRIAL	STAGE	TREATMENT	*n*	5-YEAR SURVIVAL (%)	*P*
IALT	I–III	Cisplatin-based	932	44.5	<.03
		Control	835	40.4	
BR10	IB–II	Cisplatin + vinorelbine	242	69	.03
		Control	240	54	
ANITA	IB–IIIA	Cisplatin + vinorelbine	407	60	.017
		Control	433	58	
ALPI	I–III	MVP	548	50	.49
		Control	540	45	
BLT	I–III	Cisplatin-based	192	60	.90
		Control	189	58	
CALGB	IB	Carboplatin + paclitaxel	173	59	.10
			171	57	

Abbreviations: ALPI, Adjuvant Lung Cancer Project Italy; ANITA, Adjuvant Navelbine International Trialist Association; BLT, Big Lung Trial; CALGB, Cancer and Lung Cancer Group B; IALT, International Adjuvant Lung Cancer Trial; MVP, mitomycin, vindesine, and cisplatin.

MANAGEMENT OF STAGE III NSCLC The interpretation of the results of clinical trials involving patients with stage III NSCLC has been clouded by a number of issues, including changing diagnostic techniques, different staging systems, and heterogeneous patient populations. In prior studies, patients may have had tumors ranging from nonbulky stage IIIA (clinical N1 nodes with N2 nodes discovered only at the time of surgery, despite a negative mediastinoscopy result) to bulky N2 nodes (lymph nodes >2 cm clearly visible on imaging, or multilevel ipsilateral mediastinal nodes) to clearly inoperable nodes.

Surgery followed by adjuvant chemotherapy is the treatment of choice for patients with stage IIIA disease due to hilar nodal involvement (T3N1). Surgery for N2 disease is more controversial. A randomized phase III trial demonstrated an improvement in progression-free survival but no improvement in overall survival when patients with pathologically staged N2 NSCLC were treated with concurrent chemoradiotherapy (cisplatin and etoposide) and 45 Gy of radiation followed by surgery compared with chemotherapy and 61 Gy of radiotherapy without surgery. Treatment-related mortality is greater in the surgery arm (8% vs 2%), with the majority of deaths occurring in patients undergoing pneumonectomy. In subset analysis, the investigators found survival was improved if a lobectomy was performed but not pneumonectomy compared with chemoradiotherapy alone.

Despite a careful preoperative staging evaluation, as many as a quarter of patients will be found to have metastases to N2 nodes on frozen-section examination at the time of thoracotomy or on final pathologic examination of the surgical specimen. For patients with an occult, single-station mediastinal node metastasis recognized at thoracotomy in which a complete resection of the nodes and primary tumor is technically possible, most thoracic surgeons proceed with the planned lung resection and a mediastinal lymphadenectomy. If a complete resection is not possible or there is multistation or bulky nodal disease or extracapsular nodal disease, then the planned lung resection should be aborted. These patients can then be considered for combined chemoradiotherapy as described later. Although incomplete resection rarely results in long-term survival, collected results indicate that surgery alone in stage IIIA disease (N2 disease) is associated with a 14–30% 5-year survival. The best survival rate is seen in cases with minimal N2 disease and complete resection.

Chemotherapy plus radiation therapy is the treatment of choice for patients with N3 nodal involvement or bulky stage IIIA disease. In general, patients with histologically involved lymph nodes >2 cm in short-axis diameter measured by CT, who have extranodal involvement or multistation disease along with groups of multiple smaller lymph nodes involved, are considered to have bulky, unresectable disease. Randomized phase III trials initially demonstrated an improvement in median and long-term survival for chemotherapy followed by radiation therapy compared with radiation therapy alone. Subsequent trials demonstrated administering concurrent chemotherapy and radiation therapy results in improved survival compared to sequential therapy, albeit with more side effects, such as fatigue, esophagitis, and neutropenia. Therefore, combined modality treatment with chemotherapy and radiation therapy is recommended in patients who are able to tolerate the treatment.

Superior Sulcus or Pancoast Tumors Superior sulcus tumors arise in the apex of the lung and invade adjacent structures producing Pancoast's syndrome: Horner's syndrome, shoulder and/or arm pain, and weakness and atrophy of the muscles of the hand. Patients with these tumors should undergo the same staging procedures as all patients with stage II or III NSCLC. Neoadjuvant chemotherapy or combined chemotherapy and radiation therapy is typically reserved for those patients with N0 or N1 involvement. This approach results in a 33-month median survival and 44% 5-year survival for all patients and a 94-month median survival and 54% 5-year survival in patients with an R0 resection. For patients with Pancoast tumors that have metastatic disease at the time of presentation, radiation therapy with or without chemotherapy may be offered for palliation of symptoms.

TREATMENT OF METASTATIC NSCLC Approximately two-thirds of NSCLC patients present with advanced disease (stage IIIB with a pleural effusion or stage IV) at the time of diagnosis. These patients have a median survival of 4–5 months and a 1-year survival of 10% when managed with best supportive care alone. In addition, a significant number of patients who present with early-stage NSCLC eventually relapse with distant disease. Patients who have recurrent disease have a better prognosis than those presenting with metastatic disease at the time of diagnosis. Standard medical management, the judicious use of pain medications, and the appropriate use of radiotherapy and chemotherapy form the cornerstone of management.

Chemotherapy palliates symptoms, improves the quality of life, and improves survival in patients with stage IV NSCLC, particularly in patients with good performance status. In addition, economic analysis has found chemotherapy to be cost-effective palliation for stage IV NSCLC. However, the use of chemotherapy for NSCLC requires clinical experience and careful judgment to balance potential benefits and toxicities.

First-Line Chemotherapy for Metastatic or Recurrent NSCLC The first indication of the benefit of chemotherapy in patients with advanced NSCLC came from a meta-analysis published in 1995 that reported a survival advantage in patients treated with cisplatin-based chemotherapy compared with those receiving supportive care alone (hazards ratio = 0.73; $P < .0001$). This led to a multitude of clinical trials comparing different cisplatin-based regimens in patients with advanced NSCLC all reporting a similar magnitude of benefit; 20–30% response rate and an 8- to 10-month median survival (Table 35-9).

TABLE 35-9

FIRST-LINE CHEMOTHERAPY TRIALS FOR METASTATIC NON–SMALL CELL LUNG CANCER

TRIAL	REGIMEN	*N*	RR (%)	MEDIAN SURVIVAL (MONTHS)
ECOG1594	Cisplatin + paclitaxel	288	21	7.8
	Cisplatin + gemcitabine	288	22	8.1
	Cisplatin + docetaxel	289	17	7.4
	Carboplatin + paclitaxel	290	17	8.1
TAX-326	Cisplatin + docetaxel	406	32	11.3
	Cisplatin + vinorelbine	394	25	10.1
	Carboplatin + docetaxel	404	24	9.4
EORTC	Cisplatin + paclitaxel	159	32	8.1
	Cisplatin + gemcitabine	160	37	8.9
	Paclitaxel + gemcitabine	161	28	6.7
ILCP	Cisplatin + gemcitabine	205	30	9.8
	Carboplatin + paclitaxel	204	32	9.9
	Cisplatin + vinorelbine	203	30	9.5
SWOG	Cisplatin + vinorelbine	202	28	8.0
	Carboplatin + paclitaxel	206	25	8.0
FACS	Cisplatin + irinotecan	145	31	13.9
	Carboplatin + paclitaxel	145	32	12.3
	Cisplatin + gemcitabine	146	30	14.0
	Cisplatin + vinorelbine	145	33	11.4
Scagliotti	Cisplatin + gemcitabine	863	28	10.3
	Cisplatin + pemetrexed	862	31	10.3
iPASS[a]	Carboplatin + paclitaxel	608	32	17.3
	Gefitinib	609	43	18.6

[a]Enrolled selected patients: 18 years of age or older, had histologic or cytologically confirmed stage IIIB or IV non–small cell lung cancer with histologic features of adenocarcinoma (including bronchioloalveolar carcinoma), were nonsmokers (defined as patients who had smoked <100 cigarettes in their lifetime) or former light smokers (those who had stopped smoking at least 15 years previously and had a total of ≤10 pack-years of smoking), and had had no previous chemotherapy or biologic or immunologic therapy.

Abbreviations: ECOG, Eastern Cooperative Oncology Group; EORTC, European Organization for Research and Treatment of Cancer; FACS, Follow-up After Colorectal Surgery; ILCP, Italian Lung Cancer Project; iPASS, Iressa Pan-Asian Study; RR, relative risk; SWOG, South-Western Oncology Group.

Chemotherapy was well tolerated in all studies in patients with a good performance status, ECOG PS 0–1.

An ongoing debate in the treatment of patients with NSCLC is the appropriate duration of platinum-based chemotherapy. Several large phase III randomized trials have failed to show a benefit for increasing the duration of platinum-based doublet chemotherapy beyond four to six cycles. In fact, a longer duration of chemotherapy has been associated with increased toxicities and impaired quality of life. Therefore, prolonged therapy (beyond four to six cycles) with platinum-based regimens is not recommended in patients with advanced NSCLC.

Tumor histology has emerged as an important consideration in the treatment of patients with NSCLC. A randomized phase III trial found that patients with nonsquamous NSCLC had an improved survival when treated with cisplatin and pemetrexed compared with cisplatin and gemcitabine, while patients with squamous carcinoma had an improved survival when treated with cisplatin and gemcitabine. This difference in survival is thought to be related to the differential expression of thymidylate synthase, one of the targets of pemetrexed, between tumor types. Bevacizumab, a monoclonal antibody against vascular endothelial growth factor (VEGF), when combined with chemotherapy improves response rate, progression-free survival, and overall survival in patients with advanced disease (see later discussion). However, bevacizumab cannot be given to patients with squamous cell histology NSCLC because of the risk of serious hemorrhagic effects.

Second-Line Chemotherapy and Beyond As first-line chemotherapy regimens improve, a substantial number of patients will maintain a good performance status and a desire for further therapy when they develop recurrent disease. At present, only three drugs are FDA-approved for second-line therapy of NSCLC in the United States, i.e., docetaxel, pemetrexed, and erlotinib. In general, these agents have similar overall response rates of 5–10% (depending on the patient's prior exposure to taxanes and platinum) and yield median survival times of 6–8 months. However, the available drugs have distinct toxicity profiles that can influence their use in the second-line setting. Hematologic toxicity, including febrile neutropenia, is greater for docetaxel than pemetrexed and erlotinib, whereas nonhematologic toxicity, namely rash and diarrhea, is greater with erlotinib. Most of the survival benefit for any of these agents is realized in patients who maintain a good performance status.

AGENTS THAT INHIBIT ANGIOGENESIS

Bevacizumab was the first antiangiogenic agent approved for the treatment of patients with advanced NSCLC in the United States. This drug primarily acts by sponging up VEGF and blocking the growth of new blood vessels, which are required for tumor viability.

Two randomized phase III trials of chemotherapy with or without bevacizumab had conflicting results. The first trial, conducted in North America, compared carboplatin/paclitaxel with or without bevacizumab in patients with recurrent or advanced nonsquamous NSCLC and reported a significant improvement in response rate, progression-free survival, and overall survival for chemotherapy-plus-bevacizumab–treated patients compared with chemotherapy alone. Toxicities were more frequent in bevacizumab-treated patients. The second trial, conducted in Europe, compared cisplatin/gemcitabine with or without bevacizumab in patients with recurrent or advanced nonsquamous NSCLC and reported a significant improvement in progression-free survival but no improvement in overall survival for bevacizumab-treated patients. Therefore, at this time, carboplatin–paclitaxel and bevacizumab is an approved regimen for first-line treatment of nonsquamous NSCLC in the United States but not in Europe.

AGENTS THAT INHIBIT THE EPIDERMAL GROWTH FACTOR RECEPTOR Erlotinib and gefitinib are oral small-molecule kinase inhibitors that inhibit signaling via EGF-R. These were the first EGF-R inhibitors to be approved for the treatment of patients with NSCLC. A randomized phase III trial compared erlotinib with placebo in previously treated patients with advanced NSCLC and reported an improvement in overall survival for erlotinib compared to placebo. Gefitinib received premarketing approval by the FDA after impressive results seen in phase II trials in patients with previously treated NSCLC; however, a randomized phase III trial found no difference in overall survival between patients treated with gefitinib compared with placebo. These results led to a U.S. FDA-mandated change in the gefitinib indication to include only patients who have previously benefited from this drug. However, gefitinib is still available for the treatment of NSCLC patients in Europe and Asia. Clinical features that have been shown to correlate with responsiveness to EGF-R TKI treatment include female sex, never smoking status, adenocarcinoma histology, and Asian ethnicity. Somatic mutations in the kinase domain of EGF-R and high EGF-R copy number have also been shown to correlate with response and improved survival with oral EGF-R inhibitors.

Two randomized phase III trials conducted in Asia have compared gefitinib with platinum-based chemotherapy in patients with NSCLC. The first trial compared first-line gefitinib with carboplatin–paclitaxel in never or light ex-smokers with newly diagnosed advanced NSCLC. Treatment with gefitinib was associated with a significant improvement in response rate and 12-month progression-free survival. In patients with tumors available for mutation analysis, treatment with gefitinib was favored over chemotherapy in patients with tumors that harbored an EGF-R mutation and chemotherapy was favored in patients with tumors that were EGF-R mutation negative. Quality of life favored treatment with gefitinib. The second trial enrolled only patients with tumors that were EGF-R mutation positive and reported a significant improvement in progression-free survival and disease control for patients treated with gefitinib compared with cisplatin–docetaxel. These and related results suggest standard chemotherapy regimens or gefitinib and erlotinib could be considered for first-line therapy in a subset of advanced NSCLC patients with tumors that harbor the EGF-R mutation.

Cetuximab is an intravenously administered chimeric antibody directed against EGF-R. A randomized phase III trial evaluated treatment with cisplatin–vinorelbine with or without cetuximab in patients with advanced NSCLC and at least one EGF-R–positive cell as determined by immunohistochemistry. The results showed no difference in progression-free survival but a significant improvement in response rate and overall survival in patients treated with cetuximab compared with placebo. A prespecified subgroup analysis showed no improvement in overall survival among patients of Asian ethnicity receiving cetuximab compared with placebo. However, a significant improvement in overall survival was noted among white patients receiving cetuximab; this appeared true regardless of histology. Contrary to patients with colon cancer, KRAS mutation status did not predict response to therapy with cetuximab, although the number of cases examined at the molecular level was suboptimal. Development of acneiform rash was associated with improved overall survival compared with patients with no rash. A second phase III trial in patients with advanced NSCLC with no required EGF-R testing reported no difference in overall survival between patients randomized to carboplatin–paclitaxel or docetaxel with or without cetuximab.

MAINTENANCE THERAPY Maintenance chemotherapy in nonprogressing patients (patients with a complete response, partial response, or stable disease) is a controversial topic in the treatment of NSCLC patients. Two studies have investigated maintenance single-agent chemotherapy with docetaxel or pemetrexed in nonprogressing patients following treatment with first-line platinum-based chemotherapy. Both trials randomized patients to immediate single-agent therapy versus observation and reported improvements in progression-free and overall survival. In both trials, a significant portion of patients in the observation arm did not receive therapy with the agent under investigation upon disease progression; 37% of study patients never received docetaxel in the docetaxel study, and 81% of patients never received pemetrexed in the pemetrexed study. In the trial of maintenance docetaxel versus observation, survival was identical to the treatment group in the subset of patients who received docetaxel on progression, indicating this is an active agent in NSCLC. These data are not available for the pemetrexed study. Currently, maintenance pemetrexed is the only therapy approved by the U.S. FDA following platinum-based chemotherapy in patients with advanced NSCLC. However, maintenance chemotherapy is not without toxicity and at this time should be considered on an individual patient basis.

Two randomized controlled trials have reported improvements in progression-free survival from maintenance treatment with erlotinib compared with placebo in patients with advanced NSCLC following platinum-based chemotherapy.

TREATMENT Small Cell Lung Cancer

TREATMENT OF LIMITED DISEASE SMALL CELL LUNG CANCER

Surgery SCLC is a highly aggressive disease characterized by its rapid doubling time, high growth fraction, early development of disseminated disease, and dramatic response to first-line chemotherapy and radiation. Surgical resection is not routinely recommended for patients because even those patients with LD-SCLC still have occult micrometastases. If the histologic diagnosis of SCLC is made in patients on review of a resected surgical specimen, such patients should receive standard SCLC chemotherapy as described below. If one employs classic TNM staging categories, two retrospective series have reported high cure rates for adjuvant chemotherapy following resection in patients with stage I or II SCLC.

Chemotherapy Chemotherapy significantly prolongs survival in patients with SCLC. Combination chemotherapy with a platinum agent (cisplatin or carboplatin) and etoposide for four to six cycles is the mainstay of treatment and has not changed in almost three decades. Cyclophosphamide, doxorubicin (Adriamycin), and vincristine (CAV) may be an alternative for patients who are unable to tolerate a platinum-based regimen. Despite response rates to first-line therapy as high as 80%, the median survival ranges from 12 to 20 months for patients with LD and from 7 to 11 months for patients with ED. Regardless of disease extent, the majority of patients relapse and develop chemotherapy-resistant disease. Only 6–12% of patients with LD- and 2% of patients with ED-SCLC live beyond 5 years. The prognosis is especially poor for patients who relapse within the first 3 months of therapy; these patients are said to have platinum-*resistant disease*. Patients are said to have *sensitive disease* if they relapse more than 3 months after their initial therapy and are thought to have a somewhat better overall survival. Patients with sensitive disease are thought to have the greatest potential benefit from second-line chemotherapy. Topotecan is the only FDA-approved agent with modest activity as second-line therapy in patients with SCLC.

Radiation Therapy Patients with LD-SCLC are treated with combined modality therapy with cisplatin and etoposide chemotherapy and radiation therapy. A retrospective analysis of patients with SCLC treated with once-daily fractionation found improved local control rates as the total dose delivered was increased from 30 to 50 Gy. Chemotherapy when given concurrently with radiation is more effective than sequential chemoradiation but is associated with significantly more esophagitis and hematologic toxicity. The addition of radiation therapy early on is preferred. Twice-daily (hyperfractionated) radiation has been shown to improve survival in patients with LD-SCLC but is associated with higher rates of grade 3 esophagitis and pulmonary toxicity. It is feasible to deliver once-daily radiation therapy doses up to at least 70 Gy when administered concurrently with cisplatin-based chemotherapy. This higher dose of once-daily radiotherapy may be equivalent or superior to the 45-Gy twice-daily radiotherapy dose. Patients should be carefully selected for concurrent chemoradiation therapy based on good performance status and pulmonary reserve.

Prophylactic Cranial Irradiation Prophylactic cranial irradiation (PCI) should be considered in all patients with LD- and ED-SCLC who have responded to initial therapy. A meta-analysis including 7 trials and 987 patients with LD-SCLC who had achieved a complete remission following primary chemotherapy reported a 5.4% improvement in overall survival for patients treated with PCI. In patients with ED-SCLC who had responded to first-line chemotherapy, PCI reduced the occurrence of symptomatic brain metastases and prolonged disease-free and overall survival compared with no radiation therapy. Long-term toxicities including deficits in cognition have been reported following PCI and are difficult to sort out from the effects of chemotherapy or normal aging.

Molecularly Tailored Lung Cancer Therapy In the past 40 years, clinical research in lung cancer has demonstrated that surgery, systemic chemotherapy, and radiation therapy can all be used to prolong patient survival and/or improve quality of life. However, conventional approaches, especially those that classify patients according to disease histology alone, appear to have reached a therapeutic plateau of effectiveness. One promising future approach to improve the outcome for patients with lung cancer is tailored therapy based on individualized phenotypic or genotypic tumor characteristics. Such a strategy is based on an understanding of the molecular underpinnings of the disease, recognizing that although tumors may appear similar at the histologic level, they do differ from individual to individual. It is hoped that better outcomes can be achieved by matching the most appropriate therapy to a patient at the right time.

For example, one subset of lung cancer can be defined by somatic mutations in *EGF-R*. *EGF-R* mutations are almost exclusively found in lung adenocarcinoma and are more common in females, never smokers compared with former or current smokers, and in East Asians compared with Western populations (30–70% vs 8%). These mutations, primarily in-frame deletions in exon 19 and point mutations in exon 21 (L858R), result in constitutive activation of the receptor and are associated with very high response rates (60–90%) to the specific TK inhibitors gefitinib and erlotinib. Almost all patients with these dramatic responses, however, develop acquired resistance. In about half of patients, resistance can be attributed to the emergence of clones harboring a second-site mutation in exon 20 (T790M), which alters binding of drug to the receptor. About 20% of *EGF-R* mutant tumors from patients with acquired resistance display amplification of a gene encoding a different TK, MET. As a result of these findings, many trials are being conducted in these patients using second-generation EGFR inhibitors that can overcome T790M-mediated resistance or MET inhibitors to target MET-dependent cells.

Another subset of lung adenocarcinoma can be defined by EML4-ALK fusion proteins. These translocations arise from a small inversion within chromosome 2p that leads to the formation of a fusion-gene comprising the N terminal of the echinoderm microtubule–associated protein-like 4 (EML4) gene and the intracellular TK domain of the anaplastic lymphoma kinase (ALK) gene. Patients with lung cancers harboring an ALK fusion protein have demonstrated dramatic responses to small-molecule ALK inhibitors in early clinical trials. The ALK fusion protein is relatively rare, occurring in 3–7% of NSCLCs. Clinical characteristics associated with EML4-ALK–positive lung cancer appears to be a younger age at diagnosis, minimal smoking history, male sex, and adenocarcinoma histology with signet-ring features.

Other biomarkers being explored include molecules that may predict outcomes with conventional chemotherapy. For example, low expression of the DNA repair gene excision repair cross-complementation group 1 (ERCC1) correlates with improved survival after treatment with platinum drugs, whereas tumors that have high expression of ERCC1 are less sensitive to therapy with a platinum agent. In the absence of treatment, lung cancer with low ERCC1 expression has a poorer prognosis.

Ribonucleotide reductase M1 (RRM1) encodes the regulatory subunit of ribonucleotide reductase, the rate-limiting enzyme in DNA synthesis. Ribonucleotide reductase converts ribonucleotide 5-diphosphate to deoxyribonucleotide 5-diphosphate. Notably, gemcitabine, an agent commonly used in the treatment of NSCLC, competes with ribonucleotide 5-diphosphate for incorporation into DNA. Levels of RRM1 expression are significantly and inversely correlated with disease response after two cycles of gemcitabine and carboplatin in patients with locally advanced NSCLC. In addition, low RRM1 mRNA expression levels are associated with a significantly longer median survival compared to high levels.

Thymidylate synthase (TS) catalyzes the methylation of dUMP to dTMP and is the rate-limiting irreversible step in de novo DNA synthesis. TS is one of the targets of the novel folate-based drug pemetrexed, an agent that is FDA-approved as second-line treatment in patients with NSCLC. TS expression is an independent prognostic and predictive factor in several cancers, including lung cancers, and overexpression of TS has been linked to resistance to pemetrexed, an agent commonly employed as second-line treatment in patients with nonsquamous NSCLC. TS mRNA and protein levels are significantly higher in squamous cell carcinomas and small cell carcinomas of the lung as compared with adenocarcinomas. A randomized phase III trial reported that cisplatin plus gemcitabine was more effective in squamous cell carcinomas; cisplatin plus pemetrexed was found to be more effective in adenocarcinomas and large cell carcinomas. Molecular markers are likely to play an increasing role in helping guide treatment decisions.

BENIGN LUNG NEOPLASMS

Benign tumors account for about 5% of all lung cancers. About half are hamartomas; the lungs are the site of about 90% of all hamartomas. The other half are bronchial adenomas.

HAMARTOMAS

Lung hamartomas are usually peripheral lung masses composed of normal pulmonary tissue components such as smooth muscle and collagen. They are more common in men than in women and have a peak incidence in the 60s. They are often incidental radiographic findings as solitary nodules. They have a pathognomonic "popcorn" pattern of calcification in some cases;

however, without such a finding, resection is necessary to rule out malignancy, especially in smokers.

BRONCHIAL ADENOMAS

These are centrally located slow-growing endobronchial lesions that are generally carcinoid tumors (≥80%; Chap. 49), adenocystic tumors (so called cylindromas, 10–15%), or mucoepidermoid tumors (2–3%). Mean age at presentation is 45 years (range 15–60 years). Patients often give a history of chronic cough, intermittent hemoptysis, or repeated episodes of airway obstruction with atelectasis or pneumonias with abscess formation due to endobronchial lesions obstructing the airway. They are usually visible at bronchoscopy but are highly vascular and may bleed profusely after a bronchoscopic biopsy. They are largely curable by surgical resection (local excision), but they may recur locally or become invasive and metastasize. Five-year survival after resection is 95% if the disease is localized. For bronchial adenomas that spread, the course of disease can become highly aggressive, such as SCLC, or somewhat slower, such as carcinoid tumors. Therapy is generally dictated by the pace of the disease.

CHAPTER 36
THYMOMA

Dan L. Longo

The thymus is derived from the third and fourth pharyngeal pouches and is located in the anterior mediastinum. It is composed of epithelial and stromal cells derived from the pharyngeal pouch and lymphoid precursors derived from mesodermal cells. It is the site to which bone marrow precursors that are committed to differentiate into T cells migrate to complete their differentiation. Like many organs, it is organized into functional regions, in this case the cortex and the medulla. The cortex of the thymus contains ~85% of the lymphoid cells, and the medulla contains ~15%. It appears that the primitive bone marrow progenitors enter the thymus at the corticomedullary junction and migrate first through the cortex toward the periphery of the gland and then toward the medulla as they mature. Medullary thymocytes have a phenotype that cannot be distinguished readily from that of mature peripheral blood and lymph node T cells.

Several things can go wrong with the thymus, but thymic abnormalities are very rare. If the thymus does not develop properly, serious deficiencies in T cell development ensue and severe immunodeficiency is seen (e.g., DiGeorge syndrome). If a lymphoid cell within the thymus becomes neoplastic, the disease that develops is a lymphoma. The majority of lymphoid tumors that develop in the thymus are derived from the precursor T cells, and the tumor is a precursor T cell lymphoblastic lymphoma (Chap. 15). Rare B cells exist in the thymus, and when they become neoplastic, the tumor is a mediastinal (thymic) B cell lymphoma (Chap. 15). Hodgkin's disease, particularly the nodular sclerosing subtype, often involves the anterior mediastinum. Extranodal marginal zone (MALT) lymphomas have been reported to involve the thymus in the setting of Sjögren's syndrome or other autoimmune disorders, and the lymphoma cells often express IgA instead of IgM on their surface. Castleman's disease can involve the thymus. Germ cell tumors and carcinoid tumors occasionally may arise in the thymus. If the epithelial cells of the thymus become neoplastic, the tumor that develops is a *thymoma*.

CLINICAL PRESENTATION AND DIFFERENTIAL DIAGNOSIS

Thymoma is the most common cause of an anterior mediastinal mass in adults, accounting for ~40% of all mediastinal masses. The other major causes of anterior mediastinal masses are lymphomas, germ cell tumors, and substernal thyroid tumors. Carcinoid tumors, lipomas, and thymic cysts also may produce radiographic masses. After combination chemotherapy for another malignancy, teenagers and young adults may develop a rebound thymic hyperplasia in the first few months after treatment. Granulomatous inflammatory diseases (tuberculosis, sarcoidosis) can produce thymic enlargement. Thymomas are most common in the fifth and sixth decades, are uncommon in children, and are distributed evenly between men and women.

About 40–50% of patients are asymptomatic; masses are detected incidentally on routine chest radiographs. When symptomatic, patients may have cough, chest pain, dyspnea, fever, wheezing, fatigue, weight loss, night sweats, or anorexia. Occasionally, thymomas may obstruct the superior vena cava. About 40% of patients with thymoma have another systemic autoimmune illness related to the thymoma. About 30% of patients with thymoma have myasthenia gravis, 5–8% have pure red cell aplasia, and ~5% have hypogammaglobulinemia. Thymoma with hypogammaglobulinemia also is called Good's syndrome. Among patients with myasthenia gravis, ~10–15% have a thymoma. Thymoma more rarely may be associated with polymyositis, systemic lupus erythematosus, thyroiditis, Sjögren's syndrome, ulcerative colitis, pernicious anemia, Addison's disease, scleroderma, and panhypopituitarism. In one series, 70%

of patients with thymoma were found to have another systemic illness.

DIAGNOSIS AND STAGING

Once a mediastinal mass is detected, a surgical procedure is required for definitive diagnosis. An initial mediastinoscopy or limited thoracotomy can be undertaken to get sufficient tissue to make an accurate diagnosis. Fine-needle aspiration is poor at distinguishing between lymphomas and thymomas but is more reliable in diagnosing germ cell tumors and metastatic carcinoma. Thymomas and lymphomas require sufficient tissue to examine the tumor architecture to ensure an accurate diagnosis and obtain prognostic information.

Once a diagnosis of thymoma is defined, subsequent staging generally occurs at surgery. However, chest computed tomography (CT) scans can assess local invasiveness in some instances. Magnetic resonance imaging has a defined role in the staging of posterior mediastinal tumors, but it is not clear that it adds important information to the CT scan in anterior mediastinal tumors. Somatostatin receptor imaging with indium-labeled somatostatin analogues may be of value. If invasion is not distinguished by noninvasive testing, an effort to resect the entire tumor should be undertaken. If invasion is present, neoadjuvant chemotherapy may be warranted before surgery (see "Treatment" later in this chapter).

Some 90% of thymomas are in the anterior mediastinum, but some may be in other mediastinal sites or even the neck, based on aberrant migration of the developing thymic enlage.

The staging system for thymoma was developed by Masaoka and colleagues (Table 36-1). It is an anatomic system in which the stage is increased on the basis of the degree of invasiveness. The 5-year survival of patients in the various stages is as follows: stage I, 96%; stage II, 86%; stage III, 69%; and stage IV, 50%. The French Study Group on Thymic Tumors (GETT) has proposed modifications to the Masaoka scheme based on the degree of surgical removal because the extent of surgery has been noted to be a prognostic indicator. In their system, stage I tumors are divided into A and B on the basis of whether the surgeon suspects adhesions to adjacent structures; stage III tumors are divided into A and B based on whether disease was subtotally resected or only biopsied. The concurrence between the two systems is high.

TABLE 36-1

MASAOKA STAGING SYSTEM FOR THYMOMAS

STAGE	DIAGNOSTIC CRITERIA
I	Macroscopically and microscopically completely encapsulated; no invasion through capsule
II	
IIA	Microscopic invasion outside the capsule
IIB	Macroscopic invasion into surrounding fat or grossly adherent to pleura or pericardium
III	
IIIA	Macroscopic invasion into neighboring organs, pericardium, or pleura but not great vessels
IIIB	Macroscopic invasion into neighboring organs that includes great vessels
IV	
IVA	Pleural or pericardial dissemination
IVB	Lymphatic or hematogenous metastases

	STAGE DISTRIBUTION, %	5-YEAR SURVIVAL, %	10-YEAR SURVIVAL, %
I	36	95–100	86–100
II	26	70–100	50–100
III	22	68–89	47–60
IV	10	47–69	0–11

Source: From A Masaoka et al: Cancer 48:2485, 1981. Updated from S Tomaszek et al: Ann Thorac Surg 87:1973, 2009, and CB Falkson et al: J Thorac Oncol 4:911, 2009.

PATHOLOGY AND ETIOLOGY

Thymomas are epithelial tumors, and all of them have malignant potential. It is not worthwhile to try to divide them into benign and malignant forms; the key prognostic feature is whether they are noninvasive or invasive. About 65% of thymomas are encapsulated and noninvasive, and about 35% are invasive. They may have a variable percentage of lymphocytes within the tumor, but genetic studies suggest that the lymphocytes are benign polyclonal cells. The epithelial component of the tumor may consist primarily of round or oval cells derived mainly from the cortex or spindle-shaped cells derived mainly from the medulla or combinations of the two types (Table 36-2). Cytologic features are not reliable predictors of biologic behavior. About 90% of A, AB, and B1 tumors are localized. A very small number of patients have aggressive histology features characteristic of carcinomas. Thymic carcinomas are invasive and have a poor prognosis.

The genetic lesions in thymomas are not well characterized. Some data suggest that Epstein-Barr virus may be associated with thymomas. Some tumors overexpress the p21 *ras* gene product. However, molecular pathogenesis remains undefined. A thymoma susceptibility locus has been defined on *rat* chromosome 7, but the relationship between this gene locus, termed *Tsr1*, and human thymoma has not been examined.

TABLE 36-2

WORLD HEALTH ORGANIZATION HISTOLOGIC CLASSIFICATION OF THYMUS TUMORS

TYPE	HISTOLOGIC DESCRIPTION
A	Medullary thymoma
AB	Mixed thymoma
B1	Predominantly cortical thymoma
B2	Cortical thymoma
B3	Well-differentiated thymic carcinoma
C	Thymic carcinoma

TYPE	DISTRIBUTION, %	PROGNOSIS (10-YEAR DISEASE-FREE SURVIVAL), %
A	8	100
AB	26	90–100
B1	15	78–94
B2	28	83
B3	15	36
C	8	0–35

Source: From S Tomaszek et al: Ann Thorac Surg 87:1973, 2009.

TREATMENT Thymoma

Treatment is determined by the stage of disease. For patients with encapsulated tumors and stage I disease, complete resection is sufficient to cure 96% of patients. For patients with stage II disease, complete resection may be followed by 30–60 Gy of postoperative radiation therapy to the site of the primary tumor. However, the value of radiation therapy in this setting has not been established. The main predictors of long-term survival are Masaoka stage and completeness of resection. For patients with stage III and IV disease, the use of neoadjuvant chemotherapy followed by radical surgery, with or without additional radiation therapy, and additional consolidation chemotherapy has been associated with excellent survival. Chemotherapy regimens that are most effective generally include a platinum compound (either cisplatin or carboplatin) and an anthracycline. Addition of cyclophosphamide, vincristine, and prednisone seems to improve response rates. Response rates of 50–93% have been reported in series of patients; each study involved fewer than 40 patients. A single most effective regimen has not been defined. If surgery after neoadjuvant chemotherapy fails to produce a complete resection of residual disease, radiation therapy (50–60 Gy) may help reduce recurrence rates.

This multimodality approach appears to be superior to the use of surgery followed by radiation therapy alone, which produces a 5-year survival rate of ≤50% in patients with advanced-stage disease.

Some thymic carcinomas express *c-kit*, and one patient whose *c-kit* locus was mutated responded dramatically to imatinib. Many thymomas express epidermal growth factor receptors, but the antibodies to the receptor and the kinase inhibitors that block its action have not been evaluated systematically. Octreotide plus prednisone produces responses in about one-third of patients.

INFLUENCE OF THYMECTOMY ON THE COURSE OF ACCOMPANYING DISEASES

Patients with myasthenia gravis have a high incidence of thymic abnormalities (~80%), but overt thymoma is present in only ~10–15% of patients with myasthenia gravis. It is thought that the thymus plays a role in breaking self-tolerance and generating T cells that recognize the acetylcholine receptor as a foreign antigen. Although patients with thymoma and myasthenia gravis are less likely to have a remission in the myasthenia as a consequence of thymectomy than are patients with thymic abnormalities other than thymoma, the course of myasthenia gravis is not significantly different in patients with or without thymoma. Thymectomy produces at least some symptomatic improvement in ~65% of patients with myasthenia gravis. In one large series, thymoma patients with myasthenia gravis had a better long-term survival from thymoma resection than did those without myasthenia gravis.

About 30–50% of patients with pure red cell aplasia have a thymoma. Thymectomy results in the resolution of pure red cell aplasia in ~30% of patients. About 10% of patients with hypogammaglobulinemia have a thymoma, but hypogammaglobulinemia rarely responds to thymectomy.

CHAPTER 37

BREAST CANCER

Marc E. Lippman

Breast cancer is a malignant proliferation of epithelial cells lining the ducts or lobules of the breast. In the year 2010, about 180,000 cases of invasive breast cancer and 40,000 deaths were predicted to occur in the United States. In addition, about 2000 men would be diagnosed with breast cancer. Epithelial malignancies of the breast are the most common cause of cancer in women (excluding skin cancer), accounting for about one-third of all cancer in women. As a result of improved treatment and earlier detection, the mortality rate from breast cancer has begun to decrease very substantially in the United States. This chapter will not consider rare malignancies presenting in the breast, such as sarcomas and lymphomas, but will focus on the epithelial cancers. Human breast cancer is a clonal disease; a single transformed cell—the product of a series of somatic (acquired) or germ-line mutations—is eventually able to express full malignant potential. Thus, breast cancer may exist for a long period as either a noninvasive disease or an invasive but nonmetastatic disease. These facts have significant clinical ramifications.

GENETIC CONSIDERATIONS

Not more than 10% of human breast cancers can be linked directly to germ-line mutations. Several genes have been implicated in familial cases. The Li-Fraumeni syndrome is characterized by inherited mutations in the p53 tumor-suppressor gene, which lead to an increased incidence of breast cancer, osteogenic sarcomas, and other malignancies. Inherited mutations in *PTEN* have also been reported in breast cancer.

Another tumor-suppressor gene, *BRCA-1*, has been identified at the chromosomal locus 17q21; this gene encodes a zinc finger protein, and the product therefore may function as a transcription factor. The gene appears to be involved in gene repair. Women who inherit a mutated allele of this gene from either parent have at least a 60–80% lifetime chance of developing breast cancer and about a 33% chance of developing ovarian cancer. The risk is higher among women born after 1940, presumably due to promotional effects of hormonal factors. Men who carry a mutant allele of the gene have an increased incidence of prostate cancer and breast cancer. A fourth gene, termed *BRCA-2*, which has been localized to chromosome 13q12, is also associated with an increased incidence of breast cancer in men and women.

Germ-line mutations in *BRCA-1* and *BRCA-2* can be readily detected; patients with these mutations can be counseled appropriately. All women with strong family histories for breast cancer should be referred to genetic screening programs, particularly women of Ashkenazi Jewish descent who have a high likelihood of a specific *BRCA-1* mutation (substitution of adenine for guanine at position 185).

Even more important than the role these genes play in inherited forms of breast cancer may be their role in sporadic breast cancer. A p53 mutation is present in nearly 40% of human breast cancers as an acquired defect. Acquired mutations in *PTEN* occur in about 10% of the cases. *BRCA-1* mutation in sporadic primary breast cancer has not been reported. However, decreased expression of *BRCA-1* mRNA (possibly via gene methylation) and abnormal cellular location of the *BRCA-1* protein have been found in some breast cancers. Loss of heterozygosity of *BRCA-1* and *BRCA-2* suggests that tumor-suppressor activity may be inactivated in sporadic cases of human breast cancer. Finally, increased expression of a dominant oncogene plays a role in about a quarter of human breast cancer cases. The product of this gene, a member of the epidermal growth factor receptor superfamily, is called *erbB2* (HER/2 neu) and is overexpressed in these breast cancers due to gene amplification; this overexpression can contribute to transformation of human breast epithelium and is the target of effective systemic therapy in adjuvant and metastatic disease settings.

EPIDEMIOLOGY

Breast cancer is a hormone-dependent disease. Women without functioning ovaries who never receive estrogen replacement therapy (ERT) do not develop breast cancer. The female-to-male ratio is about 150:1. For most epithelial malignancies, a log-log plot of incidence versus age shows a single-component straight-line increase with every year of life. A similar plot for breast cancer shows two components: a straight-line increase with age but with a decrease in slope beginning at the age of menopause. The three dates in a woman's life that have a major impact on breast cancer incidence are age at menarche, age at first full-term pregnancy, and age at menopause. Women who experience menarche at age 16 years have only 50–60% of the breast cancer risk of a woman having menarche at age 12 years; the lower risk persists throughout life. Similarly, menopause occurring 10 years before the median age of menopause (52 years), whether natural or surgically induced, reduces lifetime breast cancer risk by about 35%. Women who have a first full-term pregnancy by age 18 years have a 30–40% lower risk of breast cancer compared with nulliparous women. Thus, length of menstrual life—particularly the fraction occurring before first full-term pregnancy—is a substantial component of the total risk of breast cancer. These three factors (menarche, age of first full-term pregnancy, and menopause) can account for 70–80% of the variation in breast cancer frequency in different countries. A meta-analysis has shown that duration of maternal nursing correlates with substantial risk reduction independent of either parity or age at first full-term pregnancy.

International variation in incidence has provided some of the most important clues on hormonal carcinogenesis. A woman living to age 80 years in North America has one chance in nine of developing invasive breast cancer. Asian women have one-fifth to one-tenth the risk of breast cancer of women in North America or Western Europe. Asian women have substantially lower concentrations of estrogens and progesterone. These differences cannot be explained on a genetic basis because Asian women living in a Western environment have sex steroid hormone concentrations and risks identical to those of their Western counterparts. These migrant women, and more notably their daughters, also differ markedly in height and weight from Asian women in Asia; height and weight are critical regulators of age of menarche and have substantial effects on plasma concentrations of estrogens.

The role of diet in breast cancer etiology is controversial. While there are associative links between total caloric and fat intake and breast cancer risk, the exact role of fat in the diet is unproven. Increased caloric intake contributes to breast cancer risk in multiple ways: earlier menarche, later age at menopause, and increased postmenopausal estrogen concentrations reflecting enhanced aromatase activities in fatty tissues. Moderate alcohol intake also increases the risk by an unknown mechanism. Folic acid supplementation appears to modify risk in women who use alcohol but is not additionally protective in abstainers. Recommendations favoring abstinence from alcohol must be weighed against other social pressures and the possible cardioprotective effect of moderate alcohol intake. Chronic low-dose aspirin use also appears associated with a decreased incidence of breast cancer.

Understanding the potential role of exogenous hormones in breast cancer is of extraordinary importance because millions of American women regularly use oral contraceptives and postmenopausal hormone replacement therapy (HRT). The most credible meta-analyses of oral contraceptive use suggest that these agents cause a small increased risk of breast cancer. By contrast, oral contraceptives offer a substantial protective effect against ovarian epithelial tumors and endometrial cancers. HRT has a powerful effect on breast cancer risk. Data from the Women's Health Initiative (WHI) trial showed that conjugated equine estrogens plus progestins increased the risk of breast cancer and adverse cardiovascular events but with decreases in bone fractures and colorectal cancer. On balance, there were more negative events with HRT; 6 to 7 years of HRT nearly doubled the risk of breast cancer. A parallel WHI trial with >12,000 women enrolled testing conjugated estrogens alone (ERT in women who have had hysterectomies) showed no significant increase in breast cancer incidence. A meta-analysis of nonrandomized HRT studies suggests that most of the previously attributed benefit of HRT can be accounted for by higher socioeconomic status among users, which is presumably associated with better access to health care and healthier behaviors. Certain potential benefits of HRT were not assessed in WHI. HRT is an area of rapid reevaluation, but it would appear (at least from breast cancer and cardiovascular disease vantage points) that there are serious concerns about long-term HRT use. HRT in women previously diagnosed with breast cancer increases recurrence rates. A rapid decrease in the number of women on HRT has already led to a coincident decrease in breast cancer incidence.

In addition to the other factors, radiation is a risk factor in younger women. Women who have been exposed before age 30 years to radiation in the form of multiple fluoroscopies (200–300 cGy) or treatment for Hodgkin's disease (>3600 cGy) have a substantial increase in risk of breast cancer, whereas radiation exposure after age 30 years appears to have a minimal carcinogenic effect on the breast.

EVALUATION OF BREAST MASSES IN MEN AND WOMEN

Because the breasts are a common site of potentially fatal malignancy in women, examination of the breasts is an essential part of the physical examination. Unfortunately, internists frequently do not examine the breasts in men, and in women, they are apt to defer this evaluation to gynecologists. Because of the plausible association between early detection and improved outcome, it is the duty of every physician to identify breast abnormalities at the earliest possible stage and to institute a diagnostic workup. Women should be trained in breast self-examination (BSE). Although breast cancer in men is unusual, unilateral lesions should be evaluated in the same manner as in women, with the recognition that gynecomastia in men can sometimes begin unilaterally and is often asymmetric.

Virtually all breast cancer is diagnosed by biopsy of a nodule detected either on a mammogram or by palpation. Algorithms have been developed to enhance the likelihood of diagnosing breast cancer and reduce the frequency of unnecessary biopsy (Fig. 37-1).

THE PALPABLE BREAST MASS

Women should be strongly encouraged to examine their breasts monthly. A potentially flawed study from China has suggested that BSE does not alter survival, but given its safety, the procedure should still be encouraged. At worst, this practice increases the likelihood of detecting a mass at a smaller size when it can be treated with more limited surgery. Breast examination by the physician should be performed in good light so as to see retractions and other skin changes. The nipple and areolae should be inspected, and an attempt should be made to elicit nipple discharge. All regional lymph node groups should be examined, and any lesions should be measured. Physical examination alone cannot exclude malignancy. Lesions with certain features are more likely to be cancerous (hard, irregular, tethered or fixed, or painless lesions). A negative mammogram result in the presence of a persistent lump in the breast does not exclude malignancy. Palpable lesions require additional diagnostic procedures, including biopsy.

In premenopausal women, lesions that are either equivocal or nonsuspicious on physical examination should be reexamined in 2–4 weeks, during the follicular phase of the menstrual cycle. Days 5–7 of the cycle are the best time for breast examination. A dominant mass in a postmenopausal woman or a dominant mass that persists through a menstrual cycle in a premenopausal woman should be aspirated by fine-needle biopsy or referred to a surgeon. If nonbloody fluid is aspirated, the diagnosis (cyst) and therapy have been accomplished together. Solid lesions that are persistent, recurrent, complex, or bloody cysts require mammography and biopsy, although in selected patients, the so-called triple diagnostic techniques (palpation, mammography, aspiration) can be used to avoid biopsy (Figs. 37-1, 37-2, and 37-3). Ultrasound can be used in place of fine-needle aspiration (FNA) to distinguish cysts from solid lesions. Not all solid masses are detected by ultrasound; thus, a palpable mass that is not visualized on ultrasound must be presumed to be solid.

Several points are essential in pursuing these management decision trees. First, risk-factor analysis is not part of the decision structure. No constellation of risk

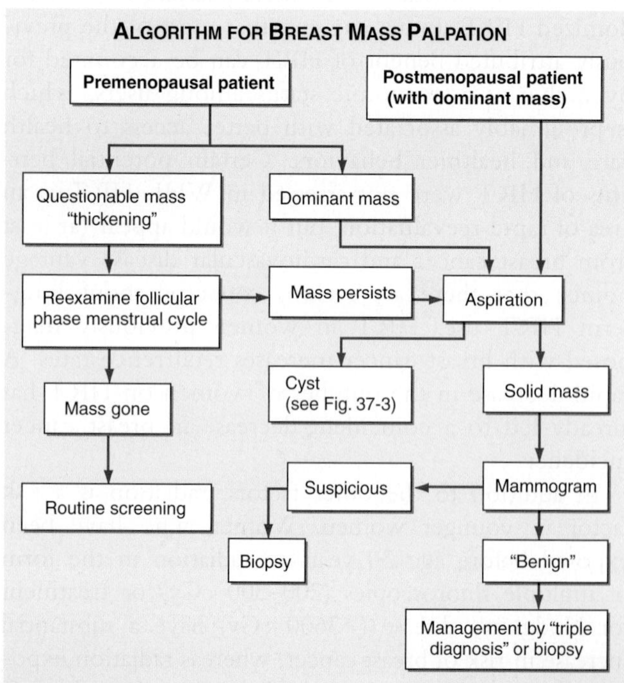

FIGURE 37-1
Approach to a palpable breast mass.

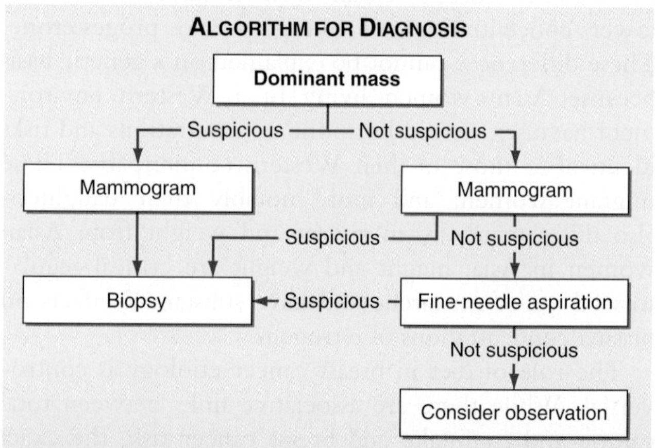

FIGURE 37-2
The "triple diagnosis" technique.

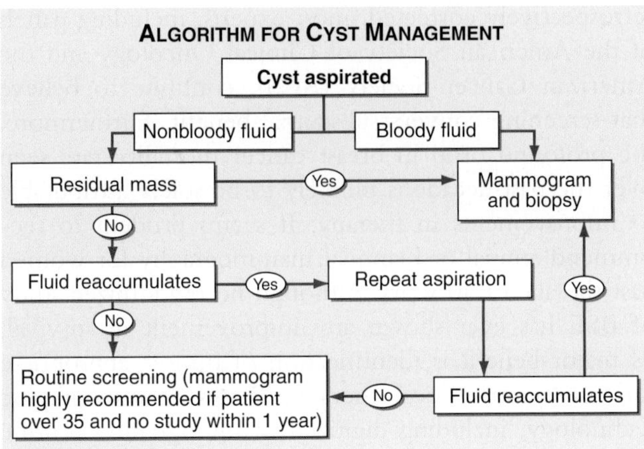

FIGURE 37-3
Management of a breast cyst.

factors, by their presence or absence, can be used to exclude biopsy. Second, FNA should be used only in centers that have proven skill in obtaining such specimens and analyzing them. The likelihood of cancer is low in the setting of a "triple negative" (benign-feeling lump, negative mammogram, and negative FNA), but it is not zero. The patient and physician must be aware of a 1% risk of false-negative results. Third, additional technologies such as magnetic resonance imaging (MRI), ultrasound, and sestamibi imaging cannot be used to exclude the need for biopsy, although in unusual circumstances, they may provoke a biopsy.

THE ABNORMAL MAMMOGRAM

Diagnostic mammography should not be confused with *screening mammography*, which is performed after a palpable abnormality has been detected. Diagnostic mammography is aimed at evaluating the rest of the breast before biopsy is performed or occasionally is part of the triple-test strategy to exclude immediate biopsy.

Subtle abnormalities that are first detected by screening mammography should be evaluated carefully by compression or magnified views. These abnormalities include clustered microcalcifications, densities (especially if spiculated), and new or enlarging architectural distortion. For some nonpalpable lesions, ultrasound may be helpful either to identify cysts or to guide biopsy. If there is no palpable lesion and detailed mammographic studies are unequivocally benign, the patient should have routine follow-up appropriate to the patient's age. It cannot be stressed too strongly that in the presence of a breast lump, a negative mammogram result does not rule out cancer.

If a nonpalpable mammographic lesion has a low index of suspicion, mammographic follow-up in 3–6 months is reasonable. Workup of indeterminate and suspicious lesions has been rendered more complex by the advent of stereotactic biopsies. Morrow and colleagues have suggested that these procedures are indicated for lesions that require biopsy but are likely to be benign—that is, for cases in which the procedure probably will eliminate additional surgery. When a lesion is more probably malignant, open biopsy should be performed with a needle localization technique. Others have proposed more widespread use of stereotactic core biopsies for nonpalpable lesions on economic grounds and because diagnosis leads to earlier treatment planning. However, stereotactic diagnosis of a malignant lesion does not eliminate the need for definitive surgical procedures, particularly if breast conservation is attempted. For example, after a breast biopsy with needle localization (i.e., local excision) of a stereotactically diagnosed malignancy, reexcision may still be necessary to achieve negative margins. To some extent, these issues are decided on the basis of referral pattern and the availability of the resources for stereotactic core biopsies. A reasonable approach is shown in Fig. 37-4.

BREAST MASSES IN A PREGNANT OR LACTATING WOMAN

During pregnancy, the breast grows under the influence of estrogen, progesterone, prolactin, and human placental lactogen. Lactation is suppressed by progesterone, which blocks the effects of prolactin. After delivery, lactation is promoted by the fall in progesterone levels, which leaves the effects of prolactin unopposed. The development of a dominant mass during pregnancy or lactation should never be attributed to hormonal changes. A dominant mass must be treated with the same concern in a pregnant woman as any other. Breast cancer develops in 1 in every 3000–4000 pregnancies. Stage for stage, breast cancer in pregnant patients is no

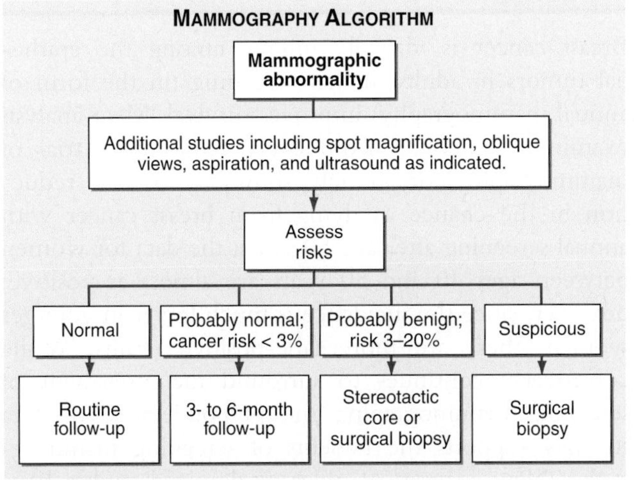

FIGURE 37-4
Approaches to abnormalities detected by mammogram.

different from premenopausal breast cancer in nonpregnant patients. However, pregnant women often have more advanced disease because the significance of a breast mass was not fully considered and/or because of endogenous hormone stimulation. Persistent lumps in the breast of pregnant or lactating women *cannot* be attributed to benign changes based on physical findings; such patients should be promptly referred for diagnostic evaluation.

BENIGN BREAST MASSES

Only about 1 in every 5–10 breast biopsies leads to a diagnosis of cancer, although the rate of positive biopsies varies in different countries and clinical settings. (These differences may be related to interpretation, medicolegal considerations, and availability of mammograms.) The vast majority of benign breast masses are due to "fibrocystic" disease, a descriptive term for small fluid-filled cysts and modest epithelial cell and fibrous tissue hyperplasia. However, fibrocystic disease is a histologic, not a clinical, diagnosis, and women who have had a biopsy with benign findings are at greater risk of developing breast cancer than those who have not had a biopsy. The subset of women with ductal or lobular cell proliferation (about 30% of patients), particularly the small fraction (3%) with atypical hyperplasia, have a fourfold greater risk of developing breast cancer than women who have not had a biopsy, and the increase in the risk is about ninefold for women in this category who also have an affected first-degree relative. Thus, careful follow-up of these patients is required. By contrast, patients with a benign biopsy without atypical hyperplasia are at little risk and may be followed routinely.

SCREENING

Breast cancer is virtually unique among the epithelial tumors in adults in that screening (in the form of annual mammography) improves survival. Meta-analysis examining outcomes from every randomized trial of mammography conclusively shows a 25–30% reduction in the chance of dying from breast cancer with annual screening after age 50 years; the data for women between ages 40 and 50 years are almost as positive; however, since the incidence is much lower in younger women, there are more false-positive results. While controversy continues to surround the assessment of screening mammography, the preponderance of data strongly supports the benefits of screening mammography. New analyses of older randomized studies have occasionally suggested that screening may not work. While the design defects in some older studies cannot be retrospectively corrected, most experts, including panels of the American Society of Clinical Oncology and the American Cancer Society (ACS), continue to believe that screening conveys substantial benefit. Furthermore, the profound drop in breast cancer mortality rate seen over the past decade is unlikely to be solely attributable to improvements in therapy. It seems prudent to recommend annual or biannual mammography for women past the age of 40 years. Although no randomized study of BSE has ever shown any improvement in survival, its major benefit is identification of tumors appropriate for conservative local therapy. Better mammographic technology, including digitized mammography, routine use of magnified views, and greater skill in mammographic interpretation, combined with newer diagnostic techniques (MRI, magnetic resonance spectroscopy, positron emission tomography, etc.) may make it possible to identify breast cancers even more reliably and earlier. Screening by any technique other than mammography is not indicated; however, the ACS recommends younger women who are *BRCA-1* or *BRCA-2* carriers or their untested first-degree relative; history of radiation therapy to the chest between ages 10 and 30 years; a lifetime risk of breast cancer of at least 20%; or a history of Li-Fraumeni, Cowden, or Bannayan-Riley-Ruvalcaba syndromes benefit from MRI screening, in which the higher sensitivity may outweigh the loss of specificity.

STAGING

Correct staging of breast cancer patients is of extraordinary importance. Not only does it permit an accurate prognosis, but in many cases therapeutic decision-making is based largely on the TNM (primary tumor, regional nodes, metastasis) classification (Table 37-1). Comparison with historic series should be undertaken with caution, as the staging has changed several times in the past 20 years. The current staging is complex and results in significant changes in outcome by stage compared with prior staging systems.

TREATMENT Breast Cancer

One of the most exciting aspects of breast cancer biology has been its recent subdivision into at least five subtypes based on gene expression profiling.

1. **Luminal A:** The luminal tumors express cytokeratins 8 and 18, have the highest levels of estrogen receptor (ER) expression, tend to be low grade, are most likely to respond to endocrine therapy, and have a favorable prognosis. They tend to be less responsive to chemotherapy.

TABLE 37-1

STAGING OF BREAST CANCER

Primary Tumor (T)	
T0	No evidence of primary tumor
TIS	Carcinoma in situ
T1	Tumor ≤2 cm
T1a	Tumor >0.1 cm but ≤0.5 cm
T1b	Tumor >0.5 but ≤1 cm
T1c	Tumor >1 cm but ≤2 cm
T2	Tumor >2 cm but ≤5 cm
T3	Tumor >5 cm
T4	Extension to chest wall, inflammation, satellite lesions, ulcerations
Regional Lymph Nodes (N)	
PN0(i−)	No regional lymph node metastasis histologically, negative IHC
PN0(i+)	No regional lymph node metastasis histologically, positive IHC, no IHC cluster greater than 0.2 mm
PN0(mol−)	No regional lymph node metastasis histologically, negative molecular findings (RT-PCR)
PN0(mol+)	No regional lymph node metastasis histologically, positive molecular findings (RT-PCR)
PN1	Metastasis in one to three axillary lymph nodes or in internal mammary nodes with microscopic disease detected by sentinel lymph node dissection but not clinically apparent
PN1mi	Micrometastasis (>0.2 mm, none >2 mm)
PN1a	Metastasis in one to three axillary lymph nodes
PN1b	Metastasis in internal mammary nodes with microscopic disease detected by sentinel lymph node dissection but not *clinically apparent*[a]
PN1c	Metastasis in one to three axillary lymph nodes and in internal mammary lymph nodes with microscopic disease detected by sentinel lymph node dissection but not clinically apparent.[a] (If associated with greater than three positive axillary lymph nodes, the internal mammary nodes are classified as pN3b to reflect increased tumor burden.)
pN2	Metastasis in four to nine axillary lymph nodes or in clinically apparent internal mammary lymph nodes in the *absence* of axillary lymph node metastasis
pN3	Metastasis in 10 or more axillary lymph nodes, or in infraclavicular lymph nodes, or in clinically apparent[a] ipsilateral internal mammary lymph nodes in the *presence* of one or more positive axillary lymph nodes; or in more than 3 axillary lymph nodes with clinically negative microscopic metastasis in internal mammary lymph nodes; or in ipsilateral subcarinal lymph nodes
Distant Metastasis (M)	
M0	No distant metastasis
M1	Distant metastasis (includes spread to ipsilateral supraclavicular nodes)

Stage Grouping			
Stage 0	TIS	N0	M0
Stage I	T1	N0	M0
Stage IIA	T0	N1	M0
	T1	N1	M0
	T2	N0	M0
Stage IIB	T2	N1	M0
	T3	N0	M0
Stage IIIA	T0	N2	M0
	T1	N2	M0
	T2	N2	M0
	T3	N1, N2	M0
Stage IIIB	T4	Any N	M0
	Any T	N3	M0
Stage IIIC	Any T	N3	M0
Stage IV	Any T	Any N	M1

[a]Clinically apparent is defined as detected by imaging studies (excluding lymphoscintigraphy) or by clinical examination.

Abbreviations: IHC, immunohistochemistry; RT-PCR, reverse transcriptase/polymerase chain reaction.

Source: Used with permission of the American Joint Committee on Cancer (AJCC), Chicago, Illinois. The original source for this material is the *AJCC Cancer Staging Manual*, 7th ed. New York: Springer, 2010; *www.springeronline.com.*

2. **Luminal B:** Tumor cells are also of luminal epithelial origin but with a gene expression pattern distinct from luminal A. Prognosis is somewhat worse that luminal A.
3. **Normal breast–like:** These tumors have a gene expression profile reminiscent of nonmalignant "normal" breast epithelium. Prognosis is similar to the luminal B group.
4. ***HER2* amplified:** These tumors have amplification of the *HER2* gene on chromosome 17q and frequently exhibit coamplification and overexpression of other genes adjacent to *HER2*. Historically, the clinical prognosis of such tumors was poor. However, with the advent of trastuzumab, the clinical outcome of *HER2*-positive patients is markedly improving.
5. **Basal:** These ER/progesterone receptor-negative and *HER2*-negative tumors (so-called triple negative) are characterized by markers of basal/myoepithelial cells. They tend to be high grade, and express cytokeratins 5/6 and 17 as well as vimentin, p63, CD10, α-smooth muscle actin, and epidermal growth factor receptor (EGF-R). Patients with *BRCA* mutations also fall within this molecular subtype. They also have stem cell characteristics.

PRIMARY BREAST CANCER Breast-conserving treatments, consisting of the removal of the primary tumor by some form of lumpectomy with or without irradiating the breast, result in a survival that is as good as (or slightly superior to) that after extensive surgical procedures, such as mastectomy or modified radical mastectomy, with or without further irradiation. Post-lumpectomy breast irradiation greatly reduces the risk of recurrence in the breast. While breast conservation is associated with a possibility of recurrence in the breast, 10-year survival is at least as good as that after more extensive surgery. Postoperative radiation to regional nodes following mastectomy is also associated with an improvement in survival. Since radiation therapy can also reduce the rate of local or regional recurrence, it should be strongly considered following mastectomy for women with high-risk primary tumors (i.e., T2 in size, positive margins, positive nodes). At present, nearly one-third of women in the United States are managed by lumpectomy. Breast-conserving surgery is not suitable for all patients: it is not generally suitable for tumors >5 cm (or for smaller tumors if the breast is small), for tumors involving the nipple areola complex, for tumors with extensive intraductal disease involving multiple quadrants of the breast, for women with a history of collagen vascular disease, and for women who either do not have the motivation for breast conservation or do not have convenient access to radiation therapy. However, these groups probably do not account for more than one-third of patients who are treated with mastectomy. Thus, a great many women still undergo mastectomy who could safely avoid this procedure and probably would if appropriately counseled.

An extensive intraductal component is a predictor of recurrence in the breast, and so are several clinical variables. Both axillary lymph node involvement and involvement of vascular or lymphatic channels by metastatic tumor in the breast are associated with a higher risk of relapse in the breast but are not contraindications to breast-conserving treatment. When these patients are excluded and when lumpectomy with negative tumor margins is achieved, breast conservation is associated with a recurrence rate in the breast of substantially <10%. The survival rate of patients who have recurrence in the breast is somewhat worse than that of women who do not. Thus, recurrence in the breast is a negative prognostic variable for long-term survival. However, recurrence in the breast is not the *cause* of distant metastasis. If recurrence in the breast caused metastatic disease, then women treated with lumpectomy, who have a higher rate of recurrence in the breast, should have poorer survival rate than women treated with mastectomy, and they do not. Most patients should consult with a radiation oncologist before making a final decision concerning local therapy. However, a multimodality clinic in which the surgeon, radiation oncologist, medical oncologist, and other caregivers cooperate to evaluate the patient and develop a treatment is usually considered a major advantage by patients.

Adjuvant Therapy The use of systemic therapy after local management of breast cancer substantially improves survival. More than half of the women who would otherwise die of metastatic breast cancer remain disease-free when treated with the appropriate systemic regimen. These data have grown more and more impressive with longer follow-up and more effective regimens.

Prognostic Variables The most important prognostic variables are provided by *tumor staging*. The size of the tumor and the status of the axillary lymph nodes provide reasonably accurate information on the likelihood of tumor relapse. The relation of pathologic stage to 5-year survival is shown in Table 37-2. For most women, the need for adjuvant therapy can be readily defined on this basis alone. In the absence of lymph node involvement, involvement of microvessels (either capillaries or lymphatic channels) in tumors is nearly equivalent to lymph node involvement. The greatest controversy concerns women with intermediate prognoses. *There is rarely justification for adjuvant chemotherapy in most women with tumors <1 cm in size whose axillary lymph nodes are negative.* HER2-*positive tumors are a potential exception.* Detection of breast cancer cells either in the circulation or bone marrow is associated with an increased relapse rate. The most exciting development in this area is the use of gene expression

TABLE 37-2

5-YEAR SURVIVAL RATE FOR BREAST CANCER BY STAGE

STAGE	5-YEAR SURVIVAL, %
0	99
I	92
IIA	82
IIB	65
IIIA	47
IIIB	44
IV	14

Source: Modified from data of the National Cancer Institute: Surveillance, Epidemiology, and End Results (SEER).

arrays to analyze patterns of tumor gene expression. Several groups have independently defined gene sets that reliably predict disease-free and overall survival far more accurately than any single prognostic variable, including the Oncotype DX analysis of 21 genes. Also, the use of such standardized risk assessment tools such as Adjuvant! Online (*www.adjuvantonline.com*) is very helpful. These tools are highly recommended in otherwise ambiguous circumstances. *Estrogen and progesterone receptor status* are of prognostic significance. Tumors that lack either or both of these receptors are more likely to recur than tumors that have them.

Several *measures of tumor growth rate* correlate with early relapse. S-phase analysis using flow cytometry is the most accurate measure. Indirect S-phase assessments using antigens associated with the cell cycle, such as PCNA (Ki67), are also valuable. Tumors with a high proportion (more than the median) of cells in S-phase pose a greater risk of relapse; chemotherapy offers the greatest survival benefit for these tumors. Assessment of DNA content in the form of ploidy is of modest value, with nondiploid tumors having a somewhat worse prognosis.

Histologic classification of the tumor has also been used as a prognostic factor. Tumors with a poor nuclear grade have a higher risk of recurrence than tumors with a good nuclear grade. Semiquantitative measures such as the Elston score improve the reproducibility of this measurement.

Molecular changes in the tumor are also useful. Tumors that overexpress *erbB2* (HER2/neu) or have a mutated p53 gene have a worse prognosis. Particular interest has centered on *erbB2* overexpression as measured by histochemistry or by fluorescence in situ hybridization. Tumors that overexpress *erbB2* are more likely to respond to higher doses of doxorubicin-containing regimens and predict those tumors that will respond to HER2/neu antibodies (trastuzumab) (herceptin) and HER2/neu kinase inhibitors.

To grow, tumors must generate a neovasculature (Chap. 25). The presence of more microvessels in a tumor, particularly when localized in so-called hot spots, is associated with a worse prognosis. This may assume even greater significance in light of blood vessel–targeting therapies such as bevacizumab (avastin). While the benefits of bevacizumab in metastatic disease have been modest, close attention should be paid to the soon-to-be reported studies evaluating its role in adjuvant therapy.

Other variables that have also been used to evaluate prognosis include proteins associated with invasiveness, such as type IV collagenase, cathepsin D, plasminogen activator, plasminogen activator receptor, and the metastasis-suppressor gene *nm23*. None of these has been widely accepted as a prognostic variable for therapeutic decision-making. One problem in interpreting these prognostic variables is that most of them have not been examined in a study using a large cohort of patients.

Adjuvant Regimens Adjuvant therapy is the use of systemic therapies in patients whose known disease has received local therapy but who are at risk of relapse. Selection of appropriate adjuvant chemotherapy or hormone therapy is highly controversial in some situations. Meta-analyses have helped to define broad limits for therapy but do not help in choosing optimal regimens or in choosing a regimen for certain subgroups of patients. A summary of recommendations is shown in Table 37-3. In general, premenopausal women for whom any form of adjuvant systemic therapy is indicated should receive multidrug chemotherapy. Antihormone therapy improves survival in premenopausal patients with positive ER and should be added following completion of chemotherapy. Prophylactic castration may also be associated with a substantial survival benefit (primarily in ER-positive patients) but is not widely used in this country.

Data on postmenopausal women are also controversial. The impact of adjuvant chemotherapy is quantitatively less clear-cut than in premenopausal patients, particularly in ER-positive cases, although survival advantages have been shown. The first decision is whether chemotherapy or endocrine therapy should be used. While adjuvant endocrine therapy (aromatase inhibitors and tamoxifen) improves survival regardless of axillary lymph node status, the improvement in survival is modest for patients in whom multiple lymph nodes are involved. For this reason, it has been usual to give chemotherapy to postmenopausal patients who have no medical contraindications and who have more than one positive lymph node; hormone therapy is commonly given subsequently. For postmenopausal women for whom systemic therapy is warranted but

TABLE 37-3

SUGGESTED APPROACHES TO ADJUVANT THERAPY

AGE GROUP	LYMPH NODE STATUS[a]	ESTROGEN RECEPTOR (ER) STATUS	TUMOR	RECOMMENDATION
Premenopausal	Positive	Any	Any	Multidrug chemotherapy + tamoxifen if ER-positive + trastuzumab in HER2/neu–positive tumors
Premenopausal	Negative	Any	>2 cm or 1–2 cm with other poor prognostic variables	Multidrug chemotherapy + tamoxifen if ER-positive + trastuzumab in HER2/neu–positive tumors
Postmenopausal	Positive	Negative	Any	Multidrug chemotherapy + trastuzumab in HER2/neu–positive tumors
Postmenopausal	Positive	Positive	Any	Aromatase inhibitors and tamoxifen with or without chemotherapy + trastuzumab in HER2/neu–positive tumors
Postmenopausal	Negative	Positive	>2 cm or 1–2 cm with other poor prognostic variables	Aromatase inhibitors and tamoxifen + trastuzumab in HER2/neu–positive tumors
Postmenopausal	Negative	Negative	>2 cm or 1–2 cm with other poor prognostic variables	Consider multidrug chemotherapy + trastuzumab in HER2/neu–positive tumors

[a]As determined by pathologic examination.

who have a more favorable prognosis (based more commonly on analysis such as the Oncotype DX methodology), hormone therapy may be used alone. Large clinical trials have shown superiority for aromatase inhibitors over tamoxifen alone in the adjuvant setting. Unfortunately, the optimal plan is unclear. Tamoxifen for 5 years followed by an aromatase inhibitor, the reverse strategy, or even switching to an aromatase inhibitor after 2–3 years of tamoxifen has been shown to be better than tamoxifen alone. No valid information currently permits selection among the three clinically approved aromatase inhibitors. Large clinical trials currently underway will help address these questions. Concomitant use of bisphosphonates is almost always warranted; however, it is not finally settled as to whether their prophylactic use increases survival in addition to just decreasing recurrences in bone.

Most comparisons of adjuvant chemotherapy regimens show little difference among them, although small advantages for doxorubicin-containing regimens and "dose-sense" regimens are usually seen.

One approach—so-called neoadjuvant chemotherapy—involves the administration of adjuvant therapy before definitive surgery and radiation therapy. Because the objective response rates of patients with breast cancer to systemic therapy in this setting exceed 75%, many patients will be "down-staged" and may become candidates for breast-conserving therapy. However, overall survival has not been improved using this approach. Patients who achieve a pathologic complete remission after neoadjuvant chemotherapy not unexpectedly have a substantially improved survival. The neoadjuvant setting also provides a wonderful opportunity for the evaluation of new agents.

Other adjuvant treatments under investigation include the use of taxanes, such as paclitaxel and docetaxel, and therapy based on alternative kinetic and biologic models. In such approaches, high doses of single agents are used separately in relatively dose-intensive cycling regimens. Node-positive patients treated with doxorubicin–cyclophosphamide for four cycles followed by four cycles of a taxane have a substantial improvement in survival as compared with women receiving doxorubicin–cyclophosphamide alone, particularly in women with ER-negative tumors. In addition, administration of the same drug combinations at the same dose but at more frequent intervals (q2 weeks with cytokine support compared with the standard q3 weeks) is even more effective. Among the 25% of women whose tumors overexpress HER2/neu, addition of trastuzumab given concurrently with a taxane and then for 1 year after chemotherapy produces significant improvement in survival. Though longer follow-up will be important, this is now the standard care for most women with HER2/neu—positive breast cancers. Cardiotoxicity, immediate and long term, remains a concern, and further efforts to exploit non—anthracycline-containing regimens are being pursued. Very-high-dose therapy with stem cell transplantation in the adjuvant setting has not proved superior to standard-dose therapy and should not be routinely used.

A variety of exciting approaches are close to adoption, and the literature needs to be followed attentively. These include the use of antiangiogenics such as bevacizumab. In addition, tyrosine kinase inhibitors such as lapatinib that target the HER2 kinase are very promising. Finally, as described in the next section, a novel class of agents targeting DNA repair—the so-called poly—ADP ribose polymerase (PARP) inhibitors—is likely to have a major impact on breast cancers either caused by *BRCA-1* or *-2* mutations or sharing similar defects in DNA repair in their etiology.

SYSTEMIC THERAPY OF METASTATIC DISEASE About one-third of patients treated for apparently localized breast cancer develop metastatic disease. Although a small number of these patients enjoy long remissions when treated with combinations of systemic and local therapy, most eventually succumb to metastatic disease. The median survival time for all patients diagnosed with mestastatic breast cancer is less than 3 years. Soft tissue, bony, and visceral (lung and liver) metastases each account for approximately one-third of sites of initial relapses. However, by the time of death, most patients will have bony involvement. Recurrences can appear at any time after primary therapy. A very cruel fact about breast cancer recurrences is that at least half of all breast cancer recurrences occur >5 years after initial therapy.

Because the diagnosis of metastatic disease alters the outlook for the patient so drastically, it should rarely be made without a confirmatory biopsy. Every oncologist has seen patients with tuberculosis, gallstones, sarcoidosis, or other nonmalignant diseases misdiagnosed and treated as though they had metastatic breast cancer or even second malignancies such as multiple myeloma thought to be recurrent breast cancer. This is a catastrophic mistake and justifies biopsy for virtually every patient at the time of initial suspicion of metastatic disease.

The choice of therapy requires consideration of local therapy needs, the overall medical condition of the patient, and the hormone receptor status of the tumor, as well as clinical judgment. Because therapy of systemic disease is palliative, the potential toxicities of therapies should be balanced against the response rates. Several variables influence the response to systemic therapy. For example, the presence of estrogen and progesterone receptors is a strong indication for endocrine therapy. On the other hand, patients with short disease-free intervals, rapidly progressive visceral disease, lymphangitic pulmonary disease, or intracranial disease are unlikely to respond to endocrine therapy.

In many cases, systemic therapy can be withheld while the patient is managed with appropriate local therapy. Radiation therapy and occasionally surgery are effective at relieving the symptoms of metastatic disease, particularly when bony sites are involved. Many patients with bone-only or bone-dominant disease have a relatively indolent course. Under such circumstances, systemic chemotherapy has a modest effect, whereas radiation therapy may be effective for long periods. Other systemic treatments, such as strontium 89 and/or bisphosphonates, may provide a palliative benefit without inducing objective responses. Most patients with metastatic disease, and certainly all who have bone involvement, should receive concurrent bisphosphonates. Since the goal of therapy is to maintain well-being for as long as possible, emphasis should be placed on avoiding the most hazardous complications of metastatic disease, including pathologic fracture of the axial skeleton and spinal cord compression. New back pain in patients with cancer should be explored aggressively on an emergent basis; to wait for neurologic symptoms is a potentially catastrophic error. Metastatic involvement of endocrine organs can cause profound dysfunction, including adrenal insufficiency and hypopituitarism. Similarly, obstruction of the biliary tree or other impaired organ function may be better managed with a local therapy than with a systemic approach.

Endocrine Therapy Normal breast tissue is estrogen dependent. Both primary and metastatic breast cancer may retain this phenotype. The best means of ascertaining whether a breast cancer is hormone dependent is through analysis of estrogen and progesterone receptor levels on the tumor. Tumors that are positive for the ER and negative for the progesterone receptor have a response rate of ~30%. Tumors that have both receptors have a response rate approaching 70%. If neither receptor is present, the objective response rates are <5%. Receptor analyses provide information as to the correct ordering of endocrine therapies as opposed to chemotherapy. Because of their lack of toxicity and because some patients whose receptor analyses are reported as negative respond to endocrine therapy, an endocrine treatment should be attempted in virtually every patient with metastatic breast cancer. Potential endocrine therapies are summarized in Table 37-4. The

TABLE 37-4

ENDOCRINE THERAPIES FOR BREAST CANCER

THERAPY	COMMENTS
Castration Surgical LHRH agonists	For premenopausal women
Antiestrogens	
Tamoxifen	Useful in pre- and postmenopausal women
"Pure" antiestrogens	Responses in tamoxifen-resistant and aromatase inhibitor–resistant patients
Surgical adrenalectomy	Rarely employed second-line choice
Aromatase inhibitors	Low toxicity; now first choice for metastatic disease
High-dose progestogens	Common fourth-line choice after AIs, tamoxifen, and fulvestrant
Hypophysectomy	Rarely used
Additive androgens or estrogens	Plausible fourth-line therapies; potentially toxic

Abbreviations: AI, aromatase inhibitor; LHRH, luteinizing hormone–releasing hormone.

choice of endocrine therapy is usually determined by toxicity profile and availability. In most patients, the initial endocrine therapy should be an aromatase inhibitor rather than tamoxifen. For the subset of postmenopausal women who are ER positive but also HER2/neu positive, response rates to aromatase inhibitors are substantially higher than to tamoxifen. Newer "pure" antiestrogens that are free of agonistic effects are also effective. Cases in which tumors shrink in response to tamoxifen withdrawal (as well as withdrawal of pharmacologic doses of estrogens) have been reported. Endogenous estrogen formation may be blocked by analogues of luteinizing hormone–releasing hormone in premenopausal women. Additive endocrine therapies, including treatment with progestogens, estrogens, and androgens, may also be tried in patients who respond to initial endocrine therapy; the mechanism of action of these latter therapies is unknown. Patients who respond to one endocrine therapy have at least a 50% chance of responding to a second endocrine therapy. It is not uncommon for patients to respond to two or three sequential endocrine therapies; however, combination endocrine therapies do not appear to be superior to individual agents, and combinations of chemotherapy with endocrine therapy are not useful. The median survival time of patients with metastatic disease is approximately 2 years, and many patients, particularly older persons and those with hormone-dependent disease, may respond to endocrine therapy for 3–5 years or longer.

Chemotherapy Unlike many other epithelial malignancies, breast cancer responds to multiple chemotherapeutic agents, including anthracyclines, alkylating agents, taxanes, and antimetabolites. Multiple combinations of these agents have been found to improve response rates somewhat, but they have had little effect on duration of response or survival. The choice among multidrug combinations frequently depends on whether adjuvant chemotherapy was administered and, if so, what type. While patients treated with adjuvant regimens such as cyclophosphamide, methotrexate, and fluorouracil (CMF regimens) may subsequently respond to the same combination in the metastatic disease setting, most oncologists use drugs to which the patients have not been previously exposed. Once patients have progressed after combination drug therapy, it is most common to treat them with single agents. Given the significant toxicity of most drugs, the use of a single effective agent will minimize toxicity by sparing the patient exposure to drugs that would be of little value. No method to select the drugs most efficacious for a given patient has been demonstrated to be useful.

Most oncologists use either an anthracycline or paclitaxel following failure with the initial regimen. However, the choice has to be balanced with individual needs. One randomized study has suggested docetaxel may be superior to paclitaxel. A nanoparticle formulation of paclitaxel (Abraxane) is also effective.

The use of a humanized antibody to *erbB2* (trastuzumab [Herceptin]) combined with paclitaxel can improve response rate and survival for women whose metastatic tumors overexpress *erbB2*. The magnitude of the survival extension is modest in patients with metastatic disease. Similarly, the use of bevacizumab (avastin) has improved the response rate and response duration to paclitaxel. Objective responses in previously treated patients may also be seen with gemcitabine, vinca alkaloids, capecitabine, Navelbine, and oral etoposide and a new class of agents (epothilones).

High-Dose Chemotherapy Including Autologous Bone Marrow Transplantation Autologous bone marrow transplantation combined with high doses of single agents can produce objective responses even in heavily pretreated patients. However, such responses are rarely durable and do not alter the clinical course for most patients with advanced metastatic disease.

STAGE III BREAST CANCER Between 10 and 25% of patients present with so-called locally advanced, or stage III, breast cancer at diagnosis. Many of these cancers are technically operable, whereas others, particularly cancers with chest wall involvement, inflammatory breast cancers, or cancers with large matted axillary lymph nodes, cannot be managed with surgery initially. Although no randomized trials have proved the efficacy of neoadjuvant chemotherapy, this approach has gained widespread use. More than 90% of patients with locally advanced breast cancer show a partial or better response to multidrug chemotherapy regimens that include an anthracycline. Early administration of this treatment reduces the bulk of the disease and frequently makes the patient a suitable candidate for salvage surgery and/or radiation therapy. These patients should be managed in multimodality clinics to coordinate surgery, radiation therapy, and systemic chemotherapy. Such approaches produce long-term disease-free survival in about 30–50% of patients.

BREAST CANCER PREVENTION Women who have one breast cancer are at risk of developing a contralateral breast cancer at a rate of approximately 0.5% per year. When adjuvant tamoxifen is administered to these patients, the rate of development of contralateral breast cancers is reduced. In other tissues of the body, tamoxifen has estrogen-like effects that are beneficial: preservation of bone mineral density and long-term lowering of cholesterol. However, tamoxifen has estrogen-like effects on the uterus, leading to an increased risk of uterine cancer (0.75% incidence after 5 years on tamoxifen). Tamoxifen also increases the risk of cataract formation. The Breast Cancer Prevention Trial (BCPT) revealed a >49% reduction in breast cancer among women with a risk of at least 1.66% taking the drug for 5 years. Raloxifene has shown similar breast cancer prevention potency but may have different effects on bone and heart. The two agents have been compared in a prospective randomized prevention trial (the Study of Tamoxifen and Raloxifene [STAR] trial). The agents are approximately equivalent in preventing breast cancer with fewer thromboembolic events and endometrial cancers with raloxifene; however, raloxifene did not reduce noninvasive cancers as effectively as tamoxifen, so no clear winner has emerged. A newer selective estrogen receptor modulator (SERM), lasofoxifene, has recently been shown to reduce cardiovascular events in addition to breast cancer and fractures, and further studies of this agent should be watched with interest. It should be recalled that prevention of contralateral breast cancers in women diagnosed with *onc* cancer is a reasonable surrogate for breast cancer prevention as these are second primaries not recurrences. In this regard, the aromatase inhibitors are all considerably more effective than tamoxifen; however, they are not approved for primary breast cancer prevention. It remains puzzling that agents with the safety profile of raloxifene, which can reduce breast cancer risk by 50% with additional benefits in preventing osteoporotic fracture, are still so infrequently prescribed.

NONINVASIVE BREAST CANCER Breast cancer develops as a series of molecular changes in the epithelial cells that lead to ever more malignant behavior. Increased use of mammography has led to more frequent diagnoses of noninvasive breast cancer. These lesions fall into two groups: ductal carcinoma in situ (DCIS) and lobular carcinoma in situ (lobular neoplasia). The management of both entities is controversial.

Ductal Carcinoma In Situ Proliferation of cytologically malignant breast epithelial cells within the ducts is termed *DCIS*. Atypical hyperplasia may be difficult to differentiate from DCIS. At least one-third of patients with untreated DCIS develop invasive breast cancer within 5 years. For many years, the standard treatment for this disease was mastectomy. However, treatment of this condition by lumpectomy and radiation therapy gives survival that is as good as the survival for invasive breast cancer treated by mastectomy. In one randomized trial, the combination of wide excision plus irradiation for DCIS caused a substantial reduction in the local recurrence rate compared with wide excision alone with negative margins, though survival was identical in the two arms. No studies have compared either of these regimens with mastectomy. Addition of tamoxifen to any DCIS surgical/radiation therapy regimen further improves local control. Data for aromatase inhibitors in this setting are not available.

Several prognostic features may help to identify patients at high risk for local recurrence after either lumpectomy alone or lumpectomy with radiation therapy. These include extensive disease; age <40 years; and cytologic features such as necrosis, poor nuclear grade, and comedo subtype with overexpression of *erbB2*. Some data suggest that adequate excision with careful determination of pathologically clear margins is associated with a low recurrence rate. When surgery is combined with radiation therapy, recurrence (which is usually in the same quadrant) occurs with a frequency of ≤10%. Given the fact that half of these recurrences will be invasive, about 5% of the initial cohort will eventually develop invasive breast cancer. A reasonable expectation of mortality for these patients is about 1%, a figure that approximates the mortality rate for DCIS managed by mastectomy. Although this train of reasoning has not formally been proved valid, it is reasonable to recommend that patients who desire breast preservation, and in whom DCIS appears to be reasonably localized, be managed by adequate surgery with meticulous pathologic evaluation, followed by breast irradiation and tamoxifen. For patients with localized DCIS, axillary lymph node dissection is unnecessary.

More controversial is the question of what management is optimal when there is any degree of invasion. Because of a significant likelihood (10–15%) of axillary lymph node involvement even when the primary lesion shows only microscopic invasion, it is prudent to do at least a level 1 and 2 axillary lymph node dissection for all patients with any degree of invasion, or sentinel node biopsy may be substituted. Further management is dictated by the presence of nodal spread.

Lobular Neoplasia Proliferation of cytologically malignant cells within the lobules is termed *lobular neoplasia.* Nearly 30% of patients who have had adequate local excision of the lesion develop breast cancer (usually infiltrating ductal carcinoma) over the next 15–20 years. Ipsilateral and contralateral cancers are equally common. Therefore, lobular neoplasia may be a premalignant lesion that suggests an elevated risk of subsequent breast cancer rather than a form of malignancy itself, and aggressive local management seems unreasonable. Most patients should be treated with an SERM for 5 years and followed with careful annual mammography and semiannual physical examinations. Additional molecular analysis of these lesions may make it possible to discriminate between patients who are at risk of further progression and require additional therapy and those in whom simple follow-up is adequate.

MALE BREAST CANCER Breast cancer is about 1/150th as frequent in men as in women; 1720 men developed breast cancer in 2006. It usually presents as a unilateral lump in the breast and is frequently not diagnosed promptly. Given the small amount of soft tissue and the unexpected nature of the problem, locally advanced presentations are somewhat more common. When male breast cancer is matched to female breast cancer by age and stage, its overall prognosis is identical. Although gynecomastia may initially be unilateral or asymmetric, any unilateral mass in a man older than age 40 years should receive a careful workup, including biopsy. On the other hand, bilateral symmetric breast development rarely represents breast cancer and is almost invariably due to endocrine disease or a drug effect. It should be kept in mind, nevertheless, that the risk of cancer is much greater in men with gynecomastia; in such men, gross asymmetry of the breasts should arouse suspicion of cancer. Male breast cancer is best managed by mastectomy and axillary lymph node dissection (modified radical mastectomy). Patients with locally advanced disease or positive nodes should also be treated with irradiation. Approximately 90% of male breast cancers contain ERs, and approximately 60% of cases with metastatic disease respond to endocrine therapy. No randomized studies have evaluated adjuvant therapy for male breast cancer. Two historic experiences suggest that the disease responds well to adjuvant systemic therapy, and, if not medically contraindicated, the same criteria for the use of adjuvant therapy in women should be applied to men.

The sites of relapse and spectrum of response to chemotherapeutic drugs are virtually identical for breast cancers in either sex.

TABLE 37-5

BREAST CANCER SURVEILLANCE GUIDELINES

TEST	FREQUENCY
Recommended	
History; eliciting symptoms; physical examination	q3–6 months × 3 years; q6–12 months × 2 years; then annually
Breast self-examination	Monthly
Mammography	Annually
Pelvic examination	Annually
Patient education about symptoms of recurrence	Ongoing
Coordination of care	Ongoing
Not Recommended	
Complete blood count	
Serum chemistry studies	
Chest radiographs	
Bone scans	
Ultrasound examination of the liver	
Computed tomography of chest, abdomen, or pelvis	
Tumor marker CA 15-3, CA 27-29	
Tumor marker CEA	

Source: Recommended Breast Cancer Surveillance Guidelines, ASCO Education Book, Fall, 1997.

Follow-Up of Breast Cancer Patients Despite the availability of sophisticated and expensive imaging techniques and a wide range of serum tumor marker tests, survival is not influenced by early diagnosis of relapse. Surveillance guidelines are given in Table 37-5. Despite pressure from patients and their families, routine computed tomography and so on are not recommended.

CHAPTER 38

GASTROINTESTINAL TRACT CANCER

Robert J. Mayer

The gastrointestinal tract is the second most common noncutaneous site for cancer and the second major cause of cancer-related mortality in the United States.

ESOPHAGEAL CANCER

INCIDENCE AND ETIOLOGY

Cancer of the esophagus is a relatively uncommon but extremely lethal malignancy. The diagnosis was made in 16,640 Americans in 2010 and led to 14,500 deaths. Worldwide, the incidence of esophageal cancer varies strikingly. It occurs frequently within a geographic region extending from the southern shore of the Caspian Sea on the west to northern China on the east and encompassing parts of Iran, Central Asia, Afghanistan, Siberia, and Mongolia. Familial increased risk has been seen in regions with high incidence, though gene associations are not yet defined. High-incidence "pockets" of the disease are also present in such disparate locations as Finland, Iceland, Curaçao, southeastern Africa, and northwestern France. In North America and western Europe, the disease is more common in blacks than whites and in males than females; it appears most often after age 50 years and seems to be associated with a lower socioeconomic status.

A variety of causative factors have been implicated in the development of the disease (Table 38-1). In the United States, esophageal cancer cases are either squamous cell carcinomas or adenocarcinomas. The etiology of squamous cell esophageal cancer is related to excess alcohol consumption and/or cigarette smoking. The relative risk increases with the amount of tobacco smoked or alcohol consumed, with these factors acting synergistically. The consumption of whiskey is linked to a higher incidence than the consumption of wine or beer. Squamous cell esophageal carcinoma has also been associated with the ingestion of nitrites, smoked opiates, and fungal toxins in pickled vegetables, as well as mucosal damage caused by such physical insults as long-term exposure to extremely hot tea, the ingestion of lye, radiation-induced strictures, and chronic achalasia. The presence of an esophageal web in association with glossitis and iron deficiency (i.e., Plummer-Vinson or Paterson-Kelly syndrome) and congenital hyperkeratosis and pitting of the palms and soles (i.e., tylosis palmaris et plantaris) have each been linked with squamous cell esophageal cancer, as have dietary deficiencies of molybdenum, zinc, selenium, and vitamin A. Bisphosphonates may increase the risk in patients with Barrett's esophagus. Patients with head and neck cancer are at increased risk of squamous cell cancer of the esophagus.

TABLE 38-1

SOME ETIOLOGIC FACTORS BELIEVED TO BE ASSOCIATED WITH ESOPHAGEAL CANCER
Excess alcohol consumption
Cigarette smoking
Other ingested carcinogens
Nitrates (converted to nitrites)
Smoked opiates
Fungal toxins in pickled vegetables
Mucosal damage from physical agents
Hot tea
Lye ingestion
Radiation-induced strictures
Chronic achalasia
Host susceptibility
Esophageal web with glossitis and iron deficiency (i.e., Plummer-Vinson or Paterson-Kelly syndrome)
Congenital hyperkeratosis and pitting of the palms and soles (i.e., tylosis palmaris et plantaris)
? Dietary deficiencies of selenium, molybdenum, zinc, and vitamin A
? Celiac sprue
Chronic gastric reflux (i.e., Barrett's esophagus) for adenocarcinoma

For unclear reasons, the incidence of squamous cell esophageal cancer has decreased somewhat in both the black and white populations in the United States over the past 30 years, while the rate of adenocarcinoma has risen dramatically, particularly in white males (M:F ratio, 6:1). Adenocarcinomas arise in the distal esophagus in the presence of chronic gastric reflux and gastric metaplasia of the epithelium (Barrett's esophagus), which is more common in obese persons. Adenocarcinomas arise within dysplastic columnar epithelium in the distal esophagus. Even before frank neoplasia is detectable, aneuploidy and p53 mutations are found in the dysplastic epithelium. These adenocarcinomas behave clinically like gastric adenocarcinoma and now account for >70% of esophageal cancers.

CLINICAL FEATURES

About 10% of esophageal cancers occur in the upper third of the esophagus (cervical esophagus), 35% in the middle third, and 55% in the lower third. Squamous cell carcinomas and adenocarcinomas cannot be distinguished radiographically or endoscopically.

Progressive dysphagia and weight loss of short duration are the initial symptoms in the vast majority of patients. Dysphagia initially occurs with solid foods and gradually progresses to include semisolids and liquids. By the time these symptoms develop, the disease is usually incurable, since difficulty in swallowing does not occur until >60% of the esophageal circumference is infiltrated with cancer. Dysphagia may be associated with pain on swallowing (odynophagia), pain radiating to the chest and/or back, regurgitation or vomiting, and aspiration pneumonia. The disease most commonly spreads to adjacent and supraclavicular lymph nodes, liver, lungs, pleura, and bone. Tracheoesophageal fistulas may develop as the disease advances, leading to severe suffering. As with other squamous cell carcinomas, hypercalcemia may occur in the absence of osseous metastases, probably from parathormone-related peptide secreted by tumor cells (Chap. 52).

DIAGNOSIS

Attempts at endoscopic and cytologic screening for carcinoma in patients with Barrett's esophagus, while effective as a means of detecting high-grade dysplasia, have not yet been shown to improve the prognosis in individuals found to have a carcinoma. Routine contrast radiographs effectively identify esophageal lesions large enough to cause symptoms. In contrast to benign esophageal leiomyomas, which result in esophageal narrowing with preservation of a normal mucosal pattern, esophageal carcinomas show ragged, ulcerating changes in the mucosa in association with deeper infiltration, producing a picture resembling achalasia. Smaller, potentially resectable tumors are often poorly visualized despite technically adequate esophagograms. Because of this, esophagoscopy should be performed in all patients suspected of having an esophageal abnormality to visualize the tumor and to obtain histopathologic confirmation of the diagnosis. Because the population of persons at risk for squamous cell carcinoma of the esophagus (i.e., smokers and drinkers) also has a high rate of cancers of the lung and the head and neck region, endoscopic inspection of the larynx, trachea, and bronchi should also be done. A thorough examination of the fundus of the stomach (by retroflexing the endoscope) is imperative as well. Endoscopic biopsies of esophageal tumors fail to recover malignant tissue in one-third of cases because the biopsy forceps cannot penetrate deeply enough through normal mucosa pushed in front of the carcinoma. Taking multiple biopsies increases the yield. Cytologic examination of tumor brushings complements standard biopsies and should be performed routinely. The extent of tumor spread to the mediastinum and para-aortic lymph nodes should be assessed by computed tomography (CT) scans of the chest and abdomen and by endoscopic ultrasound. Positron emission tomography scanning provides a useful assessment of resectability, offering accurate information regarding spread to mediastinal lymph nodes. Most patients have advanced disease at presentation.

TREATMENT Esophageal Cancer

The prognosis for patients with esophageal carcinoma is poor. Fewer than 5% of patients survive 5 years after the diagnosis; thus, management focuses on symptom control. Surgical resection of all gross tumor (i.e., total resection) is feasible in only 45% of cases, with residual tumor cells frequently present at the resection margins. Such esophagectomies have been associated with a postoperative mortality rate of approximately 5% due to anastomotic fistulas, subphrenic abscesses, and respiratory complications. About 20% of patients who survive a total resection live 5 years. The efficacy of primary radiation therapy (5500–6000 cGy) for squamous cell carcinomas is similar to that of radical surgery, sparing patients perioperative morbidity but often resulting in less satisfactory palliation of obstructive symptoms. The evaluation of chemotherapeutic agents in patients with esophageal carcinoma has been hampered by ambiguity in the definition of "response" and the debilitated physical condition of many treated individuals. Nonetheless, significant reductions in the size of measurable tumor masses have been reported in 15–25% of patients given single-agent treatment and in 30–60% of patients treated with drug combinations that include cisplatin. Combination chemotherapy and radiation therapy as the initial therapeutic approach, either alone or followed by an attempt at operative resection, seems to be beneficial. When administered along with radiation therapy, chemotherapy produces a better survival outcome than radiation therapy alone. The use of preoperative chemotherapy and radiation therapy followed by esophageal resection appears to prolong survival compared with control participants in small, randomized trials, and some reports suggest that no additional benefit accrues when surgery is added if significant shrinkage of tumor has been achieved by the chemoradiation combination.

For an incurable, surgically unresectable patient with esophageal cancer, dysphagia, malnutrition, and the management of tracheoesophageal fistulas are major issues. Approaches to palliation include repeated endoscopic dilatation, the surgical placement of a gastrostomy or jejunostomy for hydration and feeding, and endoscopic placement of an expansive metal stent to bypass the tumor. Endoscopic fulguration of the obstructing tumor with lasers is the most promising of these techniques.

TUMORS OF THE STOMACH

GASTRIC ADENOCARCINOMA

Incidence and epidemiology

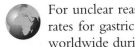

For unclear reasons, the incidence and mortality rates for gastric cancer have decreased markedly worldwide during the past 75 years. The mortality rate from gastric cancer in the United States has dropped in men from 28 to 5.8 per 100,000 persons, while in women, the rate has decreased from 27 to 2.8 per 100,000. Nonetheless, 21,000 new cases of stomach cancer were diagnosed in the United States and 10,570 Americans died of the disease in 2010. Gastric cancer incidence has decreased worldwide but remains high in Japan, China, Chile, and Ireland.

The risk of gastric cancer is greater among lower socioeconomic classes. Migrants from high- to low-incidence nations maintain their susceptibility to gastric cancer, while the risk for their offspring approximates that of the new homeland. These findings suggest that an environmental exposure, probably beginning early in life, is related to the development of gastric cancer, with dietary carcinogens considered the most likely factor(s).

Pathology

About 85% of stomach cancers are adenocarcinomas, with 15% due to lymphomas and gastrointestinal stromal tumors (GISTs) and leiomyosarcomas. Gastric adenocarcinomas may be subdivided into two categories: a *diffuse type*, in which cell cohesion is absent, so that individual cells infiltrate and thicken the stomach wall without forming a discrete mass, and an *intestinal type*, characterized by cohesive neoplastic cells that form glandlike tubular structures. The diffuse carcinomas occur more often in younger patients, develop throughout the stomach (including the cardia), result in a loss of distensibility of the gastric wall (so-called linitis plastica, or "leather bottle" appearance), and carry a poorer prognosis. Diffuse cancers have defective intercellular adhesion, mainly as a consequence of loss of expression of E-cadherin. Intestinal-type lesions are frequently ulcerative; more commonly appear in the antrum and lesser curvature of the stomach; and are often preceded by a prolonged precancerous process, often initiated by *Helicobacter pylori* infection. While the incidence of diffuse carcinomas is similar in most populations, the intestinal type tends to predominate in the high-risk geographic regions and is less likely to be found in areas where the frequency of gastric cancer is declining. Thus, different etiologic factor(s) are likely involved in these two subtypes. In the United States, ~30% of gastric cancers originate in the distal stomach, ~20% arise in the midportion of the stomach, and ~37% originate in the proximal third of the stomach. The remaining 13% involve the entire stomach.

Etiology

The long-term ingestion of high concentrations of nitrates in dried, smoked, and salted foods appears to be associated with a higher risk. The nitrates are thought to be converted to carcinogenic nitrites by bacteria (Table 38-2). Such bacteria may be introduced exogenously through the ingestion of partially decayed foods, which are consumed in abundance worldwide by the lower socioeconomic classes. Bacteria such as *H. pylori* may

TABLE 38-2

NITRATE-CONVERTING BACTERIA AS A FACTOR IN THE CAUSATION OF GASTRIC CARCINOMA[a]

Exogenous sources of nitrate-converting bacteria:
- Bacterially contaminated food (common in lower socioeconomic classes, who have a higher incidence of the disease; diminished by improved food preservation and refrigeration)
- ?*Helicobacter pylori* infection

Endogenous factors favoring growth of nitrate-converting bacteria in the stomach:
- Decreased gastric acidity
- Prior gastric surgery (antrectomy) (15- to 20-year latency period)
- Atrophic gastritis and/or pernicious anemia
- ? Prolonged exposure to histamine H_2-receptor antagonists

[a]Hypothesis: Dietary nitrates are converted to carcinogenic nitrites by bacteria.

also contribute to this effect by causing chronic gastritis, loss of gastric acidity, and bacterial growth in the stomach. The effect of *H. pylori* eradication on the subsequent risk for gastric cancer in high-incidence areas is under investigation. Loss of acidity may occur when acid-producing cells of the gastric antrum have been removed surgically to control benign peptic ulcer disease or when achlorhydria, atrophic gastritis, and even pernicious anemia develop in the elderly. Serial endoscopic examinations of the stomach in patients with atrophic gastritis have documented replacement of the usual gastric mucosa by intestinal-type cells. This process of intestinal metaplasia may lead to cellular atypia and eventual neoplasia. Since the declining incidence of gastric cancer in the United States primarily reflects a decline in distal, ulcerating, intestinal-type lesions, it is conceivable that better food preservation and the availability of refrigeration to all socioeconomic classes have decreased the dietary ingestion of exogenous bacteria. *H. pylori* has not been associated with the diffuse, more proximal form of gastric carcinoma.

Several additional etiologic factors have been associated with gastric carcinoma. Gastric ulcers and adenomatous polyps have occasionally been linked, but data on a cause-and-effect relationship are unconvincing. The inadequate clinical distinction between benign gastric ulcers and small ulcerating carcinomas may, in part, account for this presumed association. The presence of extreme hypertrophy of gastric rugal folds (i.e., Ménétrier's disease), giving the impression of polypoid lesions, has been associated with a striking frequency of malignant transformation; such hypertrophy, however, does not represent the presence of true adenomatous polyps. Individuals with blood group A have a higher incidence of gastric cancer than persons with blood group O; this observation may be related to differences in the mucous secretion, leading to altered mucosal protection from carcinogens. A germ-line mutation in the E-cadherin gene (*CDH1*), inherited in an autosomal dominant pattern and coding for a cell adhesion protein, has been linked to a high incidence of occult diffuse-type gastric cancers in young asymptomatic carriers. Duodenal ulcers are not associated with gastric cancer.

In keeping with the stepwise model of carcinogenesis, K-*ras* mutations appear to be early events in intestinal-type gastric cancer. C-met expression is amplified in about 1 in 5 cases and correlates with advanced stage. About half of intestinal-type tumors have mutations in tumor suppressor genes such as *TP53*, *TP73*, *APC* (adenomatous polyposis coli), *TFF* (trefoid factor family), *DCC* (deleted in colon cancer), and *FHIT* (fragile histidine triad). Cyclin E overexpression is associated with progression from dysplasia. Epigenetic changes (especially increased methylation) has been correlated with higher risk of invasive disease. Beta-catenin has been found in the nucleus of tumor cells at the leading edge of invasion.

Clinical features

Gastric cancers, when superficial and surgically curable, usually produce no symptoms. As the tumor becomes more extensive, patients may complain of an insidious upper abdominal discomfort varying in intensity from a vague, postprandial fullness to a severe, steady pain. Anorexia, often with slight nausea, is very common but is not the usual presenting complaint. Weight loss may eventually be observed, and nausea and vomiting are particularly prominent with tumors of the pylorus; dysphagia and early satiety may be the major symptoms caused by diffuse lesions originating in the cardia. There are no early physical signs. A palpable abdominal mass indicates long-standing growth and predicts regional extension.

Gastric carcinomas spread by direct extension through the gastric wall to the perigastric tissues, occasionally adhering to adjacent organs such as the pancreas, colon, or liver. The disease also spreads via lymphatics or by seeding of peritoneal surfaces. Metastases to intraabdominal and supraclavicular lymph nodes occur frequently, as do metastatic nodules to the ovary (Krukenberg's tumor), periumbilical region ("Sister Mary Joseph node"), or peritoneal cul-de-sac (Blumer's shelf palpable on rectal or vaginal examination); malignant ascites may also develop. The liver is the most common site for hematogenous spread of tumor.

The presence of iron-deficiency anemia in men and of occult blood in the stool in both sexes mandates a search for an occult gastrointestinal tract lesion. A careful assessment is of particular importance in patients with atrophic gastritis or pernicious anemia. Unusual clinical features associated with gastric adenocarcinomas include migratory thrombophlebitis, microangiopathic hemolytic anemia, diffuse seborrheic keratoses (so-called Leser-Trélat sign), and acanthosis nigricans.

Diagnosis

A double-contrast radiographic examination is the simplest diagnostic procedure for the evaluation of a patient with epigastric complaints. The use of double-contrast techniques helps to detect small lesions by improving mucosal detail. The stomach should be distended at some time during every radiographic examination, since decreased distensibility may be the only indication of a diffuse infiltrative carcinoma. Although gastric ulcers can be detected fairly early, distinguishing benign from malignant lesions radiographically is difficult. The anatomic location of an ulcer is not in itself an indication of the presence or absence of a cancer.

Gastric ulcers that appear benign by radiography present special problems. Some physicians believe that gastroscopy is not mandatory if the radiographic features are typically benign, if complete healing can be visualized by radiography within 6 weeks, and if a follow-up contrast radiograph obtained several months later shows a normal appearance. However, we recommend gastroscopic biopsy and brush cytology for all patients with a gastric ulcer in order to exclude a malignancy. Malignant gastric ulcers must be recognized before they penetrate into surrounding tissues because the rate of cure of early lesions limited to the mucosa or submucosa is >80%. Since gastric carcinomas are difficult to distinguish clinically or radiographically from gastric lymphomas, endoscopic biopsies should be made as deeply as possible due to the submucosal location of lymphoid tumors.

The staging system for gastric carcinoma is shown in Table 38-3.

TREATMENT Gastric Adenocarcinoma

Complete surgical removal of the tumor with resection of adjacent lymph nodes offers the only chance for cure. However, this is possible in less than one-third of patients. A subtotal gastrectomy is the treatment of choice for patients with distal carcinomas, while total or near-total gastrectomies are required for more proximal tumors. The inclusion of extended lymph node dissection in these procedures appears to confer an added risk for complications without enhancing survival. The prognosis following complete surgical resection depends on the degree of tumor penetration into the stomach wall and is adversely influenced by regional lymph node involvement, vascular invasion, and abnormal DNA content (i.e., aneuploidy), characteristics found in the vast majority of American patients. As a result, the probability of survival after 5 years for the 25–30% of patients able to undergo complete resection is ~20% for distal tumors and <10% for proximal tumors, with recurrences continuing for at least 8 years after surgery. In the absence of ascites or extensive hepatic or peritoneal metastases, even patients whose disease is believed to be incurable by surgery should be offered resection of the primary lesion. Reduction of tumor bulk is the best form of palliation and may enhance the probability of benefit from subsequent therapy.

Gastric adenocarcinoma is a relatively radioresistant tumor, and adequate control of the primary tumor requires doses of external-beam irradiation that exceed the tolerance of surrounding structures, such as bowel mucosa and spinal cord. As a result, the major role of radiation therapy in patients has been palliation of pain. Radiation therapy alone after a complete

TABLE 38-3
STAGING SYSTEM FOR GASTRIC CARCINOMA

STAGE	TNM	FEATURES	DATA FROM ACS: NO. OF CASES, %	DATA FROM ACS: 5-YEAR SURVIVAL, %
0	$T_{is}N0M0$	Node negative; limited to mucosa	1	90
IA	T1N0M0	Node negative; invasion of lamina propria or submucosa	7	59
IB	T2N0M0 T1N1M0	Node negative; invasion of muscularis propria	10	44
II	T1N2M0 T2N1M0 T3N0M0	Node positive; invasion beyond mucosa but within wall *or* Node negative; extension through wall	17	29
IIIA	T2N2M0 T3N1-2M0	Node positive; invasion of muscularis propria or through wall	21	15
IIIB	T4N0-1M0	Node negative; adherence to surrounding tissue	14	9
IIIC	T4N2-3M0 T3N3M0	>3 nodes positive; invasion of serosa or adjacent structures 7 or more positive nodes; penetrates wall without invading serosa or adjacent structures		
IV	T4N2M0 T1-4N0-2M1	Node positive; adherence to surrounding tissue *or* Distant metastases	30	3

Abbreviation: ACS, American Cancer Society; TNM, tumor, node, metastasis.

resection does not prolong survival. In the setting of surgically unresectable disease limited to the epigastrium, patients treated with 3500–4000 cGy did not live longer than similar patients not receiving radiotherapy; however, survival was prolonged slightly when 5-fluorouracil (5-FU) plus leucovorin was given in combination with radiation therapy (3-year survival rate of 50% vs 41% for radiation therapy alone). In this clinical setting, 5-FU may be functioning as a radiosensitizer.

The administration of combinations of cytotoxic drugs to patients with advanced gastric carcinoma has been associated with partial responses in 30–50% of cases; responders appear to benefit from treatment. Such drug combinations have generally included cisplatin combined with epirubicin or docetaxel and infusional 5-FU or with irinotecan. Despite this encouraging response rate, complete remissions are uncommon, the partial responses are transient, and the overall influence of multidrug therapy on survival has been unclear. The use of adjuvant chemotherapy alone following the complete resection of a gastric cancer has only minimally improved survival. However, combination chemotherapy administered before and after surgery (*perioperative treatment*) as well as postoperative chemotherapy combined with radiation therapy reduces the recurrence rate and prolongs survival.

PRIMARY GASTRIC LYMPHOMA

Primary lymphoma of the stomach is relatively uncommon, accounting for <15% of gastric malignancies and ~2% of all lymphomas. The stomach is, however, the most frequent extranodal site for lymphoma, and gastric lymphoma has increased in frequency during the past 30 years. The disease is difficult to distinguish clinically from gastric adenocarcinoma; both tumors are most often detected during the sixth decade of life; present with epigastric pain, early satiety, and generalized fatigue; and are usually characterized by ulcerations with a ragged, thickened mucosal pattern demonstrated by contrast radiographs. The diagnosis of lymphoma of the stomach may occasionally be made through cytologic brushings of the gastric mucosa but usually requires a biopsy at gastroscopy or laparotomy. Failure of gastroscopic biopsies to detect lymphoma in a given case should not be interpreted as being conclusive, since superficial biopsies may miss the deeper lymphoid infiltrate. The macroscopic pathology of gastric lymphoma may also mimic adenocarcinoma, consisting of either a bulky ulcerated lesion localized in the corpus or antrum or a diffuse process spreading throughout the entire gastric submucosa and even extending into the duodenum. Microscopically, the vast majority of gastric lymphoid tumors are non-Hodgkin's lymphomas of B cell origin; Hodgkin's disease involving the stomach is extremely uncommon. Histologically, these tumors may range from well-differentiated, superficial processes (mucosa-associated lymphoid tissue [MALT]) to high-grade, large-cell lymphomas. Like gastric adenocarcinoma, infection with *H. pylori* increases the risk for gastric lymphoma in general and MALT lymphomas in particular. Gastric lymphomas spread initially to regional lymph nodes (often to Waldeyer's ring) and may then disseminate. Gastric lymphomas are staged like other lymphomas (Chap. 15).

TREATMENT Primary Gastric Lymphoma

Primary gastric lymphoma is a far more treatable disease than adenocarcinoma of the stomach, a fact that underscores the need for making the correct diagnosis. Antibiotic treatment to eradicate *H. pylori* infection has led to regression of about 75% of gastric MALT lymphomas and should be considered before surgery, radiation therapy, or chemotherapy are undertaken in patients having such tumors. A lack of response to such antimicrobial treatment has been linked to a specific chromosomal abnormality, i.e., t(11;18). Responding patients should undergo periodic endoscopic surveillance because it remains unclear whether the neoplastic clone is eliminated or merely suppressed, although the response to antimicrobial treatment is quite durable. Subtotal gastrectomy, usually followed by combination chemotherapy, has led to 5-year survival rates of 40–60% in patients with localized high-grade lymphomas. The need for a major surgical procedure has been questioned, particularly in patients with preoperative radiographic evidence of nodal involvement, for whom chemotherapy (CHOP [cyclophosphamide, doxorubicin, vincristine, and prednisone]) plus rituximab is effective therapy. A role for radiation therapy is not defined because most recurrences develop at distant sites.

GASTRIC (NONLYMPHOID) SARCOMA

Leiomyosarcomas and GISTs make up 1–3% of gastric neoplasms. They most frequently involve the anterior and posterior walls of the gastric fundus and often ulcerate and bleed. Even lesions that appear benign on histologic examination may behave in a malignant fashion. These tumors rarely invade adjacent viscera and characteristically do not metastasize to lymph nodes, but they may spread to the liver and lungs. The treatment of choice is surgical resection. Combination chemotherapy should be reserved for patients with metastatic disease. All such tumors should be analyzed for a mutation in the c-*kit* receptor. GISTs are unresponsive to conventional chemotherapy, yet ~50% of patients experience objective response and prolonged survival when treated with imatinib mesylate (Gleevec) (400–800 mg PO daily), a selective inhibitor of the c-*kit* tyrosine kinase. Many patients with GIST whose tumors have become refractory to imatinib subsequently benefit from sunitinib (Sutent), another inhibitor of the c-*kit* tyrosine kinase.

COLORECTAL CANCER

INCIDENCE

Cancer of the large bowel is second only to lung cancer as a cause of cancer death in the United States: 142,570 new cases occurred in 2010, and 51,370 deaths were due to colorectal cancer. The incidence rate has decreased significantly during the past 20 years, likely due to enhanced and more compliantly followed screening practices. Similarly, mortality rates in the United States have decreased by approximately 25%, resulting largely from improved treatment and earlier detection.

POLYPS AND MOLECULAR PATHOGENESIS

Most colorectal cancers, regardless of etiology, arise from adenomatous polyps. A polyp is a grossly visible protrusion from the mucosal surface and may be classified pathologically as a nonneoplastic hamartoma (*juvenile polyp*), a hyperplastic mucosal proliferation (*hyperplastic polyp*), or an adenomatous polyp. Only adenomas are clearly premalignant, and only a minority of such lesions becomes cancer. Adenomatous polyps may be found in the colons of ~30% of middle-aged and ~50% of elderly people; however, <1% of polyps ever become malignant. Most polyps produce no symptoms and remain clinically undetected. Occult blood in the stool is found in <5% of patients with polyps.

A number of molecular changes are noted in adenomatous polyps, dysplastic lesions, and polyps containing microscopic foci of tumor cells (carcinoma in situ), which are thought to reflect a multistep process in the evolution of normal colonic mucosa to life-threatening invasive carcinoma. These developmental steps toward carcinogenesis include, but are not restricted to, point mutations in the K-*ras* protooncogene; hypomethylation of DNA, leading to gene activation; loss of DNA (*allelic loss*) at the site of a tumor-suppressor gene (the adenomatous polyposis coli [*APC*] gene) on the long arm of chromosome 5 (5q21); allelic loss at the site of a tumor-suppressor gene located on chromosome 18q (the deleted in colorectal cancer [*DCC*] gene); and allelic loss at chromosome 17p, associated with mutations in the p53 tumor-suppressor gene (see Fig. 24-2). Thus, the altered proliferative pattern of the colonic mucosa, which results in progression to a polyp and then to carcinoma, may involve the mutational activation of an oncogene followed by and coupled with the loss of genes that normally suppress tumorigenesis. It remains uncertain whether the genetic aberrations always occur in a defined order. Based on this model, however, cancer is believed to develop only in those polyps in which most (if not all) of these mutational events take place.

Clinically, the probability of an adenomatous polyp becoming a cancer depends on the gross appearance of the lesion, its histologic features, and its size. Adenomatous polyps may be pedunculated (stalked) or sessile (flat-based). Cancers develop more frequently in sessile polyps. Histologically, adenomatous polyps may be tubular, villous (i.e., papillary), or tubulovillous. Villous adenomas, most of which are sessile, become malignant more than three times as often as tubular adenomas. The likelihood that any polypoid lesion in the large bowel contains invasive cancer is related to the size of the polyp, being negligible (<2%) in lesions <1.5 cm, intermediate (2–10%) in lesions 1.5–2.5 cm, and substantial (10%) in lesions >2.5 cm in size.

Following the detection of an adenomatous polyp, the entire large bowel should be visualized endoscopically or radiographically, since synchronous lesions are noted in about one-third of cases. Colonoscopy should then be repeated periodically, even in the absence of a previously documented malignancy, since such patients have a 30–50% probability of developing another adenoma and are at a higher-than-average risk for developing a colorectal carcinoma. Adenomatous polyps are thought to require >5 years of growth before becoming clinically significant; colonoscopy need not be carried out more frequently than every 3 years.

ETIOLOGY AND RISK FACTORS

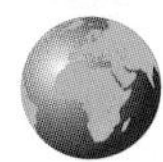

Risk factors for the development of colorectal cancer are listed in Table 38-4.

Diet

The etiology for most cases of large-bowel cancer appears to be related to environmental factors. The disease occurs more often in upper socioeconomic populations who live in urban areas. Mortality from colorectal cancer is directly correlated with per capita consumption of calories, meat protein, and dietary fat and oil as well as elevations in the serum cholesterol concentration and mortality from coronary artery disease. Geographic variations in incidence are unrelated to genetic differences, since migrant groups tend to assume the large-bowel cancer incidence rates of their adopted countries. Furthermore, population groups such as Mormons and Seventh Day Adventists, whose lifestyle and dietary

TABLE 38-4

RISK FACTORS FOR THE DEVELOPMENT OF COLORECTAL CANCER

Diet: Animal fat
Hereditary syndromes (autosomal dominant inheritance)
  Polyposis coli
  Nonpolyposis syndrome (Lynch syndrome)
Inflammatory bowel disease
Streptococcus bovis bacteremia
Ureterosigmoidostomy
? Tobacco use

habits differ somewhat from those of their neighbors, have significantly lower-than-expected incidence and mortality rates for colorectal cancer. Colorectal cancer has increased in Japan since that nation has adopted a more "Western" diet. At least three hypotheses have been proposed to explain the relationship to diet, none of which is fully satisfactory.

Animal fats

One hypothesis is that the ingestion of animal fats found in red meats and processed meat leads to an increased proportion of anaerobes in the gut microflora, resulting in the conversion of normal bile acids into carcinogens. This provocative hypothesis is supported by several reports of increased amounts of fecal anaerobes in the stools of patients with colorectal cancer. Diets high in animal (but not vegetable) fats are also associated with high serum cholesterol, which is also associated with enhanced risk for the development of colorectal adenomas and carcinomas.

Insulin resistance

The large number of calories in Western diets coupled with physical inactivity has been associated with a higher prevalence of obesity. Obese persons develop insulin resistance with increased circulating levels of insulin, leading to higher circulating concentrations of insulin-like growth factor type I (IGF-I). This growth factor appears to stimulate proliferation of the intestinal mucosa.

Fiber

Contrary to prior beliefs, the results of randomized trials and case-controlled studies have failed to show any value for dietary fiber or diets high in fruits and vegetables in preventing the recurrence of colorectal adenomas or the development of colorectal cancer. The weight of epidemiologic evidence, however, implicates diet as being the major etiologic factor for colorectal cancer, particularly diets high in animal fat and in calories.

HEREDITARY FACTORS AND SYNDROMES

Up to 25% of patients with colorectal cancer have a family history of the disease, suggesting a hereditary predisposition. Inherited large-bowel cancers can be divided into two main groups: the well-studied but uncommon polyposis syndromes and the more common nonpolyposis syndromes (Table 38-5).

Polyposis coli

Polyposis coli (familial polyposis of the colon) is a rare condition characterized by the appearance of thousands

TABLE 38-5

HEREDITABLE (AUTOSOMAL DOMINANT) GASTROINTESTINAL POLYPOSIS SYNDROMES

SYNDROME	DISTRIBUTION OF POLYPS	HISTOLOGIC TYPE	MALIGNANT POTENTIAL	ASSOCIATED LESIONS
Familial adenomatous polyposis	Large intestine	Adenoma	Common	None
Gardner's syndrome	Large and small intestines	Adenoma	Common	Osteomas, fibromas, lipomas, epidermoid cysts, ampullary cancers, congenital hypertrophy of retinal pigment epithelium
Turcot's syndrome	Large intestine	Adenoma	Common	Brain tumors
Nonpolyposis syndrome (Lynch syndrome)	Large intestine (often proximal)	Adenoma	Common	Endometrial and ovarian tumors
Peutz-Jeghers syndrome	Small and large intestines, stomach	Hamartoma	Rare	Mucocutaneous pigmentation; tumors of the ovary, breast, pancreas, endometrium
Juvenile polyposis	Large and small intestines, stomach	Hamartoma, rarely progressing to adenoma	Rare	Various congenital abnormalities

of adenomatous polyps throughout the large bowel. It is transmitted as an autosomal dominant trait; the occasional patient with no family history probably developed the condition due to a spontaneous mutation. Polyposis coli is associated with a deletion in the long arm of chromosome 5 (including the *APC* [adenomatous polyposis coli] gene) in both neoplastic (somatic mutation) and normal (germ-line mutation) cells. The loss of this genetic material (i.e., allelic loss) results in the absence of tumor-suppressor genes whose protein products would normally inhibit neoplastic growth. The presence of soft tissue and bony tumors, congenital hypertrophy of the retinal pigment epithelium, mesenteric desmoid tumors, and ampullary cancers in addition to the colonic polyps characterizes a subset of polyposis coli known as *Gardner's syndrome*. The appearance of malignant tumors of the central nervous system accompanying polyposis coli defines *Turcot's syndrome*. The colonic polyps in all these conditions are rarely present before puberty but are generally evident in affected individuals by age 25 years. If the polyposis is not treated surgically, colorectal cancer will develop in almost all patients before age 40 years. Polyposis coli results from a defect in the colonic mucosa, leading to an abnormal proliferative pattern and impaired DNA repair mechanisms. Once the multiple polyps are detected, patients should undergo a total colectomy. Medical therapy with nonsteroidal anti-inflammatory drugs (NSAIDs) such as sulindac and cyclooxygenase-2 inhibitors such as celecoxib can decrease the number and size of polyps in patients with polyposis coli; however, this effect on polyps is only temporary, and NSAIDs are not proven to reduce the risk of cancer. Colectomy remains the primary therapy and prevention. The offspring of patients with polyposis coli, who often are prepubertal when the diagnosis is made in the parent, have a 50% risk for developing this premalignant disorder and should be carefully screened by annual flexible sigmoidoscopy until age 35 years. Proctosigmoidoscopy is a sufficient screening procedure because polyps tend to be evenly distributed from cecum to anus, making more invasive and expensive techniques such as colonoscopy or barium enema unnecessary. Testing for occult blood in the stool is an inadequate screening maneuver. An alternative method for identifying carriers is testing DNA from peripheral blood mononuclear cells for the presence of a mutated *APC* gene. The detection of such a germ-line mutation can lead to a definitive diagnosis before the development of polyps.

Hereditary nonpolyposis colon cancer

Hereditary nonpolyposis colon cancer (HNPCC), also known as *Lynch syndrome*, is another autosomal dominant trait. It is characterized by the presence of three or more relatives with histologically documented colorectal cancer, one of whom is a first-degree relative of the other two; one or more cases of colorectal cancer diagnosed before age 50 years in the family; and colorectal cancer involving at least two generations. In contrast to polyposis coli, HNPCC is associated with an unusually high frequency of cancer arising in the proximal large bowel. The median age for the appearance of an adenocarcinoma is <50 years, 10–15 years younger than the median age for the general population. Despite having a poorly differentiated histologic appearance, the proximal colon tumors in HNPCC have a better prognosis than sporadic tumors from patients of similar age. Families with HNPCC often include individuals with multiple primary cancers; the association of colorectal cancer with either ovarian or endometrial carcinomas is especially strong in women. It has been recommended that members of such families undergo biennial colonoscopy beginning at age 25 years, with intermittent pelvic ultrasonography and endometrial biopsy for affected women; such a screening strategy has not yet been validated. HNPCC is associated with germline mutations of several genes, particularly *hMSH2* on chromosome 2 and *hMLH1* on chromosome 3. These mutations lead to errors in DNA replication and are thought to result in DNA instability because of defective repair of DNA mismatches resulting in abnormal cell growth and tumor development. Testing tumor cells through molecular analysis of DNA or immunohistochemical staining of paraffin-fixed tissue for "microsatellite instability" (sequence changes reflecting defective mismatch repair) in patients younger than age 50 years with colorectal cancer and a positive family history for colorectal or endometrial cancer may identify probands with HNPCC.

INFLAMMATORY BOWEL DISEASE

Large-bowel cancer is increased in incidence in patients with long-standing inflammatory bowel disease (IBD). Cancers develop more commonly in patients with ulcerative colitis than in those with granulomatous colitis, but this impression may result in part from the occasional difficulty of differentiating these two conditions. The risk of colorectal cancer in a patient with IBD is relatively small during the initial 10 years of the disease, but then it appears to increase at a rate of ~0.5–1% per year. Cancer may develop in 8–30% of patients after 25 years. The risk is higher in younger patients with pancolitis.

Cancer surveillance in patients with IBD is unsatisfactory. Symptoms such as bloody diarrhea, abdominal cramping, and obstruction, which may signal the appearance of a tumor, are similar to the complaints caused by a flare-up of the underlying disease. In patients with a history of IBD lasting ≥15 years who continue to experience exacerbations, the surgical removal of the colon can significantly reduce the risk for cancer and also eliminate the target organ for the underlying chronic gastrointestinal disorder. The value of such surveillance techniques as colonoscopy with mucosal biopsies and brushings for less symptomatic individuals with chronic IBD is uncertain. The lack of uniformity regarding the pathologic criteria that characterize dysplasia and the absence of data that such surveillance reduces the development of lethal cancers have made this costly practice an area of controversy.

OTHER HIGH-RISK CONDITIONS

Streptococcus bovis *bacteremia*

For unknown reasons, individuals who develop endocarditis or septicemia from this fecal bacterium have a high incidence of occult colorectal tumors and, possibly, upper gastrointestinal cancers as well. Endoscopic or radiographic screening appears advisable.

Tobacco use

Cigarette smoking is linked to the development of colorectal adenomas, particularly after >35 years of tobacco use. No biologic explanation for this association has yet been proposed.

PRIMARY PREVENTION

Several orally administered compounds have been assessed as possible inhibitors of colon cancer. The most effective class of chemopreventive agents is aspirin and other NSAIDs, which are thought to suppress cell proliferation by inhibiting prostaglandin synthesis. Regular aspirin use reduces the risk of colon adenomas and carcinomas as well as death from large-bowel cancer; such use also appears to diminish the likelihood of developing additional premalignant adenomas following treatment for a prior colon carcinoma. This effect of aspirin on colon carcinogenesis increases with the duration and dosage of drug use. Oral folic acid supplements and oral calcium supplements reduce the risk of adenomatous polyps and colorectal cancers in case-controlled studies. The value of vitamin D as a form of chemoprevention is under study. Antioxidant vitamins such as ascorbic acid, tocopherols, and β-carotene are ineffective at reducing the incidence of subsequent adenomas in patients who have undergone the removal of a colon adenoma. Estrogen replacement therapy has been associated with a reduction in the risk of colorectal cancer in women, conceivably by an effect on bile acid synthesis and composition or by decreasing synthesis of IGF-I. The otherwise unexplained reduction in colorectal cancer mortality rate in women may be a result of the widespread use of estrogen replacement in postmenopausal individuals.

SCREENING

The rationale for colorectal cancer screening programs is that earlier detection of localized, superficial cancers in asymptomatic individuals will increase the surgical cure rate. Such screening programs are important for individuals having a family history of the disease in first-degree relatives. The relative risk for developing colorectal cancer increases to 1.75 in such individuals and may be even higher if the relative was afflicted before age 60 years. The prior use of proctosigmoidoscopy as a screening tool was based on the observation that 60% of early lesions are located in the rectosigmoid. For unexplained reasons, however, the proportion of large-bowel cancers arising in the rectum has been decreasing during the past several decades, with a corresponding increase in the proportion of cancers in the more proximal descending colon. As such, the potential for rigid proctosigmoidoscopy to detect a sufficient number of occult neoplasms to make the procedure cost-effective has been questioned. Flexible, fiberoptic sigmoidoscopes permit trained operators to visualize the colon for up to 60 cm, which enhances the capability for cancer detection. However, this technique still leaves the proximal half of the large bowel unscreened.

Most programs directed at the early detection of colorectal cancers have focused on digital rectal examinations and fecal occult blood testing. The digital examination should be part of any routine physical evaluation in adults older than age 40 years, serving as a screening test for prostate cancer in men, a component of the pelvic examination in women, and an inexpensive maneuver for the detection of masses in the rectum. The development of the Hemoccult test has greatly facilitated the detection of occult fecal blood. Unfortunately, even when performed optimally, the Hemoccult test has major limitations as a screening technique. About 50% of patients with documented colorectal cancers have a negative fecal Hemoccult test result, consistent with the intermittent bleeding pattern of these tumors. When random cohorts of asymptomatic persons have been tested, 2–4% have Hemoccult-positive stools. Colorectal cancers have been found in <10% of these "test-positive" cases, with benign polyps being detected in an additional 20–30%. Thus, a colorectal neoplasm will not be found in most asymptomatic individuals with occult blood in their stool. Nonetheless, persons found to have Hemoccult-positive stool routinely undergo further medical evaluation, including sigmoidoscopy, barium enema, and/or colonoscopy—procedures that are not only uncomfortable and expensive but also associated with a small risk for significant complications. The added cost of these studies would appear justifiable if the small number of patients found to have occult neoplasms because of Hemoccult screening could be shown to have an improved prognosis and prolonged survival. Prospectively controlled trials showed a statistically significant reduction in mortality rate from colorectal cancer for individuals undergoing annual screening. However, this benefit only emerged after >13 years of follow-up and was extremely expensive to achieve, since all positive test results (most of which were false-positive) were followed by colonoscopy. Moreover, these colonoscopic examinations quite likely provided the opportunity for cancer prevention through the removal of potentially premalignant adenomatous polyps since the eventual development of cancer was reduced by 20% in the cohort undergoing annual screening.

Screening techniques for large-bowel cancer in asymptomatic persons remain unsatisfactory. Compliance with any screening strategy within the general population is poor. At present, the American Cancer Society suggests fecal Hemoccult screening annually and flexible sigmoidoscopy every 5 years beginning at age 50 years for asymptomatic individuals having no colorectal cancer risk factors. The American Cancer Society has also endorsed a "total colon examination" (i.e., colonoscopy or double-contrast barium enema) every 10 years as an alternative to Hemoccult testing with periodic flexible sigmoidoscopy. Colonoscopy has been shown to be superior to double-contrast barium enema and also to have a higher sensitivity for detecting villous or dysplastic adenomas or cancers than the strategy employing occult fecal blood testing and flexible sigmoidoscopy. Whether colonoscopy performed every 10 years beginning after age 50 years will prove to be cost-effective and whether it may be supplanted as a screening maneuver by sophisticated radiographic techniques ("virtual colonoscopy") remains unclear. More effective techniques for screening are needed, perhaps taking advantage of the molecular changes that have been described in these tumors. Analysis of fecal DNA for multiple mutations associated with colorectal cancer is being tested.

CLINICAL FEATURES

Presenting symptoms

Symptoms vary with the anatomic location of the tumor. Since stool is relatively liquid as it passes through the ileocecal valve into the right colon, cancers arising in the cecum and ascending colon may become quite large without resulting in any obstructive symptoms or noticeable alterations in bowel habits. Lesions of the right colon commonly ulcerate, leading to chronic, insidious blood loss without a change in the appearance of the stool. Consequently, patients with tumors of the ascending colon often present with symptoms such as fatigue, palpitations, and even angina pectoris and are found to have a hypochromic, microcytic anemia indicative of iron deficiency. Since the cancer may bleed intermittently, a random fecal occult blood test result may be negative. As a result, the unexplained presence of iron-deficiency anemia in any adult (with the possible exception of a premenopausal, multiparous woman) mandates a thorough endoscopic and/or radiographic visualization of the entire large bowel (Fig. 38-1).

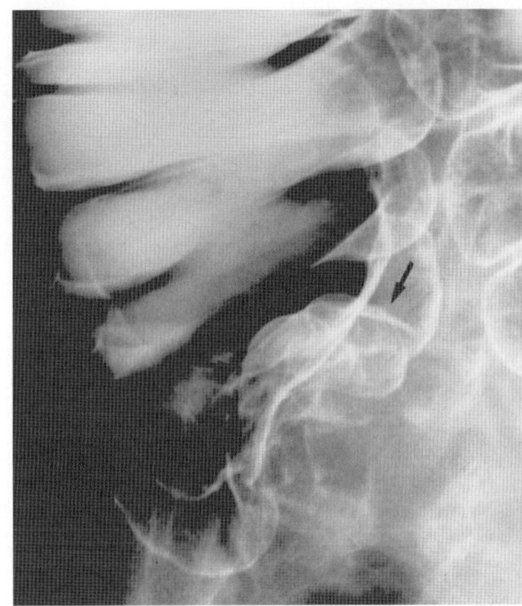

FIGURE 38-1
Double-contrast air-barium enema revealing a sessile tumor of the cecum in a patient with iron-deficiency anemia and guaiac-positive stool. The lesion at surgery was a stage II adenocarcinoma.

Since stool becomes more formed as it passes into the transverse and descending colon, tumors arising there tend to impede the passage of stool, resulting in the development of abdominal cramping, occasional obstruction, and even perforation. Radiographs of the abdomen often reveal characteristic annular, constricting lesions ("apple-core" or "napkin-ring") (Fig. 38-2).

Cancers arising in the rectosigmoid are often associated with hematochezia, tenesmus, and narrowing of the caliber of stool; anemia is an infrequent finding. While these symptoms may lead patients and their physicians to suspect the presence of hemorrhoids, the development of rectal bleeding and/or altered bowel habits demands a prompt digital rectal examination and proctosigmoidoscopy.

Staging, prognostic factors, and patterns of spread

The prognosis for individuals having colorectal cancer is related to the depth of tumor penetration into the

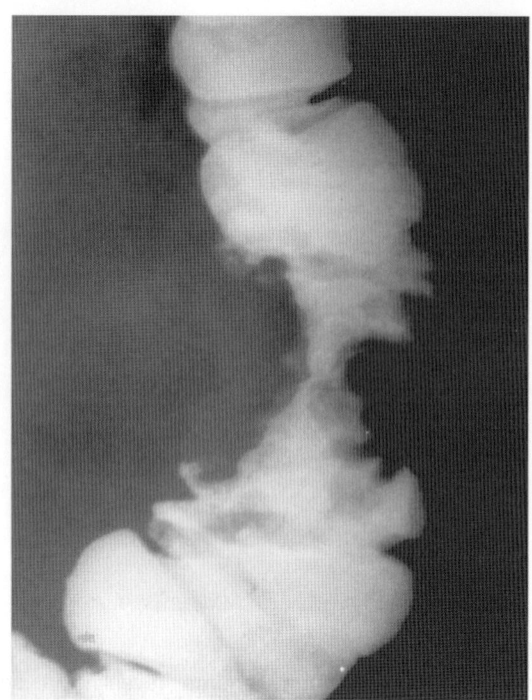

FIGURE 38-2

Annular, constricting adenocarcinoma of the descending colon. This radiographic appearance is referred to as an "apple-core" lesion and is always highly suggestive of malignancy.

bowel wall and the presence of both regional lymph node involvement and distant metastases. These variables are incorporated into the staging system introduced by Dukes and applied to a TNM classification method, in which T represents the depth of tumor penetration, N the presence of lymph node involvement, and M the presence or absence of distant metastases (Fig. 38-3). Superficial lesions that do not involve regional lymph nodes and do not penetrate through the submucosa (T1) or the muscularis (T2) are designated as *stage I* (T1–2N0M0) disease; tumors that penetrate through the muscularis but have not spread to lymph nodes are *stage II* disease (T3N0M0); regional lymph node involvement defines *stage III* (TXN_1M_0) disease; and metastatic spread to sites such as liver, lung, or bone indicates *stage IV* ($TXNXM_1$) disease. Unless gross evidence of metastatic disease is present, disease stage cannot be determined accurately before surgical resection and pathologic analysis of the operative specimens. It is not clear whether the detection of nodal metastases by special immunohistochemical molecular techniques has the same prognostic implications as disease detected by routine light microscopy.

Most recurrences after a surgical resection of a large-bowel cancer occur within the first 4 years, making 5-year survival a fairly reliable indicator of cure. The likelihood for 5-year survival in patients with colorectal cancer is stage-related (Fig. 38-3). That likelihood has improved during the past several decades when similar surgical stages have been compared. The most plausible explanation for this improvement is more thorough intraoperative and pathologic staging. In particular, more exacting attention to pathologic detail has revealed that the prognosis following the resection of a colorectal cancer is not related merely to the presence or absence of regional lymph node involvement. Prognosis may be more precisely gauged by the number of involved lymph nodes (one to three lymph nodes vs

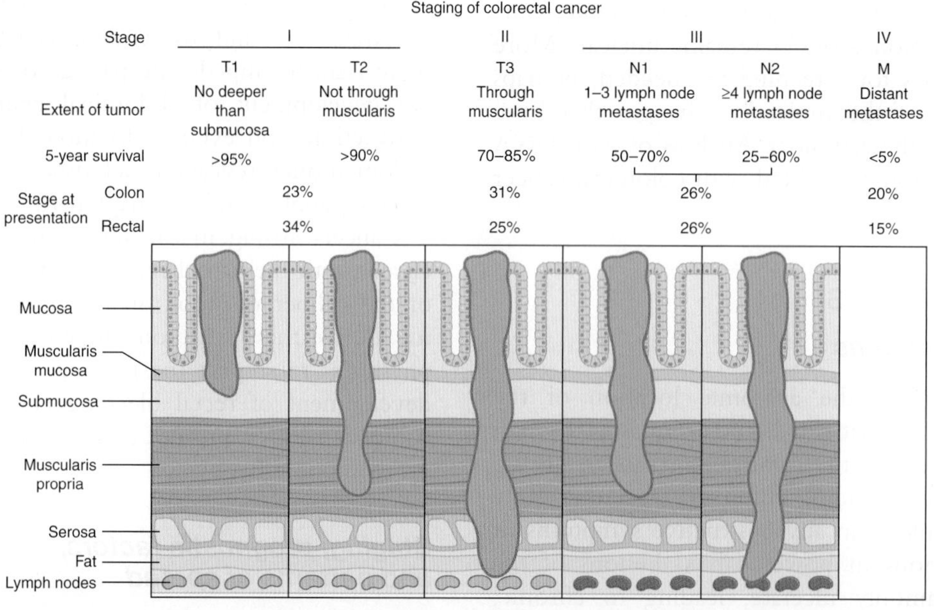

FIGURE 38-3

Staging and prognosis for patients with colorectal cancer.

TABLE 38-6

PREDICTORS OF POOR OUTCOME FOLLOWING TOTAL SURGICAL RESECTION OF COLORECTAL CANCER

Tumor spread to regional lymph nodes
Number of regional lymph nodes involved
Tumor penetration through the bowel wall
Poorly differentiated histology
Perforation
Tumor adherence to adjacent organs
Venous invasion
Preoperative elevation of CEA titer (<5 ng/mL)
Aneuploidy
Specific chromosomal deletion (e.g., allelic loss on chromosome 18q)

Abbreviation: CEA, carcinoembryonic antigen.

four or more lymph nodes) and the number of nodes examined. A minimum of 12 sampled lymph nodes is thought necessary to accurately define tumor stage, and the more nodes examined the better. Other predictors of a poor prognosis after a total surgical resection include tumor penetration through the bowel wall into pericolic fat, poorly differentiated histology, perforation and/or tumor adherence to adjacent organs (increasing the risk for an anatomically adjacent recurrence), and venous invasion by tumor (**Table 38-6**). Regardless of the clinicopathologic stage, a preoperative elevation of the plasma carcinoembryonic antigen (CEA) level predicts eventual tumor recurrence. The presence of aneuploidy and specific chromosomal deletions, such as allelic loss in chromosome 18q (involving the *DCC* gene) in tumor cells, appears to predict a higher risk for metastatic spread, particularly in patients with stage II (T3N0M0) disease. Conversely, the detection of microsatellite instability in tumor tissue indicates a more favorable outcome. In contrast to most other cancers, the prognosis in colorectal cancer is not influenced by the size of the primary lesion when adjusted for nodal involvement and histologic differentiation.

Cancers of the large bowel generally spread to regional lymph nodes or to the liver via the portal venous circulation. The liver represents the most frequent visceral site of metastasis; it is the initial site of distant spread in one-third of recurring colorectal cancers and is involved in more than two-thirds of such patients at the time of death. In general, colorectal cancer rarely spreads to the lungs, supraclavicular lymph nodes, bone, or brain without prior spread to the liver. A major exception to this rule occurs in patients having primary tumors in the distal rectum, from which tumor cells may spread through the paravertebral venous plexus, escaping the portal venous system and thereby reaching the lungs or supraclavicular lymph nodes without hepatic involvement. The median survival after the detection of distant metastases has ranged in the past from 6–9 months (hepatomegaly, abnormal liver chemistries) to 24–30 months (small liver nodule initially identified by elevated CEA level and subsequent CT scan), but effective systemic therapy is improving the prognosis.

Efforts to use gene expression profiles to identify patients at risk of recurrence or those particularly likely to benefit from adjuvant therapy have not yet yielded practice-changing results. Despite a burgeoning literature examining a host of prognostic factors, pathologic stage at diagnosis is the best predictor of long-term prognosis. Patients with lymphovascular invasion and high preoperative CEA levels are likely to have a more aggressive clinical course.

TREATMENT Colorectal Cancer

Total resection of tumor is the optimal treatment when a malignant lesion is detected in the large bowel. An evaluation for the presence of metastatic disease, including a thorough physical examination, chest radiograph, biochemical assessment of liver function, and measurement of the plasma CEA level, should be performed before surgery. When possible, a colonoscopy of the entire large bowel should be performed to identify synchronous neoplasms and/or polyps. The detection of metastases should not preclude surgery in patients with tumor-related symptoms such as gastrointestinal bleeding or obstruction, but it often prompts the use of a less radical operative procedure. At the time of laparotomy, the entire peritoneal cavity should be examined, with thorough inspection of the liver, pelvis, and hemidiaphragm and careful palpation of the full length of the large bowel. Following recovery from a complete resection, patients should be observed carefully for 5 years by semiannual physical examinations and yearly blood chemistry measurements. If a complete colonoscopy was not performed preoperatively, it should be carried out within the first several postoperative months. Some authorities favor measuring plasma CEA levels at 3-month intervals because of the sensitivity of this test as a marker for otherwise undetectable tumor recurrence. Subsequent endoscopic or radiographic surveillance of the large bowel, probably at triennial intervals, is indicated, since patients who have been cured of one colorectal cancer have a 3–5% probability of developing an additional bowel cancer during their lifetime and a >15% risk for the development of adenomatous polyps. Anastomotic ("suture-line") recurrences are infrequent in colorectal cancer patients, provided the surgical resection margins are adequate and free of tumor. The value of periodic CT scans of the abdomen, assessing for an early, asymptomatic indication of tumor recurrence, is an area of uncertainty, with some experts recommending the test be performed annually for the first 3 postoperative years.

Radiation therapy to the pelvis is recommended for patients with rectal cancer because it reduces the 20–25% probability of regional recurrences following complete surgical resection of stage II or III tumors, especially if they have penetrated through the serosa. This alarmingly high rate of local disease recurrence is believed to be due to the fact that the contained anatomic space within the pelvis limits the extent of the resection and because the rich lymphatic network of the pelvic side wall immediately adjacent to the rectum facilitates the early spread of malignant cells into surgically inaccessible tissue. The use of sharp rather than blunt dissection of rectal cancers (*total mesorectal excision*) appears to reduce the likelihood of local disease recurrence to ~10%. Radiation therapy, either pre- or postoperatively, reduces the likelihood of pelvic recurrences but does not appear to prolong survival. Combining postoperative radiation therapy with 5-FU–based chemotherapy lowers local recurrence rates and improves overall survival. Preoperative radiotherapy is indicated for patients with large, potentially unresectable rectal cancers; such lesions may shrink enough to permit subsequent surgical removal. Radiation therapy is not effective in the primary treatment of colon cancer.

Systemic therapy for patients with colorectal cancer has become more effective. 5-FU remains the backbone of treatment for this disease. Partial responses are obtained in 15–20% of patients. The probability of tumor response appears to be somewhat greater for patients with liver metastases when chemotherapy is infused directly into the hepatic artery, but intraarterial treatment is costly and toxic and does not appear to appreciably prolong survival. The concomitant administration of folinic acid (leucovorin) improves the efficacy of 5-FU in patients with advanced colorectal cancer, presumably by enhancing the binding of 5-FU to its target enzyme, thymidylate synthase. A threefold improvement in the partial response rate is noted when folinic acid is combined with 5-FU; however, the effect on survival is marginal, and the optimal dose schedule remains to be defined. 5-FU is generally administered intravenously but may also be given orally in the form of capecitabine (Xeloda) with seemingly similar efficacy.

Irinotecan (CPT-11), a topoisomerase 1 inhibitor, prolongs survival when compared to supportive care in patients whose disease has progressed on 5-FU. Furthermore, the addition of irinotecan to 5-FU and leucovorin (LV) improves response rates and survival of patients with metastatic disease. The *FOLFIRI regimen* is as follows: irinotecan, 180 mg/m^2 as a 90-min infusion on day 1; LV, 400 mg/m^2 as a 2-h infusion during irinotecan administration; immediately followed by 5-FU bolus, 400 mg/m^2, and 46-h continuous infusion of 2.4–3 g/m^2 every 2 weeks. Diarrhea is the major side effect from irinotecan. Oxaliplatin, a platinum analogue, also improves the response rate when added to 5-FU and LV as initial treatment of patients with metastatic disease. The *FOLFOX regimen* is the following: 2-h infusion of LV (400 mg/m^2 per day) followed by a 5-FU bolus (400 mg/m^2 per day) and 22-h infusion (1200 mg/m^2) every 2 weeks, together with oxaliplatin, 85 mg/m^2 as a 2-h infusion on day 1. Oxaliplatin frequently causes a dose-dependent sensory neuropathy that often resolves following the cessation of therapy. FOLFIRI and FOLFOX are equal in efficacy. In metastatic disease, these regimens may produce median survivals of 2 years.

Monoclonal antibodies are also effective in patients with advanced colorectal cancer. Cetuximab (Erbitux) and panitumumab (Vectibix) are directed against the epidermal growth factor receptor (EGF-R), a transmembrane glycoprotein involved in signaling pathways affecting growth and proliferation of tumor cells. Both cetuximab and panitumumab, when given alone, have been shown to benefit a small proportion of previously treated patients, and cetuximab appears to have therapeutic synergy with such chemotherapeutic agents as irinotecan, even in patients previously resistant to this drug; this suggests that cetuximab can reverse cellular resistance to cytotoxic chemotherapy. The antibodies are not effective in the subset of colon tumors that contain mutated *K-ras*. The use of both cetuximab and panitumumab can lead to an acne-like rash, with the development and severity of the rash being correlated with the likelihood of antitumor efficacy. Inhibitors of the EGF-R tyrosine kinase such as erlotinib (Tarceva) do not appear to be effective in colorectal cancer.

Bevacizumab (Avastin) is a monoclonal antibody directed against the vascular endothelial growth factor (VEGF) and is thought to act as an anti-angiogenesis agent. The addition of bevacizumab to irinotecan-containing combinations and to FOLFOX initially appeared to improve the outcome observed with chemotherapy alone, but subsequent studies have been less convincing. The use of bevacizumab can lead to hypertension, proteinuria, and an increased likelihood of thromboembolic events.

Patients with solitary hepatic metastases without clinical or radiographic evidence of additional tumor involvement should be considered for partial liver resection, because such procedures are associated with 5-year survival rates of 25–30% when performed on selected individuals by experienced surgeons.

The administration of 5-FU and LV for 6 months after resection of tumor in patients with stage III disease leads to a 40% decrease in recurrence rates and 30% improvement in survival. The likelihood of recurrence has been further reduced when oxaliplatin has been combined with 5-FU and LV (e.g., FOLFOX); unexpectedly, the addition of irinotecan to 5-FU and LV as well as the addition of either bevacizumab or cetuximab to FOLFOX did not enhance outcome. Patients with stage II tumors do not appear to benefit applicably from adjuvant therapy with the use of such treatment generally restricted to those patients having biologic characteristics (e.g., perforated tumors, Ty lesions, lymphovascular invasion) that place them at higher than usual risk for recurrence. In rectal cancer, the delivery of preoperative or postoperative combined modality therapy (5-FU plus radiation therapy) reduces the risk of recurrence and increases the chance of cure for patients with stages II and III tumors, with the preoperative approach being better tolerated. The 5-FU acts as a radiosensitizer when delivered together with radiation therapy. Life-extending adjuvant therapy is used in only about half of patients older than age 65 years. This age bias is completely inappropriate as the benefits and likely the tolerance of adjuvant therapy in patients age 65+ years appear similar to those seen in younger individuals.

TUMORS OF THE SMALL INTESTINE

Small-bowel tumors comprise <3% of gastrointestinal neoplasms. Because of their rarity, a correct diagnosis is often delayed. Abdominal symptoms are usually vague and poorly defined, and conventional radiographic studies of the upper and lower intestinal tract often appear normal. Small-bowel tumors should be considered in the differential diagnosis in the following situations: (1) recurrent, unexplained episodes of crampy abdominal pain; (2) intermittent bouts of intestinal obstruction, especially in the absence of IBD or prior abdominal surgery; (3) intussusception in an adult; and (4) evidence of chronic intestinal bleeding in the presence of negative conventional contrast radiographic findings. A careful small-bowel barium study is the diagnostic procedure of choice; the diagnostic accuracy may be improved by infusing barium through a nasogastric tube placed into the duodenum (enteroclysis).

BENIGN TUMORS

The histology of benign small-bowel tumors is difficult to predict on clinical and radiologic grounds alone. The symptomatology of benign tumors is not distinctive, with pain, obstruction, and hemorrhage being the most frequent symptoms. These tumors are usually discovered during the fifth and sixth decades of life, more often in the distal rather than the proximal small intestine. The most common benign tumors are adenomas, leiomyomas, lipomas, and angiomas.

Adenomas

These tumors include those of the islet cells and Brunner's glands as well as polypoid adenomas. *Islet cell adenomas* are occasionally located outside the pancreas; the associated syndromes are discussed in Chap. 49. *Brunner's gland adenomas* are not truly neoplastic but represent a hypertrophy or hyperplasia of submucosal duodenal glands. These appear as small nodules in the duodenal mucosa that secrete a highly viscous alkaline mucus. Most often, this is an incidental radiographic finding not associated with any specific clinical disorder.

Polypoid adenomas

About 25% of benign small-bowel tumors are polypoid adenomas (Table 38-5). They may present as single polypoid lesions or, less commonly, as papillary villous adenomas. As in the colon, the sessile or papillary form of the tumor is sometimes associated with a coexisting carcinoma. Occasionally, patients with Gardner's syndrome develop premalignant adenomas in the small bowel; such lesions are generally in the duodenum. Multiple polypoid tumors may occur throughout the small bowel (and occasionally the stomach and colorectum) in the Peutz-Jeghers syndrome. The polyps are usually hamartomas (juvenile polyps) having a low potential for malignant degeneration. Mucocutaneous melanin deposits as well as tumors of the ovary, breast, pancreas, and endometrium are also associated with this autosomal dominant condition.

Leiomyomas

These neoplasms arise from smooth-muscle components of the intestine and are usually intramural, affecting the overlying mucosa. Ulceration of the mucosa may cause gastrointestinal hemorrhage of varying severity. Cramping or intermittent abdominal pain is frequently encountered.

Lipomas

These tumors occur with greatest frequency in the distal ileum and at the ileocecal valve. They have a characteristic radiolucent appearance and are usually intramural and asymptomatic but on occasion cause bleeding.

Angiomas

While not true neoplasms, these lesions are important because they frequently cause intestinal bleeding. They may take the form of telangiectasia or hemangiomas. Multiple intestinal telangiectasias occur in a nonhereditary form confined to the gastrointestinal tract or as part of the hereditary Osler-Rendu-Weber syndrome. Vascular tumors may also take the form of isolated hemangiomas, most commonly in the jejunum. Angiography, especially during bleeding, is the best procedure for evaluating these lesions.

MALIGNANT TUMORS

While rare, small-bowel malignancies occur in patients with long-standing regional enteritis and celiac sprue as well as in individuals with AIDS. Malignant tumors of the small bowel are frequently associated with fever, weight loss, anorexia, bleeding, and a palpable abdominal mass. After ampullary carcinomas (many of which arise from biliary or pancreatic ducts), the most frequently occurring small-bowel malignancies are adenocarcinomas, lymphomas, carcinoid tumors, and leiomyosarcomas.

Adenocarcinomas

The most common primary cancers of the small bowel are adenocarcinomas, accounting for ~50% of malignant tumors. These cancers occur most often in the distal duodenum and proximal jejunum, where they tend to ulcerate and cause hemorrhage or obstruction. Radiologically, they may be confused with chronic duodenal ulcer disease or with Crohn's disease if the patient has long-standing regional enteritis. The diagnosis is best made by endoscopy and biopsy under direct vision. Surgical resection is the treatment of choice.

Lymphomas

Lymphoma in the small bowel may be primary or secondary. A diagnosis of a primary intestinal lymphoma requires histologic confirmation in a clinical setting in which palpable adenopathy and hepatosplenomegaly are absent and no evidence of lymphoma is seen on chest radiography, CT scan, or peripheral blood smear or on bone marrow aspiration and biopsy. Symptoms referable to the small bowel are present, usually accompanied by an anatomically discernible lesion. Secondary lymphoma of the small bowel consists of involvement of the intestine by a lymphoid malignancy extending from involved retroperitoneal or mesenteric lymph nodes (Chap. 15).

Primary intestinal lymphoma accounts for ~20% of malignancies of the small bowel. These neoplasms are non-Hodgkin's lymphomas; they usually have a diffuse, large-cell histology and are of T cell origin. Intestinal lymphoma involves the ileum, jejunum, and duodenum, in decreasing frequency—a pattern that mirrors the relative amount of normal lymphoid cells in these anatomic areas. The risk of small-bowel lymphoma is increased in patients with a prior history of malabsorptive conditions (e.g., celiac sprue), regional enteritis, and depressed immune function due to congenital immunodeficiency syndromes, prior organ transplantation, autoimmune disorders, or AIDS.

The development of localized or nodular masses that narrow the lumen results in periumbilical pain (made worse by eating) as well as weight loss, vomiting, and occasional intestinal obstruction. The diagnosis of small-bowel lymphoma may be suspected from the appearance on contrast radiographs of patterns such as infiltration and thickening of mucosal folds, mucosal nodules, areas of irregular ulceration, or stasis of contrast material. The diagnosis can be confirmed by surgical exploration and resection of involved segments. Intestinal lymphoma can occasionally be diagnosed by peroral intestinal mucosal biopsy, but since the disease mainly involves the lamina propria, full-thickness surgical biopsies are usually required.

Resection of the tumor constitutes the initial treatment modality. While postoperative radiation therapy has been given to some patients following a total resection, most authorities favor short-term (three cycles) systemic treatment with combination chemotherapy. The frequent presence of widespread intraabdominal disease at the time of diagnosis and the occasional multicentricity of the tumor often make a total resection impossible. The probability of sustained remission or cure is ~75% in patients with localized disease but is ~25% in individuals with unresectable lymphoma. In patients whose tumors are not resected, chemotherapy may lead to bowel perforation.

A unique form of small-bowel lymphoma, diffusely involving the entire intestine, was first described in oriental Jews and Arabs and is referred to as *immunoproliferative small intestinal disease* (IPSID), *Mediterranean lymphoma*, or α *heavy chain disease*. This is a B cell tumor. The typical presentation includes chronic diarrhea and steatorrhea associated with vomiting and abdominal cramps; clubbing of the digits may be observed. A curious feature in many patients with IPSID is the presence in the blood and intestinal secretions of an abnormal IgA that contains a shortened α heavy chain and is devoid of light chains. It is suspected that the abnormal α chains are produced by plasma cells infiltrating the small bowel. The clinical course of patients with IPSID is generally one of exacerbations and remissions, with death frequently resulting from either progressive malnutrition and wasting or the development of an aggressive lymphoma. The use of oral antibiotics such as tetracycline appears to be beneficial in the early phases of the disorder, suggesting a possible infectious etiology. Combination chemotherapy has been administered during later stages of the disease, with variable results. Results are better when antibiotics and chemotherapy are combined.

Carcinoid tumors

Carcinoid tumors arise from argentaffin cells of the crypts of Lieberkühn and are found from the distal duodenum to the ascending colon, areas embryologically derived from the midgut. More than 50% of intestinal carcinoids are found in the distal ileum, with most congregating close to the ileocecal valve. Most intestinal carcinoids are asymptomatic and of low malignant potential, but invasion and metastases may occur, leading to the carcinoid syndrome (Chap. 49).

Leiomyosarcomas

Leiomyosarcomas often are >5 cm in diameter and may be palpable on abdominal examination. Bleeding, obstruction, and perforation are common. Such tumors should be analyzed for the expression of mutant c-*kit* receptor (defining GIST), and in the presence of metastatic disease, justifying treatment with imatinib mesylate (Gleevec) or, in imatinib-refractory patients, sunitinib (Sutent).

CANCERS OF THE ANUS

Cancers of the anus account for 1–2% of the malignant tumors of the large bowel. Most such lesions arise in the anal canal, the anatomic area extending from the anorectal ring to a zone approximately halfway between the pectinate (or dentate) line and the anal verge. Carcinomas arising proximal to the pectinate line (i.e., in the transitional zone between the glandular mucosa of the rectum and the squamous epithelium of the distal anus) are known as *basaloid*, *cuboidal*, or *cloacogenic* tumors; about one-third of anal cancers have this histologic pattern. Malignancies arising distal to the pectinate line have squamous histology, ulcerate more frequently, and constitute ~55% of anal cancers. The prognosis for patients with basaloid and squamous cell cancers of the anus is identical when corrected for tumor size and the presence or absence of nodal spread.

The development of anal cancer is associated with infection by human papillomavirus, the same organism etiologically linked to cervical cancer. The virus is sexually transmitted. The infection may lead to anal warts (condyloma acuminata), which may progress to anal intraepithelial neoplasia and on to squamous cell carcinoma. The risk for anal cancer is increased among homosexual males, presumably related to anal intercourse. Anal cancer risk is increased in both men and women with AIDS, possibly because their immunosuppressed state permits more severe papillomavirus infection. Anal cancers occur most commonly in middle-aged persons and are more frequent in women than men. At diagnosis, patients may experience bleeding, pain, sensation of a perianal mass, and pruritus.

Radical surgery (abdominal–perineal resection with lymph node sampling and a permanent colostomy) was once the treatment of choice for this tumor type. The 5-year survival rate after such a procedure was 55–70% in the absence of spread to regional lymph nodes and <20% if nodal involvement was present. An alternative therapeutic approach combining external-beam radiation therapy with concomitant chemotherapy has resulted in biopsy-proven disappearance of all tumor in >80% of patients whose initial lesion was <3 cm in size. Tumor recurrences develop in <10% of these patients, meaning that ~70% of patients with anal cancers can be cured with nonoperative treatment. Surgery should be reserved for the minority of individuals who are found to have residual tumor after being managed initially with radiation therapy combined with chemotherapy.

CHAPTER 39

TUMORS OF THE LIVER AND BILIARY TREE

Brian I. Carr

HEPATOCELLULAR CARCINOMA

INCIDENCE

Hepatocellular carcinoma (HCC) is one of the most common malignancies worldwide. The annual global incidence is approximately 1 million cases, with a male-to-female ratio of approximately 4:1 (1:1 without cirrhosis to 9:1 in many high-incidence countries). The incidence rate equals the death rate. In the United States, approximately 22,000 new cases are diagnosed annually, with 18,000 deaths. The death rates in males in low-incidence countries such as the United States are 1.9 per 100,000 per year; in intermediate areas such as Austria and South Africa, they range from 5.1–20; and in high-incidence areas such as in Asia (China and Korea) as high as 23.1–150 per 100,000 per year (Table 39-1). The incidence of HCC in the United States is approximately 3 per 100,000 persons, with significant gender, ethnic, and geographic variations. These numbers are rapidly increasing and may be an underestimate. Approximately 4 million chronic hepatitis C virus (HCV) carriers are in the United States alone. Approximately 10% of them or 400,000 are likely to develop cirrhosis. Approximately 5% or 20,000 of these may develop HCC annually. Add to this the two other common predisposing factors—hepatitis B virus (HBV) and chronic alcohol consumption—and 60,000 new HCC cases annually seem possible. Future advances in HCC survival will likely depend in part on immunization strategies for HBV (and HCV) and earlier diagnosis by screening of patients at risk of HCC development.

Current directions

With the U.S. HCV epidemic, HCC is increasing in most states, and obesity-associated liver disease (nonalcoholic steatohepatitis [NASH]) is increasingly recognized as a cause.

TABLE 39-1

AGE-ADJUSTED INCIDENCE RATES FOR HEPATOCELLULAR CARCINOMA

	PERSONS PER 100,000 PER YEAR	
COUNTRY	**MALE**	**FEMALE**
Argentina	6.0	2.5
Brazil, Recife	9.2	8.3
Brazil, Sao Paulo	3.8	2.6
Mozambique	112.9	30.8
South Africa, Cape: black	26.3	8.4
South Africa, Cape: white	1.2	0.6
Senegal	25.6	9.0
Nigeria	15.4	3.2
Gambia	33.1	12.6
Burma	25.5	8.8
Japan	7.2	2.2
Korea	13.8	3.2
China, Shanghai	34.4	11.6
India, Bombay	4.9	2.5
India, Madras	2.1	0.7
Great Britain	1.6	0.8
France	6.9	1.2
Italy, Varese	7.1	2.7
Norway	1.8	1.1
Spain, Navarra	7.9	4.7

EPIDEMIOLOGY

There are two general types of epidemiologic studies of HCC—those of country-based incidence rates (Table 39-1) and those of migrants. Endemic hot spots occur in areas of China and sub-Saharan Africa, which are associated both with high endemic hepatitis B carrier rates as well as mycotoxin contamination of foodstuffs (aflatoxin B_1), stored grains, drinking water, and soil. Environmental factors are

TABLE 39-2

FACTORS ASSOCIATED WITH AN INCREASED RISK OF DEVELOPING HEPATOCELLULAR CARCINOMA

COMMON	UNUSUAL
Cirrhosis from any cause	Primary biliary cirrhosis
Hepatitis B or C chronic infection	Hemochromatosis
Ethanol chronic consumption	α_1 Antitrypsin deficiency
NASH/NAFL	Glycogen storage diseases
Aflatoxin B_1 or other mycotoxins	Citrullinemia
	Porphyria cutanea tarda
	Hereditary tyrosinemia
	Wilson's disease

Abbreviations: NAFL, nonalcoholic fatty liver; NASH, nonalcoholic steatohepatitis.

important, for example, Japanese in Japan have a higher incidence than those living in Hawaii, who in turn have a higher incidence than those living in California.

ETIOLOGIC FACTORS

Chemical carcinogens

Causative agents for HCC have been studied along two general lines. First are agents identified as carcinogenic in experimental animals (particularly rodents) that are thought to be present in the human environment (Table 39-2). Second is the association of HCC with various other clinical conditions. Probably the best-studied and most potent ubiquitous natural chemical carcinogen is a product of the *Aspergillus* fungus, called aflatoxin B_1. This mold and aflatoxin product can be found in a variety of stored grains in hot, humid places, where peanuts and rice are stored in unrefrigerated conditions. Aflatoxin contamination of foodstuffs correlates well with incidence rates in Africa and to some extent in China. In endemic areas of China, even farm animals such as ducks have HCC. The most potent carcinogens appear to be natural products of plants, fungi, and bacteria, such as bush trees containing pyrrolizidine alkaloids as well as tannic acid and safrole. Pollutants such as pesticides and insecticides are known rodent carcinogens.

Hepatitis

Both case-control and cohort studies have shown a strong association between chronic hepatitis B carrier rates and increased incidence of HCC. In Taiwanese male postal carriers who were hepatitis B surface antigen (HBsAg)–positive, a 98-fold greater risk for HCC was found compared with HBsAg-negative individuals. The incidence of HCC in Alaskan natives is markedly increased related to a high prevalence of HBV infection. HBV-based HCC may involve rounds of hepatic destruction with subsequent proliferation and not necessarily frank cirrhosis. The increase in Japanese HCC incidence rates in the past three decades is thought to be from hepatitis C. A large-scale World Health Organization (WHO)–sponsored intervention study is currently underway in Asia involving HBV vaccination of newborns. HCC in African blacks is not associated with severe cirrhosis but is poorly differentiated and very aggressive. Despite uniform HBV carrier rates among the South African Bantu, there is a ninefold difference in HCC incidence between Mozambicans living along the coast and inland. These differences are attributed to the additional exposure to dietary aflatoxin B_1 and other carcinogenic mycotoxins. A typical interval between HCV-associated transfusion and subsequent HCC is approximately 30 years. HCV-associated HCC patients tend to have more frequent and advanced cirrhosis, but in HBV-associated HCC, only half of patients have cirrhosis; the remainder having chronic active hepatitis.

Other etiologic conditions

The 75–85% association of HCC with underlying cirrhosis has long been recognized, more typically with macronodular cirrhosis in Southeast Asia, but also with micronodular cirrhosis (alcohol) in Europe and the United States. It is still not clear whether cirrhosis itself is a predisposing factor to the development of HCC or whether the underlying causes of the cirrhosis are actually the carcinogenic factors. However, ~20% of U.S. patients with HCC do not have underlying cirrhosis. Several underlying conditions are associated with an increased risk for cirrhosis-associated HCC (Table 39-2), including hepatitis, alcohol, autoimmune chronic active hepatitis, cryptogenic cirrhosis, and NASH. A less common association is with primary biliary cirrhosis and several metabolic diseases including hemochromatosis, Wilson disease, α_1-antitrypsin deficiency, tyrosinemia, porphyria cutanea tarda, glycogenesis types 1 and 3, citrullinemia. and orotic aciduria. The etiology of HCC in those 20% of patients who have no cirrhosis is currently unclear, and their HCC natural history is not well-defined.

Current directions

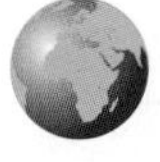

Many patients have multiple etiologies, and the interactions of either hepatitis or alcohol and smoking, or with aflatoxins, are just beginning to be explored.

CLINICAL FEATURES

Symptoms

These include abdominal pain, weight loss, weakness, abdominal fullness and swelling, jaundice, and nausea (Table 39-3). Presenting signs and symptoms differ somewhat between high- and low-incidence areas. In high-risk areas, especially in South African blacks, the most common symptom is abdominal pain; by contrast, only 40–50% of Chinese and Japanese patients present with abdominal pain. Abdominal swelling may occur as a consequence of ascites due to the underlying chronic liver disease or may be due to a rapidly expanding tumor. Occasionally, central necrosis or acute hemorrhage into the peritoneal cavity leads to death. In countries with an active surveillance program, HCC tends to be identified at an earlier stage, when symptoms may be due only to the underlying disease. Jaundice is usually due to obstruction of the intrahepatic ducts from underlying liver disease. Hematemesis may occur due to esophageal varices from the underlying portal hypertension. Bone pain is seen in 3–12% of patients, but necropsies show pathologic bone metastases in ~20% of patients. However, 25% of patients may be asymptomatic.

TABLE 39-3

HEPATOCELLULAR CARCINOMA CLINICAL PRESENTATION (*n* = 547)

SYMPTOM	PATIENT, *n* (%)
No symptom	129(24)
Abdominal pain	219(40)
Other (workup of anemia and various diseases)	64(12)
Routine physical exam finding, elevated LFTs	129(24)
Weight loss	112(20)
Appetite loss	59 (11)
Weakness/malaise	83(15)
Jaundice	30(5)
Routine CT scan screening of known cirrhosis	92(17)
Cirrhosis symptoms (ankle swelling, abdominal bloating, increased girth, pruritus, GI bleed)	98(18)
Diarrhea	7(1)
Tumor rupture	1
Patient Characteristics	
Mean age (yr)	56 ± 13
Male:female ratio	3:1
Ethnicity	
White	72%
Middle Eastern	10%
Asian	13%
African American	5%
Cirrhosis	81%
No cirrhosis	19%
Tumor Characteristics	
Hepatic tumor numbers	
1	20%
2	25%
3 or more	65%
Portal vein invasion	75%
Unilobar	25%
Bilobar	75%

Abbreviations: GI, gastrointestinal; LFT, liver function test.

Physical signs

Hepatomegaly is the most common physical sign, occurring in 50–90% of the patients. Abdominal bruits are noted in 6–25%, and ascites occurs in 30–60% of patients. Ascites should be examined by cytology. Splenomegaly is mainly due to portal hypertension. Weight loss and muscle wasting are common, particularly with rapidly growing or large tumors. Fever is found in 10–50% of patients, from unclear cause. The signs of chronic liver disease may often be present, including jaundice, dilated abdominal veins, palmar erythema, gynecomastia, testicular atrophy, and peripheral edema. Budd-Chiari syndrome can occur due to HCC invasion of the hepatic veins, with tense ascites and a large tender liver.

Paraneoplastic syndromes

Most paraneoplastic syndromes in HCC are biochemical abnormalities without associated clinical consequences. They include hypoglycemia (also caused by end-stage liver failure), erythrocytosis, hypercalcemia, hypercholesterolemia, dysfibrinogenemia, carcinoid syndrome, increased thyroxin-binding globulin, changes in secondary sex characteristics (gynecomastia, testicular atrophy, and precocious puberty), and porphyria cutanea tarda. Mild hypoglycemia occurs in rapidly growing HCC as part of terminal illness, and profound hypoglycemia may occur, although the cause is unclear. Erythrocytosis occurs in 3–12% of patients and hypercholesterolemia in 10–40%. A high percent of patients have thrombocytopenia or leukopenia, resulting from portal hypertension, and not from cancer infiltration of bone marrow, as in other tumor types.

STAGING

Multiple clinical staging systems for HCC have been described. A widely used one has been the American Joint Commission for Cancer (AJCC)/tumor, node, metastasis (TNM) classification. However, the Cancer of the Liver Italian Program (CLIP) system is now popular as it takes the cirrhosis into account, based on the Okuda system (Table 39-4). Other staging systems have been proposed, and a consensus is needed. They are all based on combining the prognostic features of liver damage with those of tumor aggressiveness and include systems from Spain (Barcelona Clinic Liver Cancer [BCLC]), Japan, Hong Kong, and others (Chinese University Prognostic Index [CUPI], Japan Integrated Staging [JIS], and SLiDe which stands for S, stage; Li, liver damage; De, des-γ-carboxy prothrombin). The best prognosis is for stage I, solitary tumors of less than 2-cm diameter without vascular invasion. Adverse prognostic features include ascites, jaundice, vascular invasion, and elevated α fetoproteins (AFPs). Vascular invasion in particular has profound effects on prognosis and may be microscopic or macroscopic (visible on computed tomography [CT] scans). Most large tumors have microscopic vascular invasion, so full staging can usually be made only after surgical resection. Stage III disease contains a mixture of lymph node–positive and –negative tumors. Stage III patients with positive lymph node disease have a poor prognosis, and few patients survive 1 year. The prognosis of stage IV is poor after either resection or transplantation, and the 1-year survival is rare. A working staging system based entirely on clinical grounds that incorporates the contribution of the underlying liver disease was originally developed by Okuda et al. (Table 39-4). Patients with Okuda stage III have a dire prognosis because they usually cannot be curatively resected, and the condition of their liver typically precludes chemotherapy.

New directions

Consensus is needed on staging. These systems will soon be upended by proteomics.

APPROACH TO THE PATIENT: Hepatocellular Carcinoma

HISTORY AND PHYSICAL EXAMINATION The history is important in evaluating putative predisposing factors, including a history of hepatitis or jaundice, blood transfusion, or use of intravenous drugs. A family history of HCC or hepatitis should be sought and a detailed social history taken to include job descriptions for industrial exposure to possible carcinogenic drugs as well as contraceptive hormones. Physical examination should include assessing stigmata of underlying liver disease such as jaundice, ascites, peripheral edema, spider nevi, palmar erythema, and weight loss. Evaluation of the abdomen for hepatic size, masses or ascites; hepatic nodularity and tenderness; and splenomegaly is needed, as is assessment of overall performance status and psychosocial evaluation.

SEROLOGIC ASSAYS AFP is a serum tumor marker for HCC; however, it is only increased in approximately half of U.S. patients. The lens culinaris agglutinin-reactive fraction of AFP (AFP-L3) assay is thought to be more specific. The other widely used assay is that for des-γ-carboxy prothrombin (DCP), a protein induced by vitamin K absence (PIVKA-2). This

TABLE 39-4

CLIP AND OKUDA STAGING SYSTEMS FOR HEPATOCELLULAR CARCINOMA

CLIP Classification

VARIABLES	POINTS 0	1	2
i. Tumor number	Single	Multiple	–
Hepatic replacement by tumor (%)	<50	<50	>50
ii. Child-Pugh score	A	B	C
iii. α Fetoprotein level (ng/mL)	<400	≥400	–
iv. Portal vein thrombosis (CT)	No	Yes	–

CLIP stages (score = sum of points): CLIP 0, 0 points; CLIP 1, 1 point; CLIP 2, 2 points; CLIP 3, 3 points.

Okuda Classification

TUMOR EXTENT[a]		ASCITES		ALBUMIN (g/L)		BILIRUBIN (mg/dL)	
≥50%	<50	+	–	≤3	>3	≥3	<3
(+)	(–)	(+)	(–)	(+)	(–)	(+)	(–)

Okuda stages: stage 1, all (–); stage 2, 1 or 2 (+); stage 3, 3 or 4 (+)

[a]Extent of liver occupied by tumor

Abbreviations: CLIP, Cancer of the Liver Italian Program; CT, computed tomography.

protein is increased in as many as 80% of HCC patients but may also be elevated in patients with vitamin K deficiency; it is always elevated after Coumadin use. It may predict for portal vein invasion. Both AFP-L3 and DCP are U.S. Food and Drug Administration (FDA) approved. Many other assays have been developed, such as glypican-3, but none has greater aggregate sensitivity and specificity. In a patient presenting with either a new hepatic mass or other indications of recent hepatic decompensation, carcinoembryonic antigen (CEA), vitamin B_{12}, AFP, ferritin, PIVKA-2, and antimitochondrial Ab should be measured, and standard liver function tests should be performed, including prothrombin time (PT), partial thromboplastin time (PTT), albumin, transaminases, γ-glutamyl transpeptidase, and alkaline phosphatase. Decreases in platelet count and white blood cell count may reflect portal hypertension and associated hypersplenism. Hepatitis A, B, and C serology should be measured. If HBV or HCV serology is positive, quantitative measurements of HBV DNA or HCV RNA are needed.

New Directions Newer biomarkers are being evaluated, especially tissue- and serum-based genomics profiling.

RADIOLOGY An ultrasound examination of the liver is an excellent screening tool. The two characteristic vascular abnormalities are hypervascularity of the tumor mass (neovascularization or abnormal tumor-feeding arterial vessels) and thrombosis by tumor invasion of otherwise normal portal veins. To determine tumor size and extent and the presence of portal vein invasion accurately, a helical/triphasic CT scan of the abdomen and pelvis with fast-contrast bolus technique should be performed to detect the vascular lesions typical of HCC. Portal vein invasion is normally detected as an obstruction and expansion of the vessel. A chest CT is used to exclude metastases. Magnetic resonance imaging (MRI) can also provide detailed information, especially with the newer contrast agents. Ethiodol (Lipiodol) is an ethiodized oil emulsion retained by liver tumors that can be delivered by hepatic artery injection (5–15 mL) for CT imaging 1 week later. For small tumors, Ethiodol injection is very helpful before biopsy because the histological presence of the dye constitutes proof that the needle biopsied the mass under suspicion. A prospective comparison of triphasic CT, gadolinium-enhanced MRI, ultrasound, and fluorodeoxyglucose positron emission tomography (FDG-PET) showed similar results for CT, MRI, and ultrasound; PET imaging was unsuccessful.

New Directions The altered tumor vascularity that is a consequence of molecularly targeted therapies is the basis for newer imaging techniques including contrast-enhanced ultrasound (CEUS) and dynamic MRI.

PATHOLOGIC DIAGNOSIS Histologic proof of the presence of HCC is obtained through a core liver biopsy of the liver mass under ultrasound guidance, as well as random biopsy of the underlying liver. Bleeding risk is increased compared with other cancers because (1) the tumors are hypervascular, and (2) patients often have thrombocytopenia and decreased liver-dependent clotting factors. Bleeding risk is further increased in the presence of ascites. Tracking of tumor has an uncommon problem. Fine-needle aspirates can provide sufficient material for diagnosis of cancer, but core biopsies are preferred. Tissue architecture allows the distinction between HCC and adenocarcinoma. Laparoscopic approaches can also be used. For patients suspected of having portal vein involvement, a core biopsy of the portal vein may be performed safely. If positive, this is regarded as an exclusion criterion for transplantation for HCC.

New Directions Immunohistochemistry has become mainstream. Prognostic subgroupings are being defined based on growth signaling pathway proteins and genotyping strategies. Furthermore, molecular profiling of the underlying liver has provided evidence for a "field effect" of cirrhosis in generating recurrent or new HCCs after primary resection.

SCREENING HIGH-RISK POPULATIONS

Screening has not been shown to save lives. Prospective studies in high-risk populations showed that ultrasound was more sensitive than AFP elevations. An Italian study in patients with cirrhosis identified a yearly HCC incidence of 3% but showed no increase in the rate of detection of potentially curable tumors with aggressive screening. Prevention strategies including universal vaccination against hepatitis are more likely to be effective than screening efforts. Despite absence of formal guidelines, most practitioners obtain 6-monthly AFP and CT (or ultrasound) when following high-risk patients (HBV carriers, HCV cirrhosis, family history of HCC).

Current directions

Cost-benefit analysis is not yet convincing, even though screening is intuitively sound. However, studies from areas of high HBV carrier rates have shown a survival benefit for screening as a result of earlier stage at diagnosis. Gamma-glutamyl transpeptidase appears useful for detecting small tumors.

TREATMENT Hepatocellular Carcinoma

Most HCC patients have two liver diseases, cirrhosis and HCC, each of which is an independent cause of death. The presence of cirrhosis usually places constraints on resection surgery, ablative therapies, and chemotherapy. Thus patient assessment and treatment planning have to take the severity of the nonmalignant liver disease into account. The clinical management choices for HCC can be complex (Fig. 39-1 and Tables 39-5, and 39-6). The natural history of HCC is highly variable. Patients presenting with advanced tumors (vascular invasion, symptoms, extrahepatic spread) have a median survival time of ~4 months, with or without treatment. Treatment results from the literature are difficult to interpret. Survival is not always a measure of the efficacy of therapy because of the adverse effects on survival of the underlying liver disease. A multidisciplinary team, including a hepatologist, interventional radiologist, surgical oncologist, transplant surgeon, and medical oncologist, is important for the comprehensive management of HCC patients.

STAGES I AND II HCC Early-stage tumors are successfully treated using various techniques, including surgical resection, local ablation (thermal or radiofrequency ablation [RFA]), and local injection therapies (Table 39-6). Because the majority of patients with HCC have a field defect in the cirrhotic liver, they are at risk for subsequent multiple primary liver tumors. Many will also have significant underlying liver disease and may not tolerate major surgical loss of hepatic parenchyma, and they may be eligible for orthotopic liver transplant (OLTX). Living related donor transplants have increased in popularity, resulting in absence of waiting for a transplant. An important principle in treating early-stage HCC is to use liver-sparing treatments and to focus on treatment of both the tumor and the cirrhosis.

Surgical Excision The risk of major hepatectomy is high (5–10% mortality rate) due to the underlying liver disease and the potential for liver failure but is acceptable in selected cases. Preoperative portal vein occlusion can sometimes be performed to cause atrophy of the HCC-involved lobe and compensatory hypertrophy of the noninvolved liver, permitting safer resection. Intraoperative ultrasound is useful for planning the surgical approach. Ultrasonography can image the proximity of major vascular structures that may be encountered during the dissection. In cirrhotic patients, any major liver surgery can result in liver failure. The Child-Pugh classification of liver failure is still a reliable prognosticator for tolerance of hepatic surgery and only Child A patients should be considered for surgical resection. Child B and C patients with stages I and II HCC should be referred for OLTX if appropriate, as well as patients with ascites or a recent history of variceal bleeding. Although open surgical excision is the most reliable, the patient may be better served with a laparoscopic approach to resection using RFA or PEI.

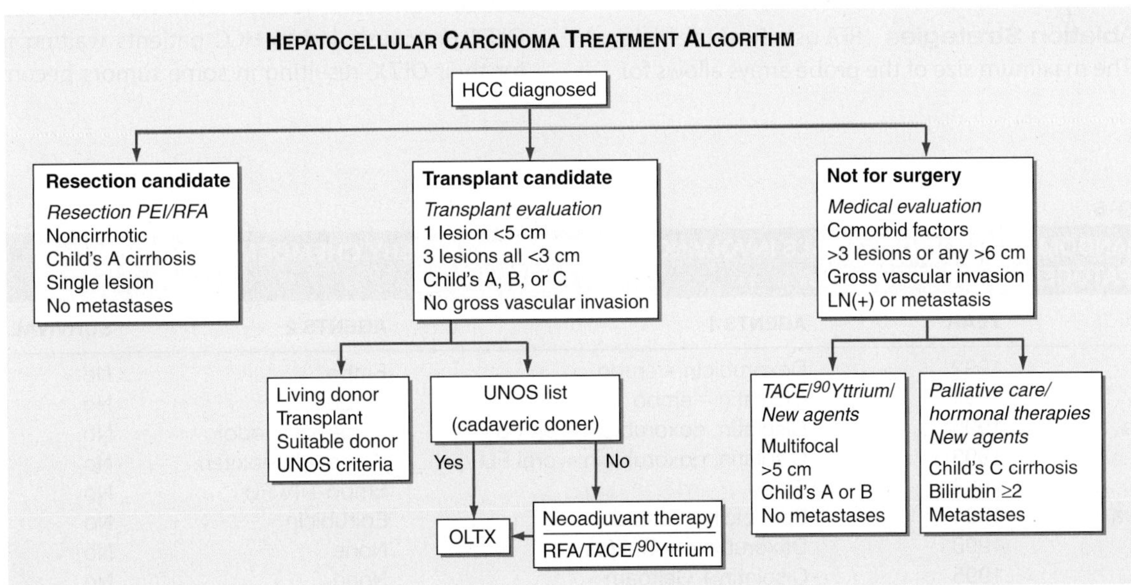

FIGURE 39-1

Hepatocellular carcinoma (HCC) treatment algorithm. Treatment approach to patients with HCC. The initial clinical evaluation is aimed at assessing the extent of the tumor and the underlying functional compromise of the liver by cirrhosis. Patients are classified as having resectable disease or unresectable disease or as transplantation candidates. LN, lymph node; OLTX, orthotopic liver transplantation; PEI, percutaneous ethanol injection; RFA, radiofrequency ablation; TACE, transarterial chemoembolization; UNOS, United Network for Organ Sharing. Child's A/B/C refers to the Child-Pugh classification of liver failure.

TABLE 39-5

TREATMENT OPTIONS FOR HEPATOCELLULAR CARCINOMA

Surgery
Resection
Liver transplantation
Local Ablative Therapies
Cryosurgery
Radiofrequency ablation
Percutaneous ethanol injection
Regional Therapies: Hepatic Artery Transcatheter Treatments
Transarterial chemotherapy
Transarterial embolization
Transarterial chemoembolization
Transarterial drug-eluting beads
Transarterial radiotherapies:
^{90}Yttrium microspheres
^{131}Iodine–Ethiodol
Conformal External-Beam Radiation
Therapy systemic therapies
Molecularly targeted therapies (sorafenib, etc.)
Chemotherapy
Immunotherapy
Hormonal therapy + growth control
Supportive therapies

No adequate comparisons of these different techniques have been undertaken and the choice of treatment is usually based on physician skill.

Local Ablation Strategies RFA uses heat to ablate tumors. The maximum size of the probe arrays allows for a 7-cm zone of necrosis, which would be adequate for a 3- to 4-cm tumor. The heat reliably kills cells within the zone of necrosis. Treatment of tumors close to the main portal pedicles can lead to bile duct injury and obstruction. This limits the location of tumors that are anatomically suited for this technique. RFA can be performed percutaneously with CT or ultrasound guidance, or at the time of laparoscopy with ultrasound guidance.

Local Injection Therapy Numerous agents have been used for local injection into tumors, most commonly, ethanol (PEI). The relatively soft HCC within the hard background cirrhotic liver allows for injection of large volumes of ethanol into the tumor without diffusion into the hepatic parenchyma or leakage out of the liver. PEI causes direct destruction of cancer cells, but it is not selective for cancer and will destroy normal cells in the vicinity. However, it usually requires multiple injections (average three), in contrast to one for RFA. The maximum size of tumor reliably treated is 3 cm, even with multiple injections.

Current Directions Resection and RFA each obtain similar results.

Liver Transplantation (OLTX) A viable option for stages I and II tumors in the setting of cirrhosis is OLTX, with survival approaching that for noncancer cases. OLTX for patients with a single lesion ≤5 cm or three or fewer nodules, each ≤3 cm (Milan criteria), resulted in excellent tumor-free survival (≥70% at 5 years). For advanced HCC, OLTX has been abandoned due to high tumor recurrence rates. Priority scoring for OLTX previously led to HCC patients waiting too long for their OLTX, resulting in some tumors becoming too

TABLE 39-6

SOME RANDOMIZED CLINICAL TRIALS INVOLVING TRANSHEPATIC ARTERY CHEMOEMBOLIZATION FOR HEPATOCELLULAR CARCINOMA

AUTHOR	YEAR	AGENTS 1	AGENTS 2	SURVIVAL EFFECT
Kawaii	1992	Doxorubicin + embo	Embo	No
Chang	1994	Cisplatin + embo	Embo	No
Hatanaka	1995	Cisplatin, doxorubicin + embo	Same + Lipiodol	No
Uchino	1993	Cisplatin, doxorubicin + oral FU	Same + tamoxifen	No
Lin	1988	Embo	Embo + IV FU	No
Yoshikawa	1994	Epirubicin + Ethiodol	Epirubicin	No
Pelletier	1990	Doxorubicin + Gelfoam	None	No
Trinchet	1995	Cisplatin + Gelfoam	None	No
Bruix	1998	Coils and Gelfoam	None	No
Pelletier	1998	Cisplatin + Ethiodol	None	No
Trinchet	1995	Cisplatin + Gelfoam	None	No
Lo	2002	Cisplatin + Ethiodol	None	Yes
Llovet	2002	Doxorubicin + Ethiodol	None	Yes

Abbreviations: Embo, embolization; FU, 5-fluorouracil; IV, intravenous.

advanced during the patient's wait for a donated liver. A variety of therapies were used as a "bridge" to OLTX, including RFA, polyethylenimine, and transcatheter arterial chemoembolization (TACE). It seems clear that these pretransplant treatments allow patients to remain on the waiting list longer, giving them greater opportunities to be transplanted. What remains unclear, however, is whether this translates into prolonged survival after transplant. Further, it is not known whether patients who have had their tumor(s) treated preoperatively follow the recurrence pattern predicted by their tumor status at the time of transplant (i.e., after local ablative therapy), or if they follow the course set by their tumor parameters present before such treatment. The United Network for Organ Sharing (UNOS) point system for priority scoring of OLTX recipients now includes additional points for patients with HCC. The success of living related donor liver transplantation programs has also led to patients receiving transplantation earlier for HCC and often with greater than minimal tumors.

Current Directions Expanded criteria for larger HCCs beyond the Milan criteria (one lesion <5 cm or three lesions, each <3 cm) are being increasingly accepted by various UNOS areas for OLTX with satisfactory longer-term survival. Furthermore, downstaging HCCs by medical therapy (TACE) is increasingly recognized as acceptable treatment before OLTX.

Adjuvant Therapy The role of adjuvant chemotherapy for patients after resection or OLTX remains unclear. Both adjuvant and neoadjuvant approaches have been studied, but no clear advantage in disease-free or overall survival has been found. However, a meta-analysis of several trials revealed a significant improvement in disease-free and overall survival. Although analysis of postoperative adjuvant systemic chemotherapy trials demonstrated no disease-free or overall survival advantage, single studies of TACE and neoadjuvant ^{131}I-Ethiodol showed enhanced survival post-resection.

Current Directions A large adjuvant trial examining resection with or without sorafenib (see later discussion) is in progress.

STAGES III AND IV HCC Fewer surgical options exist for stage III tumors involving major vascular structures. In patients without cirrhosis, a major hepatectomy is feasible, although prognosis is poor. Patients with Child's A cirrhosis may be resected, but a lobectomy is associated with significant morbidity and mortality rates, and long-term prognosis is poor. Nevertheless, a small percentage of patients will achieve long-term survival, justifying an attempt at resection when feasible. Because of the advanced nature of these tumors, even successful resection can be followed by rapid recurrence. These patients are not considered candidates for transplantation because of the high tumor recurrence rates unless their tumors can first be down-staged with neoadjuvant therapy. Decreasing the size of the primary tumor allows for less surgery, and the delay in surgery allows for extrahepatic disease to manifest on imaging studies and avoid unhelpful OLTX. The prognosis is poor for stage IV tumors, and no surgical treatment is recommended.

Systemic Chemotherapy A large number of controlled and uncontrolled clinical studies have been performed with most of the major classes of cancer chemotherapy. No single agent or combination of agents given systemically reproducibly leads to even a 25% response rate or has any effect on survival.

Regional Chemotherapy In contrast to the dismal results of systemic chemotherapy, a variety of agents given via the hepatic artery have activity for HCC confined to the liver (Table 39-6). Two randomized controlled trials have shown a survival advantage for TACE in a selected subset of patients. One used doxorubicin, and the other used cisplatin. Despite the fact that increased hepatic extraction of chemotherapy has been shown for very few drugs, some drugs such as cisplatin, doxorubicin, mitomycin C, and possibly neocarzinostatin produce substantial objective responses when administered regionally. Few data are available on continuous hepatic arterial infusion for HCC, although pilot studies with cisplatin have shown encouraging responses. Because the reports have not usually stratified responses or survival based on TNM staging, it is difficult to know long-term prognosis in relation to tumor extent. Most of the studies on regional hepatic arterial chemotherapy also use an embolizing agent such as Ethiodol, gelatin sponge particles (Gelfoam), starch (Spherex), or microspheres. Two products are composed of microspheres of defined size ranges—Embospheres (Biospheres) and Contour SE—using particles of 40–120, 100–300, 300–500, and 500–1000 μm in size. The optimal diameter of the particles for TACE has yet to be defined. Consistently higher objective response rates are reported for arterial administration of drugs together with some form of hepatic artery occlusion compared with any form of systemic chemotherapy to date. The widespread use of some form of embolization in addition to chemotherapy has added to its toxicities. These include a frequent but transient fever, abdominal pain, and anorexia (all in >60% of patients). In addition, >20% of patients have increased ascites or transient elevation of transaminases. Cystic artery spasm and cholecystitis are also not uncommon. However, higher responses have also been obtained. The hepatic toxicities associated with embolization may be ameliorated by the use of degradable starch microspheres, with 50–60% response rates. Two randomized studies of TACE versus placebo showed a survival advantage for treatment (Table 39-6). In addition, it is not clear that formal oncologic CT response criteria are adequate for HCC. A loss of vascularity on CT without size change may be an index of loss of viability and thus of response to TACE. A major problem that TACE trials have had in showing a survival advantage is that many HCC patients die of their underlying cirrhosis, not the tumor. However, improving quality of life is a legitimate goal of regional therapy.

New Therapies The major finding has been a survival advantage for oral sorafenib (Nexavar) versus placebo controls in two randomized trials, leading to its approval by the FDA. However, tumor responses were negligible, and the survival in the treatment arm in Asians was below the placebo arm in the Western trial (Table 39-7). Furthermore, prolonged survival has been reported in phase II trials using newer agents, such as bevacizumab plus erlotinib. Several forms of *radiation therapy* have been used in the treatment of HCC, including external-beam radiation and conformal radiation therapy. Radiation hepatitis remains a dose-limiting problem. The pure beta emitter ^{90}Yttrium attached to either glass or resin microspheres has been assessed in phase II trials of HCC and has encouraging survival effects with minimal toxicities. Randomized trials have yet to be performed. Vitamin K has been assessed in clinical trials at high dosage for its HCC-inhibitory actions. This idea is based on the characteristic biochemical defect in HCC of elevated plasma levels of immature prothrombin (DCP or PIVKA-2), due to a defect in the activity of prothrombin carboxylase, a vitamin K–dependent enzyme. Two vitamin K randomized controlled trials from Japan show decreased tumor occurrence.

Current Directions A number of new treatments are being evaluated for HCC (Table 39-8). These include the biologicals, such as Raf kinase and vascular endothelial growth factor (VEGF) inhibitors, ^{90}Yttrium looks promising without chemotherapy toxicities, and vitamin K_2 appears to prevent recurrences after resection. The bottleneck of liver donors for OLTX is at last widening with increasing use of living donors, and criteria for OLTX for larger HCCs are slowly expanding. Patient participation in clinical trials assessing new therapies is encouraged (*www.clinicaltrials.gov*).

TABLE 39-7

TARGETED THERAPIES IN HEPATOCELLULAR CARCINOMA TRIALS

PHASE III	TARGET	SURVIVAL (MO)
Sorafenib vs placebo	Raf, VEGFR, PDGFR	10.7 vs 7.9
Sorafenib vs placebo (Asians)	Raf, WGFR, PDGFR	6.5 vs 4.2
Phase II		
Sorafenib		9
Sorafenib (Asians)		5
Sunitinib		9.8, 8 (2 trials)
Bevacizumab	VEGF	12.4
Bevacizumab plus erlotinib	VEGF plus EGFR	15.6
Bevacizumab plus capecitabine		8
Erlotinib	EGFR	13, 10.7 (2 trials)
Linifanib	VEGFR, PDGF	9.7
Brivanib	VEGFR, FGFR	10

Abbreviations: EGFR, epidermal growth factor receptor; FGFR, fibroblast growth factor receptor; PDGF, platelet-derived growth factor; PDGFR, platelet-derived growth factor receptor; Raf, rapidly accelerated fibrosarcoma; VEGF, vascular endothelial growth factor; VEGFR vascular endothelial growth factor receptor.

SUMMARY (TABLE 39-5)

The most common modes of patient presentation

1. A patient with known history of hepatitis, jaundice, or cirrhosis, with an abnormality on ultrasonography or CT scan, or rising AFP or DCP (PIVKA-2)
2. A patient with an abnormal liver function test result as part of a routine examination
3. Radiologic workup for liver transplant for cirrhosis
4. Symptoms of HCC including cachexia, abdominal pain, or fever

TABLE 39-8

SOME NOVEL MEDICAL TREATMENTS FOR HEPATOCELLULAR CARCINOMA

EGF receptor antagonists: erlotinib, gefitinib, lapatinib, cetuximab, brivanib
Multi-kinase antagonists: sorafenib, sunitinib
VEGF antagonist: bevacizumab
VEGFR antagonist: ABT-869 (linifanib)
mTOR antagonists: sirolimus, temsirolimus, everolimus
Proteasome inhibitors: bortezomib
Vitamin K
^{131}I–Ethiodol (lipiodol)
^{131}I–Ferritin
^{90}Yttrium microspheres (TheraSphere, SIR-spheres)
^{166}Holmium, ^{188}Rhenium
Three-dimensional conformal radiation
Proton-beam high-dose radiotherapy
Gamma knife, CyberKnife
New targets: inhibitors of cyclin-dependent kinases (Cdk) and caspases

Abbreviations: EGF, epidermal growth factor; VEGF, vascular endothelial growth factor; VEGFR vascular endothelial growth factor receptor.

History and physical examination

1. Clinical jaundice, asthenia, itching (scratches), tremors, or disorientation
2. Hepatomegaly, splenomegaly, ascites, peripheral edema, skin signs of liver failure

Clinical evaluation

1. Blood tests: full blood count (splenomegaly), liver function tests, ammonia levels, electrolytes, AFP and DCP (PIVKA-2), Ca^{2+} and Mg^{2+}; hepatitis B, C, and D serology (and quantitative HBV DNA or HCV RNA, if either result is positive); neurotensin (specific for fibrolamellar HCC)
2. Triphasic dynamic helical (spiral) CT scan of liver (if inadequate, then follow with MRI); chest CT scan; upper and lower gastrointestinal endoscopy (for varices, bleeding, ulcers); and brain scan (only if symptoms suggest)
3. Core biopsy: of the tumor and separate biopsy of the underlying liver

Therapy (Tables 39-5 and 39-6)

1. HCC <2 cm: RFA, PEI, or resection
2. HCC >2 cm, no vascular invasion: liver resection, RFA, or OLTX
3. Multiple unilobar tumors or tumor with vascular invasion: TACE or sorafenib
4. Bilobar tumors, no vascular invasion: TACE with OLTX for patients with tumor response
5. Extrahepatic HCC or elevated bilirubin: sorafenib or bevacizumab plus erlotinib (combination agent trials are in progress)

OTHER PRIMARY LIVER TUMORS

FIBROLAMELLAR HCC

This rarer variant of HCC has a quite different biology than adult-type HCC. None of the known HCC causative factors seem important here. It is typically a disease of younger adults, often teenagers and predominantly females. It is AFP-negative, but patients typically have elevated blood neurotensin levels, normal liver function test results, and no cirrhosis. Radiology is similar for HCC, except that characteristic adult-type portal vein invasion is less common. Although it is often multifocal in the liver and therefore not resectable, metastases are common, especially to the lungs and locoregional lymph nodes, but survival is often much better than with adult-type HCC. Resectable tumors are associated with 5-year survival rate >50%. Patients often present with a huge liver or unexplained weight loss, fever, or elevated liver function test results on routine evaluations. These huge masses suggest quite slow growth for many tumors. Surgical resection is the best management option, even for metastases, as these tumors respond much less well to chemotherapy than adult-type HCC. Although several series of OLTX for FL-HCC have been reported, the patients seem to die from tumor recurrences, with a 2- to 5-year lag compared with OLTX for adult-type HCC. Anecdotal responses to gemcitabine plus cisplatin-TACE are reported.

Epithelioid hemangioendothelioma

This rare vascular tumor of adults is also usually multifocal and can also be associated with prolonged survival periods, even in the presence of metastases, which are commonly in the lung. There is usually no underlying cirrhosis. Histologically, these tumors are usually of borderline malignancy and express factor VIII, confirming their endothelial origin. OLTX may produce prolonged survival.

Cholangiocarcinoma

Cholangiocarcinoma (CCC) typically refers to mucin-producing adenocarcinomas (different from HCC) that arise from the bile ducts. They are grouped by their anatomic site of origin, as intrahepatic, hilar (central, ~65% of CCCs), and peripheral (or distal, ~30% of CCCs). They arise on the basis of cirrhosis less frequently than HCC, excepting primary biliary cirrhosis. Nodular tumors arising at the bifurcation of the common bile duct are called *Klatskin* tumors and are often associated with a collapsed gallbladder, a finding that mandates visualization of the entire biliary tree. The approach to management of central and peripheral CCC is quite different. Incidence is increasing. Although most CCCs have no obvious cause, a number of predisposing factors have been identified. Predisposing diseases include primary sclerosing cholangitis (10–20% of primary sclerosing cholangitis [PSC] patients); an autoimmune disease; and liver fluke in Asians, especially *Opisthorchis viverrini* and *Clonorchis sinensis*. CCC seems also to be associated with any cause of chronic biliary inflammation and injury, with alcoholic liver disease, choledocholithiasis, choledochal cysts (10%), and Caroli's disease (a rare inherited form of bile duct ectasia). CCC most typically presents as painless jaundice, often with pruritus or weight loss. Diagnosis is made by biopsy, percutaneously for peripheral liver lesions, or more commonly via endoscopic retrograde cholangiopancreatography (ERCP) under direct vision for central lesions. The tumors often stain positively for cytokeratins 7, 8, and 19 and negatively for cytokeratin 20. However, histology alone cannot usually distinguish CCC from metastases from colon or pancreas primary tumors. Serologic tumor markers appear to be nonspecific, but CEA, CA 19–9, and CA-125 are often elevated in CCC patients and are useful for following response to therapy. Radiologic evaluation typically starts with ultrasound, which is very useful in visualizing dilated bile ducts, and then proceeds with either MRI or magnetic resonance cholangiopancreatography (MRCP) or helical CT scans. Invasive cholangiopancreatography (ERCP) is then needed to define the biliary tree and obtain a biopsy or is needed therapeutically to decompress an obstructed biliary tree with internal stent placement. If that fails, then percutaneous biliary drainage will be needed, with the biliary drainage flowing into an external bag. Central tumors often invade the porta hepatis, and loco-regional lymph node involvement by tumor is frequent.

TREATMENT Cholangiocarcinoma

Hilar CCC is resectable in ~30% of patients and usually involves bile duct resection and lymphadenectomy. Typical survival is approximately 24 months, with recurrences being mainly in the operative bed but with ~30% in the lungs and liver. Distal CCC, which involves the main ducts, is normally treated by resection of the extrahepatic bile ducts, often with pancreaticoduodenectomy. Survival is similar. Due to the high rates of locoregional recurrences or positive surgical margins, many patients receive postoperative adjuvant radiotherapy. Its effect on survival has not been assessed. Intraluminal brachyradiotherapy has also shown some promise. However, photodynamic therapy enhanced survival in one study. In this technique, sodium porfimer is injected intravenously and then subjected to intraluminal red light laser photoactivation. OLTX has been assessed for treatment of unresectable CCC. The 5-year survival rate was ~20%, so enthusiasm waned. However, neoadjuvant radiotherapy with sensitizing chemotherapy has shown better survival rates for CCC treated by OLTX and is currently used by UNOS for perihilar CCC, size <3 cm with neither intrahepatic or extrahepatic metastases. Multiple chemotherapeutic agents have been assessed for activity and survival in unresectable CCC. Most have been inactive. However, both systemic and hepatic arterial gemcitabine have shown promising results. The combination of cisplatin plus gemcitabine has produced a survival advantage compared with gemcitabine alone and is considered standard therapy for unresectable CCC.

GALLBLADDER CANCER

Gallbladder cancer (GB Ca) has an even worse prognosis than CCC and with typical survival time of ~6 months or less. Women are affected much more commonly than men (4:1), unlike HCC or CCC, and GB Ca occurs more frequently than CCC. Most patients have a history of antecedent gallstones, but very few patients with gallstones develop GB Ca (~0.2%). It presents similarly to CCC and is often diagnosed unexpectedly during gallstone or cholecystitis surgery. Presentation is typically that of chronic cholecystitis, chronic right upper quadrant pain and weight loss. Useful but nonspecific serum markers include CEA and CA 19-9. CT scans or MRCP typically reveals a gallbladder mass. The mainstay of treatment is surgical, either simple or radical cholecystectomy for stages I or II disease, respectively. Survival rates are near 100% at 5 years for stage I and range from 60–90% at 5 years for stage II. More advanced GB Ca has worse survival, and many patients' disease is unresectable. Adjuvant radiotherapy, used in the presence of local lymph node disease, has not been shown to enhance survival. Chemotherapy is not useful in advanced or metastatic GB Ca.

CARCINOMA OF THE AMPULLA OF VATER

This tumor arises within 2 cm of the distal end of the common bile duct and is mainly (90%) an adenocarcinoma. Locoregional lymph nodes are commonly involved (50%), and the liver is the most frequent site for metastases. The most common clinical presentation is jaundice, and many patients also have pruritus, weight loss, and epigastric pain. Initial evaluation is performed with an abdominal ultrasound to assess vascular involvement, biliary dilation, and liver lesions. This is followed by a CT scan or MRI and especially MRCP. The most effective therapy is resection by pylorus-sparing pancreaticoduodenectomy, an aggressive procedure resulting in better survival rates than with local resection. Survival rates are ~25% at 5 years in operable patients with involved lymph nodes and ~50% in patients without involved nodes. Unlike CCC, approximately 80% of patients are thought to be resectable at diagnosis. Adjuvant chemotherapy or radiotherapy has not been shown to enhance survival. For metastatic tumors, chemotherapy is currently experimental.

TUMORS METASTATIC TO THE LIVER

These are predominantly from colon, pancreas, and breast primary tumors but can originate from any organ primary. Ocular melanomas are prone to liver metastasis. Tumor spread to the liver normally carries a poor prognosis for that tumor type. Colorectal and breast hepatic metastases were previously treated with continuous hepatic arterial infusion chemotherapy. However, more effective systemic drugs for each of these two cancers, especially the addition of oxaliplatin to colorectal cancer regimens, have reduced the use of hepatic artery infusion therapy. In a large randomized study of systemic versus infusional plus systemic chemotherapy for resected colorectal metastases to the liver, the patients receiving infusional therapy had no survival advantage, mainly due to extrahepatic tumor spread. ^{90}Yttrium resin beads are approved in the United States for treatment of colorectal hepatic metastases. The role of this modality, either alone or in combination with chemotherapy, is being evaluated in many centers. Palliation my be obtained from chemoembolization, PEI, or RFA.

BENIGN LIVER TUMORS

Three common benign tumors occur and all are found predominantly in women. They are *hemangiomas, adenomas,* and *focal nodular hyperplasia* (FNH). FNH is typically benign, and usually no treatment is needed. Hemangiomas are the most common and are entirely benign. Treatment is unnecessary unless their expansion causes symptoms. Adenomas are associated with contraceptive hormone use. They can cause pain and can bleed or rupture, causing acute problems. Their main interest for the physician is a low potential for malignant change and a 30% risk of bleeding. For this reason, considerable effort has gone into differentiating these three entities radiologically. On discovery of a liver mass, patients are usually advised to stop taking sex steroids, as adenoma regression may then occasionally occur. Adenomas can often be large masses ranging from 8–15 cm. Due to their size and definite, but low, malignant potential and potential for bleeding, adenomas are typically resected. The most useful diagnostic differentiating tool is a triphasic CT scan performed with HCC fast bolus protocol for arterial-phase imaging, together with subsequent delayed venous-phase imaging. Adenomas usually do not appear on the basis of cirrhosis, although both adenomas and HCCs are intensely vascular on the CT arterial phase and both can exhibit hemorrhage (40% of adenomas). However, adenomas have smooth, well-defined edges and enhance homogeneously, especially in the portal venous phase on delayed images, when HCCs no longer enhance. FNHs exhibit a characteristic central scar that is hypovascular on the arterial-phase and hypervascular on the delayed-phase CT images. MRI is even more sensitive in depicting the characteristic central scar of FNH.

CHAPTER 40
PANCREATIC CANCER

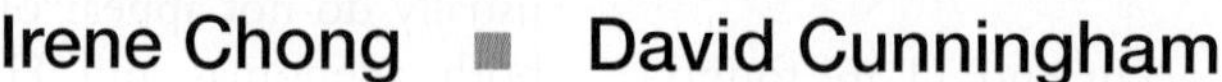
Irene Chong ■ David Cunningham

Pancreatic cancer is the fourth leading cause of cancer death in the United States and is associated with a poor prognosis. Endocrine tumors affecting the pancreas are discussed in Chap. 49. Infiltrating ductal adenocarcinomas, the subject of this chapter, account for the vast majority of cases and arise most frequently in the head of the pancreas. At the time of diagnosis, 85–90% of patients have inoperable or metastatic disease, which is reflected in the 5-year survival rate of only 5% for all stages combined. An improved 5-year survival of up to 20% may be achieved when the tumor is detected at an early stage and when complete surgical resection is accomplished.

EPIDEMIOLOGY

Pancreatic cancer represents 3% of all newly diagnosed malignancies in the United States. The most common age group at diagnosis is 60–79 years for both sexes. It was estimated that pancreatic cancer would be diagnosed in approximately 43,140 patients and account for 36,800 deaths in 2010. Over the past 30 years, 5-year survival rates have not improved substantially.

RISK FACTORS

Cigarette smoking may be the cause of up to 20–25% of all pancreatic cancers and is the most common environmental risk factor for this disease. Other risk factors are not well established due to inconsistent results from epidemiologic studies but include chronic pancreatitis and diabetes. It is difficult to evaluate whether these conditions are causally related or develop as a consequence of cancer. Alcohol does not appear to be a risk factor unless excess consumption gives rise to chronic pancreatitis.

GENETIC CONSIDERATIONS

Pancreatic cancer is associated with a number of well-defined molecular hallmarks. The most frequent genetic aberrations comprise *KRAS* mutations, mostly affecting codon 12, which are observed in 60–75% of pancreatic cancers. The tumor-suppressor genes *p16, p53,* and *SMAD4* are frequently inactivated; the *p16* gene locus on chromosome 9p21 is deleted in up to 95% of tumors, the *p53* gene is inactivated by mutation or deleted in 50–70% of tumors, and the *SMAD4* gene is deleted in 55% of pancreatic tumors. Furthermore, *SMAD4* gene inactivation is associated with poorer survival in patients with surgically resected pancreatic adenocarcinoma. *IGF-1R* and focal adhesion kinase (*FAK*) interact to promote cell proliferation and survival, and their simultaneous inhibition synergistically inhibits pancreatic cell growth. Overexpression and/or aberrant activation of *c-Src* is frequently observed, which results in cell adhesion, enhanced migration, invasion, and cell proliferation. Survivin is overexpressed in more than 80% of pancreatic tumors, which results in resistance to apoptosis, and genomic sequencing has identified *PALB2* as a susceptibility gene for pancreatic cancer.

Up to 16% of pancreatic cancers are thought to be inherited. This occurs in three separate clinical settings: (1) familial multiorgan cancer syndromes; (2) genetically driven chronic diseases; and (3) familial pancreatic cancer with as yet unidentified genetic abnormalities, which comprise the largest proportion of inherited pancreatic cancer. The familial multiorgan cancer syndromes consist of Peutz-Jeghers syndrome, familial atypical multiple mole melanoma (FAMMM), familial breast–ovarian cancer associated with germline mutations in *BRCA1* and *BRCA2*, hereditary nonpolyposis colorectal cancer (HNPCC), familial adenomatous polyposis (FAP), and Li-Fraumeni syndrome. Peutz-Jeghers syndrome, associated with mutations in the *STK11* gene, carries the highest lifetime risk of pancreatic cancer with a relative risk of approximately 132-fold above that of the general population. Genetically driven chronic causes of pancreatic cancer include hereditary pancreatitis, cystic fibrosis, and ataxia telangiectasia. The absolute number of affected first-degree relatives is also correlated with increased cancer risk, and patients with at least two first-degree relatives with pancreatic cancer should be considered to have familial pancreatic cancer until proven otherwise.

SCREENING AND EARLY DETECTION

Screening is not routinely recommended as putative tumor markers such as Ca 19-9 and CEA have insufficient sensitivity, and computed tomography (CT) has inadequate resolution to detect pancreatic dysplasia. Endoscopic ultrasound (EUS) is a more promising screening tool, and preclinical efforts are focused on identifying biomarkers that may detect pancreatic cancer at an early stage. Consensus practice recommendations based largely on expert opinion have chosen a threshold of >10-fold increased risk for developing pancreatic cancer to select individuals who may benefit from screening. This includes family members with ≥3 first-degree relatives with pancreatic cancer and patients with FAMMM, Peutz-Jeghers syndrome, or hereditary pancreatitis.

CLINICAL FEATURES

CLINICAL PRESENTATION

Obstructive jaundice occurs frequently when the cancer is located in the head of pancreas. This may be accompanied by symptoms of abdominal discomfort, pruritus, lethargy, and weight loss. Less common presenting features include epigastric pain, backache, new-onset diabetes mellitus, and acute pancreatitis caused by pressure effects on the pancreatic duct. Nausea and vomiting, resulting from gastroduodenal obstruction, may also be a symptom of this disease.

PHYSICAL SIGNS

Patients can present with jaundice and cachexia, and scratch marks may be present. Of patients with operable tumors, 25% have a palpable gallbladder (Courvoisier's sign). Physical signs related to the development of distant metastases include hepatomegaly, ascites, left supraclavicular lymphadenopathy (Virchow's node), and periumbilical lymphadenopathy (Sister Mary Joseph's nodes).

DIAGNOSIS

DIAGNOSTIC IMAGING

Patients who present with clinical features suggestive of pancreatic cancer undergo imaging to confirm the presence of a tumor and to establish whether the mass is likely to be inflammatory or malignant in nature. Other imaging objectives include the local and distant staging of the tumor, which will determine resectability and provide prognostic information. Dual-phase, contrast-enhanced spiral CT is the imaging modality of choice (Fig. 40-1). It provides accurate visualization of surrounding viscera, vessels, and lymph nodes, thus determining tumor resectability. Intestinal infiltration, and liver and lung metastases are also reliably depicted on CT. There is no advantage of magnetic resonance imaging (MRI) over CT in predicting tumor resectability, but selected cases may benefit from MRI to characterize the nature of small indeterminate liver lesions and to evaluate the cause of biliary dilatation when no obvious mass is seen on CT. Endoscopic retrograde cholangiopancreatography (ERCP) is useful for revealing small pancreatic lesions, identifying stricture or obstruction in pancreatic or common bile ducts, and facilitating stent placement (Fig. 40-2). Magnetic resonance cholangiopancreatography (MRCP) is a noninvasive method for accurately depicting the level and degree of bile and pancreatic duct dilatation. EUS is highly sensitive in detecting lesions smaller than 3 cm in size and is useful as a local staging tool for assessing vascular invasion and lymph node involvement. Positron-emission tomography with fluorodeoxyglucose positron emission tomography (FDG-PET) should be considered before surgery or radical chemoradiotherapy

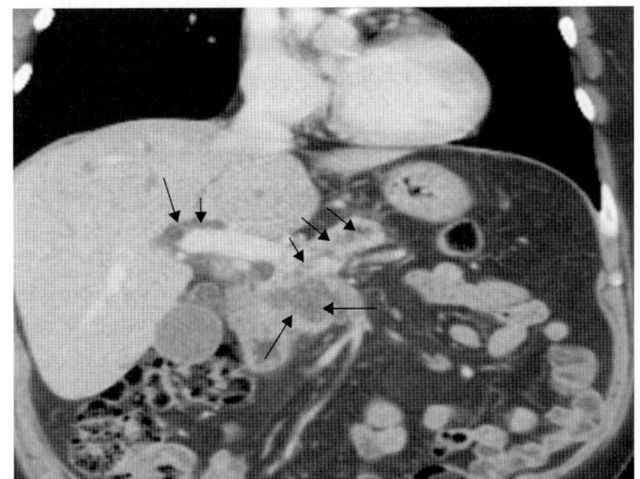

FIGURE 40-1
Coronal computed tomography scan showing pancreatic cancer and dilated intrahepatic and pancreatic ducts (*arrows*).

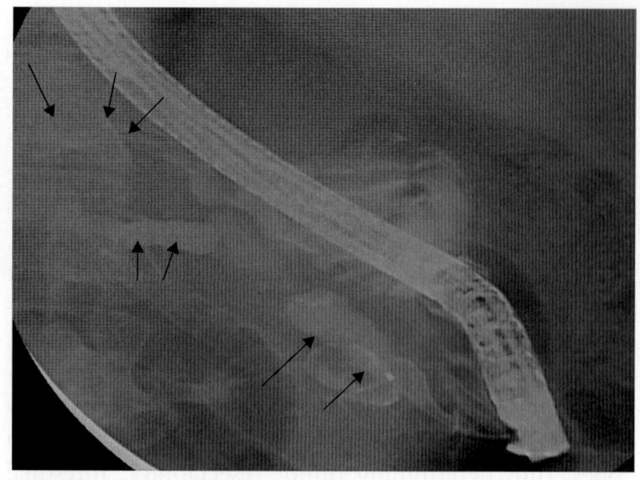

FIGURE 40-2
Endoscopic retrograde cholangiopancreatography showing contrast in dilated pancreatic duct (*arrows*).

(CRT), as it is superior to conventional imaging in detecting distant metastases.

TISSUE DIAGNOSIS AND CYTOLOGY

Preoperative confirmation of malignancy is not always necessary in patients with radiologic appearances consistent with operable pancreatic cancer. However, EUS-guided fine-needle aspiration is the technique of choice when there is any doubt and for use in patients who require neoadjuvant treatment. It has an accuracy of approximately 90% and has a smaller risk of intraperitoneal dissemination compared with the percutaneous route. Percutaneous biopsy of the pancreatic primary or liver metastases is only acceptable in patients with inoperable or metastatic disease. ERCP is a useful method for obtaining ductal brushings, but the diagnostic value of pancreatic juice sampling is only in the order of 25–30%.

SERUM MARKERS

Tumor-associated carbohydrate antigen 19-9 (CA 19-9) is elevated in approximately 70–80% of patients with pancreatic carcinoma but is not recommended as a routine diagnostic or screening test as its sensitivity and specificity are inadequate for accurate diagnosis. Preoperative CA 19-9 levels correlate with tumor stage, and postresection CA 19-9 level has prognostic value. It is an indicator of asymptomatic recurrence in patients with completely resected tumors and is used as a biomarker of response in patients with advanced disease undergoing chemotherapy. A number of studies have established a high pretreatment CA 19-9 level as an independent prognostic factor.

STAGING

The American Joint Committee on Cancer (AJCC) tumor, node, metastasis (TNM) staging of pancreatic cancer takes into account the location and size of the tumor, the involvement of lymph nodes, and distant metastasis. This information is then combined to assign a stage (Fig. 40-3). From a practical standpoint, patients are grouped according to whether the cancer is resectable, locally advanced (unresectable, but without distant spread), or metastatic.

TREATMENT Pancreatic Cancer

RESECTABLE DISEASE Approximately 10% of patients present with localized nonmetastatic disease that is potentially suitable for surgical resection. Approximately 30% of patients have R1 resection (microscopic residual disease) following surgery. Those who undergo R0 resection (no microscopic or macroscopic residual tumor) and who receive adjuvant treatment have the best chance of cure, with an estimated median survival time of 20–23 months and a 5-year survival rate of approximately 20%. Outcomes are more favorable in patients with small <3 cm, well-differentiated tumors, and lymph node–negative disease.

Patients should have surgery in dedicated pancreatic centers that have lower postoperative morbidity and mortality rates. The standard surgical procedure for patients with tumors of the pancreatic head or uncinate process is a pylorus-preserving pancreaticoduodenectomy (modified Whipple's procedure). The procedure of choice for tumors of the pancreatic body and tail is a distal pancreatectomy, which routinely includes splenectomy.

Postoperative treatment, either chemotherapy or CRT, improves long-term outcomes in this group of patients. Adjuvant chemotherapy, comprising six cycles of fluorouracil (5FU) and folinic acid (FA) or gemcitabine, is common practice in Europe based on data from three randomized controlled trials (Table 40-1). Results from the European Study Group for Pancreatic Cancer 1 trial (ESPAC-1) revealed a median survival improvement from 14.7 months with surgery alone to 20.1 months with surgery plus adjuvant 5FU/FA; patients did not benefit from CRT in this study. The Charité Onkologie trial (CONKO 001) found that the use of gemcitabine after complete resection significantly delayed the development of recurrent disease compared with surgery alone. The ESPAC-3 trial, which investigated the benefit of adjuvant 5FU/FA versus gemcitabine, revealed no survival difference between the two drugs. However, the

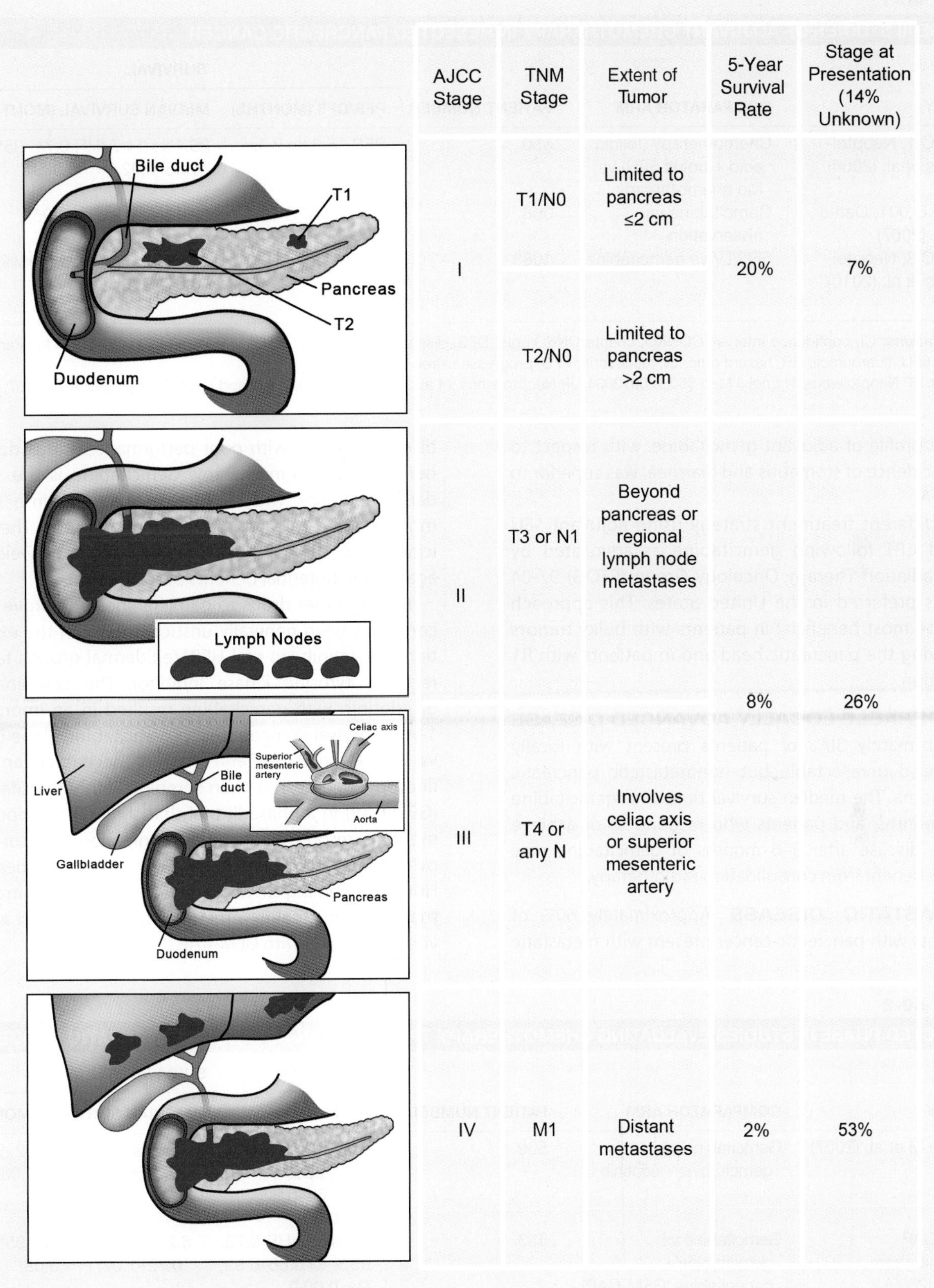

AJCC Stage	TNM Stage	Extent of Tumor	5-Year Survival Rate	Stage at Presentation (14% Unknown)
I	T1/N0	Limited to pancreas ≤2 cm	20%	7%
	T2/N0	Limited to pancreas >2 cm		
II	T3 or N1	Beyond pancreas or regional lymph node metastases	8%	26%
III	T4 or any N	Involves celiac axis or superior mesenteric artery		
IV	M1	Distant metastases	2%	53%

FIGURE 40-3
Staging of pancreatic cancer and survival according to stage. TNM, tumor, node, metastasis. (*Illustration by Stephen Millward.*)

TABLE 40-1

PHASE III STUDIES OF ADJUVANT CHEMOTHERAPY IN RESECTED PANCREATIC CANCER

			SURVIVAL	
STUDY	**COMPARATOR ARM**	**PATIENT NUMBER**	**PFS/DFS (MONTHS)**	**MEDIAN SURVIVAL (MONTHS)**
ESPAC 1, Neoptolemos et al. (2004)	Chemotherapy (folinic acid + bolus 5FU) vs mo chemotherapy	550	PFS 15.3 vs 9.4. ($P = 0.02$)	20.1 vs 14.7 (HR 0.71, 95% CI 0.55–0.92, $P = 0.009$)
CONKO 001, Oettle et al. (2007)	Gemcitabine vs observation	368	Median DFS 13.4 vs 6.9 ($P < 0.001$)	22.1 vs 20.2 ($P = 0.06$)
ESPAC 3, Neoptolemos et al. (2010)	5FU/LV vs gemcitabine	1088		23 vs 23.6 (HR 0.94, 95% CI 0.81–1.08, $P = 0.39$)

Abbreviations: CI, confidence interval; CONKO, charite ONKOlogie; DFS, disease free survival; ESPAC, European Study Group for Pancreatic Cancer; 5FU, fluorouracil; HR, hazard ratio; LV, leucovorin; PFS, progression-free survival.
Sources: JP Neoptolemos: N Engl J Med 350:1200, 2004; JP Neoptolemos, et al: JAMA 304:1073, 2010; and H Oettle et al: JAMA 297:267, 2007.

safety profile of adjuvant gemcitabine, with respect to the incidence of stomatitis and diarrhea, was superior to 5FU/FA.

A different treatment strategy using adjuvant 5FU based CRT following gemcitabine as advocated by the Radiation Therapy Oncology Group (RTOG) 97-04 trial is preferred in the United States. This approach may be most beneficial in patients with bulky tumors involving the pancreatic head and in patients with R1 resection.

INOPERABLE LOCALLY ADVANCED DISEASE

Approximately 30% of patients present with locally advanced unresectable but nonmetastatic pancreatic carcinoma. The median survival time with gemcitabine is 9 months, and patients who respond to or achieve stable disease after 3–6 months of gemcitabine may derive benefit from consolidation radiotherapy.

METASTATIC DISEASE Approximately 60% of patients with pancreatic cancer present with metastatic disease. Patients with poor performance status do not benefit from chemotherapy. Gemcitabine is the standard treatment with a median survival time of 6 months and a 1-year survival rate of only 20%. The toxicities associated with gemcitabine need to be weighed against the potential benefits of treatment.

Adding other drugs to gemcitabine to improve outcome has been generally unsuccessful with the exception of erlotinib, an oral HER1/epidermal growth factor receptor tyrosine kinase inhibitor. The combination of erlotinib with gemcitabine resulted in an improved 1-year survival compared with gemcitabine alone (23% vs 17%; $P = 0.023$) (Table 40-2). Capecitabine, an oral fluoropyrimidine, has been combined with gemcitabine (GEM-CAP) in a phase III trial that showed an improvement in response rate and progression-free survival over single-agent gemcitabine but no survival benefit. However, pooling of two other randomized controlled trials with this trial in a meta-analysis resulted in a survival advantage with GEM-CAP.

TABLE 40-2

SELECTED PHASE III STUDIES EVALUATING CHEMOTHERAPY TREATMENT IN ADVANCED PANCREATIC CANCER

			SURVIVAL	
STUDY	**COMPARATOR ARM**	**PATIENT NUMBER**	**PFS (MONTHS)**	**MEDIAN SURVIVAL (MONTHS)**
Moore M et al. (2007)	Gemcitabine vs gemcitabine + erlotinib	569	3.55 vs 3.75 (HR 0.77, 95% CI 0. 64–0.92, $P = 0.004$)	5.91 vs 6.24 (HR 0.82, 95% CI 0.69–0.99, $P = 0.038$)
GEM-CAP Cunningham, et al. (2009)	Gemcitabine vs gemcitabine + capecitabine (GEM-CAP)	533	3.8 vs 5.3 (HR 0.78, 95% CI 0.66–0.93, $P = 0.004$)	6.2 vs 7.1 (HR 0.86, 95% CI 0.72–1.02, $P = 0.08$)
GEM-CAP meta-analysis, Cunningham et al. (2009)	Gemcitabine vs GEM-CAP	935		Overall survival in favor of GEM-CAP (HR 0.86, 95% CI 0.75–0.98, $P = 0.02$)

Abbreviations: CI, confidence interval; HR, hazard ratio; PFS, progression-free survival.
Sources: D Cunningham et al: J Clin Oncol 27:5513, 2009 and MJ Moore et al: J Clin Oncol 26:1960, 2007.

A trial in good performance status patients with metastatic pancreatic cancer showed improved survival with the combination of 5FU/FA, irinotecan and oxaliplatin (FOLFIRINOX) compared with gemcitabine, but with increased toxicity. Nab-paclitaxel (Abraxane), an albumin bound nanoparticle formulation of paclitaxel, given with gemcitabine also shows promising activity.

FUTURE DIRECTIONS

The early detection and future treatment of pancreatic cancer rely on an improved understanding of molecular pathways involved in the development of this disease. This will ultimately lead to the discovery of novel agents and the identification of patient groups who are likely to benefit most from targeted therapy.

CHAPTER 41
BLADDER AND RENAL CELL CARCINOMAS

Howard I. Scher ■ Robert J. Motzer

BLADDER CANCER

A transitional cell epithelium lines the urinary tract from the renal pelvis to the ureter, urinary bladder, and the proximal two-thirds of the urethra. Cancers can occur at any point: 90% of malignancies develop in the bladder, 8% in the renal pelvis, and the remaining 2% in the ureter or urethra. Bladder cancer is the fourth most common cancer in men and the thirteenth in women; an estimated 70,530 new cases and 14,680 deaths in the United States were predicted for the year 2010. The almost 5:1 ratio of incidence to mortality reflects the higher frequency of the less lethal superficial variants compared with the more lethal invasive and metastatic variants. The incidence is three times higher in men than in women and twofold higher in whites than blacks, with a median age at diagnosis of 65 years.

Once diagnosed, urothelial tumors exhibit polychronotropism—the tendency to recur over time and in new locations in the urothelial tract. As long as urothelium is present, continuous monitoring of the tract is required.

EPIDEMIOLOGY

Cigarette smoking is believed to contribute to up to 50% of the diagnosed urothelial cancers in men and up to 40% in women. The risk of developing a urothelial malignancy in male smokers is increased two- to fourfold relative to nonsmokers and continues for 10 years or longer after cessation. Other implicated agents include the aniline dyes, the drugs phenacetin and chlornaphazine, and external-beam radiation. Chronic cyclophosphamide exposure may also increase risk, whereas vitamin A supplements appear to be protective. Exposure to *Schistosoma haematobium*, a parasite found in many developing countries, is associated with an increase in both squamous and transitional cell carcinomas of the bladder.

PATHOLOGY

Clinical subtypes are grouped into three categories: 75% are superficial, 20% invade muscle, and 5% are metastatic at presentation. Staging of the tumor within the bladder is based on the pattern of growth and depth of invasion: Ta lesions grow as exophytic lesions; carcinoma in situ (CIS) lesions start on the surface and tend to invade. The revised tumor, node, metastasis (TNM) staging system is illustrated in Fig. 41-1. About half of invasive tumors presented originally as superficial lesions that later progressed. Tumors are also rated by grade. Grade I lesions (highly differentiated tumors) rarely progress to a higher stage, whereas grade III tumors do.

More than 95% of urothelial tumors in the United States are transitional cell in origin. Pure squamous cancers with keratinization constitute 3%, adenocarcinomas 2%, and small cell tumors (with paraneoplastic syndromes) <1%. Adenocarcinomas develop primarily in the urachal remnant in the dome of the bladder or in the periurethral tissues; some assume a signet cell histology. Lymphomas and melanomas are rare. Of the transitional cell tumors, low-grade papillary lesions that grow on a central stalk are most common. These tumors are very friable, have a tendency to bleed, are at high risk for recurrence, and yet rarely progress to the more lethal invasive variety. In contrast, CIS is a high-grade tumor that is considered a precursor of the more lethal muscle-invasive disease.

PATHOGENESIS

The multicentric nature of the disease and high rate of recurrence have led to the hypothesis of a field defect in the urothelium that results in a predisposition to cancer. Molecular genetic analyses suggest that the superficial and invasive lesions develop along distinct molecular pathways in which primary tumorigenic aberrations precede secondary changes associated with progression

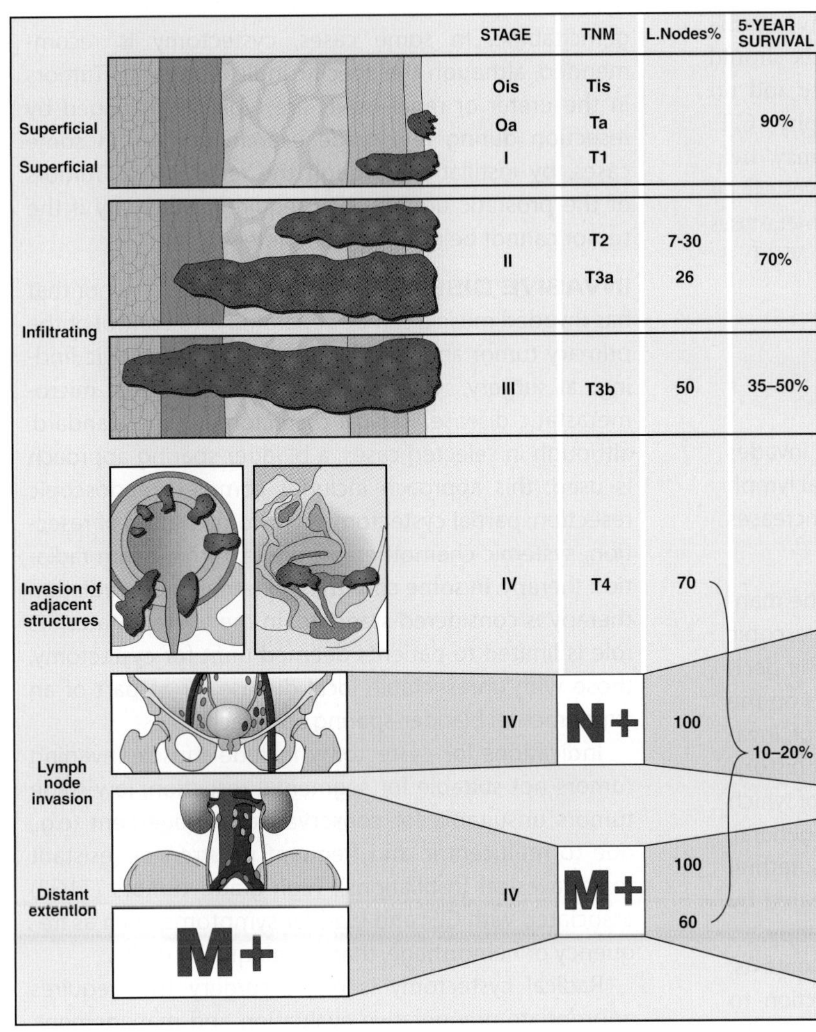

FIGURE 41-1
Bladder staging. TNM, tumor, node, metastasis.

to a more advanced stage. Low-grade papillary tumors that do not tend to invade or metastasize harbor constitutive activation of the receptor–tyrosine kinase–Ras signal transduction pathway and a high frequency of fibroblast growth factor receptor 3 (FGFR3) mutations. In contrast, CIS and invasive tumors have a higher frequency of *TP53* and *RB* gene alternations. Within all clinical stages, including Tis, T1, and T2 or greater lesions, tumors with alterations in *p53*, *p21*, and/or *RB* have a higher probability of recurrence, metastasis, and death from disease.

CLINICAL PRESENTATION, DIAGNOSIS, AND STAGING

Hematuria occurs in 80–90% of patients and often reflects exophytic tumors. The bladder is the most common source of gross hematuria (40%), but benign cystitis (22%) is a more common cause than bladder cancer (15%). Microscopic hematuria is more commonly of prostate origin (25%); only 2% of bladder cancers produce microscopic hematuria. Once hematuria is documented, a urinary cytology, visualization of the urothelial tract by computed tomography (CT) or intravenous pyelogram, and cystoscopy are recommended if no other etiology is found. Screening asymptomatic individuals for hematuria increases the diagnosis of tumors at an early stage but has not been shown to prolong life. After hematuria, irritative symptoms are the next most common presentation, which may reflect in situ disease. Obstruction of the ureters may cause flank pain. Symptoms of metastatic disease are rarely the first presenting sign.

The endoscopic evaluation includes an examination under anesthesia to determine whether a palpable mass is present. A flexible endoscope is inserted into the bladder, and bladder barbotage is performed. The visual inspection includes mapping the location, size, and number of lesions, as well as a description of the growth pattern (solid vs papillary). An intraoperative video is often recorded. All visible tumors should be resected, and a sample of the muscle underlying the tumor should be obtained to assess the depth of invasion. Normal-appearing areas are biopsied at random to ensure no field defect. A notation is made as to whether a tumor was completely or incompletely resected. Selective catheterization and visualization of the upper tracts should be performed if the cytology results are positive and no disease is visible in the bladder. Ultrasonography, CT, and/or magnetic resonance imaging (MRI) may help to determine whether a tumor extends to perivesical fat (T3) and to document nodal spread. Distant metastases are assessed by CT of the chest and abdomen, MRI, or radionuclide imaging of the skeleton.

TREATMENT Bladder Cancer

Management depends on whether the tumor invades muscle and whether it has spread to the regional lymph nodes and beyond. The probability of spread increases with increasing T stage.

SUPERFICIAL DISEASE At a minimum, the management of a superficial tumor is complete endoscopic resection with or without intravesical therapy. The decision to recommend intravesical therapy depends on the histologic subtype, number of lesions, depth of invasion, presence or absence of CIS, and antecedent history. Recurrences develop in upward of 50% of cases, of which 5–20% progress to a more advanced stage. In general, solitary papillary lesions are managed by transurethral surgery alone. CIS and recurrent disease are treated by transurethral surgery followed by intravesical therapy.

Intravesical therapies are used in two general contexts: as an adjuvant to a complete endoscopic resection to prevent recurrence or, less commonly, to eliminate disease that cannot be controlled by endoscopic resection alone. Intravesical treatments are advised for patients with recurrent disease, >40% involvement of the bladder surface by tumor, diffuse CIS, or T1 disease. The standard intravesical therapy, based on randomized comparisons, is bacillus Calmette-Guerin (BCG) in six weekly instillations followed by monthly maintenance administrations for ≥1 year. Other agents with activity include mitomycin-C, interferon (IFN), and gemcitabine. The side effects of intravesical therapies include dysuria; urinary frequency; and, depending on the drug, myelosuppression or contact dermatitis. Rarely, intravesical BCG may produce a systemic illness associated with granulomatous infections in multiple sites that requires antituberculin therapy.

Following the endoscopic resection, patients are monitored for recurrence at 3-month intervals during the first year. Recurrence may develop anywhere along the urothelial tract, including the renal pelvis, ureter, or urethra. A consequence of the "successful" treatment of tumors in the bladder is an increase in the frequency of extravesical recurrences (e.g., urethra or ureter). Those with persistent disease in the bladder or new tumors are generally considered for a second course of BCG or for intravesical chemotherapy with valrubicin or gemcitabine. In some cases, cystectomy is recommended, although the specific indications vary. Tumors in the ureter or renal pelvis are typically managed by resection during retrograde examination or, in some cases, by instillation through the renal pelvis. Tumors of the prostatic urethra may require cystectomy if the tumor cannot be resected completely.

INVASIVE DISEASE The treatment of a tumor that has invaded muscle can be separated into control of the primary tumor and, depending on the pathologic findings at surgery, systemic chemotherapy to treat micrometastatic disease. Radical cystectomy is the standard, although in selected cases, a bladder-sparing approach is used; this approach includes complete endoscopic resection; partial cystectomy; or a combination of resection, systemic chemotherapy, and external-beam radiation therapy. In some countries, external-beam radiation therapy is considered standard. In the United States, its role is limited to patients deemed unfit for cystectomy, those with unresectable local disease, or as part of an experimental bladder-sparing approach.

Indications for cystectomy include muscle-invading tumors not suitable for segmental resection; low-stage tumors unsuitable for conservative management (e.g., due to multicentric and frequent recurrences resistant to intravesical instillations); high-grade tumors (T1G3) associated with CIS; and bladder symptoms, such as frequency or hemorrhage, that impair quality of life.

Radical cystectomy is major surgery that requires appropriate preoperative evaluation and management. The procedure involves removal of the bladder and pelvic lymph nodes and creation of a conduit or reservoir for urinary flow. Grossly abnormal lymph nodes are evaluated by frozen section. If metastases are confirmed, the procedure is often aborted. In males, radical cystectomy includes the removal of the prostate, seminal vesicles, and proximal urethra. Impotence is universal unless the nerves responsible for erectile function are preserved. In females, the procedure includes removal of the bladder, urethra, uterus, fallopian tubes, ovaries, anterior vaginal wall, and surrounding fascia.

Previously, urine flow was managed by directing the ureters to the abdominal wall, where it was collected in an external appliance. Currently, most patients receive either a continent cutaneous reservoir constructed from detubularized bowel or an orthotopic neobladder. Some 70% of men receive a neobladder. With a continent reservoir, 65–85% of men will be continent at night and 85–90% during the day. Cutaneous reservoirs are drained by intermittent catheterization; orthotopic neobladders are drained more naturally. Contraindications to a neobladder include renal insufficiency, an inability to self-catheterize, or an exophytic tumor or CIS in the urethra. Diffuse CIS in the bladder is a relative

TABLE 41-1

SURVIVAL FOLLOWING SURGERY FOR BLADDER CANCER

PATHOLOGIC STAGE	5-YEAR SURVIVAL, %	10-YEAR SURVIVAL, %
T2, N0	89	87
T3a, N0	78	76
T3b, N0	62	61
T4, N0	50	45
Any T, N1	35	34

contraindication based on the risk of a urethral recurrence. Concurrent ulcerative colitis or Crohn's disease may hinder the use of resected bowel.

A partial cystectomy may be considered when the disease is limited to the dome of the bladder, a margin of at least 2 cm can be achieved, there is no CIS in other sites, and the bladder capacity is adequate after the tumor has been removed. This occurs in 5–10% of cases. Carcinomas in the ureter or in the renal pelvis are treated with nephroureterectomy with a bladder cuff to remove the tumor.

The probability of recurrence following surgery is predicted on the basis of pathologic stage, presence, or absence of lymphatic or vascular invasion, and nodal spread. Among those whose cancers recur, the recurrence develops in a median of 1 year (range, 0.04–11.1 years). Long-term outcomes vary by pathologic stage and histology (Table 41-1). The number of lymph nodes removed is also prognostic, whether or not the nodes contained tumor.

Chemotherapy (described later) has been shown to prolong the survival of patients with invasive disease but only when combined with definitive treatment of the bladder by radical cystectomy or radiation therapy. Thus, for the majority of patients, chemotherapy alone is inadequate to clear the bladder of disease. Experimental studies are evaluating bladder preservation strategies by combining chemotherapy and radiation therapy in patients whose tumors were endoscopically removed.

METASTATIC DISEASE The primary goal of treatment for metastatic disease is to achieve complete remission with chemotherapy alone or with a combined-modality approach of chemotherapy followed by surgical resection of residual disease, as is done routinely for the treatment of germ cell tumors. One can define a goal in terms of cure or palliation on the basis of the probability of achieving a complete response to chemotherapy using prognostic factors, such as Karnofsky Performance Status (KPS) (<80%), and whether the pattern of spread is nodal or visceral (liver, lung, or bone). For those with zero, one, or two risk factors, the probabilities of complete remission are 38, 25, and 5%, respectively, and median survival times are 33, 13.4, and 9.3 months, respectively. Patients who are functionally compromised or who have visceral disease or bone metastases rarely achieve long-term survival. The toxicities also vary as a function of risk, and treatment-related mortality rates are as high as 3–4% using some combinations in these poor-risk patient groups.

CHEMOTHERAPY A number of chemotherapeutic drugs have shown activity as single agents; cisplatin, paclitaxel, and gemcitabine are considered most active. Standard therapy consists of two-, three-, or four-drug combinations. Overall response rates of >50% have been reported using combinations such as methotrexate, vinblastine, doxorubicin, and cisplatin (M-VAC); cisplatin and paclitaxel (PT); gemcitabine and cisplatin (GC); or gemcitabine, paclitaxel, and cisplatin (GTC). M-VAC was considered standard, but the toxicities of neutropenia and fever, mucositis, diminished renal and auditory function, and peripheral neuropathy led to the development of alternative regimens. At present, GC is used more commonly than M-VAC, based on the results of a comparative trial of M-VAC versus GC that showed less neutropenia and fever and less mucositis for the GC regimen. Anemia and thrombocytopenia were more common with GC. GTC is not more effective than GC.

Chemotherapy has also been evaluated in the neoadjuvant and adjuvant settings. In a randomized trial, patients receiving three cycles of neoadjuvant M-VAC followed by cystectomy had significantly better median (6.2 years) and 5-year survival (57%) rates compared with cystectomy alone (median survival time, 3.8 years; 5-year survival rate, 42%). Similar results were obtained in an international study of three cycles of cisplatin, methotrexate, and vinblastine (CMV) followed by either radical cystectomy or radiation therapy. The decision to administer adjuvant therapy is based on the risk of recurrence after cystectomy. Indications for adjuvant chemotherapy include the presence of nodal disease, extravesical tumor extension, or vascular invasion in the resected specimen. Another study of adjuvant therapy found that four cycles of CMV delayed recurrence, although an effect on survival was less clear. Additional trials are studying taxane- and gemcitabine-based combinations.

The management of bladder cancer is summarized in Table 41-2.

CARCINOMA OF THE RENAL PELVIS AND URETER

About 2500 cases of renal pelvis and ureter cancer occur each year; nearly all are transitional cell carcinomas similar to bladder cancer in biology and appearance. This

TABLE 41-2

MANAGEMENT OF BLADDER CANCER

NATURE OF LESION	MANAGEMENT APPROACH
Superficial	Endoscopic removal, usually with intravesical therapy
Invasive disease	Cystectomy ± systemic chemotherapy (before or after surgery)
Metastatic disease	Curative or palliative chemotherapy (based on prognostic factors) ± surgery

tumor is also associated with chronic phenacetin abuse and with Balkan nephropathy, a chronic interstitial nephritis endemic in Bulgaria, Greece, Bosnia-Herzegovina, and Romania.

The most common symptom is painless gross hematuria, and the disease is usually detected on intravenous pyelography during the workup for hematuria. Patterns of spread are similar to those in bladder cancer. For low-grade disease localized to the renal pelvis and ureter, nephroureterectomy (including excision of the distal ureter with a portion of the bladder) is associated with a 5-year survival rate of 80–90%. More invasive or histologically poorly differentiated tumors are more likely to recur locally and to metastasize. Metastatic disease is treated with the chemotherapy used in bladder cancer, and the outcome is similar to that of metastatic transitional-cell cancer of bladder origin.

RENAL CELL CARCINOMA

Renal cell carcinomas account for 90–95% of malignant neoplasms arising from the kidney. Notable features include resistance to cytotoxic agents, infrequent responses to biologic response modifiers such as interleukin (IL) 2, robust activity to antiangiogenesis targeted agents, and a variable clinical course for patients with metastatic disease, including anecdotal reports of spontaneous regression.

EPIDEMIOLOGY

The incidence of renal cell carcinoma continues to rise and is now nearly 58,000 cases annually in the United States, resulting in 13,000 deaths. The male-to-female ratio is 2:1. Incidence peaks between the ages of 50 and 70 years, although this malignancy may be diagnosed at any age. Many environmental factors have been investigated as possible contributing causes; the strongest association is with cigarette smoking. Risk is also increased for patients who have acquired cystic disease of the kidney associated with end-stage renal disease and for those with tuberous sclerosis. Most cases are sporadic, although familial forms have been reported. One is associated with von Hippel–Lindau (VHL) syndrome. VHL syndrome is an autosomal dominant disorder. Genetic studies identified the *VHL* gene on the short arm of chromosome 3. Approximately 35% of individuals with VHL disease develop clear cell renal cell carcinoma. Other associated neoplasms include retinal hemangioma, hemangioblastoma of the spinal cord and cerebellum, pheochromocytoma, neuroendocrine tumors and cysts, and cysts in the epididymis of the testis in men and the broad ligament in women. Subtypes vary according to low risk (type 1) or high risk (type 2) of developing pheochromocytoma.

PATHOLOGY AND GENETICS

Renal cell neoplasia represents a heterogeneous group of tumors with distinct histopathologic, genetic, and clinical features ranging from benign to high-grade malignant (Table 41-3). They are classified on the basis of morphology and histology. Categories include clear cell carcinoma (60% of cases), papillary tumors (5–15%), chromophobic tumors (5–10%), oncocytomas (5–10%), and collecting or Bellini duct tumors (<1%). Papillary tumors tend to be bilateral and multifocal. Chromophobic tumors have a more indolent clinical course, and oncocytomas are considered benign neoplasms. In contrast, Bellini duct carcinomas, which are thought to

TABLE 41-3

CLASSIFICATION OF EPITHELIAL NEOPLASMS ARISING FROM THE KIDNEY

CARCINOMA TYPE	GROWTH PATTERN	CELL OF ORIGIN	CYTOGENETICS
Clear cell	Acinar or sarcomatoid	Proximal tubule	3p–
Papillary	Papillary or sarcomatoid	Proximal tubule	+7, +17, –Y
Chromophobic	Solid, tubular, or sarcomatoid	Cortical collecting duct	Hypodiploid
Oncocytic	Tumor nests	Cortical collecting duct	Undetermined
Collecting duct	Papillary or sarcomatoid	Medullary collecting duct	Undetermined

arise from the collecting ducts within the renal medulla, are very rare but very aggressive. Clear cell tumors, the predominant histology, are found in >80% of patients who develop metastases. Clear cell tumors arise from the epithelial cells of the proximal tubules and usually show chromosome 3p deletions. Deletions of 3p21–26 (where the *VHL* gene maps) are identified in patients with familial as well as sporadic tumors. *VHL* encodes a tumor-suppressor protein that is involved in regulating the transcription of vascular endothelial growth factor (VEGF), platelet-derived growth factor (PDGF), and a number of other hypoxia-inducible proteins. Inactivation of *VHL* leads to overexpression of these agonists of the VEGF and PDGF receptors, which promote tumor angiogenesis and tumor growth. Agents that inhibit proangiogenic growth factor activity show antitumor effects.

CLINICAL PRESENTATION

The presenting signs and symptoms include hematuria, abdominal pain, and a flank or abdominal mass. This classic triad occurs in 10–20% of patients. Other symptoms are fever, weight loss, anemia, and a varicocele. The tumor is most commonly detected as an incidental finding on a radiograph. Widespread use of radiologic cross-sectional imaging procedures (CT, ultrasound, MRI) contributes to earlier detection, including incidental renal masses detected during evaluation for other medical conditions. The increasing number of incidentally discovered low-stage tumors has contributed to an improved 5-year survival rate for patients with renal cell carcinoma and increased use of nephron-sparing surgery (partial nephrectomy). A spectrum of paraneoplastic syndromes has been associated with these malignancies, including erythrocytosis, hypercalcemia, nonmetastatic hepatic dysfunction (Stauffer syndrome), and acquired dysfibrinogenemia. Erythrocytosis is noted at presentation in only about 3% of patients. Anemia, a sign of advanced disease, is more common.

The standard evaluation of patients with suspected renal cell tumors includes a CT scan of the abdomen and pelvis, chest radiography, urine analysis, and urine cytology. If metastatic disease is suspected from the chest radiograph, a CT of the chest is warranted. MRI is useful in evaluating the inferior vena cava in cases of suspected tumor involvement or invasion by thrombus. In clinical practice, any solid renal masses should be considered malignant until proven otherwise; a definitive diagnosis is required. If no metastases are demonstrated, surgery is indicated, even if the renal vein is invaded. The differential diagnosis of a renal mass includes cysts, benign neoplasms (adenoma, angiomyolipoma, oncocytoma), inflammatory lesions (pyelonephritis or abscesses), and other primary or metastatic cancers. Other malignancies that may involve the kidney include transitional cell carcinoma of the renal pelvis, sarcoma, lymphoma, and Wilms' tumor. All of these are less common causes of renal masses than is renal cell cancer.

STAGING AND PROGNOSIS

Staging is based on the American Joint Committee on Cancer (AJCC) staging system (Fig. 41-2). Stage I tumors are <7 cm in greatest diameter and confined to the kidney, stage II tumors are ≥7 cm and confined to the kidney, stage III tumors extend through the renal capsule but are confined to Gerota's fascia (IIIa) or involve a single hilar lymph node (N1), and stage IV disease includes tumors that have invaded adjacent organs (excluding the adrenal gland) or involve multiple lymph nodes or distant metastases. The 5-year survival rate varies by stage: >90% for stage I, 85% for stage II, 60% for stage III, and 10% for stage IV.

TREATMENT Renal Cell Carcinoma

LOCALIZED TUMORS The standard management for stage I or II tumors and selected cases of stage III disease is radical nephrectomy. This procedure involves en bloc removal of Gerota's fascia and its contents, including the kidney, the ipsilateral adrenal gland, and adjacent hilar lymph nodes. The role of a regional lymphadenectomy is controversial. Extension into the renal vein or inferior vena cava (stage III disease) does not preclude resection even if cardiopulmonary bypass is required. If the tumor is resected, half of these patients have prolonged survival.

Nephron-sparing approaches via open or laparoscopic surgery may be appropriate for patients who have only one kidney, depending on the size and location of the lesion. A nephron-sparing approach can also be used for patients with bilateral tumors, accompanied by a radical nephrectomy on the opposite side. Partial nephrectomy techniques are applied electively to resect small masses for patients with a normal contralateral kidney. Adjuvant therapy following this surgery does not improve outcome, even in cases with a poor prognosis.

ADVANCED DISEASE Surgery has a limited role for patients with metastatic disease. However, long-term survival may occur in patients who relapse after nephrectomy in a solitary site that can be removed. One indication for nephrectomy with metastases at initial presentation is to alleviate pain or hemorrhage of a primary tumor. Also, a cytoreductive nephrectomy before systemic treatment improves survival for carefully selected patients with stage IV tumors.

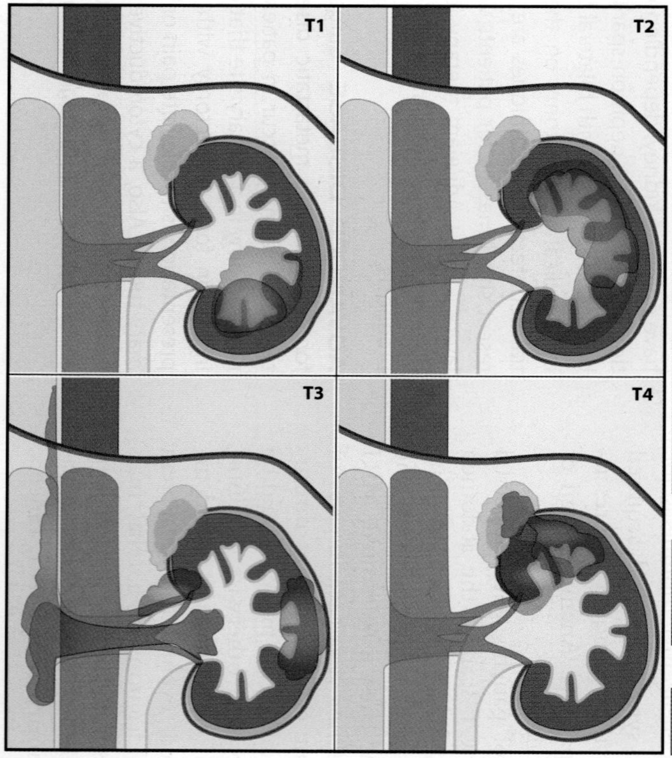

TNM	Involvement	Extent of Disease
TX	Primary not involved	
T1	≤7 cm	Limited to kidney
T1a	≤4 cm	
T1b	≥4 cm	
T2	>7 cm	Limited to kidney
T2a	>7 cm to ≤10 cm	
T2b	>10 cm	
T3	Into major veins or perinephric tissues	Not beyond Gerota's fascia
T3a	In renal vein or renal sinus fat	Not beyond Gerota's fascia
T3b	Into vena cava	Below diaphragm
T3c	Into vena cava	Above diaphragm
T4	Invasion beyond Gerota's fascia	Including contiguous extentions and into ipsilateral adrenal gland

Regional

NX	Regional lymph not assessed
N0	No lymph involvment
N1	Regional lymph involvement

Distant Metastases

M0	No distant metastases
M1	Distant metastases

Anatomic Stage or Prognostic Groups

I	T1	N0	M0
II	T2	N0	M0
III	T1 or T2,	N1	M0
	T3	N0 or N1	M0
IV	T4	Any N	M0
	Any T	Any N	M1

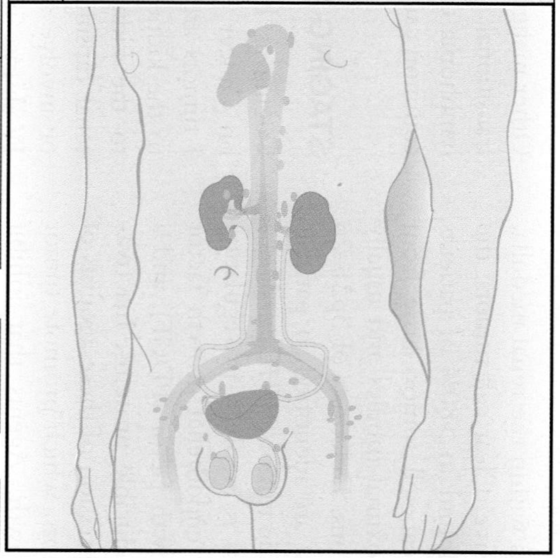

FIGURE 41-2
Renal cell carcinoma staging. TNM, tumor, node, metastasis

Metastatic renal cell carcinoma is highly refractory to chemotherapy. Cytokine therapy with IL-2 or IFN-α produces regressions in 10–20% of patients. IL-2 produces durable complete remission in a small proportion of cases. In general, cytokine therapy is considered unsatisfactory for most patients.

The situation changed dramatically when two large-scale randomized trials established a role for antiangiogenic therapy in this disease, as predicted by the genetic studies. These trials separately evaluated two orally administered antiangiogenic agents, sorafenib and sunitinib, that inhibited receptor tyrosine kinase signaling through the VEGF and PDGF receptors. Both showed efficacy as second-line treatment following progression during cytokine treatment, resulting in approval by regulatory authorities for the treatment of advanced renal cell carcinoma. A randomized phase 3 trial comparing sunitinib with IFN-α showed superior efficacy for sunitinib with an acceptable safety profile. The trial resulted in a change in the standard first-line treatment from IFN to sunitinib. Sunitinib is usually given orally at a dose of 50 mg/d for 4 weeks out of 6. Diarrhea is the main toxicity. Sorafenib is usually given orally at a dose of 400 mg twice a day. In addition to diarrhea, toxicities include rash, fatigue, and hand–foot syndrome. Temsirolimus and everolimus, inhibitors of the mammalian target of rapamycin (mTOR), show activity in patients with untreated poor-prognosis tumors and in sunitinib- and sorafenib-refractory tumors.

The prognosis of metastatic renal cell carcinoma is variable. In one analysis, no prior nephrectomy, a KPS <80, low hemoglobin, high corrected calcium, and abnormal lactate dehydrogenase level were poor prognostic factors. Patients with zero, one or two, and three or more factors had median survival times of 24, 12, and 5 months, respectively. These tumors may follow an unpredictable and protracted clinical course. It may be best to document progression before considering systemic treatment.

CHAPTER 42

BENIGN AND MALIGNANT DISEASES OF THE PROSTATE

Howard I. Scher

Benign and malignant changes in the prostate increase with age. Autopsies of men in the eighth decade of life show hyperplastic changes in >90% and malignant changes in >70% of individuals. The high prevalence of these diseases among the elderly, who often have competing causes of morbidity and mortality, mandates a risk-adapted approach to diagnosis and treatment. This can be achieved by considering these diseases as a series of states. Each state represents a distinct clinical milestone for which therapy(ies) may be recommended based on current symptoms, the risk of developing symptoms, or death from disease in relation to death from other causes within a given time frame (Fig. 42-1). For benign proliferative disorders, symptoms of urinary frequency, infection, and potential for obstruction are weighed against the side effects and complications of medical or surgical intervention. For prostate malignancies, the risks of developing the disease, symptoms, or death from cancer are balanced against the morbidities of the recommended treatments and preexisting comorbidities.

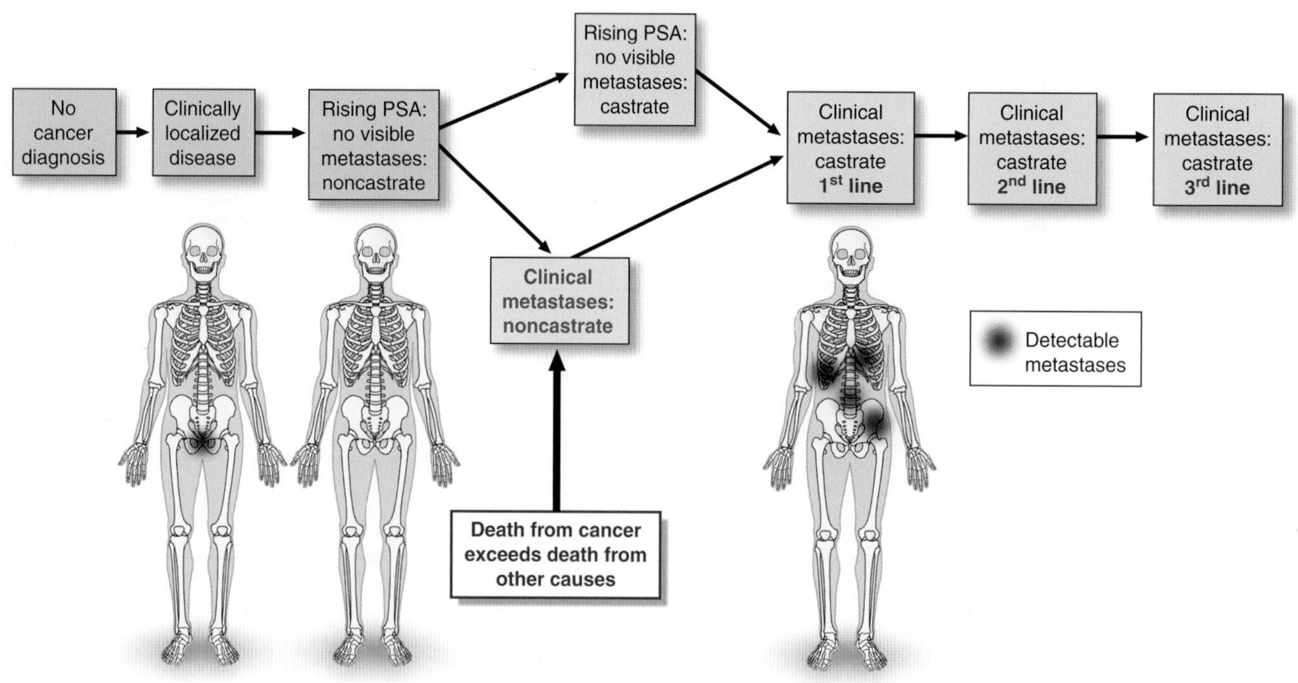

FIGURE 42-1
Clinical states of prostate cancer. PSA, prostate-specific antigen.

ANATOMY AND PATHOLOGY

The prostate is located in the pelvis and is surrounded by the rectum, the bladder, the periprostatic and dorsal vein complexes and neurovascular bundles that are responsible for erectile function, and the urinary sphincter that is responsible for passive urinary control. The prostate is composed of branching tubuloalveolar glands arranged in lobules surrounded by fibromuscular stroma. The acinar unit includes an epithelial compartment made up of epithelial, basal, and neuroendocrine cells and separated by a basement membrane, a stromal compartment that includes fibroblasts and smooth-muscle cells. Prostate-specific antigen (PSA) and prostatic acid phosphatase (PAP) are produced in the epithelial cells. Both prostate epithelial cells and stromal cells express androgen receptors (ARs) and depend on androgens for growth. Testosterone, the major circulating androgen, is converted by the enzyme 5α-reductase to dihydrotestosterone in the gland.

The periurethral portion of the gland increases in size during puberty and after the age of 55 years due to the growth of nonmalignant cells in the transition zone of the prostate that surrounds the urethra. Most cancers develop in the peripheral zone, and cancers in this location can often be palpated during a digital rectal examination (DRE).

PROSTATE CANCER

In 2010, approximately 217,730 prostate cancer cases were diagnosed, and 32,050 men died from prostate cancer in the United States. The absolute number of prostate cancer deaths has decreased in the past 5 years, which has been attributed by some to the widespread use of PSA-based detection strategies. However, the benefit of screening on survival is unclear. The paradox of management is that although 1 in 6 men will eventually be diagnosed with the disease and the disease remains the second leading cause of cancer deaths in men, only 1 man in 30 with prostate cancer will die of his disease.

EPIDEMIOLOGY

Epidemiologic studies show that the risk of being diagnosed with prostate cancer increases by a factor of two if one first-degree relative is affected and by four if two or more are affected. Current estimates are that 40% of early-onset and 5–10% of all prostate cancers are hereditary. Prostate cancer affects ethnic groups differently. Matched for age, African American males compared to white males have both a greater number of typically multifocal and highly unstable prostatic intraepithelial neoplasia (PIN) lesions, which are precursors to cancer, and larger tumors, possibly related to the higher levels of testosterone seen in African American males. Polymorphic variants of the AR, the cytochrome P450 C17, and the steroid 5α-reductase type II (SRD5A2) genes have also been implicated in the variations in incidence.

The prevalence of autopsy-detected cancers is similar around the world, while the incidence of clinical disease varies. Thus, environmental factors may play a role. High consumption of dietary fats, such as α-linoleic acid, or the polycyclic aromatic hydrocarbons that form when red meats are cooked is believed to increase risk. Similar to breast cancer in Asian women, the risk of prostate cancer in Asian men increases when they move to Western environments. Protective factors include consumption of the isoflavonoid genistein (which inhibits 5α-reductase) found in many legumes, cruciferous vegetables that contain the isothiocyanate sulforaphane, retinoids such as lycopene found in tomatoes, and inhibitors of cholesterol biosynthesis (e.g., statin drugs). The development of prostate cancer is a multistep process. One early change is hypermethylation of the GSTP1 gene promoter, which leads to loss of function of a gene that detoxifies carcinogens. The finding that many prostate cancers develop adjacent to a lesion termed PIA (proliferative inflammatory atrophy) suggests a role for inflammation.

DIAGNOSIS AND TREATMENT BY CLINICAL STATE

The prostate cancer continuum—from the appearance of a preneoplastic and invasive lesion localized to the prostate, to a metastatic lesion that results in symptoms and, ultimately, mortality—can span decades. To facilitate disease management, competing risks are considered in the context of a series of clinical states (Fig. 42-1). The states are defined operationally on the basis of whether or not a cancer diagnosis has been established and, for those with a diagnosis, whether or not metastases are detectable on imaging studies and the measured level of testosterone in the blood. With this approach, an individual resides in only one state and remains in that state until he has progressed. At each assessment, the decision to offer treatment and the specific form of treatment is based on the risk posed by the cancer relative to competing causes of mortality that may be present in that individual. It follows that the more advanced the disease, the greater the need for treatment.

For those without a cancer diagnosis, the decision to undergo testing to detect a cancer is based on the individual's estimated life expectancy and, separately, the probability that a clinically significant cancer may be present. For those with a prostate cancer diagnosis, the states model considers the probability of developing symptoms or dying from disease. Thus, a patient with localized prostate cancer who has had all cancer removed surgically remains in the state of localized disease as long as the PSA remains undetectable. The time within a state becomes a measure of the efficacy of an intervention, though the effect may not be assessable for years. As many men with active cancer are not at risk for developing metastases, symptoms, or death, the states model allows a distinction between *cure*—the elimination of all cancer cells, the primary therapeutic objective when treating most cancers—and *cancer control*, in which the tempo of the illness is altered and symptoms controlled until the patient dies of other causes. These can be equivalent therapeutically from a patient standpoint if the patient has not experienced symptoms of the disease or the treatment needed to control it. Even when a recurrence is documented, immediate therapy is not always necessary. Rather, as at the time of diagnosis, the need for intervention is based on the tempo of the illness as it unfolds in the individual, relative to the risk-to-benefit ratio of the therapy being considered.

NO CANCER DIAGNOSIS

Prevention

The results from several large double-blind, randomized chemoprevention trials have established 5α-reductase inhibitors (5ARIs) as the predominant therapy to reduce the future risk of a prostate cancer diagnosis. The Prostate Cancer Prevention Trial (PCPT), in which men older than age 55 years received the 5α-reductase inhibitor finasteride, which inhibits the type 1 isoform, or a placebo, showed a 25% (95% confidence interval, 19–31%) reduction in the period prevalence of prostate cancer across all age groups in favor of finasteride (18.4%) over placebo (24.4%). In REDUCE (Reduction by Dutasteride of Prostate Cancer Events Trial), a similar 23% reduction in the 4-year period prevalence was observed in favor of dutasteride ($P = 0.001$). Dutasteride inhibits both the type 1 and type 2 5ARI isoforms. These results contrast with those of the Selenium and Vitamin E Cancer Prevention Trial (SELECT) in which African American men ages ≥50 years and others ages ≥55 years were enrolled, which showed no difference in cancer incidence in patients receiving vitamin E (4.6%) or selenium (4.9%) alone or in combination (4.6%) relative to placebo (4.4%). A similar lack of benefit for vitamin E, vitamin C, and selenium was seen in the Physicians Health Study II.

Physical examination

The need to pursue a diagnosis of prostate cancer is based on symptoms; an abnormal DRE result; or, more typically, a change in or an elevated serum PSA. The urologic history should focus on symptoms of outlet obstruction, continence, potency, or change in ejaculatory pattern.

The DRE focuses on prostate size and consistency and abnormalities within or beyond the gland. Many cancers occur in the peripheral zone and can be palpated on DRE. Carcinomas are characteristically hard, nodular, and irregular, while induration may also be due to benign prostatic hypertrophy (BPH) or calculi. Overall, 20–25% of men with an abnormal DRE result have cancer.

Prostate-specific antigen

PSA (kallikrein-related peptidase 3; KLK3) is a kallikrein-related serine protease that causes liquefaction of seminal coagulum. It is produced by both nonmalignant and malignant epithelial cells and, as such, is prostate-specific, not prostate cancer–specific, and serum levels may also increase from prostatitis and BPH. Serum levels are not affected by DRE but the performance of a prostate biopsy can increase PSA levels up to 10-fold for 8–10 weeks. PSA circulating in the blood is inactive and mainly occurs as a complex with the protease inhibitor α_1-antichymotrypsin SERPIN A3 and as free unbound PSA forms. The formation of complexes between PSA, α_2-macroglobulin, or other protease inhibitors is less significant. Free PSA is rapidly eliminated from the blood by glomerular filtration with an estimated half-life of 12–18 hours. Elimination of PSA bound to α_1-antichymotrypsin is slow (estimated half-life of 1–2 weeks) as it is too large to be cleared by the kidneys. Levels should be undetectable after about 6 weeks if the prostate has been removed. Immunohistochemical staining for PSA can be used to establish a prostate cancer diagnosis.

PSA testing was approved by the U.S. Food and Drug Administration (FDA) in 1994 for early detection of prostate cancer, and the widespread use of the test has played a significant role in the proportion of men diagnosed with early-stage cancers: more than 70–80% of newly diagnosed cancers are organ confined. The level of PSA in blood is strongly associated with the risk and outcome of prostate cancer. A single PSA measured at age 60 years is associated (Area under the curve AUC of 0.90) with a lifetime risk of death from prostate cancer. Most (90%) prostate cancer deaths occur among men with PSA levels in top quartile (>2 ng/mL), although only a minority of men with PSA >2 ng/mL will develop lethal prostate cancer. Despite this and mortality rate reductions reported from large randomized prostate cancer screening trials, routine use of the test remains controversial. The American Cancer Society (ACS) recommends that physicians offer PSA testing and a DRE on an annual basis for men older than age 50 years with an anticipated survival of >10 years; this includes men up to age 76 years. For African Americans and men with a family history of prostate cancer, testing is advised to begin at age 45 years. The American Urologic Association recommendations are similar, with the proviso that the risks and benefits of the performance of these tests are not defined. The American College of Physicians recommends that physicians "describe the potential benefits and known harms of screening" and to "individualize the decision to screen." The National Comprehensive Cancer Network (NCCN) guidelines mirror those of the ACS, with the proviso that "physicians and potential participants must thoroughly discuss the pros and cons of screening." The NCCN also advises that men who opt to participate obtain a baseline PSA and DRE in their values and use the value to stratify future risk. As PSA values may fluctuate for no apparent reason, it is advised that isolated abnormal values should be confirmed before proceeding with further testing.

The PSA criteria used to recommend a diagnostic prostate biopsy have evolved over time. However, based on the commonly used outpoint for prostate biopsy CPSA≥4 mg/mL, most men with a PSA elevation do not have histologic widence of prostate cancer at biopsy, and commonly, many men with PSA levels below this cut point harbor cancer cells in their prostate. The goal is to increase the sensitivity of the test for younger men more likely to die of the disease and to reduce the frequency of detecting cancers of low malignant potential in elderly men more likely to die of other causes. Previously, the threshold for performance of a biopsy was 4.0 ng/mL, which has been reduced to 3 mg/mL or 2.6 ng/mL for men age <60 years by many groups based on the finding that nearly half of the men with PSAs who reached this level increased to 4 ng/mL within a relatively short (4-year) time frame and that, once diagnosed, in nearly one-third it had spread beyond the confines of the gland.

Most PSA is complexed to α_1-antichymotrypsin (ACT); only a small percentage is "free," and lower in men with cancer. Free and complexed PSA measurements are used when levels are between 4 and 10 ng/mL to decide whether a biopsy is needed. The risk of cancer is under 10% if the free PSA is >25% but as high as 56% for those with a free PSA <10%. PSA density (PSAD) measurements were developed to correct for the contribution of BPH to the total PSA level. PSAD is calculated by dividing the serum PSA by the prostate weight estimated from transrectal ultrasound (TRUS). Values <0.10 ng/mL per cm^3 are consistent with BPH, while those >0.15 ng/mL per cm^3 suggest cancer. *PSA dynamics* is the rate of change in PSA levels over time and is expressed most commonly as the PSA velocity or PSA doubling time. It is particularly useful for men with seemingly normal values that are rising. For men with a PSA level higher than 4 ng/mL, rates of rise >0.75 ng/mL per year suggest cancer, while for those with lower PSA levels, rates >0.5 ng/mL per year should be used to advise a biopsy. As an example, an increase from 2.5 to 3.2 ng/mL in a 1-year period would warrant further testing.

PSA-based detection strategies have changed the clinical spectrum of the disease. Now, 95–99% of newly diagnosed cancers are clinically localized, 40% are not palpable, and of these, 70% are pathologically organ-confined. However, the benefits of PSA screening remain controversial due to the overdetection of cancers with low malignant potential that may lead to overtreatment and unnecessary morbidity. To this end, the U.S. Prostate, Lung, Colorectal and Ovarian (PLCO) Cancer Screening trial found no mortality benefit from combined PSA screening and DRE in 76,693 randomized men (annual exam vs standard care) with a median follow-up of 11 years. However, important caveats about the PLCO study include (1) many screening participants had already undergone PSA screening before the trial, (2) contamination from PSA testing among control participants increased from 40% in year one to 52% in year 6, and (3) and the biopsy compliance was low. These factors make interpretation difficult. A subgroup analysis of this trial showed a reduction in cancer mortality among screened men with little or no comorbidity. The European Randomized Study of Screening for Prostate Cancer (ERSPC) trial followed 182,000 men a median of 9 years randomized either to PSA screening every 4 years or to a group not receiving regular PSA screening. In this study, PSA screening without DRE corresponded to a 20% relative reduction of the rate of death from prostate cancer. A report from the Swedish subgroup of this study based on 14 years of follow-up suggested that PSA screening may reduce cancer-specific mortality by nearly half with less overdiagnosis and treatment than was noted in the ERSPC as a whole. Men remain advised to make an informed decision on an individual basis about whether to undergo testing.

A diagnostic algorithm based on the DRE and PSA findings is illustrated in Fig. 42-2. In general, a biopsy is recommended if the DRE or PSA is abnormal. Twenty-five percent of men with a PSA >4 ng/mL and an abnormal DRE have cancer, as do 17% of men with a PSA of 2.5–4 ng/mL and normal DRE.

Prostate biopsy

A diagnosis of cancer is established by a TRUS-guided needle biopsy. Direct visualization by ultrasound or MRI assures that all areas of the gland are sampled. A minimum of six separate cores, three from the right and three from the left, is advised, as is a separate biopsy of the transition zone if clinically indicated. Contemporary

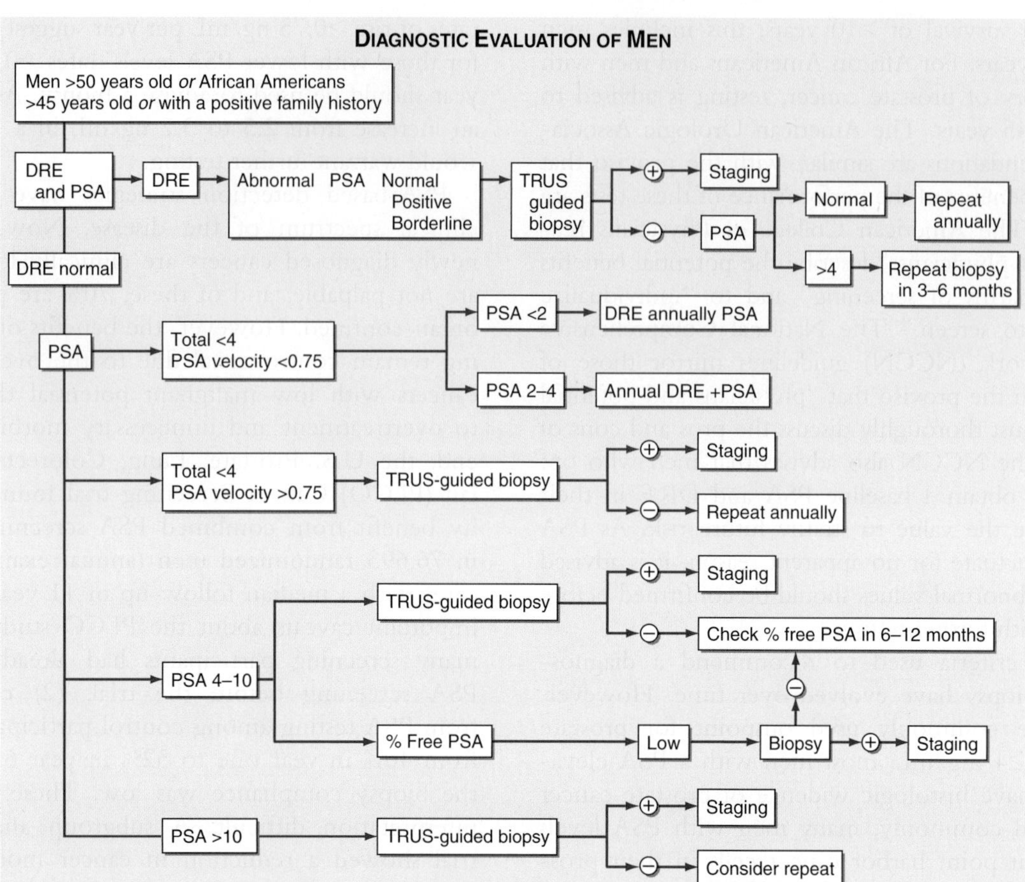

FIGURE 42-2

Algorithm for diagnostic evaluation of men based on digital rectal examination (DRE) and prostate-specific antigen (PSA) levels. TRUS, transrectal ultrasound.

schemas advise an extended-pattern 12- to 14-core biopsy that includes the sextant sampling above plus 6 cores from the lateral peripheral zones as well as a lesion-directed palpable nodule or suspicious image-guided sampling. Patients with prostatitis should have a course of antibiotics before biopsy. Men with an abnormal PSA and negative biopsy results are advised to undergo a repeat biopsy.

Each core of the biopsy is examined for the presence of cancer, and the amount of cancer is quantified based on the length of the tumor within the core and the percentage of the core involved.

Pathology

The noninvasive proliferation of epithelial cells within ducts is termed *prostatic intraepithelial neoplasia*. PIN is a precursor of cancer, but not all PIN lesions develop into invasive cancers. Of the cancers identified, >95% are adenocarcinomas; the rest are squamous or transitional cell tumors or, rarely, carcinosarcomas. Metastases to the prostate are rare, but in some cases, colon cancers or transitional cell tumors of the bladder invade the gland by direct extension.

When prostate cancer is diagnosed, a measure of histologic aggressiveness is assigned using the *Gleason grading system*, in which the dominant and secondary glandular histologic patterns are scored from 1 (well-differentiated) to 5 (undifferentiated) and summed to give a total score of 2–10 for each tumor. The most poorly differentiated area of tumor (i.e., the area with the highest histologic grade) often determines biologic behavior. The presence or absence of perineural invasion and extracapsular spread are also recorded.

Prostate cancer staging

The TNM staging system includes categories for cancers that are palpable on DRE, those identified solely on the basis of an abnormal PSA (T1c), those that are palpable but clinically confined to the gland (T2), and those that have extended outside the gland (T3 and T4) **(Table 42-1 and Fig. 42-3)**. DRE alone is inaccurate in determining the extent of disease within the gland, the

TABLE 42-1

TUMOR, NODE, METASTASIS CLASSIFICATION

TNM Staging System for Prostate Cancer[a]	
Tx	Primary tumor cannot be assessed
T0	No evidence of primary tumor
Localized Disease	
T1	Clinically inapparent tumor, neither palpable nor visible by imaging
T1a	Tumor incidental histologic finding in ≤5% of resected tissue; not palpable
T1b	Tumor incidental histologic finding in >5% of resected tissue
T1c	Tumor identified by needle biopsy (e.g., because of elevated PSA)
T2	Tumor confined within prostate[b]
T2a	Tumor involves half of one lobe or less
T2b	Tumor involves more than one half of one lobe, not both lobes
T2c	Tumor involves both lobes
Local Extension	
T3	Tumor extends through the prostate capsule[c]
T3a	Extracapsular extension (unilateral or bilateral)
T3b	Tumor invades seminal vesicles(s)
T4	Tumor is fixed or invades adjacent structures other than seminal vesicles such as external sphincter, rectum, bladder, levator muscles, and/or pelvic wall.
Metastatic Disease	
N1	Positive regional lymph nodes
M1	Distant metastases

[a]Revised from SB Edge et al (eds): *AJCC Cancer Staging Manual*, 7th ed. New York: Springer, 2010.

[b]Tumor found in one or both lobes by needle biopsy but not palpable or reliably visible by imaging is classified as T1c.

[c]Invasion into the prostatic apex or into (but not beyond) the prostatic capsule is classified not as T3 but as T2.

Abbreviations: PSA, prostate-specific antigen; TNM, tumor, node, metastasis.

presence or absence of capsular invasion, involvement of seminal vesicles, and extension of disease to lymph nodes. Because of the inadequacy of DRE for staging, the TNM staging system was modified to include the results of imaging. Unfortunately, no single test has proven to accurately indicate the stage or the presence of organ-confined disease, seminal vesicle involvement, or lymph node spread.

TRUS is the imaging technique most frequently used to assess the primary tumor, but its chief use is directing prostate biopsies, not staging. No TRUS finding consistently indicates cancer with certainty. CT lacks sensitivity and specificity to detect extraprostatic extension and is inferior to MRI in visualization of lymph nodes. In general, MRI performed with an endorectal coil is superior to CT to detect cancer in the prostate and to assess local disease extent. T1-weighted images produce a high signal in the periprostatic fat, periprostatic venous plexus, perivesicular tissues, lymph nodes, and bone marrow. T2-weighted images demonstrate the internal architecture of the prostate and seminal vesicles. Most cancers have a low signal, while the normal peripheral zone has a high signal, although the technique lacks sensitivity and specificity. MRI is also useful for the planning of surgery and radiation therapy.

Radionuclide bone scans (bone scintigraphy) are used to evaluate spread to osseous sites. This test is sensitive but relatively nonspecific because areas of increased uptake are not always related to metastatic disease. Healing fractures, arthritis, Paget's disease, and other conditions will also cause abnormal uptake. True-positive bone scans are rare if the PSA is <8 ng/mL and uncommon when the PSA is <10 ng/mL unless the tumor is high grade.

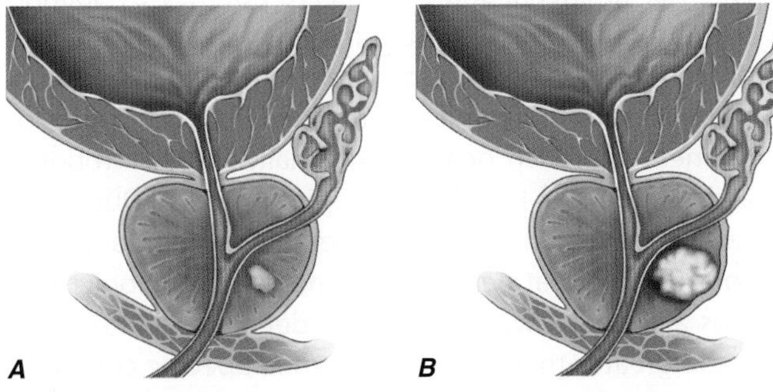

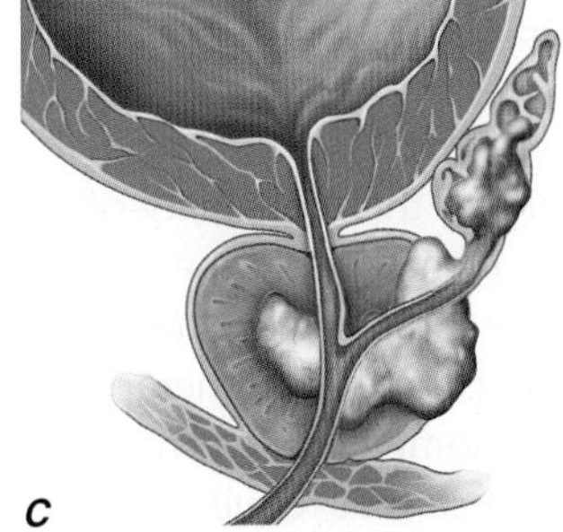

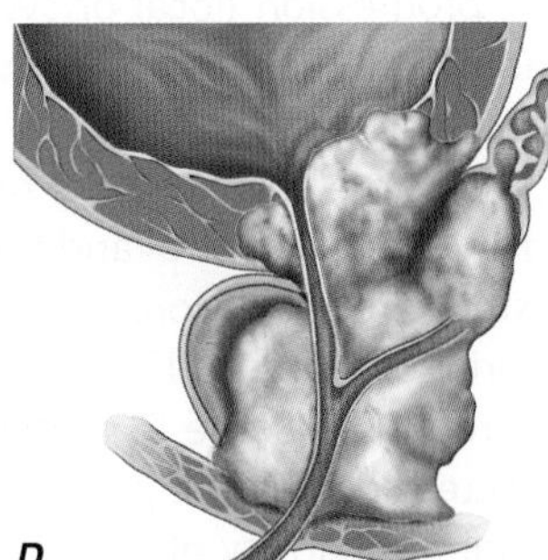

FIGURE 42-3

T stages of prostate cancer. ***(A)*** T1—clinically inapparent tumor, neither palpable nor visible by imaging; ***(B)*** T2—tumor confined within prostate; ***(C)*** T3—tumor extends through prostate capsule and may invade the seminal vesicles; ***(D)*** T4—tumor is fixed or invades adjacent structures. Eighty percent of patients present with local disease (T1 and T2), which is associated with a 5-year survival rate of 100%. An additional 12% of patients present with regional disease (T3 and T4 without metastases), which is also associated with a 100% survival rate after 5 years. Four percent of patients present with distant disease (T4 with metastases), which is associated with a 30% 5-year survival rate. (Three percent of patients are ungraded.) (*Data from AJCC, http://seer.cancer.gov/statfacts/html/prost.html. Figure © Memorial Sloan-Kettering Cancer Center Medical Graphics; used with permission.*)

TREATMENT Prostate Cancer

CLINICALLY LOCALIZED DISEASE Localized prostate cancers are those that appear to be nonmetastatic after staging studies are performed. Patients with localized disease are managed by radical prostatectomy, radiation therapy, or active surveillance. Choice of therapy requires the consideration of several factors: the presence of symptoms, the probability that the untreated tumor will adversely affect the quality or duration of survival and thus require treatment, and the probability that the tumor can be cured by single-modality therapy directed at the prostate or requires both local and systemic therapy to achieve cure. As most of the tumors detected are deemed clinically significant, most men undergo treatment.

Data from the literature do not provide clear evidence for the superiority of any one treatment relative to another. Comparison of outcomes of various forms of therapy is limited by the lack of prospective trials, referral bias, the experience of the treating teams and differences in endpoints and cancer control definitions. Often, PSA relapse–free survival is used because an effect on metastatic progression or survival may not be apparent for years. After radical surgery to remove all prostate tissue, PSA should become undetectable in the blood within 4 weeks, based on the PSA half-life in the blood of 3 days. If PSA remains detectable, the patient is considered to have persistent disease. After radiation therapy, in contrast, PSA does not become undetectable because the remaining nonmalignant elements of the gland continue to produce PSA even if all cancer cells have been eliminated. Similarly, cancer control is not well defined for a patient managed by active surveillance because PSA levels will continue to rise in the absence of therapy. Other outcomes are time to objective progression (local or systemic) and cancer-specific and overall survival; however, these outcomes may take years to assess.

The more advanced the disease, the lower the probability of local control and the higher the probability of systemic relapse. More important is that within the categories of T1, T2, and T3 disease are tumors with a range of prognoses. Some T3 tumors are curable with therapy directed solely at the prostate, and some T1 lesions have a high probability of systemic relapse that requires the integration of local and systemic therapy to achieve cure. For T1c tumors in particular, stage alone is inadequate to predict outcome and select treatment; other factors must be considered.

To better assess risk and guide treatment selection, many groups have developed prognostic models or nomograms that use a combination of the initial T stage, Gleason score, and baseline PSA. Some use discrete cut points (PSA <10 or ≥ 10 ng/mL; Gleason score of ≤ 6, 7, or ≥ 8); others employ nomograms that use PSA and Gleason score as continuous variables. More than 100 nomograms have been reported to predict the probability that a clinically significant cancer is present, disease extent (organ-confined vs non–organ-confined, node-negative or -positive), or the probability of success of treatment for specific local therapies using pretreatment variables. Considerable controversy exists over what constitutes "high risk" based on a predicted probability of success or failure. In these situations, nomograms and predictive models can only go so far. Exactly what probability of success or failure would lead a physician to recommend and a patient to seek alternative approaches is controversial. As an example, it may be appropriate to recommend radical surgery for a younger patient with a low probability of cure. Nomograms are being refined continually to incorporate additional clinical parameters, biologic determinants, and year of treatment, which can also affect outcomes, making treatment decisions a dynamic process.

The frequency of adverse events varies by treatment modality and the experience of the treating team. For example, following radical prostatectomy, incontinence rates range from 2 to 47% and impotence rates range from 25 to 89%. Part of the variability relates to how the complication is defined and whether the patient or physician is reporting the event. The time of the assessment is also important. After surgery, impotence is immediate but may reverse over time, while with radiation therapy, impotence is not immediate but may develop over time. Of greatest concern to patients are the effects on continence, sexual potency, and bowel function.

Radical Prostatectomy The goal of radical prostatectomy is to excise the cancer completely with a clear margin, to maintain continence by preserving the external sphincter, and to preserve potency by sparing the autonomic nerves in the neurovascular bundle. The procedure is advised for patients with a life expectancy of 10 years or more and is performed via a retropubic or perineal approach or via a minimally invasive robotic-assisted or hand-held laparoscopic approach. Outcomes can be predicted using postoperative nomograms that consider pretreatment factors and the pathologic findings at surgery, with PSA failure defined generally as a value greater than 0.2 or 0.4 ng/mL. Specific criteria to guide the choice of one approach over another are lacking. Minimally invasive approaches offer the advantage of a shorter hospital stay and a more rapid recovery with the trade-off of higher rates of incontinence and erectile dysfunction. Cancer control rates are comparable.

Neoadjuvant hormonal therapy has also been explored in an attempt to improve the outcomes of surgery for high-risk patients using a variety of definitions.

The results of several large trials testing 3 or 8 months of androgen depletion before surgery showed that serum PSA levels decreased by 96%, prostate volumes decreased by 34%, and margin positivity rates decreased from 41 to 17%. Unfortunately, hormones did not produce an improvement in PSA relapse–free survival. Thus, neoadjuvant hormonal therapy is not recommended.

Factors associated with incontinence include older age and urethral length, which impacts the ability to preserve the urethra beyond the apex and the distal sphincter. The specific surgical technique, open versus laparoscopic versus robotic, as well as the skill and experience of the surgeon are also factors. In a series treated at an academic center, 6% of patients had mild stress urinary incontinence (SUI) (requiring 1 pad/day), 2% moderate SUI (>1 pad/day), and 0.3% severe SUI (requiring an artificial urinary sphincter). At 1 year, 92% were completely continent. In contrast, the results in a Medicare population treated at multiple centers showed that at 3, 12, and 24 months following surgery, 58, 35, and 42%, respectively, wore pads in their underwear, and 24, 11, and 15% reported "a lot" of urine leakage.

Recovery of erectile function is associated with younger age, quality of erections before surgery, and absence of damage to the neurovascular bundles. In general, erectile function begins to return in a median of 4–6 months if both bundles are preserved. Potency is reduced by half if at least one nerve bundle is sacrificed. When cancer control requires the removal of both bundles, sural nerve grafts have shown no utility. Overall, with the availability of drugs such as sildenafil, intraurethral inserts of alprostadil, and intracavernosal injections of vasodilators, many patients recover satisfactory sexual function.

Radiation Therapy Radiation therapy is given by external beam, by radioactive sources implanted into the gland, or by a combination of the two techniques.

External-Beam Radiation Therapy Contemporary external-beam radiation therapy requires three-dimensional conformal treatment plans intensity-modulated radiation therapy (IMRT) to maximize the dose to the prostate and to minimize the exposure of the surrounding normal tissue. IMRT permits shaping of the dose, and allows the delivery of higher doses to the prostate and a further reduction in normal tissue exposure than 3D-conformal treatment alone. These advances have enabled the safe administration of doses >80 Gy, higher local control rates, and fewer side effects.

Cancer control after radiation therapy has been defined by various criteria, including a decline in PSA to <0.5 or 1 ng/mL, "nonrising" PSA values, and a negative biopsy of the prostate 2 years after completion of treatment. The current standard definition of biochemical failure (the Phoenix definition) is a rise in PSA by ≥2 ng/mL higher than the lowest PSA achieved. The date of failure is "at call" and not backdated.

Radiation dose is important and a minimum of 75.6 to 79 or 80 Gy advised. In a representative study, a PSA nadir of <1.0 ng/mL in 90% of patients receiving 75.6 or 81.0 Gy vs. 76% and 56% of those receiving 70.2 and 64.8 Gy, and positive biopsy rates at 2.5 years were 4% for those treated with 81 Gy versus 27 and 36% for those receiving 75.6 or 70.2 Gy.

Overall, radiation therapy is associated with a higher frequency of bowel complications (mainly diarrhea and proctitis) than surgery. The frequency relates directly to the volume of the anterior rectal wall receiving full-dose treatment. In one series, grade 3 rectal or urinary toxicities were seen in 2.1% of patients who received a median dose of 75.6 Gy, while grade 3 urethral strictures requiring dilation developed in 1% of cases, all of whom had undergone a transurethral resection of the prostate (TURP). Pooled data show that the frequency of grade 3 and 4 toxicities is 6.9 and 3.5%, respectively, for patients who received >70 Gy. The frequency of erectile dysfunction is related to the quality of erections pretreatment, the dose administered, and the time of assessment. Post-radiation erectile dysfunction is related to a disruption of the vascular supply and not the nerve fibers.

Neoadjuvant hormone therapy before radiation therapy has been studied. The aim is to decrease the size of the prostate and, consequently, to reduce the exposure of normal tissues to full-dose radiation, to increase local control rates, and to decrease the rate of systemic failure. Short-term hormone therapy can reduce toxicities and improve local control rates, but long-term treatment (2–3 years) is needed to prolong the time to PSA failure and lower the risk of metastatic disease. The impact on survival has been less clear. The decision to treat the pelvic lymph nodes is based on the nomogram-predicted risk of nodal spread.

Brachytherapy Brachytherapy is the direct implantation of radioactive sources (seeds) into the prostate. It is based on the principle that the deposition of radiation energy in tissues decreases as a function of the square of the distance from the source (Chap. 28). The goal is to deliver intensive irradiation to the prostate, minimizing the exposure of the surrounding tissues. The current standard technique achieves a more homogeneous dose distribution by placing seeds according to a customized template based on CT and ultrasonographic assessment of the tumor and computer-optimized dosimetry. The implantation is performed transperineally as a 1-day procedure with real-time imaging.

Improvements in brachytherapy techniques have resulted in fewer complications and a marked reduction in local failure rates. In a series of 197 patients followed for a median of 3 years, 5-year actuarial PSA relapse–free survival for patients with pretherapy PSA levels of 0–4, 4–10, and >10 ng/mL were 98, 90, and 89%, respectively. In a separate report of 201 patients who underwent posttreatment biopsies, 80% were negative, 17% were indeterminate, and 3% were positive. The results did not change with longer follow-up. Nevertheless, many physicians believe that implantation is best reserved for patients with good or intermediate prognostic features.

Brachytherapy is well tolerated, although most patients experience urinary frequency and urgency that can persist for several months. Incontinence has been seen in 2–4% of cases. Higher complication rates are observed in patients who have undergone a prior TURP, while those with obstructive symptoms at baseline are at a higher risk for retention and persistent voiding symptoms. Proctitis has been reported in <2% of patients.

Active Surveillance While prostate cancer is the most common form of cancer affecting men in the United States, patients are being diagnosed earlier and more frequently present with early-stage disease. Active surveillance, described previously as *watchful waiting* or *deferred therapy*, is the policy of monitoring the illness at fixed intervals with DREs, PSA measurements, and repeat prostate biopsies as indicated until histopathologic or serologic changes correlative of progression warrant treatment with curative intent. It evolved from studies that evaluated predominantly elderly men with well-differentiated tumors who demonstrated no clinically significant progression for protracted periods, recognition of the contrast between incidence and disease-specific mortality, the high prevalence of autopsy cancers and an effort to reduce overtreatment. A recent screening study estimated that between 50 and 100 men with low-risk disease would need to be treated to prevent one prostate cancer–specific death.

Arguing against active surveillance are the results of a Swedish randomized trial of radical prostatectomy versus active surveillance. With a median follow-up of 6.2 years, men treated by radical surgery had a lower risk of prostate cancer death relative to active surveillance patients (4.6 vs 8.9%) and a lower risk of metastatic progression (hazard ratio, 0.63). Case selection is critical, and determining clinical parameters predictive of cancer aggressiveness that can be used to reliably select men most likely to benefit from active surveillance is an area of intense study. In one prostatectomy series, it was estimated that 10–15% of those treated had "insignificant" disease. One set of criteria includes men with T1c tumors that are Gleason grade 6 or less involving 3 or fewer cores, each of them having less than 50% involvement by tumor and a PSAD of 0.15.

Concerns include the limited ability to predict pathologic findings by needle biopsy even when multiple cores are obtained, the recognized multifocality of the disease, and the possibility of a missed opportunity to cure the disease. Nomograms to help predict which patients can safely be managed by active surveillance continue to be refined, and as their predictive accuracy improves, it can be anticipated that more patients will be candidates.

RISING PSA This state consists of patients in whom the sole manifestation of disease is a rising PSA after surgery and/or radiation therapy. By definition, there is no evidence of disease on scan. For these patients, the central issue is whether the rise in PSA results from persistent disease in the primary site, systemic disease, or both. In theory, disease in the primary site may still be curable by additional local treatment: external-beam radiation for patients who had undergone surgery and prostatectomy for patients who had undergone radiation therapy.

The decision to recommend radiation therapy after prostatectomy is guided by the pathologic findings at surgery, as imaging studies such as CT and bone scan are typically uninformative. Some recommend a Prostascint scan—imaging with a radiolabeled antibody to prostate-specific membrane antigen (PSMA), which is highly expressed on prostate epithelial cells—to help with this distinction. Antibody localization to the prostatic fossa suggests local recurrence; localization to extrapelvic sites predicts failure of radiation therapy. Others recommend that a biopsy of the urethrovesical anastomosis be obtained before considering radiation. Factors that predict for response to salvage radiation therapy are a positive surgical margin, lower Gleason grade, long interval from surgery to PSA failure, slow PSA doubling time, and low (<0.5–1 ng/mL) PSA value at the time of radiation treatment. Radiation therapy is generally not recommended if the PSA was persistently elevated after surgery, which usually indicates that the disease had spread outside of the area of the prostate bed and is unlikely to be controlled with radiation therapy. As is the case for other disease states, nomograms to predict the likelihood of success are also available.

For patients with a rising PSA after radiation therapy, salvage prostatectomy can be considered if the disease was "curable" at the outset, if persistent disease has been documented by a biopsy of the prostate, and if no metastatic disease is seen on imaging studies. Unfortunately, case selection is poorly defined in most series, and morbidities are significant. As currently performed, virtually all patients are impotent after salvage radical prostatectomy, and approximately 45% have either total urinary incontinence or stress incontinence. Major bleeding, bladder neck contractures, and rectal injury are not uncommon.

More frequently, the rise in PSA after surgery or radiation therapy indicates subclinical or micrometastatic disease. In these cases, the need for treatment depends, in part, on the estimated probability that the patient will show evidence of metastatic disease on a scan and in what time frame. That immediate therapy is not always required was shown in a series in which patients received no systemic therapy until metastatic disease was documented. Overall, the median time to metastatic progression was 8 years, and 63% of the patients with rising PSA values remained free of metastases at 5 years. Factors associated with progression included the primary tumor's Gleason grade, time to recurrence, and PSA doubling time. For those with Gleason grade ≥8 tumors, the probability of metastatic progression was 37, 51, and 71% at 3, 5, and 7 years, respectively. If the time to recurrence was <2 years and PSA doubling time was long (>10 months), the proportion with metastatic disease at the same time intervals was 23, 32, and 53% versus 47, 69, and 79% if the doubling time was short (<10 months). PSA doubling times are also prognostic for survival. In one series, all patients who succumbed to disease had PSA doubling times of 3 months or less. Most physicians advise treatment when PSA doubling times are 12 months or less. A difficulty with predicting the risk of metastatic spread, symptoms, or death from disease in the rising PSA state is that most patients receive some form of therapy before the development of metastases. Nevertheless, predictive models continue to be refined.

METASTATIC DISEASE: NONCASTRATE The state of *noncastrate metastatic disease* includes men with metastases visible on an imaging study and noncastrate levels of testosterone (>150 ng/dL). The patient may be newly diagnosed or have a recurrence after treatment for localized disease. Symptoms of metastatic disease include pain from osseous spread, although many patients are asymptomatic despite extensive spread. Less common are symptoms related to marrow compromise (myelophthisis), coagulopathy, or spinal cord compression.

Standard treatment is to deplete or lower androgens by medical or surgical means and/or to block androgen binding to the AR with antiandrogens. More than 90% of male hormones originate in the testes; <10% are synthesized in the adrenal gland. Surgical orchiectomy is the "gold standard" but is least acceptable to patients (Fig. 42-4).

Testosterone-Lowering Agents Medical therapies that lower testosterone levels include the gonadotropin-releasing hormone (GnRH) agonists/antagonists, 17,20-lyase inhibitors, cyp-17 inhibitors, estrogens, and progestational agents. Estrogens such as diethylstilbestrol (DES) have fallen out of favor due to the risk of vascular complications such as fluid retention, phlebitis,

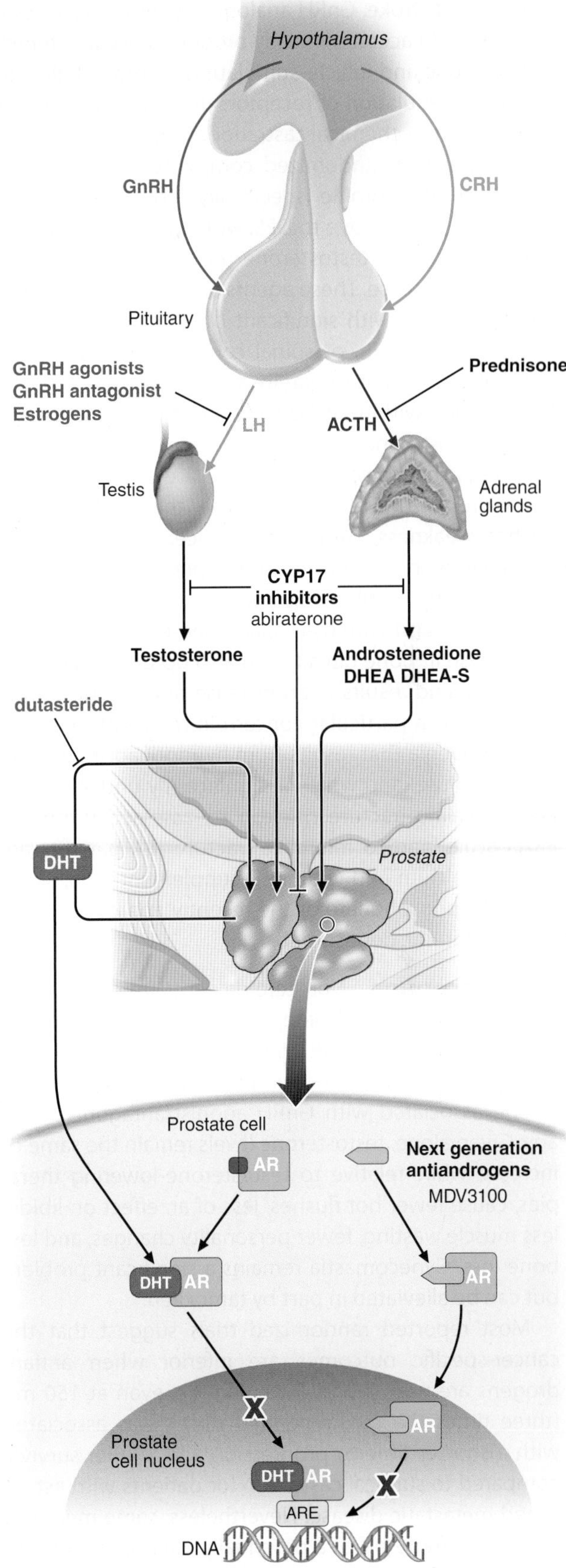

FIGURE 42-4
Sites of action of different hormone therapies.

emboli, and stroke. GnRH analogues (leuprolide acetate and goserelin acetate) initially produce a rise in luteinizing hormone and follicle-stimulating hormone followed by a downregulation of receptors in the pituitary gland, which effects a chemical castration. They were approved on the basis of randomized comparisons showing an improved safety profile (specifically, reduced cardiovascular toxicities) relative to DES, with equivalent potency. The initial rise in testosterone may result in a clinical flare of the disease. These agents are therefore contraindicated in men with significant obstructive symptoms, cancer-related pain, or spinal cord compromise. GnRH antagonists such as degarelix achieve castrate levels of testosterone within 48 hours without the initial rise in serum testosterone.

Agents that lower testosterone are associated with an androgen-depletion syndrome that includes hot flushes, weakness, fatigue, impotence, sarcopenia, anemia, change in personality, and depression. Changes in lipids, obesity, insulin resistance, and an increased risk of diabetes and cardiovascular disease can also occur. A decrease in bone density can also occur that worsens over time and results in an increase risk of clinical fractures. This is a particular concern in men with preexisting osteopenia that results from hypogonadism, steroid or alcohol use, and which is significantly underappreciated. Baseline fracture risk can be assessed using the FRAX scale, and to minimize fracture risk patients are advised calcium and vitamin D supplementation, along with a bisphosphonate or the recently approved RANK-ligand inhibitor, denosumab.

Antiandrogens Nonsteroidal antiandrogens such as flutamide, bicalutamide, and nilutamide block the ligand binding to the AR and were initially approved to block the flare associated with the rise in serum testosterone associated with GnRH agonist/antagonist therapy. Given alone, testosterone levels remain the same or increase while relative to testosterone-lowering therapies, cause fewer hot flushes, less of an effect on libido, less muscle wasting, fewer personality changes, and less bone loss. Gynecomastia remains a significant problem but can be alleviated in part by tamoxifen.

Most reported randomized trials suggest that the cancer-specific outcomes are inferior when antiandrogens are used alone. Bicalutamide, even at 150 mg (three times the recommended dose), was associated with a shorter time to progression and inferior survival compared to surgical castration for patients with established metastatic disease. Nevertheless, some men may accept the trade-off of a potentially inferior cancer outcome for an improved quality of life.

Combined androgen blockade, the administration of an antiandrogen plus a GnRH analogue or surgical orchiectomy, or triple androgen blockade, which includes the addition of a 5ARI, have not been shown to be superior to androgen depletion monotherapies, and are no longer recommended. In practice, most patients who are treated with a GnRH analogue receive an antiandrogen for the first 2–4 weeks of treatment to protect against the flare.

Intermittent Androgen Deprivation Therapy (IADT) Another way to reduce the side effects of androgen depletion is to administer antiandrogens on an intermittent basis. This was proposed as a way to prevent the selection of cells that are resistant to androgen depletion. The hypothesis is that by allowing endogenous testosterone levels to rise, the cells that survive androgen depletion will induce a normal differentiation pathway. In this way, the surviving cells that are allowed to proliferate in the presence of androgen will retain sensitivity to subsequent androgen depletion. Applied in the clinic, androgen depletion is continued for 2–6 months beyond the point of maximal response. Once treatment is stopped, endogenous testosterone levels increase, and the symptoms associated with hormone treatment abate. PSA levels also begin to rise, and at some level, treatment is restarted. With this approach, multiple cycles of regression and proliferation have been documented in individual patients. It is unknown whether the intermittent approach increases, decreases, or does not change the overall duration of sensitivity to androgen depletion. The approach is safe, but long-term data are needed to assess the course in men with low PSA levels. A trial to address this question is ongoing.

Outcomes of Androgen Depletion The anti-prostate cancer effects of the various androgen depletion strategies are similar, and the clinical course is predictable: an initial response, then a period of stability in which tumor cells are dormant and nonproliferative, followed after a variable period of time by a rise in PSA and regrowth that is visible on a scan as a castration-resistant lesion. Androgen depletion is not curative because cells that survive castration are present when the disease is first diagnosed. Considered by disease manifestation, PSA levels return to normal in 60–70% of patients, and measurable disease regression occurs in 50%; improvements in bone scan occur in 25% of cases, but the majority remains stable. Duration of survival is inversely proportional to disease extent at the time androgen depletion is first started, while the degree of PSA decline at 6 months has been shown to be prognostic. In a large-scale trial, PSA nadir proved prognostic.

An active question is whether hormones should be given in the adjuvant setting after surgery or radiation treatment of the primary tumor, or at the time that a PSA recurrence is documented, or to wait until metastatic disease or symptoms of disease are manifest. Trials in support of early therapy have often been underpowered relative to the reported benefit or have been criticized for methodologic grounds. One trial, although it showed a survival benefit for patients treated with radiation therapy and 3 years of androgen depletion relative to radiation alone, was criticized for the poor outcomes of the control group. Another showing a survival benefit for patients with positive lymph nodes who were randomized to immediate medical or surgical castration compared to observation ($P = .02$) was criticized because the confidence intervals around the 5- and 8-year survival distributions for the two groups overlapped. A large randomized study comparing early with late hormone treatment (orchiectomy or GnRH analogue) in patients with locally advanced or asymptomatic metastatic disease showed that patients treated early were less likely to progress from M0 to M1 disease, to develop pain, and to die of prostate cancer. This trial was criticized because therapy was delayed "too long" in the late-treatment group. When patients treated by radical surgery, radiation therapy, or active surveillance were randomly assigned to receive bicalutamide 150 mg or placebo, hormone treatment produced a significant reduction in the proportion of patients who developed osseous metastases at 2 years (9% for bicalutamide; 13.8% for placebo). This result has not gained acceptance in part because too many "good-risk" patients were treated and because no effect on survival was demonstrated. These criticisms are valid; however, the net influence on survival from early hormone intervention is similar to that observed in patients with breast cancer, for which adjuvant hormonal therapy is routinely given. It is of note that the American Society of Clinical Oncology Guidelines do not support immediate therapy.

METASTATIC DISEASE: CASTRATE Castration-resistant prostate cancer (CRPC), a disease that progresses despite androgen suppression by medical or surgical therapies in which the measured levels of testosterone are 50 ng/mL or lower, continues to express the AR and is dependent on signaling through the receptor for growth. CRPC can manifest in many ways. For some, it is a rise in PSA with no change in radiographs and no new symptoms. In others, it is a rising PSA and progression in bone with or without symptoms of disease. Still others show soft tissue disease with or without osseous metastases, and others have visceral spread. The prognosis, which is highly variable, can be predicted using nomograms designed for CRPC. The important point is that despite the failure of first-line hormone treatment, these tumors remain androgen driven and are not "hormone refractory": the majority of these tumors remain sensitive to second- and third-line hormonal treatments. The rising PSA is an indication of continued signaling through the AR axis.

The manifestations of disease in this patient group limit the ability to reliably assess treatment effects because the traditional measures of outcome such as tumor regression do not apply. Bone scans can be inaccurate for assessing changes in osseous disease, and no PSA-based outcome is a true surrogate for survival benefit. It is essential to define therapeutic objectives before initiating treatment, as there are defined standards of care for different disease manifestations. Therapeutic objectives need not be defined by survival only as useful endpoints also include relief of symptoms and delay of metastases or new symptoms of disease.

Management of pain secondary to osseous metastatic disease is a critical part of therapy. Optimal palliation requires assessing whether the symptoms and metastases are focal or diffuse and whether disease threatens the spinal cord, the cauda equina, or the base of the skull. Neurologic symptoms require emergency evaluation because loss of function may be permanent if not addressed quickly. Single sites of pain and areas of neurologic involvement are best treated with external beam radiation. As the disease is often diffuse, palliation at one site often is followed by the emergence of symptoms in a separate site that had not received radiation.

It is also essential to ensure that a castrate status be documented. Patients receiving an antiandrogen alone, whose serum testosterone levels are elevated, should be treated first with a GnRH analogue or orchiectomy and observed for response. Patients on an antiandrogen in combination with a GnRH analogue should have the antiandrogen discontinued, as approximately 20% will respond to the selective discontinuation of the antiandrogen. Any withdrawal response occurs within weeks of stopping flutamide but may take 8–12 weeks with nilutamide and bicalutamide because of their long terminal half-lives. Ketoconazole, 600 to 1200 mg/d in combination with hydrocortisone, which inhibits adrenal androgen production, also has activity in this setting, but has not been formally evaluated in definitive phase III trials.

Hormonal agents in late phase III development that target specific pathogenetic mechanisms of AR function reactivation include abiraterone acetate, a novel CYP17 inhibitor that blocks androgen synthesis in the adrenal gland, testis, and tumor, and MDV3100, a next-generation antiandrogen screened for activity in prostate cancer model systems with overexpressed AR. A phase III trial showed a 4-month survival benefit for abiraterone acetate plus prednisone over a placebo plus prednisone. These agents have also shown significant antitumor effects in patients who have progressed on chemotherapy.

Mitoxantrone was the first cytotoxic agent shown to provide palliation of pain secondary to castrate metastatic disease, and was approved for this indication without the demonstration of a clear survival benefit. In 2004, docetaxel was established as the first-line standard cytotoxic drug for patients in this state, based on a trial showing that q3w docetaxel was superior to weekly therapy and to mitoxantrone, results confirmed in a second trial of estramustine/docetaxel versus mitoxantrone. The addition of estramustine produced significant toxicity with no apparent improvement in survival and has been dropped from these regimens. Docetaxel and other microtubule-targeted agents produce PSA declines in 50% of patients, measurable disease regression in 25%, and both an improvement in preexisting and prevention of future cancer-related pain. Dasatinib is an oral tyrosine kinase inhibitor that targets Src and other Src family kinases that contribute to ligand-independent AR activation, and that reduces bone turnover, is under study in combination with docetaxel. Two products approved based on a survival benefit in randomized trials include cabazitaxel, a second-generation taxane FDA approved for patients who have progressed on docetaxel relative to mitoxantrone, and sipuleucel-t, a biologic approach in which antigen-presenting cells are activated ex vivo, pulsed with antigen, and reinfused.

Given the bone-dominant pattern of prostate cancer spread, two bone-seeking radioisotopes, ^{89}Sr (Metastron) and ^{153}Sm-EDTMP (Quadramet), are approved for palliation of pain, although they have no effect on PSA or survival. Fewer patients treated with one of these isotopes developed new areas of pain or required additional radiation therapy compared with patients receiving external-beam radiation therapy alone. Additionally, patients randomly assigned to a combination of ^{89}Sr and doxorubicin after induction chemotherapy had fewer skeletal events and longer survival than patients treated with doxorubicin alone. Confirmatory studies are ongoing.

An additional bone-targeting therapy, bisphosphonates inhibit osteoclasts and, in effect, protect against bone loss associated with androgen depletion and prevent skeletal events. Addition of the bisphosphonate zoledronate to "standard therapy" in patients with CRPC resulted in fewer skeletal events relative to placebo. Skeletal events included microfractures, new pain, and need for radiation therapy.

BENIGN DISEASE

SYMPTOMS

Benign proliferative disease may produce hesitancy, intermittent voiding, a diminished stream, incomplete emptying, and postvoid leakage. The severity of these symptoms can be quantitated with the self-administered American Urological Association Symptom Index (Table 42-2), although the degree of symptoms does not always relate

TABLE 42-2

AMERICAN UROLOGICAL ASSOCIATION SYMPTOM INDEX

	AUA SYMPTOM SCORE (CIRCLE 1 NUMBER ON EACH LINE)					
QUESTIONS TO BE ANSWERED	**NOT AT ALL**	**LESS THAN 1 TIME IN 5**	**LESS THAN HALF THE TIME**	**ABOUT HALF THE TIME**	**MORE THAN HALF THE TIME**	**ALMOST ALWAYS**
Over the past month, how often have you had a sensation of not emptying your bladder completely after you finished urinating?	0+	1	2	3	4	5
Over the past month, how often have you had to urinate again less than 2 h after you finished urinating?	0	1	2	3	4	5
Over the past month, how often have you found you stopped and started again several times when you urinated?	0	1	2	3	4	5
Over the past month, how often have you found it difficult to postpone urination?	0	1	2	3	4	5
Over the past month, how often have you had a weak urinary stream?	0	1	2	3	4	5
Over the past month, how often have you had to push or strain to begin urination?	0	1	2	3	4	5
Over the past month, how many times did you most typically get up to urinate from the time you went to bed at night until the time you got up in the morning?	(None)	(1 time)	(2 times)	(3 times)	(4 times)	(5 times)
Sum of 7 circled numbers (AUA symptom score): ___						

Abbreviation: AUA, American Urological Association.
Source: MJ Barry et al: J Urol 148:1549, 1992. Used with permission.

to gland size. Resistance to urine flow reduces bladder compliance, leading to nocturia; urgency; and, ultimately, urinary retention. Episodes of urinary retention may be precipitated by infection, tranquilizing drugs, antihistamines, and alcohol. Prostatitis often produces pain or induration. Typically, the symptoms remain stable over time and obstruction does not occur.

DIAGNOSTIC PROCEDURES AND TREATMENT

Asymptomatic patients do not require treatment regardless of the size of the gland, while those with an inability to urinate, gross hematuria, recurrent infection, or bladder stones may require surgery. In patients with symptoms, uroflowmetry can identify those with normal flow rates who are unlikely to benefit from surgery and those with high postvoid residuals who may need other interventions. Pressure-flow studies detect primary bladder dysfunction. Cystoscopy is recommended if hematuria is documented and to assess the urinary outflow tract before surgery. Imaging of the upper tracts is advised for patients with hematuria, a history of calculi, or prior urinary tract problems.

Medical therapies for BPH include 5α-reductase inhibitors and α-adrenergic blockers. Finasteride (10 mg/d orally) and other 5α-reductase inhibitors that block the conversion of testosterone to dihydrotestosterone decrease prostate size, increase urine flow rates, and improve symptoms. Of note is that in the REDUCE trial, a reduction in BPH outcomes including acute urinary retention and BPH-related surgery was observed. Noteworthy is that these agents lower baseline PSA levels by 50%, an important consideration when using PSA to guide biopsy recommendations. α-Adrenergic blockers such as terazosin (1–10 mg PO at bedtime) act by relaxing the smooth muscle of the bladder neck and increasing peak urinary flow rates. No data show that these agents influence the progression of the disease.

Surgical approaches include TURP; transurethral incision; or removal of the gland via a retropubic, suprapubic, or perineal approach. Also utilized are TULIP (transurethral ultrasound-guided laser-induced prostatectomy), stents, and hyperthermia.

CHAPTER 43
TESTICULAR CANCER

Robert J. Motzer ■ George J. Bosl

Primary germ cell tumors (GCTs) of the testis arising by the malignant transformation of primordial germ cells constitute 95% of all testicular neoplasms. Infrequently, GCTs arise from an extragonadal site, including the mediastinum; retroperitoneum; and, very rarely, the pineal gland. This disease is notable for the young age of the affected patients, the totipotent capacity for differentiation of the tumor cells, and its curability; approximately 95% of newly diagnosed patients are cured. Experience in the management of GCTs leads to improved outcome.

INCIDENCE AND EPIDEMIOLOGY

In 2010, 8480 new cases of testicular GCT were diagnosed in the United States, and 350 men died. The tumor occurs most frequently in men between the ages of 20 and 40 years. A testicular mass in a male ≥50 years should be regarded as a lymphoma until proved otherwise. GCT is at least four to five times more common in white than in African-American males, and a higher incidence has been observed in Scandinavia and New Zealand than in the United States.

ETIOLOGY AND GENETICS

Cryptorchidism is associated with a several-fold higher risk of GCT. Abdominal cryptorchid testes are at a higher risk than inguinal cryptorchid testes. Orchiopexy should be performed before puberty, if possible. Early orchiopexy reduces the risk of GCT and improves the ability to save the testis. An abdominal cryptorchid testis that cannot be brought into the scrotum should be removed. Approximately 2% of men with GCTs of one testis will develop a primary tumor in the other testis. Testicular feminization syndromes increase the risk of testicular GCT, and Klinefelter's syndrome is associated with mediastinal GCT.

An isochromosome of the short arm of chromosome 12 (i[12p]) is pathognomonic for GCT of all histologic types. Excess 12p copy number, either in the form of i(12p) or as increased 12p on aberrantly banded marker chromosomes, occurs in nearly all GCTs, but the gene(s) on 12p involved in the pathogenesis are not yet defined.

CLINICAL PRESENTATION

A painless testicular mass is pathognomonic for a testicular malignancy. More commonly, patients present with testicular discomfort or swelling suggestive of epididymitis and/or orchitis. In this circumstance, a trial of antibiotics is reasonable. However, if symptoms persist or a residual abnormality remains, then testicular ultrasound examination is indicated.

Ultrasound of the testis is indicated whenever a testicular malignancy is considered and for persistent or painful testicular swelling. If a testicular mass is detected, a radical inguinal orchiectomy should be performed. Because the testis develops from the gonadal ridge, its blood supply and lymphatic drainage originate in the abdomen and descend with the testis into the scrotum. An inguinal approach is taken to avoid breaching anatomic barriers and permitting additional pathways of spread.

Back pain from retroperitoneal metastases is common and must be distinguished from musculoskeletal pain. Dyspnea from pulmonary metastases occurs infrequently. Patients with increased serum levels of human chorionic gonadotropin (hCG) may present with gynecomastia. A delay in diagnosis is associated with a more advanced stage and possibly worse survival.

The staging evaluation for GCT includes a determination of serum levels of α fetoprotein (AFP), hCG, and lactate dehydrogenase (LDH). After orchiectomy, a chest radiograph and a computed tomography (CT) scan of the abdomen and pelvis should be performed. A chest CT scan is required if pulmonary nodules or mediastinal or hilar disease is suspected. Stage I disease is limited to the testis, epididymis, or spermatic cord. Stage II disease is limited to retroperitoneal (regional) lymph nodes. Stage III disease is disease outside the retroperitoneum, involving supradiaphragmatic nodal sites or viscera. The staging may be "clinical"—defined solely by physical examination, blood marker evaluation, and radiographs—or "pathologic"—defined by an operative procedure.

The regional draining lymph nodes for the testis are in the retroperitoneum and the vascular supply originates from the great vessels (for the right testis) or the renal vessels (for the left testis). As a result, the lymph nodes that are involved first by a right testicular tumor are the interaortocaval lymph nodes just below the renal vessels. For a left testicular tumor, the first involved lymph nodes are lateral to the aorta (paraaortic) and below the left renal vessels. In both cases, further nodal spread is inferior; contralateral; and, less commonly, above the renal hilum. Lymphatic involvement can extend cephalad to the retrocrural, posterior mediastinal, and supraclavicular lymph nodes. Treatment is determined by tumor histology (seminoma vs nonseminoma) and clinical stage (Fig. 43–1).

PATHOLOGY

GCTs are divided into nonseminoma and seminoma subtypes. Nonseminomatous GCTs are most frequent in the third decade of life and can display the full spectrum of embryonic and adult cellular differentiation. This entity comprises four histologies: embryonal carcinoma, teratoma, choriocarcinoma, and endodermal sinus (yolk sac) tumor. Choriocarcinoma, consisting of both cytotrophoblasts and syncytiotrophoblasts, represents malignant trophoblastic differentiation and is invariably associated with secretion of hCG. Endodermal sinus tumor is the malignant counterpart of the fetal yolk sac and is associated with secretion of AFP. Pure embryonal carcinoma may secrete AFP, hCG, or both; this pattern is biochemical evidence of differentiation. Teratoma is composed of somatic cell types derived from two or more germ layers (ectoderm, mesoderm, or endoderm). Each of these histologies may be present alone or in combination with others. Nonseminomatous GCTs tend to metastasize early to sites such as the retroperitoneal lymph nodes and lung parenchyma. One-third of patients present with disease limited to the testis (stage I), one-third with retroperitoneal metastases (stage II), and one-third with more extensive supradiaphragmatic nodal or visceral metastases (stage III).

Seminoma represents approximately 50% of all GCTs, has a median age in the fourth decade, and generally follows a more indolent clinical course. Most patients (70%) present with stage I disease, approximately 20% with stage II disease, and 10% with stage III disease; lung or other visceral metastases are rare. When a tumor contains both seminoma and nonseminoma components, patient management is directed by the more aggressive nonseminoma component.

TUMOR MARKERS

Careful monitoring of the serum tumor markers AFP and hCG is essential in the management of patients with GCT, as these markers are important for diagnosis, as prognostic indicators, in monitoring treatment response, and in the detection of early relapse. Approximately 70% of patients presenting with disseminated nonseminomatous GCT have increased serum concentrations of AFP and/or hCG. Although hCG concentrations may be increased in patients with either nonseminoma or seminoma histology, the AFP concentration is increased only in patients with nonseminoma. The presence of an increased AFP level in a patient whose tumor shows only seminoma indicates that an occult nonseminomatous component exists, and the patient should be treated for nonseminomatous GCT. LDH levels are not as specific as AFP or hCG but are increased in 50–60% patients with metastatic nonseminoma and in up to 80% of patients with advanced seminoma.

AFP, hCG, and LDH levels should be determined before and after orchiectomy. Increased serum AFP and hCG concentrations decay according to first-order kinetics; the half-life is 24–36 h for hCG and 5–7 days for AFP. AFP and hCG should be assayed serially during and after treatment. The reappearance of hCG and/or AFP or the failure of these markers to decline according to the predicted half-life is an indicator of persistent or recurrent tumor.

TREATMENT Testicular Cancer

STAGE I NONSEMINOMA If, after an orchiectomy (for clinical stage I disease), radiographs and physical examination show no evidence of disease and serum AFP and hCG concentrations are either normal or declining to normal according to the known half-life, patients may be managed by either a nerve-sparing retroperitoneal lymph node dissection (RPLND) or surveillance. The retroperitoneal lymph nodes are involved by GCT (pathologic

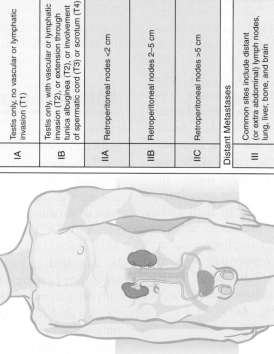

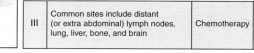

Stage	Extent of Disease
pT1	Tumor limited to the testis and epididymis without vascular or lymphatic invasion; tumor may invade into the tunica albuginea but not the tunica vaginalis
pT2	Tumor limited to the testis and epididymis with vascular or lymphatic invasion; tumor extending through the tunica albuginea with involvement of the tunica vaginalis
pT3	Tumor invades the spermatic cord with or without vascular or lymphatic invasion
pT4	Tumor invades the scrotum with or without vascular or lymphatic invasion

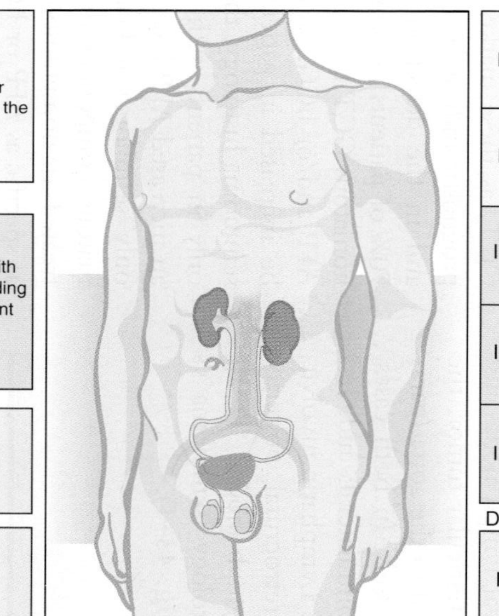
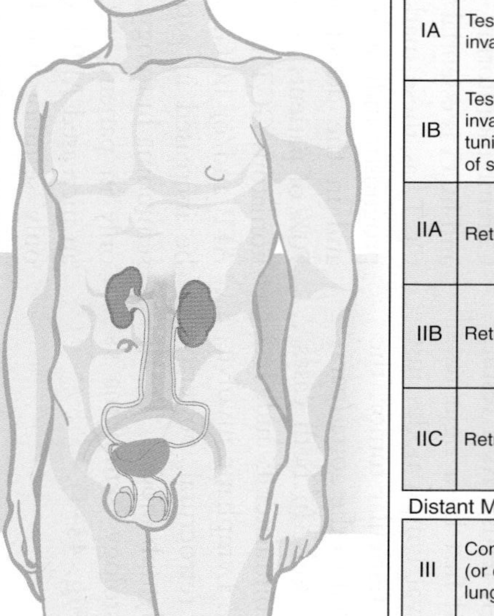

		Treatment Option	
Stage	Extent of Disease	Seminoma	Nonseminoma
IA	Testis only, no vascular or lymphatic invasion (T1)	Observation Chemotheapy or RT	RPLND or observation
IB	Testis only, with vascular or lymphatic invasion (T2), or extension through tunica albuginea (T2), or involvement of spermatic cord (T3) or scrotum (T4)	Observation Chemotheapy or RT	RPLND or chemotherapy
IIA	Retroperitoneal nodes <2 cm	RT	RPLND +/– adjuvant chemotherapy or chemotherapy followed by RPLND
IIB	Retroperitoneal nodes 2–5 cm	RT or chemotherapy	Chemotherapy, often followed by RPLND
IIC	Retroperitoneal nodes >5 cm	Chemotherapy	Chemotherapy, often followed by RPLND
Distant Metastases			
III	Common sites include distant (or extra abdominal) lymph nodes, lung, liver, bone, and brain	Chemotherapy	Chemotherapy, often followed by surgery (biopsy or resection)

FIGURE 43-1
Germ cell tumor staging and treatment.

stage II) in 20–50% of these patients. The choice of surveillance or RPLND is based on the pathology of the primary tumor. If the primary tumor shows no evidence for lymphatic or vascular invasion and is limited to the testis (T1), then either option is reasonable. If lymphatic or vascular invasion is present or the tumor extends into the tunica, spermatic cord, or scrotum (T2 through T4), then surveillance should not be offered. Either approach should cure >95% of patients.

RPLND is the standard operation for removal of the regional lymph nodes of the testis (retroperitoneal nodes). The operation removes the lymph nodes draining the primary site and the nodal groups adjacent to the primary landing zone. The standard (modified bilateral) RPLND removes all node-bearing tissue down to the bifurcation of the great vessels, including the ipsilateral iliac nodes. The major long-term effect of this operation is retrograde ejaculation and infertility. Nerve-sparing RPLND, usually accomplished by identification and dissection of individual nerve fibers, may avoid injury to the sympathetic nerves responsible for ejaculation. Normal ejaculation is preserved in ~90% of patients. Patients with pathologic stage I disease are observed, and only the <10% who relapse require additional therapy. If retroperitoneal nodes are found to be involved at RPLND, then a decision regarding adjuvant chemotherapy is made on the basis of the extent of retroperitoneal disease (see later discussion).

Surveillance is an option in the management of clinical stage I disease when no vascular or lymphatic invasion is found (T1). Only 20–30% of patients have pathologic stage II disease, implying that most RPLNDs in this situation are not therapeutic. Surveillance and RPLND lead to equivalent long-term survival rates. Patient compliance is essential if surveillance is to be successful. Patients must be carefully followed with periodic chest radiography, physical examination, CT scan of the abdomen, and serum tumor marker determinations. The median time to relapse is approximately 7 months, and late relapses (>2 years) are rare. The 70–80% of patients who do not relapse require no intervention after orchiectomy; treatment is reserved for those who do relapse. When the primary tumor is classified as T2 through T4 (extension beyond testis and epididymis or lymphatic or vascular invasion is identified), nerve-sparing RPLND is preferred. Approximately 50% of these patients have pathologic stage II disease and are destined to relapse without the RPLND.

STAGE II NONSEMINOMA Patients with limited, ipsilateral retroperitoneal adenopathy (nodes usually ≤3 cm in largest diameter) and normal levels of AFP and hCG generally undergo a modified bilateral RPLND as primary management. Increased levels of either AFP or hCG or both imply metastatic disease outside the retroperitoneum; chemotherapy is used in this setting. The local recurrence rate after a properly performed RPLND is very low. Depending on the extent of disease, the postoperative management options include either surveillance or two cycles of adjuvant chemotherapy. Surveillance is the preferred approach for patients with resected "low-volume" metastases (tumor nodes ≤2 cm in diameter *and* <6 nodes involved) because the probability of relapse is one-third or less. For those who relapse, risk-directed chemotherapy is indicated (see later discussion). Because relapse occurs in ≥50% of patients with "high-volume" metastases (>6 nodes involved, *or* any involved node >2 cm in largest diameter *or* extranodal tumor extension), two cycles of adjuvant chemotherapy should be considered, as it results in a cure in ≥98% of patients. Regimens consisting of etoposide (100 mg/m^2 daily on days 1–5) plus cisplatin (20 mg/m^2 daily on days 1–5) with or without bleomycin (30 units per day on days 2, 9, and 16) given at 3-week intervals are effective and well tolerated.

STAGES I AND II SEMINOMA Inguinal orchiectomy followed by retroperitoneal radiation therapy or surveillance cures nearly 100% of patients with stage I seminoma. Historically, radiation was the mainstay of treatment, but the reported association between radiation and secondary malignancies and the absence of a survival advantage of radiation over surveillance have led many to favor surveillance for patients committed to long-term follow-up. Studies have shown that approximately 15% of patients relapse, and rete testis involvement and size >4 cm have been associated with a higher relapse rate. The relapse is usually treated with chemotherapy. Long-term followup is essential because approximately 30% of relapses occur after 2 years and 5% after 5 years. A single dose of carboplatin has also been investigated as an alternative to radiation therapy; the outcome was similar, but long-term safety data are lacking, and the retroperitoneum remained the most frequent site of relapse.

Nonbulky retroperitoneal disease (stage IIA and most IIB) is treated with retroperitoneal radiation therapy. Approximately 90% of patients achieve relapse-free survival with retroperitoneal masses <5 cm in diameter. Because at least one-third of patients with bulkier disease relapse, initial chemotherapy is preferred for all stage IIC and some stage IIB with bulkier or multifocal disease.

CHEMOTHERAPY FOR ADVANCED GCT Regardless of histology, patients with stage IIC and stage III GCT are treated with chemotherapy. Combination chemotherapy programs based on cisplatin at doses of 100 mg/m^2 plus etoposide at doses of 500 mg/m^2 per cycle cure 70–80% of such patients, with or without bleomycin, depending on risk stratification (see later discussion).

A complete response (the complete disappearance of all clinical evidence of tumor on physical examination and radiography plus normal serum levels of AFP and hCG for ≥1 month) occurs after chemotherapy alone in ~60% of patients, and another 10–20% become disease-free with surgical resection of residual masses containing viable GCT. Lower doses of cisplatin result in inferior survival rates.

The toxicity of four cycles of the bleomycin, etoposide, and cisplatin (BEP) regimen is substantial. Nausea, vomiting, and hair loss occur in most patients, although nausea and vomiting have been markedly ameliorated by modern antiemetic regimens. Myelosuppression is frequent, and symptomatic bleomycin pulmonary toxicity occurs in ~5% of patients. Treatment-induced mortality due to neutropenia with septicemia or bleomycin-induced pulmonary failure occurs in 1–3% of patients. Dose reductions for myelosuppression are rarely indicated. Long-term permanent toxicities include nephrotoxicity (reduced glomerular filtration and persistent magnesium wasting), ototoxicity, and peripheral neuropathy. When bleomycin is administered by weekly bolus injection, Raynaud's phenomenon appears in 5–10% of patients. Other evidence of small blood vessel damage is seen less often, including transient ischemic attacks and myocardial infarction.

RISK-DIRECTED CHEMOTHERAPY Because not all patients are cured and treatment may cause significant toxicities, patients are stratified into "good-risk" and "poor-risk" groups according to pretreatment clinical features. For good-risk patients, the goal is to achieve maximum efficacy with minimal toxicity. For poor-risk patients, the goal is to identify more effective therapy with tolerable toxicity.

The International Germ Cell Cancer Consensus Group developed criteria to assign patients to three risk groups (good, intermediate, poor) (Table 43-1). The marker cut offs have been incorporated into the revised TNM (primary tumor, regional nodes, metastasis) staging of GCT. Hence, TNM stage groupings are now based on both anatomy (site and extent of disease) and biology (marker status and histology). Seminoma is either good or intermediate risk, based on the absence or presence of nonpulmonary visceral metastases. No poor-risk category exists for seminoma. Marker levels play no role in defining risk for seminoma. Nonseminomas have good-, intermediate-, and poor-risk categories based on the site of the primary tumor, the presence or absence of nonpulmonary visceral metastases, and marker levels.

For ~90% of patients with good-risk GCTs, four cycles of etoposide plus cisplatin (EP) or three cycles of BEP produce durable complete responses, with minimal acute and chronic toxicity. Pulmonary toxicity is absent when bleomycin is not used and is rare when therapy is limited to 9 weeks; myelosuppression with neutropenic fever is less frequent; and the treatment mortality rate is negligible.

TABLE 43-1

IGCCCG RISK CLASSIFICATION FOR ADVANCED GERM CELL TUMORS

RISK	NONSEMINOMA	SEMINOMA
Good	Gonadal or retroperitoneal primary site Absent nonpulmonary visceral metastases AFP <1000 ng/mL Beta-hCG <5000 mIU/mL LDH <1.5 × upper limit or normal (ULN)	Any primary site Absent nonpulmonary visceral metastases Any LDH, hCG
Intermediate	Gonadal or retroperitoneal primary site Absent nonpulmonary visceral metastases AFP 1000–10,000 ng/mL Beta-hCG 5000–50,000 mIU/mL LDH 1.5–10 × ULN	Any primary site Presence of nonpulmonary visceral metastases Any LDH, hCG
Poor	Mediastinal primary site Presence of nonpulmonary visceral metastases AFP ≥10,000 ng/mL Beta-hCG >50,000 mIU/mL LDH > 10 × ULN	No patients classified as poor prognosis

Abbreviations: AFP, α fetoprotein; hCG, human chorionic gonadotropin; IGCCCG, International Germ Cell Consensus Classification Group; LDH, lactate dehydrogenase.

Source: From International Germ Cell Cancer Consensus Group: J Clin Oncol 15:594, 1997.

Approximately 75% of intermediate-risk patients and 45% of poor-risk patients achieve durable complete remission with four cycles of BEP, and no regimen has proved superior. More effective therapy is needed.

POSTCHEMOTHERAPY SURGERY Resection of residual metastases after the completion of chemotherapy is an integral part of therapy. If the initial histology is nonseminoma and the marker values have normalized, all sites of residual disease should be resected. In general, residual retroperitoneal disease requires a modified bilateral RPLND. Thoracotomy (unilateral or bilateral) and neck dissection are less frequently required to remove residual mediastinal, pulmonary parenchymal, or cervical nodal disease. Viable tumor (seminoma, embryonal carcinoma, yolk sac tumor, or choriocarcinoma) will be present in 15%, mature teratoma in 40%, and necrotic debris and fibrosis in 45% of resected specimens. The frequency of teratoma or viable disease is highest in residual mediastinal tumors. If necrotic debris or mature teratoma is present, no further chemotherapy is necessary. If viable tumor is present but is completely excised, two additional cycles of chemotherapy are given.

If the initial histology is pure seminoma, mature teratoma is rarely present, and the most frequent finding is necrotic debris. For residual retroperitoneal disease, a complete RPLND is technically difficult owing to extensive postchemotherapy fibrosis. Observation is recommended when no radiographic abnormality exists on CT scan. Positive findings on a positron emission tomography (PET) scan correlate with viable seminoma in residua and mandate surgical excision or biopsy.

SALVAGE CHEMOTHERAPY Of patients with advanced GCT, 20–30% fail to achieve a durable complete response to first-line chemotherapy. A combination of vinblastine, ifosfamide, and cisplatin (VeIP) will cure approximately 25% of patients as a second-line therapy. Substitution of paclitaxel for vinblastine may be more effective in this setting. Patients are more likely to achieve a durable complete response if they had a testicular primary tumor and relapsed from a prior complete remission to first-line cisplatin-containing chemotherapy. In contrast, if the patient failed to achieve a complete response or has a primary mediastinal nonseminoma, then standard-dose salvage therapy is rarely beneficial. Treatment options for such patients include dose-intensive treatment, experimental therapies, and surgical resection.

Chemotherapy consisting of dose-intensive, high-dose carboplatin (≥1500 mg/m^2) plus etoposide (≥1200 mg/m^2), with or without cyclophosphamide, with peripheral blood stem cell support, induces a complete response in 25–40% of patients who have progressed after ifosfamide-containing salvage chemotherapy. Approximately half of the complete responses will be durable. High-dose therapy is standard of care for this patient population and has been suggested as treatment of choice for all patients with relapsed or refractory disease. Paclitaxel is also active in previously treated patients and shows promise in high-dose combination programs. Cure is still possible in some relapsed patients.

EXTRAGONADAL GERM CELL TUMORS AND MIDLINE CARCINOMA OF UNCERTAIN HISTOGENESIS

The prognosis and management of patients with extragonadal GCT depends on the tumor histology and site of origin. All patients with a diagnosis of extragonadal GCT should have a testicular ultrasound examination. Nearly all patients with retroperitoneal or mediastinal seminoma achieve a durable complete response to BEP or EP. The clinical features of patients with primary retroperitoneal nonseminoma GCT are similar to those of patients with a primary of testis origin, and careful evaluation will find evidence of a primary testicular GCT in about two-thirds of cases. In contrast, a primary mediastinal nonseminomatous GCT is associated with a poor prognosis; one-third of patients are cured with standard therapy (four cycles of BEP). Patients with newly diagnosed mediastinal nonseminoma are considered to have poor-risk disease and should be considered for clinical trials testing regimens of possibly greater efficacy. In addition, mediastinal nonseminoma is associated with hematologic disorders, including acute myelogenous leukemia, myelodysplastic syndrome, and essential thrombocytosis unrelated to previous chemotherapy. These hematologic disorders are very refractory to treatment. Nonseminoma of any primary site may change into other malignant histologies such as embryonal rhabdomyosarcoma or adenocarcinoma. This is called *malignant transformation*. i(12p) has been identified in the transformed cell type, indicating GCT clonal origin.

A group of patients with poorly differentiated tumors of unknown histogenesis, midline in distribution, and not associated with secretion of AFP or hCG has been described; a few (10–20%) are cured by standard cisplatin-containing chemotherapy. i(12p) is present in ~25% of such tumors (the fraction that are cisplatin-responsive), confirming their origin from primitive germ cells. This finding is also predictive of the response to cisplatin-based chemotherapy and resulting long-term survival. These tumors are heterogeneous; neuroepithelial tumors and lymphoma may also present in this fashion.

FERTILITY

Infertility is an important consequence of the treatment of GCTs. Preexisting infertility or impaired fertility is often present. Azoospermia, oligospermia, or both are present at diagnosis in at least 50% of patients with testicular GCTs. Ejaculatory dysfunction is associated with RPLND, and germ cell damage may result from cisplatin-containing chemotherapy. Nerve-sparing techniques to preserve the retroperitoneal sympathetic nerves have made retrograde ejaculation less likely in the subgroups of patients who are candidates for this operation. Spermatogenesis does recur in some patients after chemotherapy. However, because of the significant risk of impaired reproductive capacity, semen analysis and cryopreservation of sperm in a sperm bank should be recommended to all patients before treatment.

CHAPTER 44

GYNECOLOGIC MALIGNANCIES

Michael V. Seiden

OVARIAN CANCER

INCIDENCE AND PATHOLOGY

Ovarian cancer is the most lethal malignancy of gynecologic origin in the United States and other countries that have organized and effective cervical cancer screening programs. In 2010, 21,880 cases of ovarian cancer with 13,850 deaths were expected in the United States. The ovary is a complex and dynamic organ and, between the ages of approximately 11 and 50 years, is responsible for follicle maturation associated with egg maturation, ovulation, and cyclical sex steroid hormone production. These complex and linked biologic functions are coordinated through a variety of cells within the ovary, each of which possesses neoplastic potential. By far the most common and most lethal of the ovarian neoplasms arise from the ovarian epithelium found both on the surface of the ovary and in subsurface locations, known as cortical inclusion cysts, believed to be entrapped epithelium from the healing associated with prior follicle rupture during ovulation. The ovarian epithelium in good health appears as a simple epithelium, but with neoplastic transformation, it undergoes metaplastic changes into what is termed *müllerian epithelium.* The müllerian epithelium has a variety of subtypes each of which provide a specific phenotype of the tumor and in some cases different clinical presentations. Epithelial tumors are the most common ovarian neoplasm; they may be benign (50%), malignant (33%), or of borderline malignancy (16%). Age influences risk of malignancy; tumors in younger women are more likely benign. The most common of the ovarian epithelial malignancies are serous tumors (50%); tumors of mucinous (25%), endometrioid (15%), clear cell (5%), and transitional cell histology or Brenner tumor (1%) represent smaller proportions of epithelial ovarian tumors. In contrast, stromal tumors arise from the steroid hormone–producing cells and likewise have different phenotypes and clinical presentations largely dependent on the type and quantity of hormone production. Tumors arising in the germ cell are most similar in biology and behavior to testicular tumors in males (Chap. 43).

Tumors may also metastasize to the ovary from breast, colon, gastric, and pancreatic primaries. Bilateral ovarian masses from metastatic mucin-secreting gastrointestinal cancers are termed *Krukenberg tumors.*

OVARIAN CANCER OF EPITHELIAL ORIGIN

Epidemiology

A female has approximately a 1 in 72 lifetime risk (1.6%) of developing ovarian cancer, with the majority of affected women developing epithelial tumors. Epithelial tumors of the ovary have a peak incidence in women in their sixties, although age at presentation can range across the extremes of adult life, with cases being reported in women in their twenties to nineties. Known risk factors that increase the chance of subsequent ovarian cancer include epidemiologic, environmental, and genetic factors such as nulliparity, use of talc agents applied to the perineum, obesity, and probably hormone replacement therapy. Protective factors include the use of oral contraceptives, multiparity, and breastfeeding. These protective factors are thought to work through suppression of ovulation and perhaps reduction of ovarian inflammation and damage associated with the repair of the ovarian cortex associated with ovulation and perhaps suppression of gonadotropins. Other protective factors, such as fallopian tube ligation, are thought to protect the ovarian epithelium (or perhaps the distal fallopian tube fimbriae) from carcinogens that migrate from the vagina to the tubes and ovarian surface epithelium (see later discussion).

Genetic risk factors

A variety of genetic syndromes substantially increases a woman's risk of developing ovarian cancer. Approximately

10% of women with ovarian cancer have a somatic mutation in one of two DNA repair genes: *BRCA1* (chromosome 17q12-21) or *BRCA2* (chromosome 13q12-13). Individuals inheriting a single copy of a mutant allele have a very high incidence of breast and ovarian cancer. Most of these women have a family history that is notable for multiple cases of breast and/or ovarian cancer, although inheritance through male members of the family can camouflage this genotype through several generations. The most common malignancy in these women is breast carcinoma, although women harboring germ-line *BRCA1* mutations have a marked increased risk of developing ovarian malignancies in their forties and fifties with a 30–50% lifetime risk of developing ovarian cancer. Women harboring a mutation in *BRCA2* have a lower penetrance of ovarian cancer with perhaps a 20–40% chance of developing this malignancy, with onset typically in their fifties or sixties. Women with a *BRCA2* mutation also are at slightly increased risk of pancreatic cancer. Screening studies in this select population suggest that current screening techniques, including serial evaluation of the CA-125 tumor marker and ultrasound, are insufficient at detecting early-stage and curable disease, so women with these germ-line mutations are advised to undergo prophylactic removal of their ovaries and fallopian tubes typically after completing childbearing and ideally before ages 35–40 years. Early prophylactic oophorectomy also protects these women from subsequent breast cancer with a reduction of breast cancer risk of approximately 50%.

Ovarian cancer is also one form of cancer (along with colorectal and endometrial cancer) that may develop in women with Lynch syndrome, type II, caused by mutations in DNA mismatch repair genes (*MSH2, MLH1, MLH6, PMS1, PMS2*). Ovarian cancer may appear in women younger than 50 years of age in this syndrome.

Presentation

Neoplasms of the ovary tend to be painless unless they undergo torsion. Symptoms are therefore typically related to compression of local organs or due to symptoms from metastatic disease. Women with tumors localized to the ovary do have an increased incidence of symptoms including pelvic discomfort, bloating, and perhaps changes in a woman's typical urinary or bowel pattern. Unfortunately, these symptoms are frequently dismissed by either the woman or her health care team. It is believed that high-grade tumors metastasize early in the neoplastic process. Unlike other epithelial malignancies, these tumors tend to exfoliate throughout the peritoneal cavity and thus present with symptoms associated with disseminated intraperitoneal tumors. The most common symptoms at presentation include a multimonth period of progressive complaints that typically include some combination of heartburn, nausea, early satiety, indigestion, constipation, and abdominal pain. Signs include a rapid increase in abdominal girth due to the accumulation of ascites that typically alerts the patient and her physician that the concurrent gastrointestinal symptoms are likely associated with serious pathology. Radiologic evaluation typically demonstrates a complex adnexal mass and ascites. Laboratory evaluation demonstrates a markedly elevated CA-125, a shed mucin (Muc 16) associated with, but not specific for, ovarian cancer. Hematogenous and lymphatic spread are seen but are not the typical presentation. Ovarian cancers are divided into four stages, with stage I tumors confined to the ovary, stage II malignancies confined to the pelvis, and stage III confined to the peritoneal cavity (**Table 44-1**). These three stages are subdivided, with the most common presentation, stage IIIc, defined as tumors with bulky intraperitoneal disease. About 70% of

TABLE 44-1

STAGING AND SURVIVAL IN GYNECOLOGIC MALIGNANCIES

STAGE	OVARIAN	5-YEAR SURVIVAL, %	ENDOMETRIAL	5-YEAR SURVIVAL, %	CERVIX	5-YEAR SURVIVAL, %
0	—		—		Carcinoma in situ	100
I	Confined to ovary	90–95	Confined to corpus	89	Confined to uterus	85
II	Confined to pelvis	70–80	Involves corpus and cervix	73	Invades beyond uterus but not to pelvic wall	65
III	Intraabdominal spread	20–50	Extends outside the uterus but not outside the true pelvis	52	Extends to pelvic wall and/or lower third of vagina, or hydronephrosis	35
IV	Spread outside abdomen	1–5	Extends outside the true pelvis or involves the bladder or rectum	17	Invades mucosa of bladder or rectum or extends beyond the true pelvis	7

women present with stage IIIc disease. Stage IV disease includes women with parenchymal metastases (liver, lung, spleen) or, alternatively, abdominal wall or pleural disease. The 30% not presenting with stage IIIc disease are roughly evenly distributed among the other stages.

Screening

Ovarian cancer is the fifth most lethal malignancy in women in the United States, curable in early stages but seldom curable in advanced stages; hence, screening is of considerable interest. Furthermore the ovary is well visualized with a variety of imaging techniques, most notably transvaginal ultrasound. Early-stage tumors often produce proteins that can be measured in the blood such as CA-125 and HE-4. Nevertheless, the incidence of ovarian cancer in the middle-aged female population is low, with only approximately 1 in 2000 women between the ages of 50 and 60 years carrying an asymptomatic and undetected tumor. Thus effective screening techniques must be sensitive but, more importantly, highly specific so to minimize the number of false-positive test results. Even a screening test with 98% specificity and 50% sensitivity would have a positive predictive value of only about 1%. Despite these formidable barriers, ongoing studies are evaluating the utility of various screening strategies. However, screening for ovarian cancer is currently not recommended outside of a clinical trial.

TREATMENT Ovarian Cancer

In women presenting with a localized ovarian mass, the principal diagnostic and therapeutic maneuver is to determine if the tumor is benign or malignant and, in the event that the tumor is malignant, whether the tumor arises in the ovary or is a site of metastatic disease. Metastatic disease to the ovary can be seen from primary tumors of the colon, appendix, stomach (Krukenberg tumors), and breast. Typically, women undergo a unilateral salpingo-oophorectomy, and if pathology reveals a primary ovarian malignancy, then the procedure is followed by a hysterectomy, removal of the remaining tube and ovary, omentectomy, and pelvic node sampling along with some random biopsies of the peritoneal cavity. This extensive surgical procedure is performed because approximately 30% of tumors that by visual inspection appear to be confined to the ovary have already disseminated to the peritoneal cavity and/or surrounding lymph nodes.

If there is evidence of bulky intraabdominal disease, a comprehensive attempt at maximal tumor cytoreduction is attempted even if it involves partial bowel resection; splenectomy and in certain cases, more extensive upper abdominal surgery. The ability to debulk metastatic ovarian cancer to minimal visible disease is associated with an improved prognosis compared with women left with visible disease. Patients without gross residual disease after resection have a median survival time of 39 months compared with 17 months for those left with macroscopic tumor. Once tumors have been surgically debulked, women receive therapy with a platinum agent, typically with a taxane. Debate continues as to whether this therapy should be delivered intravenously or alternatively whether some of the therapy should be delivered directly into the peritoneal cavity via a catheter. Three randomized studies have demonstrated improved survival rates with intraperitoneal therapy, but this approach is still not widely accepted due to technical challenges associated with this delivery route and increased toxicity. In women who present with bulky disease, an alternative approach is to treat with platinum plus a taxane for several cycles (neoadjuvant therapy). Subsequent surgical procedures are more effective at leaving the patient without gross residual tumor, and survival is comparable to surgery followed by chemotherapy.

With optimal debulking surgery and platinum-based chemotherapy (usually carboplatin dosed to an area under the curve [AUC] of 7.5 plus paclitaxel 175 mg/m^2 by 3-h infusion in monthly cycles), 70% of women who present with advanced-stage tumors respond, and 40–50% experience a complete remission with normalization of their CA-125, computed tomography (CT) scans, and physical examination. Unfortunately, only half the complete responders remain in remission. Disease recurs within 1 to 4 years from the completion of their primary therapy in half of complete responders. CA-125 levels often increase as a first sign of relapse; however, data are not clear that early intervention influences survival. Recurrent disease is effectively managed, but not cured, with a variety of chemotherapeutic agents. Eventually, all of these women develop chemotherapy-refractory disease at which point refractory ascites, poor bowel motility, and obstruction or pseudoobstruction due to a tumor-infiltrated aperistaltic bowel are common. Limited surgery to relieve intestinal obstruction, localized radiation therapy to relieve pressure or pain from masses, or palliative chemotherapy may be helpful. Agents with >15% response rates include gemcitabine, topotecan, liposomal doxorubicin, and bevacizumab. Approximately 20% of ovarian cancers are HER2/neu positive, and trastuzumab may induce responses in this subset.

Five-year survival correlates with the stage of disease: stage I, 90–95%; stage II, 70–80%; stage III, 20–50%; and stage IV, 1–5% (Table 44-1). Prognosis is also influenced by histologic grade: 5-year survival rates are 88% for well-differentiated tumors, 58% for moderately differentiated tumors, and 27% for poorly differentiated tumors. Histologic type has less influence on outcome. Patients with tumors of low malignant potential are managed by surgery; chemotherapy and radiation therapy do not improve survival.

OVARIAN SEX CORD AND STROMAL TUMORS

Epidemiology, presentation, and predisposing syndromes

Approximately 7% of ovarian neoplasms are stromal or sex cord tumors, with approximately 1800 cases expected each year in the United States. Ovarian stromal tumors or sex cord tumors are most common in women in their fifties or sixties, but tumors can present in the extremes of age, including the pediatric population. These tumors arise from the mesenchymal components of the ovary, including steroid-producing cells as well as fibroblasts. Essentially all of these tumors are of low malignant potential and present as unilateral solid masses. Three clinical presentations are common: the detection of an abdominal mass abdominal pain due to ovarian torsion, intratumoral hemorrhage, or rupture or signs and symptoms due to hormonal production by these tumors.

The most common hormone-producing tumors include thecomas, granulosa cell tumor, and juvenile granulosa tumors in children. These estrogen-producing tumors often present with breast tenderness as well as isosexual precocious pseudopuberty in children; menometrorrhagia, oligomenorrhea, or amenorrhea in premenopausal women; or alternatively as postmenopausal bleeding in older women. In some women, estrogen-associated secondary malignancies, such as endometrial or breast cancer, may present as synchronous malignancies. Alternatively, endometrial cancer may serve as the presenting malignancy with evaluation subsequently identifying a unilateral solid ovarian neoplasm that proves to be an occult granulosa cell tumor. Sertoli-Leydig tumors often present with hirsutism, virilization, and occasionally Cushing's syndrome due to increased production of testosterone, androstenedione, or other 17-ketosteroids. Hormonally inert tumors include fibroma that presents as a solitary mass often in association with ascites and occasionally hydrothorax also known as Meigs' syndrome. A subset of these tumors present in individuals with a variety of inherited disorders that predispose them to mesenchymal neoplasia. Associations include juvenile granulosa cell tumors and perhaps Sertoli-Leydig tumors with Ollier's disease (multiple enchondromatosis) or Maffucci's syndrome, ovarian sex cord tumors with annular tubules with Peutz-Jeghers syndrome, and fibromas with Gorlin disease.

TREATMENT Sex Cord Tumors

The mainstay of treatment for sex cord tumors is surgical resection. Most women present with tumors confined to the ovary. For the small subset of women who present with metastatic disease or develop evidence of tumor recurrence after primary resection, survival is still typically long, often in excess of a decade. Because these tumors are slow growing and relatively refractory to chemotherapy, women with metastatic disease are often debulked as disease is usually peritoneal-based (as with epithelial ovarian cancer). Definitive data that surgical debulking of metastatic or recurrent disease prolongs survival are lacking, but ample data document women who have survived years or in some cases decades after resection of recurrent disease. In addition, large peritoneal-based metastases also have a proclivity for hemorrhage, sometimes with catastrophic complications. Chemotherapy is occasionally effective, and women tend to receive regimens designed to treat epithelial or germ cell tumors (GSTs). These tumors often produce high levels of müllerian inhibiting substance (MIS), inhibin, and in the case of Sertoli-Leydig tumors α fetoprotein (AFP). These proteins are detectable in serum and can be used as tumor markers to monitor women for recurrent disease as the increase and decrease of these proteins in the serum tend to reflect the changing bulk of systemic tumor.

Germ cell tumors of the ovary

GSTs like their counterparts in the testis, are cancers of germ cells. These totipotent cells contain the programming for differentiation to essentially all tissue types, and hence the GSTs include a histologic menagerie of bizarre tumors, including benign teratomas and a variety of malignant tumors, such as immature teratomas, dysgerminomas, yolk sac malignancies, and choriocarcinomas. Benign teratoma (or dermoid cyst) is the most common germ cell neoplasm of the ovary and often presents in young woman. These tumors include a complex mixture of differentiated tissue, including tissues from all three germ layers. In older women, these differentiated tumors can develop malignant transformation, most commonly squamous cell carcinomas. Malignant GSTs include dysgerminomas, yolk sac tumors, immature teratomas, and embryonal and choriocarcinomas. There are no known genetic abnormalities that unify these tumors. A subset of dysgerminomas harbors mutations in c-*Kit* oncogenes (as seen in gastrointestinal stromal tumors [GISTs]), whereas a subset of GSTs have isochromosome 12 abnormalities as seen in testicular malignancies. In addition, a subset of dysgerminomas is associated with dysgenetic ovaries. Identification of a dysgerminoma arising in genotypic XY gonads is important in that it highlights the need to identify and remove the contralateral gonad due to risk of gonadoblastoma.

Presentation

GSTs can present at all ages, but the peak age of presentation tends to be in females in their late teens or early twenties. Typically these tumors will become large ovarian masses, which eventually present as palpable low abdominal or pelvic masses. Similar to sex cord tumors, torsion or hemorrhage may present urgently or emergently as acute abdominal pain. Some of these tumors produce elevated levels of human chorionic gonadotropin (hCG) that can lead to isosexual precocious puberty when tumors present in younger girls. Unlike epithelial ovarian cancer, these tumors have a higher proclivity for nodal or hematogenous metastases. As with testicular tumors some of these tumors tend to produce AFP (yolk sac tumors) or hCG (embryonal and choriocarcinomas as well as some dysgerminomas) that are reliable tumor markers.

TREATMENT GSTs

GSTs typically present in women who are still of childbearing age, and because bilateral tumors are uncommon (except in dysgerminoma, 10–15%), the typical treatment is unilateral oophorectomy or salpingo-oophorectomy. Because nodal metastases to pelvic and para-aortic nodes are common and may affect treatment choices, these nodes should be carefully inspected, and if enlarged, should be resected if possible. Women with malignant GSTs typically receive bleomycin, etoposide, and cisplatin (BEP) chemotherapy. In the majority of women, even those with advanced-stage disease, cure is expected. Close follow-up without adjuvant therapy of women with stage I tumors is reasonable if there is high confidence that the patient and health care team are committed to compulsive and careful follow-up, as chemotherapy at the time of tumor recurrence is likely to be curative.

Dysgerminoma is the ovarian counterpart of testicular seminoma. The 5-year disease-free survival rate is 100% in early-stage patients and 61% in stage III disease. Although the tumor is highly radiation-sensitive, radiation produces infertility in many patients. BEP chemotherapy is as effective or more so without causing infertility. The use of BEP following incomplete resection is associated with 95%, 2-year disease-free survival. This chemotherapy is now the treatment of choice for dysgerminoma.

FALLOPIAN TUBE CANCER

Transport of the egg to the uterus occurs via transit through the fallopian tube, with the distal ends of these tubes composed of fimbriae that drape about the ovarian surface and capture the egg as it erupts from the ovarian cortex. Fallopian tube malignancies typically have the same histologic pattern as ovarian malignancies, with the most common epithelial malignancy being of serous histology. Previous teaching was that these malignancies were rare, but more careful histologic examination suggests that many "ovarian malignancies" might actually arise in the distal fimbria of the fallopian tube. Data supporting this theory are strongest in the population of women who carry *BRCA1* or *BRCA2* somatic mutations. These women often present with adnexal masses, and similar to ovarian cancer, these tumors spread relatively early throughout the peritoneal cavity and respond to platinum and taxane therapy and have a natural history that is essentially identical to that of ovarian cancer (Table 44-1).

CERVICAL CANCER

GLOBAL CONSIDERATIONS

Cervical cancer is the second most common and most lethal malignancy in women worldwide likely due to the widespread infection with high-risk strains of human papillomavirus (HPV) and limited utilization or access to Pap smear screening in many nations throughout the world. Nearly 500,000 cases of cervical cancer are expected worldwide with approximately 240,000 deaths annually. Cancer incidence is particularly high in women residing in Central and South America, the Caribbean, and southern and eastern Africa. The mortality rate is disproportionately high in Africa. In the United States, 12,200 women were diagnosed with cervical cancer and 4210 women died. Whereas efforts in developed countries have looked at high-technology screening techniques for HPV involving polymerase chain reaction (PCR) and other molecular technologies, there is an urgent need for high-throughput low-technology strategies to identify and treat women bearing high risk but treatable cervical dysplasia. The development of effective vaccines for high-risk HPV types makes it imperative to determine economical, socially acceptable, and logistically feasible strategies to deliver and distribute this vaccine to girls and perhaps boys before their engagement in sexual activity.

HUMAN PAPILLOMAVIRUS INFECTION AND PREVENTIVE VACCINATION

HPV is the primary neoplastic-initiating event in the vast majority of women with invasive cervical cancer. This double-strand DNA virus infects epithelium near the transformation zone of the cervix. More than 60 types of HPV are known, with approximately 20 types having the ability to generate high-grade dysplasia and malignancy. HPV16 and 18 are the types most frequently associated with high-grade dysplasia and targeted by both vaccines approved by the U.S. Food and Drug Administration. The large majority of sexually active adults are exposed to HPV, and most women clear the infection without specific intervention. The 8-kilobase HPV genome encodes seven early genes, most notably *E6* and *E7*, which can bind to *RB* and *p53*, respectively. High-risk types of HPV encode *E6* and *E7* molecules that are particularly effective at inhibiting the normal cell-cycle checkpoint functions of these regulatory proteins, leading to immortalization but not full transformation of cervical epithelium. A minority of woman fail to clear the infection with subsequent HPV integration into the host genome. Over the course of as short as months but more typically years, some of these women develop high-grade dysplasia. The time from dysplasia to carcinoma is likely years to more than a decade and almost certainly requires the acquisition of other poorly defined genetic mutations within the infected and immortalized epithelium.

Risk factors include a high number of sexual partners, young age of first intercourse, and history of venereal disease. Smoking is a cofactor; heavy smokers have a higher risk of dysplasia with HPV infection. HIV infection, especially when associated with low CD4+ T cell counts, is associated with a higher rate of high-grade dysplasia and likely a shorter latency period between infection and invasive disease.

Currently approved vaccines include the recombinant proteins to the late proteins, L1 and L2 of HPV-16 and -18. Vaccination of women before the initiation of sexual activity dramatically reduces the rate of HPV-16 and -18 infection and subsequent dysplasia. There is also partial protection against other HPV types, although vaccinated women are still at risk for HPV infection and still require standard Pap smear screening. Although no randomized trial data demonstrate the utility of Pap smears, the dramatic drop in cervical cancer incidence and death in developed countries employing wide-scale screening provides strong evidence for its effectiveness. The incorporation of HPV testing by PCR or other molecular techniques increases the sensitivity of detecting cervical pathology but at the cost of lower sensitivity in that it identifies many women with transient infections who require no specific medical intervention.

CLINICAL PRESENTATIONS

The majority of cervical malignancies are squamous cell carcinomas associated with HPV. Adenocarcinomas are also HPV-related and arise deep in the endocervical canal; they are typically not seen by visual inspection of the cervix and thus often missed by Pap smear screening. A variety of rarer malignancies, including atypical epithelial tumors, carcinoids, small cell carcinomas, sarcomas, and lymphomas, have also been reported.

The principal role of Pap smear testing is the detection of asymptomatic preinvasive cervical dysplasia of squamous epithelial lining. Invasive carcinomas often have symptoms or signs that include postcoital spotting or intermenstrual cycle bleeding or menometrorrhagia. Foul-smelling or persistent yellow discharge may also be seen. Presentations that include pelvic or sacral pain suggest lateral extension of the tumor into pelvic nerve plexus by either the primary tumor or a pelvic node and are signs of advanced-stage disease. Likewise, flank pain from hydronephrosis from ureteral compression or deep-vein thrombosis from iliac vessel compression suggests either extensive nodal disease or direct extension of the primary tumor to the pelvic sidewall. The most common finding of physical examination is a visible tumor on the cervix.

TREATMENT Cervical Cancer

Scans are not part of the formal clinical staging of cervical cancer yet are very useful in planning appropriate therapy. CT can detect hydronephrosis indicative of pelvic sidewall disease but is not accurate at evaluating other pelvic structures. Magnetic resonance imaging (MRI) is more accurate at estimating uterine extension and paracervical extension of disease into soft tissues typically bordered by broad and cardinal ligaments that support the uterus in the central pelvis. Positron emission tomography (PET) scan may be the most accurate technique for evaluating the pelvis and more importantly nodal (pelvic, para-aortic, and scalene) sites for disease. This technique seems more prognostic (and probably accurate) than CT, MRI, or lymphangiography, especially in the para-aortic region.

Stage I cervical tumors are confined to the cervix, whereas stage II tumors extend into the upper vagina or paracervical soft tissue (Fig. 44-1). Stage III tumors extend to the lower vagina or the pelvic sidewalls, whereas stage IV tumors invade the bladder or rectum or have spread to distant sites. Very small stage I cervical tumors can be treated with a variety of surgical procedures. In young women desiring to maintain fertility, radical trachelectomy removes the cervix with subsequent anastomosis of the upper vagina to the uterine corpus. Larger cervical tumors confined to the cervix

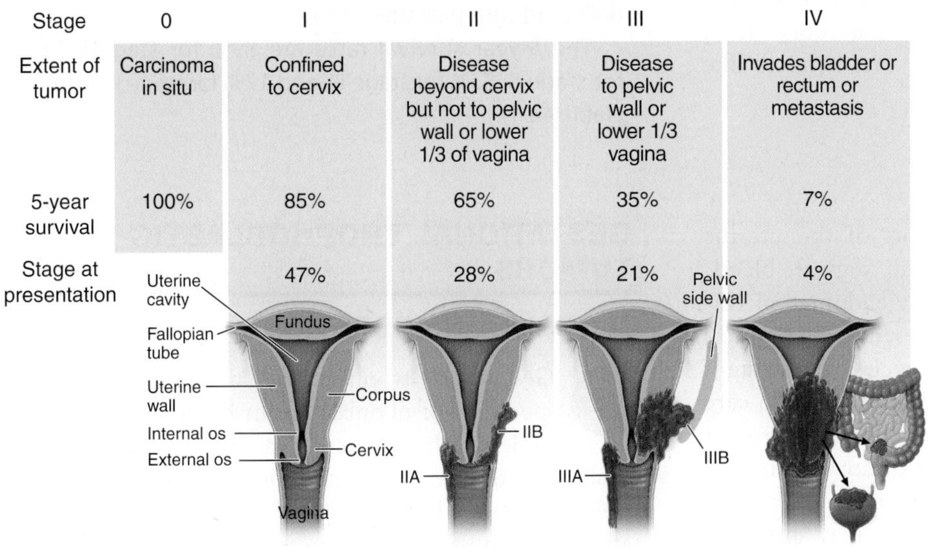

Staging of cervix cancer
Stage
0
I
II
III
IV
Extent of tumor
Carcinoma in situ
Confined to cervix
Disease beyond cervix but not to pelvic wall or lower 1/3 of vagina
Disease to pelvic wall or lower 1/3 vagina
Invades bladder or rectum or metastasis
5-year survival
100%
85%
65%
35%
7%
Stage at presentation
47%
28%
21%
4%
Uterine cavity
Fundus
Fallopian tube
Uterine wall
Corpus
Internal os
External os
Cervix
Vagina
IIA
IIB
IIIA
Pelvic side wall
IIIB

FIGURE 44-1
Anatomic display of the stages of cervix cancer defined by location, extent of tumor, frequency of presentation, and 5-year survival rate.

can be treated with either surgical resection or radiation therapy in combination with cisplatin-based chemotherapy with a high chance of cure. Larger tumors that extend down the vagina or into the paracervical soft tissues or the pelvic sidewalls are treated with combination chemotherapy and radiation therapy. The treatment of recurrent or metastatic disease is unsatisfactory due to the relative resistance of these tumors to chemotherapy and currently available biological agents.

UTERINE CANCER

EPIDEMIOLOGY

Several different tumor types arise in uterine corpus. Most tumors arise in the glandular lining and are endometrial adenocarcinomas. Tumors can also arise in the smooth muscle; most are benign (uterine leiomyoma), with a small minority of tumors being sarcomas. The endometrioid histologic subtype of endometrial cancer is the most common gynecologic malignancy in the United States. In 2010, it was diagnosed in 43,470 women and 7950 women died from the disease. Development of these tumors is a multistep process with estrogen playing an important early role in driving endometrial gland proliferation. Relative overexposure to this class of hormones is a risk factor for the subsequent development of endometrioid tumors. In contrast progestins drive glandular maturation and are protective. Hence, women with high endogenous or pharmacologic exposure to estrogens, especially if unopposed by progesterone are at high risk for endometrial cancer. Obese women, women treated with unopposed estrogens, or women with estrogen-producing tumors (such as granulosa cell tumors of the ovary) are at higher risk for endometrial cancer. In addition, treatment with tamoxifen, which has antiestrogenic effects in breast tissue but estrogenic effects in uterine epithelium, is associated with an increased risk of endometrial cancer. Secondary events such as the loss of the PTEN or Cables tumor suppressor genes likely serve as secondary events in carcinogenesis. The molecular events that underlie less common endometrial cancers such as clear cell and papillary serous tumors of the uterine corpus are unknown.

Women with mutation in one of a series of DNA mismatch repair genes associated with the Lynch syndrome, also known as hereditary nonpolyposis colon cancer (HNPCC) syndrome, are at increased risk for endometrioid endometrial carcinoma. These individuals have germ-line mutations in *MSH2*; *MLH1*; and in rare cases *PMS1* and *PMS2*. Individuals who carry these mutations typically have a family history of cancer and are at markedly increased risk for colon cancer and modestly increased risk for ovarian cancer and a variety of other tumors. Middle-aged women with HNPCC carry a 4% annual risk of endometrial cancer and a relative overall risk of approximately 200-fold compared with age-matched women without HNPCC.

PATHOLOGY

Approximately 75–80% of endometrial cancers are adenocarcinomas. The prognosis depends on stage, histologic grade, and depth of myometrial invasion. Approximately 10% of patients have tumors with areas of squamous cell differentiation. When the tumor is well differentiated, it is called *adenoacanthoma*; when poorly differentiated, *adenosquamous* carcinoma. Less common histologies include mucinous carcinoma (5%) and a papillary serous tumor (<10%) that behaves like ovarian cancer.

PRESENTATIONS

The majority of women with tumors of the uterine corpus present with postmenopausal vaginal bleeding due to shedding of the malignant endometrial lining. Premenopausal women often present with atypical bleeding between typical menstrual cycles. These signs typically bring a woman to the attention of a health care professional, and hence the majority of women present with early-stage disease in which the tumor is confined to the uterine corpus. Diagnosis is typically established by endometrial biopsy. Epithelial tumors may spread to pelvic or para-aortic lymph nodes. Pulmonary metastases can appear later in the natural history of this disease but are very uncommon at initial presentation. Serous tumors tend to have patterns of spread much more reminiscent of ovarian cancer with many patients presenting with omental disease and sometimes ascites. Some women presenting with uterine sarcomas will present with pelvic pain. Nodal metastases are uncommon with sarcomas, which are more likely to present with either intraabdominal disease or pulmonary metastases.

TREATMENT Uterine Cancer

Most women with endometrial cancer have disease that is localized to the uterus (75% are stage I, Table 44-1), and definitive treatment typically involves a hysterectomy with removal of the ovaries and fallopian tubes. The resection of lymph nodes does not improve outcome but does provide prognostic information. Node involvement defines stage III disease, present in 13% of patients. Tumor grade and depth of invasion are the two key prognostic variables in early-stage tumors, and women with low-grade and/or minimally invasive tumors are typically observed after definitive surgical therapy. Patients with high-grade tumors or tumors that are deeply invasive (stage IB, 13%) are at higher risk for pelvic recurrence or recurrence at the vaginal cuff, which is typically prevented by vaginal vault brachytherapy.

Women with regional metastases or metastatic disease (3% of patients) with low-grade tumors can be treated with progesterone. Poorly differentiated tumors are typically resistant to hormonal manipulation and thus are treated with chemotherapy. The role of chemotherapy in the adjuvant setting is currently under investigation. Chemotherapy for metastatic disease is delivered with palliative intent.

The 5-year survival rates are 89% for stage I, 73% for stage II, 52% for stage III, and 17% for stage IV disease (Table 44-1).

GESTATIONAL TROPHOBLASTIC TUMORS

GLOBAL CONSIDERATIONS

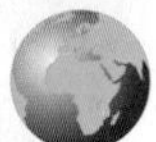

Gestational trophoblastic diseases represent a spectrum of neoplasia from benign hydatidiform mole to choriocarcinoma due to persistent trophoblastic disease associated most commonly with molar pregnancy but occasionally seen after normal gestation. The most common presentations of trophoblastic tumors are partial and complete molar pregnancies. These represent approximately 1 in 1500 conceptions in developed Western countries. The incidence widely varies globally, with areas in Southeast Asia having a much higher incidence of molar pregnancy. Regions with high molar pregnancy rates are often associated with diets low in carotene and animal fats.

RISK FACTORS

Trophoblastic tumors result from the outgrowth or persistence of placental tissue. They arise most commonly in the uterus but can also arise in other sites such as the fallopian tubes due to ectopic pregnancy. Risk factors include poorly defined dietary and environmental factors as well as conceptions at the extremes of reproductive age, with the incidence particularly high in females conceiving younger than age 16 years or older than age 50 years. In older women, the incidence of molar pregnancy might be as high as one in three, likely due to increased risk of abnormal fertilization of the aged ova. Most trophoblastic neoplasms are associated with complete moles, diploid tumors with all genetic material from the paternal donor (known as parental disomy). This is thought to occur when a single sperm fertilizes an enucleate egg that subsequently duplicates the paternal DNA. Trophoblastic proliferation occurs with exuberant villous stroma. If pseudopregnancy extends out past the twelfth week, fluid progressively accumulates within the stroma, leading to "hydropic changes." There is no fetal development in complete moles.

Partial moles arise from the fertilization of an egg with two sperm, hence two-thirds of genetic material is paternal in these triploid tumors. Hydropic changes are less dramatic, and fetal development can often occur through the late first trimester or early second trimester at which point spontaneous abortion is common. Laboratory findings will include excessively high hCG and high AFP. The risk of persistent gestational trophoblastic disease after partial mole is approximately 5%. Complete and partial moles can be noninvasive or invasive. Myometrial invasion occurs in no more than one in six complete moles and a lower portion of partial moles.

PRESENTATION OF INVASIVE TROPHOBLASTIC DISEASE

The clinical presentation of molar pregnancy is changing in developed countries due to the early detection of pregnancy with home pregnancy kits and the very early use of Doppler and ultrasound to evaluate the early fetus and uterine cavity for evidence of a viable fetus. Thus, in these countries, the majority of women presenting with trophoblastic disease have their moles detected early and have typical symptoms of early pregnancy, including nausea, amenorrhea, and breast tenderness. With uterine evacuation of early complete and partial moles, most women experience spontaneous remission of their disease as monitored by serial hCG levels. These women require no chemotherapy. Patients with persistent elevation of hCG or rising hCG postevacuation have persistent or actively growing gestational trophoblastic disease and require therapy. Most series suggest that between 15 and 25% of women will have evidence of persistent gestational trophoblastic disease after molar evacuation.

In women who lack access to prenatal care, presenting symptoms can be life threatening including the development of preeclampsia or even eclampsia. Hyperthyroidism can also be seen. Evacuation of large moles can be associated with life-threatening complications including uterine perforation, volume loss, high-output cardiac failure, and adult respiratory distress syndrome.

For women with evidence of rising hCG or radiologic confirmation of metastatic or persistent regional disease, prognosis can be estimated through a variety of scoring algorithms that identify those women at low, intermediate, and high risk for requiring multi-agent chemotherapy. In general, women with widely metastatic nonpulmonary disease, very elevated hCG, and prior normal antecedent term pregnancy are considered at high risk and typically require multi-agent chemotherapy for cure.

TREATMENT Invasive Trophoblastic Disease

The management for a persistent and rising hCG postevacuation of a molar conception is typically chemotherapy, although surgery can play an important role for disease that is persistently isolated in the uterus (especially if childbearing is complete) or to control hemorrhage. For women wishing to maintain fertility or with metastatic disease, the preferred treatment is chemotherapy. Chemotherapy is guided by the hCG level, which typically drops to undetectable levels with effective therapy. Single-agent treatment with methotrexate or actinomycin D cures 90% of women with low-risk disease. Patients with high-risk disease (high hCG levels, presentation 4 or more months after pregnancy, brain or liver metastases, failure of methotrexate therapy) are typically treated with multi-agent chemotherapy (e.g., etoposide, methotrexate, and actinomycin D alternating with cyclophosphamide and vincristine [EMA-CO]), which is typically curative even in those women with extensive metastatic disease. Cisplatin, bleomycin, and either etoposide or vinblastine are also active combinations. Survival in high-risk disease exceeds 80%. Cured women may get pregnant again without evidence of increased fetal or maternal complications.

CHAPTER 45

SOFT TISSUE AND BONE SARCOMAS AND BONE METASTASES

Shreyaskumar R. Patel ■ Robert S. Benjamin

Sarcomas are rare (<1% of all malignancies) mesenchymal neoplasms that arise in bone and soft tissues. These tumors are usually of mesodermal origin, although a few are derived from neuroectoderm, and they are biologically distinct from the more common epithelial malignancies. Sarcomas affect all age groups; 15% are found in children younger than 15 years of age, and 40% occur after age 55 years. Sarcomas are one of the most common solid tumors of childhood and are the fifth most common cause of cancer deaths in children. Sarcomas may be divided into two groups, those derived from bone and those derived from soft tissues.

SOFT TISSUE SARCOMAS

Soft tissues include muscles, tendons, fat, fibrous tissue, synovial tissue, vessels, and nerves. Approximately 60% of soft tissue sarcomas arise in the extremities, with the lower extremities involved three times as often as the upper extremities. Thirty percent arise in the trunk, the retroperitoneum accounting for 40% of all trunk lesions. The remaining 10% arise in the head and neck.

INCIDENCE

Approximately 11,000 new cases of soft tissue sarcomas occurred in the United States in 2010. The annual age-adjusted incidence is 3 per 100,000 population, but the incidence varies with age. Soft tissue sarcomas constitute 0.7% of all cancers in the general population and 6.5% of all cancers in children.

EPIDEMIOLOGY

Malignant transformation of a benign soft tissue tumor is extremely rare, with the exception that malignant peripheral nerve sheath tumors (neurofibrosarcoma, malignant schwannoma) can arise from neurofibromas in patients with neurofibromatosis. Several etiologic factors have been implicated in soft tissue sarcomas.

Environmental factors

Trauma or previous injury is rarely involved, but sarcomas can arise in scar tissue resulting from a prior operation, burn, fracture, or foreign body implantation. Chemical carcinogens such as polycyclic hydrocarbons, asbestos, and dioxin may be involved in the pathogenesis.

Iatrogenic factors

Sarcomas in bone or soft tissues occur in patients who are treated with radiation therapy. The tumor nearly always arises in the irradiated field. The risk increases with time.

Viruses

Kaposi's sarcoma (KS) in patients with HIV type 1, classic KS, and KS in HIV-negative homosexual men is caused by human herpesvirus (HHV) 8. No other sarcomas are associated with viruses.

Immunologic factors

Congenital or acquired immunodeficiency, including therapeutic immunosuppression, increases the risk of sarcoma.

GENETIC CONSIDERATIONS

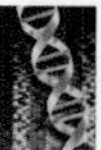

Li-Fraumeni syndrome is a familial cancer syndrome in which affected individuals have germline abnormalities of the tumor-suppressor gene p53 and an increased incidence of soft tissue sarcomas and other malignancies, including breast cancer, osteosarcoma, brain tumor, leukemia, and adrenal carcinoma (Chap. 24). Neurofibromatosis 1 (NF-1, peripheral form, von Recklinghausen's disease) is characterized by multiple neurofibromas and café au lait spots. Neurofibromas occasionally undergo malignant degeneration to become malignant peripheral nerve sheath tumors. The gene for NF-1 is located in the pericentromeric region of chromosome 17 and encodes neurofibromin, a tumor-suppressor protein with guanosine 5'-triphosphate (GTP)ase-activating activity that inhibits Ras function (Chap. 46). Germ-line mutation of the *Rb-1* locus (chromosome 13q14) in patients with inherited retinoblastoma is associated with the development of osteosarcoma in those who survive the retinoblastoma and of soft tissue sarcomas unrelated to radiation therapy. Other soft tissue tumors, including desmoid tumors, lipomas, leiomyomas, neuroblastomas, and paragangliomas, occasionally show a familial predisposition.

Ninety percent of synovial sarcomas contain a characteristic chromosomal translocation t(X;18)(p11;q11) involving a nuclear transcription factor on chromosome 18 called *SYT* and two breakpoints on X. Patients with translocations to the second X breakpoint (*SSX2*) may have longer survival than those with translocations involving *SSX1*.

Insulin-like growth factor (IGF) type II is produced by some sarcomas and may act as an autocrine growth factor and as a motility factor that promotes metastatic spread. IGF-II stimulates growth through IGF-I receptors, but its effects on motility are through different receptors. If secreted in large amounts, IGF-2 may produce hypoglycemia (Chap. 52).

CLASSIFICATION

Approximately 20 different groups of sarcomas are recognized on the basis of the pattern of differentiation toward normal tissue. For example, rhabdomyosarcoma shows evidence of skeletal muscle fibers with cross-striations, leiomyosarcomas contain interlacing fascicles of spindle cells resembling smooth muscle, and liposarcomas contain adipocytes. When precise characterization of the group is not possible, the tumors are called *unclassified sarcomas*. All of the primary bone sarcomas can also arise from soft tissues (e.g., extraskeletal osteosarcoma). The entity *malignant fibrous histiocytoma (MFH)* includes many tumors previously classified as fibrosarcomas or as pleomorphic variants of other sarcomas and is characterized by a mixture of spindle (fibrous) cells and round (histiocytic) cells arranged in a storiform pattern with frequent giant cells and areas of pleomorphism. As immunohistochemical suggestion of differentiation, particularly myogenic differentiation, may be found in a significant fraction of these patients, many are now characterized as poorly differentiated leiomyosarcomas, and the terms *undifferentiated pleomorphic sarcoma* and *myxofibrosarcoma* are replacing MFH and myxoid MFH.

For purposes of treatment, most soft tissue sarcomas can be considered together. However, some specific tumors have distinct features. For example, *liposarcoma* can have a spectrum of behaviors. Pleomorphic liposarcomas and dedifferentiated liposarcomas behave like other high-grade sarcomas; in contrast, well-differentiated liposarcomas (better termed *atypical lipomatous tumors*) lack metastatic potential, and myxoid liposarcomas metastasize infrequently, but when they do, they have a predilection for unusual metastatic sites containing fat, such as the retroperitoneum, mediastinum, and subcutaneous tissue. Rhabdomyosarcomas, Ewing's sarcoma, and other small-cell sarcomas tend to be more aggressive and are more responsive to chemotherapy than other soft tissue sarcomas.

Gastrointestinal stromal cell tumors (GISTs), previously classified as gastrointestinal leiomyosarcomas, are now recognized as a distinct entity within soft tissue sarcomas. Their cell of origin resembles the interstitial cell of Cajal, which controls peristalsis. The majority of malignant GISTs have activating mutations of the *c-kit* gene that result in ligand-independent phosphorylation and activation of the KIT receptor tyrosine kinase, leading to tumorigenesis.

DIAGNOSIS

The most common presentation is an asymptomatic mass. Mechanical symptoms referable to pressure, traction, or entrapment of nerves or muscles may be present. All new and persistent or growing masses should be biopsied, either by a cutting needle (core-needle biopsy) or by a small incision, placed so that it can be encompassed in the subsequent excision without compromising a definitive resection. Lymph node metastases occur in 5%, except in synovial and epithelioid sarcomas, clear-cell sarcoma (melanoma of the soft parts), angiosarcoma, and rhabdomyosarcoma, in which nodal spread may be seen in 17%. The pulmonary parenchyma is the most common site of metastases. Exceptions are GISTs, which metastasize to the liver; myxoid liposarcomas, which seek fatty tissue; and clear-cell sarcomas, which may metastasize to bones. Central nervous system metastases are rare, except in alveolar soft part sarcoma.

Radiographic evaluation

Imaging of the primary tumor is best with plain radiographs and magnetic resonance imaging (MRI) for tumors of the extremities or head and neck and by computed tomography (CT) for tumors of the chest, abdomen, or retroperitoneal cavity. A radiograph and CT scan of the chest are important for the detection of lung metastases. Other imaging studies may be indicated, depending on the symptoms, signs, or histology.

STAGING AND PROGNOSIS

The histologic grade, relationship to fascial planes, and size of the primary tumor are the most important prognostic factors. The current American Joint Commission on Cancer (AJCC) staging system is shown in Table 45-1. Prognosis is related to the stage. Cure is common in the absence of metastatic disease, but a small number of patients with metastases can also be cured. Most patients with stage IV disease die within 12 months, but some patients may live with slowly progressive disease for many years.

TREATMENT Soft Tissue Sarcomas

AJCC stage I patients are adequately treated with surgery alone. Stage II patients are considered for adjuvant radiation therapy. Stage III patients may benefit from adjuvant chemotherapy. Stage IV patients are managed primarily with chemotherapy with or without other modalities.

SURGERY Soft tissue sarcomas tend to grow along fascial planes, with the surrounding soft tissues compressed to form a pseudocapsule that gives the sarcoma the appearance of a well-encapsulated lesion. This is invariably deceptive because "shelling out," or marginal excision, of such lesions results in a 50–90% probability of local recurrence. Wide excision with a negative margin, incorporating the biopsy site, is the standard surgical procedure for local disease. The adjuvant use of radiation therapy and/or chemotherapy improves the local control rate and permits the use of limb-sparing surgery with a local control rate (85–90%) comparable to that achieved by radical excisions and amputations. Limb-sparing approaches are indicated except when negative margins are not obtainable, when the risks of radiation are prohibitive, or when neurovascular structures are involved so that resection will result in serious functional consequences to the limb.

RADIATION THERAPY External-beam radiation therapy is an adjuvant to limb-sparing surgery for improved local control. Preoperative radiation therapy allows the use of smaller fields and smaller doses but results in a higher rate of wound complications. Postoperative radiation therapy must be given to larger fields, as the entire surgical bed must be encompassed, and in higher doses to compensate for hypoxia in the operated field. This results in a higher rate of late complications. Brachytherapy or interstitial therapy, in which the radiation source is inserted into the tumor bed, is comparable in efficacy (except in low-grade lesions), less time consuming, and less expensive.

ADJUVANT CHEMOTHERAPY Chemotherapy is the mainstay of treatment for Ewing's primitive neuroectodermal tumors (PNETs) and rhabdomyosarcomas. Meta-analysis of 14 randomized trials revealed a significant improvement in local control and disease-free survival in favor of doxorubicin-based chemotherapy. Overall survival improvement was 4% for all sites and

TABLE 45-1

AMERICAN JOINT COMMISSION ON CANCER STAGING SYSTEM FOR SARCOMAS

HISTOLOGIC GRADE (G)	TUMOR SIZE (T)	NODE STATUS (N)	METASTASES (M)
Well differentiated (G1)	≤5 cm (T1)	Not involved (N0)	Absent (M0)
Moderately differentiated (G2)	>5 cm (T2)	Involved (N1)	Present (M1)
Poorly differentiated (G3)	Superficial fascial involvement (Ta)		
Undifferentiated (G4)	Deep fascial involvement (Tb)		

DISEASE STAGE	5-YEAR SURVIVAL RATE, %
Stage I	98.8
A: G1,2; T1a,b; N0; M0	
B: G1,2; T2a; N0; M0	
Stage II	81.8
A: G1,2; T2b; N0; M0	
B: G3,4; T1; N0; M0	
C: G3,4; T2a; N0; M0	
Stage III G3,4; T2b; N0; M0	51.7
Stage IV	<20
A: any G; any T; N1; M0	
B: any G; any T; any N; M1	

7% for the extremity site. An updated meta-analysis including four additional trials with doxorubicin and ifosfamide combination has reported a statistically significant 6% survival advantage in favor of chemotherapy. A chemotherapy regimen including an anthracycline and ifosfamide with growth factor support improved overall survival by 19% for high-risk (high-grade, ≥5 cm primary, or locally recurrent) extremity soft tissue sarcomas.

ADVANCED DISEASE Metastatic soft tissue sarcomas are largely incurable, but up to 20% of patients who achieve a complete response become long-term survivors. The therapeutic intent, therefore, is to produce a complete remission with chemotherapy (<10%) and/or surgery (30–40%). Surgical resection of metastases, whenever possible, is an integral part of the management. Some patients benefit from repeated surgical excision of metastases. The two most active chemotherapeutic agents are doxorubicin and ifosfamide. These drugs show a steep dose-response relationship in sarcomas. Gemcitabine with or without docetaxel has become an established second-line regimen and is particularly active in patients with leiomyosarcomas. Dacarbazine also has some modest activity. Taxanes have selective activity in angiosarcomas, and vincristine, etoposide, and irinotecan are effective in rhabdomyosarcomas and Ewing's sarcomas. Imatinib targets the KIT and platelet-derived growth factor (PDGF) tyrosine kinase activity and is standard therapy for advanced/metastatic GISTs and dermatofibrosarcoma protuberans. Imatinib is now also indicated as adjuvant therapy for completely resected primary GISTs.

BONE SARCOMAS

INCIDENCE AND EPIDEMIOLOGY

Bone sarcomas are rarer than soft tissue sarcomas; they accounted for only 0.2% of all new malignancies and 2600 new cases in the United States in 2010. Several benign bone lesions have the potential for malignant transformation. Enchondromas and osteochondromas can transform into chondrosarcoma; fibrous dysplasia, bone infarcts, and Paget's disease of bone can transform into either malignant fibrous histiocytoma or osteosarcoma.

CLASSIFICATION

Benign tumors

The common benign bone tumors include enchondroma, osteochondroma, chondroblastoma, and chondromyxoid fibroma of cartilage origin; osteoid osteoma and osteoblastoma of bone origin; fibroma and desmoplastic fibroma of fibrous tissue origin; hemangioma of vascular origin; and giant cell tumor of unknown origin.

Malignant tumors

The most common malignant tumors of bone are plasma cell tumors (Chap. 17). The four most common malignant nonhematopoietic bone tumors are osteosarcoma, chondrosarcoma, Ewing's sarcoma, and malignant fibrous histiocytoma. Rare malignant tumors include chordoma (of notochordal origin), malignant giant cell tumor and adamantinoma (of unknown origin), and hemangioendothelioma (of vascular origin).

Musculoskeletal Tumor Society staging system

Sarcomas of bone are staged according to the Musculoskeletal Tumor Society staging system based on grade and compartmental localization. A Roman numeral reflects the tumor grade: stage I is low grade, stage II is high grade, and stage III includes tumors of any grade that have lymph node or distant metastases. In addition, the tumor is given a letter reflecting its compartmental localization. Tumors designated A are intracompartmental (i.e., confined to the same soft tissue compartment as the initial tumor), and tumors designated B are extracompartmental (i.e., extending into the adjacent soft tissue compartment or into bone). The tumor, node, metastasis (TNM) staging system is shown in Table 45-2.

OSTEOSARCOMA

Osteosarcoma, accounting for almost 45% of all bone sarcomas, is a spindle cell neoplasm that produces osteoid (unmineralized bone) or bone. Approximately 60% of all osteosarcomas occur in children and adolescents in the second decade of life, and approximately 10% occur in the third decade of life. Osteosarcomas in the fifth and sixth decades of life are frequently secondary to either radiation therapy or transformation in a preexisting benign condition, such as Paget's disease. Males are affected 1.5–2 times as often as females. Osteosarcoma has a predilection for metaphyses of long bones; the most common sites of involvement are the distal femur, proximal tibia, and proximal humerus. The classification of osteosarcoma is complex, but 75% of osteosarcomas fall into the "classic" category, which include osteoblastic, chondroblastic, and fibroblastic osteosarcomas. The remaining 25% are classified as "variants" on the basis of (1) clinical characteristics, as in the case of osteosarcoma of the jaw, postradiation osteosarcoma, or Paget's osteosarcoma; (2) morphologic characteristics, as in the case of telangiectatic osteosarcoma, small cell osteosarcoma, or epithelioid osteosarcoma; or (3) location, as in

TABLE 45-2

STAGING SYSTEM FOR BONE SARCOMAS

Primary tumor (T)	TX	Primary tumor cannot be assessed
	T0	No evidence of primary tumor
	T1	Tumor ≤8 cm in greatest dimension
	T2	Tumor >8 cm in greatest dimension
	T3	Discontinuous tumors in the primary bone site
Regional lymph nodes (N)	NX	Regional lymph nodes cannot be assessed
	N0	No regional lymph node metastasis
	N1	Regional lymph node metastasis
Distant metastasis (M)	MX	Distant metastasis cannot be assessed
	M0	No distant metastasis
	M1	Distant metastasis
	M1a	Lung
	M1b	Other distant sites
Histologic grade (G)	GX	Grade cannot be assessed
	G1	Well differentiated—low grade
	G2	Moderately differentiated—low grade
	G3	Poorly differentiated—high grade
	G4	Undifferentiated—high grade (Ewing's is always classed G4)

Stage Grouping

Stage IA	T1	N0	M0	G1,2 low grade
Stage IB	T2	N0	M0	G1,2 low grade
Stage IIA	T1	N0	M0	G3,4 high grade
Stage IIB	T2	N0	M0	G3,4 high grade
Stage III	T3	N0	M0	Any G
Stage IVA	Any T	N0	M1a	Any G
Stage IVB	Any T	N1	Any M	Any G
	Any T	Any N	M1b	Any G

parosteal or periosteal osteosarcoma. Diagnosis usually requires a synthesis of clinical, radiologic, and pathologic features. Patients typically present with pain and swelling of the affected area. A plain radiograph reveals a destructive lesion with a moth-eaten appearance, a spiculated periosteal reaction (sunburst appearance), and a cuff of periosteal new bone formation at the margin of the soft tissue mass (Codman's triangle). A CT scan of the primary tumor is best for defining bone destruction and the pattern of calcification, whereas MRI is better for defining intramedullary and soft tissue extension. A chest radiograph and CT scan are used to detect lung metastases. Metastases to the bony skeleton should be imaged by a bone scan or by fluorodeoxyglucose positron emission tomography (FDG-PET). Almost all osteosarcomas are hypervascular. Angiography is not helpful for diagnosis, but it is the most sensitive test for assessing the response to preoperative chemotherapy. Pathologic diagnosis is established either with a core-needle biopsy, when feasible, or with an open biopsy with an appropriately placed incision that does not compromise future limb-sparing resection. Most osteosarcomas are high-grade. The most important prognostic factor for long-term survival is response to chemotherapy. Preoperative chemotherapy followed by limb-sparing surgery (which can be accomplished in >80% of patients) followed by postoperative chemotherapy is standard management. The effective drugs are doxorubicin, ifosfamide, cisplatin, and high-dose methotrexate with leucovorin rescue. The various combinations of these agents that have been used have all been about equally successful. Long-term survival rates in extremity osteosarcoma range from 60 to 80%. Osteosarcoma is radioresistant; radiation therapy has no role in the routine management. Malignant fibrous histiocytoma is considered a part of the spectrum of osteosarcoma and is managed similarly.

CHONDROSARCOMA

Chondrosarcoma, which constitutes ~20–25% of all bone sarcomas, is a tumor of adulthood and old age with a peak incidence in the fourth to sixth decades of life. It has a predilection for the flat bones, especially the shoulder and pelvic girdles, but can also affect the diaphyseal portions of long bones. Chondrosarcomas can arise de novo or as a malignant transformation of an enchondroma or, rarely, of the cartilaginous cap of an osteochondroma. Chondrosarcomas have an indolent natural history and typically present as pain and swelling. Radiographically, the lesion may have a lobular appearance with mottled or punctate or annular calcification of the cartilaginous matrix. It is difficult to distinguish low-grade chondrosarcoma from benign lesions by radiographic or histologic examination. The diagnosis is therefore influenced by clinical history and physical examination. A new onset of pain, signs of inflammation, and a progressive increase in the size of the mass suggest malignancy. The histologic classification is complex, but most tumors fall within the classic category. Like other bone sarcomas, high-grade chondrosarcomas spread to the lungs. Most chondrosarcomas are resistant to chemotherapy, and surgical resection of primary or recurrent tumors, including pulmonary metastases, is the mainstay of therapy. This rule does not hold for two histologic variants. Dedifferentiated chondrosarcoma has a high-grade osteosarcoma or a malignant fibrous histiocytoma component that responds to chemotherapy. Mesenchymal chondrosarcoma, a rare variant composed of a small cell element, also is responsive to systemic chemotherapy and is treated like Ewing's sarcoma.

EWING'S SARCOMA

Ewing's sarcoma, which constitutes ~10–15% of all bone sarcomas, is common in adolescence and has a peak incidence in the second decade of life. It typically involves the diaphyseal region of long bones and also has an affinity for flat bones. The plain radiograph may show a characteristic "onion peel" periosteal reaction with a generous soft tissue mass, which is better demonstrated by CT or MRI. This mass is composed of sheets of monotonous, small, round, blue cells and can be confused with lymphoma, embryonal rhabdomyosarcoma, and small-cell carcinoma. The presence of p30/32, the product of the *mic-2* gene (which maps to the pseudoautosomal region of the X and Y chromosomes) is a cell-surface marker for Ewing's sarcoma (and other members of the Ewing's family of tumors, sometimes called PNETs). Most PNETs arise in soft tissues; they include peripheral neuroepithelioma, Askin's tumor (chest wall), and esthesioneuroblastoma. Glycogen-filled cytoplasm detected by staining with periodic acid–Schiff is also characteristic of Ewing's sarcoma cells. The classic cytogenetic abnormality associated with this disease (and other PNETs) is a reciprocal translocation of the long arms of chromosomes 11 and 22, t(11;22), which creates a chimeric gene product of unknown function with components from the *fli-1* gene on chromosome 11 and *ews* on 22. This disease is very aggressive, and it is therefore considered a systemic disease. Common sites of metastases are lung, bones, and bone marrow. Systemic chemotherapy is the mainstay of therapy, often being used before surgery. Doxorubicin, cyclophosphamide or ifosfamide, etoposide, vincristine, and dactinomycin are active drugs. Topotecan or irinotecan in combination with an alkylating agent are often used in relapsed patients. Targeted therapy with an anti-IGF1 receptor antibody appears to have promising activity in refractory cases. Local treatment for the primary tumor includes surgical resection, usually with limb salvage or radiation therapy. Patients with lesions below the elbow and below the mid-calf have a 5-year survival rate of 80% with effective treatment. Ewing's sarcoma at first presentation is a curable tumor, even in the presence of obvious metastatic disease, especially in children younger than 11 years old.

TUMORS METASTATIC TO BONE

Bone is a common site of metastasis for carcinomas of the prostate, breast, lung, kidney, bladder, and thyroid and for lymphomas and sarcomas. Prostate, breast, and lung primaries account for 80% of all bone metastases. Metastatic tumors of bone are more common than primary bone tumors. Tumors usually spread to bone hematogenously, but local invasion from soft tissue masses also occurs. In descending order of frequency, the sites most often involved are the vertebrae, proximal femur, pelvis, ribs, sternum, proximal humerus, and skull. Bone metastases may be asymptomatic or may produce pain, swelling, nerve root or spinal cord compression, pathologic fracture, or myelophthisis (replacement of the marrow). Symptoms of hypercalcemia may be noted in cases of bony destruction.

Pain is the most frequent symptom. It usually develops gradually over weeks, is usually localized, and often is more severe at night. When patients with back pain develop neurologic signs or symptoms, emergency evaluation for spinal cord compression is indicated (Chap. 54). Bone metastases exert a major adverse effect on quality of life in cancer patients.

Cancer in the bone may produce osteolysis, osteogenesis, or both. Osteolytic lesions result when the tumor produces substances that can directly elicit bone resorption (vitamin D–like steroids, prostaglandins, or parathyroid hormone–related peptide) or cytokines that can induce the formation of osteoclasts (interleukin 1 and tumor necrosis factor). Osteoblastic lesions result when the tumor produces cytokines that activate osteoblasts. In general, purely osteolytic lesions are best detected by plain radiography, but they may not be apparent until they are >1 cm. These lesions are more commonly associated with hypercalcemia and with the excretion of hydroxyproline-containing peptides indicative of matrix destruction. When osteoblastic activity is prominent, the lesions may be readily detected using radionuclide bone scanning (which is sensitive to new bone formation), and the radiographic appearance may show increased bone density or sclerosis. Osteoblastic lesions are associated with higher serum levels of alkaline phosphatase and, if extensive, may produce hypocalcemia. Although some tumors may produce mainly osteolytic lesions (e.g., kidney cancer) and others mainly osteoblastic lesions (e.g., prostate cancer), most metastatic lesions produce both types of lesion and may go through stages when one or the other predominates.

In older patients, particularly women, it may be necessary to distinguish metastatic disease of the spine from osteoporosis. In osteoporosis, the cortical bone may be preserved, whereas cortical bone destruction is usually noted with metastatic cancer.

TREATMENT Metastatic Bone Disease

Treatment of metastatic bone disease depends on the underlying malignancy and the symptoms. Some metastatic bone tumors are curable (lymphoma, Hodgkin's disease), and others are treated with palliative intent. Pain may be relieved by local radiation therapy.

Hormonally responsive tumors are responsive to hormone inhibition (antiandrogens for prostate cancer, antiestrogens for breast cancer). Strontium 89 and samarium 153 are bone-seeking radionuclides that can exert antitumor effects and relieve symptoms. Bisphosphonates such as pamidronate may relieve pain and inhibit bone resorption, thereby maintaining bone mineral density and reducing risk of fractures in patients with osteolytic metastases from breast cancer and multiple myeloma. Careful monitoring of serum electrolytes and creatinine is recommended. Monthly administration prevents bone-related clinical events and may reduce the incidence of bone metastases in women with breast cancer. When the integrity of a weight-bearing bone is threatened by an expanding metastatic lesion that is refractory to radiation therapy, prophylactic internal fixation is indicated. Overall survival is related to the prognosis of the underlying tumor. Bone pain at the end of life is particularly common; an adequate pain relief regimen including sufficient amounts of narcotic analgesics is required.

CHAPTER 46

PRIMARY AND METASTATIC TUMORS OF THE NERVOUS SYSTEM

Lisa M. DeAngelis ■ Patrick Y. Wen

INTRODUCTION

Primary brain tumors are diagnosed in approximately 52,000 people each year in the United States. At least half of these tumors are malignant and associated with a high mortality rate. Glial tumors account for about 60% of all primary brain tumors, and 80% of those are malignant neoplasms. Meningiomas account for 25%, vestibular schwannomas 10%, and central nervous system (CNS) lymphomas about 2%. Brain metastases are three times more common than all primary brain tumors combined and are diagnosed in approximately 150,000 people each year. Metastases to the leptomeninges and epidural space of the spinal cord each occur in approximately 3–5% of patients with systemic cancer and are also a major cause of neurologic disability in this population.

APPROACH TO THE PATIENT: Primary and Metastatic Tumors of the Nervous System

CLINICAL FEATURES Brain tumors of any type can present with a variety of symptoms and signs that fall into two categories: general and focal; patients often have a combination of the two (Table 46-1). General or nonspecific symptoms include headache, cognitive difficulties, personality change, and gait disorder. Generalized symptoms arise when the enlarging tumor and its surrounding edema cause an increase in intracranial pressure or direct compression of cerebrospinal fluid (CSF) circulation leading to hydrocephalus. The classic headache associated with a brain tumor is most evident in the morning and improves during the day, but this particular pattern is actually seen in a minority of patients. Headache may be accompanied by nausea or vomiting when intracranial pressure is elevated. Headaches are often holocephalic but can be ipsilateral to the side of a tumor. Occasionally, headaches have features of a typical migraine with unilateral throbbing pain associated with visual scotoma. Personality changes may include apathy and withdrawal from social circumstances, mimicking depression. Focal or lateralizing findings include hemiparesis, aphasia, or visual field defect. Lateralizing symptoms such as hemiparesis are typically subacute and progressive. A visual field defect is often not noticed by the patient; its presence may only be revealed after it leads to an injury such as an automobile accident occurring in the blind visual field. Language difficulties may be mistaken for confusion. Seizures are a common presentation of brain tumors, occurring in about 25% of patients with brain metastases or malignant gliomas but can be the presenting symptom in up to 90% of patients with low-grade gliomas. Most seizures have a focal signature that reflects their location in the brain and many proceed to secondary generalization. All generalized seizures that arise from a brain tumor will have a focal onset whether or not it is apparent clinically.

NEUROIMAGING Cranial magnetic resonance imaging (MRI) is the preferred diagnostic test for any patient suspected of having a brain tumor and should be performed with gadolinium contrast administration. Computed tomography (CT) should be reserved for patients unable to undergo MRI (e.g., pacemaker). Malignant brain tumors—whether primary or metastatic—typically enhance with gadolinium and may have central areas of necrosis; they are characteristically surrounded by edema of the neighboring white matter. Low-grade gliomas typically do not enhance with gadolinium and are best appreciated on fluid-attenuated inversion recovery (FLAIR) MRIs. Meningiomas have a characteristic appearance on MRI as they are dural-based with a dural tail and compress but do not invade the brain. Dural metastases or a dural lymphoma can have a similar

TABLE 46-1

SYMPTOMS AND SIGNS AT PRESENTATION OF BRAIN TUMORS

	HIGH-GRADE GLIOMA (%)	LOW-GRADE GLIOMA (%)	MENINGIOMA (%)	METASTASES (%)
Generalized				
Impaired cognitive function	50	10	30	60
Hemiparesis	40	10	36	60
Headache	50	40	37	50
Lateralizing				
Seizures	20	70+	17	18
Aphasia	20	<5		18
Visual field deficit	—	—	—	7

appearance. Imaging is characteristic for many primary and metastatic tumors, but occasionally there is diagnostic uncertainty based on imaging alone. In such patients, a brain biopsy may be helpful in determining a definitive diagnosis. However, when a tumor is strongly suspected, the biopsy can be obtained as an intraoperative frozen section before a definitive resection is performed.

Functional MRI is useful in presurgical planning and defining eloquent sensory, motor, and language cortex. Positron emission tomography (PET) is useful in determining the metabolic activity of the lesions seen on MRI; MR perfusion and spectroscopy can provide information on blood flow or tissue composition. These techniques may help distinguish tumor progression from necrotic tissue as a consequence of treatment with radiation and chemotherapy or identify foci of high-grade tumor in an otherwise low-grade–appearing glioma.

Neuroimaging is the only test necessary to diagnose a brain tumor. Laboratory tests are rarely useful, although patients with metastatic disease may have elevation of a tumor marker in their serum that reflects the presence of brain metastases (e.g., human chorionic gonadotropin [βhCG] from testicular cancer). Additional testing such as cerebral angiogram, electroencephalogram (EEG), or lumbar puncture is rarely indicated or helpful.

TREATMENT Brain Tumors

Therapy of any intracranial malignancy requires both symptomatic and definitive treatments. Definitive treatment is based on the specific tumor type and includes surgery, radiotherapy (RT), and chemotherapy. However, symptomatic treatments apply to brain tumors of any type. Most high-grade malignancies are accompanied by substantial surrounding edema, which contributes to neurologic disability and raised intracranial pressure. Glucocorticoids are highly effective at reducing perilesional edema and improving neurologic function, often within hours of administration. Dexamethasone has been the glucocorticoid of choice because of its relatively low mineralocorticoid activity. Initial doses are typically 12 mg to 16 mg a day in divided doses given orally or intravenously (both are equivalent). While glucocorticoids rapidly ameliorate symptoms and signs, their long-term use causes substantial toxicity, including insomnia, weight gain, diabetes mellitus, steroid myopathy, and personality changes. Consequently, a taper is indicated as definitive treatment is administered and the patient improves.

Patients with brain tumors who present with seizures require anticonvulsant drug therapy. There is no role for prophylactic anticonvulsant drugs in patients who have not had a seizure; thus, their use should be restricted to those who have had a convincing ictal event. The agents of choice are those drugs that do not induce the hepatic microsomal enzyme system. These include levetiracetam, topiramate, lamotrigine, valproic acid, anad lacosamide. Other drugs such as phenytoin and carbamazepine are used less frequently because they are potent enzyme inducers that can interfere with both glucocorticoid metabolism and the metabolism of chemotherapeutic agents needed to treat the underlying systemic malignancy or the primary brain tumor.

Venous thromboembolic disease occurs in 20–30% of patients with high-grade gliomas and brain metastases. Therefore, anticoagulants should be used prophylactically during hospitalization and in patients who are nonambulatory. Those who have had either a deep-vein thrombosis or pulmonary embolus can receive therapeutic doses of anticoagulation safely and without increasing the risk for hemorrhage into the tumor. Inferior vena cava filters are reserved for patients with absolute contraindications to anticoagulation such as recent craniotomy.

PRIMARY BRAIN TUMORS

PATHOGENESIS

No underlying cause has been identified for the majority of primary brain tumors. The only established risk factors are exposure to ionizing radiation (meningiomas, gliomas, and schwannomas) and immunosuppression (primary CNS lymphoma). Evidence for an association with exposure to electromagnetic fields, including cellular telephones, head injury, foods containing N-nitroso compounds, or occupational risk factors, are unproven. A small minority of patients have a family history of brain tumors. Some of these familial cases are associated with genetic syndromes (Table 46-2).

As with other neoplasms, brain tumors arise as a result of a multistep process driven by the sequential acquisition of genetic alterations. These include loss of tumor suppressor genes (e.g., p53 and phosphatase and tensin homolog on chromosome 10 [PTEN]) and amplification and overexpression of protooncogenes such as the epidermal growth factor receptor (EGF-R) and the platelet-derived growth factor receptors (PDGFRs). The accumulation of these genetic abnormalities results in uncontrolled cell growth and tumor formation.

TABLE 46-2

GENETIC SYNDROMES ASSOCIATED WITH PRIMARY BRAIN TUMORS

SYNDROME	INHERITANCE	GENE/PROTEIN	ASSOCIATED TUMORS
Cowden's syndrome	AD	Mutations of PTEN (ch10p23)	**Dysplastic cerebellar gangliocytoma (Lhermitte-Duclos disease), meningioma, astrocytoma** Breast, endometrial, thyroid cancer, trichilemmomas
Familial schwannomatosis	Sporadic Hereditary	Mutations in INI1/SNF5 (ch22q11)	**Schwannomas, gliomas**
Gardner's syndrome	AD	Mutations in APC (ch5q21)	**Medulloblastoma, glioblastoma, craniopharyngioma** Familial polyposis, multiple osteomas, skin and soft tissue tumors
Gorlin syndrome (Basal cell nevus syndrome)	AD	Mutations in Patched 1 gene (ch9q22.3)	**Medulloblastomas** Basal cell carcinoma
Li-Fraumeni syndrome	AD	Mutations in p53 (ch17p13.1)	**Gliomas, medulloblastomas** Sarcomas, breast cancer, leukemias, others
Multiple Endocrine Neoplasia 1 (Werner's syndrome)	AD	Mutations in Menin (ch11q13)	**Pituitary adenoma, malignant schwannomas** Parathyroid and pancreatic islet cell tumors
Neurofibromatosistype 1 (NF1)	AD	Mutations in NF1/Neurofibromin (ch17q12-22)	**Schwannomas, astrocytomas, optic nerve gliomas, meningiomas** Neurofibromas, neurofibrosarcomas, others
Neurofibromatosis type 2 (NF2)	AD	Mutations in NF2/Merlin (ch22q12)	**Bilateral vestibular schwannomas, astrocytomas, multiple meningiomas, ependymomas**
Tuberous sclerosis (TSC) (Bourneville's disease)	AD	Mutations in TSC1/TSC2 (ch9q34/16)	**Subependymal giant cell astrocytoma, ependymomas, glioma, ganglioneuroma, hamartoma**
Turcot's syndrome	AD AR	Mutations in APC[a] (ch5) hMLH1 (ch3p21)	**Gliomas, medulloblastomas** Adenomatous colon polyps, adenocarcinoma
Von Hippel–Lindau (VHL) syndrome	AD	Mutations in VHL gene (ch3p25)	**Hemangioblastomas** Retinal angiomas, renal cell carcinoma, pheochromocytoma, pancreatic tumors and cysts, endolymphatic sac tumors of the middle ear

[a]Various DNA mismatch repair gene mutations may cause a similar clinical phenotype, also referred to as Turcot's syndrome, in which there is a predisposition to nonpolyposis colon cancer and brain tumors.

Abbreviations: AD, autosomal dominant; APC, adenomatous polyposis coli; AR, autosomal recessive; ch, chromosome; PTEN, phosphatase and tensin homologue; TSC, tuberous sclerosis complex.

Important progress has been made in understanding the molecular pathogenesis of several types of brain tumors, including glioblastomas and medulloblastomas. Glioblastomas can be separated into two main subtypes based on genetic and biologic differences (Fig. 46-1). The majority are primary glioblastomas. These arise de novo and are characterized by EGF-R amplification and mutations, and deletion or mutation of PTEN. Secondary glioblastomas arise in younger patients as lower-grade tumors and transform over a period of several years into glioblastomas. These tumors have inactivation of the p53 tumor suppressor gene, overexpression of PDGFR, and mutations of the isocitrate dehydrogenase 1 and 2 genes. Despite their genetic differences, primary and secondary glioblastomas are morphologically indistinguishable, although they are likely to respond differently to molecular therapies. The molecular subtypes of medulloblastomas are also being elucidated. Approximately 25% of medulloblastomas have activating mutations of the sonic hedgehog signaling pathway, raising the possibility that inhibitors of this pathway may have therapeutic potential.

The adult nervous system contains neural stem cells that are capable of self-renewal, proliferation, and differentiation into distinctive mature cell types. There is increasing evidence that neural stem cells, or related progenitor cells, can be transformed into tumor stem cells and give rise to primary brain tumors, including gliomas and medulloblastomas. These stem cells appear to be more resistant to standard therapies than the tumor cells themselves and contribute to the difficulty in eradicating these tumors. There is intense interest in developing therapeutic strategies that effectively target tumor stem cells.

INTRINSIC "MALIGNANT" TUMORS

ASTROCYTOMAS

These are infiltrative tumors with a presumptive glial cell of origin. The World Health Organization (WHO) classifies astrocytomas into four prognostic grades based on histologic features: grade I (pilocytic astrocytoma, subependymal giant cell astrocytoma); grade II (diffuse astrocytoma); grade III (anaplastic astrocytoma); and grade IV (glioblastoma). Grades I and II are considered low-grade, and grades III and IV high-grade, astrocytomas.

Low-grade astrocytoma

These tumors occur predominantly in children and young adults.

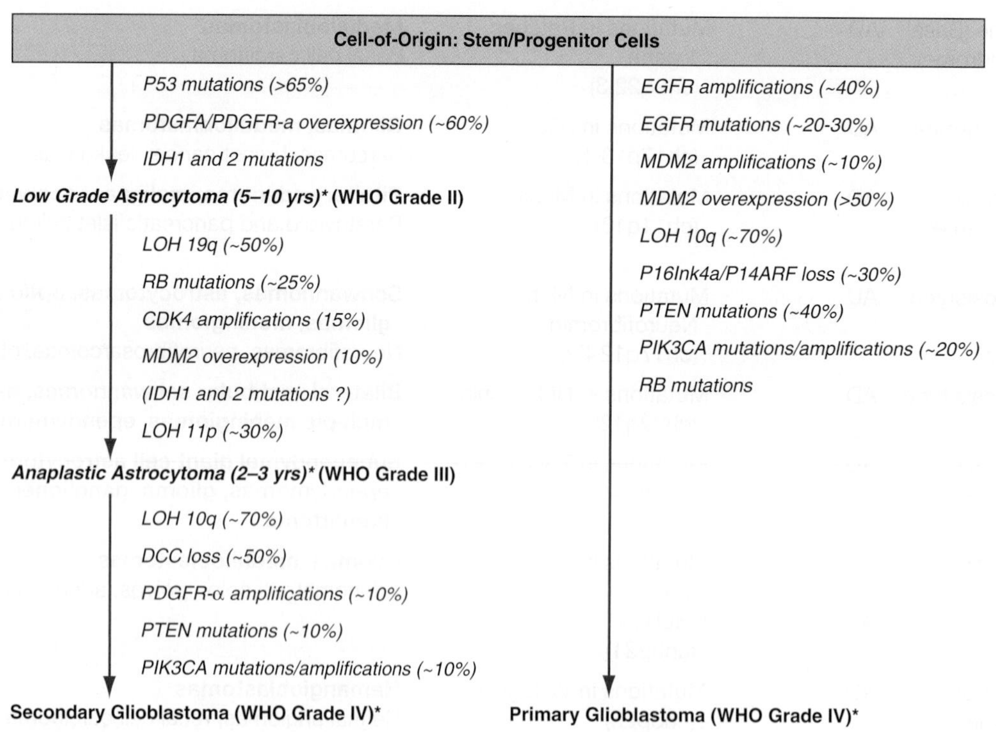

FIGURE 46-1

Genetic and chromosomal alterations involved in the development of primary and secondary glioblastomas. A *slash* indicates one or the other or both. DCC, deleted in colorectal carcinoma; EGF-R, epidermal growth factor receptor; IDH, isocitrate dehydrogenase; LOH, loss of heterozygosity; MDM2, murine double minute 2; PDGF, platelet-derived growth factor; PDGFR, platelet-derived growth factor receptor; PIK3CA, phosphatidylinositol 3-kinase, catalytic; PTEN, phosphatase and tensin homologue; RB, retinoblastoma; WHO, World Health Organization.

Grade I astrocytomas

Pilocytic astrocytomas (WHO grade I) are the most common tumor of childhood. They occur typically in the cerebellum but may also be found elsewhere in the neuraxis, including the optic nerves and brainstem. Frequently they appear as cystic lesions with an enhancing mural nodule. They are potentially curable if they can be completely resected. Giant cell subependymal astrocytomas are usually found in the ventricular wall of patients with tuberous sclerosis. They often do not require intervention but can be treated surgically or with inhibitors of the mammalian target of rapamycin (mTOR).

Grade II astrocytomas

These are infiltrative tumors that usually present with seizures in young adults. They appear as nonenhancing tumors with increased T2/FLAIR signal (Fig. 46-2). If feasible, patients should undergo maximal surgical resection, although complete resection is rarely possible because of the invasive nature of the tumor. Radiotherapy is helpful, but there is no difference in overall survival between radiotherapy administered postoperatively or delayed until the time of tumor progression. There is increasing evidence that chemotherapeutic agents such as temozolomide, an oral alkylating agent, can be helpful in some patients.

High-grade astrocytoma

Grade III (anaplastic) astrocytoma

These account for approximately 15–20% of high-grade astrocytomas. They generally present in the fourth and fifth decades of life as variably enhancing tumors. Treatment is the same as for glioblastoma, consisting of maximal safe surgical resection followed by radiotherapy with concurrent and adjuvant temozolomide or with radiotherapy and adjuvant temozolomide alone.

Grade IV astrocytoma (glioblastoma)

Glioblastoma accounts for the majority of high-grade astrocytomas. They are the most common cause of malignant primary brain tumors, with over 10,000 cases diagnosed each year in the United States. Patients usually present in the sixth and seventh decades of life with headache, seizures, or focal neurologic deficits. The tumors appear as ring-enhancing masses with central necrosis and surrounding edema (Fig. 46-3). These are highly infiltrative tumors, and the areas of increased T2/FLAIR signal surrounding the main tumor mass contain invading tumor cells. Treatment involves maximal surgical resection followed by partial-field external-beam radiotherapy (6000 cGy in thirty 200-cGy fractions) with concomitant temozolomide followed by 6–12 months of adjuvant temozolomide. With this regimen, median survival is increased to 14.6 months compared with only 12 months with radiotherapy alone, and 2-year survival is increased to 27% compared with 10% with radiotherapy alone. Patients whose tumor contains the DNA repair enzyme O^6-methylguanine-DNA methyltransferase (MGMT) are relatively resistant to temozolomide and have a worse prognosis compared with those whose tumors contain low levels of MGMT as a result of silencing of the MGMT gene by promoter hypermethylation. Implantation of biodegradable polymers containing the chemotherapeutic agent carmustine

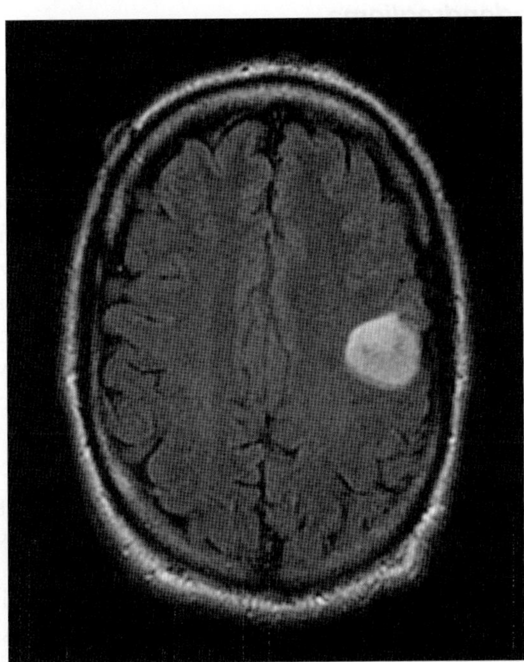

FIGURE 46-2
Fluid-attenuated inversion recovery (FLAIR) magnetic resonance image of a left frontal low-grade astrocytoma. This lesion did not enhance.

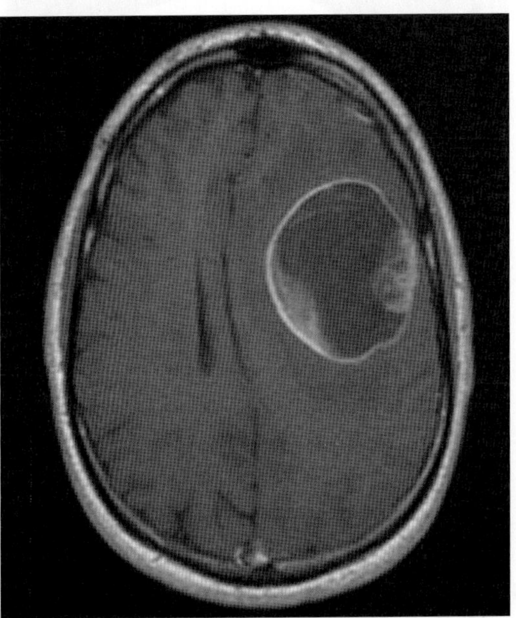

FIGURE 46-3
Postgadolinium T1 magnetic resonance image of a large cystic left frontal glioblastoma.

into the tumor bed after resection of the tumor also produces a modest improvement in survival.

Despite optimal therapy, glioblastomas invariably recur. Treatment options for recurrent disease may include reoperation, carmustine wafers, and alternate chemotherapeutic regimens. Reirradiation is rarely helpful. Bevacizumab, a humanized vascular endothelial growth factor (VEGF) monoclonal antibody, has activity in recurrent glioblastoma, increasing progression-free survival and reducing peritumoral edema and glucocorticoid use (Fig. 46-4). Treatment decisions for patients with recurrent glioblastoma must be made on an individual basis, taking into consideration such factors as previous therapy, time to relapse, performance status, and quality of life. Whenever feasible, patients with recurrent disease should be enrolled in clinical trials. Novel therapies undergoing evaluation in patients with glioblastoma include targeted molecular agents directed at receptor tyrosine kinases and signal transduction pathways; anti angiogenic agents, especially those directed at the VEGF receptors; chemotherapeutic agents that cross the blood–brain barrier more effectively than currently available drugs; gene therapy; immunotherapy; and infusion of radiolabeled drugs and targeted toxins into the tumor and surrounding brain by means of convection-enhanced delivery.

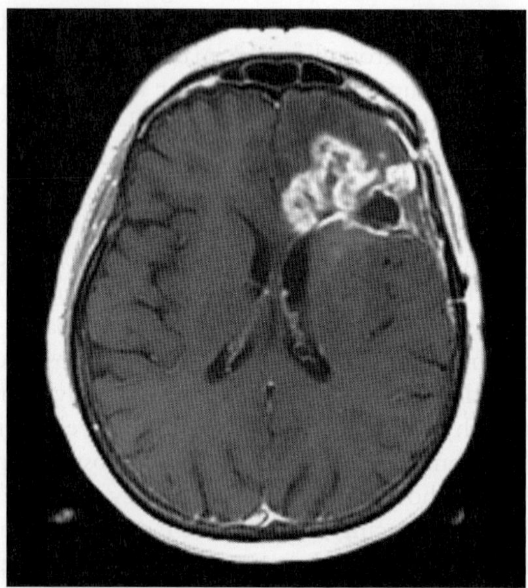

A

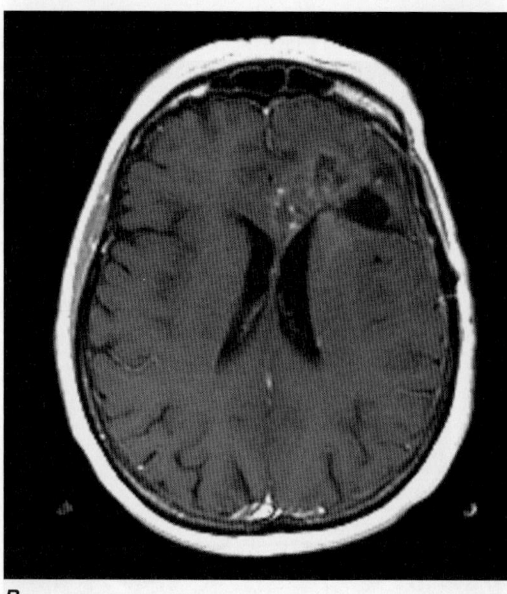

B

FIGURE 46-4

Postgadolinium T1 magnetic resonance image of a recurrent glioblastoma before (***A***) and after (***B***) administration of bevacizumab. Note the decreased enhancement and mass effect.

The most important adverse prognostic factors in patients with high-grade astrocytomas are older age, histologic features of glioblastoma, poor Karnofsky performance status, and unresectable tumor. Patients with unmethylated MGMT promoter resulting in the presence of the repair enzyme in tumor cells and resistance to temozolomide also have a worse prognosis.

Gliomatosis cerebri

Rarely, patients may present with a highly infiltrating, nonenhancing tumor involving more than two lobes. These tumors do not qualify for the histologic diagnosis of glioblastoma but behave aggressively and have a similarly poor outcome. Treatment involves radiotherapy and temozolomide chemotherapy.

Oligodendroglioma

Oligodendrogliomas account for approximately 15–20% of gliomas. They are classified by the WHO into well-differentiated oligodendrogliomas (grade II) or anaplastic oligodendrogliomas (AOs) (grade III). Tumors with oligodendroglial components have distinctive features such as perinuclear clearing—giving rise to a "fried-egg" appearance—and a reticular pattern of blood vessel growth. Some tumors have both an oligodendroglial as well as an astrocytic component. These mixed tumors, or oligoastrocytomas (OAs), are also classified into well-differentiated OA (grade II) or anaplastic oligoastrocytomas (AOAs) (grade III).

Grade II oligodendrogliomas and OAs are generally more responsive to therapy and have a better prognosis than pure astrocytic tumors. These tumors present similarly to grade II astrocytomas in young adults. The tumors are nonenhancing and often partially calcified. They should be treated with surgery and, if necessary, radiotherapy and chemotherapy. Patients with oligodendrogliomas have a median survival in time excess of 10 years.

Anaplastic oligodendrogliomas and AOAs present in the fourth and fifth decades as variably enhancing tumors. They are more responsive to therapy than grade III astrocytomas. Co-deletion of chromosomes 1p and 19q, mediated by an unbalanced translocation of 19p to 1q, occurs in 61–89% of patients with AO and 14 to 20% of patients with AOA. Tumors with the 1p and 19q co-deletion are particularly sensitive to chemotherapy with procarbazine, lomustine (cyclohexylchloroethylnitrosourea [CCNU]), and vincristine (PCV) or temozolomide, as well as to radiotherapy. Median survival of patients with AO or AOA is approximately 3–6 years.

Ependymomas

Ependymomas are tumors derived from ependymal cells that line the ventricular surface. They account for approximately 5% of childhood tumors and frequently arise from the wall of the fourth ventricle in the posterior fossa. Although adults can have intracranial ependymomas, they occur more commonly in the spine, especially in the filum terminale of the spinal cord, where they have a myxopapillary histology. Ependymomas that can be completely resected are potentially curable. Partially resected ependymomas will recur and require irradiation. The less common anaplastic ependymomas are more aggressive but can be treated in the same way as ependymomas. Subependymomas are slow-growing benign lesions arising in the wall of ventricles that often do not require treatment.

Other less common gliomas

Gangliogliomas and pleomorphic xanthoastrocytomas occur in young adults. They behave as more indolent forms of grade II gliomas and are treated in the same way. Brainstem gliomas usually occur in children and young adults. Despite treatment with radiotherapy and chemotherapy, the prognosis is poor with median survival of only 1 year. Gliosarcomas contain both an astrocytic as well as a sarcomatous component and are treated in the same way as glioblastomas.

PRIMARY CENTRAL NERVOUS SYSTEM LYMPHOMA

Primary central nervous system lymphoma (PCNSL) is a rare non-Hodgkin's lymphoma accounting for fewer than 3% of primary brain tumors. For unclear reasons, its incidence is increasing, particularly in immunocompetent individuals.

PCNSL in immunocompetent patients usually consists of diffuse large B cell lymphomas. PCNSL may also occur in immunocompromised patients, usually those infected with the human immunodeficiency virus (HIV) or organ transplant recipients on immunosuppressive therapy. PCNSL in immunocompromised patients is typically large cell with immunoblastic and more aggressive features. These patients are usually severely immunocompromised with CD4 counts of less than 50/mL. The Epstein-Barr virus (EBV) frequently plays an important role in the pathogenesis of HIV-related PCNSL.

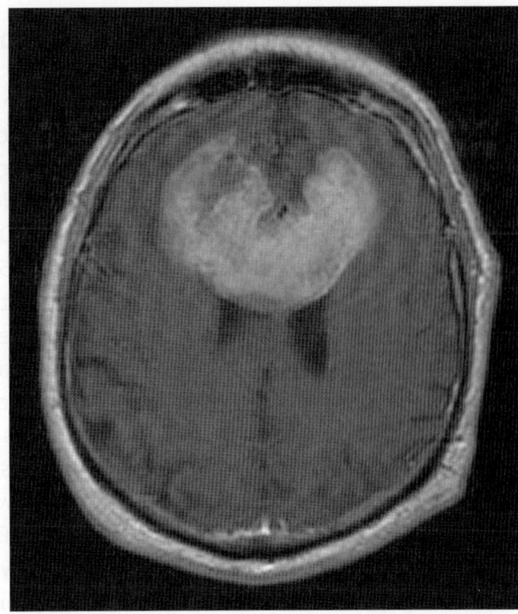

FIGURE 46-5
Postgadolinium T1 magnetic resonance image demonstrating a large bifrontal primary central nervous system lymphoma. The periventricular location and diffuse enhancement pattern are characteristic of lymphoma.

Immunocompetent patients are older (median, 60 years) compared to HIV-related PCNSL (median, 31 years). PCNSL usually presents as a mass lesion, with neuropsychiatric symptoms, symptoms of increased intracranial pressure, lateralizing signs, or seizures.

On contrast-enhanced MRI, PCNSL usually appears as a densely enhancing tumor (Fig. 46-5). Immunocompetent patients have solitary lesions more often than immunosuppressed patients. Frequently, there is involvement of the basal ganglia, corpus callosum, or periventricular region. Although the imaging features are often characteristic, PCNSL can sometimes be difficult to differentiate from high-grade gliomas, infections, or demyelination. Stereotactic biopsy is necessary to obtain a histologic diagnosis. Whenever possible, glucocorticoids should be withheld until after the biopsy has been obtained, since they have a cytolytic effect on lymphoma cells and may lead to nondiagnostic tissue. In addition, patients should be tested for HIV and the extent of disease assessed by performing PET or CT of the body, MRI of the spine, CSF analysis, and slit-lamp examination of the eye. Bone marrow biopsy and testicular ultrasound are occasionally performed.

TREATMENT **Primary Central Nervous System Lymphoma**

Unlike other primary brain tumors, PCNSL is relatively sensitive to glucocorticoids, chemotherapy, and radiotherapy. Durable complete responses and long-term survival are possible with these treatments. High-dose methotrexate, a folate antagonist that interrupts DNA synthesis, produces response rates ranging from 35 to 80% and median survival up to 50 months. Combination of methotrexate with other chemotherapeutic agents such as cytarabine, as well as whole-brain radiotherapy, increases the response rate to 70–100%. However, radiotherapy is associated with delayed neurotoxicity, especially in patients over the age of 60 years. As a result, radiotherapy is frequently omitted in older patients with PCNSL. There is emerging evidence that the anti-CD20 monoclonal antibody rituximab may have activity in PCNSL, although there remain concerns about its ability to pass through the blood–brain barrier as it becomes reconstituted with therapy. For some patients, high-dose chemotherapy with autologous stem cell rescue may offer the best chance of preventing relapse.

At least 50% of patients will eventually develop recurrent disease. Treatment options include radiotherapy for patients who have not had prior irradiation, retreatment with methotrexate, as well as other agents such as temozolomide, rituximab, procarbazine, topotecan, and pemetrexed. High-dose chemotherapy with autologous stem cell rescue may have a role in selected patients with relapsed disease.

PCNSL IN IMMUNOCOMPROMISED PATIENTS
PCNSL in immunocompromised patients often produces multiple-ring enhancing lesions that can be difficult to differentiate from metastases and infections such as toxoplasmosis. The diagnosis is usually established by examination of the cerebrospinal fluid for cytology and EBV DNA; toxoplasmosis serologic testing; brain PET imaging for hypermetabolism of the lesions consistent with tumor instead of infection; and, if necessary, brain biopsy. Since the advent of highly active antiretroviral drugs, the incidence of HIV-related PCNSL has declined. These patients may be treated with whole-brain radiotherapy, high-dose methotrexate, and initiation of highly active antiretroviral therapy. In organ transplant recipients, reduction of immunosuppression may improve outcome.

MEDULLOBLASTOMAS

Medulloblastomas are the most common malignant brain tumor of childhood, accounting for approximately 20% of all primary CNS tumors among children. They arise from granule cell progenitors or from multipotent progenitors from the ventricular zone. Approximately 5% of children have inherited disorders with germ-line mutations of genes that predispose to the development of medulloblastoma. The Gorlin syndrome, the most common of these inherited disorders, is due to mutations in the patched-1 (PTCH-1) gene, a key component in the sonic hedgehog pathway. Turcot's syndrome, caused by mutations in the adenomatous polyposis coli (APC) gene and familial adenomatous polyposis, has also been associated with an increased incidence of medulloblastoma. Histologically, medulloblastomas appear as highly cellular tumors with abundant dark staining, round nuclei, and rosette formation (Homer-Wright rosettes). They present with headache, ataxia, and signs of brainstem involvement. On MRI, they appear as densely enhancing tumors in the posterior fossa, sometimes associated with hydrocephalus. Seeding of the CSF is common. Treatment involves maximal surgical resection, craniospinal irradiation, and chemotherapy with agents such as cisplatin, lomustine, cyclophosphamide, and vincristine. Approximately 70% of patients have long-term survival but usually at the cost of significant neurocognitive impairment. A major goal of current research is to improve survival while minimizing long-term complications.

PINEAL REGION TUMORS

A large number of tumors can arise in the region of the pineal gland. These typically present with headache, visual symptoms, and hydrocephalus. Patients may have Parinaud's syndrome characterized by impaired upgaze and accommodation. Some pineal tumors such as pineocytomas and benign teratomas can be treated simply by surgical resection. Germinomas respond to irradiation, while pineoblastomas and malignant germ cell tumors require craniospinal radiation and chemotherapy.

EXTRINSIC "BENIGN" TUMORS

MENINGIOMAS

Meningiomas are diagnosed with increasing frequency as more people undergo neuroimaging studies for various indications. They are now the most common primary brain tumor, accounting for approximately 32% of the total. Their incidence increases with age. They tend to be more common in women and in patients with neurofibromatosis type 2 (NF2). They also occur more commonly in patients with a history of cranial irradiation.

Meningiomas arise from the dura mater and are composed of neoplastic meningothelial (arachnoidal cap) cells. They are most commonly located over the cerebral convexities, especially adjacent to the sagittal sinus,

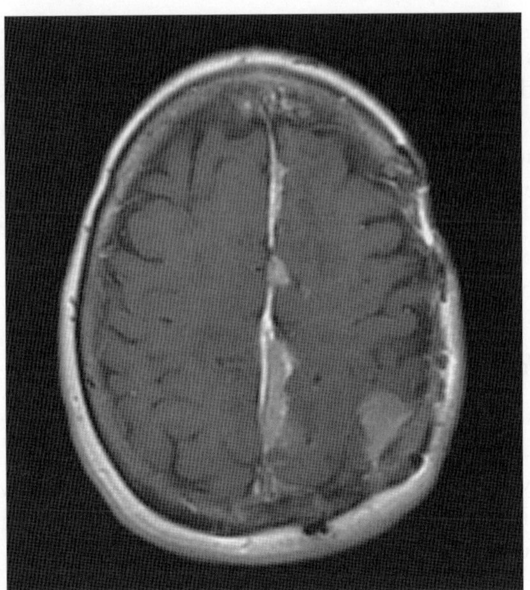

FIGURE 46-6

Postgadolinium T1 magnetic resonance image demonstrating multiple meningiomas along the falx and left parietal cortex.

but can also occur in the skull base and along the dorsum of the spinal cord. Meningiomas are classified by the WHO into three histologic grades of increasing aggressiveness: grade I (benign meningiomas), grade II (atypical meningiomas), and grade III (malignant meningiomas).

Many meningiomas are found incidentally following neuroimaging for unrelated reasons. They can also present with headaches, seizures, or focal neurologic deficits. On imaging studies, they have a characteristic appearance usually consisting of a partially calcified, densely enhancing extraaxial tumor arising from the dura (Fig. 46-6). Occasionally, they may have a dural tail, consisting of thickened, enhanced dura extending like a tail from the mass. The main differential diagnosis of meningioma is a dural metastasis.

If the meningioma is small and asymptomatic, no intervention is necessary, and the lesion can be observed with serial MRI studies. Larger, symptomatic lesions should be resected surgically. If complete resection is achieved, the patient is cured. Incompletely resected tumors tend to recur, although the rate of recurrence can be very slow with grade I tumors. Tumors that cannot be resected or can only be partially removed may benefit from treatment with external-beam radiotherapy or stereotactic radiosurgery (SRS). These treatments may also be helpful in patients whose tumor has recurred after surgery. Hormonal therapy and chemotherapy are currently unproven.

Rarer tumors that resemble meningiomas include hemangiopericytomas and solitary fibrous tumors. These are treated with surgery and radiotherapy but have a higher propensity to recur.

SCHWANNOMAS

These are generally benign tumors arising from the Schwann cells of cranial and spinal nerve roots. The most common schwannomas, termed *vestibular schwannomas* or *acoustic neuromas*, arise from the vestibular portion of the eighth cranial nerve and account for approximately 9% of primary brain tumors. Patients with NF2 have a high incidence of vestibular schwannomas that are frequently bilateral. Schwannomas arising from other cranial nerves, such as the trigeminal nerve (cranial nerve V), occur with much lower frequency. Neurofibromatosis type 1 (NF1) is associated with an increased incidence of schwannomas of the spinal nerve roots.

Vestibular schwannomas may be found incidentally on neuroimaging or present with progressive unilateral hearing loss; dizziness; tinnitus; or less commonly, symptoms resulting from compression of the brainstem and cerebellum. On MRI, they appear as densely enhancing lesions, enlarging the internal auditory canal and often extending into the cerebellopontine angle (Fig. 46-7). The differential diagnosis includes meningioma. Very small, asymptomatic lesions can be observed with serial MRIs. Larger lesions should be treated with surgery or stereotactic radiosurgery. The optimal treatment will depend on the size of the tumor, symptoms, and the patient's preference. In patients with small vestibular schwannomas and relatively intact hearing, early surgical intervention increases the chance of preserving hearing.

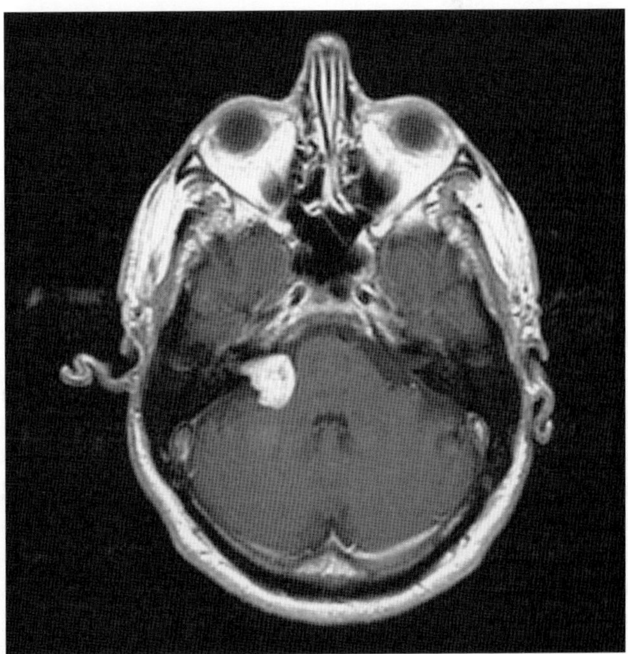

FIGURE 46-7

Postgadolinium magnetic resonance image of a right vestibular schwannoma. The tumor can be seen to involve the internal auditory canal.

PITUITARY TUMORS

These account for approximately 9% of primary brain tumors. They can be divided into functioning and nonfunctioning tumors. Functioning tumors are usually microadenomas (<1 cm in diameter) that secrete hormones and produce specific endocrine syndromes (e.g., acromegaly for growth hormone–secreting tumors, Cushing's syndrome for adrenocorticotropic hormone [ACTH]–secreting tumors, and galactorrhea, amenorrhea, and infertility for prolactin-secreting tumors). Nonfunctioning pituitary tumors tend to be macroadenomas (>1 cm) that produce symptoms by mass effect, giving rise to headaches, visual impairment (such as bitemporal hemianopia), and hypopituitarism. Prolactin-secreting tumors respond well to dopamine agonists such as bromocriptine and cabergoline. Other pituitary tumors usually require treatment with surgery and sometimes radiotherapy or radiosurgery and hormonal therapy.

CRANIOPHARYNGIOMAS

Craniopharyngiomas are rare, usually suprasellar, partially calcified, solid, or mixed solid–cystic benign tumors that arise from remnants of Rathke's pouch. They have a bimodal distribution, occurring predominantly in children but also between the ages of 55 and 65 years. They present with headaches, visual impairment, and impaired growth in children and hypopituitarism in adults. Treatment involves surgery, radiotherapy, or the combination of the two.

OTHER BENIGN TUMORS

Dysembryoplastic neuroepithelial tumors

These are benign, supratentorial tumors, usually in the temporal lobes. They typically occur in children and young adults with a long-standing history of seizures. If the seizures are refractory, surgical resection is curative.

Epidermoid cysts

These consist of squamous epithelium surrounding a keratin-filled cyst. They are usually found in the cerebellopontine angle and the intrasellar and suprasellar regions. They may present with headaches, cranial nerve abnormalities, seizures, or hydrocephalus. Imaging studies demonstrate extraaxial lesions with characteristics that are similar to CSF but have restricted diffusion. Treatment involves surgical resection.

Dermoid cysts

Like epidermoid cysts, dermoid cysts arise from epithelial cells that are retained during closure of the neural tube. They contain both epidermal and dermal structures such as hair follicles, sweat glands, and sebaceous glands. Unlike epidermoid cysts, these tumors usually have a midline location. They occur most frequently in the posterior fossa, especially the vermis, fourth ventricle, and suprasellar cistern. Radiographically, dermoid cysts resemble lipomas, demonstrating T1 hyperintensity and variable signal on T2. Symptomatic dermoid cysts can be treated with surgery.

Colloid cysts

These usually arise in the anterior third ventricle and may present with headaches, hydrocephalus, and very rarely sudden death. Surgical resection is curative or a third ventriculostomy may relieve the obstructive hydrocephalus and be sufficient therapy.

NEUROCUTANEOUS SYNDROMES (PHAKOMATOSES)

A number of genetic disorders are characterized by cutaneous lesions and an increased risk of brain tumors. Most of these disorders have an autosomal dominance inheritance with variable penetrance.

NEUROFIBROMATOSIS TYPE 1 (VON RECKLINGHAUSEN'S DISEASE)

NF1 is an autosomal dominant disorder with an incidence of approximately 1 in 2600–3000. Approximately half the cases are familial; the remainder are new mutations arising in patients with unaffected parents. The NF1 gene on chromosome 17q11.2 encodes a protein, *neurofibromin*, a guanosine triphosphatase (GTPase)–activating protein (GAP) that modulates signaling through the ras pathway. Mutations of the NF1 gene result in a large number of nervous system tumors, including neurofibromas, plexiform neurofibromas, optic nerve gliomas, astrocytomas, and meningiomas. In addition to neurofibromas, which appear as multiple, soft, rubbery cutaneous tumors, other cutaneous manifestations of NF1 include café au lait spots and axillary freckling. NF1 is also associated with hamartomas of the iris termed Lisch nodules, pheochromocytomas, pseudoarthrosis of the tibia, scoliosis, epilepsy, and mental retardation.

NEUROFIBROMATOSIS TYPE 2

NF2 is less common than NF1, with an incidence of 1 in 25,000–40,000. It is an autosomal dominant disorder with full penetrance. As with NF1, approximately half the cases arise from new mutations. The NF2 gene on 22q encodes a cytoskeletal protein "merlin" (moesin, ezrin, radixin-like protein) that functions as a tumor suppressor. NF2 is characterized by bilateral vestibular schwannomas in over 90% of patients, multiple meningiomas, and spinal ependymomas and astrocytomas. Treatment of bilateral vestibular schwannomas can be challenging because the goal is to preserve hearing for as long as possible. These patients may also have posterior subcapsular lens opacities and retinal hamartomas.

TUBEROUS SCLEROSIS (BOURNEVILLE'S DISEASE)

This is an autosomal dominant disorder with an incidence of approximately 1 in 5000 to 10,000 live births. It is caused by mutations in either the TSC1 gene, which maps to chromosome 9q34, and encodes a protein termed *hamartin*, or the TSC2 gene, which maps to chromosome 16p13.3 and encodes the tuberin protein. Hamartin forms a complex with tuberin, which inhibits cellular signaling through mTOR, and acts as a negative regulator of the cell cycle. Patients with tuberous sclerosis have seizures, mental retardation, adenoma sebaceum (facial angiofibromas), shagreen patch, hypomelanotic macules, periungual fibromas, renal angiomyolipomas, and cardiac rhabdomyomas. These patients have an increased incidence of subependymal nodules, cortical tubers, and subependymal giant cell astrocytomas (SEGA). Patients frequently require anticonvulsants for seizures. SEGAs often do not need treatment but occasionally require surgical resection. There is emerging evidence that mTOR inhibitors may have activity in SEGAs.

TUMORS METASTATIC TO THE BRAIN

Brain metastases arise from hematogenous spread and frequently arise from either a lung primary or are associated with pulmonary metastases. Most metastases develop at the gray matter–white matter junction in the watershed distribution of the brain where intravascular tumor cells lodge in terminal arterioles. The distribution of metastases in the brain approximates the proportion of blood flow such that about 85% of all metastases are supratentorial and 15% occur in the posterior fossa. The most common sources of brain metastases are lung and breast carcinomas; melanoma has the greatest propensity to metastasize to the brain, being found in 80% of patients at autopsy (Table 46-3). Other tumor types such as ovarian and esophageal carcinoma rarely metastasize to the brain. Prostate and breast cancer also have a propensity to metastasize to the dura and can mimic meningioma. Leptomeningeal metastases are common from hematologic malignancies and also breast and lung cancers. Spinal cord compression primarily arises in patients with prostate and breast cancer, tumors with a strong propensity to metastasize to the axial skeleton.

TABLE 46-3

FREQUENCY OF NERVOUS SYSTEM METASTASES BY COMMON PRIMARY TUMORS

	BRAIN %	LM %	ESCC %
Lung	41	17	15
Breast	19	58	22
Melanoma	10	12	4
Prostate	1	1	10
GIT	7	—	5
Renal	3	2	7
Lymphoma	<1	10	10
Sarcoma	7	1	9
Other	11	—	18

Abbreviations: ESCC, epidural spinal cord compression; GIT, gastrointestinal tract; LM, leptomeningeal metastases.

DIAGNOSIS OF METASTASES

Brain metastases are best visualized on MRI, where they usually appear as well-circumscribed lesions (Fig. 46-8). The amount of perilesional edema can be highly variable with large lesions causing minimal edema and sometimes very small lesions causing extensive edema. Enhancement may be in a ring pattern or diffuse. Occasionally, intracranial metastases will hemorrhage; although melanoma, thyroid, and kidney cancer have the greatest propensity to hemorrhage, the most common cause of a hemorrhagic metastasis is lung cancer because it accounts for the majority of brain metastases. The radiographic appearance of brain metastasis is nonspecific, and similar appearing lesions can occur with infection, including brain abscesses and also with demyelinating lesions, sarcoidosis, radiation necrosis in a previously treated patient, or a primary brain tumor that may be a second malignancy in a patient with systemic cancer. However, biopsy is rarely necessary for diagnosis in most patients because imaging alone in the appropriate clinical situation usually suffices. This is straightforward for the majority of patients with brain metastases because they have a known systemic cancer. However, in approximately 10% of patients, a systemic cancer may present with a brain metastasis, and if there is not an easily accessible systemic site to biopsy, then a brain lesion must be removed for diagnostic purposes.

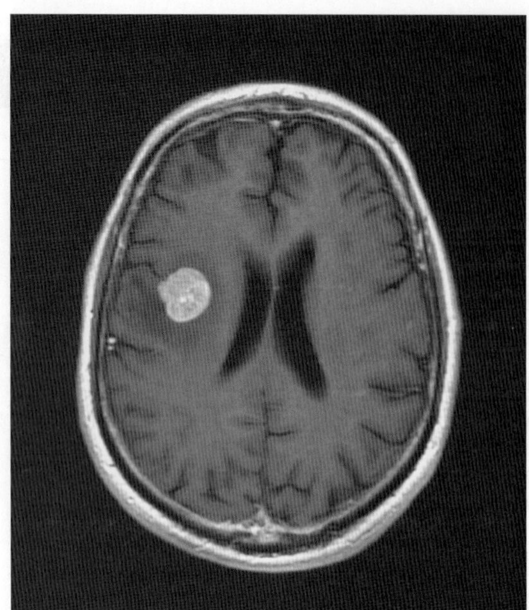

A

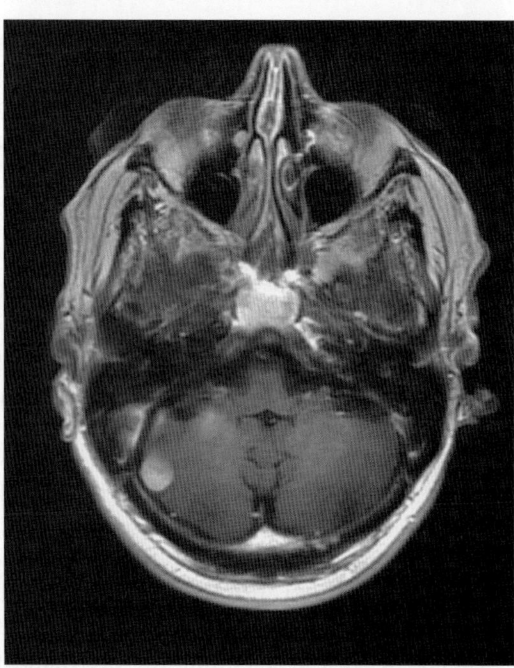

B

FIGURE 46-8

Postgadolinium T1 magnetic resonance images of multiple brain metastases from non–small cell lung cancer involving the right frontal (***A***) and right cerebellar (***B***) hemispheres. Note the diffuse enhancement pattern and absence of central necrosis.

TREATMENT Tumors Metastatic to the Brain

DEFINITIVE TREATMENT The number and location of brain metastases often determine the therapeutic options. The patient's overall condition and the current or potential control of the systemic disease are also major determinants. Brain metastases are single in approximately half of patients and multiple in the other half.

RADIATION THERAPY The standard treatment for brain metastases has been whole-brain radiotherapy (WBRT) usually administered to a total dose of 3000 cGy in 10 fractions. This affords rapid palliation, and approximately 80% of patients improve with glucocorticoids and radiation therapy. However, it is not curative. Median survival is only 4–6 months. More recently, stereotactic radiosurgery (SRS) delivered through a variety of techniques, including the gamma knife, linear accelerator, proton beam, and CyberKnife, all can deliver highly focused doses of RT, usually in a single fraction. SRS can effectively sterilize the visible lesions and afford local disease control in 80–90% of patients. In addition, there are some patients who have clearly been cured of their brain metastases using SRS, whereas this is distinctly rare with WBRT. However, SRS can be used only for lesions 3 cm or less in diameter and should be confined to patients with only 1–3 metastases. The addition of WBRT to SRS improves disease control in the nervous system but does not prolong survival.

SURGERY Randomized controlled trials have demonstrated that surgical extirpation of a single brain metastasis followed by WBRT is superior to WBRT alone. Removal of two lesions or a single symptomatic mass, particularly if compressing the ventricular system, can also be useful. This is particularly useful in patients who have highly radioresistant lesions such as renal carcinoma. Surgical resection can afford rapid symptomatic improvement and prolonged survival. RT administered after complete resection of a brain metastasis improves disease control but does not prolong survival.

CHEMOTHERAPY Chemotherapy is rarely useful for brain metastases. Metastases from certain tumor types that are highly chemosensitive, such as germ cell tumors or small cell lung cancer, may respond to chemotherapeutic regimens chosen according to the underlying malignancy. Increasingly, there are data demonstrating responsiveness of brain metastases to chemotherapy including small molecule–targeted therapy when the lesion possesses the target. This has been best illustrated in patients with lung cancer harboring EGF-R mutations that sensitize them to EGF-R inhibitors. Antiangiogenic agents such as bevacizumab may also prove efficacious in the treatment of CNS metastases.

LEPTOMENINGEAL METASTASES

Leptomeningeal metastases are also identified as carcinomatous meningitis; meningeal carcinomatosis; or in the case of specific tumors, leukemic or lymphomatous meningitis. Among the hematologic malignancies, acute leukemia is the most common to metastasize to the subarachnoid space, and in lymphomas the aggressive diffuse lymphomas can metastasize to the subarachnoid space frequently as well. Among solid tumors, breast and lung carcinomas and melanoma most frequently spread in this fashion. Tumor cells reach the subarachnoid space via the arterial circulation or occasionally through retrograde flow in venous systems that drain metastases along the bony spine or cranium. In addition, leptomeningeal metastases may develop as a direct consequence of prior brain metastases and can develop in almost 40% of patients who have a metastasis resected from the cerebellum.

CLINICAL FEATURES

Leptomeningeal metastases are characterized clinically by multilevel symptoms and signs along the neuraxis. Combinations of lumbar and cervical radiculopathies, cranial neuropathies, seizures, confusion, and encephalopathy from hydrocephalus or raised intracranial pressure can be present. Focal deficits such as hemiparesis or aphasia are rarely due to leptomeningeal metastases unless there is direct brain infiltration and are more often associated with coexisting brain lesions. New-onset limb pain in patients with breast, lung cancer, or melanoma should prompt consideration of leptomeningeal spread.

LABORATORY AND IMAGING DIAGNOSIS

Leptomeningeal metastases are particularly challenging to diagnose as identification of tumor cells in the subarachnoid compartment may be elusive. MRI can be definitive in patients when there are clear tumor nodules adherent to the cauda equina or spinal cord, enhancing cranial nerves, or subarachnoid enhancement on brain imaging (Fig. 46-9). Imaging is diagnostic in approximately 75% of patients and is more often positive in patients with solid tumors. Demonstration of tumor cells in the CSF is definitive and often considered the gold standard. However, CSF cytologic examination is positive in only 50% of patients on the first lumbar puncture and still misses 10% after three CSF samples. CSF cytologic examination is most useful in hematologic malignancies. Accompanying CSF abnormalities include an elevated protein concentration and an elevated white count. Hypoglycorrhachia is noted in fewer than 25% of patients but is useful when present. Identification of tumor markers or molecular confirmation of clonal proliferation with techniques such as flow cytometry within the CSF can also be definitive when present. Tumor markers are usually specific to solid tumors, and chromosomal or molecular markers are most useful in patients with hematologic malignancies.

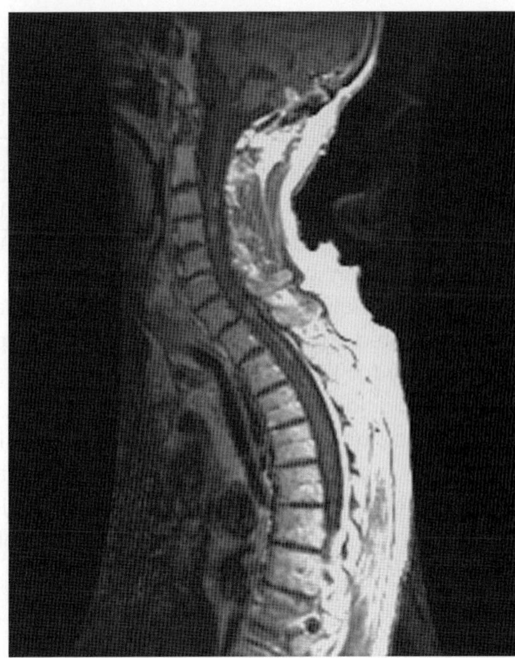

A

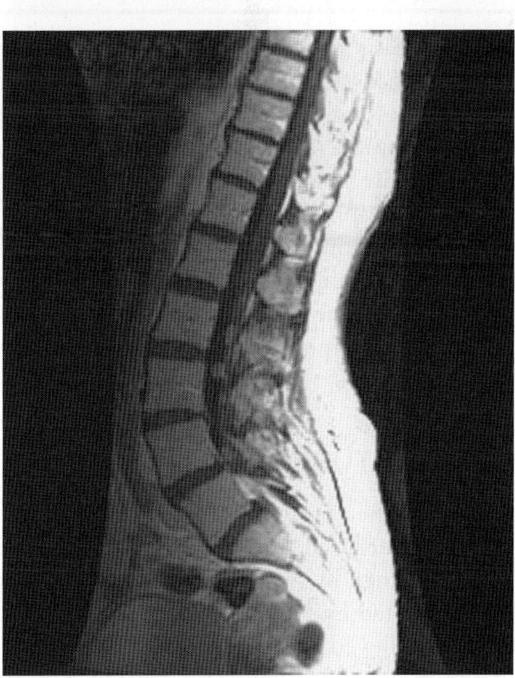

B

FIGURE 46-9
Postgadolinium magnetic resonance images of extensive leptomeningeal metastases from breast cancer. Nodules along the dorsal surface of the spinal cord (***A***) and cauda equina (***B***) are seen.

TREATMENT **Leptomeningeal Metastases**

The treatment of leptomeningeal metastasis is palliative as there is no curative therapy. RT to the symptomatically involved areas, such as skull base for cranial neuropathy, can relieve pain and sometimes improve function.

Whole neuraxis RT has extensive toxicity with myelosuppression and gastrointestinal irritation as well as limited effectiveness. Systemic chemotherapy with agents that can penetrate the blood–CSF barrier may be helpful. Alternatively, intrathecal chemotherapy can be effective, particularly in hematologic malignancies. This is optimally delivered through an intraventricular cannula (Ommaya reservoir) rather than by lumbar puncture. Few drugs can be delivered safely into the subarachnoid space, and they have a limited spectrum of antitumor activity, perhaps accounting for the relatively poor response to this approach. In addition, impaired CSF flow dynamics can compromise intrathecal drug delivery. Surgery has a limited role in the treatment of leptomeningeal metastasis, but placement of a ventriculoperitoneal shunt can relieve raised intracranial pressure. However, it compromises delivery of chemotherapy into the CSF.

EPIDURAL METASTASIS

Epidural metastasis occurs in 3–5% of patients with a systemic malignancy and causes neurologic compromise by compressing the spinal cord or cauda equina. The most common cancers that metastasize to the epidural space are malignancies that spread to bone, such as breast and prostate. Lymphoma can cause bone involvement and compression, but it can also invade the intervertebral foramens and cause spinal cord compression without bone destruction. The thoracic spine is affected most commonly followed by the lumbar and then cervical spine.

CLINICAL FEATURES

Back pain is the presenting symptom of epidural metastasis in virtually all patients; the pain may precede neurologic findings by weeks or months. The pain is usually exacerbated by lying down; by contrast, arthritic pain is often relieved by recumbency. Leg weakness is seen in about 50% of patients as is sensory dysfunction. Sphincter problems are present in about 25% of patients at diagnosis.

DIAGNOSIS

Diagnosis is established by imaging, with MRI of the complete spine being the best test (Fig. 46-10). Contrast is not needed to identify spinal or epidural lesions. Any patient with cancer who has severe back pain should undergo an MRI. Plain films, bone scans, or even CT scans may show bone metastases, but only MRI can reliably delineate epidural tumor. For patients unable to have an MRI, CT myelography should be performed to outline the epidural space. The differential diagnosis of epidural tumor includes epidural abscess, acute or chronic hematomas, and rarely, extramedullary hematopoiesis.

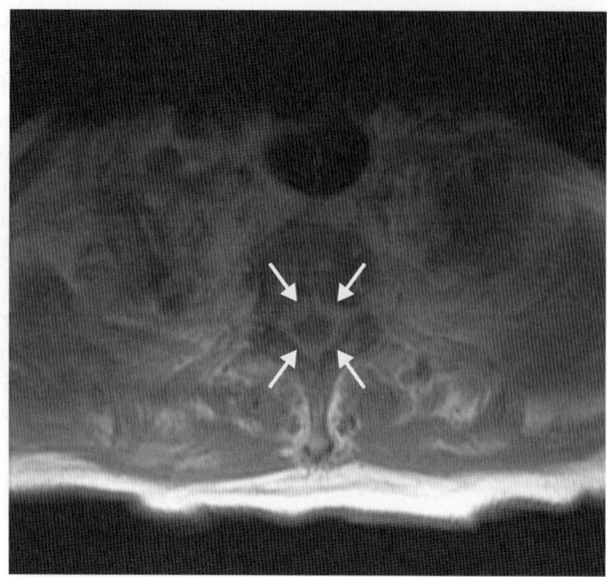

FIGURE 46-10
Postgadolinium T1 magnetic resonance image showing circumferential epidural tumor around the thoracic spinal cord from esophageal cancer.

TREATMENT Epidural Metastasis

Epidural metastasis requires immediate treatment. A randomized controlled trial demonstrated the superiority of surgical resection followed by RT compared with RT alone. However, patients must be able to tolerate surgery, and the surgical procedure of choice is a complete removal of the mass, which is typically anterior to the spinal canal, necessitating an extensive approach and resection. Otherwise, RT is the mainstay of treatment and can be used for patients with radiosensitive tumors, such as lymphoma, or for those unable to undergo surgery. Chemotherapy is rarely used for epidural metastasis unless the patient has minimal to no neurologic deficit and a highly chemosensitive tumor such as lymphoma or germinoma. Patients generally fare well if treated before there is severe neurologic deficit. Recovery after paraparesis is better after surgery than with RT alone, but survival is often short due to widespread metastatic tumor.

NEUROLOGIC TOXICITY OF THERAPY

TOXICITY FROM RADIOTHERAPY

Radiotherapy can cause a variety of toxicities in the CNS. These are usually described based on their relationship in time to the administration of RT, e.g., they can be acute (occurring within days of RT), early delayed (months), or late delayed (years). In general, the acute and early delayed syndromes resolve and do not result in persistent deficits, whereas the late delayed toxicities are usually permanent and sometimes progressive.

Acute toxicity

Acute cerebral toxicity usually occurs during RT to the brain. RT can cause a transient disruption of the blood–brain barrier, resulting in increased edema and elevated intracranial pressure. This is usually manifest as headache, lethargy, nausea, and vomiting and can be both prevented and treated with the administration of glucocorticoids. There is no acute RT toxicity that affects the spinal cord.

Early delayed toxicity

Early delayed toxicity is usually apparent weeks to months after completion of cranial irradiation and is likely due to focal demyelination. Clinically, it may be asymptomatic or take the form of worsening or reappearance of a preexisting neurologic deficit. At times a contrast-enhancing lesion can be seen on MRI or CT that can mimic the tumor for which the patient received the RT. For patients with a malignant glioma, this has been described as "pseudoprogression" because it mimics tumor recurrence on MRI but actually represents inflammation and necrotic debris engendered by effective therapy. This is seen with increased frequency when chemotherapy, particularly temozolomide, is given concurrently with RT. Pseudoprogression can resolve on its own or, if very symptomatic, may require resection. A rare form of early delayed toxicity is the somnolence syndrome that occurs primarily in children and is characterized by marked sleepiness.

In the spinal cord, early delayed RT toxicity is manifest as a Lhermitte symptom with paresthesias of the limbs or along the spine when the patient flexes the neck. Although frightening, it is benign, resolves on its own, and does not portend more serious problems.

Late delayed toxicity

Late delayed toxicities are the most serious as they are often irreversible and cause severe neurologic deficits. In the brain, late toxicities can take several forms, the most common of which include radiation necrosis and leukoencephalopathy. Radiation necrosis is a focal mass of necrotic tissue that is contrast enhancing on CT or MRI and may be associated with significant edema. This may appear identical to pseudoprogression but is seen months to years after RT and is always symptomatic. Clinical symptoms and signs include seizure and lateralizing findings referable to the location of the necrotic mass. The necrosis is caused by the effect of RT on cerebral vasculature with resultant fibrinoid necrosis and occlusion of the blood vessels. It can mimic tumor radiographically, but unlike tumor, it is typically hypometabolic on a PET scan and has reduced perfusion on perfusion MR sequences. It may require resection for diagnosis and treatment unless it can be managed with glucocorticoids. There are rare reports of improvement with hyperbaric oxygen or anticoagulation but the usefulness of these approaches is questionable.

Leukoencephalopathy is seen most commonly after WBRT as opposed to focal RT. On T2 or FLAIR MR sequences, there is diffuse increased signal seen throughout the hemispheric white matter, often bilaterally and symmetrically. There tends to be a periventricular predominance that may be associated with atrophy and ventricular enlargement. Clinically, patients develop cognitive impairment, gait disorder, and later urinary incontinence, all of which can progress over time. These symptoms mimic those of normal-pressure hydrocephalus, and placement of a ventriculoperitoneal shunt can improve function in some patients but does not reverse the deficits completely. Increased age is a risk factor for leukoencephalopathy but not for radiation necrosis. Necrosis appears to depend on an as yet unidentified predisposition.

Other late neurologic toxicities include endocrine dysfunction if the pituitary or hypothalamus was included in the RT port. A radiation-induced neoplasm can occur many years after therapeutic RT for either a prior CNS tumor or a head and neck cancer; accurate diagnosis requires surgical resection or biopsy. In addition, RT causes accelerated atherosclerosis, which can cause stroke either from intracranial vascular disease or carotid plaque from neck irradiation.

The peripheral nervous system is relatively resistant to RT toxicities. Peripheral nerves are rarely affected by RT, but the plexus is more vulnerable. Plexopathy develops more commonly in the brachial distribution than in the lumbosacral distribution. It must be differentiated from tumor progression in the plexus, which is usually accomplished with CT or MRI of the area or PET scan demonstrating tumor infiltrating the region. Clinically, tumor progression is usually painful, whereas radiation-induced plexopathy is painless. Radiation plexopathy is also more commonly associated with lymphedema of the affected limb. Sensory loss and weakness are seen in both.

TOXICITY FROM CHEMOTHERAPY

Neurotoxicity is second to myelosuppression as the dose-limiting toxicity of chemotherapeutic agents (Table 46-4). Chemotherapy causes peripheral neuropathy from a number of commonly used agents, and

TABLE 46-4

NEUROLOGIC SIGNS CAUSED BY AGENTS COMMONLY USED IN PATIENTS WITH CANCER

Acute encephalopathy (delirium)	Seizures
Methotrexate (high-dose IV, IT)	Methotrexate
Cisplatin	Etoposide (high-dose)
Vincristine	Cisplatin
Asparaginase	Vincristine
Procarbazine	Asparaginase
5-Flourouracil (±levamisole)	Nitrogen mustard
Cytarabine (high-dose)	Carmustine
Nitrosoureas (high-dose or arterial)	Dacarbazine (intraarterial or high-dose)
Ifosfamide	Busulfan (high-dose)
Etoposide (high-dose)	Myelopathy (intrathecal drugs)
Bevacizumab (PRES)	Methotrexate
Chronic encephalopathy (dementia)	Cytarabine
Methotrexate	Thiotepa
Carmustine	Peripheral neuropathy
Cytarabine	Vinca alkaloids
Fludarabine	Cisplatin
Visual loss	Procarbazine
Tamoxifen	Etoposide
Gallium nitrate	Teniposide
Cisplatin	Cytarabine
Fludarabine	Taxanes
Cerebellar dysfunction/ataxia	Suramin
5-Fluorouracil (± levamisole)	Bortezomib
Cytarabine	
Procarbazine	

Abbreviations: IT, intrathecal; IV, intravenous; PRES, posterior reversible encephalopathy syndrome.

the type of neuropathy can differ, depending on the drug. Vincristine causes paresthesias but little sensory loss and is associated with motor dysfunction, autonomic impairment (frequently ileus), and rarely cranial nerve compromise. Cisplatin causes large fiber sensory loss resulting in sensory ataxia but little cutaneous sensory loss and no weakness. The taxanes also cause a predominately sensory neuropathy. Agents such as bortezomib and thalidomide also cause neuropathy.

Encephalopathy and seizures are common toxicities from chemotherapeutic drugs. Ifosfamide can cause a severe encephalopathy, which is reversible with discontinuation of the drug and the use of methylene blue for severely affected patients. Fludarabine also causes a severe global encephalopathy that may be permanent. Bevacizumab and other anti-VEGF agents can cause posterior reversible encephalopathy syndrome. Cisplatin can cause hearing loss and less frequently vestibular dysfunction.

CHAPTER 47

CARCINOMA OF UNKNOWN PRIMARY

Gauri R. Varadhachary ■ James L. Abbruzzese

Carcinoma of unknown primary (CUP) is a biopsy-proven (mainly epithelial) malignancy for which the anatomic site of origin remains unidentified after an intensive search. CUP is one of the 10 most frequently diagnosed cancers worldwide, accounting for approximately 3–5% of all cancers. Most investigators do not include lymphomas, metastatic melanomas, and metastatic sarcomas that present without a known primary tumor as CUP because these cancers have specific stage- and histology-based treatments that guide management.

With the increasing availability of additional sophisticated imaging, invasive diagnostic techniques, and the emergence of effective targeted therapies in several cancers, an individualized management algorithm with an impact on quality of life and survival is critical. The reasons cancers present as CUP remain unclear. One hypothesis is that the primary tumor either regresses after seeding the metastasis or remains so small that it is not detected. It is possible that CUP falls on the continuum of cancer presentation in which the primary has been contained or eliminated by the natural body defenses. Alternatively, CUP may represent a specific malignant event that results in an increase in metastatic spread or survival relative to the primary. Whether the CUP metastases truly define a clone that is genetically and phenotypically unique to this diagnosis remains to be determined.

BIOLOGY OF CARCINOMA OF UNKNOWN PRIMARY

No characteristics that are unique to CUP relative to metastases from known primaries have been identified. Abnormalities in chromosomes 1 and 12 and other complex cytogenetic abnormalities have been reported. Aneuploidy has been described in 70% of CUP patients with metastatic adenocarcinoma or undifferentiated carcinoma. The overexpression of various genes, including *Ras, bcl-2* (40%), *her-2* (11%), and *p53* (26–53%), has been studied in CUP samples, but they have no effect on response to therapy or survival. The extent of angiogenesis in CUP relative to that in metastases from known primaries has also been evaluated, but no consistent findings have emerged.

CLINICAL EVALUATION

Obtaining a thorough medical history from CUP patients is essential, paying particular attention to previous surgeries, removed lesions, and family medical history to assess potential hereditary cancers. Physical examination, including a digital rectal examination in men and breast and pelvic examinations in women, should be performed. Determining the patient's performance status, nutritional status, comorbid illnesses, and cancer-induced complications is essential since these may affect treatment planning.

Role of serum tumor markers and cytogenetics

Most tumor markers, including CEA, CA-125, CA 19-9, and CA 15-3, when elevated, are nonspecific and not helpful in determining the primary tumor site. Men who present with adenocarcinoma and osteoblastic metastasis should undergo a prostate-specific antigen (PSA) test. In patients with undifferentiated or poorly differentiated carcinoma (especially with a midline tumor), elevated β-human chorionic gonadotropin (βhCG) and α fetoprotein (AFP) levels suggest the possibility of an extragonadal germ cell (testicular) tumor. Cytogenetic studies had a larger role in the past, although interpretation of these older studies can be challenging. In our opinion, with the availability of immunohistochemical stains, cytogenetic analyses are indicated only occasionally. We reserve them for undifferentiated neoplasms with inconclusive immunohistochemical stains and those for which a high suspicion of lymphoma exists.

Role of imaging studies

Chest radiographs are always obtained in CUP workups but findings are often negative, especially with low-volume disease. A computed tomography (CT) scan of the chest, abdomen, and pelvis is indicated in the search for the primary, evaluate the extent of disease, and select the most favorable biopsy site. Older studies suggested that the primary tumor site is detected in 20–35% of patients who undergo a CT scan of the abdomen and pelvis, although by current definition these patients would not be considered as having CUP. Older studies also suggest a latent primary tumor prevalence of 20%; with more sophisticated imaging, this prevalence is <5% today.

Mammography should be performed in all women who present with metastatic adenocarcinoma, especially in those with adenocarcinoma and isolated axillary lymphadenopathy. Magnetic resonance imaging (MRI) of the breast is a recognized follow-up modality in patients with suspected occult primary breast carcinoma following negative mammography and sonography results. The results of these imaging modalities can influence surgical management; a negative breast MRI result predicts a low tumor yield at mastectomy.

A conventional workup for a squamous cell carcinoma and cervical CUP (neck lymphadenopathy with no known primary tumor) includes a CT scan or MRI and invasive studies, including indirect and direct laryngoscopy, bronchoscopy, and upper endoscopy. Ipsilateral (or bilateral) tonsillectomy (with histopathology) has been recommended for these patients. Fluorodeoxyglucose positron emission tomography (FDG-PET) scans are useful in this patient population and may help guide the biopsy; determine the extent of disease; facilitate the appropriate treatment, including planning radiation fields; and help with disease surveillance. A smaller radiation field encompassing the primary (when found) and metastatic adenopathy decreases the risk of chronic xerostomia. Several studies have evaluated the utility of positron emission tomography (PET) in patients with cervical CUP. These trials have included a small number of patients; primary tumors were identified in ~21–30%.

The diagnostic contribution of PET to the evaluation of other CUP (outside of the neck adenopathy indication) is controversial. PET-CT can be helpful for patients who are candidates for surgical intervention for solitary metastatic disease because the presence of disease outside the primary site may affect surgical planning.

Invasive studies, including upper endoscopy, colonoscopy, and bronchoscopy, should be limited to symptomatic patients or those with laboratory, imaging or pathologic abnormalities that suggest that these techniques will result in a high yield in search for a primary cancer.

PATHOLOGIC DIAGNOSIS OF CARCINOMA OF UNKNOWN PRIMARY

A detailed pathologic examination of the most accessible biopsied tissue specimen is mandatory in CUP patients. Pathologic evaluation typically consists of hematoxylin-and-eosin stains and immunohistochemical tests. Electron microscopy and cytogenetics are rarely useful.

Light microscopy evaluation

Adequate tissue obtained by fine-needle aspiration or core-needle biopsy should first be stained with hematoxylin and eosin and subjected to light microscopic examination. On light microscopy, 60–65% of CUPs are adenocarcinoma, and 5% are squamous cell carcinoma. The remaining 30–35% are poorly differentiated adenocarcinoma, poorly differentiated carcinoma, poorly differentiated neoplasm. A small percentage of lesions are diagnosed as neuroendocrine cancers (2%), mixed tumors (adenosquamous, or sarcomatoid carcinomas), or undifferentiated neoplasm (Table 47-1).

Role of immunohistochemical analysis

Immunohistochemical stains are peroxidase-labeled antibodies against specific tumor antigens that are used to define tumor lineage. The number of available immunohistochemical stains is ever-increasing. However, in CUP cases, more is not necessarily better, and immunohistochemical stains should be used in conjunction with the patient's clinical presentation and imaging studies to select the best therapy. Communication between the clinician and pathologist is essential. No stain is 100% specific, and overinterpretation should be avoided. PSA and thyroglobulin tissue markers, which are positive in prostate and thyroid cancer, respectively, are the most specific of the current marker panel. However, these

TABLE 47-1

MAJOR HISTOLOGIES IN CARCINOMA OF UNKNOWN PRIMARY

HISTOLOGY	PROPORTION, %
Well- to moderately differentiated adenocarcinoma	60
Squamous cell cancer	5
Poorly differentiated adenocarcinoma, poorly differentiated carcinoma	30
Neuroendocrine	2
Undifferentiated malignancy	3

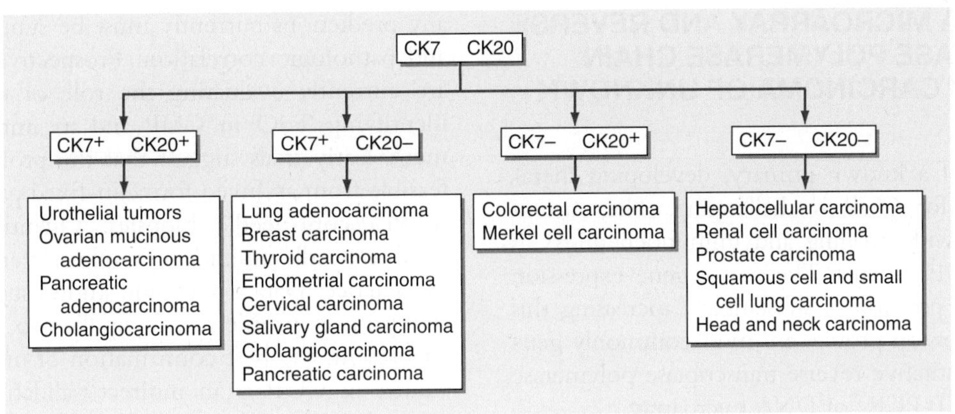

FIGURE 47-1
Approach to cytokeratin (CK7 and CK20) markers used in carcinoma of unknown primary.

cancers rarely present as CUP, so the yield of these tests may be low. Figure 47-1 delineates a simple algorithm for immunohistochemical staining in CUP cases. Table 47-2 lists additional tests that may be useful to further define the tumor lineage. A more comprehensive algorithm may improve the diagnostic accuracy but can make the process complex. With the use of immunohistochemical markers, electron microscopic analysis, which is time-consuming and expensive, is rarely needed.

TABLE 47-2

ADDITIONAL IMMUNOHISTOCHEMICAL STAINS USEFUL IN THE DIAGNOSIS OF CARCINOMA OF UNKNOWN PRIMARY

TISSUE MARKER	DIAGNOSIS
Estrogen and progesterone receptors	Breast cancer
BRST-1	Breast cancer
Gross cystic disease fibrous protein-15	Breast cancer
Thyroid transcription factor 1	Lung and thyroid cancer
Thyroglobulin	Thyroid cancer
Chromogranin, synaptophysin, CD56	Neuroendocrine cancer
CDX-2	Gastrointestinal cancer
Calretinin, mesothelin	Mesothelioma
Leukocyte common antigen	Lymphoma
HMB-45, tyrosinase, Melan-A	Melanoma
URO-III, thrombomodulin	Bladder cancer
α Fetoprotein	Hepatocellular cancer, germ cell cancer
β-Human chronic gonadotropin	Germ cell cancer
Prostate specific antigen	Prostate cancer
WT-1, estrogen receptor (ER)	Müllerian or ovarian cancer
RCC, CD 10	Renal cell carcinoma

There are >20 subtypes of cytokeratin (CK) intermediate filaments with different molecular weights and differential expression in various cell types and cancers. Monoclonal antibodies to specific CK subtypes have been used to help classify tumors according to their sites of origin; commonly used CK stains in CUP are CK7 and CK20. CK7 is found in tumors of the lung, ovary, endometrium, and breast and not in those of the lower gastrointestinal tract, whereas CK20 is normally expressed in the gastrointestinal epithelium, urothelium, and Merkel cells. CK20+/CK7– strongly suggests a primary tumor of the colon; 75–95% of colon tumors show this pattern of staining. CK20–/CK7+ suggests cancer of the lung, breast, ovary, endometrium, and pancreaticobiliary tract; some of these can also be CK20+. The nuclear CDX-2 transcription factor, which is the product of a homeobox gene necessary for intestinal organogenesis, is often used to aid in the diagnosis of gastrointestinal adenocarcinomas.

Thyroid transcription factor 1 (TTF-1) is a 38-kDa homeodomain-containing nuclear protein that plays a role in transcriptional activation during embryogenesis in the thyroid, diencephalon, and respiratory epithelium. TTF-1 nuclear staining results are typically positive in lung and thyroid cancers. Approximately 68% of adenocarcinomas and 25% of squamous cell lung cancers stain positive for TTF-1, which helps differentiate a lung primary tumor from metastatic adenocarcinoma in a pleural effusion, the mediastinum, or the lung parenchyma.

Distinguishing pleural mesothelioma from lung adenocarcinoma can be challenging. Calretinin, Wilms' tumor gene-1 (WT-1), and mesothelin have been suggested as useful markers for mesothelioma.

Gross cystic disease fibrous protein-15, a 15-kDa monomer protein, is a marker of apocrine differentiation that is detected in 62–72% of breast carcinomas. UROIII, high-molecular-weight cytokeratin, thrombomodulin, and CK20 are the markers used to diagnose lesions of urothelial origin.

ROLE OF DNA MICROARRAY AND REVERSE TRANSCRIPTASE POLYMERASE CHAIN REACTION IN CARCINOMA OF UNKNOWN PRIMARY

In the absence of a known primary, developing therapeutic strategies for CUP is challenging. The current diagnostic yield with imaging and immunochemistry is ~20–30% for CUP patients. The use of gene expression studies holds the promise of substantially increasing this yield. Gene expression profiles are most commonly generated using quantitative reverse transcriptase polymerase chain reaction (RT-PCR) or DNA microarray.

Neural network programs have been used to develop predictive algorithms from the gene expression profiles. Typically, a training set of gene profiles from known cancers (preferably from metastatic sites) are used to train the software. The program can then be used to predict the putative origin of a test tumor and presumably of true CUP. Comprehensive gene expression databases that have become available for common malignancies may also be useful in CUP. Investigators have used expression data from normal differentiated tissues to identify conserved expression profiles found in malignant tissue as a basis for predicting the tissue of origin (ToO). These approaches have been effective in blind testing against known primary cancers and their metastasis. However, because, by definition, the primary tumor site is not identifiable in CUP, validation of site prediction in this setting can be challenging, and any predictions currently must be supported by clinical and pathologic correlation. Prospective validation trials are currently evaluating the role of molecular studies identifying ToO in CUP and its impact on management. Early trials suggest that the profiling approach is feasible from archived formalin-fixed paraffin-embedded (FFPE) core-needle biopsies. Quantitative RT-PCR on fine-needle aspiration samples is very useful in clinical practice. Data from some studies suggest that a putative primary profile can be applied to 80–85% of cases. At present, the best confirmation of molecular profiling studies in CUP is an indirect validation based on the patient's presentation and clinical course. Current studies are geared to understanding profiling tools' accuracy, clinical effectiveness, and how these assays complement immunohistochemistry and help guide therapy.

TREATMENT Carcinoma of Unknown Primary

GENERAL CONSIDERATIONS The treatment of CUP continues to evolve, albeit slowly. The median survival duration of most patients with disseminated CUP is ~6–10 months. Systemic chemotherapy is the primary treatment modality in most cases, but the careful integration of surgery, radiation therapy, and even periods of observation are important in the overall management of this condition (Figs. 47-2 and 47-3). Prognostic factors include performance status, site and number of metastases, response to chemotherapy, and

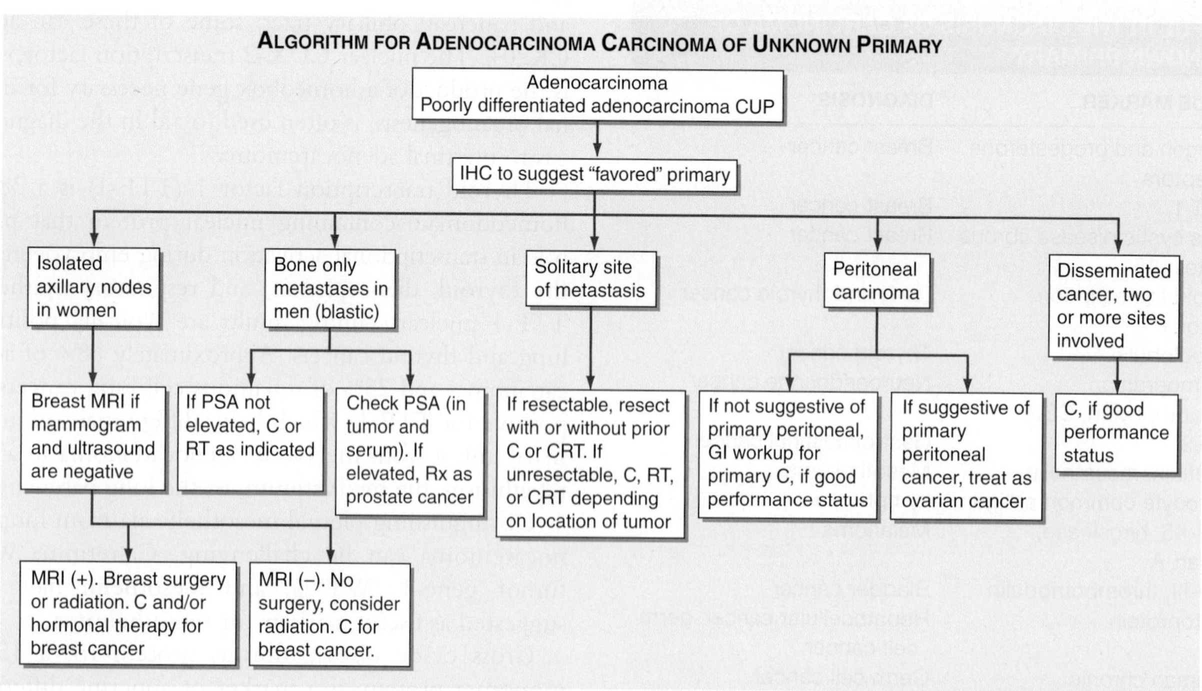

FIGURE 47-2
Treatment algorithm for adenocarcinoma and poorly differentiated adenocarcinoma carcinoma of unknown primary (CUP). C, chemotherapy; CRT, chemoradiation; CT, computed tomography; GI, gastrointestinal; IHC, immunohistochemistry; MRI, magnetic resonance imaging; PSA, prostate-specific antigen; RT, radiation; Rx, prescription.

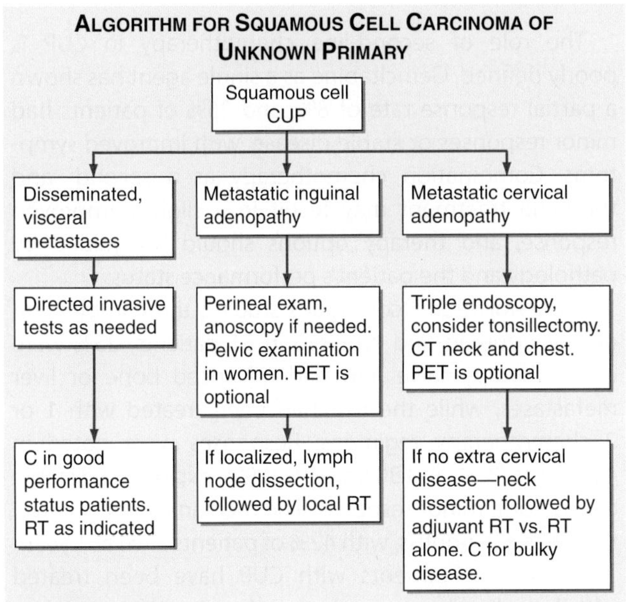
ALGORITHM FOR SQUAMOUS CELL CARCINOMA OF UNKNOWN PRIMARY
Squamous cell CUP
Disseminated, visceral metastases
Metastatic inguinal adenopathy
Metastatic cervical adenopathy
Directed invasive tests as needed
Perineal exam, anoscopy if needed. Pelvic examination in women. PET is optional
Triple endoscopy, consider tonsillectomy. CT neck and chest. PET is optional
C in good performance status patients. RT as indicated
If localized, lymph node dissection, followed by local RT
If no extra cervical disease—neck dissection followed by adjuvant RT vs. RT alone. C for bulky disease.

FIGURE 47-3

Treatment algorithm for squamous cell carcinoma of unknown primary (CUP). C, chemotherapy; CT, computed tomography; PET, positron emission tomography; RT, radiation.

serum lactate dehydrogenase (LDH) levels. Culine and colleagues developed a prognostic model using performance status and serum LDH levels, which allowed the assignment of patients into two subgroups with divergent outcomes. Future prospective trials using this prognostic model are warranted. Clinically, several CUP diagnoses fall into a favorable prognostic subset. Others, including those with disseminated CUP that do not fit a subset, have a more unfavorable prognosis.

TREATMENT OF FAVORABLE SUBSETS OF CUP

Women with isolated axillary adenopathy

Women with isolated axillary adenopathy with adenocarcinoma or carcinoma are usually treated for stage II or III breast cancer based on pathologic findings. These patients should undergo a breast MRI if mammogram and ultrasound findings are negative. Radiation therapy to the ipsilateral breast is indicated if the breast MRI is positive. Chemotherapy and/or hormonal therapy is indicated based on patient's age (premenopausal or postmenopausal), nodal disease bulk, and hormone receptor status (Chap. 37). It is important to verify that the pathology does represent a breast cancer profile (morphology, immunohistochemical markers including HER-2, gene expression) before embarking on a breast cancer therapeutic program.

Women with peritoneal carcinomatosis The term *primary peritoneal papillary serous carcinoma* (PPSC) has been used to describe CUP with carcinomatosis with the pathologic and laboratory (elevated CA-125 antigen) characteristics of ovarian cancer but no ovarian primary tumor identified on transvaginal sonography or laparotomy. Studies suggest that ovarian cancer and PPSC, which are both of müllerian origin, have similar gene expression profiles. Similar to patients with ovarian cancer, patients with PPSC are candidates for cytoreductive surgery, followed by adjuvant taxane and platinum-based chemotherapy. In one retrospective study of 258 women with peritoneal carcinomatosis who had undergone cytoreductive surgery and chemotherapy, 22% of patients had a complete response to chemotherapy; the median survival duration was 18 months (range, 11–24 months). However, not all peritoneal carcinomatosis in women is PPSC. Careful pathologic evaluation can help diagnose a colon cancer profile (CDX-2+, CK-20+, CK7–) or a pancreaticobiliary cancer.

Poorly differentiated carcinoma with midline adenopathy Men with poorly differentiated or undifferentiated carcinoma that presents as a midline adenopathy should be evaluated for extragonadal germ cell malignancy. If diagnosed and treated as such, they often experience a good response to treatment with platinum-based combination chemotherapy. Response rates of >50% have been noted, and 10–15% long-term survivors have been reported. Older patients (especially smokers) who present with mediastinal adenopathy are more likely to have a lung or head and neck cancer profile.

Neuroendocrine carcinoma Low-grade neuroendocrine carcinoma often has an indolent course, and treatment decisions are based on symptoms and tumor bulk. Urine 5-hydroxyindoleacetic acid (5-HIAA) and serum chromogranin may be elevated and can be followed as markers. Often the patient is treated with somatostatin analogues alone for hormone-related symptoms (diarrhea, flushing, nausea). Specific local therapies or systemic therapy would only be indicated if the patient is symptomatic with local pain secondary to significant growth of the metastasis or the hormone-related symptoms are not controlled with endocrine therapy. Patients with high-grade neuroendocrine carcinoma are treated as having small cell lung cancer and are responsive to chemotherapy; 20–25% show a complete response, and up to 10% patients survive more than 5 years.

Squamous cell carcinoma presenting as neck adenopathy Patients with early-stage squamous cell carcinoma involving the cervical lymph nodes are candidates for node dissection and radiation therapy, which can result in long-term survival. The role of chemotherapy in these patients is undefined, although chemoradiation therapy or induction chemotherapy is often used and is beneficial in bulky N2/N3 lymph node disease.

Solitary metastatic site Patients with solitary metastases can also experience good treatment outcomes. Some patients who present with locoregional disease are candidates for aggressive trimodality management; both prolonged disease-free interval and occasionally cure are possible.

Men with blastic skeletal metastases and elevated PSA Blastic bone-only metastasis is a rare presentation, and elevated serum PSA or tumor staining with PSA may provide confirmatory evidence of prostate cancer in these patients. Those with elevated levels are candidates for hormonal therapy for prostate cancer, although it is important to rule out other primary tumors (lung most common).

Management of Disseminated CUP Patients who present with liver, brain, and adrenal metastatic disease usually have a poor prognosis. Beside primary peritoneal carcinoma, carcinomatosis presenting as CUP in other settings is not uncommon. Gastric, appendicular, colon, pancreas, and cholangiocarcinoma are all possible primaries, and imaging, endoscopy, and pathologic data help in the evaluation.

Traditionally, platinum-based combination chemotherapy regimens have been used to treat patients with CUP. In a phase II study by Hainsworth and colleagues, 55 mostly chemotherapy-naive patients were treated with paclitaxel, carboplatin, and oral etoposide every 3 weeks. The overall response rate was 47%, with a median overall survival duration of 13.4 months. Briasoulis and colleagues reported similar response rates and survival durations in 77 patients with CUP who had been treated with paclitaxel and carboplatin. In this study, patients with nodal or pleural disease and women with peritoneal carcinomatosis had higher response rates and overall survival durations of 13 and 15 months, respectively. Studies incorporating newer agents, including gemcitabine, irinotecan, and targeted agents, are showing higher response rates. In a phase II randomized trial by Culine and colleagues, 80 patients were randomly assigned to receive gemcitabine with cisplatin or irinotecan with cisplatin; 78 patients were assessable for efficacy and toxicity. Objective responses were observed in 21 patients (55%) in the gemcitabine and cisplatin arm and in 15 patients (38%) in the irinotecan and cisplatin arm. The median survival durations were 8 months for gemcitabine and cisplatin and 6 months for irinotecan and cisplatin.

The role of second-line chemotherapy in CUP is poorly defined. Gemcitabine as a single agent has shown a partial response rate of 8%, and 25% of patients had minor responses or stable disease, with improved symptoms. Combination chemotherapy as a second- and third-line treatment may result in a slightly improved response, and therapy options should be guided by pathology and the patient's performance status.

Hainsworth and colleagues studied the combination of bevacizumab and erlotinib in 51 patients; 25% were chemotherapy-naive and had advanced bone or liver metastases, while the rest had been treated with 1 or 2 chemotherapy regimens. Responses were noted in 4 patients (8%), and 30 patients (59%) experienced stable disease or a minor response. The median overall survival time was 8.9 months, with 42% of patients alive at 1 year.

Historically, patients with CUP have been treated with broad-spectrum regimens that work for a variety of primary cancers, a "one treatment fits all" approach. With incremental improved responses over the past decade in known cancer types, we anticipate overall better response rates with newer regimens for selected CUP patients. With a more robust immunohistochemical panel (directed approach) and new molecular profiling tools, one may hope to create a more tailored treatment algorithm for CUP patients.

SUMMARY

Patients with CUP should undergo a directed diagnostic search for the primary tumor on the basis of clinical and pathologic data. Subsets of patients have prognostically favorable disease, as defined by clinical or histologic criteria, and may substantially benefit from aggressive treatment and expect prolonged survival. However, for most patients who present with advanced CUP, the prognosis remains poor, with early resistance to available cytotoxic therapy. The current focus has shifted away from empirical chemotherapeutic trials to understanding the metastatic phenotype, ToO profiling, and evaluating molecular targets in CUP patients. Our understanding of this challenging disease is growing steadily in the era of sophisticated diagnostics and therapeutics. A strategy that integrates information from a patient's clinical presentation including imaging and pathology with directed immunohistochemistry and molecular profiling in selected cases will help us select the best treatment for our patients.

SECTION X

ENDOCRINE NEOPLASIA

CHAPTER 48

THYROID CANCER

J. Larry Jameson ■ Anthony P. Weetman

APPROACH TO THE PATIENT A Thyroid Nodule

Palpable thyroid nodules are found in about 5% of adults, but the prevalence varies considerably worldwide. Given this high prevalence rate, practitioners commonly identify thyroid nodules. The main goal of this evaluation is to identify, in a cost-effective manner, the small subgroup of individuals with malignant lesions.

Nodules are more common in iodine-deficient areas, in women, and with aging. Most palpable nodules are >1 cm in diameter, but the ability to feel a nodule is influenced by its location within the gland (superficial versus deeply embedded), the anatomy of the patient's neck, and the experience of the examiner. More sensitive methods of detection, such as computed tomography (CT), thyroid ultrasound, and pathologic studies, reveal thyroid nodules in >20% of glands. The presence of these thyroid incidentalomas has led to much debate about how to detect nodules and which nodules to investigate further. Most authorities still rely on physical examination to detect thyroid nodules, reserving ultrasound for monitoring nodule size or as an aid in thyroid biopsy.

An approach to the evaluation of a solitary nodule is outlined in Fig. 48-1. Most patients with thyroid nodules have normal thyroid function tests. Nonetheless, thyroid function should be assessed by measuring a

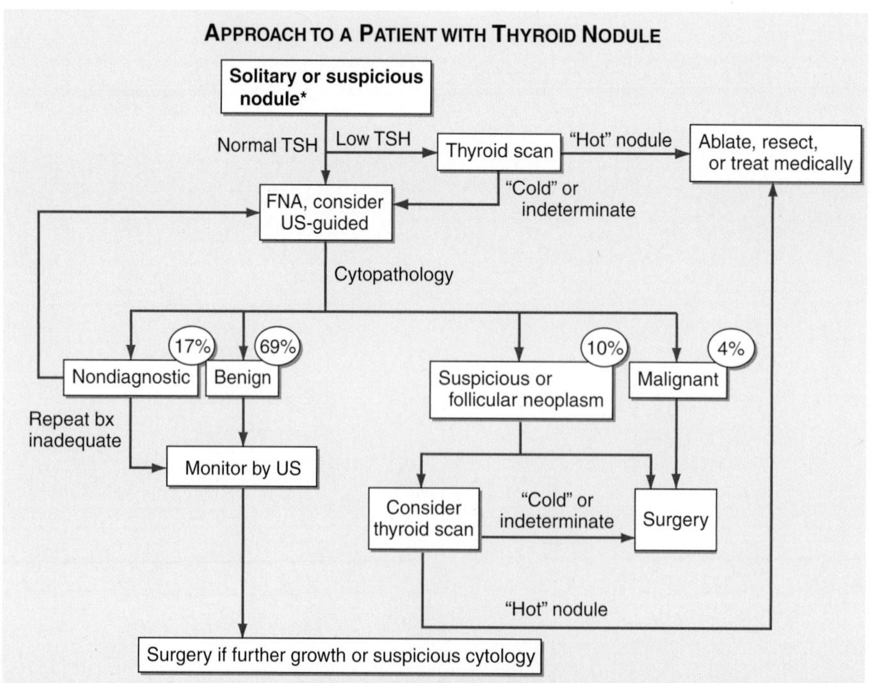

FIGURE 48-1
Approach to the patient with a thyroid nodule. See text and references for details. *About one-third of nodules are cystic or mixed solid and cystic. FNA, fine-needle aspiration; TSH, thyroid-stimulating hormone; US, ultrasound.

thyroid-stimulating hormone (TSH) level, which may be suppressed by one or more autonomously functioning nodules. If the TSH is suppressed, a radionuclide scan is indicated to determine if the identified nodule is "hot," as lesions with increased uptake are almost never malignant and fine-needle aspiration (FNA) is unnecessary. Otherwise, FNA biopsy, ideally performed with ultrasound guidance, should be the first step in the evaluation of a thyroid nodule. FNA has good sensitivity and specificity when performed by physicians familiar with the procedure and when the results are interpreted by experienced cytopathologists. The technique is particularly useful for detecting papillary thyroid cancer (PTC). The distinction between benign and malignant follicular lesions is often not possible using cytology alone.

In several large studies, FNA biopsies yielded the following findings: 70% benign, 10% malignant or suspicious for malignancy, and 20% nondiagnostic or yielding insufficient material for diagnosis. Characteristic features of malignancy mandate surgery. A diagnosis of follicular neoplasm also warrants surgery, as benign and malignant lesions cannot be distinguished based on cytopathology or frozen section. The management of patients with benign lesions is more variable. Many authorities advocate TSH suppression, but others monitor nodule size without suppression. With either approach, thyroid nodule size should be monitored, ideally using ultrasound. Repeat FNA is indicated if a nodule enlarges, and a second biopsy should be performed within 2–5 years to confirm the benign status of the nodule.

BENIGN NEOPLASMS

The various types of benign thyroid nodules are listed in Table 48-1. These lesions are common (5–10% adults), particularly when assessed by sensitive techniques such as ultrasound. The risk of malignancy is very low for *macrofollicular adenomas* and *normofollicular adenomas*. *Microfollicular, trabecular, and Hürthle cell variants* raise greater concern, and the histology is more difficult to interpret. About one-third of palpable nodules are *thyroid cysts*. These may be recognized by their ultrasound appearance or based on aspiration of large amounts of pink or straw-colored fluid (colloid). Many are mixed cystic and solid lesions, in which case it is desirable to aspirate cellular components under ultrasound or harvest cells after cytospin of cyst fluid. Cysts frequently recur, even after repeated aspiration, and may require surgical excision if they are large or if the cytology is suspicious. Sclerosis has been used with variable success but is often painful and may be complicated by infiltration of the sclerosing agent.

The treatment approach for benign nodules is similar to that for multinodular goitermultinodular goiter

TABLE 48-1

CLASSIFICATION OF THYROID NEOPLASMS

BENIGN	
Follicular epithelial cell adenomas	
Macrofollicular (colloid)	
Normofollicular (simple)	
Microfollicular (fetal)	
Trabecular (embryonal)	
Hürthle cell variant (oncocytic)	
MALIGNANT	**APPROXIMATE PREVALENCE, %**
Follicular epithelial cell	
Well-differentiated carcinomas	
Papillary carcinomas	80–90
Pure papillary	
Follicular variant	
Diffuse sclerosing variant	
Tall cell, columnar cell variants	
Follicular carcinomas	5–10
Minimally invasive	
Widely invasive	
Hürthle cell carcinoma (oncocytic)	
Insular carcinoma	
Undifferentiated (anaplastic) carcinomas	
C cell (calcitonin-producing)	
Medullary thyroid cancer	<10
Sporadic	
Familial	
MEN 2	
Other malignancies	
Lymphomas	1–2
Sarcomas	
Metastases	
Others	

Abbreviation: MEN, multiple endocrine neoplasia.

(MNG). TSH suppression with levothyroxine decreases the size of about 30% of nodules and may prevent further growth. If a nodule has not decreased in size after 6–12 months of suppressive therapy, treatment should be discontinued because little benefit is likely to accrue from long-term treatment; the risk of iatrogenic subclinical thyrotoxicosis should also be considered.

THYROID CANCER

Thyroid carcinoma is the most common malignancy of the endocrine system. Malignant tumors derived from the follicular epithelium are classified according to histologic features. Differentiated tumors, such as PTC or follicular thyroid cancer (FTC), are often curable, and the prognosis is good for patients identified with early-stage disease. In contrast, anaplastic thyroid cancer (ATC) is aggressive, responds poorly to treatment, and is associated with a bleak prognosis.

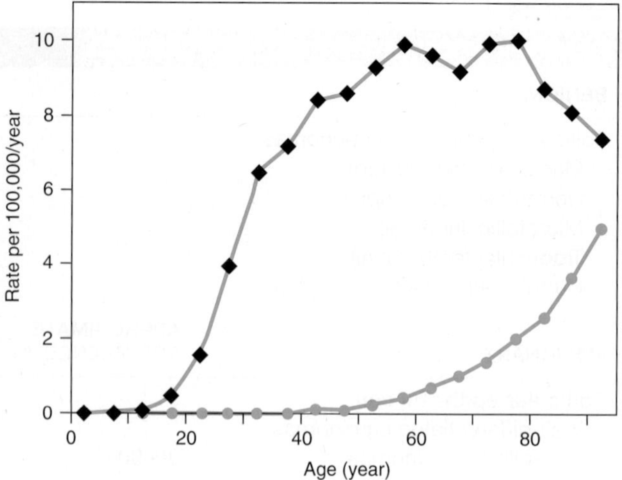

FIGURE 48-2
Age-associated incidence (—♦—) and mortality (—•—) rates for invasive thyroid cancer. (*Adapted from LAG Ries et al [eds]: SEER Cancer Statistics Review, 1973–1996, Bethesda, National Cancer Institute, 1999.*)

The incidence of thyroid cancer (~9/100,000 per year) increases with age, plateauing after about age 50 years (Fig. 48-2). Age is also an important prognostic factor—thyroid cancer at a young age (<20 years) or in older persons (>45 years) is associated with a worse prognosis. Thyroid cancer is twice as common in women as men, but male gender is associated with a worse prognosis. Additional important risk factors include a history of childhood head or neck irradiation, large nodule size (≥4 cm), evidence for local tumor fixation or invasion into lymph nodes, and the presence of metastases (Table 48-2). Several unique features of thyroid cancer facilitate its management: (1) thyroid nodules are readily palpable, allowing early detection and biopsy by FNA; (2) iodine radioisotopes can be used to diagnose (^{123}I) and treat (^{131}I) differentiated thyroid cancer, reflecting the unique uptake of this anion by the thyroid gland; and (3) serum markers allow the detection of residual or recurrent disease, including the use of thyroglobulin (Tg) levels for PTC and FTC and calcitonin for medullary thyroid cancer (MTC).

TABLE 48-2

RISK FACTORS FOR THYROID CARCINOMA IN PATIENTS WITH THYROID NODULE

History of head and neck irradiation age <20 or >45 years	Family history of thyroid cancer or MEN 2
Bilateral disease	Vocal cord paralysis, hoarse voice
Increased nodule size (>4 cm)	Nodule fixed to adjacent structures
New or enlarging neck mass	Extrathyroidal extension
Male gender	Suspected lymph node involvement Iodine deficiency (follicular cancer)

Abbreviation: MEN, multiple endocrine neoplasia.

CLASSIFICATION

Thyroid neoplasms can arise in each of the cell types that populate the gland, including thyroid follicular cells, calcitonin-producing C cells, lymphocytes, and stromal and vascular elements, as well as metastases from other sites (Table 48-1). The American Joint Committee on Cancer (AJCC) has designated a staging system using the TNM (tumor, node, metastasis) classification (Table 48-3). Several other classification and staging systems are also widely used, some of which place greater emphasis on histologic features or risk factors such as age or gender.

PATHOGENESIS AND GENETIC BASIS

RADIATION

Early studies of the pathogenesis of thyroid cancer focused on the role of external radiation, which predisposes to chromosomal breaks, leading to genetic rearrangements and loss of tumor-suppressor genes. External radiation of the mediastinum, face, head, and neck region was administered in the past to treat an array of conditions, including acne and enlargement of

TABLE 48-3

THYROID CANCER CLASSIFICATION[a]

Papillary or Follicular Thyroid Cancers		
	<45 years	>45 years
Stage I	Any T, any N, M0	T1, N0, M0
Stage II	Any T, any N, M1	T2 or T3, N0, M0
Stage III	—	T4, N0, M0 Any T, N1, M0
Stage IV	—	Any T, any N, M1
Anaplastic Thyroid Cancer		
Stage IV	All cases are stage IV	
Medullary Thyroid Cancer		
Stage I	T1, N0, M0	
Stage II	T2–T4, N0, M0	
Stage III	Any T, N1, M0	
Stage IV	Any T, any N, M1	

[a]Criteria include: T, the size and extent of the primary tumor (T1 ≤ 1 cm; 1 cm <T2 ≤ 4 cm; T3 >4 cm; T4 direct invasion through the thyroid capsule); N, the absence (N0) or presence (N1) of regional node involvement; M, the absence (M0) or presence (M1) of metastases.
Source: American Joint Committee on Cancer staging system for thyroid cancers using the TNM classification.

the thymus, tonsils, and adenoids. Radiation exposure increases the risk of benign and malignant thyroid nodules, is associated with multicentric cancers, and shifts the incidence of thyroid cancer to an earlier age group. Radiation from nuclear fallout also increases the risk of thyroid cancer. Children seem more predisposed to the effects of radiation than adults. Of note, radiation derived from ^{131}I therapy appears to contribute minimal increased risk of thyroid cancer.

THYROID-STIMULATING HORMONE AND GROWTH FACTORS

Many differentiated thyroid cancers express TSH receptors and, therefore, remain responsive to TSH. This observation provides the rationale for levothyroxine (T_4) suppression of TSH in patients with thyroid cancer. Residual expression of TSH receptors also allows TSH-stimulated uptake of ^{131}I therapy (see later discussion).

ONCOGENES AND TUMOR-SUPPRESSOR GENES

Thyroid cancers are monoclonal in origin, consistent with the idea that they originate as a consequence of mutations that confer a growth advantage to a single cell. In addition to increased rates of proliferation, some thyroid cancers exhibit impaired apoptosis and features that enhance invasion, angiogenesis, and metastasis. Thyroid neoplasms have been analyzed for a variety of genetic alterations but without clear evidence of an ordered acquisition of somatic mutations as they progress from the benign to the malignant state. On the other hand, certain mutations are relatively specific for thyroid neoplasia, some of which correlate with histologic classification (Table 48-4).

As described earlier, activating mutations of the TSH-R and the $G_{S\alpha}$ subunit are associated with autonomously functioning nodules. Though these mutations induce thyroid cell growth, this type of nodule is almost always benign.

Activation of the RET-RAS-BRAF signaling pathway is seen in most PTCs, though the types of mutations are heterogeneous. A variety of rearrangements involving the *RET* gene on chromosome 10 brings this receptor tyrosine kinase under the control of other promoters, leading to receptor overexpression. *RET* rearrangements occur in 20–40% of PTCs in different series and were observed with increased frequency in tumors developing after the Chernobyl radiation accident. Rearrangements in PTC have also been observed for another tyrosine kinase gene, *TRK1*, which is located on chromosome 1. To date, the identification of PTC with *RET* or *TRK1* rearrangements has not proven useful for predicting prognosis or treatment responses. *BRAF* mutations appear to be the most common genetic alteration in PTC. These mutations activate the kinase, which stimulates the mitogen-activated protein MAP kinase (MAPK) cascade. *RAS* mutations, which also stimulate the MAPK cascade, are found in about 20–30% of thyroid neoplasms, including both PTC and FTC. Of note, simultaneous *RET, BRAF,* and *RAS* mutations do not occur in the same tumor, suggesting that activation of the MAPK cascade is critical for tumor development, independent of the step that initiates the cascade.

RAS mutations also occur in FTCs. In addition, a rearrangement of the thyroid developmental transcription factor PAX8 with the nuclear receptor PPARγ is identified in a significant fraction of FTCs. Loss of heterozygosity of 3p or 11q, consistent with deletions of tumor-suppressor genes, is also common in FTCs.

Most of the mutations seen in differentiated thyroid cancers have also been detected in ATCs. *BRAF* mutations are seen in up to 50% of ATCs. Mutations in CTNNB1, which encodes β-catenin, occur in about two-thirds of ATCs, but not in PTC or FTC. Mutations of the tumor suppressor p53 also play an important role in the development of ATC. Because p53 plays a role in cell cycle surveillance, DNA repair, and apoptosis, its loss may contribute to the rapid acquisition of genetic instability as well as poor treatment responses (Chap. 25) (Table 48-4).

The role of molecular diagnostics in the clinical management of thyroid cancer is under investigation. In principle, analyses of specific mutations might aid in classification, prognosis, or choice of treatment. However, there is no clear evidence to date that this information alters clinical decision making.

MTC, when associated with multiple endocrine neoplasia (MEN) type 2, harbors an inherited mutation of the *RET* gene. Unlike the rearrangements of *RET* seen in PTC, the mutations in MEN2 are point mutations that induce constitutive activity of the tyrosine kinase (Chap. 50). MTC is preceded by hyperplasia of the C cells, raising the likelihood that as-yet-unidentified "second hits" lead to cellular transformation. A subset of sporadic MTC contain somatic mutations that activate *RET*.

WELL-DIFFERENTIATED THYROID CANCER

PAPILLARY

PTC is the most common type of thyroid cancer, accounting for 70–90% of well-differentiated thyroid malignancies. Microscopic PTC is present in up to 25% of thyroid glands at autopsy, but most of these lesions are very small (several millimeters) and are not clinically significant. Characteristic cytologic features of PTC help make the diagnosis by FNA or after surgical

TABLE 48-4

GENETIC ALTERATIONS IN THYROID NEOPLASIA

GENE/PROTEIN	TYPE OF GENE	CHROMOSOMAL LOCATION	GENETIC ABNORMALITY	TUMOR
TSH receptor	GPCR receptor	14q31	Point mutations	Toxic adenoma, differentiated carcinomas
$G_{S\alpha}$	G protein	20q13.2	Point mutations	Toxic adenoma, differentiated carcinomas
RET/PTC	Receptor tyrosine kinase	10q11.2	Rearrangements PTC1: (inv(10) q11.2q21) PTC2: (t(10;17) (q11.2;q23)) PTC3: ELE1/TK	PTC
RET	Receptor tyrosine kinase	10q11.2	Point mutations	MEN 2, medullary thyroid cancer
BRAF	MEK kinase	7q24	Point mutations, rearrangements	PTC, ATC
TRK	Receptor tyrosine kinase	1q23-24	Rearrangements	Multinodular goiter, papillary thyroid cancer
RAS	Signal transducing p21	Hras 11p15.5Kras12p12.1; Nras 1p13.2	Point mutations	Differentiated thyroid carcinoma, adenomas
p53	Tumor suppressor, cell cycle control, apoptosis	17p13	Point mutations Deletion, insertion	Anaplastic cancer
APC	Tumor suppressor, adenomatous polyposis coli gene	5q21-q22	Point mutations	Anaplastic cancer, also associated with familial polyposis coli
p16 (MTS1, CDKN2A)	Tumor suppressor, cell cycle control	9p21	Deletions	Differentiated carcinomas
p21/WAF	Tumor suppressor, cell cycle control	6p21.2	Overexpression	Anaplastic cancer
MET	Receptor tyrosine kinase	7q31	Overexpression	Follicular thyroid cancer
c-MYC	Receptor tyrosine kinase	8q24.12.-13	Overexpression	Differentiated carcinoma
PTEN	Phosphatase	10q23	Point mutations	PTC in Cowden's syndrome(multiple hamartomas breast tumors, gastrointestinal polyps, thyroid tumors)
CTNNB1	β-Catenin	3p22	Point mutations	Anaplastic cancer
Loss of heterozygosity (LOH)	?Tumor suppressors	3p; 11q13, other loci	Deletions	Differentiated thyroid carcinomas, anaplastic cancer
PAX8-PPARγ 1	Transcription factor Nuclear receptor fusion	t(2;3)(q13;p25)	Translocation	Follicular adenoma or carcinoma

Abbreviations: APC, adenomatous polyposis coli; BRAF, v-raf homologue, B1; CDKN2A, cyclin-dependent kinase inhibitor 2A; c-MYC, cellular homologue of myelocytomatosis virus proto-oncogene; ELE1/TK, RET-activating gene ele1/tyrosine kinase; GPCR, G protein–coupled receptor; $G_{S\alpha}$, G-protein stimulating α-subunit; MEK, mitogen extracellular signal-regulated kinase; MEN 2, multiple endocrine neoplasia-2; MET, met proto-oncogene (hepatocyte growth factor receptor); MTS, multiple tumor suppressor; P21, p21 tumor suppressor; p53, p53 tumor suppressor gene; PAX8, paired domain transcription factor; PPARγ1, peroxisome-proliferator activated receptorγ1; PTC, papillary thyroid cancer; PTEN, phosphatase and tensin homologue; RAS, rat sarcoma proto-oncogene; RET, rearranged during transfection proto-oncogene; TRK, tyrosine kinase receptor; TSH, thyroid-stimulating hormone; WAF, wild-type p53 activated fragment.

Source: Adapted with permission from P Kopp, JL Jameson, in JL Jameson (ed): *Principles of Molecular Medicine*. Totowa, NJ, Humana Press, 1998.

resection; these include psammoma bodies, cleaved nuclei with an "orphan-Annie" appearance caused by large nucleoli, and the formation of papillary structures.

PTC tends to be multifocal and to invade locally within the thyroid gland as well as through the thyroid capsule and into adjacent structures in the neck. It has a propensity to spread via the lymphatic system but can metastasize hematogenously as well, particularly to bone and lung. Because of the relatively slow growth of the tumor, a significant burden of pulmonary metastases may accumulate, sometimes with remarkably few symptoms. The prognostic implication of lymph node spread is debated. Lymph node involvement by thyroid cancer can be well tolerated but appears to increase the risk of recurrence and mortality, particularly in older patients. The staging of PTC by the TNM system is outlined in Table 48-3. Most papillary cancers are identified in the early stages (>80% stages I or II) and have an excellent prognosis, with survival curves similar to expected survival (Fig. 48-3*A*). Mortality is markedly increased in stage IV disease (distant metastases), but this group comprises only about 1% of patients. The treatment of PTC is described later.

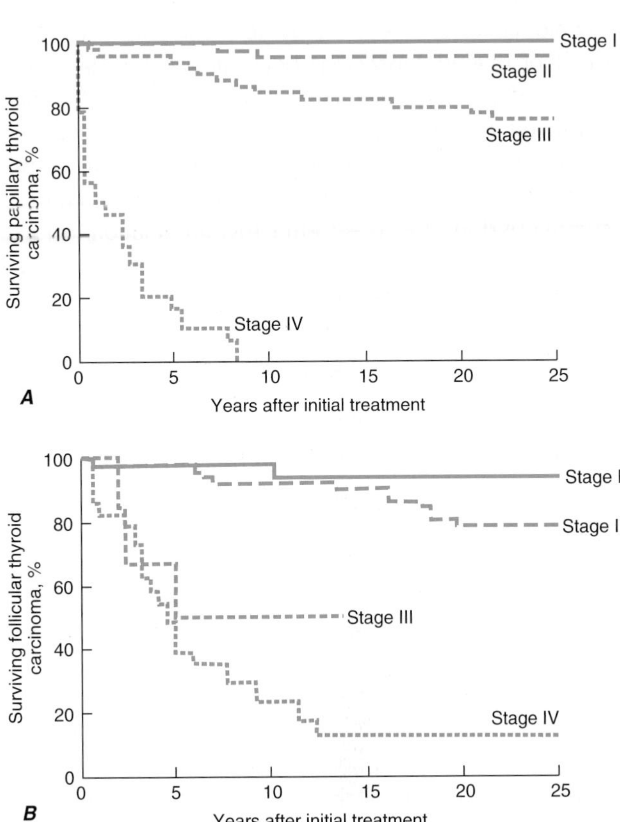

FIGURE 48-3

Survival rates in patients with differentiated thyroid cancer. ***A***. Papillary cancer, cohort of 1851 patients. I, 1107 (60%); II, 408 (22%); III, 312 (17%); IV, 24 (1%); *n* = 1185. ***B***. Follicular cancer, cohort of 153 patients. I, 42 (27%); II, 82 (54%); III, 6 (4%); IV, 23 (15%); *n* = 153. (*Adapted from PR Larsen et al: William's Textbook of Endocrinology, 9th ed, JD Wilson et al [eds]: Philadelphia, Saunders, 1998, pp 389–575, with permission.*)

FOLLICULAR

The incidence of FTC varies widely in different parts of the world; it is more common in iodine-deficient regions. FTC is difficult to diagnose by FNA because the distinction between benign and malignant follicular neoplasms rests largely on evidence of invasion into vessels, nerves, or adjacent structures. FTC tends to spread by hematogenous routes leading to bone, lung, and central nervous system metastases. Mortality rates associated with FTC are less favorable than for PTC, in part because a larger proportion of patients present with stage IV disease (Fig. 48-3*B*). Poor prognostic features include distant metastases, age >50 years, primary tumor size >4 cm, Hürthle cell histology, and the presence of marked vascular invasion.

TREATMENT Well-Differentiated Thyroid Cancer

SURGERY All well-differentiated thyroid cancers should be surgically excised. In addition to removing the primary lesion, surgery allows accurate histologic diagnosis and staging, and multicentric disease is commonly found in the contralateral thyroid lobe. Lymph node spread can also be assessed at the time of surgery, and involved nodes can be removed. Recommendations about the extent of surgery vary for stage I disease, as survival rates are similar for lobectomy and near-total thyroidectomy. Lobectomy is associated with a lower incidence of hypoparathyroidism and injury to the recurrent laryngeal nerves. However, it is not possible to monitor Tg levels or to perform whole-body ^{131}I scans in the presence of the residual lobe. Moreover, if final staging or subsequent follow-up indicates the need for radioiodine scanning or treatment, repeat surgery is necessary to remove the remaining thyroid tissue. Therefore, near-total thyroidectomy is preferable in almost all patients; complication rates are acceptably low if the surgeon is highly experienced in the procedure. Postsurgical radioablation of the remnant thyroid tissue is increasingly being used because it may destroy remaining or multifocal thyroid carcinoma, and it facilitates the use of Tg determinations and radioiodine scanning for long-term follow-up by eliminating residual normal or neoplastic tissue.

TSH SUPPRESSION THERAPY As most tumors are still TSH-responsive, levothyroxine suppression of TSH is a mainstay of thyroid cancer treatment. Though TSH suppression clearly provides therapeutic benefit, there are no prospective studies that identify the optimal level of TSH suppression. A reasonable goal is to suppress TSH as much as possible without subjecting the patient to unnecessary side effects from excess thyroid hormone, such as atrial fibrillation, osteopenia, anxiety, and other manifestations of thyrotoxicosis. For patients at low risk of recurrence, TSH should be suppressed into the low but detectable range (0.1–0.5 mIU/L). For patients at high risk of recurrence or with known metastatic disease, complete TSH suppression is indicated if there are no strong contraindications to mild thyrotoxicosis. In this instance, unbound T_4 must also be monitored to avoid excessive treatment.

RADIOIODINE TREATMENT Well-differentiated thyroid cancer still incorporates radioiodine, though less efficiently than normal thyroid follicular cells. Radioiodine uptake is determined primarily by expression of the sodium iodide symporter (NIS) and is stimulated by TSH, requiring expression of the TSH-R. The retention time for radioactivity is influenced by the extent to which the tumor retains differentiated functions such as iodide trapping and organification. After near-total thyroidectomy, substantial thyroid tissue often remains, particularly in the thyroid bed and surrounding the parathyroid glands. Consequently, ^{131}I ablation is necessary to eliminate remaining normal thyroid tissue and to treat residual tumor cells.

Indications The use of therapeutic doses of radioiodine remains an area of controversy in thyroid cancer management. However, postoperative thyroid ablation and radioiodine treatment of known residual PTC or FTC clearly reduces recurrence rates but has a smaller impact on mortality, particularly in patients at relatively low risk. This low-risk group includes most patients with stage 1 PTC with primary tumors <1.5 cm in size. For patients with larger papillary tumors, spread to the adjacent lymph nodes, FTC, or evidence of metastases, thyroid ablation and radioiodine treatment are generally indicated.

^{131}I Thyroid Ablation and Treatment As noted earlier, the decision to use ^{131}I for thyroid ablation should be coordinated with the surgical approach, as radioablation is much more effective when there is minimal remaining normal thyroid tissue. A typical strategy is to treat the patient for several weeks postoperatively with liothyronine (25 μg bid or tid), followed by thyroid hormone withdrawal. Ideally, the TSH level should increase to >50 mU/L over 3–4 weeks. The level to which TSH rises is dictated largely by the amount of normal thyroid tissue remaining postoperatively. Recombinant human TSH (rhTSH) has also been used to enhance ^{131}I uptake for postsurgical ablation. It appears to be at least as effective as thyroid hormone withdrawal and should be particularly useful as residual thyroid tissue prevents an adequate endogenous TSH rise.

A pretreatment scanning dose of ^{131}I (usually 111–185 MBq [3–5 mCi]) can reveal the amount of residual tissue and provides guidance about the dose needed to accomplish ablation. However, because of concerns about radioactive "stunning" that impairs subsequent treatment, there is a trend to avoid pretreatment scanning and to proceed directly to ablation, unless there is suspicion that the amount of residual tissue will alter therapy. A maximum outpatient ^{131}I dose is 1110 MBq (29.9 mCi) in the United States, though ablation is often more complete using greater doses (1850–3700 MBq [50–100 mCi]). Patients should be placed on a low-iodine diet (<50 μg/d urinary iodine) to increase radioiodine uptake. In patients with known residual cancer, the larger doses ensure thyroid ablation and may destroy remaining tumor cells. A whole-body scan following the high-dose radioiodine treatment is useful to identify possible metastatic disease.

Follow-Up Whole-Body Thyroid Scanning and Thyroglobulin Determinations An initial whole-body scan should be performed about 6 months after thyroid ablation. The strategy for follow-up management of thyroid cancer has been altered by the availability of rhTSH to stimulate ^{131}I uptake and by the improved sensitivity of Tg assays to detect residual or recurrent disease. A scheme for using either rhTSH or thyroid hormone withdrawal for thyroid scanning is summarized in Fig. 48-4. After thyroid ablation, rhTSH can be used in follow-up to stimulate Tg and ^{131}I uptake without subjecting patients to thyroid hormone withdrawal and its associated symptoms of hypothyroidism as well as the risk of tumor growth after prolonged TSH stimulation. Alternatively, in patients who are likely to require ^{131}I treatment, the traditional approach of thyroid hormone withdrawal can be used to increase TSH. This involves switching patients from T_4 to the more rapidly cleared hormone liothyronine (T_3), thereby allowing TSH to increase more quickly. Because TSH stimulates Tg levels, Tg measurements should be obtained after administration of rhTSH or when TSH levels have risen after thyroid hormone withdrawal.

In low-risk patients who have no clinical evidence of residual disease after ablation and a basal Tg <1 ng/mL, increasing evidence supports the use of rhTSH-stimulated Tg levels 1 year after ablation, without the need for radioiodine scanning. If stimulated Tg levels are low (<2 ng/ml) and, ideally, undetectable, these patients can be managed with suppressive therapy and measurements of unstimulated Tg every 6–12 months. The absence of Tg antibodies should be confirmed in these patients. On the other hand, patients with residual disease on whole-body scanning or those with elevated Tg levels require additional ^{131}I therapy. In addition, most authorities advocate radioiodine treatment for scan-negative, Tg-positive (Tg >5–10 ng/mL)

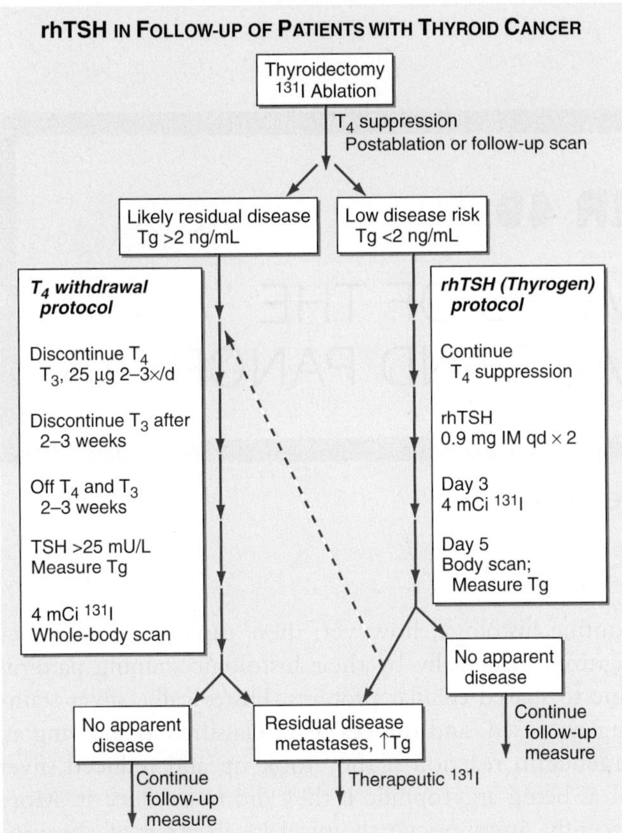

FIGURE 48-4

Use of recombinant human thyroid-stimulating hormone (TSH) in the follow-up of patients with thyroid cancer. rhTSH, recombinant human TSH; Tg, thyroglobulin; T_3, liothyronine; T_4, levothyroxine.

patients, as many derive therapeutic benefit from a large dose of ^{131}I.

In addition to radioiodine, external-beam radiotherapy is also used to treat specific metastatic lesions, particularly when they cause bone pain or threaten neurologic injury (e.g., vertebral metastases).

New Potential Therapies Kinase inhibitors are being explored as a means to target pathways known to be active in thyroid cancer, including the Ras, BRAF, epidermal growth factor receptor, vascular endothelial growth receptor, and angiogenesis pathways. Partial responses have been seen in small trials using motesaniv, sorafenib, and other agents, but the efficacy of these agents awaits larger studies.

ANAPLASTIC AND OTHER FORMS OF THYROID CANCER

ANAPLASTIC THYROID CANCER

As noted earlier, ATC is a poorly differentiated and aggressive cancer. The prognosis is poor, and most patients die within 6 months of diagnosis. Because of the undifferentiated state of these tumors, the uptake of radioiodine is usually negligible, but it can be used therapeutically if there is residual uptake. Chemotherapy has been attempted with multiple agents, including anthracyclines and paclitaxel, but it is usually ineffective. External-beam radiation therapy can be attempted and continued if tumors are responsive.

THYROID LYMPHOMA

Lymphoma in the thyroid gland often arises in the background of Hashimoto's thyroiditis. A rapidly expanding thyroid mass suggests the possibility of this diagnosis. Diffuse large-cell lymphoma is the most common type in the thyroid. Biopsies reveal sheets of lymphoid cells that can be difficult to distinguish from small cell lung cancer or ATC. These tumors are often highly sensitive to external radiation. Surgical resection should be avoided as initial therapy because it may spread disease that is otherwise localized to the thyroid. If staging indicates disease outside of the thyroid, treatment should follow guidelines used for other forms of lymphoma (Chap. 15).

MEDULLARY THYROID CARCINOMA

MTC can be sporadic or familial and accounts for about 5% of thyroid cancers. There are three familial forms of MTC: MEN 2A, MEN 2B, and familial MTC without other features of MEN (Chap. 50). In general, MTC is more aggressive in MEN 2B than in MEN 2A, and familial MTC is more aggressive than sporadic MTC. Elevated serum calcitonin provides a marker of residual or recurrent disease. It is reasonable to test all patients with MTC for *RET* mutations, as genetic counseling and testing of family members can be offered to those individuals who test positive for mutations.

The management of MTC is primarily surgical. Unlike tumors derived from thyroid follicular cells, these tumors do not take up radioiodine. External radiation treatment and chemotherapy may provide palliation in patients with advanced disease (Chap. 50).

CHAPTER 49

ENDOCRINE TUMORS OF THE GASTROINTESTINAL TRACT AND PANCREAS

Robert T. Jensen

GENERAL FEATURES OF GASTROINTESTINAL NEUROENDOCRINE TUMORS

Gastrointestinal (GI) neuroendocrine tumors (NETs) are tumors derived from the diffuse neuroendocrine system of the GI tract; that system is composed of amine- and acid-producing cells with different hormonal profiles, depending on the site of origin. The tumors historically are divided into carcinoid tumors and pancreatic endocrine tumors (PETs), although recent pathologic classifications have proposed that they all be classified as gastrointestinal NETs. In this chapter, the term *carcinoid tumor* is retained because it is widely used. These tumors originally were classified as APUDomas (for *a*mine *p*recursor *u*ptake and *d*ecarboxylation), as were pheochromocytomas, melanomas, and medullary thyroid carcinomas because they share certain cytochemical features as well as various pathologic, biologic, and molecular features (Table 49-1). It was originally proposed that APUDomas had a similar embryonic origin from neural crest cells, but it is now known the peptide-secreting cells are not of neuroectodermal origin. Nevertheless, the concept of APUDomas is useful because the tumors from the cells have important similarities as well as some differences (Table 49-1). In this section, the areas of similarity between PETs and carcinoids will be discussed together and areas in which there are important differences will be discussed separately.

CLASSIFICATION, PATHOLOGY, TUMOR BIOLOGY OF NEUROENDOCRINE TUMORS

NETs generally are composed of monotonous sheets of small round cells with uniform nuclei, and mitoses are uncommon. They can be identified tentatively on routine histology; however, these tumors are now recognized principally by their histologic staining patterns due to shared cellular proteins. Historically, silver staining was used, and tumors were classified as showing an argentaffin reaction if they took up and reduced silver or as being argyrophilic if they did not reduce it. More recently, immunocytochemical localization of chromogranins (A, B, C), neuron-specific enolase, and synaptophysin, which are all neuroendocrine cell markers, is used (Table 49-1). Chromogranin A is currently the most widely used.

Ultrastructurally, these tumors possess electron-dense neurosecretory granules and frequently contain small clear vesicles that correspond to synaptic vesicles of neurons. NETs synthesize numerous peptides, growth factors, and bioactive amines that may be ectopically secreted, giving rise to a specific clinical syndrome (Table 49-2). The diagnosis of the specific syndrome requires the clinical features of the disease (Table 49-2) and cannot be made from the immunocytochemistry results alone. The presence or absence of a specific clinical syndrome also cannot be predicted from the immunocytochemistry alone (Table 49-1). Furthermore, pathologists cannot distinguish between benign and malignant NETs unless metastases or invasion is present.

Carcinoid tumors frequently are classified according to their anatomic area of origin (i.e., foregut, midgut, hindgut) because tumors with similar areas of origin share functional manifestations, histochemistry, and secretory products (Table 49-3). Foregut tumors generally have a low serotonin (5-HT) content; are argentaffin-negative but argyrophilic; occasionally secrete adrenocorticotropic hormone (ACTH) or 5-hydroxytryptophan (5-HTP), causing an atypical carcinoid syndrome (Fig. 49-1); are often multihormonal; and may metastasize to bone. They uncommonly produce a clinical syndrome due to the secreted

TABLE 49-1

GENERAL CHARACTERISTICS OF GASTROINTESTINAL NEUROENDOCRINE TUMORS (CARCINOIDS, PANCREATIC ENDOCRINE TUMORS)

A. Share general neuroendocrine cell markers (identification used for diagnosis)
   1. Chromogranins (A, B, C) are acidic monomeric soluble proteins found in the large secretory granules. Chromogranin A is the most widely used.
   2. Neuron-specific enolase (NSE) is the γ-γ dimer of the enzyme enolase and is a cytosolic marker of neuroendocrine differentiation.
   3. Synaptophysin is an integral membrane glycoprotein of 38,000 molecular weight found in small vesicles of neurons and neuroendocrine tumors.

B. Pathologic similarities
   1. All are APUDomas showing *a*mine *p*recursor *u*ptake and *d*ecarboxylation.
   2. Ultrastructurally, they have dense-core secretory granules (>80 nm).
   3. Histologically, generally appear similar with few mitoses and uniform nuclei.
   4. Frequently synthesize multiple peptides or amines, which can be detected immunocytochemically but may not be secreted.
   5. Presence or absence of clinical syndrome or type cannot be predicted by immunocytochemical studies.
   6. Histologic classifications increasingly predictive of biologic behavior. Only invasion or metastases establish malignancy

C. Similarities of biologic behavior
   1. Generally slow growing, but a proportion are aggressive.
   2. Secrete biologically active peptides or amines, which can cause clinical symptoms.
   3. Generally have high densities of somatostatin receptors, which are used for both localization and treatment.

D. Similarities and differences in molecular abnormalities
   1. Similarities
      a. Uncommon—alterations in common oncogenes (*ras, jun, fos,* etc).
      b. Uncommon—alterations in common tumor-suppressor genes (p53, retinoblastoma).
      c. Alterations at MEN 1 locus (11q13) and p16^{INK4a} (9p21) occur in a proportion (10–45%).
      d. Methylation of various genes occurs in 40–87% (*ras*-associated domain family I, p14, p16, O^6 methyl guanosine methyltransferases, retinoic acid receptor β)
   2. Differences
      a. PETs—loss of 1p (21%), 3p (8–47%), 3q (8–41%), 11q (21–62%), 6q (18–68%). Gains at 17q (10–55%), 7q (16–68%), 4q (33%).
      b. Carcinoids—loss of 18q (38–67%) >18p (33–43%) > 9p, 16q21(21–23%). Gains at 17q, 19p (57%), 4q (33%), 14q (20%).

Abbreviation: MEN 1, multiple endocrine neoplasia type 1; PET, pancreatic endocrine tumor.

TABLE 49-2

GASTROINTESTINAL NEUROENDOCRINE TUMOR SYNDROME

NAME	BIOLOGICALLY ACTIVE PEPTIDE(S) SECRETED	INCIDENCE (NEW CASES/10^6 POPULATION/ YEAR)	TUMOR LOCATION	MALIGNANT, %	ASSOCIATED WITH MEN 1, %	MAIN SYMPTOMS AND SIGNS
I. Established Specific Functional Syndrome						
A. Carcinoid tumor						
Carcinoid syndrome	Serotonin, possibly tachykinins, motilin, prostaglandins	0.5–2	Midgut (75–87%) Foregut (2–33%) Hindgut (1–8%) Unknown (2–15%)	95–100	Rare	Diarrhea (32–84%) Flushing (63–75%) Pain (10–34%) Asthma (4–18%) Heart disease (11–41%)

(*continued*)

TABLE 49-2

GASTROINTESTINAL NEUROENDOCRINE TUMOR SYNDROME (*CONTINUED*)

NAME	BIOLOGICALLY ACTIVE PEPTIDE(S) SECRETED	INCIDENCE (NEW CASES/10^6 POPULATION/ YEAR)	TUMOR LOCATION	MALIGNANT, %	ASSOCIATED WITH MEN 1, %	MAIN SYMPTOMS AND SIGNS
B. Pancreatic endocrine tumor						
Zollinger-Ellison syndrome	Gastrin	0.5–1.5	Duodenum (70%) Pancreas (25%) Other sites (5%)	60–90	20–25	Pain (79–100%) Diarrhea (30–75%) Esophageal symptoms (31–56%)
Insulinoma	Insulin	1–2	Pancreas (>99%)	<10	4–5	Hypoglycemic symptoms (100%)
VIPoma (Verner-Morrison syndrome, pancreatic cholera, WDHA)	Vasoactive intestinal peptide	0.05–0.2	Pancreas (90%, adult) Other (10%, neural,adrenal, periganglionic)	40–70	6	Diarrhea (90–100%) Hypokalemia (80–100%) Dehydration (83%)
Glucagonoma	Glucagon	0.01–0.1	Pancreas (100%)	50–80	1–20	Rash (67–90%) Glucose intolerance (38–87%) Weight loss (66–96%)
Somatostatinoma	Somatostatin	Rare	Pancreas (55%) Duodenum/ jejunum (44%)	>70	45	Diabetes mellitus (63–90%) Cholelithiases (65–90%) Diarrhea (35–90%)
GRFoma	Growth hormone–releasing hormone	Unknown	Pancreas (30%) Lung (54%) Jejunum (7%) Other (13%)	>60	16	Acromegaly (100%)
ACTHoma	ACTH	Rare	Pancreas (4–16% all ectopic Cushing's)	>95	Rare	Cushing's syndrome (100%)
PET causing carcinoid syndrome	Serotonin, ?tachykinins	Rare (43 cases)	Pancreas (<1% all carcinoids)	60–88	Rare	Same as carcinoid syndrome above
PET causing hypercalcemia	PTHrP Others unknown	Rare	Pancreas (rare cause of hypercalcemia)	84	Rare	Abdominal pain due to hepatic metastases
II. Possible Specific Functional Syndrome						
PET secreting calcitonin	Calcitonin	Rare	Pancreas (rare cause of hypercalcitonemia)	>80	16	Diarrhea (50%)
PET secreting renin	Renin	Rare	Pancreas	Unknown	No	Hypertension
PET secreting luteinizing hormone	Luteinizing hormone	Rare	Pancreas	Unknown	No	Anovulation, virilization (female); reduced libido (male)
PET secreting erythropoietin	Erythropoietin	Rare	Pancreas	100	No	Polycythemia
PET secreting IF-II	Insulin-like growth growth factor II	Rare	Pancreas	Unknown	No	Hypoglycemia

(*continued*)

TABLE 49-2

GASTROINTESTINAL NEUROENDOCRINE TUMOR SYNDROME (*CONTINUED*)

NAME	BIOLOGICALLY ACTIVE PEPTIDE(S) SECRETED	INCIDENCE (NEW CASES/10^6 POPULATION/ YEAR)	TUMOR LOCATION	MALIGNANT, %	ASSOCIATED WITH MEN 1, %	MAIN SYMPTOMS AND SIGNS
III. No Functional Syndrome						
PPoma/ nonfunctional	None	1–2	Pancreas (100%)	>60	18–44	Weight loss (30–90%) Abdominal mass (10–30%) Pain (30–95%)

Abbreviations: ACTH, adrenocorticotropic hormone; GRFoma, growth hormone-releasing factor secreting pancreatic endocrine tumor; IF-II, insulin-like growth factor 2; MEN, multiple endocrine neoplasia; PET, pancreatic endocrine tumor; PPoma, tumor secreting pancreatic polypeptide; PTHrP, parathyroid hormone–related peptide; VIPoma, tumor secreting vasoactive intestinal peptide; WDHA, watery diarrhea, hypokalemia, and achlorhydria syndrome.

products. Midgut carcinoids are argentaffin-positive, have a high serotonin content, most frequently cause the typical carcinoid syndrome when they metastasize (Table 49-3 and Fig. 49-1), release serotonin and tachykinins (substance P, neuropeptide K, substance K), rarely secrete 5-HTP or ACTH, and less commonly metastasize to bone. Hindgut carcinoids (rectum, transverse and descending colon) are argentaffin-negative, are often argyrophilic, rarely contain serotonin or cause the carcinoid syndrome (Fig. 49-1 and Table 49-3),

TABLE 49-3

CARCINOID TUMOR LOCATION, FREQUENCY OF METASTASES, AND ASSOCIATION WITH THE CARCINOID SYNDROME

	LOCATION (% OF TOTAL)	INCIDENCE OF METASTASES	INCIDENCE OF CARCINOID SYNDROME
Foregut			
Esophagus	<0.1	—	—
Stomach	4.6	10	9.5
Duodenum	2.0	—	3.4
Pancreas	0.7	71.9	20
Gallbladder	0.3	17.8	5
Bronchus, lung, trachea	27.9	5.7	13
Midgut			
Jejunum	1.8	{58.4	9
Ileum	14.9		9
Meckel's diverticulum	0.5	—	13
Appendix	4.8	38.8	<1
Colon	8.6	51	5
Liver	0.4	32.	—
Ovary	1.0	2 32	50
Testis	<0.1	—	50
Hindgut			
Rectum	13.6	3.9	—

Source: Location is from the PAN-SEER data (1973–1999), and incidence of metastases from the SEER data (1992–1999), reported by IM Modlin et al: Cancer 97:934, 2003. Incidence of carcinoid syndrome is from 4349 cases studied from 1950–1971, reported by JD Godwin: Cancer 36:560, 1975.

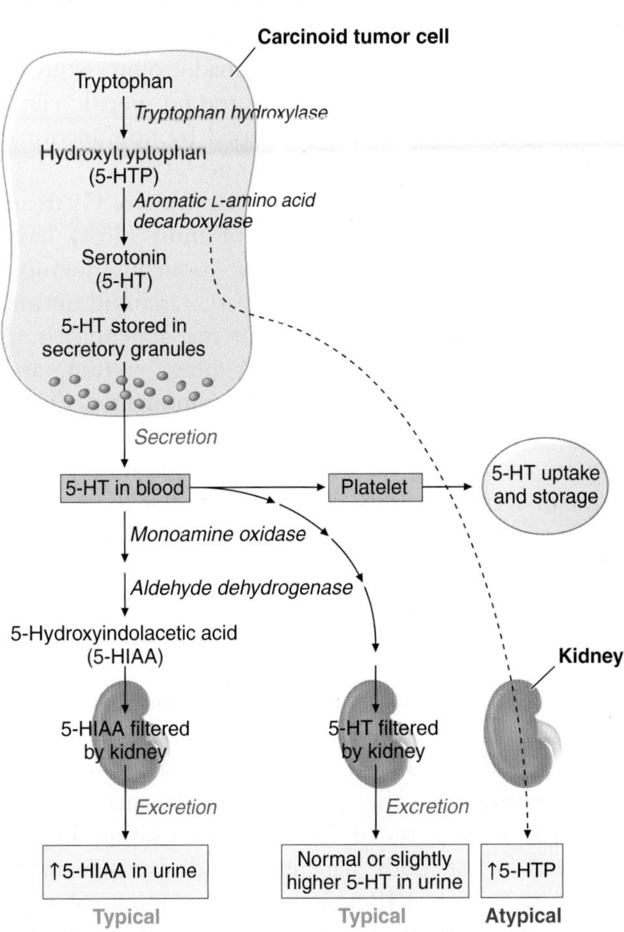

FIGURE 49-1

Synthesis, secretion, and metabolism of serotonin (5-HT) in patients with typical and atypical carcinoid syndromes. 5-HIAA, 5-hydroxyindolacetic acid.

rarely secrete 5-HTP or ACTH, contain numerous peptides, and may metastasize to bone.

Pancreatic endocrine tumors can be classified into nine well-established specific functional syndromes (Table 49-2), five possible specific functional syndromes (PETs secreting calcitonin, renin, luteinizing hormone, erythropoietin, or insulin-like growth factor II) (Table 49-2) and nonfunctional PETs (pancreatic polypeptide-secreting tumors; PPomas). Other functional hormonal syndromes due to nonpancreatic tumors (usually intraabdominal in location) have been described only rarely and are not included in Table 49-2. They include secretion of glucagon-like peptide-2 (GLP-2) that causes intestinal villus hypertrophy (enteroglucagonomas), secretion of GLP-1 that causes hypoglycemia and delayed transit, and intestinal and ovarian tumors secreting peptide tyrosine tyrosine (PYY) that result in altered motility and constipation. Each of the functional syndromes listed in Table 49-2 is associated with symptoms due to the specific hormone released. In contrast, nonfunctional PETs release no products that cause a specific clinical syndrome. "Nonfunctional" is a misnomer in the strict sense because those tumors frequently ectopically secrete a number of peptides (pancreatic polypeptide [PP], chromogranin A, ghrelin, neurotensin, α subunits of human chorionic gonadotropin, neuron-specific enolase); however, they cause no specific clinical syndrome. The symptoms caused by nonfunctional PETs are entirely due to the tumor per se.

Carcinoid tumors can occur in almost any GI tissue (Table 49-3); however, at present most (70%) have their origin in one of three sites: bronchus, jejunoileum, or colon or rectum. In the past, carcinoid tumors most frequently were reported in the appendix (i.e., 40%); however, the bronchus or lung, rectum, and small intestine are now the most common sites. Overall, the GI tract is the most common site for these tumors, accounting for 64%, with the respiratory tract a distant second at 28%. Both race and sex can affect the frequency as well as the distribution of carcinoid tumors. African Americans have a high incidence of carcinoids, and rectal carcinoids are the most common. Females have a lower incidence of small-intestinal and pancreatic carcinoids.

The term *pancreatic endocrine tumor*, although widely used and therefore retained here, is also a misnomer, strictly speaking, because these tumors can occur either almost entirely in the pancreas (insulinomas, glucagonomas, nonfunctional PETs, PETs causing hypercalcemia) or at both pancreatic and extrapancreatic sites (gastrinomas, VIPomas [vasoactive intestinal peptide], somatostatinomas, GRFomas [growth hormone–releasing factor]). PETs are also called islet cell tumors; however, the use of this term is discouraged because it is not established that they originate from the islets and many can occur at extrapancreatic sites.

A number of new classification systems have been proposed for both carcinoids and PETs. In the World Health Organization (WHO) classification it has been proposed that these tumors all be classified as GI neuroendocrine tumors (including carcinoids and PETs), which divides them into three general categories: (1a) well-differentiated NETs, (1b) well-differentiated neuroendocrine carcinomas that have low-grade malignancy, and (2) poorly differentiated neuroendocrine carcinomas that are usually small cell neuroendocrine carcinomas of high-grade malignancy. The term *carcinoid* is synonymous with *well-differentiated NETs* (1a). This classification is further divided on the basis of tumor location and biology. In addition, for the first time, a standard TNM (tumor, node, metastasis) classification and grading system has been proposed for GI neuroendocrine tumors. The new WHO classification and the TNM classification and grading system were proposed to facilitate the comparison and evaluation of clinical, pathologic, and prognostic features and results of treatment in GI NETs from different studies. These classification systems may provide important prognostic information that can guide treatment **(Table 49-4)**.

The exact incidence of carcinoid tumors or PETs varies according to whether only symptomatic tumors or all tumors are considered. The incidence of clinically significant carcinoids is 7–13 cases/million population per year, whereas any malignant carcinoids at autopsy are reported in 21–84 cases/million population per year. The incidence of GI NETs is approximately 25–50 cases per million in the United States, which makes them less common than adenocarcinomas of the GI tract. However, their incidence has increased sixfold in the past 30 years. Clinically significant PETs have a prevalence of 10 cases/million population, with insulinomas, gastrinomas, and nonfunctional PETs having an incidence of 0.5–2 cases/million population per year (Table 49-2). VIPomas are two to eight times less common, glucagonomas are 17 to 30 times less common, and somatostatinomas are the least common. In autopsy studies, 0.5–1.5% of all cases have a PET; however, in fewer than 1 in 1000 cases was a functional tumor thought to occur.

Both carcinoid tumors and PETs commonly show malignant behavior (Tables 49-2 and 49-3). With PETs, except for insulinomas in which <10% are malignant, 50–100% in different series are malignant. With carcinoid tumors, the percentage showing malignant behavior varies in different locations. For the three most common sites of occurrence, the incidence of metastases varies greatly from jejunoileum (58%) > lung/bronchus (6%) > rectum (4%) (Table 49-3). With both carcinoid tumors and PETs, a number of factors, summarized in Table 49-4, are important prognostic factors in determining survival and the aggressiveness of the tumor. Patients with PETs (excluding insulinomas)

TABLE 49-4

PROGNOSTIC FACTORS IN NEUROENDOCRINE TUMORS

I. Both carcinoid tumors and PETs
- Presence of liver metastases ($P < .001$)
- Extent of liver metastases ($P < .001$)
- Presence of lymph node metastases ($P < .001$)
- Depth of invasion ($P < .001$)
- Rapid rate of tumor growth
- Elevated serum alkaline phosphatase levels ($P = .003$)
- Primary tumor site ($P < .001$)
- Primary tumor size ($P < .005$)
- Various histologic features
  - Tumor differentiation ($P < .001$)
  - High growth indices (high $K_{i\text{-}67}$ index, PCNA expression)
  - High mitotic counts ($P < .001$)
  - Necrosis present
  - Presence of cytokeratin 19 ($P < .02$)
  - Vascular or perineural invasion
  - Vessel density (low microvessel density, increased lymphatic density)
  - High CD10 metalloproteinase expression (in series with all grades of NETs)
  - Flow cytometric features (i.e., aneuploidy)
  - High VEGF expression (in low-grade or well-differentiated NETs only)
- WHO, TNM, and grading classification
- Presence of a pancreatic NET rather than GI NET associated with poorer prognosis ($P = .0001$)
- Older age ($P < .01$)

II. Carcinoid tumors
- Presence of carcinoid syndrome
- Laboratory results [urinary 5-HIAA levels ($P < .01$), plasma neuropeptide K ($P < .05$), serum chromogranin A ($P < .01$)]
- Presence of a second malignancy
- Male sex ($P < .001$)
- Mode of discovery (incidental > symptomatic)
- Molecular findings (TGF-α expression [$P < .05$], chr 16q LOH or gain chr 4p [$P < .05$])
- WHO, TNM, and grading classification
- Molecular findings (gain in chr 14, loss of 3p13 [ileal carcinoid], upregulation of Hoxc6)

III. PETs
- Ha-*ras* oncogene or p53 overexpression
- Female gender
- MEN 1 syndrome absent
- Presence of nonfunctional tumor (some studies, not all)
- WHO, TNM, and grading classification
- Laboratory findings (increased chromogranin A in some studies; gastrinomas—increased gastrin level)
- Molecular findings [increased HER2/*neu* expression ($P = .032$), chr 1q, 3p, 3q, or 6q LOH ($P = .0004$), EGF receptor overexpression ($P = .034$), gains in chr 7q, 17q, 17p, 20q; alterations in the VHL gene (deletion, methylation)

Abbreviations: 5-HIAA, 5-hydroxyindoleacetic acid; chr, chromosome; EGF, epidermal growth factor; Ki-67, proliferation-associated nuclear antigen recognized by Ki-67 monoclonal antibody; LOH, loss of heterozygosity; MEN, multiple endocrine neoplasia; NET, neuroendocrine tumors; PCNA, proliferating cell nuclear antigen; PET, pancreatic endocrine tumor; TGF-α, transforming growth factor α; TNM, tumor, node, metastasis; VEGF, vascular endothelial growth factor; WHO, World Health Organization.

generally have a poorer prognosis than do patients with GI NETs (carcinoids). The presence of liver metastases is the single most important prognostic factor in single and multivariate analyses for both carcinoid tumors and PETs. Particularly important in the development of liver metastases is the size of the primary tumor. For example, with small-intestinal carcinoids, which are the most common cause of the carcinoid syndrome due to metastatic disease in the liver (Table 49-2), metastases occur in 15–25% if the tumor diameter is <1 cm, 58–80% if it is 1–2 cm in diameter, and >75% if it is >2 cm in diameter. Similar data exist for gastrinomas and other PETs in which the size of the primary tumor is an independent predictor of the development of liver metastases. The presence of lymph node metastases; the depth of invasion; the rapid rate of growth; various histologic features (differentiation, mitotic rates, growth indices, vessel density, vascular endothelial growth factor [VEGF], and CD10 metalloproteinase expression); necrosis; presence of cytokeratin; elevated serum alkaline phosphatase levels; older age; advanced stages in WHO, TNM, or grading classification systems; and flow cytometric results such as the presence of aneuploidy are all important prognostic factors for the development of metastatic disease (Table 49-4). For patients with carcinoid tumors, additional associations with a worse prognosis include the development of the carcinoid syndrome (especially the development of carcinoid heart disease), male sex, the presence of a symptomatic tumor or greater increases in a number of tumor markers (5-hydroxyindolacetic acid [5-HIAA], neuropeptide K, chromogranin A), and the presence of various molecular features. With PETs or gastrinomas, which have been the best studied PET long-term, a worse prognosis is associated with female sex, overexpression of the Ha-ras oncogene or p53, the absence of multiple endocrine neoplasia type 1 (MEN 1), higher levels of various tumor markers (i.e., chromogranin A, gastrin), and various molecular features (Table 49-4).

A number of diseases due to various genetic disorders are associated with an increased incidence of neuroendocrine tumors (Table 49-5). Each one is caused by

TABLE 49-5

GENETIC SYNDROMES ASSOCIATED WITH AN INCREASED INCIDENCE OF NEUROENDOCRINE TUMORS (CARCINOIDS OR PANCREATIC ENDOCRINE TUMORS)

SYNDROME	LOCATION OF GENE MUTATION AND GENE PRODUCT	NETS SEEN/FREQUENCY
Multiple endocrine neoplasia type 1 (MEN 1)	11q13 (encodes 610-amino-acid protein, menin)	80–100% develop PETs (microscopic), 20–80% (clinical): (nonfunctional > gastrinoma > insulinoma) Carcinoids: gastric (13–30%), bronchial or thymic (8%)
von Hippel–Lindau disease	3q25 (encodes 213-amino-acid protein)	12–17% develop PETs (almost always nonfunctional)
von Recklinghausen's disease (neurofibromatosis 1 [NF-1])	17q11.2 (encodes 2485-amino-acid protein, neurofibromin)	0–10% develop PETs, primarily duodenal somatostatinomas (usually nonfunctional) Rarely insulinoma, gastrinoma
Tuberous sclerosis	9q34 (TSCI) encodes 1164-amino-acid protein, hamartin) 16p13 (TSC2) (encodes 1807-amino-acid protein, tuberin)	Uncommonly develop PETs (nonfunctional and functional [insulinoma, gastrinoma])

Abbreviations: NET, neuroendocrine tumor; PET, pancreatic endocrine tumor.

a loss of a possible tumor-suppressor gene. The most important is MEN 1, which is an autosomal dominant disorder due to a defect in a 10-exon gene on 11q13, which encodes for a 610-amino-acid nuclear protein, menin (Chap. 50). Patients with MEN 1 develop hyperparathyroidism due to parathyroid hyperplasia in 95–100% of cases, PETs in 80–100%, pituitary adenomas in 54–80%, adrenal adenomas in 27–36%, bronchial carcinoids in 8%, thymic carcinoids in 8%, gastric carcinoids in 13–30% of patients with Zollinger-Ellison syndrome (ZES), skin tumors (angiofibromas [88%], collagenomas [72%]), central nervous system (CNS) tumors (meningiomas [<8%]), and smooth-muscle tumors (leiomyomas, leiomyosarcomas [1–7%]). Among patients with MEN 1, 80–100% develop nonfunctional PETs (most are microscopic with 0–13% large or symptomatic), functional PETs occur in 20–80% in different series with a mean of 54% developing ZES, 18% insulinomas, 3% glucagonomas, 3% VIPomas, and <1% GRFomas or somatostatinomas. MEN 1 is present in 20–25% of all patients with ZES, 4% of patients with insulinomas, and a low percentage (<5%) of patients with the other PETs.

Three phacomatoses associated with neuroendocrine tumors are von Hippel–Lindau disease (VHL), von Recklinghausen's disease (neurofibromatosis type 1 [NF-1]), and tuberous sclerosis (Bourneville's disease) (Table 49-5). VHL is an autosomal dominant disorder due to defects on chromosome 3p25, which encodes for a 213-amino-acid protein that interacts with the elongin family of proteins as a transcriptional regulator (Chaps. 46, 50, and 51). In addition to cerebellar hemangioblastomas, renal cancer, and pheochromocytomas, 10–17% develop a PET. Most are nonfunctional, although insulinomas and VIPomas have been reported. Patients with NF-1 (von Recklinghausen's disease) have defects in a gene on chromosome 17q11.2 that encodes for a 2845-amino-acid protein, neurofibromin, which functions in normal cells as a suppressor of the ras signaling cascade (Chap. 46). Up to 10% of these patients develop an upper GI carcinoid tumor, characteristically in the periampullary region (54%). Many are classified as somatostatinomas because they contain somatostatin immunocytochemically; however, they uncommonly secrete somatostatin and rarely produce a clinical somatostatinoma syndrome. NF-1 has rarely been associated with insulinomas and ZES. NF-1 accounts for 48% of all duodenal somatostastinomas and 23% of all ampullary carcinoid tumors. Tuberous sclerosis is caused by mutations that alter either the 1164-amino-acid protein hamartin (TSC1) or the 1807-amino-acid protein tuberin (TSC2) (Chap. 46). Both hamartin and tuberin interact in a pathway related to phosphatidylinositol 3-kinases and mTor signaling cascades. A few cases including nonfunctional and functional PETs (insulinomas and gastrinomas) have been reported in these patients (Table 49-5).

In contrast to most common nonendocrine tumors, such as carcinoma of the breast, colon, lung, or stomach, in neither PETs nor carcinoid tumors have alterations in common oncogenes (*ras, myc, fos, src, jun*) or common tumor-suppressor genes (p53, retinoblastoma susceptibility gene) been found to be generally important in their molecular pathogenesis (Table 49-1). Alterations that may be important in their pathogenesis include changes in the *MEN 1* gene, p16/MTS1 tumor-suppressor gene, and *DPC 4/Smad 4 gene*; amplification of the HER-2/*neu* protooncogene; alterations in transcription factors (Hoxc6 [GI carcinoids]), growth factors, and their receptor expression; methylation of a number of genes that probably results in their inactivation; and deletions of unknown tumor-suppressor genes as well as gains in other unknown genes (Table 49-1). Comparative genomic hybridization, genome-wide allelotyping studies, and genome-wide single-nucleotide polymorphism analyses have shown that chromosomal losses and gains are common in PETs and carcinoids, but they differ between these two NETs and some have prognostic significance (Table 49-4). Mutations in the *MEN 1* gene are probably particularly important. There is loss of heterozygosity at the MEN 1 locus on chromosome 11q13 in 93% of sporadic PETs (i.e., in patients without MEN 1) and in 26–75% of sporadic carcinoid tumors. Mutations in the *MEN 1* gene are reported in 31–34% of sporadic gastrinomas. The presence of a number of these molecular alterations (PET or carcinoid) correlates with tumor growth, tumor size, and disease extent or invasiveness and may have prognostic significance.

CARCINOID TUMORS AND CARCINOID SYNDROME

CHARACTERISTICS OF THE MOST COMMON GI CARCINOID TUMORS

Appendiceal carcinoids

Appendiceal carcinoids occur in 1 in every 200–300 appendectomies, usually in the appendiceal tip. Most (i.e., >90%) are <1 cm in diameter without metastases in older studies, but more recently 2–35% have had metastases (Table 49-3). In the SEER data of 1570 appendiceal carcinoids, 62% were localized, 27% had regional metastases, and 8% had distant metastases. Approximately 50% between 1 and 2 cm metastasized to lymph nodes. Their percentage of the total number of carcinoids decreased from 43.9% (1950–1969) to 2.4% (1992–1999).

Small-intestinal carcinoids

Small-intestinal carcinoids account for approximately one-third of all small-bowel tumors in various surgical series. These are frequently multiple; 70–80% are present in the ileum, and 70% within 6 cm (24 in) of the ileocecal valve. Forty percent are <1 cm in diameter, 32% are 1–2 cm, and 29% are >2 cm. Between 35 and 70% are associated with metastases (Table 49-3). They characteristically cause a marked fibrotic reaction, which can lead to intestinal obstruction. Distant metastases occur to liver in 36–60%, to bone in 3%, and to lung in 4%. As discussed previously, tumor size is an important variable in the frequency of metastases. However, even a proportion of small carcinoid tumors of the small intestine (<1 cm) have metastases in 15–25% of cases, whereas the proportion increases to 58–100% for tumors 1–2 cm in diameter. Carcinoids also occur in the duodenum, with 31% having metastases. No duodenal tumor <1 cm in two series metastasized, whereas 33% of those >2 cm had metastases. Small-intestinal carcinoids are the most common cause (60–87%) of the carcinoid syndrome and are discussed in a later section (Table 49-6).

TABLE 49-6

CLINICAL CHARACTERISTICS IN PATIENTS WITH CARCINOID SYNDROME

	AT PRESENTATION	DURING COURSE OF DISEASE
Symptoms and signs		
Diarrhea	32–73%	68–84%
Flushing	23–65%	63–74%
Pain	10%	34%
Asthma/wheezing	4–8%	3–18%
Pellagra	2%	5%
None	12%	22%
Carcinoid heart disease present	11%	14–41%
Demographics		
Male	46–59%	46–61%
Age		
Mean	57 yr	52–54 yr
Range	25–79 yr	9-91 yr
Tumor location		
Foregut	5-9%	2–33%
Midgut	78–87%	60–87%
Hindgut	1–5%	1–8%
Unknown	2–11%	2–15%

Rectal carcinoids

Rectal carcinoids represent 1–2% of all rectal tumors. They are found in approximately 1 in every 2500 proctoscopies. Nearly all occur between 4 and 13 cm above the dentate line. Most are small, with 66–80% being <1 cm in diameter, and rarely metastasize (5%). Tumors between 1 and 2 cm can metastasize in 5–30%, and those >2 cm, which are uncommon, in >70%.

Bronchial carcinoids

Bronchial carcinoids account for 1–2% of primary lung tumors. The frequency of bronchial carcinoids has increased more than fivefold over the past 30 years. A number of different classifications of bronchial carcinoid tumors have been proposed. In some studies, lung NETs are classified into four categories: typical carcinoid (also called bronchial carcinoid tumor, Kulchitsky cell carcinoma I [KCC-I]), atypical carcinoid (also called well-differentiated neuroendocrine carcinoma [KC-II]), intermediate small cell neuroendocrine carcinoma, and small cell neuroendocarcinoma (KC-III). Another proposed classification includes three categories of lung NETs: benign or low-grade malignant (typical carcinoid), low-grade malignant (atypical carcinoid), and high-grade malignant (poorly differentiated carcinoma of the large cell or small cell type). The WHO classification includes four general categories: typical carcinoid, atypical carcinoid, large cell neuroendocrine carcinoma, and small cell carcinoma. These different categories of lung NETs have different prognoses, varying from excellent for typical carcinoid to poor for small cell neuroendocrine carcinomas. The occurrence of large cell and small cell lung carcinoids, but not typical or atypical lung carcinoids, is related to tobacco use.

Gastric carcinoids

Gastric carcinoids account for 3 of every 1000 gastric neoplasms. Three different subtypes of gastric carcinoids are proposed to occur. Each originates from gastric enterochromaffin-like cells (ECL cells), one of the six types of gastric neuroendocrine cells, in the gastric mucosa. Two subtypes are associated with hypergastrinemic states, either chronic atrophic gastritis (type I) (80% of all gastric carcinoids) or ZES, which is almost always a part of the MEN 1 syndrome (type II) (6% of all cases). These tumors generally pursue a benign course, with type 1 uncommonly (<10%) associated with metastases, whereas type II tumors are slightly more aggressive with 10–30% percentage associated with metastases. They are usually multiple and small and infiltrate only to the submucosa. The third subtype of gastric carcinoid (type III) (sporadic) occurs without hypergastrinemia (14–25% of all gastric carcinoids) and has an aggressive course, with 54–66% developing metastases. Sporadic carcinoids are usually single, large tumors; 50% have atypical histology, and they can be a cause of the carcinoid syndrome. Gastric carcinoids as a percentage of all carcinoids are increasing in frequency (1.96% [1969–1971], 3.6% [1973–1991], 5.8% [1991–1999]).

CARCINOID TUMORS WITHOUT THE CARCINOID SYNDROME

The age of patients at diagnosis ranges from 10 to 93 years, with a mean age of 63 years for the small intestine and 66 years for the rectum. The presentation is diverse and is related to the site of origin and the extent of malignant spread. In the appendix, carcinoid tumors usually are found incidentally during surgery for suspected appendicitis. Small-intestinal carcinoids in the jejunoileum present with periodic abdominal pain (51%), intestinal obstruction with ileus or invagination (31%), an abdominal tumor (17%), or GI bleeding (11%). Because of the vagueness of the symptoms, the diagnosis usually is delayed approximately 2 years from onset of the symptoms, with a range up to 20 years. Duodenal, gastric, and rectal carcinoids are most frequently found by chance at endoscopy. The most common symptoms of rectal carcinoids are melena or bleeding (39%), constipation (17%), and diarrhea (12%). Bronchial carcinoids frequently are discovered as a lesion on a chest radiograph, and 31% of the patients are asymptomatic. Thymic carcinoids present as anterior mediastinal masses, usually on chest radiograph or CT scan. Ovarian and testicular carcinoids usually present as masses discovered on physical examination or ultrasound. Metastatic carcinoid tumor in the liver frequently presents as hepatomegaly in a patient who may have minimal symptoms and nearly normal liver function test results.

CARCINOID TUMORS WITH SYSTEMIC SYMPTOMS DUE TO SECRETED PRODUCTS

Carcinoid tumors immunocytochemically can contain numerous GI peptides: gastrin, insulin, somatostatin, motilin, neurotensin, tachykinins (substance K, substance P, neuropeptide K), glucagon, gastrin-releasing peptide, vasoactive intestinal peptide (VIP), PP, ghrelin, other biologically active peptides (ACTH, calcitonin, growth hormone), prostaglandins, and bioactive amines (serotonin). These substances may or may not be released in sufficient amounts to cause symptoms. In various studies of patients with carcinoid tumors, elevated serum levels of PP were found in 43%, motilin in 14%, gastrin in 15%, and VIP in 6%. Foregut carcinoids are more likely to produce various GI peptides than are midgut carcinoids. Ectopic ACTH production causing Cushing's syndrome is seen increasingly with foregut carcinoids (respiratory tract primarily) and in some series has been the most common cause of the ectopic ACTH syndrome, accounting for 64% of all cases. Acromegaly due to growth hormone–releasing factor release occurs with foregut carcinoids, as does the somatostatinoma syndrome, but rarely occurs with duodenal carcinoids. The most common systemic syndrome with carcinoid tumors is the carcinoid syndrome, which is discussed in detail in the next section.

CARCINOID SYNDROME

Clinical features

The cardinal features from a number of series at presentation as well as during the disease course are shown in Table 49-6. Flushing and diarrhea are the two most common symptoms, occurring in up to 73% initially and in up to 89% during the course of the disease. The characteristic flush is of sudden onset; it is a deep red or violaceous erythema of the upper body, especially the neck and face, often associated with a feeling of warmth and occasionally associated with pruritus, lacrimation, diarrhea, or facial edema. Flushes may be precipitated by stress; alcohol; exercise; certain foods, such as cheese; or certain agents, such as catecholamines, pentagastrin, and serotonin reuptake inhibitors. Flushing episodes may be brief, lasting 2 to 5 min, especially initially, or may last hours, especially later in the disease course. Flushing usually is associated with metastastic midgut carcinoids but can also occur with foregut carcinoids. With bronchial carcinoids, the flushes frequently are prolonged for hours to days, reddish in color, and associated with salivation, lacrimation, diaphoresis, diarrhea, and hypotension. The flush associated with gastric carcinoids can also be reddish in color, but with a patchy distribution over the face and neck, although the classic flush seen with midgut carcinoids can also be seen with gastric carcinoids. It may be provoked by food and have accompanying pruritus.

Diarrhea is present in 32–73% initially and 68–84% at some time in the disease course. Diarrhea usually occurs with flushing (85% of cases). The diarrhea usually is described as watery, with 60% of patients having <1 L/d of diarrhea. Steatorrhea is present in 67%, and in 46%, it is greater than 15 g/d (normal <7 g). Abdominal pain may be present with the diarrhea or independently in 10–34% of cases.

Cardiac manifestations occur initially in 11–20% of patients with carcinoid syndrome and in 17–56% (mean, 40%) at some time in the disease course. The cardiac disease is due to the formation of fibrotic plaques (composed of smooth-muscle cells, myofibroblasts, and elastic tissue) involving the endocardium, primarily on the right side, although lesions on the left side also occur occasionally, especially if a patent foramen ovale exists. The dense fibrous deposits are most commonly on the ventricular aspect of the tricuspid valve and less commonly on the pulmonary valve cusps. They can result in constriction of the valves, and pulmonic stenosis is usually predominant, whereas the tricuspid valve is often fixed open, resulting in regurgitation predominating. Overall, in patients with carcinoid heart disease, 97% have tricuspid insufficiency, 59% tricuspid stenosis, 50% pulmonary insufficiency, 25% pulmonary stenosis, and 11% (0–25%) left-side lesions. Up to 80% of patients with cardiac lesions develop heart failure. Lesions on the left side are much less extensive, occur in 30% at autopsy, and most frequently affect the mitral valve.

Other clinical manifestations include wheezing or asthma-like symptoms (8–18%) and pellagra-like skin lesions (2–25%). A variety of noncardiac problems due to increased fibrous tissue have been reported, including retroperitoneal fibrosis causing urethral obstruction, Peyronie's disease of the penis, intraabdominal fibrosis, and occlusion of the mesenteric arteries or veins.

Pathobiology

Carcinoid syndrome occurred in 8% of 8876 patients with carcinoid tumors, with a rate of 1.4–18.4% in different studies. It occurs only when sufficient concentrations of products secreted by the tumor reach the systemic circulation. In 91% of cases, this occurs after distant metastases to the liver. Rarely, primary gut carcinoids with nodal metastases with extensive retroperitoneal invasion, pancreatic carcinoids with retroperitoneal lymph nodes, or carcinoids of the lung or ovary with direct access to the systemic circulation can cause the carcinoid syndrome without hepatic metastases. All carcinoid tumors do not have the same propensity to metastasize and cause the carcinoid syndrome (Table 49-3). Midgut carcinoids account for 60–67% of cases of carcinoid syndrome, foregut tumors for 2–33%, hindgut for 1–8%, and an unknown primary location for 2–15%.

One of the main secretory products of carcinoid tumors involved in the carcinoid syndrome is serotonin (5-hydroxytryptamine [5-HT]) (Fig. 49-1), which is synthesized from tryptophan. Up to 50% of dietary tryptophan can be used in this synthetic pathway by tumor cells, and this can result in inadequate supplies for conversion to niacin; hence, some patients (2.5%) develop pellagra-like lesions. Serotonin has numerous biologic effects, including stimulating intestinal secretion with inhibition of absorption, stimulating increases in intestinal motility, and stimulating fibrogenesis. In various studies, 56–88% of all carcinoid tumors were associated with serotonin overproduction; however, 12–26% of the patients did not have the carcinoid syndrome. In one study, platelet serotonin was elevated in 96% of patients with midgut carcinoids, 43% with foregut tumors, and 0% with hindgut tumors. In 90–100% of patients with the carcinoid syndrome, there is evidence of serotonin overproduction. Serotonin is thought to be predominantly responsible for the diarrhea because of its effects on gut motility and intestinal secretion, primarily through 5-HT_3 and, to a lesser degree, 5-HT_4 receptors. Serotonin receptor antagonists (especially 5-HT_3 antagonists) relieve the diarrhea in many, but not all, patients. Additional studies suggest that prostaglandin E_2 (PGE_2) and tachykinins may be important mediators of diarrhea in some patients. In one study, plasma tachykinin levels correlated with symptoms of both flushing and diarrhea. Serotonin does not appear to be involved in the flushing because serotonin receptor antagonists do not relieve flushing. In patients with gastric carcinoids, the characteristic red, patchy pruritic flush probably is due to histamine release because H_1 and H_2 receptor antagonists can prevent it. Numerous studies have shown that tachykinins are stored in carcinoid tumors and released during flushing. However, some studies have demonstrated that octreotide can relieve the flushing induced by pentagastrin in these patients without altering the stimulated increase in plasma substance P, suggesting that other mediators must be involved in the flushing. A correlation between plasma tachykinin levels, but not substance P levels, and flushing has been reported. Both histamine and serotonin may be responsible for the wheezing as well as the fibrotic reactions involving the heart, causing Peyronie's disease and intraabdominal fibrosis. The exact mechanism of the heart disease has remained unclear, although increasing evidence supports a central role for serotonin. The valvular heart disease caused by the appetite-suppressant drug dexfenfluramine is histologically indistinguishable from that observed in carcinoid disease. Furthermore, ergot-containing dopamine receptor agonists used for Parkinson's disease (pergolide, cabergoline) cause valvular heart disease that closely resembles that seen in the carcinoid syndrome. Metabolites of fenfluramine, as well as the dopamine receptor agonists, have high affinity for serotonin receptor subtype 5-HT_{2B} receptors, whose activation is known to cause fibroblast mitogenesis. Serotonin receptor subtypes 5-$HT_{1B,1D,2A,2B}$ normally are expressed in human heart valve interstitial cells. High levels of 5-HT_{2B} receptors are known to occur in heart valves and occur in cardiac fibroblasts and cardiomyocytes. Studies of cultured interstitial cells from human cardiac valves have demonstrated that these valvulopathic drugs induce mitogenesis by activating 5-HT_{2B} receptors and stimulating upregulation of transforming growth factor β and collagen biosynthesis. These observations support the conclusion that serotonin overproduction by carcinoid tumors is important in mediating the valvular changes, possibly by activating 5-HT_{2B} receptors in the endocardium. Both the magnitude of serotonin overproduction and prior chemotherapy are important predictors of progression of the heart disease. Atrial natriuretic peptide (ANP) overproduction also has been reported in patients with cardiac disease, but its role in the pathogenesis is unknown. However, high plasma levels of ANP have a worse prognosis. Plasma connective tissue growth factor levels are elevated in many fibrotic conditions; elevated levels occur in patients with carcinoid heart disease and correlate with the presence of right-ventricular dysfunction and the extent of valvular regurgitation in patients with carcinoid tumors.

Patients may develop either a typical or, rarely, an atypical carcinoid syndrome. In patients with the typical form, which characteristically is caused by a midgut carcinoid tumor, the conversion of tryptophan to 5-HTP is the rate-limiting step (Fig. 49-1). Once 5-HTP is formed, it is rapidly converted to 5-HT and stored in secretory granules of the tumor or in platelets. A small amount remains in plasma and is converted to 5-HIAA, which appears in large amounts in the urine. These patients have an expanded serotonin pool size, increased blood and platelet serotonin, and increased urinary 5-HIAA. Some carcinoid tumors cause an atypical carcinoid syndrome that is thought to be due to a deficiency in the enzyme dopa decarboxylase; thus, 5-HTP cannot be converted to 5-HT (serotonin), and 5-HTP is secreted into the bloodstream (Fig. 49-1). In these patients, plasma serotonin levels are normal, but urinary levels may be increased because some 5-HTP is converted to 5-HT in the kidney. Characteristically, urinary 5-HTP and 5-HT are increased, but urinary 5-HIAA levels are only slightly elevated. Foregut carcinoids are the most likely to cause an atypical carcinoid syndrome.

One of the most immediate life-threatening complications of the carcinoid syndrome is the development of a carcinoid crisis. This is more common in patients who have intense symptoms or have greatly increased urinary 5-HIAA levels (i.e., >200 mg/d). The crises may occur spontaneously or be provoked by stress, anesthesia, chemotherapy, or a biopsy. Patients develop intense flushing, diarrhea, abdominal pain, cardiac abnormalities including tachycardia, hypertension, or hypotension. If not adequately treated, this can be a terminal event.

DIAGNOSIS OF THE CARCINOID SYNDROME AND CARCINOID TUMORS

The diagnosis of carcinoid syndrome relies on measurement of urinary or plasma serotonin or its metabolites in the urine. The measurement of 5-HIAA is used most frequently. False-positive elevations may occur if the patient is eating serotonin-rich foods such as bananas, pineapples, walnuts, pecans, avocados, or hickory nuts or is taking certain medications (cough syrup containing guaifenesin, acetaminophen, salicylates, serotonin reuptake inhibitors, or L-dopa). The normal range in daily urinary 5-HIAA excretion is 2–8 mg/d. Serotonin overproduction was noted in 92% of patients with carcinoid syndrome in one study, and in another study, 5-HIAA had 73% sensitivity and 100% specificity for carcinoid syndrome.

Most physicians use only the urinary 5-HIAA excretion rate; however, plasma and platelet serotonin levels, if available, may provide additional information. Platelet serotonin levels are more sensitive than urinary 5-HIAA but are not generally available. Because patients with foregut carcinoids may produce an atypical carcinoid syndrome, if this syndrome is suspected and the urinary 5-HIAA is minimally elevated or normal, other urinary metabolites of tryptophan, such as 5-HTP and 5-HT, should be measured (Fig. 49-1).

Flushing occurs in a number of other diseases, including systemic mastocytosis, chronic myeloid leukemia with increased histamine release, menopause, reactions to alcohol or glutamate, side effects of chlorpropamide, calcium channel blockers, and nicotinic acid. None of these conditions cause increased urinary 5-HIAA.

The diagnosis of carcinoid tumor can be suggested by the carcinoid syndrome, recurrent abdominal symptoms in a healthy-appearing individual, or the discovery of hepatomegaly or hepatic metastases associated with minimal symptoms. Ileal carcinoids, which make up 25% of all clinically detected carcinoids, should be suspected in patients with bowel obstruction, abdominal pain, flushing, or diarrhea.

Serum chromogranin A levels are elevated in 56–100% of patients with carcinoid tumors, and the level correlates with tumor bulk. Serum chromogranin A levels are not specific for carcinoid tumors because they are also elevated in patients with PETs and other neuroendocrine tumors. Plasma neuron-specific enolase levels are also used as a marker of carcinoid tumors but are less sensitive than chromogranin A, being increased in only 17–47% of patients.

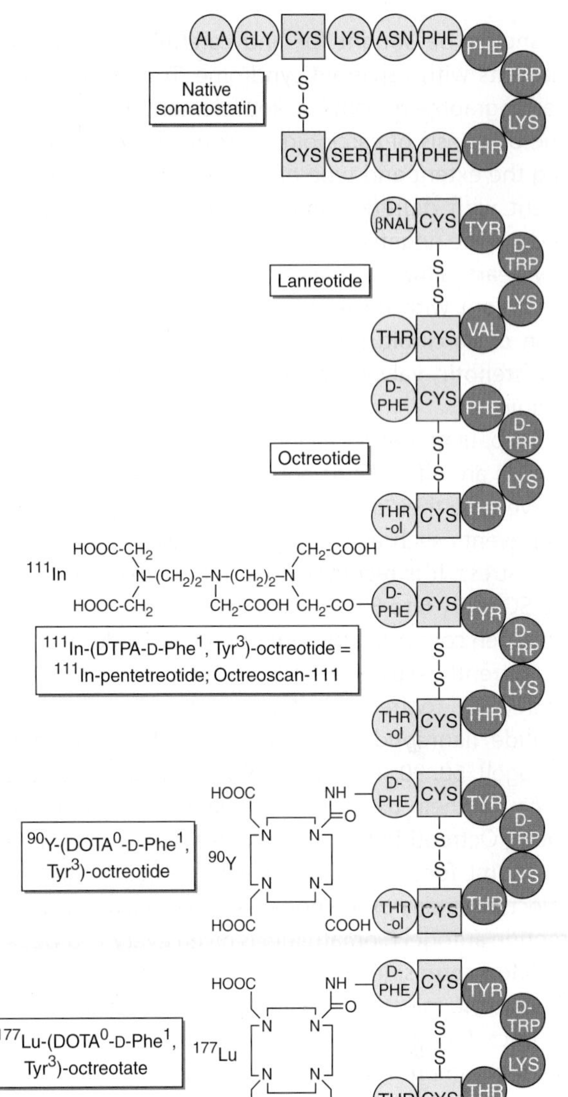

FIGURE 49-2

Structure of somatostatin and synthetic analogues used for diagnostic or therapeutic indications.

TREATMENT Carcinoid Syndrome and Nonmetastatic Carcinoid Tumors

CARCINOID SYNDROME Treatment includes avoiding conditions that precipitate flushing, dietary supplementation with nicotinamide, treatment of heart failure with diuretics, treatment of wheezing with oral bronchodilators, and control of the diarrhea with antidiarrheal agents such as loperamide and diphenoxylate. If patients still have symptoms, serotonin receptor antagonists or somatostatin analogues (Fig. 49-2) are the drugs of choice.

There are 14 subclasses of serotonin receptors, and antagonists for many are not available. The 5-HT$_1$ and 5-HT$_2$ receptor antagonists methylsergide, cyproheptadine, and ketanserin have all been used to control the diarrhea but usually do not decrease flushing. The use of methylsergide is limited because it can cause or enhance retroperitoneal fibrosis. Ketanserin diminishes diarrhea in 30–100% of patients. 5-HT$_3$ receptor antagonists (ondansetron, tropisetron, alosetron) can control diarrhea and nausea in up to 100% of patients and occasionally ameliorate the flushing. A combination of histamine H$_1$ and H$_2$ receptor antagonists (i.e., diphenhydramine and cimetidine or ranitidine) may control flushing in patients with foregut carcinoids.

Synthetic analogues of somatostatin (octreotide, lanreotide) are now the most widely used agents to control the symptoms of patients with carcinoid syndrome (Fig. 49-2). These drugs are effective at relieving symptoms and decreasing urinary 5-HIAA levels in patients with this syndrome. Octreotide-LAR (long-acting release) and lanreotide-SR/autogel (Somatuline) control symptoms in 74% and 68%, respectively, of patients with carcinoid syndrome and show a biochemical response in 51% and 39%. Patients with mild to moderate symptoms usually are treated initially with octreotide 100 μg subcutaneously (SC) every 8 h and begun on long-acting monthly depot forms (octreotide-LAR or lanreotide-autogel). Forty percent of patients escape control after a median time of 4 months, and the depot dosage may have to be increased as well as supplemented with the shorter-acting formulation, SC octreotide.

Carcinoid heart disease is associated with a decreased mean survival time (3.8 years), and therefore it should be sought for and carefully assessed in all patients with carcinoid syndrome. Transthoracic echocardiography remains a key element in establishing the diagnosis of carcinoid heart disease and determining the extent and type of cardiac abnormalities. Treatment with diuretics and somatostatin analogues can reduce the negative hemodynamic effects and secondary heart failure. It remains unclear whether long-term treatment with these drugs will decrease the progression of carcinoid heart disease. Balloon valvuloplasty for stenotic valves or cardiac valve surgery may be required.

In patients with carcinoid crises, somatostatin analogues are effective at both treating the condition and preventing their development during known precipitating events such as surgery, anesthesia, chemotherapy, and stress. It is recommended that octreotide 150–250 μg SC every 6 to 8 h be used 24–48 h before anesthesia and then continued throughout the procedure.

Currently, sustained-release preparations of both octreotide (octreotide-LAR, 10, 20, 30 mg) and lanreotide (lanreotide-PR [prolonged release, lanreotide-autogel], 60, 90, 120 mg) are available and widely used because their use greatly facilitates long-term treatment. Octreotide-LAR (30 mg/mo) gives a plasma level ≥1 ng/mL for 25 days, whereas this requires three to six injections a day of the non–sustained-release form. Lanreotide autogel (Somatuline) is given every 4–6 weeks.

Short-term side effects occur in up to half of patients. Pain at the injection site and side effects related to the GI tract (59% discomfort, 15% nausea, diarrhea) are the most common. They are usually short-lived and do not interrupt treatment. Important long-term side effects include gallstone formation, steatorrhea, and deterioration in glucose tolerance. The overall incidence of gallstones or biliary sludge in one study was 52%, with 7% having symptomatic disease that required surgical treatment.

Interferon α is reported to be effective in controlling symptoms of the carcinoid syndrome either alone or combined with hepatic artery embolization. With interferon α alone the response rate is 42%, and with interferon α with hepatic artery embolization, diarrhea was controlled for 1 year in 43%, and flushing was controlled in 86%.

Hepatic artery embolization alone or with chemotherapy (chemoembolization) has been used to control the symptoms of carcinoid syndrome. Embolization alone is reported to control symptoms in up to 76% of patients and chemoembolization (5-fluorouracil, doxorubicin, cisplatin, mitomycin) in 60–75% of patients. Hepatic artery embolization can have major side effects, including nausea, vomiting, pain, and fever. In two studies, 5–7% of patients died from complications of hepatic artery occlusion.

Other drugs have been used successfully in small numbers of patients to control the symptoms of carcinoid syndrome. Parachlorophenylanine can inhibit tryptophan hydroxylase and therefore the conversion of tryptophan to 5-HTP. However, its severe side effects, including psychiatric disturbances, make it intolerable for long-term use. α-Methyldopa inhibits the conversion of 5-HTP to 5-HT, but its effects are only partial.

Peptide radioreceptor therapy (using radiotherapy with radiolabeled somatostatin analogues), the use of radiolabeled microspheres, and other methods for treatment of advanced metastatic disease may facilitate control of the carcinoid syndrome and are discussed in a later section dealing with treatment of advanced disease.

CARCINOID TUMORS (NONMETASTATIC)

Surgery is the only potentially curative therapy. Because with most carcinoids the probability of metastatic disease increases with increasing size, the extent of surgical resection is determined accordingly. With appendiceal carcinoids <1 cm, simple appendectomy was curative in 103 patients followed for up to 35 years. With rectal carcinoids <1 cm, local resection is curative. With small-intestinal carcinoids <1 cm, there is not complete agreement. Because 15–69% of small-intestinal carcinoids this size have metastases in different studies, some recommend a wide resection with en bloc resection of the adjacent lymph-bearing mesentery. If the carcinoid tumor is >2 cm for rectal, appendiceal, or small-intestinal carcinomas, a full cancer operation should be done. This includes a right hemicolectomy for appendiceal carcinoid, an abdominoperineal resection or low anterior resection for rectal carcinoids, and an en bloc resection of adjacent lymph nodes for small-intestinal carcinoids. For carcinoids 1–2 cm in diameter for appendiceal tumors, a simple appendectomy is proposed by some, whereas others favor a formal right hemicolectomy. For rectal carcinoids 1–2 cm, it is recommended that a wide local full-thickness excision be performed.

With type I or II gastric carcinoids, which are usually <1 cm, endoscopic removal is recommended. In type I or II gastric carcinoids, if the tumor is >2 cm or if there is local invasion, some recommend total gastrectomy, whereas others recommend antrectomy in type I to reduce the hypergastrinemia, which led to regression of the carcinoids in a number of studies. For types I and II gastric carcinoids of 1–2 cm, there is no agreement, with some recommending endoscopic treatment followed by chronic somatostatin treatment and careful follow-up and others recommending surgical treatment. With type III gastric carcinoids >2 cm, excision and regional lymph node clearance are recommended. Most tumors <1 cm are treated endoscopically.

Resection of isolated or limited hepatic metastases may be beneficial and will be discussed in a later section on treatment of advanced disease.

PANCREATIC ENDOCRINE TUMORS

Functional PETs usually present clinically with symptoms due to the hormone-excess state. Only late in the course of the disease does the tumor per se cause prominent symptoms such as abdominal pain. In contrast, all the symptoms due to nonfunctional PETs are due to the tumor per se. The overall result of this is that some functional PETs may present with severe symptoms with a small or undetectable primary tumor, whereas nonfunctional tumors usually present late in the disease course with large tumors, which are frequently metastatic. The mean delay between onset of continuous symptoms and diagnosis of a functional PET syndrome is 4–7 years. Therefore, the diagnoses frequently are missed for extended periods.

TREATMENT Pancreatic Endocrine Tumor

Treatment of PETs requires two different strategies. First, treatment must be directed at the hormone-excess state such as the gastric acid hypersecretion in gastrinomas or the hypoglycemia in insulinomas. Ectopic hormone secretion usually causes the presenting symptoms and can cause life-threatening complications. Second, with all the tumors except insulinomas, >50% are malignant (Table 49-2); therefore, treatment must also be directed against the tumor per se. Because in many patients these tumors are not surgically curable due to the presence of advanced disease at diagnosis, surgical resection for cure, which addresses both treatment aspects, is often not possible.

GASTRINOMA (ZOLLINGER-ELLISON SYNDROME)

A gastrinoma is a neuroendocrine tumor that secretes gastrin; the resultant hypergastrinemia causes gastric acid hypersecretion (ZES). The chronic hypergastrinemia results in marked gastric acid hypersecretion and growth of the gastric mucosa with increased numbers of parietal cells and proliferation of gastric ECL cells. The gastric acid hypersecretion characteristically causes peptic ulcer disease, often refractory and severe, as well as diarrhea. The most common presenting symptoms are abdominal pain (70–100%), diarrhea (37–73%), and gastroesophageal reflux disease (GERD) (30–35%); 10–20% have diarrhea only. Although peptic ulcers may occur in unusual locations, most patients have a typical duodenal ulcer. Important observations that should suggest this diagnosis include peptic ulcer disease (PUD); with diarrhea; PUD in an unusual location or with multiple ulcers; PUD refractory to treatment or persistent; PUD associated with prominent gastric folds; PUD associated with findings suggestive of MEN 1 (endocrinopathy, family history of ulcer or endocrinopathy, nephrolithiases); and PUD without *Helicobacter pylori* present. *H. pylori* is present in >90% of idiopathic peptic ulcers but is present in <50% of patients with gastrinomas. Chronic unexplained diarrhea also should suggest gastrinoma.

Approximately 20–25% of patients with ZES have MEN 1, and in most cases, hyperparathyroidism is present before the gastrinoma. These patients are treated differently from those without MEN 1; therefore, MEN 1 should be sought in all patients by family history and by measuring plasma ionized calcium and prolactin levels and plasma hormone levels (parathormone, growth hormone).

Most gastrinomas (50–70%) are present in the duodenum, followed by the pancreas (20–40%) and other intraabdominal sites (mesentery, lymph nodes, biliary tract, liver, stomach, ovary). Rarely, the tumor may involve extraabdominal sites. In MEN 1 the gastrinomas are also usually in the duodenum (70–90%), followed by the pancreas (10–30%), and are almost always multiple. About 60–90% of gastrinomas are malignant (Table 49-2) with metastatic spread to the lymph nodes and liver. Distant metastases to bone occur in 12–30% of patients with liver metastases.

Diagnosis

The diagnosis of ZES requires the demonstration of inappropriate fasting hypergastrinemia, usually by demonstrating hypergastrinemia occurring with an increased basal gastric acid output (BAO) (hyperchlorhydria). More than 98% of patients with gastrinomas have fasting hypergastrinemia, although in 40–60% the level may be elevated less than 10-fold. Therefore, when the diagnosis is suspected, a fasting gastrin should be determined first. It is important to remember that potent gastric acid suppressant drugs such as proton pump inhibitors (omeprazole, esomeprazole, pantoprazole, lansoprazole, rabeprazole) can suppress acid secretion sufficiently to cause hypergastrinemia; because of their prolonged duration of action, these drugs have to be discontinued for a week before the gastrin determination. Withdrawal of proton pump inhibitors (PPIs) should be performed carefully and is best done in consultation with GI units with experience in this area. The widespread use of PPIs can confound the diagnosis of ZES by raising a false-positive diagnosis by causing hypergastrinemia in a patient being treated with idiopathic peptic disease (without ZES) and lead to a false-negative diagnosis because at routine doses used to treat patients with idiopathic peptic disease, PPIs control symptoms in most ZES patients and thus mask the diagnosis. If ZES is suspected and the gastrin level is elevated, it is important to show that it is increased when gastric pH is ≤2.0 because physiologically hypergastrinemia secondary to achlorhydria (atrophic gastritis, pernicious anemia) is one of the most common causes of hypergastrinemia. Nearly all gastrinoma patients have a fasting pH ≤2 when the patient is off antisecretory drugs. If the fasting gastrin is >1000 pg/mL (increased 10-fold) and the pH is ≤2.0, which occurs in 40–60% of patients with gastrinoma, the diagnosis of ZES is established after the possibility of retained antrum syndrome has been ruled out by history. In patients with hypergastrinemia with fasting gastrins <1000 pg/mL and gastric pH ≤2.0, other conditions, such as *H. pylori* infections, antral G-cell hyperplasia or hyperfunction, gastric outlet obstruction, and, rarely, renal failure, can masquerade as ZES. To establish the diagnosis in this group, a determination of BAO and a secretin provocative test should be done. In patients with ZES without previous gastric acid–reducing surgery, the BAO is usually (>90%) elevated (i.e., >15 mEq/h). The secretin provocative test result is usually positive, with the criterion of a >120-pg/mL increase over the basal level having the highest sensitivity (94%) and specificity (100%).

TREATMENT Gastrinomas

Gastric acid hypersecretion in patients with gastrinomas can be controlled in almost every case by oral gastric antisecretory drugs. Because of their long duration of action and potency, which allows dosing once or twice a day, the PPIs (H^+,K^+-ATPase inhibitors) are the drugs of choice. Histamine H_2-receptor antagonists are also effective, although more frequent dosing (q 4–8 h) and high doses are required. In patients with MEN 1 with hyperparathyroidism, correction of the hyperparathyroidism increases the sensitivity to gastric antisecretory drugs and decreases the basal acid output. Long-term treatment with PPIs (>15 years) has proved to be safe and effective, without development of tachyphylaxis. Although patients with ZES, especially those with MEN 1, more frequently develop gastric carcinoids, no data suggest that the long-term use of PPIs increases this risk in these patients. With long-term PPI use in ZES patients, vitamin B_{12} deficiency can develop; thus, vitamin B_{12} levels should be assessed during follow-up.

With the increased ability to control acid hypersecretion, more than 50% of patients who are not cured (>60% of patients) will die from tumor-related causes. At presentation, careful imaging studies are essential to localize the extent of the tumor. A third of patients present with hepatic metastases, and in <15% of those patients the disease is limited, so that surgical resection may be possible. Surgical short-term cure is possible in 60% of all patients without MEN 1 or liver metastases (40% of all patients) and in 30% of patients long-term. In patients with MEN 1, long-term surgical cure is rare because the tumors are multiple, frequently with lymph node metastases. Therefore, all patients with gastrinomas without MEN 1 or a medical condition that limits life expectancy should undergo surgery by a surgeon experienced in the treatment of these disorders.

INSULINOMAS

An insulinoma is an endocrine tumor of the pancreas that is thought to be derived from beta cells that ectopically secrete insulin, which results in hypoglycemia. The average age of occurrence is 40–50 years old. The most common clinical symptoms are due to the effect of the hypoglycemia on the CNS (neuroglycemic symptoms) and include confusion, headache, disorientation, visual difficulties, irrational behavior, and even coma. Also, most patients have symptoms due to excess catecholamine release secondary to the hypoglycemia, including sweating, tremor, and palpitations. Characteristically, these attacks are associated with fasting.

Insulinomas are generally small (>90% <2 cm) and usually not multiple (90%); only 5–15% are malignant, and they almost invariably occur only in the pancreas, distributed equally in the pancreatic head, body, and tail.

Insulinomas should be suspected in all patients with hypoglycemia, especially when there is a history suggesting that attacks are provoked by fasting, or with a family history of MEN 1. Insulin is synthesized as proinsulin, which consists of a 21-amino-acid α chain and a 30-amino-acid β chain connected by a 33-amino-acid connecting peptide (C peptide). In insulinomas, in addition to elevated plasma insulin levels, elevated plasma proinsulin levels are found, and C-peptide levels can be elevated.

Diagnosis

The diagnosis of insulinoma requires the demonstration of an elevated plasma insulin level at the time of hypoglycemia. A number of other conditions may cause fasting hypoglycemia, such as the inadvertent or surreptitious use of insulin or oral hypoglycemic agents, severe liver disease, alcoholism, poor nutrition, and other extrapancreatic tumors. Furthermore, postprandial hypoglycemia can be caused by a number of conditions that confuse the diagnosis of insulinoma. Particularly important here is the increased occurrence of hypoglycemia after gastric bypass surgery for obesity, which is now widely performed. The most reliable test to diagnose insulinoma is a fast up to 72 h with serum glucose, C-peptide, proinsulin, and insulin measurements every 4–8 h. If at any point the patient becomes symptomatic or glucose levels are persistently below <2.2 mmol/L (40 mg/dL), the test should be terminated and repeat samples for the above studies should be obtained before glucose is given. Some 70–80% of patients will develop hypoglycemia during the first 24 h, and 98% by 48 h. In nonobese normal subjects, serum insulin levels should decrease to <43 pmol/L (<6 μU/mL) when blood glucose decreases to <2.2 mmol/L (<40 mg/dL) and the ratio of insulin to glucose is <0.3 (in mg/dL). In addition to having an insulin level >6 μU/mL when blood glucose is <40 mg/dL, some investigators also require an elevated C-peptide and serum proinsulin level, an insulin/glucose ratio >0.3, and a decreased plasma β-hydroxybutyrate level for the diagnosis of insulinomas. Surreptitious use of insulin or hypoglycemic agents may be difficult to distinguish from insulinomas. The combination of proinsulin levels (normal in exogenous insulin/hypoglycemic agent users), C-peptide levels (low in exogenous insulin users), antibodies to insulin (positive in exogenous insulin users), and measurement of sulfonylurea levels in serum or plasma will allow the correct diagnosis to be made. The diagnosis of insulinoma has been complicated by the introduction of specific insulin assays that do not also interact with proinsulin, as do many of the older radioimmunoassays (RIAs), and therefore give lower plasma insulin levels. The increased use of these specific insulin assays has resulted in increased numbers of patients with insulinomas having lower plasma insulin values than the 6 μU/mL levels proposed to be characteristic of insulinomas by RIA. In these patients, the assessment of proinsulin and C-peptide levels at the time of hypoglycemia is particularly helpful for establishing the correct diagnosis. An elevated proinsulin level when the fasting glucose level is <45 mg/dL is sensitive and specific.

TREATMENT Insulinomas

Only 5–15% of insulinomas are malignant; therefore, after appropriate imaging (see later), surgery should be performed. In different studies, 75–100% of patients are cured by surgery. Before surgery, the hypoglycemia can be controlled by frequent small meals and the use of diazoxide (150–800 mg/d). Diazoxide is a benzothiadiazide whose hyperglycemic effect is attributed to inhibition of insulin release. Its side effects are sodium retention and GI symptoms such as nausea. Approximately 50–60% of patients respond to diazoxide. Other agents effective in some patients to control the hypoglycemia include verapamil and diphenylhydantoin. Long-acting somatostatin analogues such as octreotide and lanreotide are acutely effective in 40% of patients. However, octreotide must be used with care because it inhibits growth hormone secretion and can alter plasma glucagon levels; therefore, in some patients, it can worsen the hypoglycemia.

For the 5–15% of patients with malignant insulinomas, these drugs or somatostatin analogues are used initially. In a small number of patients with insulinomas, some with malignant tumors, mammalian target of rapamycin (mTor) inhibitors (everolimus, rapamycin) are reported to control the hypoglycemia. If they are not effective, various antitumor treatments such as hepatic arterial embolization, chemoembolization, chemotherapy, and peptide receptor radiotherapy have been used (see later discussion).

Insulinomas, which are usually benign (>90%) and intrapancreatic in location, are increasingly resected using a laparoscopic approach, which has lower morbidity rates. This approach requires that the insulinoma be localized on preoperative imaging studies.

GLUCAGONOMAS

A glucagonoma is an endocrine tumor of the pancreas that secretes excessive amounts of glucagon, which causes a distinct syndrome characterized by dermatitis, glucose intolerance or diabetes, and weight loss. Glucagonomas principally occur between 45 and 70 years of age. The tumor is clinically heralded by a characteristic dermatitis (migratory necrolytic erythema) (67–90%), accompanied by glucose intolerance (40–90%), weight loss (66–96%), anemia (33–85%), diarrhea (15–29%), and thromboembolism (11–24%). The characteristic rash usually starts as an annular erythema at intertriginous and periorificial sites, especially in the groin or buttock. It subsequently becomes raised, and bullae form; when the bullae rupture, eroded areas form. The lesions can wax and wane. The development of a similar rash in patients receiving glucagon therapy suggests that the rash is a direct effect of the hyperglucagonemia. A characteristic laboratory finding is hypoaminoacidemia, which occurs in 26–100% of patients.

Glucagonomas are generally large tumors at diagnosis (5–10 cm). Some 50–80% occur in the pancreatic tail. From 50 to 82% have evidence of metastatic spread at presentation, usually to the liver. Glucagonomas are rarely extrapancreatic and usually occur singly.

Diagnosis

The diagnosis is confirmed by demonstrating an increased plasma glucagon level. Characteristically, plasma glucagon levels exceed 1000 pg/mL (normal is <150 pg/mL) in 90%; 7% are between 500 and 1000 pg/mL, and 3% are <500 pg/mL. A trend toward lower levels at diagnosis has been noted in the past decade. A plasma glucagon level >1000 pg/mL is considered diagnostic of glucagonoma. Other diseases causing increased plasma glucagon levels include renal insufficiency, acute pancreatitis, hypercorticism, hepatic insufficiency, severe stress, and prolonged fasting or familial hyperglucagonemia, as well as danazol treatment. With the exception of cirrhosis, these disorders do not increase plasma glucagon >500 pg/mL.

Necrolytic migratory erythema is not pathognomonic for glucagonoma and occurs in myeloproliferative disorders, hepatitis B infection, malnutrition, short-bowel syndrome, inflammatory bowel disease, and malabsorption disorders.

TREATMENT Glucagonomas

In 50–80% of patients, hepatic metastases are present, so curative surgical resection is not possible. Surgical debulking in patients with advanced disease or other antitumor treatments may be beneficial (see later discussion). Long-acting somatostatin analogues such as octreotide and lanreotide improve the skin rash in 75% of patients and may improve the weight loss, pain, and diarrhea but usually do not improve the glucose intolerance.

SOMATOSTATINOMA SYNDROME

The somatostatinoma syndrome is due to an NET that secretes excessive amounts of somatostatin, which causes a distinct syndrome characterized by diabetes mellitus, gallbladder disease, diarrhea, and steatorrhea. There is no general distinction in the literature between a tumor that contains somatostatin-like immunoreactivity (somatostatinoma) and does (11–45%) or does not (55–90%) produce a clinical syndrome (somatostatinoma syndrome) by secreting somatostatin. In a review of 173 cases of somatostatinomas, only 11% were associated with the somatostatinoma syndrome. The mean age is 51 years. Somatostatinomas occur primarily in the pancreas and small intestine, and the frequency of the symptoms and occurrence of the somatostatinoma syndrome differ in each. Each of the usual symptoms is more common in pancreatic than in intestinal somatostatinomas: diabetes mellitus (95% vs 21%), gallbladder disease (94% vs 43%), diarrhea (92% vs 38%), steatorrhea (83% vs 12%), hypochlorhydria (86% vs 12%), and weight loss (90% vs 69%). The somatostatinoma syndrome occurs in 30–90% of pancreatic and 0–5% of small-intestinal somatostatinomas. In various series, 43% of all duodenal NETs contain somatostatin; however, the somatostatinoma syndrome is rarely present (<2%). Somatostatinomas occur in the pancreas in 56–74% of cases, with the primary location being the pancreatic head. The tumors are usually solitary (90%) and large (mean size, 4.5 cm). Liver metastases are common, being present in 69–84% of patients. Somatostatinomas are rare in patients with MEN 1, occurring in only 0.65%.

Somatostatin is a tetradecapeptide that is widely distributed in the CNS and GI tract, where it functions as a neurotransmitter or has paracrine and autocrine actions. It is a potent inhibitor of many processes, including release of almost all hormones, acid secretion, intestinal and pancreatic secretion, and intestinal absorption. Most of the clinical manifestations are directly related to these inhibitory actions.

Diagnosis

In most cases, somatostatinomas have been found by accident either at the time of cholecystectomy or during endoscopy. The presence of psammoma bodies in a duodenal tumor should particularly raise suspicion. Duodenal somatostatin-containing tumors are increasingly associated with von Recklinghausen's disease. Most of these tumors (>98%) do not cause the somatostatinoma syndrome. The diagnosis of the somatostatinoma syndrome requires the demonstration of elevated plasma somatostatin levels.

TREATMENT Somatostatinomas

Pancreatic tumors are frequently (70–92%) metastatic at presentation, whereas 30–69% of small-intestinal somatostatinomas have metastases. Surgery is the treatment of choice for those without widespread hepatic metastases. Symptoms in patients with the somatostatinoma syndrome are also improved by octreotide treatment.

VIPOMAS

VIPomas are endocrine tumors that secrete excessive amounts of vasoactive intestinal peptide, which causes a distinct syndrome characterized by large-volume diarrhea, hypokalemia, and dehydration. This syndrome also is called Verner-Morrison syndrome, pancreatic cholera, and WDHA syndrome for *w*atery *d*iarrhea, *h*ypokalemia, and *a*chlorhydria, which some patients develop. The mean age of patients with this syndrome is 49 years; however, it can occur in children, and when it does, it is usually caused by a ganglioneuroma or ganglioneuroblastoma.

The principal symptoms are large-volume diarrhea (100%) severe enough to cause hypokalemia (80–100%), dehydration (83%), hypochlorhydria (54–76%), and flushing (20%). The diarrhea is secretory in nature, persisting during fasting, and is almost always >1 L/d and in 70% is >3 L/d. In a number of studies, the diarrhea was intermittent initially in up to half of patients. Most patients do not have accompanying steatorrhea (16%), and the increased stool volume is due to increased excretion of sodium and potassium, which, with the anions, accounts for the osmolality of the stool. Patients frequently have hyperglycemia (25–50%) and hypercalcemia (25–50%).

VIP is a 28-amino-acid peptide that is an important neurotransmitter, ubiquitously present in the CNS and GI tract. Its known actions include stimulation of small-intestinal chloride secretion as well as effects on smooth muscle contractility, inhibition of acid secretion, and vasodilatory effects, which explain most features of the clinical syndrome.

In adults, 80–90% of VIPomas are pancreatic in location, with the rest due to VIP-secreting pheochromocytomas, intestinal carcinoids, and rarely ganglioneuromas. These tumors are usually solitary, 50–75% are in the pancreatic tail, and 37–68% have hepatic metastases at diagnosis. In children <10 years old, the syndrome is usually due to ganglioneuromas or ganglioblastomas and is less often malignant (10%).

Diagnosis

The diagnosis requires the demonstration of an elevated plasma VIP level and the presence of large-volume diarrhea. A stool volume <700 mL/d is proposed to exclude the diagnosis of VIPoma. When the patient fasts, a number of diseases can be excluded that can cause marked diarrhea. Other diseases that can produce a secretory large-volume diarrhea include gastrinomas, chronic laxative abuse, carcinoid syndrome, systemic mastocytosis, rarely medullary thyroid cancer, diabetic diarrhea, sprue, and AIDS. Among these conditions, only VIPomas caused a marked increase in plasma VIP. Chronic surreptitious use of laxatives or diuretics can be particularly difficult to detect clinically. Hence, in a patient with unexplained chronic diarrhea, screens for laxatives should be performed; they will detect many, but not all, laxative abusers.

TREATMENT **Vasoactive Intestinal Peptidomas**

The most important initial treatment in these patients is to correct their dehydration, hypokalemia, and electrolyte losses with fluid and electrolyte replacement. These patients may require 5 L/d of fluid and >350 mEq/d of potassium. Because 37–68% of adults with VIPomas have metastatic disease in the liver at presentation, a significant number of patients cannot be cured surgically. In these patients, long-acting somatostatin analogues such as octreotide and lanreotide are the drugs of choice.

Octreotide–lanreotide will control the diarrhea short- and long-term in 75–100% of patients. In nonresponsive patients, the combination of glucocorticoids and octreotide–lanreotide has proved helpful in a small number of patients. Other drugs reported to be helpful in small numbers of patients include prednisone (60–100 mg/d), clonidine, indomethacin, phenothiazines, loperamide, lidamidine, lithium, propranolol, and metoclopramide. Treatment of advanced disease with embolization, chemoembolization, chemotherapy, radiotherapy, radiofrequency ablation, and peptide receptor radiotherapy may be helpful (see later discussion).

NONFUNCTIONAL PANCREATIC ENDOCRINE TUMORS

Nonfunctional PETs (NF-PETs) are endocrine tumors that originate in the pancreas and secrete no products, or their products do not cause a specific clinical syndrome. The symptoms are due entirely to the tumor per se. NF-PETs secrete chromogranin A (90–100%), chromogranin B (90–100%), PP (58%), α-HCG (human chorionic gonadotropin) (40%), and β-HCG (20%). Because the symptoms are due to the tumor mass, patients with NF-PETs usually present late in the disease course with invasive tumors and hepatic metastases (64–92%), and the tumors are usually large (72% >5 cm). NF-PETs are usually solitary except in patients with MEN 1, in which case they are multiple. They occur primarily in the pancreatic head. Even though these tumors do not cause a functional syndrome, immunocytochemical studies show that they synthesize numerous peptides and cannot be distinguished from functional tumors by immunocytochemistry. In MEN 1, 80–100% of patients have microscopic NF-PETs, but they become large or symptomatic in only a minority (0–13%) of cases. In VHL, 12–17% develop NF-PETs, and in 4%, they are ≥3 cm in diameter.

The most common symptoms are abdominal pain (30–80%); jaundice (20–35%); and weight loss, fatigue, or bleeding. About 10–30% are found incidentally. The average time from the beginning of symptoms to diagnosis is 5 years.

Diagnosis

The diagnosis is established by histologic confirmation in a patient without either the clinical symptoms or the elevated plasma hormone levels of one of the established syndromes. The principal difficulty in diagnosis is to distinguish an NF-PET from a nonendocrine pancreatic tumor, which is more common. Even though chromogranin A levels are elevated in almost every patient, this is not specific for this disease as it can be found in functional PETs, carcinoids, and other neuroendocrine disorders. Plasma PP is increased in 22–71% of patients and should strongly suggest the diagnosis in a patient with a pancreatic mass because it is usually normal in patients with pancreatic adenocarcinomas. Elevated plasma PP is not diagnostic of this tumor because it is elevated in a number of other conditions, such as chronic renal failure, old age, inflammatory conditions, and diabetes. A positive somatostatin receptor scan in a patient with a pancreatic mass should suggest the presence of PET or NF-PET rather than a nonendocrine tumor.

TREATMENT Nonfunctional Pancreatic Endocrine Tumors

Overall survival in patients with sporadic NF-PET is 30–63% at 5 years, with a median survival of 6 years. Unfortunately, surgical curative resection can be considered only in a minority of these patients because 64–92% present with metastatic disease. Treatment needs to be directed against the tumor per se using the various modalities discussed later for advanced disease. The treatment of NF-PETs in either MEN 1 patients or patients with VHL is controversial. Most recommend surgical resection for any tumor >2–3 cm in diameter; however, there is no consensus on smaller NF-PETs, with most recommending careful surveillance of these patients.

GRFOMAS

GRFomas are endocrine tumors that secrete excessive amounts of growth hormone–releasing factor (GRF) that cause acromegaly. GRF is a 44-amino-acid peptide, and 25–44% of PETs have GRF immunoreactivity, although it is uncommonly secreted. GRFomas are lung tumors in 47–54% of cases, PETs in 29–30%, and small-intestinal carcinoids in 8–10%; up to 12% occur at other sites. Patients have a mean age of 38 years, and the symptoms usually are due to either acromegaly or the tumor per se. The acromegaly caused by GRFomas is indistinguishable from classic acromegaly. The pancreatic tumors are usually large (>6 cm), and liver metastases are present in 39%. They should be suspected in any patient with acromegaly and an abdominal tumor; a patient with MEN 1 with acromegaly; or a patient without a pituitary adenoma with acromegaly; or associated with hyperprolactinemia, which occurs in 70% of GRFomas. GRFomas are an uncommon cause of acromegaly. GRFomas occur in <1% of MEN 1 patients. The diagnosis is established by performing plasma assays for GRF and growth hormone. Most GRFomas have a plasma GRF level >300 pg/mL (normal <5 pg/mL men, <10 pg/mL women). Patients with GRFomas also have increased plasma levels of insulin-like growth factor type I (IGF-I) levels similar to those in classic acromegaly. Surgery is the treatment of choice if diffuse metastases are not present. Long-acting somatostatin analogues such as octreotide and lanreotide are the agents of choice, with 75–100% of patients responding.

OTHER RARE PANCREATIC ENDOCRINE TUMOR SYNDROMES

Cushing's syndrome (ACTHoma) due to a PET occurs in 4–16% of all ectopic Cushing's syndrome cases. It occurs in 5% of cases of sporadic gastrinomas, almost invariably in patients with hepatic metastases, and is an independent poor prognostic factor. Paraneoplastic hypercalcemia due to PETs releasing parathyroid hormone–related peptide (PTHrP), a PTH-like material, or unknown factor, is rarely reported. The tumors are usually large, and liver metastases are usually present. Most (88%) appear to be due to release of PTHrP. PETs occasionally can cause the carcinoid syndrome. PETs secreting calcitonin have been proposed as a specific clinical syndrome. Half of the patients have diarrhea, which disappears with resection of the tumor. The proposal that this could be a discrete syndrome is supported by the finding that 25–42% of patients with medullary thyroid cancer with hypercalcitonemia develop diarrhea, probably secondary to a motility disorder. This is classified in Table 49-2 as a possible specific disorder because so few cases have been described. Similarly classified with only a few cases described are a renin-producing PET in a patient presenting with hypertension; PETs secreting luteinizing hormone, resulting in masculinization or decreased libido; a PET-secreting erythropoietin resulting in polycythemia; and PETs secreting insulin-like growth factor II causing hypoglycemia (Table 49-2). Ghrelin is a 28-amino-acid peptide with a number of metabolic functions. Even though it is detectable immunohistochemically in most PETs, no specific syndrome is associated with release of ghrelin by the PET.

TUMOR LOCALIZATION

Localization of the primary tumor and knowledge of the extent of the disease are essential to the proper management of all carcinoids and PETs. Without proper localization studies, it is not possible to determine whether the patient is a candidate for curative resection or cytoreductive surgery or requires antitumor treatment or to predict the patient's prognosis reliably.

Numerous tumor localization methods are used in both types of NETs, including conventional imaging studies (computed tomographic [CT] scanning, magnetic resonance imaging [MRI], transabdominal ultrasound, selective angiography), somatostatin receptor scintigraphy (SRS), and positron emission tomographic (PET) scanning. In PETs, endoscopic ultrasound (EUS) and functional localization by measuring venous hormonal gradients are also reported to be useful. Bronchial carcinoids are usually detected by standard chest radiography and assessed by CT. Rectal, duodenal, colonic, and gastric carcinoids are usually detected by GI endoscopy.

PETs, as well as carcinoid tumors, frequently overexpress high-affinity somatostatin receptors in both their primary tumors and their metastases. Of the five types of somatostatin receptors (sst_{1-5}), radiolabeled octreotide binds with high affinity to sst_2 and sst_5, has a lower affinity for sst_3, and has a very low affinity for sst_1 and sst_4. Between 90 and 100% of carcinoid tumors and PETs possess sst_2, and many also have the other four sst subtypes. Interaction with these receptors can be used to localize NETs by using (^{111}In-DTPA-d-Phe^1)octreotide and radionuclide scanning (SRS) as well as for treatment of the hormone-excess state with octreotide or lanreotide, as discussed earlier. Because of its sensitivity and ability to localize tumor throughout the body, SRS is the initial imaging modality of choice for localizing both the primary and metastatic NETs. SRS localizes tumor in 73–89% of patients with carcinoids and in 56–100% of patients with PETs, except insulinomas. Insulinomas are usually small and have low densities of sst receptors, resulting in SRS being positive in only 12–50% of patients with insulinomas. Figure 49-3 shows an example of the increased sensitivity of SRS in a patient with a carcinoid tumor. The CT scan showed a single liver metastasis, whereas the SRS demonstrated three metastases in the liver in multiple locations. Occasional false-positive responses with SRS can occur (12% in one study) because numerous other normal tissues as well as diseases can have high densities of sst receptors, including granulomas (sarcoid, tuberculosis, etc.), thyroid diseases (goiter, thyroiditis), and activated lymphocytes (lymphomas, wound infections). For PETs in the pancreas, EUS is highly sensitive, localizing 77–100% of insulinomas, which occur almost exclusively within the pancreas. Endoscopic ultrasound is less sensitive for extrapancreatic tumors. It is increasingly used in patients with MEN 1 and to a lesser extent VHL to detect small PETs not seen with other modalities or for serial PET assessments to determine size changes or rapid growth in patients in whom surgery is deferred. EUS with cytologic evaluation also is used frequently to distinguish an NF-PET from a pancreatic adenocarcinoma or another nonendocrine pancreatic tumor.

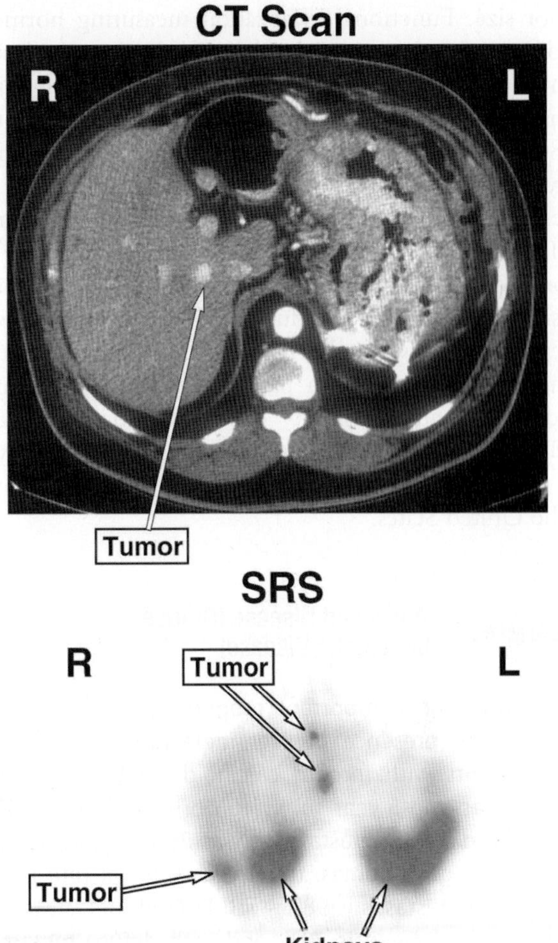

FIGURE 49-3
Ability of computed tomography (CT) scanning (*top*) or somatostatin receptor scintigraphy (SRS) (*bottom*) to localize metastatic carcinoid in the liver.

Insulinomas overexpress receptors for GLP-1; a radiolabeled GLP-1 analogue can detect occult insulinomas not localized by other imaging modalities. Functional localization by measuring hormonal gradients is now uncommonly used with gastrinomas (after intraarterial secretin injections) but is still frequently used in insulinoma patients in whom other imaging study results are negative (assessing hepatic vein insulin concentrations post-intraarterial calcium injections). The intraarterial calcium test may also allow differentiation of the cause of the hypoglycemia and indicate whether it is due to an insulinoma or a nesidioblastosis. The latter entity is becoming increasingly important because hypoglycemia after gastric bypass surgery for obesity is increasing in frequency, and it is primarily due to nesidioblastosis, although it can occasionally be due to an insulinoma.

If liver metastases are identified by SRS, to plan the proper treatment either a CT or an MRI is recommended to assess the size and exact location of the metastases because SRS does not provide information on tumor size. Functional localization measuring hormone gradients after intraarterial calcium injections in insulinomas (insulin) or gastrin gradients after secretin injections in gastrinoma is a sensitive method, being positive in 80–100% of patients. However, this method provides only regional localization and therefore is reserved for cases in which the other imaging modalities are negative.

Two newer imaging modalities (PET and use of hybrid scanners such as CT and SRS) may have increased sensitivity. PET with ^{18}F-fluoro-DOPA in patients with carcinoids or with ^{11}C-5-HTP or ^{68}gallium-labeled somatostatin analogues in patients with PETs or carcinoids has greater sensitivity than conventional imaging studies or SRS and probably will be used increasingly in the future. PET for GI NETs is not currently approved in the United States.

TREATMENT Advanced Disease (Diffuse Metastatic Disease)

The single most important prognostic factor for survival is the presence of liver metastases (Fig. 49-4). For patients with foregut carcinoids without hepatic metastases, the 5-year survival in one study was 95%, and with distant metastases, it was 20% (Fig. 49-4, bottom). With gastrinomas, the 5-year survival rate without liver metastases is 98%; with limited metastases in one hepatic lobe, it is 78%; and with diffuse metastases, 16% (Fig. 49-4, top). In a large study of 156 patients (67 PETs, rest carcinoids), the overall 5-year survival rate was 77%; it was 96% without liver metastases, 73% with liver metastases, and 50% with distant disease. Therefore, treatment for advanced metastatic disease is an important challenge. A number of different modalities are reported to be effective, including cytoreductive surgery (surgically or by radiofrequency ablation [RFA]), treatment with chemotherapy, somatostatin analogues, interferon α, hepatic embolization alone or with chemotherapy (chemoembolization), radiotherapy with radiolabeled beads/microspheres, peptide radio-receptor therapy, and liver transplantation.

SPECIFIC ANTITUMOR TREATMENTS Cytoreductive surgery, unfortunately, is possible in only 9–22% of patients who present with limited hepatic metastases. Although no randomized studies have proved that it extends life, results from a number of studies suggest that it probably increases survival; therefore, it is recommended, if possible. RFA can be applied to GI NET liver metastases if they are limited in number (usually <5) and size (usually <3.5 cm in diameter). Response rates are >80%, the morbidity rate is low, and this procedure may be particularly helpful in patients with functional PETs that are difficult to control medically.

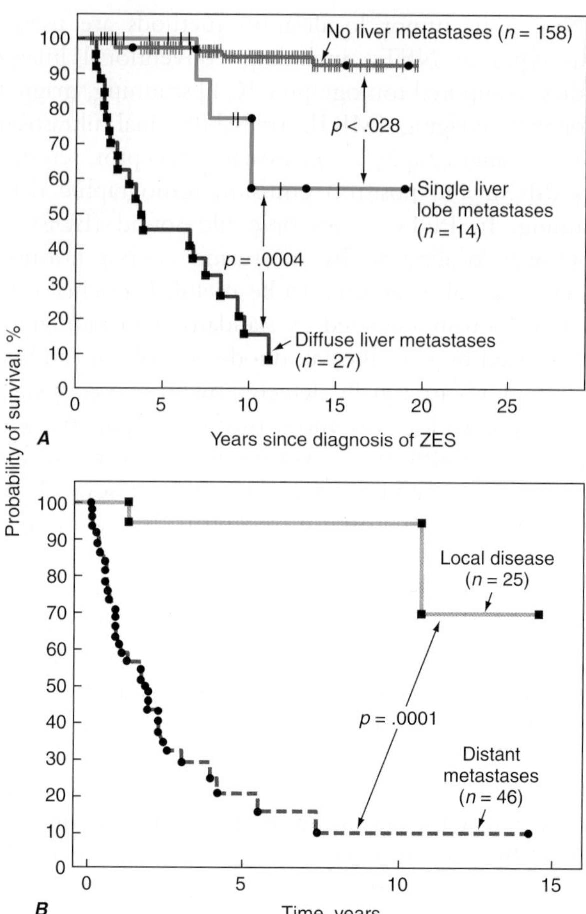

FIGURE 49-4
Effect of the presence and extent of liver metastases on survival in patients with gastrinomas ***(A)*** or carcinoid tumors ***(B)***. ZES, Zollinger-Ellison syndrome. (*Top panel is drawn from data from 199 patients with gastrinomas modified from F Yu et al: J Clin Oncol 17:615, 1999. Bottom panel is drawn from data from 71 patients with foregut carcinoid tumors from EW McDermott et al: Br J Surg 81:1007, 1994.*)

Chemotherapy for metastatic carcinoid tumors has generally been disappointing, with response rates of 0–40% with various two- and three-drug combinations. Chemotherapy for PETs has been more successful, with tumor shrinkage reported in 30–70% of patients. The current regimen of choice is streptozotocin and doxorubicin. In poorly differentiated PETs, chemotherapy with cisplatin, etoposide, or their derivatives is the recommended treatment, with response rates of 40–70%; however, responses are generally short-lived. Some newer combinations of chemotherapeutic agents show promise in small numbers of patients, including temozolomide (TMZ) alone, especially in PETs, which frequently have O^6-methylguanine DNA methyltransferase deficiency, which increases their TMZ sensitivity (34% response rate), and TMZ plus capecitabine (response rate, 59–71%, in retrospective studies).

Long-acting somatostatin analogues such as octreotide, lanreotide, and interferon α rarely decrease tumor size (i.e., 0–17%); however, these drugs have tumoristatic effects, stopping additional growth in 26–95% of patients with NETs. A randomized, double-blind study in patients with metastatic midgut carcinoids demonstrated a marked lengthening of time to progression (14.3 vs 6 months, $P = .000072$) from the use of octreotide-LAR. This improvement was seen in patients with limited liver involvement. Whether this change will result in extended survival has not been proved. Somatostatin analogues can induce apoptosis in carcinoid tumors, and interferon α can decrease Bcl-2 protein expression, which probably contributes to its antiproliferative effects.

Hepatic embolization and chemoembolization (with dacarbazine, cisplatin, doxorubicin, 5-fluorouracil, or streptozotocin) have been reported to decrease tumor bulk and help control the symptoms of the hormone-excess state. These modalities generally are reserved for liver-directed therapy in cases in which treatment with somatostatin analogues, interferon (carcinoids), or chemotherapy (PETs) fails. Embolization, when combined with treatment with octreotide and interferon α, significantly reduces tumor progression ($P = .008$) compared with treatment with embolization and octreotide alone in patients with advanced midgut carcinoids.

Radiotherapy with radiolabeled somatostatin analogues that are internalized by the tumors is being investigated. Three different radionuclides are being used. High doses of ^{111}In-DTPA-d-Phe^{1}octreotide, which emits γ-rays, internal conversion, and Auger electrons; yttrium-90, which emits high-energy β-particles coupled by a DOTA chelating group to octreotide or octreotate; and ^{177}lutetium-coupled analogues, which emit both, are all in clinical studies. ^{111}Indium-, ^{90}yttrium-, and ^{177}lutetium-labeled compounds caused tumor stabilization in 41–81%, 44–88%, and 23–40%, respectively, and a decrease in tumor size in 8–30%, 6–37%, and 38%, respectively, of patients with advanced metastatic NETs. Use of ^{177}Lu-labeled analogues to treat 504 patients with malignant NETs produced a reduction of tumor size of >50% in 30% of patients (2% complete) and tumor stabilization in 51%. An effect on survival has not been established. These results suggest that this novel therapy may be helpful, especially in patients with widespread metastatic disease.

Selective internal radiation therapy using ^{90}yttrium glass or resin microspheres is being evaluated in patients with unresectable NET liver metastases. The treatment requires careful evaluation for vascular shunting before treatment and generally is reserved for patients without extrahepatic metastatic disease and with adequate hepatic reserve. The ^{90}Y-microspheres are delivered to the liver by intraarterial injection from percutaneous placed catheters. In four studies involving metastatic NETs, the response rate varied from 50–61% (partial or complete), tumor stabilization occurred in 22–41%, and overall survival varied from 25–70 months. In the largest study (148 patients), no radiation-induced liver failure occurred and the most common side effect was fatigue (6.5%).

The use of liver transplantation has been abandoned for treatment of most metastatic tumors to the liver. However, for metastatic NETs, it is still a consideration. In a review of 103 cases of malignant NETs (48 PETs, 43 carcinoids) the 2- and 5-year survival rates were 60% and 47%, respectively. However, recurrence-free survival was low (<24%). For younger patients with metastatic NETs limited to the liver, liver transplantation may be justified.

Newer approaches show some promise in the treatment of advanced GI NETs. They include the use of growth factor inhibitors or inhibitors of their receptors (using tyrosine kinase inhibitors, monoclonal antibodies), inhibitors of mTor signaling (everolimus, temsirolimus), angiogenesis inhibitors, and VEGF or VEGF receptor tyrosine kinase inhibitors. A number of these agents, particularly sunitinib (tyrosine kinase inhibitor), various mTor inhibitors, and bevacizumub (monoclonal antibody against VEGF), show impressive activity. Additional value may result from selected combinations of agents.

CHAPTER 50

MULTIPLE ENDOCRINE NEOPLASIA

Camilo Jimenez Vasquez ■ Robert F. Gagel

NEOPLASTIC DISORDERS AFFECTING MULTIPLE ENDOCRINE ORGANS

Multiple endocrine neoplasia (MEN) syndrome is defined as a disorder with neoplasms in two or more different hormonal tissues in several members of a family. Several distinct genetic disorders predispose to endocrine gland neoplasia and cause hormone excess syndromes (Table 50-1). DNA-based genetic testing is available for these disorders, but effective management requires an understanding of endocrine neoplasia and the range of clinical features that may be manifested in an individual patient.

MULTIPLE ENDOCRINE NEOPLASIA TYPE 1

MEN 1, or Wermer's syndrome, is inherited as an autosomal dominant trait. This syndrome is characterized by neoplasia of the parathyroid glands, enteropancreatic tumors, anterior pituitary adenomas, and other neuroendocrine tumors with variable penetrance (Table 50-1). Although rare, MEN 1 is the most common MEN syndrome, with an estimated prevalence of 2–20 per 100,000 in the general population. It is caused by inactivating mutations of the tumor-suppressor gene *MEN1* located at chromosome 11q13. The *MEN1* gene codes for a nuclear protein called Menin. Menin

TABLE 50-1

DISEASE ASSOCIATIONS IN THE MULTIPLE ENDOCRINE NEOPLASIA (MEN) SYNDROMES

MEN 1	MEN 2	MIXED SYNDROMES
Parathyroid hyperplasia or adenoma	**MEN 2A**	**Von Hippel–Lindau syndrome**
Islet cell hyperplasia, adenoma, or carcinoma	MTC	Pheochromocytoma
Pituitary hyperplasia or adenoma	Pheochromocytoma	Islet cell tumor
Other, less common manifestations: foregut carcinoid, pheochromocytoma, visceral subcutaneous or lipomas	Parathyroid hyperplasia or adenoma	Renal cell carcinoma
	MEN 2A with cutaneous lichen amyloidosis	Hemangioblastoma of central nervous system
	MEN 2A with Hirschsprung disease	Retinal angiomas
	Familial MTC	**Neurofibromatosis with features of MEN 1 or 2**
	MEN 2B	**Carney complex**
	MTC	Myxomas of heart, skin, and breast
	Pheochromocytoma	Spotty cutaneous pigmentation
	Mucosal and gastrointestinal neuromas	Testicular, adrenal, and GH-producing pituitary tumors
	Marfanoid features	Peripheral nerve schwannomas
		Familial growth hormone or prolactin-producing pituitary tumors

Abbreviations: GH, growth hormone; MTC, medullary thyroid carcinoma.

interacts with JunD, suppressing JunD-dependent transcriptional activation. It is unclear how this accounts for Menin growth regulatory activity, since JunD is associated with inhibition of cell growth. Each child born to an affected parent has a 50% probability of inheriting the gene. The variable penetrance of the several neoplastic components can make the differential diagnosis and treatment challenging.

CLINICAL MANIFESTATIONS

Primary hyperparathyroidism is the most common manifestation of MEN 1, with an estimated penetrance of 95–100%. Hypercalcemia may develop during the teenage years, and most individuals are affected by age 40 years (Fig. 50-1). Hyperparathyroidism is the earliest manifestation of the syndrome in most MEN 1 patients. The neoplastic changes in hyperparathyroidism provide a specific example of one of the cardinal features of endocrine tumors in MEN 1: multicentricity. The neoplastic changes inevitably affect multiple parathyroid glands, making surgical cure difficult. Screening for hyperparathyroidism involves measurement of either an albumin-adjusted or an ionized serum calcium level. The diagnosis is established by demonstrating elevated levels of serum calcium and intact parathyroid hormone. Manifestations of hyperparathyroidism in MEN 1 do not differ substantially from those in sporadic hyperparathyroidism and include calcium-containing kidney stones, kidney failure, nephrocalcinosis, bone abnormalities (i.e., osteoporosis, osteitis fibrosa cystica), and gastrointestinal and musculoskeletal complaints. Management is challenging because of early onset, significant recurrence rates, and the multiplicity of parathyroid gland involvement. Differentiation of hyperparathyroidism of MEN 1 from other forms of familial primary hyperparathyroidism usually is based on family history, histologic features of resected parathyroid tissue, the presence of a *MEN1* mutation, and sometimes long-term observation to determine whether other manifestations of MEN 1 develop. Parathyroid hyperplasia is the most common cause of hyperparathyroidism in MEN 1, although single and multiple adenomas have been described. Hyperplasia of one or more parathyroid glands is common in younger patients; adenomas usually are found in older patients or those with long-standing disease.

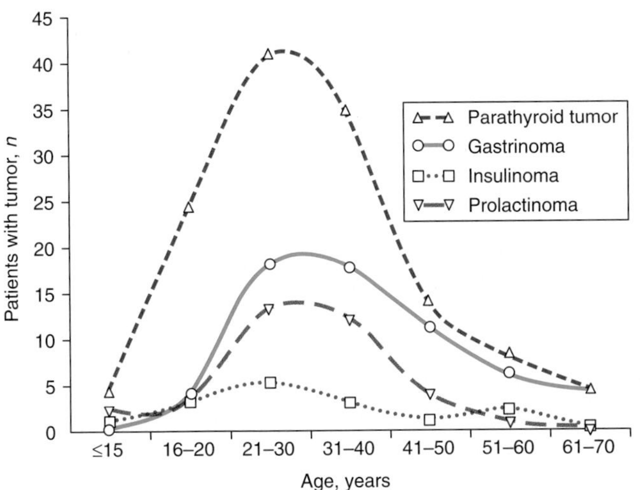

FIGURE 50-1
Age at onset of endocrine tumor expression in multiple endocrine neoplasia type 1 (MEN 1). Data derived from retrospective analysis for each endocrine organ hyperfunction in 130 cases of MEN 1. Age at onset is the age at first symptom or, with tumors not causing symptoms, age at the time of the first abnormal finding on a screening test result. The rate of diagnosis of hyperparathyroidism increased sharply between ages 16 and 20 years. (*Reprinted with permission from S Marx et al: Ann Intern Med 129:484, 1998.*)

Enteropancreatic tumors are the second most common manifestation of MEN 1, with an estimated penetrance of 50%. They tend to occur in parallel with hyperparathyroidism (Fig. 50-1); 30% are malignant. Most of these tumors secrete peptide hormones that cause specific clinical syndromes. Those syndromes, however, may have an insidious onset and a slow progression, making their diagnosis difficult and in many cases delayed. Some enteropancreatic tumors do not secrete hormones. Those "silent" tumors usually are found during radiographic screening. Metastasis, most commonly to the liver, occurs in about a third of patients.

Gastrinomas are the most common enteropancreatic tumors observed in MEN 1 patients and result in the Zollinger-Ellison syndrome (ZES). ZES is caused by excessive gastrin production and occurs in more than half of MEN 1 patients with small carcinoid-like tumors in the duodenal wall or, less often, by pancreatic islet cell tumors. There may be more than one gastrin-producing tumor, making localization difficult. The robust acid production may cause esophagitis, duodenal ulcers throughout the duodenum, ulcers involving the proximal jejunum, and diarrhea. The ulcer diathesis is commonly refractory to conservative therapy such as antacids. The diagnosis is made by finding increased gastric acid secretion, elevated basal gastrin levels in the serum (generally >115 pmol/L [200 pg/mL]), and an exaggerated response of serum gastrin to either secretin or calcium. Other causes of elevated serum gastrin levels, such as achlorhydria, treatment with H_2 receptor antagonists or proton pump inhibitors, retained gastric antrum, small-bowel resection, gastric outlet obstruction, and hypercalcemia, should be excluded (Fig. 50-1). High-resolution, early-phase computed tomography (CT) scanning, abdominal magnetic resonance imaging (MRI) with contrast, octreotide scan, and endoscopic ultrasound are the best preoperative techniques for identification of the primary and metastatic gastrinoma; intraoperative ultrasonography is the most sensitive method for detection of small tumors. Approximately one-fourth of all cases of ZES occur in the context of MEN 1.

Insulinomas are the second most common enteropancreatic tumors in patients who have MEN 1. Unlike gastrinomas, most insulinomas originate in the pancreas bed, becoming the most common pancreatic tumor in MEN 1. Hypoglycemia caused by insulinomas is observed in about one-third of MEN 1 patients with pancreatic islet cell tumors (Fig. 50-1). The tumors may be benign or malignant (25%). The diagnosis can be suggested by documenting hypoglycemia during a short fast with simultaneous inappropriate elevation of serum insulin and C-peptide levels. More commonly, it is necessary to subject the patient to a supervised 12- to 72-h fast to provoke hypoglycemia. Large insulinomas may be identified by CT or MRI scanning; small tumors not detected by conventional radiographic techniques may be localized by endoscopic ultrasound or selective arteriographic injection of calcium into each of the arteries that supply the pancreas and sampling of the hepatic vein for insulin to determine the anatomic region containing the tumor. Intraoperative ultrasonography is used frequently to localize these tumors. The trend toward earlier diagnosis of, hence, smaller tumors has reduced the usefulness of octreotide scanning, which is positive in a minority of these patients.

Glucagonoma, which is seen occasionally in MEN 1, causes a syndrome of hyperglycemia, skin rash (necrolytic migratory erythema), anorexia, glossitis, anemia, depression, diarrhea, and venous thrombosis. In about half of these patients, the plasma glucagon level is high, leading to its designation as the *glucagonoma syndrome,* although elevation of the plasma glucagon level in MEN 1 patients is not necessarily associated with these symptoms. Some patients with this syndrome also have elevated plasma ghrelin levels. The glucagonoma syndrome may represent a complex interaction between glucagon and ghrelin overproduction and the nutritional status of the patient.

The *Verner-Morrison,* or *watery diarrhea, syndrome* consists of watery diarrhea, hypokalemia, hypochlorhydria, and metabolic acidosis. The diarrhea can be voluminous and almost always is found in association with an islet cell tumor in the context of MEN 1, prompting use of the term *pancreatic cholera.* However, when not associated with MEN 1, the syndrome outside of MEN 1 is not restricted to pancreatic islet tumors and has been observed with carcinoids or other tumors. This syndrome is believed to be due to overproduction of vasoactive intestinal peptide (VIP), although plasma VIP levels may not be elevated. Hypercalcemia may be induced by the effects of VIP to stimulate osteoclastic bone resorption as well as by hyperparathyroidism. Other disorders that should be considered in the differential diagnosis of chronic diarrhea include infectious or parasitic diseases, inflammatory bowel disease, sprue, and other endocrine causes such as ZES, carcinoid, and medullary thyroid carcinoma.

The pancreatic neoplasms differ from the other components of MEN 1 in that approximately one-third of the tumors display malignant features, including hepatic metastases. The pancreatic neoplasms also can be used to highlight another characteristic of MEN 1: the specific impact of a hormone produced by one component of MEN 1 on another neoplastic component of this syndrome. Specific examples include the effects of either corticotropin-releasing hormone (CRH) or growth hormone–releasing hormone (GHRH) production by an islet cell tumor to cause a syndrome of excess adrenocorticotropin (ACTH) (Cushing's disease) or growth hormone (GH) (acromegaly) production by the pituitary gland. These secondary interactions add complexity to the diagnosis and management of these tumor syndromes. Pancreatic islet cell tumors are diagnosed by identification of a characteristic clinical syndrome, hormonal assays with or without provocative stimuli, or radiographic techniques. One approach involves annual screening of individuals at risk with measurement of basal and meal-stimulated levels of pancreatic polypeptide to identify the tumors as early as possible; the rationale for this screening strategy is the concept that surgical removal of islet cell tumors at an early stage will be curative. Other approaches to screening include measurement of serum gastrin and pancreatic polypeptide levels every 2–3 years, with the rationale that pancreatic neoplasms will be detected at a later stage but can be managed medically, if possible, or by surgery. High-resolution, early-phase CT scanning or endoscopic ultrasound provides the best preoperative technique for identification of these tumors; intraoperative ultrasonography is the most sensitive method for detection of small tumors. Although fluorodeoxyglucose–positron emission tomography (FDG-PET) scanning detects ~50% of pancreatic islet cell tumors, most of these tumors are large; as most of these tumors can be identified by CT or ultrasound, the lack of sensitivity for small tumors makes FDG-PET scanning unhelpful for early diagnosis.

Pituitary tumors occur in 20–30% of patients with MEN 1 and tend to be multicentric. These tumors can exhibit aggressive behavior and local invasiveness that makes them difficult to resect. Prolactinomas are the most common (Fig. 50-1) and are diagnosed by finding serum prolactin levels >200 μg/L with or without a pituitary mass evident on MRI. Values <200 μg/L may be due to a prolactin-secreting neoplasm or to compression of the pituitary stalk by a different type of pituitary tumor. Acromegaly due to excessive GH production is the second most common syndrome caused by pituitary tumors in MEN 1 and can rarely be due to production of

GHRH by an islet cell tumor (see earlier discussion). The possibility of hereditary growth hormone– or prolactin-secreting tumors (discussed in "Other Genetic Endocrine Tumor Syndromes" later in this chapter) should be considered in the differential diagnosis. Cushing's disease can be caused by ACTH-producing pituitary tumors or by ectopic production of ACTH or CRH by other components of the MEN 1 syndrome, including islet cell or carcinoid tumors or adrenal adenomas. Diagnosis of pituitary Cushing's disease is generally best accomplished by a high-dose dexamethasone suppression test or by petrosal venous sinus sampling for ACTH after IV injection of CRH. Differentiation of a primary pituitary tumor from an ectopic CRH-producing tumor may be difficult because the pituitary is the source of ACTH in both disorders; documentation of CRH production by a pancreatic islet or carcinoid tumor may be the only method of proving ectopic CRH production.

Adrenal cortical tumors are found in almost half of gene carriers but are rarely functional; malignancy in cortical adenomas is uncommon. Rare cases of pheochromocytoma have been described in the context of MEN 1. Due to their rarity, screening for these tumors is indicated only when there are suggestive symptoms.

Carcinoid tumors in MEN 1 are of the foregut type and are derived from thymus, lung, stomach, or duodenum; they may metastasize or be locally invasive. These tumors usually produce serotonin, calcitonin, or CRH; the typical carcinoid syndrome with flushing, diarrhea, and bronchospasm is rare (Chap. 49). Mediastinal carcinoid tumors (an upper mediastinal mass) are more common in men; bronchial carcinoid tumors are more common in women. Carcinoid tumors are a late manifestation of MEN 1; some reports have emphasized the importance of routine chest CT screening for mediastinal carcinoid tumors because of their high rate of malignant transformation and aggressive behavior.

Unusual manifestations of MEN 1

Subcutaneous or visceral lipomas and cutaneous leiomyomas also may be present but rarely undergo malignant transformation. Skin angiofibromas or collagenomas are seen in most patients with MEN 1 when carefully sought.

GENETIC CONSIDERATIONS

MEN1 gene mutations are found in >90% of families with the syndrome (Fig. 50-2). Genetic testing can be performed in individuals at risk for the development of MEN 1 and is commercially available in the United States and Europe. The major value of genetic testing in a kindred with an identifiable mutation is the assignment or exclusion of gene carrier status. In those identified as carrying the mutant gene, routine screening for individual manifestations of MEN 1 should be performed as outlined earlier. Those with negative genetic test results in a kindred with a known germ-line mutation can be excluded from further screening for MEN 1. A significant percentage of sporadic parathyroid, islet cell, and carcinoid tumors also have loss or mutation of *MEN1*. There is no correlation between a particular germ-line mutation and a clinical phenotype. It is presumed that these mutations are somatic and occur in a single cell, leading to subsequent transformation.

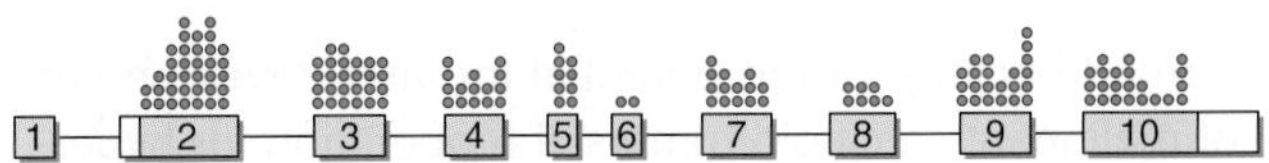

FIGURE 50-2
Schematic depiction of the MEN1 gene and the distribution of mutations. The shaded areas show coding sequence. The closed circles show the relative distribution of mutations, mostly inactivating, in each exon. Mutation data are derived from the Human Gene Mutation Database, from which more detailed information can be obtained at *www.uwcm.ac.uk/uwcm/mg/hgmd0.html*. *(From M Krawczak, DN Cooper: Trends Genet 13:1321, 1998.)*

TREATMENT Multiple Endocrine Neoplasia Type 1

Almost everyone who inherits a mutant *MEN1* gene develops at least one clinical manifestation of the syndrome. Most develop hyperparathyroidism, 80% develop pancreatic islet cell tumors, and more than half develop pituitary tumors. For most of these tumors, initial surgery is not curative and patients frequently require multiple surgical procedures and surgery on two or more endocrine glands during a lifetime. For this reason, it is essential to establish clear goals for management of these patients rather than to recommend surgery casually each time a tumor is discovered. Ranges for acceptable management are discussed below.

HYPERPARATHYROIDISM Individuals with serum calcium levels >3.0 mmol/L (12 mg/dL), evidence of calcium nephrolithiasis or renal dysfunction, neuropathic or muscular symptoms, or bone involvement (including osteopenia) and individuals <50 years of age should undergo parathyroid exploration. There is less agreement about the necessity for parathyroid exploration in individuals who do not meet these criteria, and observation may be appropriate in MEN 1 patients with asymptomatic hyperparathyroidism.

When parathyroid surgery is indicated in MEN 1, there are two approaches. In the first, all parathyroid tissue is identified and removed at the time of primary operation, and parathyroid tissue is implanted in the nondominant forearm. Thymectomy also should be performed because of the potential for later development of malignant carcinoid tumors. If reoperation for hyperparathyroidism is necessary at a later date, transplanted parathyroid tissue can be resected from the forearm with titration of tissue removal to lower the intact parathyroid hormone (PTH) to <50% of basal.

Another approach is to remove 3–3.5 parathyroid glands from the neck (leaving ~50 mg of parathyroid tissue), carefully marking the location of residual tissue so that the remaining tissue can be located easily during subsequent surgery. If this approach is used, intraoperative PTH measurements should be utilized to monitor adequacy of removal of parathyroid tissue with a goal of reducing postoperative serum intact PTH to ≤50% of basal values.

The use of high-resolution CT scanning (1 mm) and imaging during three phases of contrast flow has substantially improved the ability to identify aberrantly located parathyroid tissue. As this issue arises with some frequency in the context of parathyroid disease in MEN 1, this technique should be utilized to locate parathyroid tissue before reoperation for a failed exploration, and it may be useful before the initial operation.

PANCREATIC ISLET CELL TUMORS **(See Chap. 49 for discussion of pancreatic islet cell tumors not associated with MEN 1.)** Two features of pancreatic islet cell tumors in MEN 1 complicate management. First, the tumors are multicentric, are malignant about one-third of the time, and cause death in 10–20% of patients. Second, performance of a total pancreatectomy to prevent malignancy causes diabetes mellitus, a disease with significant long-term complications that include neuropathy, retinopathy, and nephropathy. These features make it difficult to formulate clear-cut guidelines, but some general concepts appear to be valid. (1) Islet cell tumors producing insulin, glucagon, VIP, GHRH, or CRH should be resected because medical therapy for the hormonal effects of these tumors are generally ineffective. (2) Gastrin-producing islet cell tumors that cause ZES are frequently multicentric. Recent experience suggests that a high percentage of ZES in MEN 1 is caused by duodenal wall carcinoid tumors and that resection of these tumors improves the cure rate. Treatment with H_2 receptor antagonists (cimetidine or ranitidine) or proton pump inhibitors (omeprazole, lansoprazole, esomeprazole, etc.) provides an alternative, and some think preferable, therapy to surgery for control of ulcer disease in patients with multicentric tumors or hepatic metastases. (3) In families with a high incidence of malignant islet cell tumors that cause death, total pancreatectomy at an early age may be considered to prevent malignancy, although it should be noted that this surgical intervention does not prevent the development of neuroendocrine tumors outside the pancreatoduodenal region.

Management of metastatic islet cell carcinoma is unsatisfactory. Hormonal abnormalities sometimes can be controlled. For example, ZES can be treated with H_2 receptor antagonists or proton pump inhibitors; the somatostatin analogues octreotide and lanreotide are useful in the management of carcinoid, glucagonoma, and the watery diarrhea syndrome. Bilateral adrenalectomy may be required for ectopic ACTH syndrome if medical therapy is ineffective. Islet cell carcinomas frequently metastasize to the liver but may grow slowly. Hepatic artery embolization, radiofrequency ablation, or chemotherapy (5-fluorouracil, streptozocin, chlorozotocin, doxorubicin, or dacarbazine) may reduce tumor streptozotocin mass, control symptoms of hormone excess, and prolong life; however, these treatments are never curative. There is evolving evidence that everolimus, an inhibitor of mTor (mammalian target of rapamycin) causes regression of tumor size; 2 of 13 islet cell carcinomas and 2 of 12 carcinoid tumors had a >30% reduction in size and >60% had stable disease.

PITUITARY TUMORS Treatment of prolactinomas with dopamine agonists (bromocriptine, cabergoline, or quinagolide) usually returns the serum prolactin level to normal and prevents further tumor growth. Surgical resection of a prolactinoma is rarely curative but may relieve mass effects. Transsphenoidal resection is appropriate for neoplasms that secrete ACTH, GH, or the α subunit of the pituitary glycoprotein hormones. Octreotide reduces tumor mass in one-third of GH-secreting tumors and reduces GH and insulin-like growth factor I levels in >75% of patients. Pegvisomant, a GH antagonist, rapidly lowers insulin-like growth factor levels in patients with acromegaly. Radiation therapy may be useful for large or recurrent tumors.

Improvements in the management of MEN 1, particularly the earlier recognition of islet cell and pituitary tumors, have improved outcomes in these patients. As a result, other neoplastic manifestations that develop later in the course of this disorder, such as carcinoid syndrome, are now seen with increased frequency.

MULTIPLE ENDOCRINE NEOPLASIA TYPE 2

CLINICAL MANIFESTATIONS

Medullary thyroid carcinoma (MTC) and pheochromocytoma are associated in two major syndromes: MEN type 2A and MEN type 2B (Table 50-1). MEN 2A is the combination of MTC, hyperparathyroidism, and pheochromocytoma. Three subvariants of MEN 2A are familial medullary thyroid carcinoma (FMTC), MEN 2A with cutaneous lichen amyloidosis, and MEN 2A with Hirschsprung disease. MEN 2B is the combination of MTC, pheochromocytoma, mucosal neuromas, intestinal ganglioneuromatosis, and marfanoid features.

Multiple endocrine neoplasia type 2A

MTC is the most common manifestation. This tumor usually develops in childhood, beginning as hyperplasia of the calcitonin-producing cells (C cells) of the thyroid. MTC typically is located at the junction of the upper one-third and lower two-thirds of each lobe of the thyroid, reflecting the high density of C cells in this location; tumors >1 cm in size frequently are associated with local or distant metastases.

Pheochromocytoma occurs in ~50% of patients with MEN 2A and causes palpitations, nervousness, headaches, and sometimes sweating (Chap. 51). About half of the tumors are bilateral, and >50% of patients who have had unilateral adrenalectomy develop a pheochromocytoma in the contralateral gland within a decade. A second feature of these tumors is a disproportionate increase in the secretion of epinephrine relative to norepinephrine. This characteristic differentiates the MEN 2 pheochromocytomas from sporadic pheochromocytoma and those associated with von Hippel–Lindau (VHL) syndrome, hereditary paraganglioma, or neurofibromatosis. Capsular invasion is common, but metastasis is uncommon. Finally, the pheochromocytomas almost always are found in the adrenal gland, differentiating the pheochromocytomas in MEN 2 from the extraadrenal tumors more commonly found in hereditary paraganglioma syndromes.

Hyperparathyroidism occurs in 15–20% of patients, with the peak incidence in the third or fourth decade. The manifestations of hyperparathyroidism do not differ from those in other forms of primary hyperparathyroidism (Chap. 51). Diagnosis is established by finding hypercalcemia, hypophosphatemia, hypercalciuria, and an inappropriately high serum level of intact PTH. Multiglandular parathyroid hyperplasia is the most common histologic finding, although with long-standing disease adenomatous changes may be superimposed on hyperplasia.

The most common subvariant of MEN 2A is familial MTC, an autosomal dominant syndrome in which MTC is the only manifestation (Table 50-1). The clinical diagnosis of FMTC is established by the identification of MTC in multiple generations without a pheochromocytoma. Since the penetrance of pheochromocytoma is 50% in MEN 2A, it is possible that MEN 2A could masquerade as FMTC in small kindreds. It is important to consider this possibility carefully before classifying a kindred as having FMTC; failure to do so could lead to death or serious morbidity from pheochromocytoma in an affected kindred member. The difficulty of differentiating MEN 2A and FMTC is discussed further later.

Multiple endocrine neoplasia type 2B

The association of MTC, pheochromocytoma, mucosal neuromas, and a marfanoid habitus is designated MEN 2B. MTC in MEN 2B develops earlier and is more aggressive than in MEN 2A. Metastatic disease has been described before 1 year of age, and death may occur in the second or third decade of life. However, the prognosis is not invariably bad even in patients with metastatic disease, as evidenced by a number of multigenerational families with this disease.

Pheochromocytoma occurs in more than half of MEN 2B patients and does not differ from that in MEN 2A. Hypercalcemia is rare in MEN 2B, and there are no well-documented examples of hyperparathyroidism.

The mucosal neuromas and marfanoid body habitus are the most distinctive features and are recognizable in childhood. Neuromas are present on the tip of the tongue, under the eyelids, and throughout the gastrointestinal tract and are true neuromas, distinct from neurofibromas. The most common presentation in children relates to gastrointestinal symptomatology, including intermittent colic, pseudoobstruction, and diarrhea.

GENETIC CONSIDERATIONS

Mutations of the *RET* protooncogene have been identified in most patients with MEN 2 (Fig. 50-3). *RET* encodes a tyrosine kinase receptor that in combination with a co-receptor, GFRα, normally is activated by glial cell–derived neurotrophic factor (GDNF) or other members of this transforming growth factor β–like family of peptides, including artemin, persephin, and neurturin. In the C cell there is evidence that persephin normally activates the *RET*/GFRα-4 receptor complex and is partially responsible for migration of the C cells into the thyroid gland, whereas in the developing neuronal system of the gastrointestinal tract, GDNF activates the *RET*/GFRα-1 complex. *RET* mutations induce constitutive activity of the receptor, explaining the autosomal dominant transmission of the disorder.

Naturally occurring mutations localize to two regions of the *RET* tyrosine kinase receptor. The first is a cysteine-rich extracellular domain; point mutations in the coding sequence for one of six cysteines (codons 609, 611, 618, 620, 630, and 634) cause amino acid substitutions that induce receptor dimerization and activation in the absence of its ligand. Codon 634 mutations occur in 80% of MEN 2A kindreds and are most commonly associated with classic MEN 2A features (Figs. 50-3 and 50-2); an arginine substitution at this codon accounts for half of all MEN 2A mutations. All reported families with MEN 2A and cutaneous lichen amyloidosis have a codon 634 mutation. Mutations of codon 609, 611, 618, or 620 occur in 10–15% of MEN 2A kindreds and

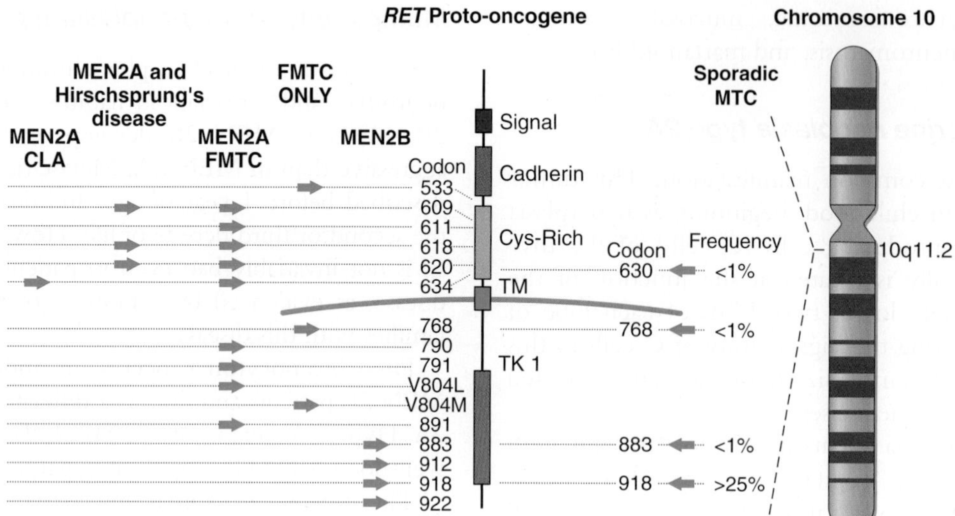

FIGURE 50-3

Schematic diagram of the RET protooncogene showing mutations found in multiple endocrine neoplasia (MEN) type 2 and sporadic medullary thyroid carcinoma (MTC). The *RET* protooncogene is located on the proximal arm of chromosome 10q (10q11.2). Activating mutations of two functional domains of RET tyrosine kinase receptor have been identified. The first affects a cysteine-rich (Cys-Rich) region in the extracellular portion of the receptor. Each germ-line mutation changes a cysteine at codons 609, 611, 618, 620, or 634 to another amino acid. The second region is the intracellular tyrosine kinase (TK) domain. Codon 634 mutations account for ~80% of all germ-line mutations. Mutations of codons 630, 768, 883, and 918 have been identified as somatic (non–germ-line) mutations that occur in a single parafollicular or C cell within the thyroid gland in sporadic MTC. A codon 918 mutation is the most common somatic mutation. Cadherin, a cadherin-like region in the extracellular domain; CLA, cutaneous lichen amyloidosis; FMTC, familial medullary thyroid carcinoma; MEN2, multiple endocrine neoplasia type 2; Signal, the signal peptide; TK, tyrosine kinase domain; TM, transmembrane domain.

are more commonly associated with FMTC (Fig. 50-3). Mutations in codons 609, 618, and 620 also have been identified in a variant of MEN 2A that includes Hirschsprung disease (Fig. 50-3). The second region of the *RET* tyrosine kinase that is mutated in MEN 2 is in the substrate recognition pocket at codon 918 (Fig. 50-3). This activating mutation is present in ~95% of patients with MEN 2B and accounts for 5% of all *RET* protooncogene mutations in MEN 2. Mutations of codon 883 and 922 also have been identified in a few patients with MEN 2B.

Uncommon mutations (<5% of the total) include those of codons 533 (exon 8), 666, 768, 777, 790, 791, 804, 891, and 912. Mutations associated with only FMTC include codons 533, 768, and 912. With greater experience, mutations that once were associated with FMTC only (666, 791, V804L, V804M, and 891) have been found in MEN 2A as there have been occasional descriptions of pheochromocytoma. At present it is reasonable to conclude that only kindreds with codon 533, 768, or 912 mutations are consistently associated with FMTC; in kindreds with all other *RET* mutations, pheochromocytoma is a possibility. The recognition that germ-line mutations occur in at least 6% of patients with apparently sporadic MTC has led to the firm recommendation that all patients with MTC should be screened for these mutations. The effort to screen patients with sporadic MTC, combined with the fact that new kindreds with classic MEN 2A are being recognized less frequently has led to a shift in the mutation frequencies. These findings mirror results in other malignancies in which germ-line mutations of cancer-causing genes contribute to a greater percentage of apparently sporadic cancer than was considered previously. The recognition of new *RET* mutations suggests that more will be identified in the future.

Somatic mutations (found only in the tumor and not transmitted in the germ line) of the *RET* protooncogene have been identified in sporadic MTC; 25–60% of sporadic tumors have codon 918 mutations, and somatic mutations in codons 630, 768, and 804 have been identified (Fig. 50-3).

TREATMENT Multiple Endocrine Neoplasia Type 2

SCREENING FOR MULTIPLE ENDOCRINE NEOPLASIA TYPE 2 Death from MTC can be prevented by early thyroidectomy. The identification of *RET* protooncogene mutations and the application of DNA-based molecular diagnostic techniques to identify these mutations have simplified the screening process. During the initial evaluation of a kindred, a *RET* protooncogene analysis should be performed on an individual with proven MEN 2A. Establishment of the specific germ-line mutation facilitates the subsequent analysis of other family members. Each family member at risk should be tested twice for the presence of the specific mutation; the second analysis should be performed on a new DNA sample and, ideally, in a second laboratory to exclude sample mix-up or technical error (see *www.genetests.org* for an up-to-date list of laboratory testing sites). Both false-positive and false-negative analyses have been described. A false-negative test result is of the greatest concern because calcitonin testing is now rarely performed as a diagnostic backup study; if there is a genetic test error, a child may present in the second or third decade with metastatic MTC. Individuals in a kindred with a known mutation who have two normal analyses can be excluded from further screening.

There is a consensus that children with codon 883, 918, and 922 mutations, those associated with MEN 2B, should have a total thyroidectomy and central lymph node dissection (level VI) performed during the first months of life or soon after identification of the syndrome. If local metastasis is discovered, a more extensive lymph node dissection (levels II to V) is generally indicated. In children with codon 611, 618, 620, 630, 634, and 891 mutations, thyroidectomy should be performed before age 6 years because of reports of local metastatic disease in children this age. Finally, there are kindreds with codon 609, 768, 790, 791, 804, and 912 mutations in which the phenotype of MTC appears to be less aggressive. A clinician caring for children with one of these mutations faces a dilemma. In many kindreds, there has never been a death from MTC caused by one of these mutations. However, in other kindreds, there are examples of metastatic disease occurring early in life. For example, metastatic disease before age 6 years has been described with codon 609 and 804 mutations and before age 14 years in a patient with a codon 912 mutation. In kindreds with these mutations, two management approaches have been suggested: (1) perform a total thyroidectomy with or without central node dissection at some arbitrary age (perhaps 6–10 years of age) or (2) continue annual or biannual calcitonin provocative testing with performance of total thyroidectomy with or without central neck dissection when the test becomes abnormal. The pentagastrin test involves measurement of serum calcitonin basally and 2, 5, 10, and 15 min after a bolus injection of 5 μg pentagastrin per kilogram of body weight. Patients should be warned before pentagastrin injection of epigastric tightness, nausea, warmth, and tingling of extremities and reassured that the symptoms will last ~2 min. If pentagastrin is unavailable, an alternative is a short calcium infusion performed by obtaining a baseline serum calcitonin and then infusing 150 mg calcium salt IV over 10 min with measurement of serum calcitonin at 5, 10, 15, 30 min after initiation of the infusion.

The *RET* protooncogene analysis should be performed in patients with suspected MEN 2B to detect codon 883, 918, and 922 mutations, especially in newborn children in whom the diagnosis is suspected but the clinical phenotype is not fully developed. Other family members at risk for MEN 2B also should be tested because the mucosal neuromas can be subtle. Most MEN 2B mutations represent de novo mutations derived from the paternal allele. In the rare families with proven germ-line transmission of MTC but no identifiable *RET* protooncogene mutation (sequencing of the entire *RET* gene should be performed), annual pentagastrin or calcium testing should be performed on members at risk.

Annual screening for pheochromocytoma in patients with germ-line *RET* mutations should be performed by measuring basal plasma or 24-h urine catecholamines and metanephrines. The goal is to identify a pheochromocytoma before it causes significant symptoms or is likely to cause sudden death, an event most commonly associated with large tumors. Although there are kindreds with FMTC and specific *RET* mutations in which no pheochromocytomas have been identified (Fig. 50-3), clinical experience is insufficient to exclude pheochromocytoma screening in these individuals. Radiographic studies such as MRI or CT scans generally are reserved for individuals with abnormal screening tests or symptoms suggestive of pheochromocytoma (Chap. 51). Women should be tested during pregnancy because undetected pheochromocytoma can cause maternal death during childbirth.

Measurement of serum calcium and parathyroid hormone levels every 2–3 years provides an adequate screen for hyperparathyroidism, except in families in which hyperparathyroidism is a prominent component, in which measurements should be made annually.

MEDULLARY THYROID CARCINOMA Hereditary MTC is a multicentric disorder. Total thyroidectomy with a central lymph node dissection should be performed in children who carry the mutant gene. Incomplete thyroidectomy leaves the possibility of later transformation of residual C cells. The goal of early therapy is cure, and a strategy that does not accomplish this goal is shortsighted. Long-term follow-up studies indicate an excellent outcome, with ~90% of children free of disease 15–20 years after surgery. In contrast, 15–25% of patients in whom the diagnosis is made on the basis of a palpable thyroid nodule die from the disease within 15–20 years.

In adults with MTC >1 cm in size, metastases to regional lymph nodes are common (>75%). Total thyroidectomy with central lymph node dissection and selective dissection of other regional chains provides the best chance for cure. In patients with extensive local metastatic disease in the neck, external radiation may prevent local recurrence or reduce tumor mass but is not curative. Chemotherapy with combinations of adriamycin, vincristine, cyclophosphamide, and dacarbazine may provide palliation. Clinical trials with small compounds (tyrosine kinase inhibitors) that interact with the ATP-binding pocket of the RET, vascular endothelial receptor, and type 2 and epidermal growth factor receptors and prevent phosphorylation have shown promise for treatment of hereditary and sporadic MTC. A phase I trial of vandetanib has shown that 45% of patients have a 30% or greater reduction of tumor size and prolongation of progression-free survival by at least 11 months. Similar phase II results have been observed for XL184, sunitinib, tipifarnib, and sorafenib, and phase II trials of E7080 and pazopanib are under way. It seems likely that one or more of these compounds will be approved for treatment of metastatic MTC within the next few years.

PHEOCHROMOCYTOMA The long-term goal for management of pheochromocytoma is to prevent death and cardiovascular complications. Improvements in radiographic imaging of the adrenals make direct examination of the apparently normal contralateral gland during surgery less important, and the rapid evolution of laparoscopic abdominal or retroperitoneal surgery has simplified management of early pheochromocytoma. The major question is whether to remove both adrenal glands or remove only the affected adrenal at the time of primary surgery. Issues to be considered in making this decision include the possibility of malignancy (<15 reported cases), the high probability of developing pheochromocytoma in the apparently unaffected gland over an 8- to 10-year period, and the risks of adrenal insufficiency caused by removal of both glands (at least two deaths related to adrenal insufficiency have occurred in MEN 2 patients). Most clinicians recommend removing only the affected gland. If both adrenals are removed, glucocorticoid and mineralocorticoid replacement is mandatory. An alternative approach is to perform a cortical-sparing adrenalectomy, removing the pheochromocytoma and adrenal medulla and leaving the adrenal cortex behind. This approach is usually successful and eliminates the necessity for steroid hormone replacement in most patients, although the pheochromocytoma recurs in a small percentage.

HYPERPARATHYROIDISM Hyperparathyroidism has been managed by one of two approaches. Removal of 3.5 glands with maintenance of the remaining half gland in the neck is the usual procedure. In families in which hyperparathyroidism is a prominent manifestation (almost always associated with a codon 634 *RET* mutation) and recurrence is common, total parathyroidectomy with transplantation of parathyroid tissue into the nondominant forearm is preferred. This approach is discussed earlier in the context of hyperparathyroidism associated with MEN 1.

OTHER GENETIC ENDOCRINE TUMOR SYNDROMES

A number of mixed syndromes exist in which the neoplastic associations differ from those in MEN 1 or 2 (Table 50-1).

The cause of VHL syndrome—the association of central nervous system tumors, renal cell carcinoma, pheochromocytoma, and islet cell neoplasms—is a mutation in the *VHL* tumor-suppressor gene. Germ-line-inactivating mutations of the *VHL* gene cause tumor formation when there is additional loss or somatic mutation of the normal *VHL* allele in brain, kidney, pancreatic islet, or adrenal medullary cells. Missense mutations been identified in >40% of VHL families with pheochromocytoma, suggesting that families with this type of mutation should be surveyed routinely for pheochromocytoma. A point that may be useful in differentiating VHL from MEN 1 (overlapping features include islet cell tumor and rare pheochromocytoma) or MEN 2 (overlapping feature is pheochromocytoma) is that hyperparathyroidism rarely occurs in VHL.

The molecular defect in type 1 neurofibromatosis inactivates neurofibromin, a cell membrane–associated protein that normally activates a GTPase. Inactivation of this protein impairs GTPase and causes continuous activation of p21 Ras and its downstream tyrosine kinase pathway. Endocrine tumors also form in less common neoplastic genetic syndromes. These include Cowden disease, Carney complex, familial growth hormone and prolactin tumors, and familial carcinoid syndrome. Carney complex includes myxomas of the heart, skin, and breast; peripheral nerve schwannomas; spotty skin pigmentation; and testicular, adrenal, and GH-secreting pituitary tumors. Linkage analysis has identified two loci: chromosome 2p in half of the families and 17q in the others. The 17q gene has been identified as the regulatory subunit (type IA) of protein kinase A (*PRKA1A*). Familial growth hormone–or prolactin-producing neoplasms without other manifestations of MEN 1 are caused by germ-line–inactivating mutation of the aryl hydrocarbon receptor interacting protein (AIP). It is transmitted in an autosomal dominant manner. Other types of endocrine tumors have not, to date, been associated with AIP mutations.

CHAPTER 51

PHEOCHROMOCYTOMA AND ADRENOCORTICAL CARCINOMA

Hartmut P. H. Neumann ■ Wiebke Arlt ■ Dan L. Longo

Pheochromocytomas and paragangliomas are catecholamine-producing tumors derived from the sympathetic or parasympathetic nervous system. These tumors may arise sporadically or be inherited as features of multiple endocrine neoplasia type 2 (MEN 2) or several other pheochromocytoma-associated syndromes. The diagnosis of pheochromocytomas provides a potentially correctable cause of hypertension, and their removal can prevent hypertensive crises that can be lethal. The clinical presentation is variable, ranging from an adrenal incidentaloma to a patient in hypertensive crisis with associated cerebrovascular or cardiac complications.

EPIDEMIOLOGY

Pheochromocytoma is estimated to occur in 2–8 of 1 million persons per year, and about 0.1% of hypertensive patients harbor a pheochromocytoma. Autopsy series reveal prevalence of 0.2%. The mean age at diagnosis is about 40 years, although the tumors can occur from early childhood until late in life. The "rule of 10s" for pheochromocytomas states that about 10% are bilateral, 10% are extraadrenal, and 10% are malignant. However, these percentages are higher in the inherited syndromes.

ETIOLOGY AND PATHOGENESIS

Pheochromocytomas and paragangliomas are well-vascularized tumors that arise from cells derived from the sympathetic (e.g., adrenal medulla) or parasympathetic (e.g., carotid body, glomus vagale) paraganglia (Fig. 51-1). The name *pheochromocytoma* reflects the black-colored staining caused by chromaffin oxidation of catecholamines. Although a variety of terms have been used to describe these tumors, most clinicians use the term *pheochromocytoma* to describe symptomatic catecholamine-producing tumors, including those in extraadrenal retroperitoneal, pelvic, and thoracic sites. The term *paraganglioma* is used to describe catecholamine-producing tumors in the head and neck. These tumors may secrete little or no catecholamines.

The etiology of sporadic pheochromocytomas and paragangliomas is unknown. However, about 25% of patients have an inherited condition, including germline mutations in the *RET, VHL, NF1, SDHB, SDHC, SDHD,* or *SDHAF2* genes. Biallelic gene inactivation has been demonstrated for the *VHL, NF1,* and *SDH* genes, whereas *RET* mutations activate the receptor tyrosine kinase activity. SDH is an enzyme of the Krebs cycle and the mitochondrial respiratory chain. The VHL protein is a component of a ubiquitin E3 ligase. *VHL* mutations reduce protein degradation, resulting in upregulation of components involved in cell cycle progression, glucose metabolism, and oxygen sensing.

CLINICAL FEATURES

The clinical presentation is so variable that pheochromocytoma has been termed "the great masquerader" (Table 51-1). Among the presenting symptoms, episodes of palpitations, headaches, and profuse sweating are typical and constitute a classic triad. The presence of all three symptoms in association with hypertension makes pheochromocytoma a likely diagnosis. However, a pheochromocytoma can be asymptomatic for years, and some tumors grow to a considerable size before patients note symptoms.

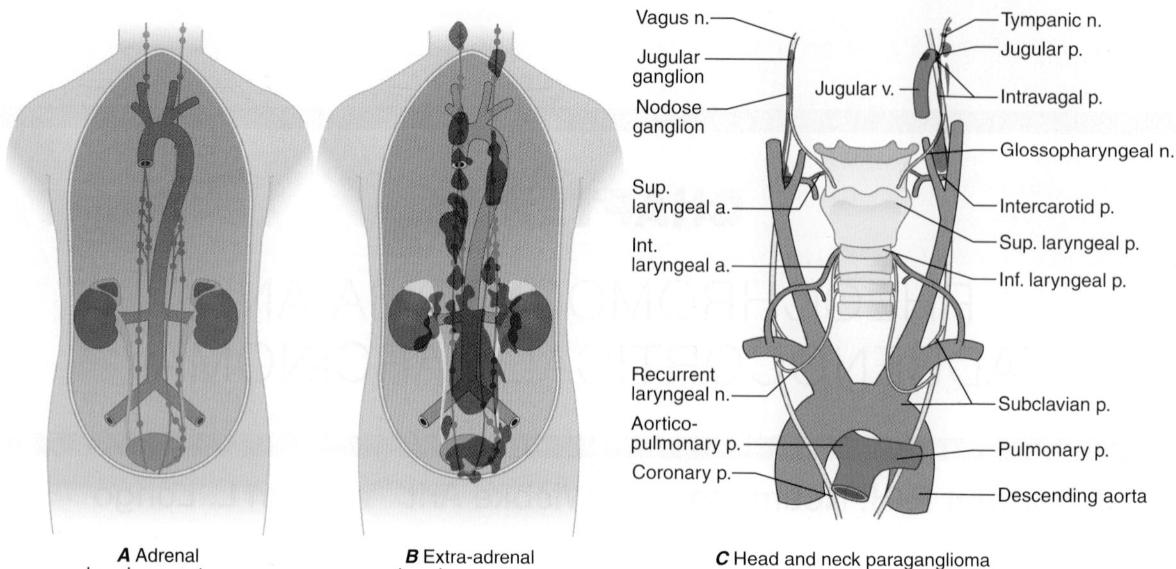

FIGURE 51-1

The paraganglial system and topographic sites (in red) of pheochromocytomas and paragangliomas. *(Parts A, and B from WM Manger, RW Gifford: Clinical and Experimental Pheochromocytoma. Cambridge: Blackwell Science, 1996; part C from GG Glenner, PM Grimley: Tumors of the Extra-adrenal Paraganglion System [Including Chemoreceptors], Atlas of Tumor Pathology, 2nd Series, Fascicle 9. Washington, DC: AFIP, 1974.)*

The dominant sign is hypertension. Classically, patients have episodic hypertension, but sustained hypertension is also common. Catecholamine crises can lead to heart failure, pulmonary edema, arrhythmias, and intracranial hemorrhage. During episodes of hormone release, which can occur at very divergent intervals, patients are anxious and pale, and they experience tachycardia and palpitations. These paroxysms generally last less than an hour and may be precipitated by surgery, positional changes, exercise, pregnancy, urination (particularly bladder pheochromocytomas), and various medications (e.g., tricyclic antidepressants, opiates, metoclopramide).

TABLE 51-1

CLINICAL FEATURES ASSOCIATED WITH PHEOCHROMOCYTOMA

HEADACHES	WEIGHT LOSS
Sweating attacks	Paradoxical response to antihypertensive drugs
Palpitations and tachycardia	Polyuria and polydipsia
Hypertension, sustained or paroxysmal	Constipation
Anxiety and panic attacks	Orthostatic hypotension
Pallor	Dilated cardiomyopathy
Nausea	Erythrocytosis
Abdominal pain	Elevated blood sugar
Weakness	Hypercalcemia

DIAGNOSIS

The diagnosis is based on documentation of catecholamine excess by biochemical testing and localization of the tumor by imaging. Both are of equal importance, although measurement of catecholamines is traditionally the first step.

BIOCHEMICAL TESTING

Pheochromocytomas and paragangliomas synthesize and store catecholamines, which include norepinephrine (noradrenaline), epinephrine (adrenaline), and dopamine. Elevated plasma and urinary levels of catecholamines and the methylated metabolites, metanephrines, are the cornerstone for the diagnosis. The hormonal activity of tumors fluctuates, resulting in considerable variation in serial catecholamine measurements. Thus, there is some value in obtaining tests during or soon after a symptomatic crisis. However, most tumors continuously leak O-methylated metabolites, which are detected by measurements of metanephrines.

Catecholamines and metanephrines can be measured by using different methods (e.g., high-performance liquid chromatography, enzyme-linked immunosorbent assay, and liquid chromatography/mass spectrometry).

In a clinical context suspicious for pheochromocytoma, when values are increased three times the upper limit of normal, a pheochromocytoma is highly likely regardless of the assay used. However, as summarized in Table 51-2, the sensitivity and specificity of available biochemical tests vary greatly, and these differences are important in assessing patients with borderline elevations of different compounds. Urinary tests for vanillylmandelic acid (VMA), metanephrines (total or fractionated), and catecholamines are widely available and are used commonly for initial testing. Among these tests, the fractionated metanephrines and catecholamines are the most sensitive. Plasma tests are more convenient and include measurements of catecholamines and metanephrines. Measurements of plasma metanephrine are the most sensitive and are less susceptible to false-positive elevations from stress, including venipuncture. Although the incidence of false-positive test results has been reduced by the introduction of newer assays, physiologic stress responses and medications that increase catecholamines still can confound testing. Because the tumors are relatively rare, borderline elevations are likely to be false positives. In this circumstance, it is important to exclude diet or drug exposure (withdrawal of levodopa, sympathomimetics, diuretics, tricyclic antidepressants, alpha and beta blockers) that might cause false positives and then repeat testing or perform a clonidine suppression test (measurement of plasma metanephrines 3 h after oral administration of 300 μg of clonidine). Other pharmacologic tests, such as the phentolamine test and the glucagon provocation test, are of relatively low sensitivity and are not recommended.

DIAGNOSTIC IMAGING

A variety of methods have been used to localize pheochromocytomas and paragangliomas (Table 51-2). Computed tomography (CT) and magnetic resonance imaging (MRI) are similar in sensitivity. CT should be performed with contrast. T2-weighted MRI with gadolinium contrast is optimal for detecting pheochromocytomas and is somewhat better than CT for imaging extra-adrenal pheochromocytomas and paragangliomas. About 5% of adrenal incidentalomas, which usually are detected by CT or MRI, prove to be pheochromocytomas after endocrinologic evaluation.

Tumors also can be localized by using radioactive tracers, including ^{131}I- or ^{123}I-metaiodobenzylguanidine (MIBG), ^{111}In-somatostatin analogues, or 18F-dopa (or dopamine) positron emission tomography (PET). Because these agents exhibit selective uptake in paragangliomas, nuclear imaging is particularly useful in the hereditary syndromes.

DIFFERENTIAL DIAGNOSIS

When one is entertaining the possibility of a pheochromocytoma, other disorders to consider include essential hypertension, anxiety attacks, use of cocaine or amphetamines, mastocytosis or carcinoid syndrome (usually lacking hypertension), intracranial lesions, clonidine withdrawal, autonomic epilepsy, and factitious crises (usually from sympathomimetic amines). When an asymptomatic adrenal mass is identified, likely diag-noses other than pheochromocytoma include a nonfunctioning adrenal adenoma, aldosteronoma, and cortisol-producing adenoma (Cushing's syndrome).

TABLE 51-2

BIOCHEMICAL AND IMAGING METHODS USED FOR PHEOCHROMOCYTOMA AND PARAGANGLIOMA DIAGNOSIS

DIAGNOSTIC METHOD	SENSITIVITY	SPECIFICITY
24-h urinary tests		
Vanillylmandelic acid	++	++++
Catecholamines	+++	+++
Fractionated metanephrines	++++	++
Total metanephrines	+++	++++
Plasma tests		
Catecholamines	+++	++
Free metanephrines	++++	+++
CT	++++	+++
MRI	++++	+++
MIBG scintigraphy	+++	++++
Somatostatin receptor scintigraphy*	++	++
Dopa (dopamine) PET	+++	++++

*Particularly high in head and neck paragangliomas.

Abbreviations: CT, computed tomography; MIBG, metaiodobenzylguanidine; PET, positron emission tomography.

TREATMENT Pheochromocytoma

Complete tumor removal is the ultimate therapeutic goal. Preoperative patient preparation is essential for safe surgery. α-Adrenergic blockers (phenoxybenzamine) should be initiated at relatively low doses (e.g., 5–10 mg orally three times per day) and increased as tolerated every few days. Because patients are volume-constricted, liberal salt intake and hydration are necessary to avoid orthostasis. Adequate alpha blockade generally requires 7 days, with a typical final dose of 20–30 mg phenoxybenzamine three times per day. Oral prazosin or intravenous phentolamine can be used to manage paroxysms while awaiting adequate alpha blockade. Before surgery, blood pressure should be consistently below 160/90 mmHg, with moderate orthostasis. Beta blockers (e.g., 10 mg propranolol three to four times per day) can be added after starting alpha blockers and increased as needed if tachycardia persists. Other antihypertensives, such as calcium channel blockers or angiotensin-converting enzyme inhibitors, have been used when blood pressure is difficult to control with phenoxybenzamine alone.

Surgery should be performed by teams of anesthesiologists and surgeons with experience in the management of pheochromocytomas. Blood pressure can be labile during surgery, particularly at the onset of intubation or when the tumor is manipulated. Nitroprusside infusion is useful for intraoperative hypertensive crises, and hypotension usually responds to volume infusion. Although laparotomy was the traditional surgical approach, endoscopic surgery, using either a transperitoneal or a retroperitoneal approach, is associated with fewer complications, a faster recovery, and optimal cosmetic results. Atraumatic endoscopic surgery has become the method of choice. It may be possible to preserve the normal adrenal cortex, particularly in hereditary disorders in which bilateral pheochromocytomas are more likely. Extra-adrenal abdominal as well as most thoracic pheochromocytomas also can be removed endoscopically. Postoperatively, catecholamine normalization should be documented. An adrenocorticotropic hormone test should be used to exclude cortisol deficiency when bilateral adrenal cortex–sparing surgery is performed.

MALIGNANT PHEOCHROMOCYTOMA

About 5–10% of pheochromocytomas and paragangliomas are malignant. The diagnosis of malignant pheochromocytoma is problematic. Typical histologic criteria of cellular atypia, presence of mitoses, and invasion of vessels or adjacent tissues do not reliably identify which tumors have the capacity to metastasize. Thus, the term *malignant pheochromocytoma* generally is restricted to tumors with distant metastases, most commonly found in lungs, bone, or liver, suggesting a vascular pathway of spread. Because hereditary syndromes are associated with multifocal tumor sites, these features should be anticipated in patients with germ-line mutations of *RET, VHL, SDHD, or SDHB*. However, distant metastases also occur in these syndromes, especially in carriers of *SDHB* mutations.

Treatment of malignant pheochromocytoma or paraganglioma is challenging. Options include tumor mass reduction, alpha blockers for symptoms, chemotherapy, and nuclear medicine radiotherapy. Averbuch's chemotherapy protocol includes dacarbazine (600 mg/m^2 on days 1 and 2), cyclophosphamide (750 mg/m^2 on day 1), and vincristine (1.4 mg/m^2 on day 1) repeated every 21 days for three to six cycles. Palliation (stable disease to shrinkage) is achieved in about half of patients. Other chemotherapeutic protocols remain in the experimental stage. An alternative is 1^{31} I-MIBG treatment using 200-mCi doses at monthly intervals over three to six cycles. The prognosis of metastatic pheochromocytoma or paraganglioma is variable, with a 5-year survival rate of 30–60%.

PHEOCHROMOCYTOMA IN PREGNANCY

Pheochromocytomas occasionally are diagnosed in pregnancy. Endoscopic removal, preferably in the forth to sixth month of gestation, is possible and can be followed by uneventful childbirth. Regular screening in families with inherited pheochromocytomas provides an opportunity to identify and remove asymptomatic tumors in women of reproductive age.

PHEOCHROMOCYTOMA-ASSOCIATED SYNDROMES

About 25–33% of patients with a pheochromocytoma or paraganglioma have an inherited syndrome. The mean age at diagnosis is about 15 years lower in patients with inherited syndromes compared with patients with sporadic tumors.

Neurofibromatosis type 1 (NF 1) was the first described pheochromocytoma-associated syndrome (Chap. 46). The *NF1* gene functions as a tumor suppressor by regulating the Ras signaling cascade. Classic features of neurofibromatosis include multiple neurofibromas, café au lait spots, axillary freckling of the skin, and Lisch nodules of the iris (Fig. 51-2). Pheochromocytomas occur in only about 1% of these patients and are located

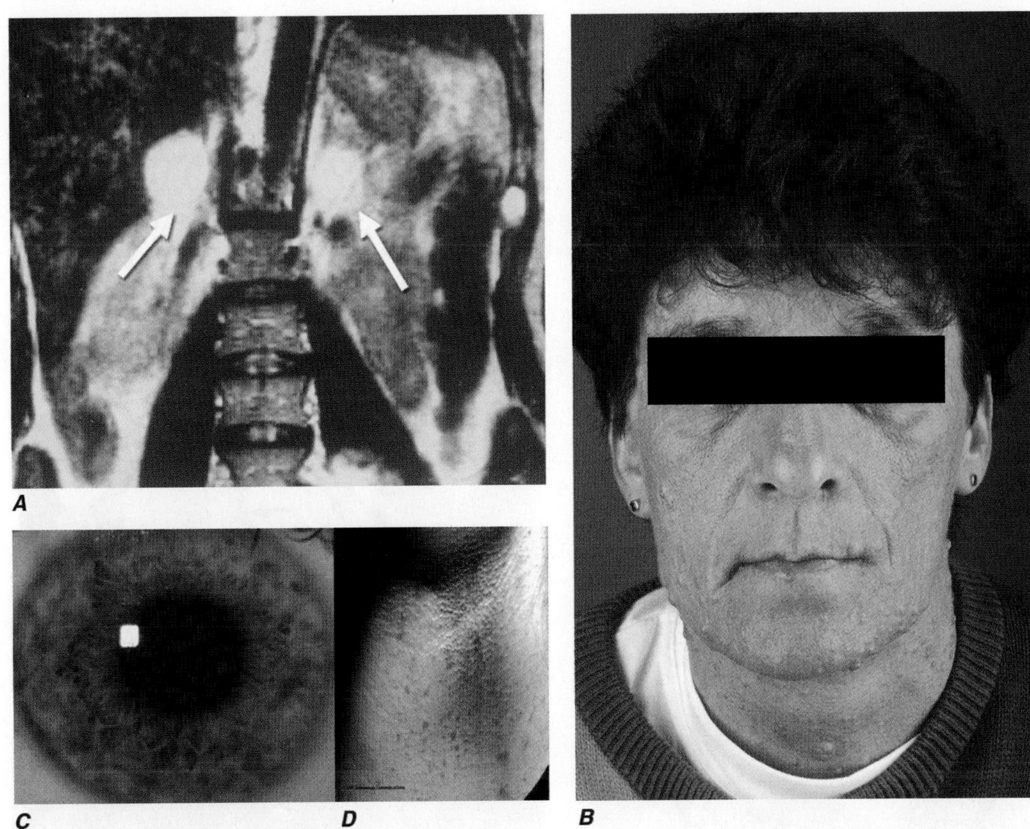

FIGURE 51-2
Neurofibromatosis. ***A.*** Magnetic resonance image of bilateral adrenal pheochromocytoma. ***B.*** Cutaneous neurofibromas. ***C.*** Lisch nodules of the iris. ***D.*** Axillary freckling. *(Part A from HPH Neumann et al: Keio J Med 54:15, 2005; with permission.)*

predominantly in the adrenals. Malignant pheochromocytoma is not uncommon.

The best-known pheochromocytoma-associated syndrome is the autosomal dominant disorder *multiple endocrine neoplasia type 2A and type 2B (MEN 2A, MEN 2B)* (Chap. 50). Both types of MEN 2 are caused by mutations in *RET* (*RE*arranged during *T*ransfection), which encodes a tyrosine kinase. The locations of RET mutations correlate with the severity of disease and the type of MEN 2 (Chap. 50). MEN 2A is characterized by medullary thyroid carcinoma (MTC), pheochromocytoma, and hyperparathyroidism; MEN 2B also includes MTC and pheochromocytoma, as well as multiple mucosal neuromas, marfanoid habitus, and other developmental disorders, though it typically lacks hyperparathyroidism. MTC is seen in virtually all patients with MEN 2, but pheochromocytoma occurs in only about 50% of these patients. Nearly all pheochromocytomas are benign and located in the adrenals, often bilateral (Fig. 51-3). Pheochromocytoma may be symptomatic before MTC. Prophylactic thyroidectomy is being performed in many carriers of *RET* mutations; pheochromocytomas should be excluded before any surgery in these patients.

Von Hippel-Lindau syndrome (VHL) is an autosomal dominant disorder that predisposes to retinal and cerebellar hemangioblastomas, which also occur in the brainstem and spinal cord (Fig. 51-4). Other important features of VHL are clear cell renal carcinomas, pancreatic islet cell tumors, endolymphatic sac tumors (ELSTs) of the inner ear, cystadenomas of the epididymis and broad ligament, and multiple pancreatic or renal cysts.

The *VHL* gene encodes an E3 ubiquitin ligase that regulates expression of hypoxia-inducible factor-1 (HIF-1), among other genes. Loss of *VHL* is associated with increased expression of vascular endothelial growth factor (VEGF) that induces angiogenesis. Although the *VHL* gene can be inactivated by all types of mutations, patients with pheochromocytoma predominantly have missense mutations. About 20–30% of patients with VHL have pheochromocytomas, but in some families the incidence can reach 90%. The recognition of pheochromocytoma as a VHL-associated feature provides an opportunity to diagnose retinal, central nervous system, renal, and pancreatic tumors at a stage when effective treatment may still be possible

The *paraganglioma syndromes (PGL)* have been classified by genetic analyses of families with head and neck

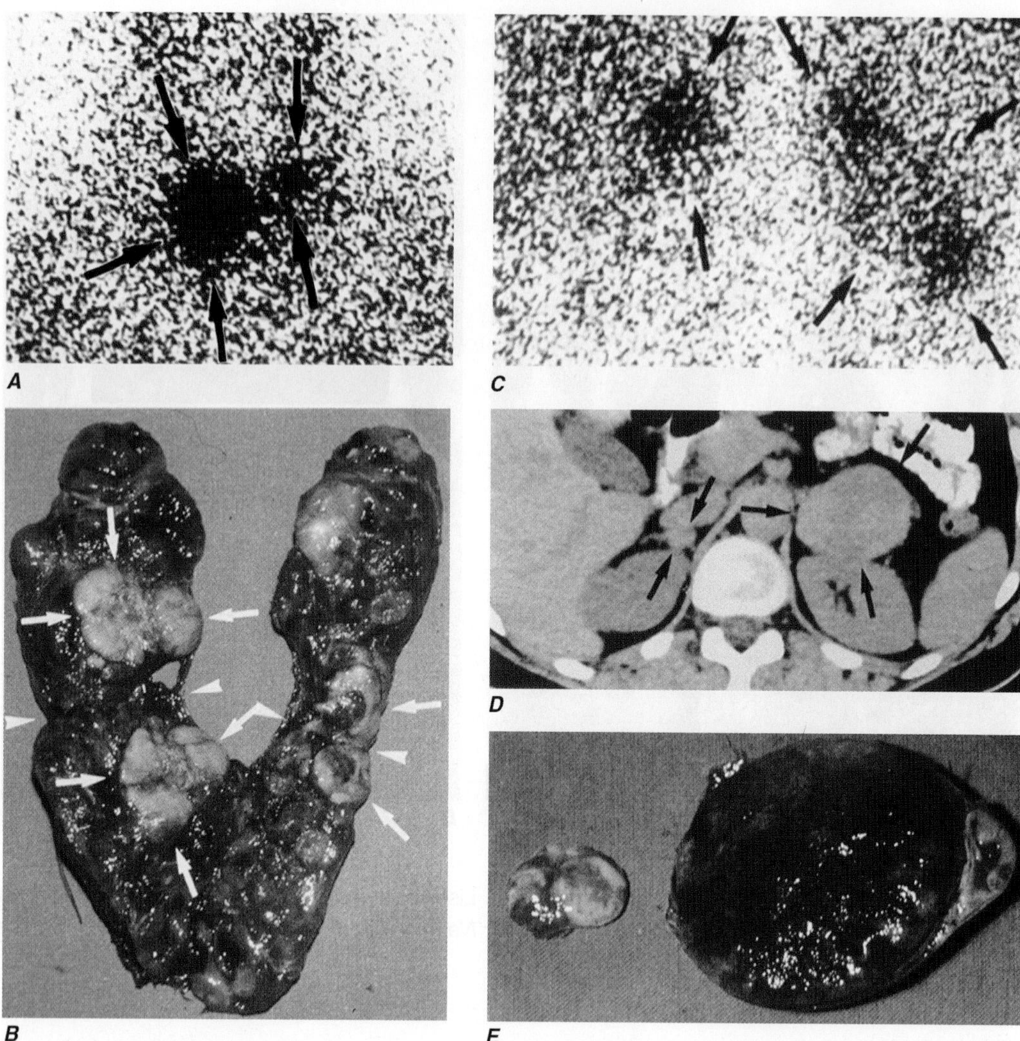

FIGURE 51-3
Multiple endocrine neoplasia type 2. Multifocal medullary thyroid carcinoma shown by metaiodobenzylguanidine (MIBG) scintigraphy (***A***) and operative specimen (***B***). Arrows demonstrate the tumors; arrowheads show the tissue bridge of the cut specimen. Bilateral adrenal pheochromocytoma shown by MIBG scintigraphy (***C***), computed tomography imaging (***D***), and operative specimens. (***E***) (*From HPH Neumann et al: Keio J Med 54:15, 2005; with permission.*)

paragangliomas. The susceptibility genes encode subunits of the enzyme succinate dehydrogenase (SDH), a component in the Krebs cycle and the mitochondrial electron transport chain. SDH is formed by four subunits (A–D). Mutations of *SDHB* (PGL4), *SDHC* (PGL3), *SDHD* (PGL1), and *SDHAF2* (PGL2) predispose to the paraganglioma syndromes. Mutations of SDHA do not predispose to paraganglioma tumors but instead cause Leigh's disease, a form of encephalopathy. The transmission of the disease in carriers of *SDHB, SDHC,* and *SDHAF2* germ-line mutations is autosomal dominant. In contrast, in SDHD families, only the progeny of affected fathers develop tumors if they inherit the mutation. In a small number of patients with familial pheochromocytoma, a mutation has not been identified. PGL1 is most common, followed by PGL4; PGL2 and PGL3 are rare. Adrenal, extra-adrenal abdominal, and thoracic pheochromocytomas that are components of PGL1 and PGL4, are rare in PGL3 but, absent in PGL2 (Fig. 51-5). About one-third of the patients with PGL4 develop metastases.

Familial pheochromocytoma (FP) has been attributed to hereditary, exclusively adrenal tumors in patients with germline mutations in the *TMEM127* gene.

GUIDELINES FOR GENETIC SCREENING IN PATIENTS WITH PHEOCHROMOCYTOMA OR PARAGANGLIOMA

In addition to family history, general features suggesting an inherited syndrome include young age, multifocal tumors, extra-adrenal tumors, and malignant tumors

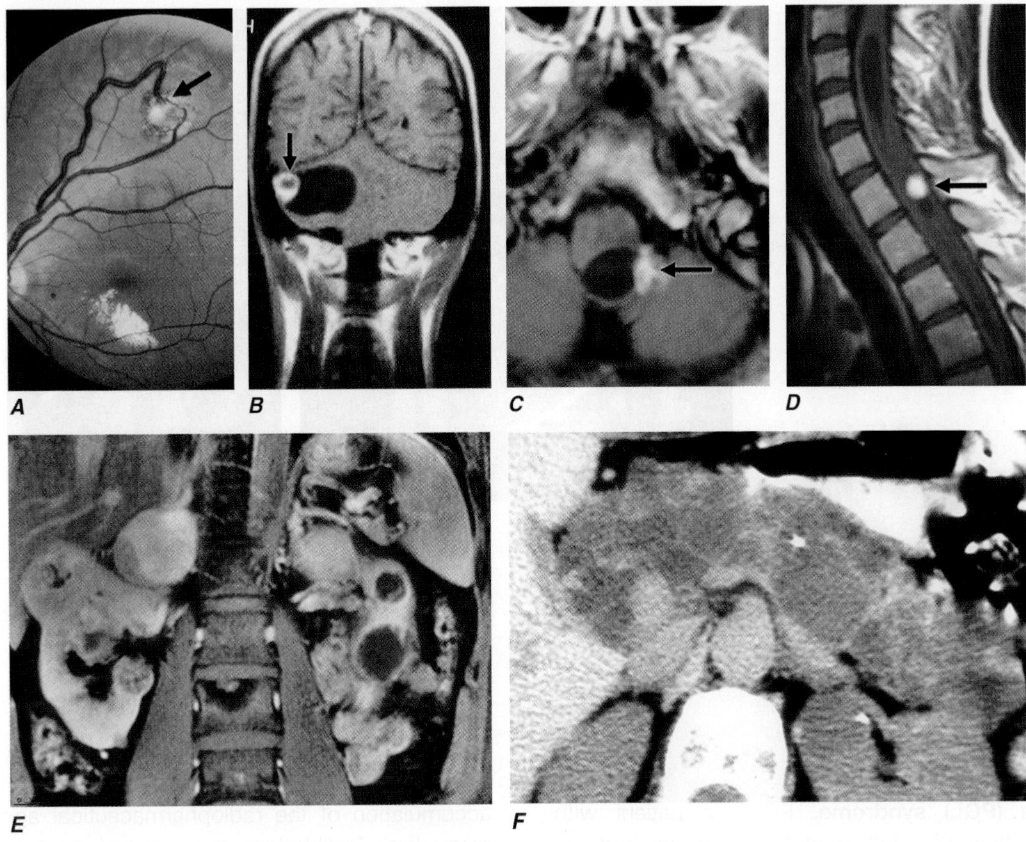

FIGURE 51-4
Von Hippel-Lindau disease. Retinal angioma (***A***), hemangioblastomas of cerebellum are shown by magnetic resonance imaging in the brainstem (***B***) and spinal cord (***C*** and ***D***), bilateral pheochromocytomas and bilateral renal clear cell carcinomas (***E***), and multiple pancreatic cysts (***F***). (*Parts A and D from HPH Neumann et al: Adv Nephrol Necker Hosp 27:361, 1997. Copyright Elsevier. Part B from SH Morgan, J-P Grunfeld [eds]:* Inherited Disorders of the Kidney. Oxford, UK: *Oxford University Press, 1998. Part F from HPH Neumann et al: Contrib Nephrol 136:193, 2001. Copyright S. Karger AG, Basel.*)

(Fig. 51-6). Because of the relatively high prevalence of familial syndromes among patients who present with pheochromocytoma or paraganglioma, it is useful to identify germline mutations even in patients without a known family history. A first step is to search for clinical features of inherited syndromes and to perform an in-depth, multigenerational family history. Each of these syndromes exhibits autosomal dominant transmission with variable penetrance, but a proband with a mother affected by paraganglial tumors is not predisposed to PLG1 (*SDHD* mutation carrier). Cutaneous neurofibromas, café au lait spots, and axillary freckling suggest neurofibromatosis. Germ-line mutations in *NF1* have not been reported in patients with sporadic pheochromocytomas. Thus, *NF1* testing does not have to be performed in the absence of other clinical features of neurofibromatosis. A personal or family history of medullary thyroid cancer or elevation of serum calcitonin strongly suggest MEN 2 and should prompt testing for *RET* mutations. A history of visual impairment, or tumors of the cerebellum, kidney, brainstem, or spinal cord, suggests the possibility of VHL. A personal or family history of head and neck paraganglioma suggests PGL1 or PGL4.

A single adrenal pheochromocytoma in a patient with an otherwise unremarkable history may still be associated with mutations of *VHL, RET, SDHB*, or *SDHD* (in decreasing order of frequency). Two-thirds of extra-adrenal tumors are associated with one of these syndromes, and multi focal tumors occur with decreasing frequency in carriers of *RET, SDHD, VHL*, and *SDHB* mutations. About 30% of head and neck paragangliomas are associated with germ-line mutations of one of the SDH subunit genes (particularly *SDHD*) and are rare in carriers of *VHL* and *RET* mutations.

Once the underlying syndrome is diagnosed, the benefit of genetic testing can be extended to relatives. For this purpose, it is necessary to identify the germline mutation in the proband and, after genetic counseling, perform DNA sequence analyses of the responsible gene in relatives to determine whether they are affected. Other family members may benefit from biochemical screening for paraganglial tumors in individuals who carry a germ-line mutation.

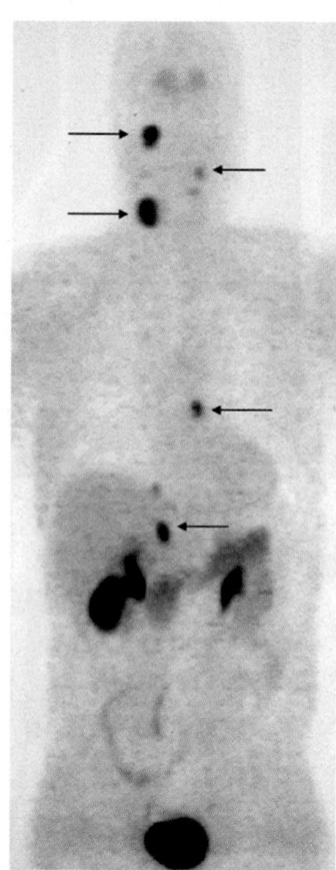

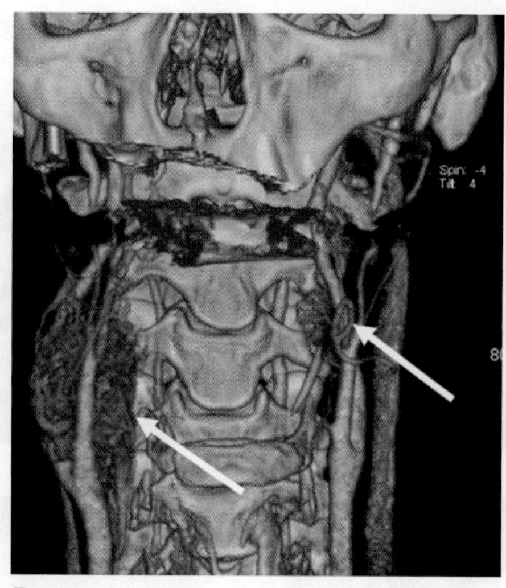

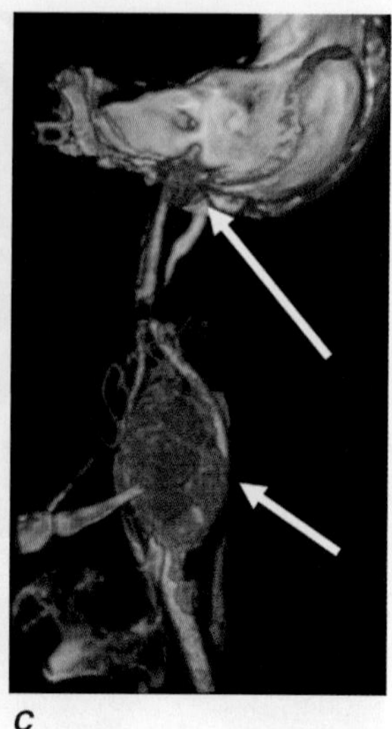

FIGURE 51-5

Paraganglioma (PGL) syndrome. PGL1, a patient with incomplete resection of a left carotid body tumor and the SDHD W5X mutation. ***A.*** 18F-dopa positron emission tomography demonstrating tumor uptake in the right jugular glomus, the right carotid body, the left carotid body, the left coronary glomus, and the right adrenal gland. Note the physiologic accumulation of the radiopharmaceutical agent in the kidneys, liver, gallbladder, renal pelvis, and urinary bladder. ***B*** and ***C.*** Computed tomography angiography with three-dimensional reconstruction. Arrows point to the paraganglial tumors. (*From S Hoegerle et al: Eur J Nucl Med Mol Imaging 30:689, 2003; with permission.*)

ADRENOCORTICAL CARCINOMA

Adrenocortical carcinoma (ACC) is a rare malignancy with an annual incidence of 1–2 per million population. ACC is generally considered a highly malignant tumor; however, it presents with broad interindividual variability with regard to biologic characteristics and clinical behavior. Somatic mutations in the tumor suppressor gene *TP53* are found in 25% of apparently sporadic ACC. Germline *TP53* mutations are the cause of the Li-Fraumeni syndrome associated with multiple solid organ cancers, including ACC, and are found in 25% of pediatric ACC cases; the *TP53* mutation R337H is found in almost all pediatric ACC in Brazil. Other genetic changes identified in ACC include alterations in the Wnt/β-catenin pathway and in the insulin-like growth factor 2 (IGF2) cluster; IGF2 overexpression is found in 90% of ACC.

Patients with large adrenal tumors suspicious of malignancy should be managed by a multidisciplinary specialist team, including an endocrinologist, an oncologist, a surgeon, a radiologist, and a histopathologist.Fine-needle aspiration (FNA) is not indicated in suspected ACC: first, cytology and also histopathology of a core biopsy cannot differentiate between benign and malignant primary adrenal masses (Fig. 51-7); second, FNA violates the tumor capsule and may even cause needle canal metastasis. Even when the entire tumor specimen is available, the histopathologic differentiation between benign and malignant lesions is a diagnostic challenge. The most common histopathologic classification is the Weiss score, taking into account high nuclear grade; mitotic rate (>5/high-power field); atypical mitosis; <25% clear cells; diffuse architecture; and presence of necrosis, venous invasion, and invasion of sinusoidal structures and tumor capsule. The presence of three or more elements suggests ACC.

Although 60–70% of ACCs are biochemically found to overproduce hormones, this is not clinically apparent in many patients due to the relatively inefficient steroid production by the adrenocortical cancer cells. Excess production of glucocorticoids and adrenal androgen precursors are most common. Mixed excess production of several corticosteroid classes by an adrenal tumor is generally indicative of malignancy.

Tumor staging at diagnosis (Table 51-3) has important prognostic implications and requires scanning of the

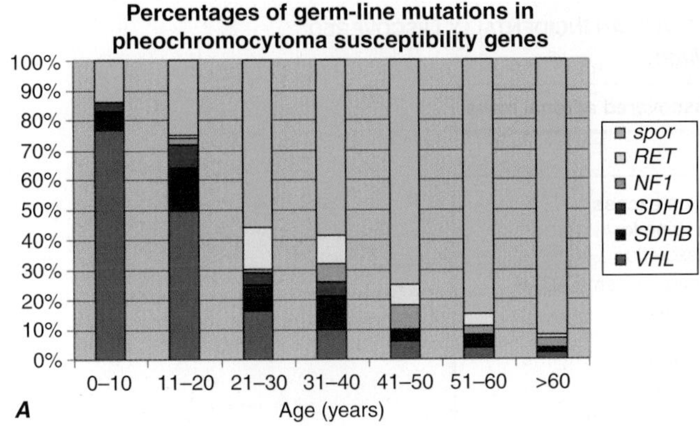

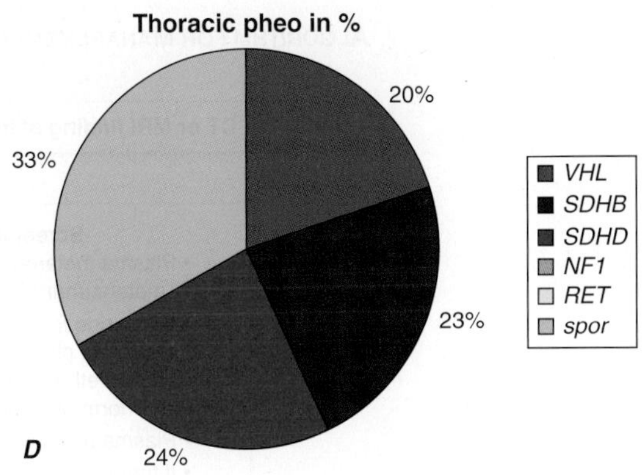

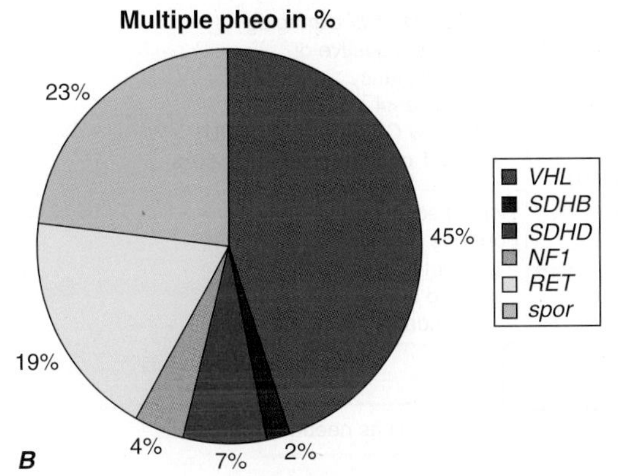

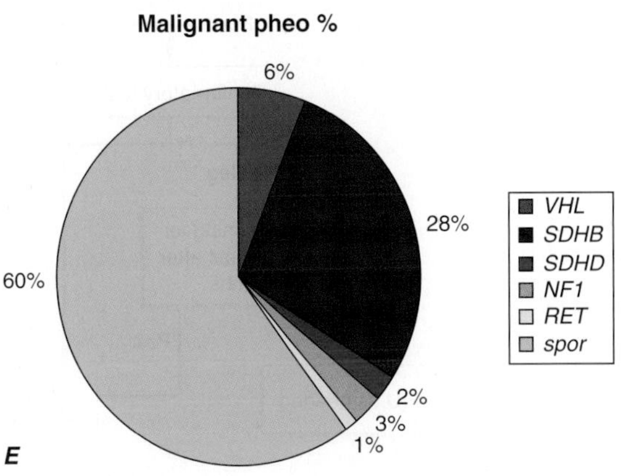

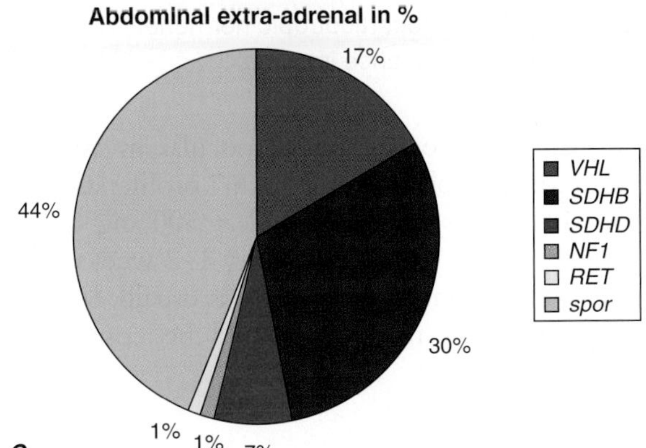

FIGURE 51-6

Mutation distribution in the RET, VHL, NF1, SDHB, and SDHD genes. (***A***). Correlation with age. The bars depict the frequency of sporadic or various inherited forms of pheochromocytoma in different age groups. The inherited disorders are much more common among younger individuals presenting with pheochromocytoma. Germ-line mutations according to (***B***) multiple, (***C***) extraadrenal retroperitoneal, (***D***) thoracic, and (***E***) malignant pheochromocytomas (*Data from the Freiburg International Pheochromocytoma and Paraganglioma Registry in 2009.*)

chest and abdomen for local organ invasion, lymphadenopathy, and metastases. Intravenous contrast medium is necessary for maximum sensitivity for hepatic metastases. An adrenal origin may be difficult to determine on standard axial CT imaging if the tumors are large and invasive, but CT reconstructions or MRI is more informative (Fig. 51-8) using multiple planes and different sequences. Vascular and adjacent organ invasion is diagnostic of malignancy. 18-Fluoro-2-deoxy-D-glucose positron emission tomography (18-FDG PET) is highly sensitive for the detection of malignancy and can be used to detect small metastases or local recurrence that may not be obvious on CT (Fig. 51-8). However, FDG PET is not specific and therefore cannot be used for differentiating benign from malignant adrenal lesions. Metastasis in ACC most frequently occurs to liver and lung.

ACC carries a poor prognosis and cure can be achieved only by complete surgical removal. Capsule violation during primary surgery, metastasis at diagnosis, and primary treatment in a non-specialist center are major determinants of poor survival. If the primary tumor invades adjacent organs, en bloc removal of kidney and spleen should be considered to reduce the risk of recurrence. Surgery can also be considered in a patient with metastases if there is severe tumor-related hormone excess. This indication needs to be carefully weighed against surgical risk, including

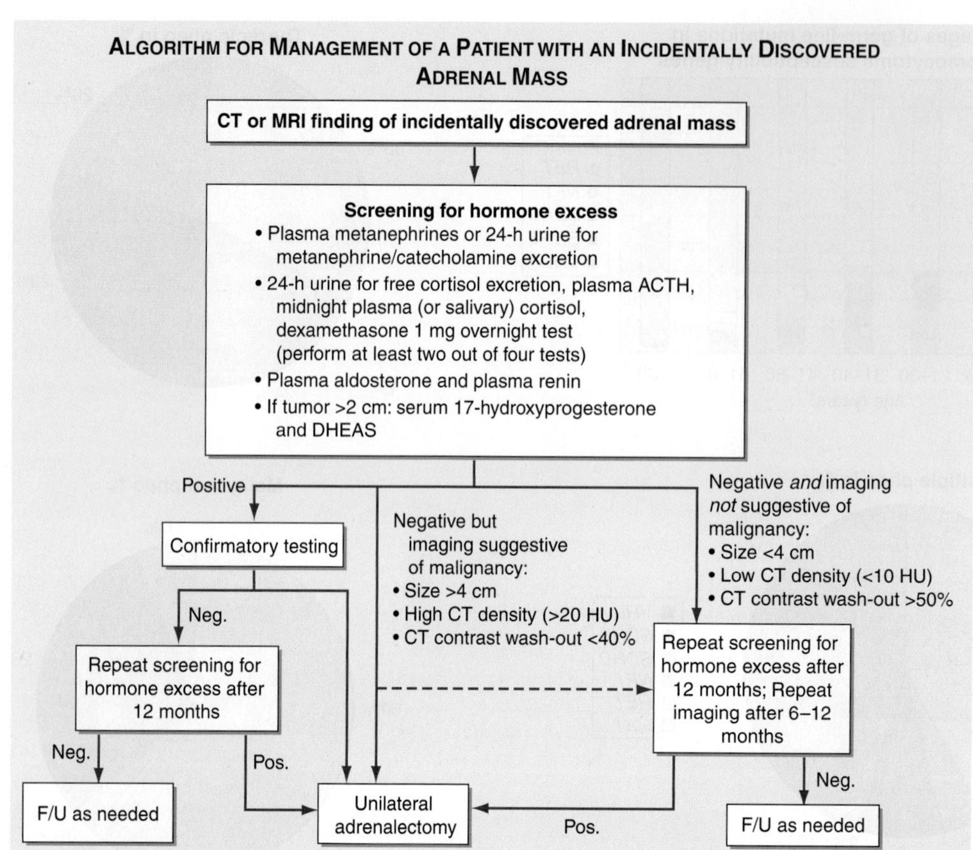

FIGURE 51-7

Management of a patient with an incidentally discovered adrenal mass. ACTH, adrenocorticotropic hormone; CT, computed tomography; DHEAS, dehydroepiandrosterone sulfate; F/U, follow-up; MRI, magnetic resonance imaging.

thromboembolic complications, and the resulting delay in the introduction of other therapeutic options. Patients with confirmed ACC and successful removal of the primary tumor should receive adjuvant treatment with mitotane (o,p'DDD), particularly in patients with a high risk of recurrence as determined by tumor size >8 cm, histopathologic signs of vascular invasion, capsule invasion or violation, and a Ki67 proliferation index ≥10%. Mitotane is usually started at 500 mg qid, with doses increased by 1000 mg/d every 1–2 weeks as tolerated. The maximum tolerated dose is usually 8–10 g/m^2 per day. Adjuvant mitotane should be continued for

TABLE 51-3

CLASSIFICATION SYSTEM FOR STAGING OF ADRENOCORTICAL CARCINOMA

STAGE	ENSAT STAGE	TNM DEFINITIONS
I	**T1, N0, M0**	T1, tumor ≤5 cm N0, no positive lymph node M0, no distant metastases
II	**T2, N0, M0**	T2, tumor >5 cm N0, no positive lymph node M0, no distant metastases
III	**T1–T2, N1, M0** **T3–T4, N0–N1, M0**	N1, positive lymph node(s) M0, no distant metastases T3, tumor infiltration into surrounding tissue T4, tumor invasion into adjacent organs ***or*** venous tumor thrombus in vena cava or renal vein
IV	**T1–T4, N0–N1, M1**	M1, presence of distant metastases

Abbreviation: ENSAT, European Network for the Study of Adrenal Tumors ; TNM, tumor, node, metastasis.

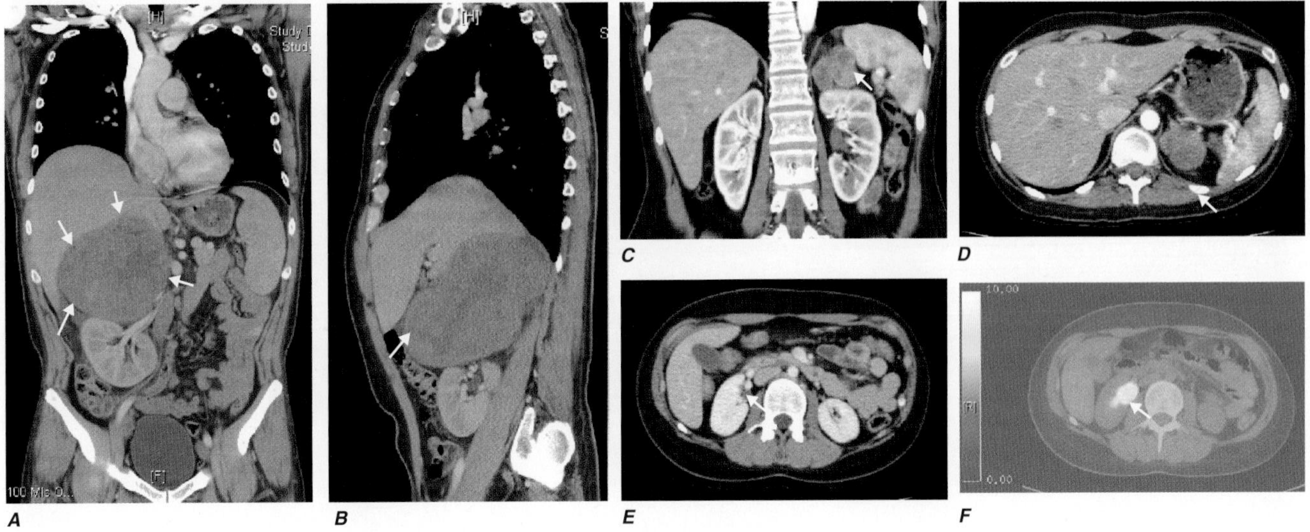

FIGURE 51-8

Imaging in adrenocortical carcinoma. Magnetic resonance imaging scan with (***A***) frontal and (***B***) lateral views of a right adrenocortical carcinoma that was detected incidentally. Computed tomography (CT) scan with (***C***) coronal and (***D***) transverse views depicting a right-sided adrenocortical carcinoma. Note the irregular border and inhomogeneous structure. CT scan (***E***) and positron emission tomography–computed tomography (***F***) visualizing a peritoneal metastasis of an adrenocortical carcinoma in close proximity to the right kidney (*arrow*).

at least 2 years, if the patient can tolerate side effects. Regular monitoring of plasma mitotane levels is mandatory (therapeutic range 14–20 mg/L; neurotoxic complications more frequent >20 mg/L), as is concurrent replacement with hydrocortisone. The latter should be given at higher doses than usually employed in adrenal insufficiency (e.g., 20 mg tid), as mitotane increases glucocorticoid inactivation due to the induction of hepatic CYP3A4 activity. It also increases circulating cortisol-binding globulin, thereby decreasing the available free cortisol fraction. Single metastases can be addressed surgically or with radiofrequency ablation as appropriate. If the tumor recurs or progresses during mitotane treatment, chemotherapy should be considered (e.g., cisplatin, etoposide, doxorubicin plus continuing mitotane, the so-called Berrutti regimen); painful bone metastasis responds to irradiation. Overall survival in ACC is still poor, with 5-year survival rates of 30–40%.

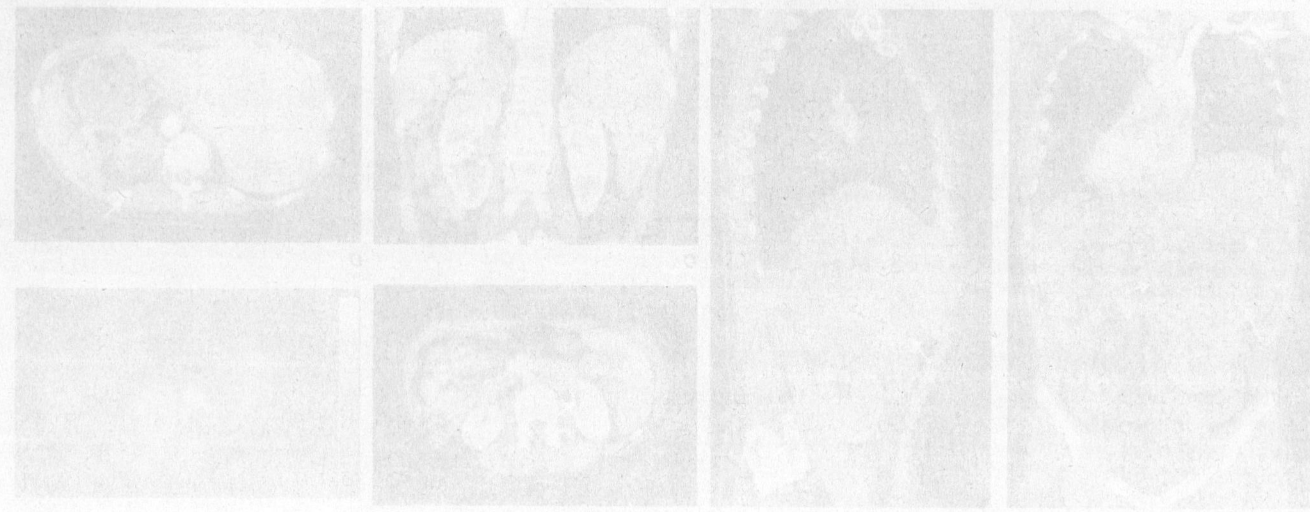

SECTION XI

REMOTE EFFECTS OF CANCER

CHAPTER 52

PARANEOPLASTIC SYNDROMES: ENDOCRINOLOGIC AND HEMATOLOGIC

J. Larry Jameson ■ Dan L. Longo

In addition to local tissue invasion and metastasis, neoplastic cells can produce a variety of products that can stimulate hormonal, hematologic, dermatologic, and neurologic responses. *Paraneoplastic syndromes* is the term used to refer to the disorders that accompany benign or malignant tumors but are not directly related to mass effects or invasion. Tumors of neuroendocrine origin, such as small cell lung carcinoma (SCLC) and carcinoids, produce a wide array of peptide hormones and are common causes of paraneoplastic syndromes. However, almost every type of tumor has the potential to produce hormones or cytokines or to induce immunologic responses. Careful studies of the prevalence of paraneoplastic syndromes indicate that they are more common than is generally appreciated. The signs, symptoms, and metabolic alterations associated with paraneoplastic disorders may be overlooked in the context of a malignancy and its treatment. Consequently, atypical clinical manifestations in a patient with cancer should prompt consideration of a paraneoplastic syndrome. The most common endocrinologic and hematologic syndromes associated with underlying neoplasia will be discussed here.

ENDOCRINE PARANEOPLASTIC SYNDROMES

Etiology

Hormones can be produced from eutopic or ectopic sources. *Eutopic* refers to the expression of a hormone from its normal tissue of origin, whereas *ectopic* refers to hormone production from an atypical tissue source. For example, adrenocorticotropic hormone (ACTH) is expressed eutopically by the corticotrope cells of the anterior pituitary, but it can be expressed ectopically in SCLC. Many hormones are produced at low levels from a wide array of tissues in addition to the classic endocrine source. Thus, ectopic expression is often a quantitative change rather than an absolute change in tissue expression. Nevertheless, the term *ectopic expression* is firmly entrenched and conveys the abnormal physiology associated with hormone production by neoplastic cells. In addition to high levels of hormones, ectopic expression typically is characterized by abnormal regulation of hormone production (e.g., defective feedback control) and peptide processing (resulting in large, unprocessed precursors).

A diverse array of molecular mechanisms has been suggested to cause ectopic hormone production. In rare instances, genetic rearrangements explain aberrant hormone expression. For example, translocation of the *parathyroid hormone (PTH)* gene can result in high levels of PTH expression in tissues other than the parathyroid gland, apparently because the genetic rearrangement brings the *PTH* gene under the control of atypical regulatory elements. A related phenomenon is well documented in many forms of leukemia and lymphoma, in which somatic genetic rearrangements confer a growth advantage and alter cellular differentiation and function (Chap. 15). Although genetic rearrangements may cause selected cases of ectopic hormone production, this mechanism is probably rare, as many tumors are associated with excessive production of numerous peptides. Cellular dedifferentiation probably underlies most cases of ectopic hormone production. Many cancers are poorly differentiated, and certain tumor products, such as human chorionic gonadotropin (hCG), parathyroid hormone–related protein (PTHrP), and α fetoprotein, are characteristic of gene expression at earlier developmental stages. In contrast, the propensity of certain cancers to produce particular hormones (e.g., squamous cell carcinomas produce PTHrP) suggests that dedifferentiation is partial or that selective pathways are derepressed.

These expression profiles probably reflect alterations in transcriptional repression, changes in DNA methylation, or other factors that govern cell differentiation.

In SCLC, the pathway of differentiation has been relatively well defined. The neuroendocrine phenotype is dictated in part by the basic-helix-loop-helix (bHLH) transcription factor human achaete-scute homologue 1 (hASH-1), which is expressed at abnormally high levels in SCLC associated with ectopic ACTH. The activity of hASH-1 is inhibited by hairy enhancer of split 1 (HES-1) and by Notch proteins, which also are capable of inducing growth arrest. Thus, abnormal expression of these developmental transcription factors appears to provide a link between cell proliferation and differentiation.

Ectopic hormone production would only be an epiphenomenon associated with cancer if it did not result in clinical manifestations. Excessive and unregulated production of hormones such as ACTH, PTHrP, and vasopressin can lead to substantial morbidity and complicate the cancer treatment plan. Moreover, the paraneoplastic endocrinopathies are sometimes the presenting feature of underlying malignancy and may prompt the search for an unrecognized tumor.

A large number of paraneoplastic endocrine syndromes have been described, linking overproduction of particular hormones with specific types of tumors. However, certain recurring syndromes emerge from this group (Table 52-1). The most common paraneoplastic endocrine syndromes include hypercalcemia from overproduction of PTHrP and other factors, hyponatremia from excess vasopressin, and Cushing's syndrome from ectopic ACTH.

HYPERCALCEMIA CAUSED BY ECTOPIC PRODUCTION OF PARATHYROID HORMONE–RELATED PROTEIN

Etiology

Humoral hypercalcemia of malignancy (HHM) occurs in up to 20% of patients with cancer. HHM is most common in cancers of the lung, head and neck, skin, esophagus, breast, and genitourinary tract and in multiple myeloma and lymphomas. Although several distinct humoral causes of HHM occur, it is caused most commonly by overproduction of PTHrP. In addition to acting as a circulating humoral factor, bone metastases (e.g., breast, multiple myeloma) may produce PTHrP, leading to local osteolysis and hypercalcemia.

PTHrP is structurally related to PTH and binds to the PTH receptor, explaining the similar biochemical features of HHM and hyperparathyroidism. PTHrP plays a key role in skeletal development and regulates cellular proliferation and differentiation in other tissues, including skin, bone marrow, breast, and hair follicles. The mechanism of PTHrP induction in malignancy is incompletely understood; however, tumor-bearing tissues commonly associated with HHM normally produce PTHrP during development or cell renewal. PTHrP expression is stimulated by hedgehog pathways and Gli transcription factors that are active in many malignancies. Transforming growth factor β (TGF-β), which is produced by many tumors, also stimulates PTHrP, in part by activating the Gli pathway. Mutations in certain oncogenes, such as *Ras*, also can activate PTHrP expression. In adult T cell lymphoma, the transactivating Tax protein produced by human T cell lymphotropic virus I (HTLV-I) stimulates PTHrP promoter activity. Metastatic lesions to bone are more likely to produce PTHrP than are metastases in other tissues, suggesting that bone produces factors (e.g., TGF-β) that enhance PTHrP production or that PTHrP-producing metastases have a selective growth advantage in bone. Thus, PTHrP production can be stimulated by mutations in oncogenes, altered expression of viral or cellular transcription factors, and local growth factors.

Another relatively common cause of HHM is excess production of 1,25-dihydroxyvitamin D. Like granulomatous disorders associated with hypercalcemia, lymphomas can produce an enzyme that converts 25-hydroxyvitamin D to the more active 1,25-dihydroxyvitamin D, leading to enhanced gastrointestinal calcium absorption. Other causes of HHM include tumor-mediated production of osteolytic cytokines and inflammatory mediators.

Clinical manifestations

The typical presentation of HHM is a patient with a known malignancy who is found to be hypercalcemic on routine laboratory tests. Less often, hypercalcemia is the initial presenting feature of malignancy. Particularly when calcium levels are markedly increased (>3.5 mmol/L [>14 mg/dL]), patients may experience fatigue, mental status changes, dehydration, or symptoms of nephrolithiasis.

Diagnosis

Features that favor HHM, as opposed to primary hyperparathyroidism, include known malignancy, recent onset of hypercalcemia, and very high serum calcium levels. Like hyperparathyroidism, hypercalcemia caused by PTHrP is accompanied by hypercalciuria and hypophosphatemia. Patients with HHM typically have metabolic alkalosis rather than hyperchloremic acidosis, as is seen in hyperparathyroidism. Measurement of PTH is useful to exclude primary hyperparathyroidism; the PTH level should be suppressed in HHM. An elevated PTHrP level confirms the diagnosis, and it is increased in ~80% of hypercalcemic patients with cancer.

TABLE 52-1

PARANEOPLASTIC SYNDROMES CAUSED BY ECTOPIC HORMONE PRODUCTION

PARANEOPLASTIC SYNDROME	ECTOPIC HORMONE	TYPICAL TUMOR TYPES[a]
Common		
Hypercalcemia of malignancy	Parathyroid hormone-related protein (PTHrP)	Squamous cell (head and neck, lung, skin), breast, genitourinary, gastrointestinal
	1,25 dihydroxyvitamin D	Lymphomas
	Parathyroid hormone (PTH) (rare)	Lung, ovary
	Prostaglandin E2 (PGE2) (rare)	Renal, lung
Syndrome of inappropriate antidiuretic hormone secretion (SIADH)	Vasopressin	Lung (squamous, small cell), gastrointestinal, genitourinary, ovary
Cushing's syndrome	Adrenocorticotropic hormone (ACTH)	Lung (small cell, bronchial carcinoid, adenocarcinoma, squamous), thymus, pancreatic islet, medullary thyroid carcinoma
	Corticotropin-releasing hormone (CRH) (rare)	Pancreatic islet, carcinoid, lung, prostate
	Ectopic expression of gastric inhibitory peptide (GIP), luteinizing hormone (LH)/human chorionic gonadotropin (hCG), other G protein–coupled receptors (rare)	Macronodular adrenal hyperplasia
Less Common		
Non-islet cell hypoglycemia	Insulin-like growth factor (IGF-II)	Mesenchymal tumors, sarcomas, adrenal, hepatic, gastrointestinal, kidney, prostate
	Insulin (rare)	Cervix (small cell carcinoma)
Male feminization	hCG[b]	Testis (embryonal, seminomas), germinomas, choriocarcinoma, lung, hepatic, pancreatic islet
Diarrhea or intestinal hypermotility	Calcitonin[c]	Lung, colon, breast, medullary thyroid carcinoma
	Vasoactive intestinal peptide (VIP)	Pancreas, pheochromocytoma, esophagus
Rare		
Oncogenic osteomalacia	Phosphatonin (fibroblast growth factor 23 [FGF23])	Hemangiopericytomas, osteoblastomas, fibromas, sarcomas, giant cell tumors, prostate, lung
Acromegaly	Growth hormone–releasing hormone (GHRH)	Pancreatic islet, bronchial and other carcinoids
	Growth hormone (GH)	Lung, pancreatic islet
Hyperthyroidism	Thyroid-stimulating hormone (TSH)	Hydatidiform mole, embryonal tumors, struma ovarii
Hypertension	Renin	Juxtaglomerular tumors, kidney, lung, pancreas, ovary

[a]Only the most common tumor types are listed. For most ectopic hormone syndromes, an extensive list of tumors has been reported to produce one or more hormones.

[b]hCG is produced eutopically by trophoblastic tumors. Certain tumors produce disproportionate amounts of the hCG α or hCG β subunit. High levels of hCG rarely cause hyperthyroidism because of weak binding to the TSH receptor.

[c]Calcitonin is produced eutopically by medullary thyroid carcinoma and is used as a tumor marker.

1,25-Dihydroxyvitamin D levels may be increased in patients with lymphoma.

TREATMENT Humoral Hypercalcemia of Malignancy

The management of HHM begins with removal of excess calcium in the diet, medications, or intravenous (IV) solutions. Oral phosphorus (e.g., 250 mg Neutra-Phos 3–4 times daily) should be given until serum phosphorus is >1 mmol/L (>3 mg/dL). Saline rehydration is used to dilute serum calcium and promote calciuresis. Forced diuresis with furosemide or other loop diuretics can enhance calcium excretion but provides relatively little value except in life-threatening hypercalcemia. When used, loop diuretics should be administered only after complete rehydration and with careful monitoring of fluid balance. Bisphosphonates such as pamidronate (60–90 mg IV), zoledronate (4–8 mg IV), and etidronate (7.5 mg/kg per day orally (PO) for 3–7 consecutive days) can reduce serum calcium within 1–2 days and suppress calcium release for several weeks. Bisphosphonate infusions can be repeated, or oral bisphosphonates can be used for chronic treatment. Dialysis should be considered in severe hypercalcemia when saline hydration and bisphosphonate treatments are not possible or are too slow in onset. Previously used agents such as calcitonin and mithramycin have little utility now that bisphosphonates are available. Calcitonin (2–8 U/kg subcutaneously every 6–12 h) should be considered when rapid correction of severe hypercalcemia is needed. Hypercalcemia associated with lymphomas, multiple myeloma, or leukemia may respond to glucocorticoid treatment (e.g., prednisone 40–100 mg PO in four divided doses).

ECTOPIC VASOPRESSIN: TUMOR-ASSOCIATED SIADH

Etiology

Vasopressin is an antidiuretic hormone normally produced by the posterior pituitary gland. Ectopic vasopressin production by tumors is a common cause of the syndrome of inappropriate antidiuretic hormone (SIADH), occurring in at least half of patients with SCLC. SIADH also can be caused by a number of nonneoplastic conditions, including central nervous system (CNS) trauma, infections, and medications. Compensatory responses to SIADH, such as decreased thirst, may mitigate the development of hyponatremia. However, with prolonged production of excessive vasopressin, the osmostat controlling thirst and hypothalamic vasopressin secretion may become reset. In addition, intake of free water, orally or intravenously, can quickly worsen hyponatremia because of reduced renal diuresis.

Tumors with neuroendocrine features, such as SCLC and carcinoids, are the most common sources of ectopic vasopressin production, but they also occur in other forms of lung cancer and with CNS lesions, head and neck cancer, and genitourinary, gastrointestinal, and ovarian cancers. The mechanism of activation of the vasopressin gene in these tumors is unknown but often involves concomitant expression of the adjacent oxytocin gene, suggesting derepression of this locus.

Clinical manifestations

Most patients with ectopic vasopressin secretion are asymptomatic and are identified because of the presence of hyponatremia on routine chemistry testing. Symptoms may include weakness, lethargy, nausea, confusion, depressed mental status, and seizures. The severity of symptoms reflects the rapidity of onset as well as the extent of hyponatremia. Hyponatremia usually develops slowly but may be exacerbated by the administration of IV fluids or the institution of new medications.

Diagnosis

The diagnostic features of ectopic vasopressin production are the same as those of other causes of SIADH. Hyponatremia and reduced serum osmolality occur in the setting of an inappropriately normal or increased urine osmolality. Urine sodium excretion is normal or increased unless volume depletion is present. Other causes of hyponatremia should be excluded, including renal, adrenal, or thyroid insufficiency. Physiologic sources of vasopressin stimulation (CNS lesions, pulmonary disease, nausea); adaptive circulatory mechanisms (hypotension, heart failure, hepatic cirrhosis); and medications, including many chemotherapeutic agents, also should be considered as possible causes of hyponatremia. Vasopressin measurements are not usually necessary to make the diagnosis.

TREATMENT Ectopic Vasopressin: Tumor-Associated SIADH

Most patients with ectopic vasopressin production develop hyponatremia over several weeks or months. The disorder should be corrected gradually unless mental status is altered or there is risk of seizures. Treatment of the underlying malignancy may reduce ectopic vasopressin production, but this response is slow if it occurs at all. Fluid restriction to less than urine output, plus insensible losses, is often sufficient to correct hyponatremia partially. However, strict monitoring of the amount and types of liquids consumed or administered intravenously is required for fluid restriction to be effective. Salt tablets and saline are not helpful unless volume depletion is also present. Demeclocycline (150–300 mg orally three to four times daily) can be used to inhibit vasopressin action on the renal distal tubule, but its onset of action is relatively slow (1–2 weeks). Conivaptan, a nonpeptide V_2-receptor antagonist, can be administered either PO (20–120 mg bid) or IV (10–40 mg) and is particularly effective when used in combination with fluid restriction in euvolemic hyponatremia. Severe hyponatremia (Na <115 mEq/L) or mental status changes may require treatment with hypertonic (3%) or normal saline infusion together with furosemide to enhance free water clearance. The rate of sodium correction should be slow (0.5–1 mEq/L per h) to prevent rapid fluid shifts and the possible development of central pontine myelinolysis.

CUSHING'S SYNDROME CAUSED BY ECTOPIC ACTH PRODUCTION

See also Chap. 51.

Etiology

Ectopic ACTH production accounts for 10–20% of cases of Cushing's syndrome. The syndrome is particularly common in neuroendocrine tumors. SCLC (>50%) is by far the most common cause of ectopic ACTH followed by thymic carcinoid (15%), islet cell tumors (10%), bronchial carcinoid (10%), other carcinoids (5%), and pheochromocytomas (2%). Ectopic ACTH production is caused by increased expression of the proopiomelanocortin (POMC) gene, which encodes ACTH, along with melanocyte-stimulating hormone (MSH), β lipotropin, and several other peptides. In many tumors, there is abundant but aberrant expression of the POMC gene from an internal promoter, proximal to the third exon, which encodes ACTH. However, because this product lacks the signal sequence necessary for protein processing, it is not secreted. Increased production of ACTH arises instead from less abundant, but unregulated, POMC expression from the same promoter site used in the pituitary. However, because the tumors lack many of the enzymes needed to process the POMC polypeptide, it is typically released as multiple large, biologically inactive fragments along with relatively small amounts of fully processed, active ACTH.

Rarely, corticotropin-releasing hormone (CRH) is produced by pancreatic islet cell tumors, SCLC, medullary thyroid cancer, carcinoids, or prostate cancer. When levels are high enough, CRH can cause pituitary corticotrope hyperplasia and Cushing's syndrome. Tumors that produce CRH sometimes also produce ACTH, raising the possibility of a paracrine mechanism for ACTH production.

A distinct mechanism for ACTH-independent Cushing's syndrome involves ectopic expression of various G protein–coupled receptors in the adrenal nodules. Ectopic expression of the gastric inhibitory peptide (GIP) receptor is the best-characterized example of this mechanism. In this case, meals induce GIP secretion, which inappropriately stimulates adrenal growth and glucocorticoid production.

Clinical manifestations

The clinical features of hypercortisolemia are detected in only a small fraction of patients with documented ectopic ACTH production. Patients with ectopic ACTH syndrome generally exhibit less marked weight gain and centripetal fat redistribution, probably because the exposure to excess glucocorticoids is relatively short and because cachexia reduces the propensity for weight gain and fat deposition. The ectopic ACTH syndrome is associated with several clinical features that distinguish it from other causes of Cushing's syndrome (e.g., pituitary adenomas, adrenal adenomas, iatrogenic glucocorticoid excess). The metabolic manifestations of ectopic ACTH syndrome are dominated by fluid retention and hypertension, hypokalemia, metabolic alkalosis, glucose intolerance, and occasionally steroid psychosis. The very high ACTH levels often cause increased pigmentation, and MSH activity derived from the POMC precursor peptide is also increased. The extraordinarily high glucocorticoid levels in patients with ectopic sources of ACTH can lead to marked skin fragility and easy bruising. In addition, the high cortisol levels often overwhelm the renal 11β-hydroxysteroid dehydrogenase type II enzyme, which normally inactivates cortisol and prevents it from binding to renal mineralocorticoid receptors. Consequently, in addition to the excess mineralocorticoids produced by ACTH stimulation of the adrenal gland, high levels of cortisol exert activity through the mineralocorticoid receptor, leading to severe hypokalemia.

Diagnosis

The diagnosis of ectopic ACTH syndrome is usually not difficult in the setting of a known malignancy. Urine free cortisol levels fluctuate but are typically greater than two to four times normal, and the plasma ACTH level is usually >22 pmol/L (>100 pg/mL). A suppressed ACTH level excludes this diagnosis and indicates an ACTH-independent cause of Cushing's syndrome (e.g., adrenal or exogenous glucocorticoid). In contrast to pituitary sources of ACTH, most ectopic sources of ACTH do not respond to glucocorticoid suppression. Therefore, high-dose dexamethasone (8 mg PO) suppresses 8:00 A.M. serum cortisol (50% decrease from baseline) in ~80% of pituitary ACTH-producing adenomas but fails to suppress ectopic ACTH in ~90% of cases. Bronchial and other carcinoids are well-documented exceptions to these general guidelines, as these ectopic sources of ACTH may exhibit feedback regulation indistinguishable from pituitary adenomas, including suppression by high-dose dexamethasone, and ACTH responsiveness to adrenal blockade with metyrapone. If necessary, petrosal sinus catheterization can be used to evaluate a patient with ACTH-dependent Cushing's syndrome when the source of ACTH is unclear. After CRH stimulation, a 3:1 petrosal sinus:peripheral ACTH ratio strongly suggests a pituitary ACTH source. Imaging studies are also useful in the evaluation of suspected carcinoid lesions, allowing biopsy and characterization of hormone production using special stains.

TREATMENT Cushing's Syndrome Caused by Ectopic ACTH Production

The morbidity associated with the ectopic ACTH syndrome can be substantial. Patients may experience depression or personality changes because of extreme cortisol excess. Metabolic derangements, including diabetes mellitus and hypokalemia, can worsen fatigue. Poor wound healing and predisposition to infections can complicate the surgical management of tumors, and opportunistic infections caused by organisms such as *Pneumocystis carinii* and mycoses are often the cause of death in patients with ectopic ACTH production. Depending on prognosis and treatment plans for the underlying malignancy, measures to reduce cortisol levels are often indicated. Treatment of the underlying malignancy may reduce ACTH levels but is rarely sufficient to reduce cortisol levels to normal. Adrenalectomy is not practical for most of these patients but should be considered if the underlying tumor is not resectable and the prognosis is otherwise favorable (e.g., carcinoid). Medical therapy with ketoconazole (300–600 mg PO twice a day), metyrapone (250–500 mg PO every 6 h), mitotane (3–6 g PO in four divided doses, tapered to maintain low cortisol production), or other agents that block steroid synthesis or action is often the most practical strategy for managing the hypercortisolism associated with ectopic ACTH production. Glucocorticoid replacement should be provided to prevent adrenal insufficiency. Unfortunately, many patients eventually progress despite medical blockade.

TUMOR-INDUCED HYPOGLYCEMIA CAUSED BY EXCESS PRODUCTION OF INSULIN GROWTH FACTOR TYPE II

Mesenchymal tumors, hemangiopericytomas, hepatocellular tumors, adrenal carcinomas, and a variety of other large tumors have been reported to produce excessive amounts of insulin-like growth factor type II (IGF-II) precursor, which binds weakly to insulin receptors and strongly to IGF-I receptors, leading to insulin-like actions. The gene encoding IGF-II resides on a chromosome 11p15 locus that is normally imprinted (that is, expression is exclusively from a single parental allele). Biallelic expression of the IGF-II gene occurs in a subset of tumors, suggesting loss of methylation and loss of imprinting as a mechanism for gene induction. In addition to increased IGF-II production, IGF-II bioavailability is increased due to complex alterations in circulating binding proteins. Increased IGF-II suppresses growth hormone (GH) and insulin, resulting in reduced IGF binding protein 3 (IGFBP-3), IGF-I, and acid-labile subunit (ALS). The reduction in ALS and IGFBP-3, which normally sequester IGF-II, causes it to be displaced to a small circulating complex that has greater access to insulin target tissues. For this reason, circulating IGF-II levels may not be markedly increased despite causing hypoglycemia. In addition to IGF-II–mediated hypoglycemia, tumors may occupy enough of the liver to impair gluconeogenesis.

In most cases, the tumor causing hypoglycemia is clinically apparent (usually >10 cm in size), and hypoglycemia develops in association with fasting. The diagnosis is made by documenting low serum glucose and suppressed insulin levels in association with symptoms of hypoglycemia. Serum IGF-II levels may not be increased (IGF-II assays may not detect IGF-II precursors). Increased IGF-II mRNA expression is found in most of these tumors. Any medications associated with hypoglycemia should be eliminated. Treatment of the underlying malignancy, if possible, may reduce the predisposition to hypoglycemia. Frequent meals and IV glucose, especially during sleep or fasting, are often necessary to prevent hypoglycemia. Glucagon and glucocorticoids have also been used to enhance glucose production.

HUMAN CHORIONIC GONADOTROPIN

hCG is composed of α and β subunits and can be produced as intact hormone, which is biologically active, or as uncombined biologically inert subunits. Ectopic production of intact hCG occurs most often in association with testicular embryonal tumors, germ cell tumors, extragonadal germinomas, lung cancer, hepatoma, and pancreatic islet tumors. Eutopic production of hCG occurs with trophoblastic malignancies. hCG α subunit production is particularly common in lung cancer and pancreatic islet cancer. In men, high hCG levels stimulate steroidogenesis and aromatase activity in testicular Leydig cells, resulting in increased estrogen production and the development of gynecomastia. Precocious puberty in boys or gynecomastia in men should prompt measurement of hCG and consideration of a testicular tumor or another source of ectopic hCG production. Most women are asymptomatic. hCG is easily measured. Treatment should be directed at the underlying malignancy.

ONCOGENIC OSTEOMALACIA

Hypophosphatemic oncogenic osteomalacia, also called tumor-induced osteomalacia (TIO), is characterized by markedly reduced serum phosphorus and renal phosphate wasting, leading to muscle weakness, bone pain, and osteomalacia. Serum calcium and PTH levels are normal, and 1,25-dihydroxyvitamin D is low. Oncogenic osteomalacia is usually caused by benign mesenchymal tumors, such as hemangiopericytomas, fibromas, and giant cell tumors, often of the skeletal extremities or head. It has also been described in sarcomas and in patients with prostate and lung cancer. Resection of the tumor reverses the disorder, confirming its humoral basis. The circulating phosphaturic factor is called *phosphatonin*—a factor that inhibits renal tubular reabsorption of phosphate and renal conversion of 25-hydroxyvitamin D to 1,25-dihydroxyvitamin D. Phosphatonin has been identified as fibroblast growth factor 23 (FGF23). FGF23 levels are increased in some, but not all, patients with osteogenic osteomalacia. The disorder exhibits biochemical features similar to those seen with inactivating mutations in the *PHEX* gene, the cause of hereditary X-linked hypophosphatemia. The *PHEX* gene encodes a protease that inactivates FGF23. Treatment involves removal of the tumor, if possible, and supplementation with phosphate and vitamin D. Octreotide treatment reduces phosphate wasting in some patients with tumors that express somatostatin receptor subtype 2. Octreotide scans may also be useful in detecting these tumors.

HEMATOLOGIC SYNDROMES

The elevation of granulocyte, platelet, and eosinophil counts in most patients with myeloproliferative disorders is caused by the proliferation of the myeloid elements due to the underlying disease rather than to a paraneoplastic syndrome. The paraneoplastic hematologic syndromes in patients with solid tumors are less well characterized than are the endocrine syndromes because the ectopic hormone(s) or cytokines responsible have not been identified in most of these tumors (Table 52-2). The extent of the paraneoplastic syndromes parallels the course of the cancer.

ERYTHROCYTOSIS

Ectopic production of erythropoietin by cancer cells causes most paraneoplastic erythrocytosis. The ectopically produced erythropoietin stimulates the production of red blood cells (RBCs) in the bone marrow and raises the hematocrit. Other lymphokines and hormones produced by cancer cells may stimulate erythropoietin release but have not been proved to cause erythrocytosis.

Most patients with erythrocytosis have an elevated hematocrit (>52% in men, >48% in women) that is detected on a routine blood count. Approximately 3% of patients with renal cell cancer, 10% of patients with hepatoma, and 15% of patients with cerebellar hemangioblastomas have erythrocytosis. In most cases, the erythrocytosis is asymptomatic.

TABLE 52-2

PARANEOPLASTIC HEMATOLOGIC SYNDROMES

SYNDROME	PROTEINS	CANCERS TYPICALLY ASSOCIATED WITH SYNDROME
Erythrocytosis	Erythropoietin	Renal cancers Hepatocarcinoma, cerebellar hemangioblastomas
Granulocytosis	G-CSFGM-CSFIL-6	Lung cancer, gastrointestinal cancer, ovarian cancer Genitourinary cancer Hodgkin's disease
Thrombocytosis	IL-6	Lung cancer, gastrointestinal cancer, breast cancer Ovarian cancer, lymphoma
Eosinophilia	IL-5	Lymphoma leukemia, lung cancer
Thrombophlebitis	Unknown	Lung cancer, pancreatic cancer, gastrointestinal cancer, breast cancer Genitourinary cancer Ovarian cancer, prostate cancer, lymphoma

Abbreviations: G-CSF, granulocyte colony-stimulating factor; GM-CSF, granulocyte-macrophage colony-stimulating factor; IL, interleukin.

Patients with erythrocytosis due to a renal cell cancer, hepatoma, or CNS cancer should have measurement of red cell mass. If the red cell mass is elevated, the serum erythropoietin level should be measured. Patients with an appropriate cancer, elevated erythropoietin levels, and no other explanation for erythrocytosis (e.g., hemoglobinopathy that causes increased O_2 affinity; Chap. 2) have the paraneoplastic syndrome.

TREATMENT Erythrocytosis

Successful resection of the cancer usually resolves the erythrocytosis. If the tumor cannot be resected or treated effectively with radiation therapy or chemotherapy, phlebotomy may control any symptoms related to erythrocytosis.

GRANULOCYTOSIS

Approximately 30% of patients with solid tumors have granulocytosis (granulocyte count >8000/μL). In about half of patients with granulocytosis and cancer, the granulocytosis has an identifiable nonparaneoplastic etiology (infection, tumor necrosis, glucocorticoid administration, etc.). The other patients have proteins in urine and serum that stimulate the growth of bone marrow cells. Tumors and tumor cell lines from patients with lung, ovarian, and bladder cancers have been documented to produce granulocyte colony-stimulating factor (G-CSF), granulocyte-macrophage colony-stimulating factor (GM-CSF), and/or interleukin 6 (IL-6). However, the etiology of granulocytosis has not been characterized in most patients.

Patients with granulocytosis are nearly all asymptomatic, and the differential white blood cell count does not have a shift to immature forms of neutrophils. Granulocytosis occurs in 40% of patients with lung and gastrointestinal cancers, 20% of patients with breast cancer, 30% of patients with brain tumors and ovarian cancers, 20% of patients with Hodgkin's disease, and 10% of patients with renal cell carcinoma. Patients with advanced-stage disease are more likely to have granulocytosis than are those with early-stage disease.

Paraneoplastic granulocytosis does not require treatment. The granulocytosis resolves when the underlying cancer is treated.

THROMBOCYTOSIS

Some 35% of patients with thrombocytosis (platelet count >400,000/μL) have an underlying diagnosis of cancer. IL-6, a candidate molecule for the etiology of paraneoplastic thrombocytosis, stimulates the production of platelets in vitro and in vivo. Some patients with cancer and thrombocytosis have elevated levels of IL-6 in plasma. Another candidate molecule is thrombopoietin, a peptide hormone that stimulates megakaryocyte proliferation and platelet production. The etiology of thrombocytosis has not been established in most cases.

Patients with thrombocytosis are nearly all asymptomatic. Thrombocytosis is not clearly linked to thrombosis in patients with cancer. Thrombocytosis is present in 40% of patients with lung and gastrointestinal cancers; 20% of patients with breast, endometrial, and ovarian cancers; and 10% of patients with lymphoma. Patients with thrombocytosis are more likely to have advanced-stage disease and have a poorer prognosis than do patients without thrombocytosis. Paraneoplastic thrombocytosis does not require treatment.

EOSINOPHILIA

Eosinophilia is present in ~1% of patients with cancer. Tumors and tumor cell lines from patients with lymphomas or leukemia may produce IL-5, which stimulates eosinophil growth. Activation of IL-5 transcription in lymphomas and leukemias may involve translocation of the long arm of chromosome 5, to which the genes for IL-5 and other cytokines map.

Patients with eosinophilia are typically asymptomatic. Eosinophilia is present in 10% of patients with lymphoma; 3% of patients with lung cancer; and occasional patients with cervical, gastrointestinal, renal, and breast cancer. Patients with markedly elevated eosinophil counts (>5000/μL) can develop shortness of breath and wheezing. A chest radiograph may reveal diffuse pulmonary infiltrates from eosinophil infiltration and activation in the lungs.

TREATMENT Eosinophilia

Definitive treatment is directed at the underlying malignancy: Tumors should be resected or treated with radiation or chemotherapy. In most patients who develop shortness of breath related to eosinophilia, symptoms resolve with the use of oral or inhaled glucocorticoids.

THROMBOPHLEBITIS

Deep-vein thrombosis (DVT) and pulmonary embolism are the most common thrombotic conditions in patients with cancer. Migratory or recurrent thrombophlebitis may be the initial manifestation of cancer. Nearly 15% of patients who develop DVT or pulmonary embolism have a diagnosis of cancer (Chap. 21). The coexistence of peripheral venous thrombosis with visceral carcinoma, particularly pancreatic cancer, is called *Trousseau's syndrome*.

Pathogenesis

Patients with cancer are predisposed to thromboembolism because they are often at bed rest or immobilized, and tumors may obstruct or slow blood flow. Chronic IV catheters also predispose to clotting. In addition, clotting may be promoted by release of procoagulants or cytokines from tumor cells or associated inflammatory cells or by platelet adhesion or aggregation. The specific molecules that promote thromboembolism have not been identified.

In addition to cancer causing secondary thrombosis, primary thrombophilic diseases may be associated with cancer. For example, the antiphospholipid antibody syndrome is associated with a wide range of pathologic manifestations. About 20% of patients with this syndrome have cancers. Among patients with cancer and antiphospholipid antibodies, 35–45% develop thrombosis.

Clinical Manifestations

Patients with cancer who develop DVT usually develop swelling or pain in the leg, and physical examination reveals tenderness, warmth, and redness. Patients who present with pulmonary embolism develop dyspnea, chest pain, and syncope, and physical examination shows tachycardia, cyanosis, and hypotension. Some 5% of patients with no history of cancer who have a diagnosis of DVT or pulmonary embolism will have a diagnosis of cancer within 1 year. The most common cancers associated with thromboembolic episodes include lung, pancreatic, gastrointestinal, breast, ovarian, and genitourinary cancers; lymphomas; and brain tumors. Patients with cancer who undergo surgical procedures requiring general anesthesia have a 20–30% risk of DVT.

Diagnosis

The diagnosis of DVT in patients with cancer is made by impedance plethysmography or bilateral compression ultrasonography of the leg veins. Patients with a noncompressible venous segment have deep venous thrombosis. If compression ultrasonography is normal and there is a high clinical suspicion for DVT, venography should be done to look for a luminal filling defect. Elevation of D-dimer is not as predictive of DVT in patients with cancer as it is in patients without cancer; elevations are seen in people over age 65 years without concomitant evidence of thrombosis, probably as a consequence of increased thrombin deposition and turnover in aging.

Patients with symptoms and signs suggesting a pulmonary embolism should be evaluated with a chest radiograph, electrocardiogram, arterial blood gas analysis, and ventilation–perfusion scan. Patients with mismatched segmental perfusion defects have a pulmonary embolus. Patients with equivocal ventilation–perfusion findings should be evaluated as described above for DVT in their legs. If DVT is detected, they should be anticoagulated. If DVT is not detected, they should be considered for a pulmonary angiogram.

Patients without a diagnosis of cancer who present with an initial episode of thrombophlebitis or pulmonary embolus need no additional tests for cancer other than a careful history and physical examination. In light of the many possible primary sites, diagnostic testing in asymptomatic patients is wasteful. However, if the clot is refractory to standard treatment or is in an unusual site or if the thrombophlebitis is migratory or recurrent, efforts to find an underlying cancer are indicated.

TREATMENT Thrombophlebitis

Patients with cancer and a diagnosis of DVT or pulmonary embolism should be treated initially with IV unfractionated heparin or low-molecular-weight heparin for at least 5 days, and warfarin should be started within 1 or 2 days. The warfarin dose should be adjusted so that the international normalized ratio (INR) is 2–3. Patients with proximal DVT and a relative contraindication to heparin anticoagulation (hemorrhagic brain metastases or pericardial effusion) should be considered for placement of a filter in the inferior vena cava (Greenfield filter) to prevent pulmonary embolism. Warfarin should be administered for 3–6 months. An alternative approach is to use low-molecular-weight heparin for 6 months. Patients with cancer who undergo a major surgical procedure should be considered for heparin prophylaxis or pneumatic boots. Breast cancer patients undergoing chemotherapy and patients with implanted catheters should be considered for prophylaxis (1 mg/d warfarin).

Neurologic paraneoplastic syndromes are discussed in Chap. 53.

ACKNOWLEDGMENT

The authors acknowledge the contributions of Bruce E. Johnson to prior versions of this chapter in Harrison's Principles of Internal Medicine.

CHAPTER 53

PARANEOPLASTIC NEUROLOGIC SYNDROMES

Josep Dalmau ■ Myrna R. Rosenfeld

Paraneoplastic neurologic disorders (PNDs) are cancer-related syndromes that can affect any part of the nervous system (Table 53-1). They are caused by mechanisms other than metastasis or by any of the complications of cancer such as coagulopathy, stroke, metabolic and nutritional conditions, infections, and side effects of cancer therapy. In 60% of patients, the neurologic symptoms precede the cancer diagnosis. Clinically disabling PNDs occur in 0.5–1% of all cancer patients, but they affect 2–3% of patients with neuroblastoma or small cell lung cancer (SCLC) and 30–50% of patients with thymoma or sclerotic myeloma.

TABLE 53-1

PARANEOPLASTIC SYNDROMES OF THE NERVOUS SYSTEM

CLASSIC SYNDROMES: USUALLY OCCUR WITH CANCER ASSOCIATION	NONCLASSIC SYNDROMES: MAY OCCUR WITH AND WITHOUT CANCER ASSOCIATION
Encephalomyelitis	Brainstem encephalitis
Limbic encephalitis	Stiff-person syndrome
Cerebellar degeneration (adults)	Necrotizing myelopathy
Opsoclonus–myoclonus	Motor neuron disease
Subacute sensory neuronopathy	Guillain-Barré syndrome
Gastrointestinal paresis or pseudo-obstruction	Subacute and chronic mixed sensory-motor neuropathies
Dermatomyositis (adults)	Neuropathy associated with plasma cell dyscrasias and lymphoma
Lambert-Eaton myasthenic syndrome	Vasculitis of nerve
Cancer or melanoma associated retinopathy	Pure autonomic neuropathy
	Acute necrotizing myopathy
	Polymyositis
	Vasculitis of muscle
	Optic neuropathy
	BDUMP

Abbreviation: BDUMP, bilateral diffuse uveal melanocytic proliferation.

PATHOGENESIS

Most PNDs are mediated by immune responses triggered by neuronal proteins (onconeuronal antigens) expressed by tumors. In PNDs of the central nervous system (CNS), many antibody-associated immune responses have been identified (Table 53-2). These antibodies react with the patient's tumor, and their detection in serum or cerebrospinal fluid (CSF) usually predicts the presence of cancer. When the antigens are intracellular, most syndromes are associated with extensive infiltrates of CD4+ and CD8+ T cells, microglial activation, gliosis, and variable neuronal loss. The infiltrating T cells are often in close contact with neurons undergoing degeneration, suggesting a primary pathogenic role. T cell-mediated cytotoxicity may contribute directly to cell death in these PNDs. Thus, both humoral and cellular immune mechanisms participate in the pathogenesis of many PNDs. This complex immunopathogenesis may underlie the resistance of many of these conditions to therapy.

In contrast to the disorders associated with immune responses against intracellular antigens, those associated with antibodies to antigens expressed on the neuronal cell surface of the CNS or at neuromuscular synapses are more responsive to immunotherapy (Table 53-3, and Fig. 53-1). These disorders occur with and without a cancer association, and there is increasing evidence that they are mediated by the antibodies.

Other PNDs are likely immune-mediated, although their antigens are unknown. These include several syndromes of inflammatory neuropathies and myopathies.

TABLE 53-2

ANTIBODIES TO INTRACELLULAR ANTIGENS, SYNDROMES, AND ASSOCIATED CANCERS

ANTIBODY	ASSOCIATED NEUROLOGIC SYNDROME(S)	TUMORS
Anti-Hu	Encephalomyelitis, subacute sensory neuronopathy	SCLC
Anti-Yo	Cerebellar degeneration	Ovary, breast
Anti-Ri	Cerebellar degeneration, opsoclonus	Breast, gynecologic, SCLC
Anti-Tr	Cerebellar degeneration	Hodgkin lymphoma
Anti-CV_2/CRMP5	Encephalomyelitis, chorea, optic neuritis, uveitis, peripheral neuropathy	SCLC, thymoma, other
Anti-Ma proteins	Limbic, hypothalamic, brainstem encephalitis	Testicular (Ma2), other (Ma)
Anti-amphiphysin	Stiff-person syndrome, encephalomyelitis	Breast, SCLC
Recoverin, bipolar cell antibodies, others[a]	Cancer-associated retinopathy (CAR) Melanoma-associated retinopathy (MAR)	SCLC (CAR), melanoma (MAR)
Anti-GAD	Stiff-person, cerebellar syndromes	Infrequent tumor association (thymoma)

[a]A variety of target antigens have been identified.

Abbreviations: CRMP, collapsing response-mediator protein; SCLC, small cell lung cancer.

In addition, many patients with typical PND syndromes are antibody-negative. For still other PNDs, the cause remains quite obscure. These include, among others, several neuropathies that occur in the terminal stages of cancer and a number of neuropathies associated with plasma cell dyscrasias or lymphoma without evidence of inflammatory infiltrates or deposits of immunoglobulin, cryoglobulin, or amyloid.

APPROACH TO THE PATIENT

Paraneoplastic Neurologic Disorders

Three key concepts are important for the diagnosis and management of PNDs. First, it is common for symptoms to appear before the presence of a tumor is known; second, the neurologic syndrome usually develops rapidly, producing severe deficits in a short period of

TABLE 53-3

ANTIBODIES TO CELL SURFACE OR SYNAPTIC ANTIGENS, SYNDROMES, AND ASSOCIATED TUMORS

ANTIBODY	NEUROLOGIC SYNDROME	TUMOR TYPE WHEN ASSOCIATED
Anti-AChR (muscle)[a]	Myasthenia gravis	Thymoma
Anti-AChR (neuronal)[a]	Autonomic neuropathy	SCLC
Anti-VGKC- related proteins[b] (LGI1, Caspr2)	Neuromyotonia, limbic encephalitis	Thymoma, SCLC
Anti-VGCC[c]	LEMS, cerebellar degeneration	SCLC
Anti-NMDAR[d]	Anti-NMDAR encephalitis	Teratoma
Anti-AMPAR[d]	Limbic encephalitis with relapses	SCLC, thymoma, breast
Anti-$GABA_BR$[d]	Limbic encephalitis, seizures	SCLC, neuroendocrine
Glycine receptor[d]	Encephalomyelitis with rigidity, stiff-person syndrome	Lung cancer

[a]A direct pathogenic role of these antibodies has been demonstrated.

[b]Anti-VGKC-related proteins are pathogenic for some types of neuromyotonia.

[c]Anti-VGCC antibodies are pathogenic for LEMS.

[d] These antibodies are strongly suspected to be pathogenic.

Abbreviations: AChR, acetylcholine receptor; AMPAR, α-amino-3-hydroxy-5-methylisoxazole-4-propionic acid receptor; $GABA_BR$, gamma-amino-butyric acid B receptor; GAD, glutamic acid decarboxylase; LEMS, Lambert-Eaton myasthenic syndrome; NMDAR, *N*-methyl-D-aspartate receptor; SCLC, small cell lung cancer; VGCC, voltage-gated calcium channel; VGKC, voltage-gated potassium channel.

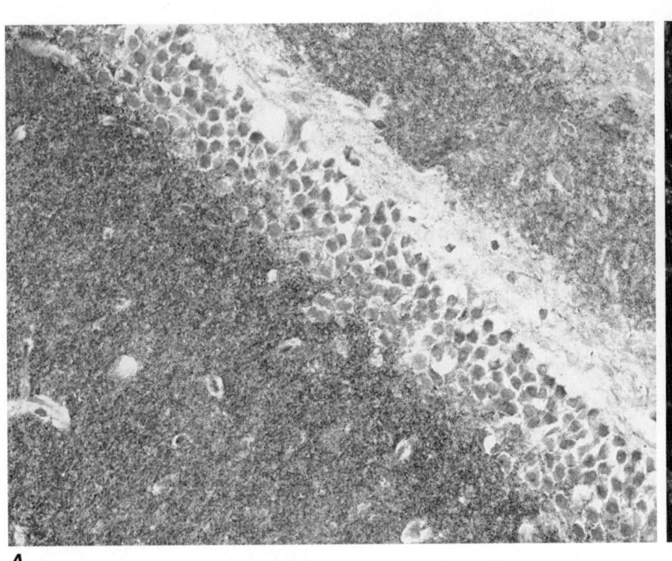

A

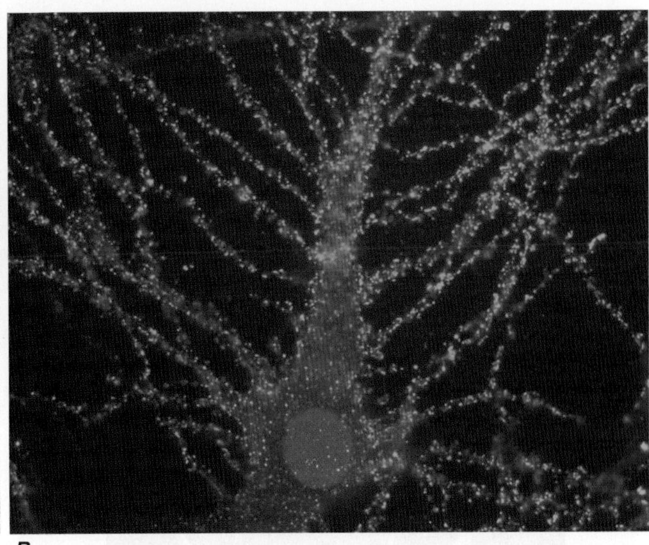

B

FIGURE 53-1

Antibodies to NR1/NR2 subunits of the N-methyl-d-aspartate receptor (NMDA) receptor in a patient with paraneoplastic encephalitis and ovarian teratoma. ***A*** is a section of dentate gyrus of rat hippocampus immunolabeled (brown staining) with the patient's antibodies. The reactivity predominates in the molecular layer, which is highly enriched in dendritic processes. ***B*** shows the antibody reactivity with cultures of rat hippocampal neurons; the intense green immunolabeling is due to the antibodies against the NR1 subunits of NMDA receptors.

time; and third, there is evidence that prompt tumor control improves the neurologic outcome. Therefore, the major concern of the physician is to recognize a disorder promptly as paraneoplastic to identify and treat the tumor.

PND OF THE CENTRAL NERVOUS SYSTEM AND DORSAL ROOT GANGLIA When symptoms involve brain, spinal cord, or dorsal root ganglia, the suspicion of PND is usually based on a combination of clinical, radiologic, and CSF findings. In these cases, a biopsy of the affected tissue is often difficult to obtain, and although useful to rule out other disorders (e.g., metastasis, infection), neuropathologic findings are not specific for PND. Furthermore, there are no specific radiologic or electrophysiologic tests that are diagnostic of PND. The presence of antineuronal antibodies (Tables 53-2 and 53-3) may help in the diagnosis, but only 60–70% of PNDs of the CNS and less than 20% of those involving the peripheral nervous system have neuronal or neuromuscular antibodies that can be used as diagnostic tests. Magnetic resonance imaging (MRI) and CSF studies are important to rule out neurologic complications due to the direct spread of cancer, particularly metastatic and leptomeningeal disease. In most PNDs, the MRI findings are nonspecific. Paraneoplastic limbic encephalitis is usually associated with characteristic MRI abnormalities in the mesial temporal lobes (see later discussion), but similar findings can occur with other disorders (e.g., nonparaneoplastic autoimmune limbic encephalitis, human herpesvirus type 6 [HHV-6] encephalitis) (Fig. 53-2). The CSF profile of patients with PND of the CNS or dorsal root ganglia typically consists of mild to moderate pleocytosis (<200 mononuclear cells, predominantly lymphocytes), an increase in the protein concentration, intrathecal synthesis of IgG, and a variable presence of oligoclonal bands.

PND OF NERVE AND MUSCLE If symptoms involve peripheral nerve, neuromuscular junction, or muscle, the diagnosis of a specific PND is usually established on clinical, electrophysiologic, and pathologic grounds. The clinical history, accompanying symptoms (e.g., anorexia, weight loss), and type of syndrome dictate the studies and degree of effort needed to demonstrate a neoplasm. For example, the frequent association of Lambert-Eaton myasthenic syndrome (LEMS) with SCLC should lead to a chest and abdomen computed tomography (CT) or body positron emission tomography (PET) scan and, if findings are negative, periodic tumor screening for at least 3 years after the neurologic diagnosis. In contrast, the weak association of polymyositis with cancer calls into question the need for repeated cancer screenings in this situation. Serum and urine immunofixation studies should be considered in patients with peripheral neuropathy of unknown cause; detection of a monoclonal gammopathy suggests the need for additional studies to uncover a B cell

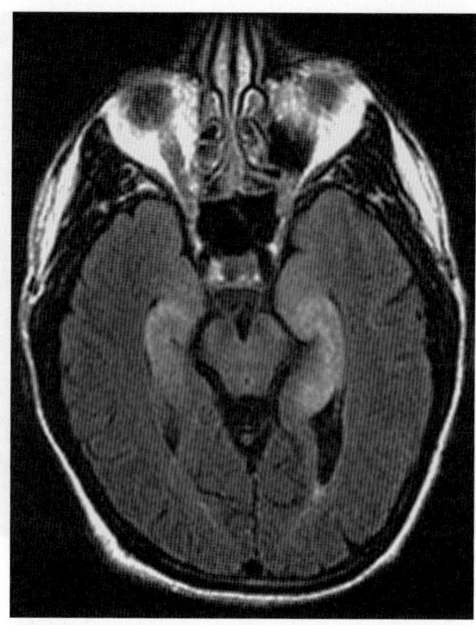

FIGURE 53-2
Fluid-attenuated inversion recovery sequence magnetic resonance image of a patient with limbic encephalitis and LGI1 antibodies. Note the abnormal hyperintensity involving the medial aspect of the temporal lobes.

or plasma cell malignancy. In paraneoplastic neuropathies, diagnostically useful antineuronal antibodies are limited to anti-CV_2/CRMP5 and anti-Hu.

For any type of PND, if antineuronal antibodies are negative, the diagnosis relies on the demonstration of cancer and the exclusion of other cancer-related or independent neurologic disorders. Combined CT and PET scans often uncover tumors undetected by other tests. For germ-cell tumors of the testis and teratomas of the ovary ultrasound and MRI may reveal tumors undetectable by PET.

SPECIFIC PARANEOPLASTIC NEUROLOGIC SYNDROMES

PARANEOPLASTIC ENCEPHALOMYELITIS AND FOCAL ENCEPHALITIS

The term *encephalomyelitis* describes an inflammatory process with multifocal involvement of the nervous system, including the brain, brainstem, cerebellum, and spinal cord. It is often associated with dorsal root ganglia and autonomic dysfunction. For any given patient, the clinical manifestations are determined by the areas predominantly involved, but pathologic studies almost always reveal abnormalities beyond the symptomatic regions. Several clinicopathologic syndromes may occur alone or in combination: (1) *cortical encephalitis*, which may present as "epilepsia partialis continua"; (2) *limbic encephalitis*, characterized by confusion, depression, agitation, anxiety, severe short-term memory deficits, partial complex seizures, and sometimes dementia (the MRI usually shows unilateral or bilateral medial temporal lobe abnormalities, best seen with T2 and fluid-attenuated inversion recovery sequences, and occasionally enhancing with gadolinium); (3) *brainstem encephalitis*, resulting in eye movement disorders (nystagmus, opsoclonus, supranuclear or nuclear paresis), cranial nerve paresis, dysarthria, dysphagia, and central autonomic dysfunction; (4) *cerebellar gait and limb ataxia*; (5) *myelitis*, which may cause lower or upper motor neuron symptoms, myoclonus, muscle rigidity, and spasms; and (6) *autonomic dysfunction* as a result of involvement of the neuraxis at multiple levels, including hypothalamus, brainstem, and autonomic nerves (see autonomic neuropathy). Cardiac arrhythmias, postural hypotension, and central hypoventilation are frequent causes of death in patients with encephalomyelitis.

Paraneoplastic encephalomyelitis and focal encephalitis are usually associated with SCLC, but many other cancers have also been reported. Patients with SCLC and these syndromes usually have anti-Hu antibodies in serum and CSF. Anti-CV_2/CRMP5 antibodies occur less frequently; some of these patients may develop chorea, uveitis, or optic neuritis. Antibodies to Ma proteins are associated with limbic, hypothalamic, and brainstem encephalitis and occasionally with cerebellar symptoms (Fig. 53-3); some patients develop hypersomnia, cataplexy, and severe hypokinesia. MRI abnormalities are frequent, including those described with limbic encephalitis and variable involvement of the hypothalamus, basal ganglia, or upper brainstem. The oncologic associations of these antibodies are shown in Table 53-2.

TREATMENT Encephalomyelitis and Focal Encephalitis

Most types of paraneoplastic encephalitis and encephalomyelitis respond poorly to treatment. Stabilization of symptoms or partial neurologic improvement may occasionally occur, particularly if there is a satisfactory response of the tumor to treatment. The roles of plasma exchange, intravenous immunoglobulin (IVIg), and immunosuppression have not been established. Approximately 30% of patients with anti-Ma2-associated encephalitis respond to treatment of the tumor (usually a germ-cell neoplasm of the testis) and immunotherapy.

ENCEPHALITIDES WITH ANTIBODIES TO CELL-SURFACE OR SYNAPTIC PROTEINS (TABLE 53-3)

These disorders are important for three reasons: (1) they can occur with and without tumor association; (2) some

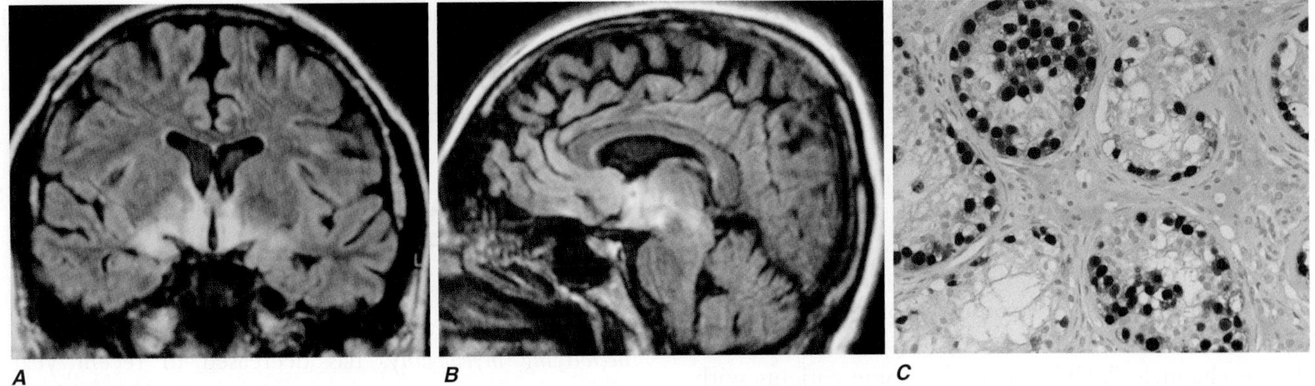

FIGURE 53-3

Magnetic resonance image (MRI) and tumor of a patient with anti-Ma2-associated encephalitis. ***A*** and ***B*** are fluid-attenuated inversion recovery MRI sequences showing abnormal hyperintensities in the medial temporal lobes, hypothalamus, and upper brainstem. ***C*** corresponds to a section of the patient's orchiectomy incubated with a specific marker (Oct4) of germ-cell tumors. The positive (brown) cells correspond to an intratubular germ-cell neoplasm.

syndromes predominate in young individuals and children; and (3) despite the severity of the symptoms, patients usually respond to treatment of the tumor, if found, and immunotherapy (glucocorticoids, plasma exchange, IVIg, rituximab, or cyclophosphamide).

Encephalitis with antibodies to voltage-gated potassium channels (VGKC)-related proteins (LGI1, Caspr2) predominates in men and frequently presents with memory loss and seizures (limbic encephalopathy) along with hyponatremia and sleep and autonomic dysfunction. Less commonly, patients develop neuromyotonia or a mixed clinical picture (Morvan's syndrome). Approximately 20% of patients with antibodies to VGKC-related proteins have an underlying tumor, usually SCLC or thymoma.

Encephalitis with N-methyl-D-aspartate (NMDA) receptor antibodies (Fig. 53-1) usually occurs in young women and children, but men and older patients of both sexes can be affected. The disorder has a characteristic pattern of symptom progression that includes a prodrome resembling a viral process, followed in a few days by the onset of severe psychiatric symptoms, memory loss, seizures, decreased level of consciousness, abnormal movements (orofacial, limb, and trunk dyskinesias, dystonic postures), autonomic instability, and frequent hypoventilation. The syndrome is often misdiagnosed as a viral or idiopathic encephalitis, neuroleptic malignant syndrome, or encephalitis lethargica, and many patients are initially evaluated by psychiatrists with the suspicion of drug abuse or an acute psychosis. The detection of an associated ovarian teratoma is age-dependent; 50% of female patients older than age 18 years have uni- or bilateral ovarian teratomas, while fewer than 9% of girls younger than 14 years have a teratoma. In male patients, the detection of a tumor is rare.

Encephalitis with α-amino-3-hydroxy-5-methylisoxazole-4-propionate (AMPA) receptor antibodies affects middle-aged women, who develop acute limbic dysfunction or less frequently prominent psychiatric symptoms; 70% of the patients have an underlying tumor in the lung, breast, or thymus. The neurologic disorder responds to treatment of the tumor and immunotherapy. Neurologic relapses may occur; these also respond to immunotherapy and are not necessarily associated with tumor recurrence.

Encephalitis with γ-aminobutyric acid type B ($GABA_B$) receptor antibodies usually presents with limbic encephalitis and seizures; 50% of the patients have SCLC or a neuroendocrine tumor of the lung. Neurologic symptoms often respond to immunotherapy and treatment of the tumor if found. Patients may have additional antibodies to glutamic acid decarboxylase (GAD), of unclear significance. Other antibodies to nonneuronal proteins are often found in these patients as well as in patients with AMPA receptor antibodies, indicating a general tendency to autoimmunity.

PARANEOPLASTIC CEREBELLAR DEGENERATION

This disorder is often preceded by a prodrome that may include dizziness, oscillopsia, blurry or double vision, nausea, and vomiting. A few days or weeks later, patients develop dysarthria, gait and limb ataxia, and variable dysphagia. The examination usually shows downbeating nystagmus and, rarely, opsoclonus. Brainstem dysfunction, upgoing toes, or a mild neuropathy may occur, but more often the clinical features are restricted to the cerebellum. Early in the course, MRI studies are usually normal; later, the MRI typically reveals cerebellar atrophy. The disorder results from extensive degeneration of Purkinje cells, with variable involvement of other cerebellar cortical neurons, deep cerebellar nuclei, and spinocerebellar tracts. The tumors more frequently involved are SCLC, cancer of the breast and ovary, and Hodgkin lymphoma.

Anti-Yo antibodies in patients with breast and gynecologic cancers and anti-Tr antibodies in patients with Hodgkin lymphoma are the two immune responses typically associated with prominent or pure cerebellar degeneration. Antibodies to P/Q-type voltage-gated calcium channels (VGCC) occur in some patients with SCLC and cerebellar dysfunction; only some of these patients develop LEMS. A variable degree of cerebellar dysfunction can be associated with virtually any of the antibodies and PND of the CNS shown in Table 53-2. A number of single case reports have described neurologic improvement after tumor removal, plasma exchange, IVIg, cyclophosphamide, rituximab, or glucocorticoids. However, large series of patients with antibody-positive paraneoplastic cerebellar degeneration show that this disorder rarely improves with any treatment.

PARANEOPLASTIC OPSOCLONUS–MYOCLONUS SYNDROME

Opsoclonus is a disorder of eye movement characterized by involuntary, chaotic saccades that occur in all directions of gaze; it is frequently associated with myoclonus and ataxia. Opsoclonus–myoclonus may be cancer-related or idiopathic. When the cause is paraneoplastic, the tumors involved are usually cancer of the lung and breast in adults and neuroblastoma in children. The pathologic substrate of opsoclonus–myoclonus is unclear, but studies suggest that disinhibition of the fastigial nucleus of the cerebellum is involved. Most patients do not have detectable antineuronal antibodies. A small subset of patients with ataxia, opsoclonus, and other eye-movement disorders develop anti-Ri antibodies; in rare instances, muscle rigidity, autonomic dysfunction, and dementia also occur. The tumors most frequently involved in anti-Ri-associated syndromes are breast and ovarian cancer. If the tumor is not successfully treated, the neurologic syndrome in adults often progresses to encephalopathy, coma, and death. In addition to treating the tumor, symptoms may respond to immunotherapy (glucocorticoids, plasma exchange, and/or IVIg).

At least 50% of children with opsoclonus–myoclonus have an underlying neuroblastoma. Hypotonia, ataxia, behavioral changes, and irritability are frequent accompanying symptoms. Neurologic symptoms often improve with treatment of the tumor and glucocorticoids, adrenocorticotropic hormone (ACTH), plasma exchange, IVIg, and rituximab. Many patients are left with psychomotor retardation and behavioral and sleep problems.

PARANEOPLASTIC SYNDROMES OF THE SPINAL CORD

The number of reports of paraneoplastic spinal cord syndromes, such as *subacute motor neuronopathy* and *acute necrotizing myelopathy*, has decreased in recent years. This may represent a true decrease in incidence due to improved and prompt oncologic interventions or the identification of nonparaneoplastic etiologies.

Some patients with cancer develop *upper* or *lower motor neuron dysfunction* or both, resembling amyotrophic lateral sclerosis. It is unclear whether these disorders have a paraneoplastic etiology or simply coincide with the presence of cancer. There are isolated case reports of cancer patients with motor neuron dysfunction who had neurologic improvement after tumor treatment. A search for lymphoma should be undertaken in patients with a rapidly progressive motor neuron syndrome and a monoclonal protein in serum or CSF.

Paraneoplastic myelitis may present with upper or lower motor neuron symptoms, segmental myoclonus, and rigidity and can be the first manifestation of encephalomyelitis.

Paraneoplastic myelopathy can also produce several syndromes characterized by prominent muscle stiffness and rigidity. The spectrum ranges from focal symptoms in one or several extremities (*stiff-limb syndrome* or *stiff-person syndrome*) to a disorder that also affects the brainstem (known as *encephalomyelitis with rigidity*) and likely has a different pathogenesis. Some patients with encephalomyelitis and rigidity have glycine receptor antibodies.

PARANEOPLASTIC STIFF-PERSON SYNDROME

This disorder is characterized by progressive muscle rigidity, stiffness, and painful spasms triggered by auditory, sensory, or emotional stimuli. Rigidity mainly involves the lower trunk and legs, but it can affect the upper extremities and neck. Symptoms improve with sleep and general anesthetics. Electrophysiologic studies demonstrate continuous motor unit activity. Antibodies associated with the stiff-person syndrome target proteins (GAD, amphiphysin) involved in the function of inhibitory synapses utilizing γ-aminobutyric acid (GABA) or glycine as neurotransmitters. Paraneoplastic stiff-person syndrome and amphiphysin antibodies are often related to SCLC and breast cancer. By contrast, antibodies to GAD may occur in some cancer patients but are much more frequently present in the nonparaneoplastic disorder.

TREATMENT Stiff-Person Syndrome

Optimal treatment of stiff-person syndrome requires therapy of the underlying tumor, glucocorticoids, and symptomatic use of drugs that enhance GABA-ergic transmission (diazepam, baclofen, sodium valproate, tiagabine, vigabatrin). A benefit of IVIg has been demonstrated for the nonparaneoplastic disorder but remains to be established for the paraneoplastic syndrome.

PARANEOPLASTIC SENSORY NEURONOPATHY OR DORSAL ROOT GANGLIONOPATHY

This syndrome is characterized by sensory deficits that may be symmetric or asymmetric, painful dysesthesias, radicular pain, and decreased or absent reflexes. All modalities of sensation and any part of the body, including face and trunk, can be involved. Specialized sensations such as taste and hearing can also be affected. Electrophysiologic studies show decreased or absent sensory nerve potentials with normal or near-normal motor conduction velocities. Symptoms result from an inflammatory, likely immune-mediated, process that targets the dorsal root ganglia, causing neuronal loss, proliferation of satellite cells, and secondary degeneration of the posterior columns of the spinal cord. The dorsal and less frequently the anterior nerve roots and peripheral nerves may also be involved. This disorder often precedes or is associated with encephalomyelitis and autonomic dysfunction and has the same immunologic and oncologic associations, e.g., anti-Hu antibodies and SCLC.

TREATMENT Sensory Neuronopathy

As with anti-Hu-associated encephalomyelitis, the therapeutic approach focuses on prompt treatment of the tumor. Glucocorticoids occasionally produce clinical stabilization or improvement. The benefit of IVIg and plasma exchange is not proved.

PARANEOPLASTIC PERIPHERAL NEUROPATHIES

These disorders may develop any time during the course of the neoplastic disease. Neuropathies occurring at late stages of cancer or lymphoma usually cause mild to moderate sensorimotor deficits due to axonal degeneration of unclear etiology. These neuropathies are often masked by concurrent neurotoxicity from chemotherapy and other cancer therapies. In contrast, the neuropathies that develop in the early stages of cancer frequently show a rapid progression, sometimes with a relapsing and remitting course, and evidence of inflammatory infiltrates and axonal loss or demyelination in biopsy studies. If demyelinating features predominate, IVIg, plasma exchange, or glucocorticoids may improve symptoms. Occasionally, anti-CV_2/CRMP5 antibodies are present; detection of anti-Hu suggests concurrent dorsal root ganglionitis.

Guillain-Barré syndrome and *brachial plexitis* have occasionally been reported in patients with lymphoma, but there is no clear evidence of a paraneoplastic association.

Malignant monoclonal gammopathies include (1) multiple myeloma and sclerotic myeloma associated with IgG or IgA monoclonal proteins and (2) Waldenström's macroglobulinemia, B cell lymphoma, and chronic B cell lymphocytic leukemia associated with IgM monoclonal proteins. These disorders may cause neuropathy by a variety of mechanisms, including compression of roots and plexuses by metastasis to vertebral bodies and the pelvis, deposits of amyloid in peripheral nerves, and paraneoplastic mechanisms. The paraneoplastic variety has several distinctive features. Approximately half of patients with sclerotic myeloma develop a sensorimotor neuropathy with predominantly motor deficits, resembling a chronic inflammatory demyelinating neuropathy; some patients develop elements of the POEMS syndrome (*p*olyneuropathy, *o*rganomegaly, *e*ndocrinopathy, *M* protein, *s*kin changes). Treatment of the plasmacytoma or sclerotic lesions usually improves the neuropathy. In contrast, the sensorimotor or sensory neuropathy associated with multiple myeloma rarely responds to treatment. Between 5 and 10% of patients with Waldenström's macroglobulinemia develop a distal symmetric sensorimotor neuropathy with predominant involvement of large sensory fibers. These patients may have IgM antibodies in their serum against myelin-associated glycoprotein and various gangliosides. In addition to treating the Waldenström's macroglobulinemia, other therapies may improve the neuropathy, including plasma exchange, IVIg, chlorambucil, cyclophosphamide, fludarabine, or rituximab.

Vasculitis of the nerve and muscle causes a painful symmetric or asymmetric distal axonal sensorimotor neuropathy with variable proximal weakness. It predominantly affects elderly men and is associated with an elevated erythrocyte sedimentation rate and increased CSF protein concentration. SCLC and lymphoma are the primary tumors involved. Glucocorticoids and cyclophosphamide often result in neurologic improvement.

Peripheral nerve hyperexcitability (*neuromyotonia,* or *Isaacs' syndrome*) is characterized by spontaneous and continuous muscle fiber activity of peripheral nerve origin. Clinical features include cramps, muscle twitching (fasciculations or myokymia), stiffness, delayed muscle relaxation (pseudomyotonia), and spontaneous or evoked carpal or pedal spasms. The involved muscles may be hypertrophic, and some patients develop paresthesias and hyperhidrosis. CNS dysfunction, including mood changes, sleep disorder, or hallucinations, may occur. The electromyogram shows fibrillations; fasciculations; and doublet, triplet, or multiplet single-unit (myokymic) discharges that have a high intraburst frequency. Approximately 20% of patients have serum antibodies to Caspr2-related proteins. The disorder often occurs without cancer; if paraneoplastic, benign, and malignant thymomas and SCLC are the usual tumors. Phenytoin, carbamazepine, and plasma exchange improve symptoms.

Paraneoplastic autonomic neuropathy usually develops as a component of other disorders, such as LEMS and encephalomyelitis. It may rarely occur as a pure or predominantly autonomic neuropathy with adrenergic or cholinergic dysfunction at the pre- or postganglionic levels. Patients can develop several life-threatening complications, such as gastrointestinal paresis with pseudoobstruction, cardiac dysrhythmias, and postural hypotension. Other clinical features include abnormal pupillary responses, dry mouth, anhidrosis, erectile dysfunction, and problems in sphincter control. The disorder occurs in association with several tumors, including SCLC, cancer of the pancreas or testis, carcinoid tumors, and lymphoma. Because autonomic symptoms can be the presenting feature of encephalomyelitis, serum anti-Hu and anti-CV_2/CRMP5 antibodies should be sought. Antibodies to ganglionic (α3-type) neuronal acetylcholine receptors are the cause of autoimmune autonomic ganglionopathy, a disorder that frequently occurs without cancer association.

LAMBERT-EATON MYASTHENIC SYNDROME

LEMS is a presynaptic disorder that usually affects the proximal muscles of the lower limbs together with cranial nerve findings in 70% of patients mimicking myasthenia gravis (MG). In contrast to MG, LEMS patients have depressed or absent reflexes and autonomic symptoms such as dry mouth. LEMS is caused by autoantibodies to the P/Q-type calcium channels at the motor nerve terminals.

MYASTHENIA GRAVIS

Muscle weakness and fatigue commonly occur in a characteristic pattern. Diplopia and ptosis are early findings; changes in voice, fatigue on chewing, tongue weakness occur that increases with longer effort and improves with rest. Antibodies to the acetylcholine receptor are etiologic and it is most commonly seen in thymoma.

POLYMYOSITIS-DERMATOMYOSITIS

Cancer can be associated with dermatomyositis, a progressive, symmetric muscle weakness generally affecting proximal muscles that is associated with a rash, usually a flat red rash on the face and upper trunk. The rash may be pruritic. Humoral immune mechanisms are implicated. Muscle enzymes are elevated. Glucocorticoids or other immunosuppressive drugs may produce some improvement at least transiently.

ACUTE NECROTIZING MYOPATHY

Patients with this syndrome develop myalgias and rapid progression of weakness involving the extremities and the pharyngeal and respiratory muscles, often resulting in death. Serum muscle enzymes are elevated, and muscle biopsy shows extensive necrosis with minimal or absent inflammation and sometimes deposits of complement. The disorder occurs as a paraneoplastic manifestation of a variety of cancers including SCLC and cancer of the gastrointestinal tract, breast, kidney, and prostate, among others. Glucocorticoids and treatment of the underlying tumor rarely control the disorder.

PARANEOPLASTIC VISUAL SYNDROMES

This group of disorders involves the retina and, less frequently, the uvea and optic nerves. The term *cancer-associated retinopathy* is used to describe paraneoplastic cone and rod dysfunction characterized by photosensitivity, progressive loss of vision and color perception, central or ring scotomas, night blindness, and attenuation of photopic and scotopic responses in the electroretinogram (ERG). The most commonly associated tumor is SCLC. Melanoma-associated retinopathy affects patients with metastatic cutaneous melanoma. Patients develop acute onset of night blindness and shimmering, flickering, or pulsating photopsias that often progress to visual loss. The ERG shows reduced b waves with normal dark adapted a waves. Paraneoplastic optic neuritis and uveitis are very uncommon and can develop in association with encephalomyelitis. Some patients with paraneoplastic uveitis harbor anti-CV_2/CRMP5 antibodies.

Some paraneoplastic retinopathies are associated with serum antibodies that specifically react with the subset of retinal cells undergoing degeneration, supporting an immune-mediated pathogenesis (Table 53-2). Paraneoplastic retinopathies usually fail to improve with treatment, although rare responses to glucocorticoids, plasma exchange, and IVIg have been reported.

SECTION XII

ONCOLOGIC EMERGENCIES AND LATE EFFECTS COMPLICATIONS

CHAPTER 54
ONCOLOGIC EMERGENCIES

Rasim Gucalp ■ Janice Dutcher

Emergencies in patients with cancer may be classified into three groups: pressure or obstruction caused by a space-occupying lesion, metabolic or hormonal problems (paraneoplastic syndromes, Chap. 52), and treatment-related complications.

STRUCTURAL-OBSTRUCTIVE ONCOLOGIC EMERGENCIES

SUPERIOR VENA CAVA SYNDROME

Superior vena cava syndrome (SVCS) is the clinical manifestation of superior vena cava (SVC) obstruction, with severe reduction in venous return from the head, neck, and upper extremities. Malignant tumors, such as lung cancer, lymphoma, and metastatic tumors, are responsible for the majority of SVCS cases. With the expanding use of intravascular devices (e.g., permanent central venous access catheters, pacemaker/defibrillator leads), the prevalence of benign causes of SVCS is increasing now, accounting for at least 40% of cases. Lung cancer, particularly of small cell and squamous cell histologies, accounts for approximately 85% of all cases of malignant origin. In young adults, malignant lymphoma is a leading cause of SVCS. Hodgkin's lymphoma involves the mediastinum more commonly than other lymphomas but rarely causes SVCS. When SVCS is noted in a young man with a mediastinal mass, the differential diagnosis is lymphoma vs primary mediastinal germ cell tumor. Metastatic cancers to the mediastinum, such as testicular and breast carcinomas, account for a small proportion of cases. Other causes include benign tumors, aortic aneurysm, thyromegaly, thrombosis, and fibrosing mediastinitis from prior irradiation, histoplasmosis, or Behçet's syndrome. SVCS as the initial manifestation of Behçet's syndrome may be due to inflammation of the SVC associated with thrombosis.

Patients with SVCS usually present with neck and facial swelling (especially around the eyes), dyspnea, and cough. Other symptoms include hoarseness, tongue swelling, headaches, nasal congestion, epistaxis, hemoptysis, dysphagia, pain, dizziness, syncope, and lethargy. Bending forward or lying down may aggravate the symptoms. The characteristic physical findings are dilated neck veins; an increased number of collateral veins covering the anterior chest wall; cyanosis; and edema of the face, arms, and chest. More severe cases include proptosis, glossal and laryngeal edema, and obtundation. The clinical picture is milder if the obstruction is located above the azygos vein. Symptoms are usually progressive, but in some cases, they may improve as collateral circulation develops.

Signs and symptoms of cerebral and/or laryngeal edema, though rare, are associated with a poorer prognosis and require urgent evaluation. Seizures are more likely related to brain metastases than to cerebral edema from venous occlusion. Patients with small cell lung cancer and SVCS have a higher incidence of brain metastases than those without SVCS.

Cardiorespiratory symptoms at rest, particularly with positional changes, suggest significant airway and vascular obstruction and limited physiologic reserve. Cardiac arrest or respiratory failure can occur, particularly in patients receiving sedatives or undergoing general anesthesia.

Rarely, esophageal varices may develop. These are "downhill" varices based on the direction of blood flow from cephalad to caudad (in contrast to "uphill" varices associated with caudad to cephalad flow from portal hypertension). If the obstruction to the SVC is proximal to the azygous vein, varices develop in the upper one-third of the esophagus. If the obstruction involves or is distal to the azygous vein, varices occur in the entire length of the esophagus. Variceal bleeding may be a late complication of chronic SVCS.

The diagnosis of SVCS is a clinical one. The most significant chest radiographic finding is widening of the superior mediastinum, most commonly on the right side. Pleural effusion occurs in only 25% of patients, often on the right side. The majority of these effusions are exudative and occasionally chylous. However, a normal chest radiograph is still compatible with the diagnosis if other characteristic findings are present. Computed tomography (CT) provides the most reliable view of the mediastinal anatomy. The diagnosis of SVCS requires diminished or absent opacification of central venous structures with prominent collateral venous circulation. Magnetic resonance imaging (MRI) has no advantages over CT. Invasive procedures, including bronchoscopy, percutaneous needle biopsy, mediastinoscopy, and even thoracotomy, can be performed by a skilled clinician without any major risk of bleeding. For patients with a known cancer, a detailed workup usually is not necessary, and appropriate treatment may be started after obtaining a CT scan of the thorax. For those with no history of malignancy, a detailed evaluation is essential to rule out benign causes and determine a specific diagnosis to direct the appropriate therapy.

TREATMENT Superior Vena Cava Syndrome

The one potentially life-threatening complication of a superior mediastinal mass is tracheal obstruction. Upper airway obstruction demands emergent therapy. Diuretics with a low-salt diet, head elevation, and oxygen may produce temporary symptomatic relief. Glucocorticoids may be useful at shrinking lymphoma masses; they are of no benefit in patients with lung cancer.

Radiation therapy is the primary treatment for SVCS caused by non-small cell lung cancer (NSCLC) and other metastatic solid tumors. Chemotherapy is effective when the underlying cancer is small cell carcinoma of the lung, lymphoma, or germ cell tumor. SVCS recurs in 10–30% of patients; it may be palliated with the use of intravascular self-expanding stents (Fig. 54-1). Early stenting may be necessary in patients with severe symptoms; however, the prompt increase in venous return after stenting may precipitate heart failure and pulmonary edema. Surgery may provide immediate relief for patients in whom a benign process is the cause.

Clinical improvement occurs in most patients, although this improvement may be due to the development of adequate collateral circulation. The mortality associated with SVCS does not relate to caval obstruction but rather to the underlying cause.

SVCS AND CENTRAL VENOUS CATHETERS IN ADULTS The use of long-term central venous catheters has become common practice in patients with cancer. Major vessel thrombosis may occur. In these cases, catheter removal should be combined with anticoagulation to prevent embolization. SVCS in this setting, if detected early, can be treated by fibrinolytic therapy without sacrificing the catheter. The routine use of low-dose warfarin or low-molecular-weight heparin to prevent thrombosis related to permanent central venous access catheters in cancer patients is not recommended.

PERICARDIAL EFFUSION OR TAMPONADE

Malignant pericardial disease is found at autopsy in 5–10% of patients with cancer, most frequently with lung cancer, breast cancer, leukemias, and lymphomas. Cardiac tamponade as the initial presentation of extrathoracic malignancy is rare. The origin is not malignancy in about 50% of cancer patients with symptomatic pericardial disease, but it can be related to irradiation, drug-induced pericarditis, hypothyroidism, idiopathic pericarditis, infection, or autoimmune diseases. Two types of radiation pericarditis occur: an acute inflammatory, effusive pericarditis occurring within months of irradiation, which usually resolves spontaneously, and a chronic effusive pericarditis that may appear up to 20 years after radiation therapy and is accompanied by a thickened pericardium.

Most patients with pericardial metastasis are asymptomatic. However, the common symptoms are dyspnea, cough, chest pain, orthopnea, and weakness. Pleural effusion, sinus tachycardia, jugular venous distention, hepatomegaly, peripheral edema, and cyanosis are the most frequent physical findings. Relatively specific diagnostic findings, such as paradoxical pulse, diminished heart sounds, pulsus alternans (pulse waves alternating between those of greater and lesser amplitude with successive beats), and friction rub are less common than with nonmalignant pericardial disease. Chest radiographs and electrocardiography reveal abnormalities in 90% of patients, but half of these abnormalities are nonspecific. Echocardiography is the most helpful diagnostic test. Pericardial fluid may be serous, serosanguineous, or hemorrhagic, and cytologic examination of pericardial fluid is diagnostic in most patients. Cancer patients with pericardial effusion containing malignant cells on cytology have a very poor survival, about 7 weeks.

TREATMENT Pericardial Effusion or Tamponade

Pericardiocentesis with or without the introduction of sclerosing agents, the creation of a pericardial window, complete pericardial stripping, cardiac irradiation, or systemic chemotherapy are effective treatments. Acute pericardial tamponade with life-threatening hemodynamic instability requires immediate drainage of fluid.

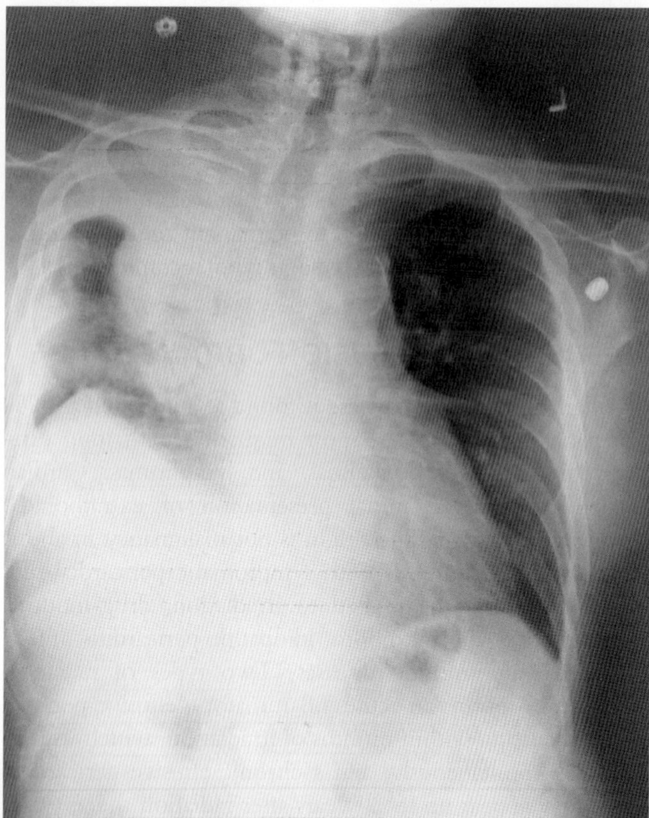

A

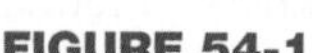

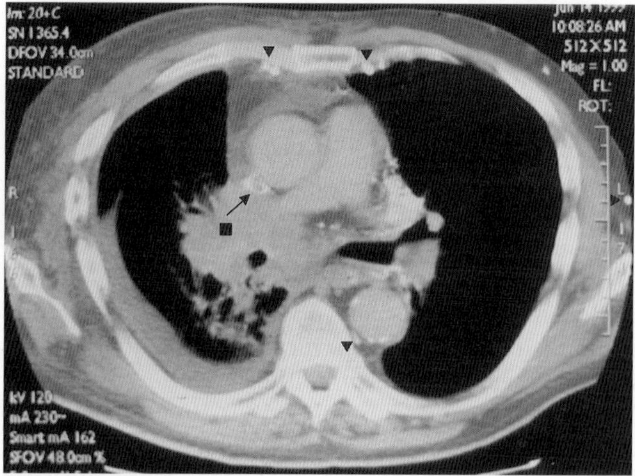

B

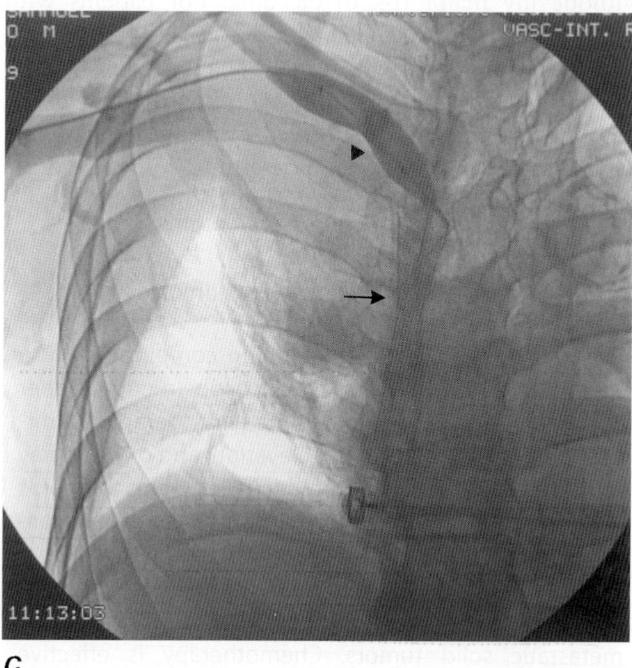

C

FIGURE 54-1

Superior vena cava syndrome (SVCS). ***A.*** Chest radiographs of a 59-year-old man with recurrent SVCS caused by non-small cell lung cancer showing right paratracheal mass with right pleural effusion. ***B.*** Computed tomography of same patient demonstrating obstruction of SVC with thrombosis (*arrow*) by the lung cancer (*square*) and collaterals (*arrowheads*). ***C.*** Balloon angioplasty (*arrowhead*) with Wallstent (*arrow*) in same patient.

This can be quickly achieved by pericardiocentesis. The recurrence rate after percutaneous catheter drainage is about 20%. Sclerotherapy (pericardial instillation of bleomycin, mitomycin C, or tetracycline) may decrease recurrences. Alternatively, subxiphoid pericardiotomy can be performed in 45 min under local anesthesia. Thoracoscopic pericardial fenestration can be employed for benign causes; however, 60% of malignant pericardial effusions recur after this procedure.

INTESTINAL OBSTRUCTION

Intestinal obstruction and reobstruction are common problems in patients with advanced cancer, particularly colorectal or ovarian carcinoma. However, other cancers, such as lung or breast cancer and melanoma, can metastasize within the abdomen, leading to intestinal obstruction. Typically, obstruction occurs at multiple sites in peritoneal carcinomatosis. Melanoma has a predilection to involve the small bowel; this involvement may be isolated and resection may result in prolonged survival. Intestinal pseudoobstruction is caused by infiltration of the mesentery or bowel muscle by tumor, involvement of the celiac plexus, or paraneoplastic neuropathy in patients with small cell lung cancer. Paraneoplastic neuropathy is associated with IgG antibodies reactive to neurons of the myenteric and submucosal plexuses of the jejunum and stomach. Ovarian cancer can lead to authentic luminal obstruction or to pseudoobstruction that results when circumferential invasion of a bowel segment arrests the forward progression of peristaltic contractions.

The onset of obstruction is usually insidious. Pain is the most common symptom and is usually colicky in nature. Pain can also be due to abdominal distention, tumor masses, or hepatomegaly. Vomiting can be intermittent or continuous. Patients with complete obstruction usually have constipation. Physical examination may reveal abdominal distention with tympany, ascites, visible peristalsis, high-pitched bowel sounds, and tumor masses. Erect plain abdominal films may reveal multiple air-fluid levels and dilation of the small or large bowel. Acute cecal dilation to >12–14 cm is considered a surgical emergency because of the high likelihood of rupture. CT scan is useful in differentiating benign from malignant causes of obstruction in patients who have undergone surgery for malignancy. Malignant obstruction is suggested by a mass at the site of obstruction or prior surgery, adenopathy, or an abrupt transition zone and irregular bowel thickening at the obstruction site. Benign obstruction is more likely when CT shows mesenteric vascular changes, a large volume of ascites, or a smooth transition zone and smooth bowel thickening at the obstruction site. The prognosis for the patient with cancer who develops intestinal obstruction is poor; median survival is 3–4 months. About 25–30% of patients are found to have intestinal obstruction due to causes other than cancer. Adhesions from previous operations are a common benign cause. Ileus induced by vinca alkaloids, narcotics, or other drugs is another reversible cause.

TREATMENT Intestinal Obstruction

The management of intestinal obstruction in patients with advanced malignancy depends on the extent of the underlying malignancy and the functional status of the major organs. The initial management should include surgical evaluation. Operation is not always successful and may lead to further complications with a substantial mortality rate (10–20%). Laparoscopy can diagnose and treat malignant bowel obstruction in some cases. Self-expanding metal stents placed in the gastric outlet, duodenum, proximal jejunum, colon, or rectum may palliate obstructive symptoms at those sites without major surgery. Patients known to have advanced intraabdominal malignancy should receive a prolonged course of conservative management, including nasogastric decompression. Percutaneous endoscopic or surgical gastrostomy tube placement is an option for palliation of nausea and vomiting, the so-called "venting gastrostomy." Treatment with antiemetics, antispasmodics, and analgesics may allow patients to remain outside the hospital. Octreotide may relieve obstructive symptoms through its inhibitory effect on gastrointestinal secretion.

URINARY OBSTRUCTION

Urinary obstruction may occur in patients with prostatic or gynecologic malignancies, particularly cervical carcinoma; metastatic disease from other primary sites such as carcinomas of the breast, stomach, lung, colon, and pancreas; or lymphomas. Radiation therapy to pelvic tumors may cause fibrosis and subsequent ureteral obstruction. Bladder outlet obstruction is usually due to prostate and cervical cancers and may lead to bilateral hydronephrosis and renal failure.

Flank pain is the most common symptom. Persistent urinary tract infection, persistent proteinuria, or hematuria in patients with cancer should raise suspicion of ureteral obstruction. Total anuria and/or anuria alternating with polyuria may occur. A slow, continuous rise in the serum creatinine level necessitates immediate evaluation. Renal ultrasound is the safest and cheapest way to identify hydronephrosis. The function of an obstructed kidney can be evaluated by a nuclear scan. CT scan can reveal the point of obstruction and identify a retroperitoneal mass or adenopathy.

TREATMENT Urinary Obstruction

Obstruction associated with flank pain, sepsis, or fistula formation is an indication for immediate palliative urinary diversion. Internal ureteral stents can be placed under local anesthesia. Percutaneous nephrostomy offers an alternative approach for drainage. In the case of bladder outlet obstruction due to malignancy, a suprapubic cystostomy can be used for urinary drainage.

MALIGNANT BILIARY OBSTRUCTION

This common clinical problem can be caused by a primary carcinoma arising in the pancreas, ampulla of Vater, bile duct, or liver or by metastatic disease to the periductal lymph nodes or liver parenchyma. The most common metastatic tumors causing biliary obstruction are gastric, colon, breast, and lung cancers. Jaundice, light-colored stools, dark urine, pruritus, and weight loss due to malabsorption are usual symptoms. Pain and secondary infection are uncommon in malignant biliary obstruction. Ultrasound, CT scan, or percutaneous transhepatic or endoscopic retrograde cholangiography will identify the site and nature of the biliary obstruction.

TREATMENT Malignant Biliary Obstruction

Palliative intervention is indicated only in patients with disabling pruritus resistant to medical treatment, severe malabsorption, or infection. Stenting under radiographic control, surgical bypass, or radiation therapy with or without chemotherapy may alleviate the obstruction. The choice of therapy should be based on the site of obstruction (proximal vs distal), the type of tumor (sensitive to radiotherapy, chemotherapy, or neither), and the general condition of the patient. In the absence of pruritus, biliary obstruction may be a largely asymptomatic cause of death.

SPINAL CORD COMPRESSION

Malignant spinal cord compression (MSCC) is defined as compression of the spinal cord and/or cauda equina by an extradural tumor mass. The minimum radiologic evidence for cord compression is indentation of the theca at the level of clinical features. Spinal cord compression occurs in 5–10% of patients with cancer. Epidural tumor is the first manifestation of malignancy in about 10% of patients. The underlying cancer is usually identified during the initial evaluation; lung cancer is the most common cause of MSCC.

Metastatic tumor involves the vertebral column more often than any other part of the bony skeleton. Lung, breast, and prostate cancer are the most frequent offenders. Multiple myeloma also has a high incidence of spine involvement. Lymphomas, melanoma, renal cell cancer, and genitourinary cancers also cause cord compression. The thoracic spine is the most common site (70%), followed by the lumbosacral spine (20%) and the cervical spine (10%). Involvement of multiple sites is most frequent in patients with breast and prostate carcinoma. Cord injury develops when metastases to the vertebral body or pedicle enlarge and compress the underlying dura. Another cause of cord compression is direct extension of a paravertebral lesion through the intervertebral foramen. These cases usually involve a lymphoma, myeloma, or pediatric neoplasm. Parenchymal spinal cord metastasis due to hematogenous spread is rare. Intramedullary metastases can be seen in lung cancer, multiple myeloma, renal cell cancer, and breast cancer and are frequently associated with brain metastases and leptomeningeal disease.

Expanding extradural tumors induce injury through several mechanisms. Obstruction of the epidural venous plexus leads to edema. Local production of inflammatory cytokines enhances blood flow and edema formation. Compression compromises blood flow leading to ischemia. Production of vascular endothelial growth factor is associated with spinal cord hypoxia and has been implicated as a potential cause of damage after spinal cord injury.

The most common initial symptom in patients with spinal cord compression is localized back pain and tenderness due to involvement of vertebrae by tumor. Pain is usually present for days or months before other neurologic findings appear. It is exacerbated by movement and by coughing or sneezing. It can be differentiated from the pain of disk disease by the fact that it worsens when the patient is supine. Radicular pain is less common than localized back pain and usually develops later. Radicular pain in the cervical or lumbosacral areas may be unilateral or bilateral. Radicular pain from the thoracic roots is often bilateral and is described by patients as a feeling of tight, band-like constriction around the thorax and abdomen. Typical cervical radicular pain radiates down the arm; in the lumbar region, the radiation is down the legs. *Lhermitte's sign*, a tingling or electric sensation down the back and upper and lower limbs upon flexing or extending the neck, may be an early sign of cord compression. Loss of bowel or bladder control may be the presenting symptom but usually occurs late in the course. Occasionally, patients present with ataxia of gait without motor and sensory involvement due to involvement of the spinocerebellar tract.

On physical examination, pain induced by straight leg raising, neck flexion, or vertebral percussion may help to determine the level of cord compression. Patients develop numbness and paresthesias in the extremities or trunk. Loss of sensibility to pinprick is as common as loss of sensibility to vibration or position. The upper limit of the zone of sensory loss is often one or two vertebrae below the site of compression. Motor findings include weakness, spasticity, and abnormal muscle stretching. An extensor plantar reflex reflects significant compression. Deep tendon reflexes may be brisk. Motor and sensory loss usually precedes sphincter disturbance. Patients with autonomic dysfunction may present with decreased anal tonus, decreased perineal sensibility, and a distended bladder. The absence of the anal wink reflex or the bulbocavernosus reflex confirms cord involvement. In doubtful cases, evaluation of postvoiding urinary residual volume can be helpful. A residual volume of >150 mL suggests bladder dysfunction. Autonomic dysfunction is an unfavorable prognostic factor. Patients with progressive neurologic symptoms should have frequent neurologic examinations and rapid therapeutic intervention. Other illnesses that may mimic cord compression include osteoporotic vertebral collapse, disk disease, pyogenic abscess or vertebral tuberculosis, radiation myelopathy, neoplastic leptomeningitis, benign tumors, epidural hematoma, and spinal lipomatosis.

Cauda equina syndrome is characterized by low back pain; diminished sensation over the buttocks, posterior-superior thighs, and perineal area in a saddle distribution; rectal and bladder dysfunction; sexual impotence; absent bulbocavernous, patellar, and Achilles' reflexes; and variable amount of lower-extremity weakness. This reflects compression of nerve roots as they form the cauda equina after leaving the spinal cord.

Patients with cancer who develop back pain should be evaluated for spinal cord compression as quickly as

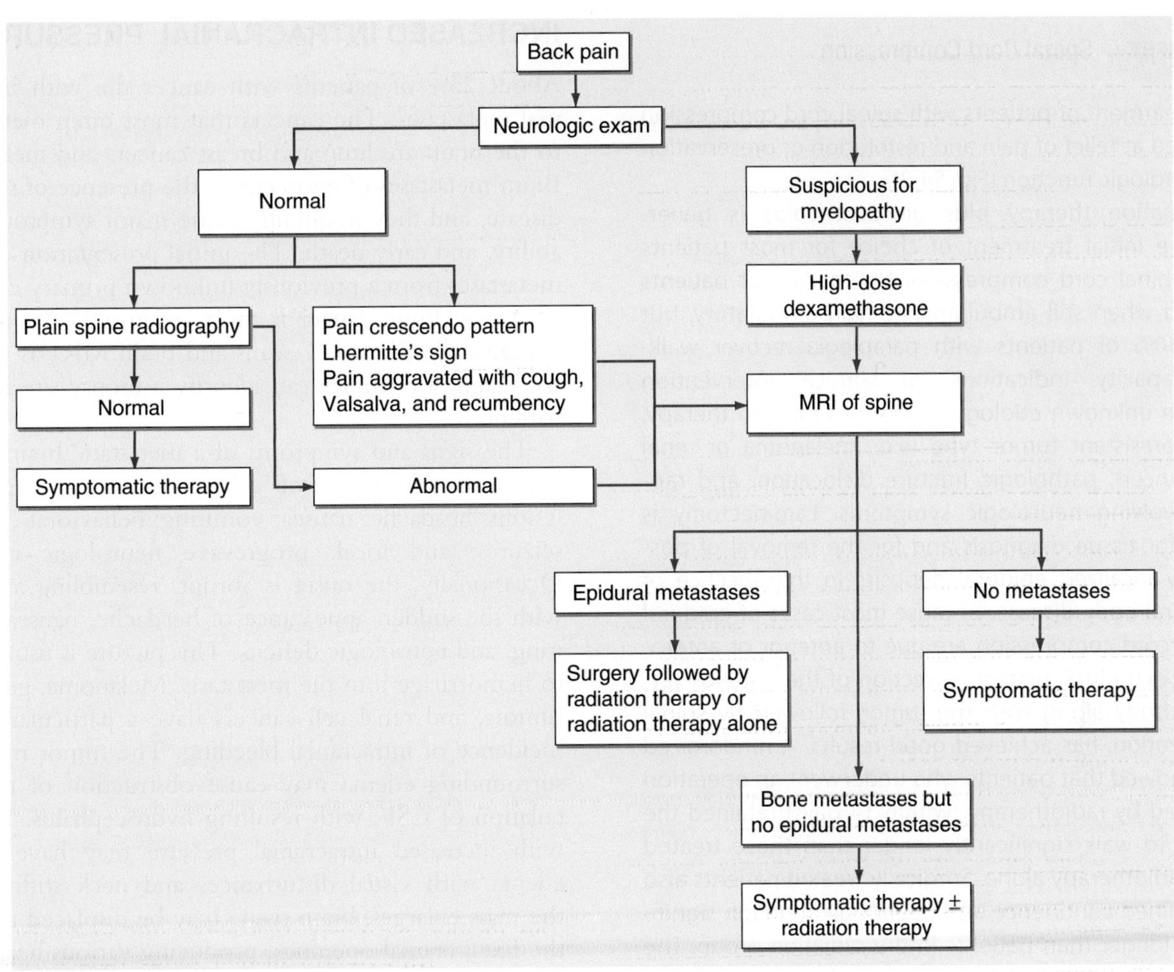

FIGURE 54-2

Management of cancer patients with back pain. MRI, magnetic resonance imaging.

possible (Fig. 54-2). Treatment is more often successful in patients who are ambulatory and still have sphincter control at the time treatment is initiated. Patients should have a neurologic examination and plain films of the spine. Those whose physical examination suggests cord compression should receive dexamethasone (6 mg intravenously every 6 h), starting immediately.

Erosion of the pedicles (the "winking owl" sign) is the earliest radiologic finding of vertebral tumor. Other radiographic changes include increased intrapedicular distance, vertebral destruction, lytic or sclerotic lesions, scalloped vertebral bodies, and vertebral body collapse. Vertebral collapse is not a reliable indicator of the presence of tumor; about 20% of cases of vertebral collapse, particularly those in older patients and postmenopausal women, are due not to cancer but to osteoporosis. Also, a normal appearance on plain films of the spine does not exclude the diagnosis of cancer. The role of bone scans in the detection of cord compression is not clear; this method is sensitive but less specific than spinal radiography.

The full-length image of the cord provided by MRI is the imaging procedure of choice. Multiple epidural metastases are noted in 25% of patients with cord compression, and their presence influences treatment plans. On T1-weighted images, good contrast is noted between the cord, cerebrospinal fluid (CSF), and extradural lesions. Owing to its sensitivity in demonstrating the replacement of bone marrow by tumor, MRI can show which parts of a vertebra are involved by tumor. MRI also visualizes intraspinal extradural masses compressing the cord. T2-weighted images are most useful for the demonstration of intramedullary pathology. Gadolinium-enhanced MRI can help to delineate intramedullary disease. MRI is as good as or better than myelography plus postmyelogram CT scan in detecting metastatic epidural disease with cord compression. Myelography should be reserved for patients who have poor MR images or who cannot undergo MRI promptly. CT scan in conjunction with myelography enhances the detection of small areas of spinal destruction.

In patients with cord compression and an unknown primary tumor, a simple workup including chest radiography, mammography, measurement of prostate-specific antigen, and abdominal CT usually reveals the underlying malignancy.

TREATMENT Spinal Cord Compression

The treatment of patients with spinal cord compression is aimed at relief of pain and restoration or preservation of neurologic function (Fig. 54-2).

Radiation therapy plus glucocorticoids is generally the initial treatment of choice for most patients with spinal cord compression. Up to 75% of patients treated when still ambulatory remain ambulatory, but only 10% of patients with paraplegia recover walking capacity. Indications for surgical intervention include unknown etiology, failure of radiation therapy, a radioresistant tumor type (e.g., melanoma or renal cell cancer), pathologic fracture dislocation, and rapidly evolving neurologic symptoms. Laminectomy is done for tissue diagnosis and for the removal of posteriorly localized epidural deposits in the absence of vertebral body disease. Because most cases of epidural spinal cord compression are due to anterior or anterolateral extradural disease, resection of the anterior vertebral body along with the tumor, followed by spinal stabilization, has achieved good results. A randomized trial showed that patients who underwent an operation followed by radiotherapy (within 14 days) retained the ability to walk significantly longer than those treated with radiotherapy alone. Surgically treated patients also maintained continence and neurologic function significantly longer than patients in the radiation group. The length of survival was not significantly different in the two groups, although there was a trend toward longer survival in the surgery group. The study drew some criticism for the poorer than expected results in the patients who did not go to surgery. However, patients should be evaluated for surgery if they are expected to survive longer than 3 months. Conventional radiotherapy has a role after surgery. Chemotherapy may have a role in patients with chemosensitive tumors who have had prior radiotherapy to the same region and who are not candidates for surgery. Most patients with prostate cancer who develop cord compression have already had hormonal therapy; however, for those who have not, androgen deprivation is combined with surgery and radiotherapy.

Patients with metastatic vertebral tumors may benefit from percutaneous vertebroplasty or kyphoplasty, the injection of acrylic cement into a collapsed vertebra to stabilize the fracture. Pain palliation is common, and local antitumor effects have been noted. Cement leakage may cause symptoms in about 10% of patients. Bisphosphonates may be helpful in prevention of spinal cord compression (SCC) in patients with bony involvement.

The histology of the tumor is an important determinant of both recovery and survival. Rapid onset and progression of signs and symptoms are poor prognostic features.

INCREASED INTRACRANIAL PRESSURE

About 25% of patients with cancer die with intracranial metastases. The cancers that most often metastasize to the brain are lung and breast cancers and melanoma. Brain metastases often occur in the presence of systemic disease, and they frequently cause major symptoms, disability, and early death. The initial presentation of brain metastases from a previously unknown primary cancer is common. Lung cancer is most commonly the primary malignancy. Chest CT scans and brain MRI as the initial diagnostic studies can identify a biopsy site in most patients.

The signs and symptoms of a metastatic brain tumor are similar to those of other intracranial expanding lesions: headache; nausea; vomiting; behavioral changes; seizures; and focal, progressive neurologic changes. Occasionally, the onset is abrupt, resembling a stroke, with the sudden appearance of headache, nausea, vomiting, and neurologic deficits. This picture is usually due to hemorrhage into the metastasis. Melanoma, germ cell tumors, and renal cell cancers have a particularly high incidence of intracranial bleeding. The tumor mass and surrounding edema may cause obstruction of the circulation of CSF, with resulting hydrocephalus. Patients with increased intracranial pressure may have papilledema with visual disturbances and neck stiffness. As the mass enlarges, brain tissue may be displaced through the fixed cranial openings, producing various herniation syndromes.

CT scan and MRI are equally effective in the diagnosis of brain metastases. CT scan with contrast should be used as a screening procedure. The CT scan shows brain metastases as multiple enhancing lesions of various sizes with surrounding areas of low-density edema. If a single lesion or no metastases are visualized by contrast-enhanced CT, MRI of the brain should be performed. Gadolinium-enhanced MRI is more sensitive than CT at revealing meningeal involvement and small lesions, particularly in the brainstem or cerebellum.

Intracranial hypertension secondary to tretinoin therapy has been reported.

TREATMENT Increased Intracranial Pressure

Dexamethasone is the best initial treatment for all symptomatic patients with brain metastases. If signs and symptoms of brain herniation (particularly headache, drowsiness, and papilledema) are present, the patient should be intubated and hyperventilated to maintain P_{CO_2} between 25 and 30 mmHg and should receive infusions of mannitol (1–1.5 g/kg) every 6 h. Other measures include head elevation, fluid restriction, and hypertonic saline with diuretics. Patients with multiple lesions should receive whole-brain radiation.

Patients with a single brain metastasis and with controlled extracranial disease may be treated with surgical excision followed by whole-brain radiation therapy, especially if they are younger than 60 years. Radioresistant tumors should be resected if possible. Stereotactic radiosurgery is an effective treatment for inaccessible or recurrent lesions. With a gamma knife or linear accelerator, multiple small, well-collimated beams of ionizing radiation destroy lesions seen on MRI. Some patients with increased intracranial pressure associated with hydrocephalus may benefit from shunt placement. If neurologic deterioration is not reversed with medical therapy, ventriculotomy to remove CSF or craniotomy to remove tumors or hematomas may be necessary.

NEOPLASTIC MENINGITIS

Tumor involving the leptomeninges is a complication of both primary central nervous system (CNS) tumors and tumors that metastasize to the CNS. The incidence is estimated at 3–8% of patients with cancer. Melanoma, breast and lung cancer, lymphoma (including AIDS-associated), and acute leukemia are the most common causes. Synchronous intraparenchymal brain metastases are evident in 11–31% of patients with neoplastic meningitis.

Patients typically present with multifocal neurologic signs and symptoms, including headache, gait abnormality, mental changes, nausea, vomiting, seizures, back or radicular pain, and limb weakness. Signs include cranial nerve palsies, extremity weakness, paresthesia, and decreased deep tendon reflexes.

Diagnosis is made by demonstrating malignant cells in the CSF; however, up to 40% of patients may have false-negative CSF cytology. An elevated CSF protein level is nearly always present (except in human T-lymphotropic virus type I associated adult T cell leukemia). Patients with neurologic signs and symptoms consistent with neoplastic meningitis who have a negative CSF cytology but an elevated CSF protein level should have the spinal tap repeated at least three times for cytologic examination before the diagnosis is rejected. MRI findings suggestive of neoplastic meningitis include leptomeningeal, subependymal, dural, or cranial nerve enhancement; superficial cerebral lesions; and communicating hydrocephalus. Spinal cord imaging by MRI is a necessary component of the evaluation of nonleukemia neoplastic meningitis as ~20% of patients have cord abnormalities, including intradural enhancing nodules that are diagnostic for leptomeningeal involvement. Cauda equina lesions are common, but lesions may be seen anywhere in the spinal canal. Radiolabeled CSF flow study results are abnormal in up to 70% of patients with neoplastic meningitis; ventricular outlet obstruction, abnormal flow in the spinal canal, or impaired flow over the cerebral convexities may affect distribution of intrathecal chemotherapy, resulting in decreased efficacy or increased toxicity. Radiation therapy may correct CSF flow abnormalities before use of intrathecal chemotherapy. Neoplastic meningitis can also lead to intracranial hypertension and hydrocephalus. Placement of a ventriculoperitoneal shunt may effectively palliate symptoms in these patients.

The development of neoplastic meningitis usually occurs in the setting of uncontrolled cancer outside the CNS; thus, prognosis is poor (median survival time, 10–12 weeks). However, treatment of the neoplastic meningitis may successfully alleviate symptoms and control the CNS spread.

TREATMENT Neoplastic Meningitis

Intrathecal chemotherapy, usually methotrexate, cytarabine, or thiotepa, is delivered by lumbar puncture or by an intraventricular reservoir (Ommaya) three times a week until the CSF is free of malignant cells. Injections are given twice a week for a month and then weekly for a month. An extended-release preparation of cytarabine (Depocyte) has a longer half-life and is more effective than other formulations. Among solid tumors, breast cancer responds best to therapy. Patients with neoplastic meningitis from either acute leukemia or lymphoma may be cured of their CNS disease if the systemic disease can be eliminated.

SEIZURES

Seizures occurring in a patient with cancer can be caused by the tumor itself, by metabolic disturbances, by radiation injury, by cerebral infarctions, by chemotherapy-related encephalopathies, or by CNS infections. Metastatic disease to the CNS is the most common cause of seizures in patients with cancer. However, seizures occur more frequently in those with primary brain tumors than in those with metastatic brain lesions. Seizures are a presenting symptom of CNS metastasis in 6–29% of cases. Approximately 10% of patients with CNS metastasis eventually develop seizures. Tumors that affect the frontal, temporal, and parietal lobes are more commonly associated with seizures than are occipital lesions. The presence of frontal lesions correlates with early seizures, and the presence of hemispheric symptoms increases the risk for late seizures. Both early and late seizures are uncommon in patients with posterior fossa and sellar lesions. Seizures are common in patients with CNS metastases from melanoma and low-grade primary brain tumors.

Very rarely, cytotoxic drugs such as etoposide, busulfan, and chlorambucil cause seizures. Another cause of seizures related to drug therapy is reversible posterior leukoencephalopathy syndrome (RPLS). RPLS is associated with administration of cisplatin, 5-fluorouracil, bleomycin, vinblastine, vincristine, etoposide, paclitaxel, ifosfamide, cyclophosphamide, doxorubicin, cytarabine, methotrexate, oxaliplatin, cyclosporine, tacrolimus, and bevacizumab. RPLS is characterized by headache, altered consciousness, generalized seizures, visual disturbances, hypertension, and posterior cerebral white matter vasogenic edema on CT or MRI. Seizures may begin focally but are typically generalized.

TREATMENT **Seizures**

Patients in whom seizures due to CNS metastases have been demonstrated should receive anticonvulsive treatment with phenytoin. Prophylactic anticonvulsant therapy is not recommended unless the patient is at high risk for late seizures (melanoma primary, hemorrhagic metastases, treatment with radiosurgery). Serum phenytoin levels should be monitored closely and the dosage adjusted according to serum levels. Phenytoin induces the hepatic metabolism of dexamethasone, reducing its half-life, while dexamethasone may decrease phenytoin levels. Most antiseizure medications induce CYP450, which alters the metabolism of antitumor agents, including irinotecan, taxanes, and etoposide as well as molecular targeted agents, including imatinib, gefitinib, erlotinib, and tipifarnib. Levetiracetam and topiramate are anticonvulsant agents not metabolized by the hepatic cytochrome P450 system and do not alter the metabolism of antitumor agents.

PULMONARY AND INTRACEREBRAL LEUKOSTASIS

Hyperleukocytosis and the leukostasis syndrome associated with it is a potentially fatal complication of acute leukemia (particularly myeloid leukemia) that can occur when the peripheral blast cell count is >100,000/mL. The frequency of hyperleukocytosis is 5–13% in acute myelid leukemia (AML) and 10–30% in acute lymphoid leukemia; however, leukostasis is rare in lymphoid leukemia. At such high blast cell counts, blood viscosity is increased, blood flow is slowed by aggregates of tumor cells, and the primitive myeloid leukemic cells are capable of invading through the endothelium and causing hemorrhage. Brain and lung are most commonly affected. Patients with brain leukostasis may experience stupor, headache, dizziness, tinnitus, visual disturbances, ataxia, confusion, coma, or sudden death. Administration of 600 cGy of whole-brain irradiation can protect against this complication and can be followed by rapid institution of antileukemic therapy. Hydroxyurea, 3-5 g, can rapidly reduce a high blast cell count while the accurate diagnostic workup is in progress. Pulmonary leukostasis may present as respiratory distress, hypoxemia, and progress to respiratory failure. Chest radiographs may be normal but usually show interstitial or alveolar infiltrates. Arterial blood gas results should be interpreted cautiously. Rapid consumption of plasma oxygen by the markedly increased number of white blood cells can cause spuriously low arterial oxygen tension. Pulse oximetry is the most accurate way of assessing oxygenation in patients with hyperleukocytosis. Leukapheresis may be helpful in decreasing circulating blast counts. Treatment of the leukemia can result in pulmonary hemorrhage from lysis of blasts in the lung, called *leukemic cell lysis pneumopathy*. Intravascular volume depletion and unnecessary blood transfusions may increase blood viscosity and worsen the leukostasis syndrome. Leukostasis is very rarely a feature of the high white cell counts associated with chronic lymphoid or chronic myeloid leukemia.

When acute promyelocytic leukemia is treated with differentiating agents like tretinoin and arsenic trioxide, cerebral or pulmonary leukostasis may occur as tumor cells differentiate into mature neutrophils. This complication can be largely avoided by using cytotoxic chemotherapy together with the differentiating agents.

HEMOPTYSIS

Hemoptysis may be caused by nonmalignant conditions, but lung cancer accounts for a large proportion of cases. Up to 20% of patients with lung cancer have hemoptysis some time in their course. Endobronchial metastases from carcinoid tumors, breast cancer, colon cancer, kidney cancer, and melanoma may also cause hemoptysis. The volume of bleeding is often difficult to gauge. Massive hemoptysis is defined as >200–600 mL of blood produced in 24 h. However, any hemoptysis should be considered massive if it threatens life. When respiratory difficulty occurs, hemoptysis should be treated emergently. The first priorities are to maintain the airway, optimize oxygenation, and stabilize the hemodynamic status. *Often patients can tell where the bleeding is occurring.* They should be placed bleeding side down and given supplemental oxygen. If large-volume bleeding continues or the airway is compromised, the patient should be intubated and undergo emergency bronchoscopy. If the site of bleeding is detected, either the patient undergoes a definitive surgical procedure or the lesion is treated with a neodymium:yttrium-aluminum-garnet (Nd:YAG) laser. The surgical option is preferred. Bronchial artery embolization may control brisk bleeding in 75–90% of patients, permitting the definitive surgical procedure to be done more safely. Embolization without definitive surgery is associated with rebleeding in 20–50% of patients. Recurrent hemoptysis usually responds to a second embolization procedure. A postembolization syndrome characterized by pleuritic pain, fever, dysphagia, and leukocytosis may occur; it lasts 5–7 days and resolves with symptomatic treatment. Bronchial or esophageal wall necrosis, myocardial infarction, and spinal cord infarction are rare complications.

Pulmonary hemorrhage with or without hemoptysis in hematologic malignancies is often associated with fungal infections, particularly *Aspergillus* spp. After granulocytopenia resolves, the lung infiltrates in aspergillosis may cavitate and cause massive hemoptysis. Thrombocytopenia and coagulation defects should be corrected, if possible. Surgical evaluation is recommended in patients with aspergillosis-related cavitary lesions.

Bevacizumab, an antibody to vascular endothelial growth factor that inhibits angiogenesis, has been associated with life-threatening hemoptysis in patients with NSCLC, particularly squamous cell histology. NSCLC patients with cavitary lesions have higher risk for pulmonary hemorrhage.

AIRWAY OBSTRUCTION

Airway obstruction refers to a blockage at the level of the mainstem bronchi or above. It may result either from intraluminal tumor growth or from extrinsic compression of the airway. The most common cause of malignant upper airway obstruction is invasion from an adjacent primary tumor, most commonly lung cancer, followed by esophageal, thyroid, and mediastinal malignancies. Extrathoracic primary tumors such as renal, colon, or breast cancer can cause airway obstruction through endobronchial and/or mediastinal lymph node metastases. Patients may present with dyspnea, hemoptysis, stridor, wheezing, intractable cough, postobstructive pneumonia, or hoarseness. Chest radiographs usually demonstrate obstructing lesions. CT scans reveal the extent of tumor. Cool, humidified oxygen; glucocorticoids; and ventilation with a mixture of helium and oxygen (Heliox) may provide temporary relief. If the obstruction is proximal to the larynx, a tracheostomy may be lifesaving. For more distal obstructions, particularly intrinsic lesions incompletely obstructing the airway, bronchoscopy with laser treatment, photodynamic therapy, or stenting can produce immediate relief in most patients (Fig. 54-3). However, radiation therapy (either external-beam irradiation or brachytherapy) given together with glucocorticoids may also open the airway. Symptomatic extrinsic compression may be palliated by stenting. Patients with primary airway tumors such as squamous cell carcinoma, carcinoid tumor, adenocystic carcinoma, or NSCLC should have surgery.

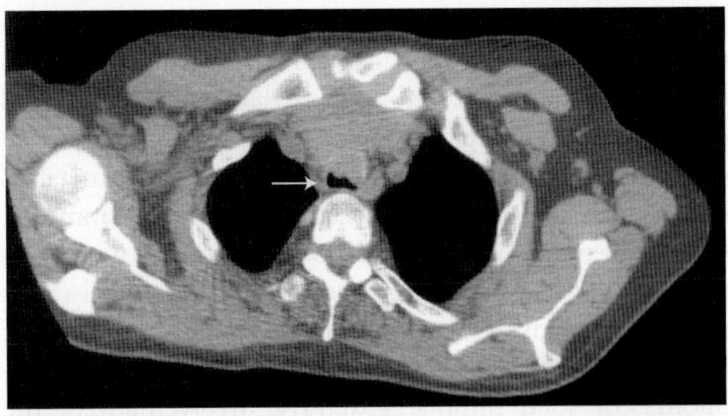

A

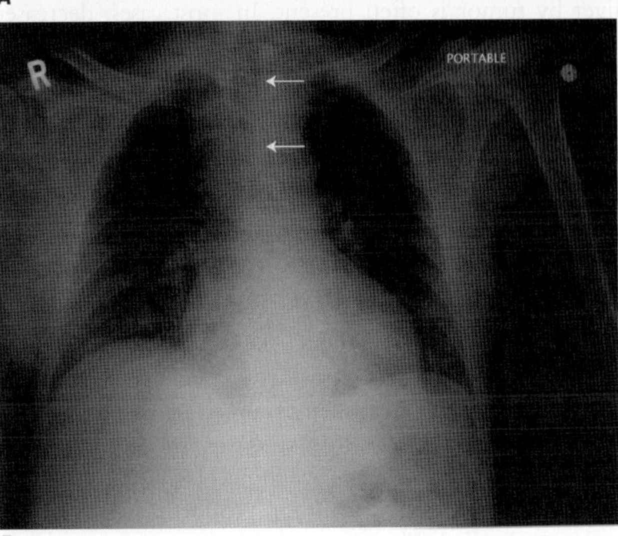

B

FIGURE 54-3

Airway obstruction. *A.* CT scan of a 62-year-old man with tracheal obstruction caused by renal carcinoma showing paratracheal mass (***A***) with tracheal invasion/obstruction (*arrow*). ***B.*** Chest x-ray of same patient after stent (*arrows*) placement.

METABOLIC EMERGENCIES

HYPERCALCEMIA

Hypercalcemia is the most common paraneoplastic syndrome. Its pathogenesis and management are discussed fully in Chap 52.

SYNDROME OF INAPPROPRIATE SECRETION OF ANTIDIURETIC HORMONE

Hyponatremia is a common electrolyte abnormality in cancer patients, and the syndrome of inappropriate secretion of antidiuretic hormone (SIADH) is the most common cause among patients with cancer. SIADH is discussed fully in Chap. 52.

LACTIC ACIDOSIS

Lactic acidosis is a rare and potentially fatal metabolic complication of cancer. The body produces about 1500 mmol of lactic acid per day, most of which is metabolized by the liver. Normally, this lactate is generated by the skin (25%), muscle (25%), red cells (20%), brain (20%), and gut (10%). Lactic acidosis may occur as a consequence of increased production or decreased hepatic metabolism. Normal venous levels of lactate are 0.5–2.2 mmol/L (4.5–19.8 mg/dL). Lactic acidosis associated with sepsis and circulatory failure is a common preterminal event in many malignancies. Lactic acidosis in the absence of hypoxemia may occur in patients with leukemia, lymphoma, or solid tumors. Extensive involvement of the liver by tumor is often present. In most cases, decreased metabolism and increased production by the tumor both contribute to lactate accumulation. Tumor cell overexpression of certain glycolytic enzymes and mitochondrial dysfunction can contribute to its increased lactate production. HIV-infected patients have an increased risk of aggressive lymphoma; lactic acidosis that occurs in such patients may be related either to the rapid growth of the tumor or from toxicity of nucleoside reverse transcriptase inhibitors. Symptoms of lactic acidosis include tachypnea, tachycardia, change of mental status, and hepatomegaly. The serum level of lactic acid may reach 10–20 mmol/L (90–180 mg/dL). Treatment is aimed at the underlying disease. *The danger from lactic acidosis is from the acidosis, not the lactate.* Sodium bicarbonate should be added if acidosis is very severe or if hydrogen ion production is very rapid and uncontrolled. The prognosis is poor.

HYPOGLYCEMIA

Persistent hypoglycemia is occasionally associated with tumors other than pancreatic islet cell tumors. Usually these tumors are large; tumors of mesenchymal origin, hepatomas, or adrenocortical tumors may cause hypoglycemia. Mesenchymal tumors are usually located in the retroperitoneum or thorax. Obtundation, confusion, and behavioral aberrations occur in the postabsorptive period and may precede the diagnosis of the tumor. These tumors often secrete incompletely processed insulin-like growth factor II (IGF-II), a hormone capable of activating insulin receptors and causing hypoglycemia. Tumors secreting incompletely processed big IGF-II are characterized by an increased IGF-II to IGF-I ratio, suppressed insulin and C-peptide level, and inappropriately low growth hormone and β-hydroxybutyrate concentrations. Rarely, hypoglycemia is due to insulin secretion by a non-islet cell carcinoma. The development of hepatic dysfunction from liver metastases and increased glucose consumption by the tumor can contribute to hypoglycemia. If the tumor cannot be resected, hypoglycemia symptoms may be relieved by the administration of glucose, glucocorticoids, or glucagon.

Hypoglycemia can be artifactual; hyperleukocytosis from leukemia, myeloproliferative diseases, leukemoid reactions, or colony-stimulating factor treatment can increase glucose consumption in the test tube after blood is drawn, leading to pseudohypoglycemia.

ADRENAL INSUFFICIENCY

In patients with cancer, adrenal insufficiency may go unrecognized because the symptoms, such as nausea, vomiting, anorexia, and orthostatic hypotension, are nonspecific and may be mistakenly attributed to progressive cancer or to therapy. Primary adrenal insufficiency may develop owing to replacement of both glands by metastases (lung, breast, colon, or kidney cancer; lymphoma), removal of both glands, or hemorrhagic necrosis in association with sepsis or anticoagulation. Impaired adrenal steroid synthesis occurs in patients being treated for cancer with mitotane, ketoconazole, or aminoglutethimide or undergoing a rapid reduction in glucocorticoid therapy. Rarely, metastatic replacement causes primary adrenal insufficiency as the first manifestation of an occult malignancy. Metastasis to the pituitary or hypothalamus is found at autopsy in up to 5% of patients with cancer, but associated secondary adrenal insufficiency is rare. Megestrol acetate, used to manage cancer and HIV-related cachexia, may suppress plasma levels of cortisol and adrenocorticotropic hormone (ACTH). Patients taking megestrol may develop adrenal insufficiency, and even those whose adrenal dysfunction is not symptomatic may have inadequate adrenal reserve if they become seriously ill. Paradoxically, some patients may develop Cushing's syndrome and/or hyperglycemia because of the glucocorticoid-like activity of megestrol acetate. Cranial irradiation for childhood brain tumors may affect the hypothalamus-pituitary-adrenal axis, resulting in secondary adrenal insufficiency.

Acute adrenal insufficiency is potentially lethal. Treatment of suspected adrenal crisis is initiated after the sampling of serum cortisol and ACTH levels (Chap. 51).

TREATMENT-RELATED EMERGENCIES

TUMOR LYSIS SYNDROME

Tumor lysis syndrome (TLS) is characterized by hyperuricemia, hyperkalemia, hyperphosphatemia, and hypocalcemia and is caused by the destruction of a large number of rapidly proliferating neoplastic cells. Acidosis may also develop. Acute renal failure occurs frequently.

TLS is most often associated with the treatment of Burkitt's lymphoma, acute lymphoblastic leukemia, and other rapidly proliferating lymphomas, but it also may be seen with chronic leukemias and, rarely, with solid tumors. This syndrome has been seen in patients with chronic lymphocytic leukemia after treatment with nucleosides like fludarabine. TLS has been observed with administration of glucocorticoids, hormonal agents such as letrozole and tamoxifen, and monoclonal antibodies such as rituximab and gemtuzumab. TLS usually occurs during or shortly (1–5 days) after chemotherapy. Rarely, spontaneous necrosis of malignancies causes TLS.

Hyperuricemia may be present at the time of chemotherapy. Effective treatment kills malignant cells and leads to increased serum uric acid levels from the turnover of nucleic acids. Owing to the acidic local environment, uric acid can precipitate in the tubules, medulla, and collecting ducts of the kidney, leading to renal failure. Lactic acidosis and dehydration may contribute to the precipitation of uric acid in the renal tubules. The finding of uric acid crystals in the urine is strong evidence for uric acid nephropathy. The ratio of urinary uric acid to urinary creatinine is >1 in patients with acute hyperuricemic nephropathy and <1 in patients with renal failure due to other causes.

Hyperphosphatemia, which can be caused by the release of intracellular phosphate pools by tumor lysis, produces a reciprocal depression in serum calcium, which causes severe neuromuscular irritability and tetany. Deposition of calcium phosphate in the kidney and hyperphosphatemia may cause renal failure. Potassium is the principal intracellular cation, and massive destruction of malignant cells may lead to hyperkalemia. Hyperkalemia in patients with renal failure may rapidly become life-threatening by causing ventricular arrhythmias and sudden death.

The likelihood that TLS will occur in patients with Burkitt's lymphoma is related to the tumor burden and renal function. Hyperuricemia and high serum levels of lactate dehydrogenase (LDH >1500 U/L), both of which correlate with total tumor burden, also correlate with the risk of TLS. In patients at risk for TLS, pretreatment evaluations should include a complete blood count, serum chemistry evaluation, and urine analysis. High leukocyte and platelet counts may artificially elevate potassium levels ("pseudohyperkalemia") due to lysis of these cells after the blood is drawn. In these cases, plasma potassium instead of serum potassium should be followed. In pseudohyperkalemia, no electrocardiographic abnormalities are present. In patients with abnormal baseline renal function, the kidneys and retroperitoneal area should be evaluated by sonography and/or CT to rule out obstructive uropathy. Urine output should be watched closely.

TREATMENT Tumor Lysis Syndrome

Recognition of risk and prevention are the most important steps in the management of this syndrome (Fig. 54-4). The standard preventive approach consists of allopurinol, urinary alkalinization, and aggressive hydration. Intravenous allopurinol may be given in patients who cannot tolerate oral therapy. In some cases, uric acid levels cannot be lowered sufficiently with the standard preventive approach. Rasburicase (recombinant urate oxidase) can be effective in these instances. Urate oxidase is missing from primates and catalyzes the conversion of poorly soluble uric acid to readily soluble allantoin. Rasburicase acts rapidly, decreasing uric acid levels within hours; however, it may cause hypersensitivity reactions such as bronchospasm, hypoxemia, and hypotension. Rasburicase should also be administered to high-risk patients for TLS prophylaxis. Rasburicase is contraindicated in patients with glucose-6-phosphate dehydrogenase deficiency who are unable to break down hydrogen peroxide, an end product of the urate oxidase reaction. Despite aggressive prophylaxis, TLS and/or oliguric or anuric renal failure may occur. Care should be taken to prevent worsening of symptomatic hypocalcemia by induction of alkalosis during bicarbonate infusion. Administration of sodium bicarbonate may also lead to urinary precipitation of calcium phosphate, which is less soluble at alkaline pH. Dialysis is often necessary and should be considered early in the course. Hemodialysis is preferred. Hemofiltration offers a gradual, continuous method of removing cellular by-products and fluid. The prognosis is excellent, and renal function recovers after the uric acid level is lowered to ≤10 mg/dL.

HUMAN ANTIBODY INFUSION REACTIONS

The initial infusion of human or humanized antibodies (e.g., rituximab, gemtuzumab, trastuzumab) is associated with fever, chills, nausea, asthenia, and headache in up to half of treated patients. Bronchospasm and hypotension occur in 1% of patients. Severe manifestations, including pulmonary infiltrates, acute respiratory distress syndrome, and cardiogenic shock, occur rarely. Laboratory manifestations include elevated hepatic aminotransferase levels, thrombocytopenia, and prolongation of prothrombin time. The pathogenesis is thought to be activation of immune effector processes (cells and complement) and release of inflammatory cytokines, such as tumor necrosis factor α and interleukin 6 (cytokine release syndrome). Severe reactions from rituximab have occurred with high numbers (more than 50×10^9 lymphocytes) of circulating cells bearing the target antigen (CD 20) and have been associated with a rapid fall in circulating tumor cells, mild electrolyte evidence of TLS, and very rarely, with death. In addition, increased liver enzymes, D-dimer, LDH, and prolongation of the prothrombin time may occur. Diphenhydramine, hydrocortisone, and acetaminophen can often

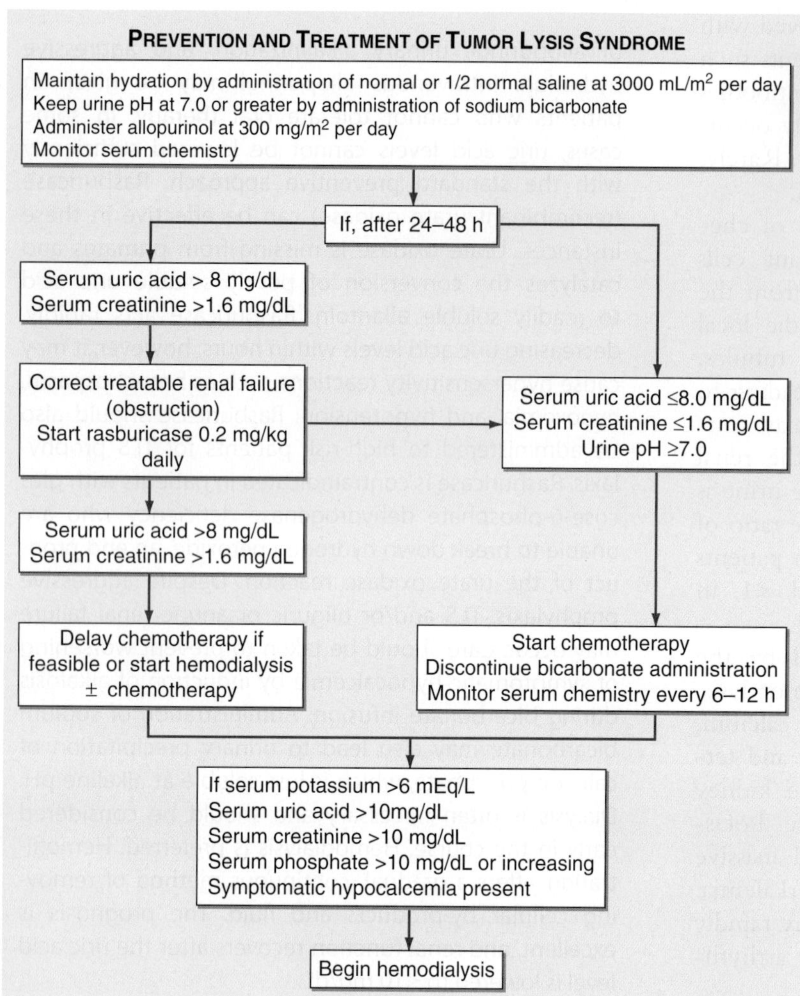

PREVENTION AND TREATMENT OF TUMOR LYSIS SYNDROME
Maintain hydration by administration of normal or 1/2 normal saline at 3000 mL/m² per day
Keep urine pH at 7.0 or greater by administration of sodium bicarbonate
Administer allopurinol at 300 mg/m² per day
Monitor serum chemistry
If, after 24–48 h
Serum uric acid > 8 mg/dL
Serum creatinine >1.6 mg/dL
Correct treatable renal failure (obstruction)
Start rasburicase 0.2 mg/kg daily
Serum uric acid ≤8.0 mg/dL
Serum creatinine ≤1.6 mg/dL
Urine pH ≥7.0
Serum uric acid >8 mg/dL
Serum creatinine >1.6 mg/dL
Delay chemotherapy if feasible or start hemodialysis ± chemotherapy
Start chemotherapy
Discontinue bicarbonate administration
Monitor serum chemistry every 6–12 h
If serum potassium >6 mEq/L
Serum uric acid >10mg/dL
Serum creatinine >10 mg/dL
Serum phosphate >10 mg/dL or increasing
Symptomatic hypocalcemia present
Begin hemodialysis

FIGURE 54-4
Management of patients at high risk for the tumor lysis syndrome.

prevent or suppress the infusion-related symptoms. If they occur, the infusion is stopped and restarted at half the initial infusion rate after the symptoms have abated. Severe "cytokine release syndrome" may require intensive support for acute respiratory distress syndrome (ARDS) and resistant hypotension.

HEMOLYTIC-UREMIC SYNDROME

Hemolytic-uremic syndrome (HUS) and, less commonly, thrombotic thrombocytopenic purpura (TTP) may rarely occur after treatment with antineoplastic drugs, including mitomycin, cisplatin, bleomycin, and gemcitabine. It occurs most often in patients with gastric, lung, colorectal, pancreatic, and breast carcinoma. In one series, 35% of patients were without evident cancer at the time this syndrome appeared. Secondary HUS/TTP has also been reported as a rare but sometimes fatal complication of bone marrow transplantation.

HUS usually has its onset 4–8 weeks after the last dose of chemotherapy, but it is not rare to detect it several months later. HUS is characterized by microangiopathic hemolytic anemia, thrombocytopenia, and renal failure. Dyspnea, weakness, fatigue, oliguria, and purpura are also common initial symptoms and findings. Systemic hypertension and pulmonary edema frequently occur. Severe hypertension, pulmonary edema, and rapid worsening of hemolysis and renal function may occur after a blood or blood product transfusion. Cardiac findings include atrial arrhythmias, pericardial friction rub, and pericardial effusion. Raynaud's phenomenon is part of the syndrome in patients treated with bleomycin.

Laboratory findings include severe to moderate anemia associated with red blood cell fragmentation and numerous schistocytes on peripheral smear. Reticulocytosis, decreased plasma haptoglobin, and an LDH level document hemolysis. The serum bilirubin level is usually normal or slightly elevated. The Coombs' test is negative. The white cell count is usually normal, and thrombocytopenia (<100,000/μL) is almost always present. Most patients have a normal coagulation profile, although some have mild elevations in thrombin time and in levels of fibrin degradation products. The serum creatinine level is elevated at presentation and shows a pattern of subacute worsening within weeks of the initial azotemia. The urinalysis reveals hematuria, proteinuria, and granular or hyaline casts, and circulating immune complexes may be present.

The basic pathologic lesion appears to be deposition of fibrin in the walls of capillaries and arterioles, and these deposits are similar to those seen in HUS due to other causes. These microvascular abnormalities involve mainly the kidneys and rarely occur in other organs. The pathogenesis of chemotherapy-related HUS is unknown. Other forms of HUS/TTP are related to a decrease in processing of von Willebrand factor by a protease called ADAMTS13.

The case fatality rate is high; most patients die within a few months. There is no consensus on the optimal treatment for chemotherapy-induced HUS. Treatment modalities for HUS/TTP including immunocomplex removal (plasmapheresis, immunoadsorption, or exchange transfusion), antiplatelet/anticoagulant therapies, immunosuppressive therapies, and plasma exchange lead to varying degrees of success. Rituximab is successfully used in patients with chemotherapy-induced HUS as well as in ADAMTS13-deficient TTP.

NEUTROPENIA AND INFECTION

These remain the most common serious complications of cancer therapy. They are covered in detail in Chap. 29.

PULMONARY INFILTRATES

Patients with cancer may present with dyspnea associated with diffuse interstitial infiltrates on chest radiographs. Such infiltrates may be due to progression of the underlying malignancy, treatment-related toxicities, infection, or unrelated diseases. The cause may be multifactorial; however, most commonly, they occur as a consequence of treatment. Infiltration of the lung by malignancy has been described in patients with leukemia, lymphoma, and breast and other solid cancers. Pulmonary lymphatics may be involved diffusely by neoplasm (pulmonary lymphangitic carcinomatosis), resulting in a diffuse increase in interstitial markings on chest radiographs. The patient is often mildly dyspneic at the onset, but pulmonary failure develops over a period of weeks. In some patients, dyspnea precedes changes on the chest radiographs and is accompanied by a nonproductive cough. This syndrome is characteristic of solid tumors. In patients with leukemia, diffuse microscopic neoplastic peribronchial and peribronchiolar infiltration is frequent but may be asymptomatic. However, some patients present with diffuse interstitial infiltrates, an alveolar capillary block syndrome, and respiratory distress. In these situations, glucocorticoids can provide symptomatic relief, but specific chemotherapy should always be started promptly.

Several cytotoxic agents, such as bleomycin, methotrexate, busulfan, nitrosoureas, gemcitabine, mitomycin, vinorelbine, docetaxel, and ifosfamide may cause pulmonary damage. The most frequent presentations are interstitial pneumonitis, alveolitis, and pulmonary fibrosis. Some cytotoxic agents, including methotrexate and procarbazine, may cause an acute hypersensitivity reaction. Cytosine arabinoside has been associated with noncardiogenic pulmonary edema. Administration of multiple cytotoxic drugs, as well as radiotherapy and preexisting lung disease, may potentiate the pulmonary toxicity. Supplemental oxygen may potentiate the effects of drugs and radiation injury. Patients should always be managed with the lowest forced expiratory volume in 1 second (FIO_2) that is sufficient to maintain hemoglobin saturation.

The onset of symptoms may be insidious, with symptoms including dyspnea, nonproductive cough, and tachycardia. Patients may have bibasilar crepitant rales, end-inspiratory crackles, fever, and cyanosis. The chest radiograph generally shows an interstitial and sometimes an intraalveolar pattern that is strongest at the lung bases and may be symmetric. A small effusion may occur. Hypoxemia with decreased carbon monoxide diffusing capacity is always present. Glucocorticoids may be helpful in patients in whom pulmonary toxicity is related to radiation therapy or to chemotherapy. Treatment is otherwise supportive.

Molecular targeted agents, imatinib, erlotinib, and gefitinib are potent inhibitors of tyrosine kinases. These drugs may cause interstitial lung disease. In the case of gefitinib, preexisting fibrosis, poor performance status, and prior thoracic irradiation are independent risk factors; this complication has a high fatality rate. In Japan, incidence of interstitial lung disease associated with gefitinib was about 4.5% compared to 0.5% in the United States. Temsirolimus, a derivative of rapamycin, is an agent that blocks the effects of mTOR, an enzyme that has an important role in regulating the synthesis of proteins that control cell division. It may cause ground-glass opacities in the lung with or without diffuse interstitial disease and lung parenchymal consolidation.

Radiation pneumonitis and/or fibrosis is a relatively frequent side effect of thoracic radiation therapy. It may be acute or chronic. Radiation-induced lung toxicity is a function of the irradiated lung volume, dose per fraction, and radiation dose. The larger the irradiated lung field, the higher the risk for radiation pneumonitis. The use of concurrent chemoradiation increases pulmonary toxicity. Radiation pneumonitis usually develops from 2 to 6 months after completion of radiotherapy. The clinical syndrome, which varies in severity, consists of dyspnea, cough with scanty sputum, low-grade fever, and an initial hazy infiltrate on chest radiographs. The infiltrate and tissue damage usually are confined to the radiation field. The patients subsequently may develop a patchy alveolar infiltrate and air bronchograms, which may progress to acute respiratory failure that is sometimes fatal. A lung biopsy may be necessary to make the diagnosis. Asymptomatic infiltrates found incidentally after radiation therapy need not be treated. However, prednisone should be administered to patients with fever or other symptoms. The dosage should be tapered slowly after the resolution of radiation pneumonitis, as abrupt withdrawal of glucocorticoids may cause an exacerbation of pneumonia. Delayed radiation fibrosis may occur years after radiation therapy and is signaled by dyspnea on exertion. Often it is mild, but it can progress to chronic respiratory failure. Therapy is supportive.

Classical radiation pneumonitis that leads to pulmonary fibrosis is due to radiation-induced production of local cytokines such as platelet-derived growth factor β, tumor necrosis factor, interleukins, and transforming growth factor β in the radiation field. An immunologically mediated sporadic radiation pneumonitis occurs in about 10% of patients; bilateral alveolitis mediated by T cells results in infiltrates outside the radiation field. This form of radiation pneumonitis usually resolves without sequelae.

Pneumonia is a common problem in patients undergoing treatment for cancer. Bacterial pneumonia typically causes a localized infiltrate on chest radiographs. Therapy is tailored to the causative organism. When diffuse interstitial infiltrates appear in a febrile patient, the differential diagnosis is extensive and includes pneumonia due to infection with *Pneumocystis carinii*; viral infections including cytomegalovirus, adenovirus, herpes simplex virus, herpes zoster, respiratory syncytial virus, or intracellular pathogens such as *Mycoplasma* and *Legionella* spp.; effects of drugs or radiation; tumor progression; nonspecific pneumonitis; and fungal disease. Detection of opportunistic pathogens in pulmonary infections is still a challenge. Diagnostic tools include chest radiographs, CT scans, bronchoscopy with bronchoalveolar lavage, brush cytology, transbronchial biopsy, fine-needle aspiration, and open lung biopsy. In addition to the culture, evaluation of bronchoalveolar lavage fluid for *P. carinii* by polymerase chain reaction (PCR) and serum galactomannan test improve the diagnostic yield. Patients with cancer who are neutropenic and have fever and local infiltrates on chest radiograph should be treated initially with broad-spectrum antibiotics. A new or persistent focal infiltrate not responding to broad-spectrum antibiotics argues for initiation of empiric antifungal therapy. When diffuse bilateral infiltrates develop in patients with febrile neutropenia, broad-spectrum antibiotics plus trimethoprim-sulfamethoxazole, with or without erythromycin, should be initiated. Addition of an antiviral agent is necessary in some settings, such as patients undergoing allogeneic hematopoietic stem cell transplantation. If the patient does not improve in 4 days, open lung biopsy is the procedure of choice. Bronchoscopy with bronchoalveolar lavage may be used in patients who are poor candidates for surgery.

In patients with pulmonary infiltrates who are afebrile, heart failure and multiple pulmonary emboli are in the differential diagnosis.

NEUTROPENIC ENTEROCOLITIS

Neutropenic enterocolitis (typhlitis) is the inflammation and necrosis of the cecum and surrounding tissues that may complicate the treatment of acute leukemia. Nevertheless, it may involve any segment of the gastrointestinal tract including small intestine, appendix, and colon. This complication has also been seen in patients with other forms of cancer treated with taxanes and in patients receiving high-dose chemotherapy (Fig. 54-5). The patient develops right lower quadrant abdominal

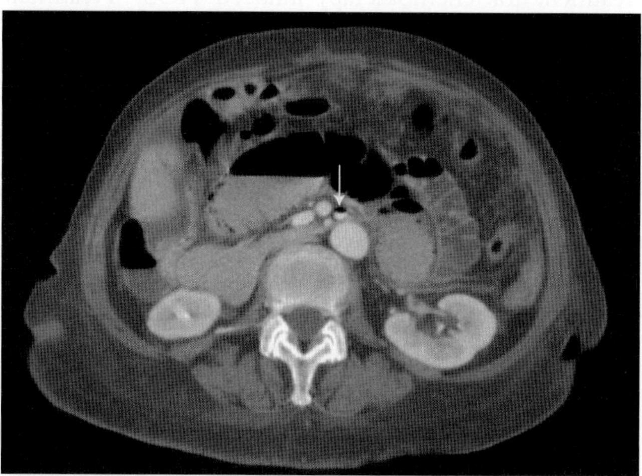

A

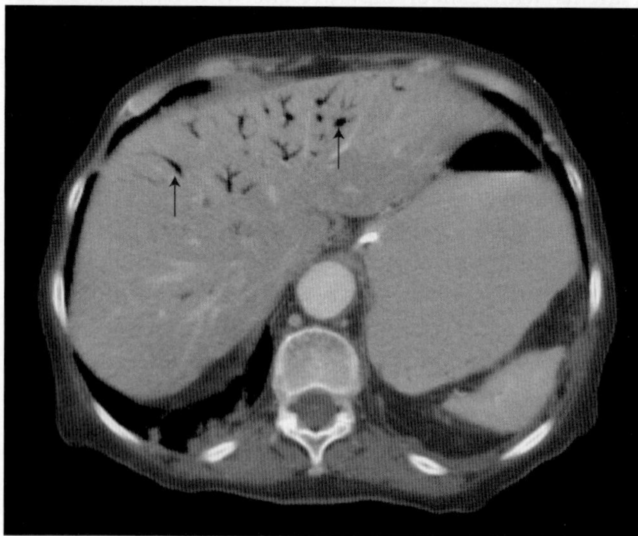

B

FIGURE 54-5

Abdominal computed tomography (CT) scans of a 72-year-old woman with neutropenic enterocolitis secondary to chemotherapy. *A.* Air in inferior mesenteric vein (*arrow*) and bowel wall with pneumatosis intestinalis. ***B.*** CT scans of upper abdomen demonstrating air in portal vein (*arrows*).

pain, often with rebound tenderness and a tense, distended abdomen, in a setting of fever and neutropenia. Watery diarrhea (often containing sloughed mucosa) and bacteremia are common, and bleeding may occur. Plain abdominal films are generally of little value in the diagnosis; CT scan may show marked bowel wall thickening, particularly in the cecum, with bowel wall edema, mesenteric stranding, and ascites. Patients with bowel wall thickness >10 mm on ultrasonogram have higher mortality rates. However, bowel wall thickening is significantly more prominent in patients with *Clostridium difficile* colitis. Pneumatosis intestinalis is a more specific finding, seen only in those with neutropenic enterocolitis and ischemia. The combined involvement of the small and large bowel suggests a diagnosis of neutropenic enterocolitis. Rapid institution of broad-spectrum antibiotics and nasogastric suction may reverse the process. Surgical intervention is reserved for severe cases of neutropenic enterocolitis with evidence of perforation, peritonitis, gangrenous bowel, or gastrointestinal hemorrhage despite correction of any coagulopathy.

C. difficile colitis is increasing in incidence. Newer strains of *C. difficile* produce about 20 times more of toxins A and B compared to previously studied strains. *C. difficile* risk is also increased with chemotherapy. Antibiotic coverage for *C. difficile* should be added if pseudomembranous colitis cannot be excluded.

HEMORRHAGIC CYSTITIS

Hemorrhagic cystitis can develop in patients receiving cyclophosphamide or ifosfamide. Both drugs are metabolized to acrolein, which is a strong chemical irritant that is excreted in the urine. Prolonged contact or high concentrations may lead to bladder irritation and hemorrhage. Symptoms include gross hematuria, frequency, dysuria, burning, urgency, incontinence, and nocturia. The best management is prevention. Maintaining a high rate of urine flow minimizes exposure. In addition, 2-mercaptoethanesulfonate (mesna) detoxifies the metabolites and can be coadministered with the instigating drugs. Mesna usually is given three times on the day of ifosfamide administration in doses that are each 20% of the total ifosfamide dose. If hemorrhagic cystitis develops, the maintenance of a high urine flow may be sufficient supportive care. If conservative management is not effective, irrigation of the bladder with a 0.37–0.74% formalin solution for 10 min stops the bleeding in most cases. *N*-acetylcysteine may also be an effective irrigant. Prostaglandin (carboprost) can inhibit the process. In extreme cases, ligation of the hypogastric arteries, urinary diversion, or cystectomy may be necessary.

Hemorrhagic cystitis also occurs in patients who undergo bone marrow transplantation (BMT). In the BMT setting, early-onset hemorrhagic cystitis is related to drugs in the treatment regimen (e.g., cyclophosphamide), and late-onset hemorrhagic cystitis is usually due to the polyoma virus BKV or adenovirus type 11. BKV load in urine alone or in combination with acute graft-versus-host disease correlate with development of hemorrhagic cystitis. Viral causes are usually detected by PCR-based diagnostic tests. Treatment of viral hemorrhagic cystitis is largely supportive, with reduction in doses of immunosuppressive agents, if possible. No antiviral therapy is approved, though cidofovir is reported to be effective in small series.

HYPERSENSITIVITY REACTIONS TO ANTINEOPLASTIC DRUGS

Many antineoplastic drugs may cause hypersensitivity reaction (HSR). These reactions are unpredictable and potentially life-threatening. Most reactions occur during or within hours of parenteral drug administration. Taxanes, platinum compounds, asparaginase, etoposide, and biologic agents, including rituximab, bevacizumab, trastuzumab, gemtuzumab, cetuximab, and alemtuzumab, are more commonly associated with acute HSR than are other agents. Acute hypersensitivity reactions to some drugs, such as taxanes, occur during the first or second dose administered. HSR from platinum compounds occurs after prolonged exposure. Skin testing may identify patients with high risk for HSR after carboplatin exposure. Premedication with histamine H_1 and H_2 receptor antagonists and glucocorticoids reduce the incidence of hypersensitivity reaction to taxanes, particularly paclitaxel. Despite premedication, HSR may still occur. In these cases, retreatment may be attempted with care, but use of alternative agents may be required.

CHAPTER 55

LATE CONSEQUENCES OF CANCER AND ITS TREATMENT

Carl E. Freter ■ Dan L. Longo

Over 10 million Americans are cancer survivors. The vast majority of these people will bear some mark of their cancer and/or its treatment, and a large proportion will experience long-term consequences that include medical problems, psychosocial dysfunction, economic hardship, sexual dysfunction, and discrimination in employment and insurance. Many of these problems are directly related to cancer treatment. As patients with more types of malignancies survive longer, the biologic toll that very imperfect therapies take in terms of morbidity and mortality rates is being recognized increasingly. These consequences of therapy confront the patients and the cancer specialists and general internists who manage them every day. Although long-term survivors of childhood leukemias, Hodgkin's lymphoma, and testicular cancer have increased knowledge about the consequences of cancer treatment, researchers and physicians keep learning more as patients survive longer with newer therapies. The pace of the development of therapies that mitigate treatment-related consequences has been slow, partly due to an understandable aversion to altering regimens that work and partly due to a lack of new, effective, less toxic therapeutic agents with less "collateral damage" to replace known agents with known toxicities. The types of damage from cancer treatment vary. Often, a final common pathway is irreparable damage to DNA. Surgery can create dysfunction, including blind gut loops that lead to absorption problems and loss of function of removed body parts. Radiation may damage end-organ function, for example, loss of potency in prostate cancer patients, pulmonary fibrosis, neurocognitive impairment, acceleration of atherosclerosis, and second cancers. Cancer chemotherapy may act as a carcinogen and has a kaleidoscope of other toxicities, as discussed in this chapter. Table 55-1 lists the long-term effects of treatment.

The first goal of therapy is to eradicate or control the malignancy. Late treatment consequences are, indeed, testimony to the increasing success of such treatment. Their occurrence sharply underlines the necessity to develop more effective therapies with less long-term morbidity and mortality. At the same time, a sense of perspective and relative risk is necessary; fear of long-term complications should not prevent the application of effective (particularly curative) cancer treatment.

CARDIOVASCULAR DYSFUNCTION

CHEMOTHERAPEUTIC AGENTS

The cardiovascular toxicity of cancer chemotherapeutic agents includes dysrhythmias, cardiomyopathic congestive heart failure (CHF), pericardial disease, and peripheral vascular disease. Because these cardiac toxicities are difficult to distinguish from disease that is not associated with cancer treatment, determining the clear etiologic implication of cancer chemotherapeutic agents may be difficult. Cardiovascular complications occurring in an unexpected clinical setting in patients who have undergone cancer therapy is often important in raising suspicion. Dose-dependent myocardial toxicity of anthracyclines with characteristic myofibrillar dropout is pathologically pathagnomonic on endomyocardial biopsy. Anthracycline cardiotoxity occurs through a root mechanism of chemical free-radical damage. Fe(III)–doxorubicin complexes damage DNA, nuclear and cytoplasmic membranes, and mitochondria. About 5% of patients receiving >450–550 mg/m^2 doxorubicin will develop CHF. Cardiotoxicity in relation to the dose of anthracycline is clearly not a step function but rather a continuous function, and occasional patients are

TABLE 55-1

LATE EFFECTS OF CANCER THERAPY

SURGICAL PROCEDURE		EFFECT
Amputation		Functional loss
Lymph node dissection		Risk of lymphedema
Ostomy		Psychosocial impact
Splenectomy		Risk of sepsis
Adhesions		Risk of obstruction
Bowel anastomoses		Malabsorption syndromes
RADIATION THERAPY		**EFFECT**
Organ		
Bone		Premature termination of growth, osteonecrosis
Soft tissues		Atrophy, fibrosis
Brain		Neuropsychiatric deficits, cognitive dysfunction
Thyroid		Hypothyroidism, Graves' disease, cancer
Salivary glands		Dry mouth, caries, dysgeusia
Eyes		Cataracts
Heart		Pericarditis, myocarditis, coronary artery disease
Lung		Pulmonary fibrosis
Kidney		Decreased function, hypertension
Liver		Decreased function
Intestine		Malabsorption, stricture
Gonads		Infertility, premature menopause
Any		Secondary neoplasia
CHEMOTHERAPY		**EFFECT**
Organ	**Drug**	
Bone	Glucocorticoids	Osteoporosis, avascular necrosis
Brain	Methotrexate, cytarabine (Ara-C), others	Neuropsychiatric deficits, cognitive decline?
Peripheral nerves	Vincristine, platinum, taxanes	Neuropathy, hearing loss
Eyes	Glucocorticoids	Cataracts
Heart	Anthracyclines, trastuzumab	Cardiomyopathy
Lung	Bleomycin	Pulmonary fibrosis
	Methotrexate	Pulmonary hypersensitivity
Kidney	Platinum, others	Decreased function, hypomagnesemia
Liver	Various	Altered function
Gonads	Alkylating agents, others	Infertility, premature menopause
Bone marrow	Various	Aplasia, myelodysplasia, secondary leukemia

seen with CHF at substantially lower doses. Advanced age, other concomitant cardiac disease, hypertension, diabetes, and thoracic radiation therapy are all important cofactors in promoting anthracycline-associated CHF. Anthracycline-related CHF is difficult to reverse; the mortality rate is as high as 50%, making prevention crucial. Some anthracyclines, such as mitoxantrone, are associated with less cardiotoxicity, and continuous infusion regimens or doxorubicin encapsulated in liposomes are associated with less cardiotoxicity. Dexrazoxane, an intracellular iron chelator, may limit anthracycline toxicity, but concern about limiting chemotherapeutic efficacy has limited its use. Monitoring patients for cardiac toxicity typically involves periodic gated nuclear cardiac blood pool ejection fraction testing (multi gated acquisition scan [MUGA]) or cardiac ultrasonography. Cardiac magnetic resonance imaging (MRI) has been used but is not standard or widespread. Testing is performed more frequently at higher cumulative doses, with additional risk factors, certainly for any newly developing CHF or other symptoms of cardiac dysfunction.

Trastuzumab after anthracyclines is currently the next most commonly used cardiotoxic drug. Trastuzumab is commonly used in adjuvant therapy or for advanced HER2-positive breast cancer, sometimes in conjunction with anthracyclines, and is believed to result in additive or possibly synergistic toxicity. In contrast to anthracyclines, cardiotoxicity from trastuzumab is not dose-related, is usually reversible, is not associated with pathologic changes of anthracyclines on cardiac myofibrils, and has a different biochemical mechanism inhibiting intrinsic cardiac repair mechanisms. Toxicity is monitored routinely every three to four doses with functional cardiac testing as described earlier for anthracyclines.

Other cardiotoxic drugs include lapatinib, phosphoramide mustards (cyclophosphamide), ifosfamide, interleukin 2, imatinib, and sunitinib.

RADIATION THERAPY

Radiation therapy that includes the heart can cause interstitial myocardial fibrosis, acute and chronic pericarditis, valvular disease, and accelerated premature atherosclerotic coronary artery disease. Repeated or high (>6000 cGy) radiation doses are associated with greater risk, as is concomitant or distant cardiotoxic cancer chemotherapy exposure. Symptoms of acute pericarditis, which peaks about 9 months after treatment, include dyspnea, chest pain, and fever. Chronic constrictive pericarditis may develop 5–10 years after radiation therapy. Cardiac valvular disease includes aortic insufficiency from fibrosis and papillary muscle dysfunction that results in mitral regurgitation. A threefold increased risk of fatal myocardial infarction is associated with mantle field radiation, with accelerated coronary artery disease. Carotid radiation similarly increases the risk of embolic stroke.

TREATMENT Chemotherapeutic and Radiation-Induced Cardiovascular Disease

Therapy for chemotherapeutic and radiation-induced cardiovascular disease is essentially the same as therapy for disease that is not associated with cancer treatment. Discontinuation of the offending agent is the first step. Diuretics, fluid and sodium restriction, and antiarylthmic agents are often useful for treating acute symptoms. Afterload reduction with angiotensin-converting enzyme (ACE) inhibitors or, in some cases, β-adrenergic blockers (carvedilol) often is of significant benefit, and digitalis may be helpful as well.

PULMONARY DYSFUNCTION

CHEMOTHERAPEUTIC AGENTS

Bleomycin generates activated free-radical oxygen species and causes pneumonitis associated with a radiographic or interstitial ground-glass appearance diffusely throughout both lungs, often worse in the lower lobes. This toxicity is dose-related and dose-limiting. The diffusion capacity of the lungs for carbon dioxide (DL^{CO}) is a sensitive measure of toxicity and recovery, and a baseline value generally is obtained for future comparison before bleomycin therapy. Additive or synergistic risk factors include age, prior lung disease, and concomitant use of other chemotherapy, along with lung irradiation and high concentrations of inspired oxygen. Other chemotherapeutic agents notable for pulmonary toxicity include mitomycin, nitrosoureas, doxorubicin with radiation, gemcitabine combined with weekly docetaxel, methotrexate, and fludarabine. High-dose alkylating agents, cyclophosphamide, ifosfamide, and melphalan are used frequently in the hematopoietic stem cell transplant setting, often with whole-body radiation. This therapy may result in severe pulmonary fibrosis and/or pulmonary venoocclusive disease.

RADIATION THERAPY

Risk factors for radiation pneumonitis include advanced age, poor performance status, preexisting compromised pulmonary function, radiation volume, and dose. The dose "threshold" for lung damage is thought to be in the range of 5–20 Gy. Hypoxemia and dyspnea on exertion are characteristic. Fine, high-pitched "Velcro rales" may be an accompanying physical finding, and fever, cough, and pleuritic chest pain are common symptoms. The DL^{CO} is the most sensitive measure of pulmonary functional impairment, and ground-glass infiltrates often correspond with relatively sharp edges to the irradiated volume, although the pneumonitis may progress beyond the field and occasionally involve the contralateral unirradiated lung.

TREATMENT Pulmonary Dysfunction

Chemotherapy-and radiation-induced pneumonitis are generally glucocorticoid-responsive, except in the case of nitrosoureas. Prednisone, 1 mg/kg, often is used to control acute symptoms and pulmonary dysfunction, with a generally slow taper. Prolonged glucocorticoid therapy requires gastrointestinal protection with proton pump inhibitors, management of hyperglycemia, heightened infection management, and prevention or treatment of steroid-induced osteoporosis. Antibiotics, bronchodilators, oxygen in only necessary doses, and diuretics may all play an important role in management of pneumonitis, and consultation with a pulmonologist should be undertaken routinely. Amifostine has been studied as a pulmonary radioprotectant, with inconclusive results, and is associated with skin rash, fatigue, and nausea; hence, it is not considered standard therapy at this time. Transforming growth factor β (TGF-β) is believed to be a major inducer of radiation fibrosis and represents a therapeutic target for development of anti-TGF-β therapies. As a general rule, patients who have received chest radiation therapy or bleomycin should receive supplemental O_2 when only absolutely necessary and at the lowest FiO_2 possible.

NEUROLOGIC DYSFUNCTION

CHEMOTHERAPEUTIC AGENTS

Chemotherapy-and radiation-induced neurologic dysfunction are increasing in both incidence and severity as a result of improved supportive care leading to more aggressive regimens and longer cancer survival allowing the development of late toxicity. Direct effects on myelin, glial cells, and neurons have been implicated, with alterations in cellular cytoskeleton, axonal transport, and cellular metabolism as mechanisms.

Vinca alkaloids produce a characteristic "stocking-glove" neuropathy, with numbness and tingling advancing to loss of motor function, which is highly dose-related. Distal sensorimotor polyneuropathy prominently involves loss of deep tendon reflexes with initially loss of pain and temperature sensation, followed by proprioceptive and vibratory loss. This requires a careful patient history and physical examination by experienced oncologists to decide when the drug must be stopped due to toxicity. Milder toxicity often slowly resolves completely. Vinca alkaloids may be associated with jaw claudication, autonomic neuropathy, ileus, cranial nerve palsies, and, in severe cases, encephalopathy, seizures, and coma.

Cisplatin is associated with sensorimotor neuropathy as well as hearing loss, especially at doses >400 mg/m^2, requiring audiometry in patients with preexisting hearing compromise. Carboplatin often is substituted in such cases because of its lesser effect on hearing.

Neurocognitive dysfunction has been well described in childhood survivors of acute lymphocytic leukemia (ALL) treatment, including intrathecal methotrexate or cytarabine in conjunction with prophylactic cranial irradiation. Methotrexate alone may cause acute leucoencephalopathy characterized by somnolence and confusion that is often reversible. Acute toxicity is dose-related, especially at doses >3 g/m^2, with younger patients being at greater risk. Subacute methotrexate toxicity occurs weeks after therapy and often is ameliorated with glucocorticoid therapy. Chronic methotrexate toxicity (leucoencephalopathy) develops months or years after treatment and is characterized clinically as progressive loss of cognitive function and focal neurologic signs that are irreversible, are promoted by synchronous or metachronous radiation therapy, and are more pronounced at a younger age.

Neurocognitive decline after chemotherapy alone occurs notably in breast cancer patients receiving adjuvant chemotherapy; this has been referred to as "chemo brain." It is clinically associated with impaired memory, learning, attention, and speed of information processing. The magnitude of the problem has been difficult to assess in light of the fact that cognitive decline is a normal feature of aging. It is not entirely clear that women receiving adjuvant therapy for breast cancer have a more rapid cognitive decline than do age-matched control participants. Furthermore, its causes are unexplained given the poor penetrance of chemotherapy agents into the central nervous system (CNS). No prevention or therapy has been developed. This entity is attracting the attention of investigators.

Many cancer patients experience intrusive or debilitating concerns about cancer recurrence after successful therapy. In addition, these patients may experience job, insurance, stress, relationship, financial, and sexual difficulties. Physicians need to ask about and address these issues explicitly with cancer survivors, with referral to the appropriate counseling or support systems. Suicidal ideation and suicide have an increased incidence in cancer patients and survivors.

RADIATION THERAPY

Acute radiation CNS toxicity occurs within weeks and is characterized by nausea, drowsiness, hypersomnia, and ataxia, symptoms that most often abate with time. Early-delayed toxicity occurring weeks to 3 months after therapy is associated with symptoms similar to those of acute toxicity and is pathologically associated with reversible demyelination. Chronic, late radiation injury occurs 9 months to up to 10 years after therapy. Focal necrosis is a common pathologic finding, and glucocorticoid therapy may be helpful. Diffuse radiation injury is associated with global CNS neurologic dysfunction and diffuse white matter changes on computed tomography or MRI. Pathologically, small vessel changes are prominent. Glucocorticoids may be symptomatically useful but do not alter the course. Necrotizing encephalopathy is the most severe form of radiation injury and almost always is associated with chemotherapy, notably methotrexate.

Cranial radiation also may be associated with an array of endocrine abnormalities with disruption of normal pituitary–hypothalamic axis function. A high index of suspicion needs to be maintained to identify and treat this toxicity.

Radiation-associated spinal cord injury (myelopathy) is highly dose-dependent and rarely occurs with modern radiation therapy. An early, self-limited form involving electric sensations down the spine on neck flexion (Lhermitte's sign) is seen 6–12 weeks after treatment and generally resolves over weeks. Peripheral nerve toxicity is quite rare owing to relative radiation resistance.

HEPATIC DYSFUNCTION

CHEMOTHERAPEUTIC AGENTS

Long-term hepatic damage from standard chemotherapy regimens is rare. Long-term methotrexate or high-dose chemotherapy alone or with radiation therapy—e.g., in preparative regimens for bone marrow transplantation—may result in venoocclusive disease of the liver. This potentially lethal complication classically presents with anicteric ascites, elevated alkaline phosphatase, and hepatosplenomegaly. Pathologically, venous congestion, epithelial cell proliferation, and hepatocyte atrophy progressing to frank fibrosis are noted. Frequent monitoring of liver function tests during any type of chemotherapy is necessary to avoid both idiosyncratic and expected toxicities. Ursodiol may prevent cholestasis in the setting of high-dose therapy before bone marrow transplant.

RADIATION THERAPY

Hepatic radiation damage depends on dose, volume, fractionation, preexisting liver disease, and synchronous or metachronous chemotherapy. In general, radiation doses to the liver >1500 cGy can produce hepatic dysfunction with a steep dose-injury curve. Radiation-induced liver disease closely mimics hepatic venoocclusive disease.

RENAL AND BLADDER DYSFUNCTION

Cisplatin produces reversible decrements in renal function but also may produce severe irreversible toxicity in the presence of renal disease and may predispose to accentuated damage with subsequent renal insults. Magnesium wasting with hypomagnesemia may be seen. Cyclophosphamide and ifosphamide, as prodrugs primarily activated in the liver, have cleavage products (acrolein) that can produce hemorrhagic cystitis. This can be prevented with the free-radical scavenger 2-mercaptoethane sulfonate (MESNA), which is required for ifosfamide administration. Hemorrhagic cystitis caused by these agents may predispose these patients to bladder cancer.

REPRODUCTIVE AND ENDOCRINE DYSFUNCTION

CHEMOTHERAPEUTIC AGENTS

Alkylating agents are associated with the highest rates of male and female infertility, which is directly dependent on age, dose, and duration of treatment. The age at treatment is an important determinant of fertility outcome, with prepubertal patients having the highest tolerance. Ovarian failure is age-related, and females who resume menses after treatment are still at increased risk for premature menopause. Males generally have reversible azospermia during lower-intensity alkylator chemotherapy, and long-term infertility is associated with total doses of cyclophosphamide >9 g/m^2 and with high-intensity therapy such as that used in hematopoietic stem cell transplantation. Males undergoing potentially sterilizing chemotherapy should be offered sperm banking. However, some cancers are associated with defective spermatogenesis. Gonadotropin-releasing hormone (GnRH) analogues to preserve ovarian function remain experimental. Assisted reproductive technologies may be helpful to couples with chemotherapy-induced infertility.

RADIATION THERAPY

The testicles and ovaries of prepubertal patients are less sensitive to radiation damage; spermatogenesis is affected by low doses of radiation, and complete azospermia occurs at 600–700 cGy. Leydig cell dysfunction, in contrast, occurs at <2000 cGy; hence, endocrine function is lost at much higher radiation doses than spermatogenesis. Erectile dysfunction occurs in up to 80% of men treated with external-beam radiation therapy for prostate cancer. Sildenafil (and congeners) may be useful in reversing erectile dysfunction. Ovarian function damage with radiation is age-related and occurs at doses of 150–500 cGY. Premature induction of menopause can have serious medical and psychological sequelae. Hormone replacement therapy often is contraindicated, as in estrogen receptor–positive breast cancer. Attention must be paid to maintenance of bone mass with calcium and vitamin D supplements and oral bisphosphonates; this is monitored by bone density determinations. Paroxetine, clonidine, pregabalin, and other drugs may be useful in symptomatically controlling hot flashes. In those without contraindications, estrogen may be used for periods <5 years at the lowest dose that relieves symptoms.

Long-term survivors of childhood cancer (e.g., ALL) who have received cranial radiation may have altered leptin biology and growth hormone deficiency, leading to obesity and reduced strength, exercise tolerance, and bone density.

Radiation therapy to the neck, for example, in Hodgkin's lymphoma, may lead to hypothyroidism, Graves' disease, thyroiditis, and thyroid malignancies. Thyroid-stimulating hormone (TSH) is followed routinely in these patients and suppressed with synthroid when elevated to prevent hypothyroidism and suppress the TSH drive, which may cause thyroid cancer.

OCULAR COMPLICATIONS

Cataracts may be caused by glucocorticoids, depending on the duration and dose; radiation therapy; and, uncommonly, tamoxifen. Orbital radiation therapy may cause blindness.

ORAL COMPLICATIONS

Radiation therapy can produce xerostomia (dry mouth) with an attendant increase in caries and poor dentition. Taste and appetite may be suppressed. Bisphosphonate use may result in osteonecrosis of the jaw.

RAYNAUD'S PHENOMENON

Up to 40% of patients treated with bleomycin may develop Raynaud's phenomenon. The mechanism is unknown.

SECOND MALIGNANCIES

Second malignancies in patients cured of cancer are a major cause of death, and treated cancer patients must be monitored for their occurrence. The induction of second malignancies is governed by the complex interplay of a number of factors, including age, sex, environmental exposures, genetic susceptibility, and cancer treatment itself. In a number of settings, the events leading to the primary cancer themselves increase the risk of second malignancies. Patients with lung cancer are at increased risk of esophageal and head and neck cancers, and vice versa, due to shared risk factors, including alcohol and tobacco abuse. Indeed, the risk of developing a second primary head and neck, esophageal, or lung cancer is also increased in these patients. Patients with breast cancer are at increased risk of cancer in the opposite breast. Patients with Hodgkin's lymphoma are at risk for non-Hodgkin's lymphomas. Genetic cancer syndromes, for example, multiple endocrine neoplasia and Li-Fraumeni, Lynch, Cowden, and Gardner's syndromes, are examples of genetically based second malignancies of specific types. Cancer treatment itself does not appear to be responsible for the risk of these secondary malignancies. Deficient DNA repair can greatly increase the risk of cancers from DNA-damaging agents, as in ataxia-telangectasia. Importantly, the risk of treatment-related second malignancies is at least additive and often is synergistic with combined chemotherapy and radiation therapy; hence, for such combined therapy treatment approaches, it is important to establish the necessity of each modality in the treatment program. All these patients require special surveillance or in some cases prophylactic surgery as part of appropriate treatment and follow-up.

CHEMOTHERAPEUTIC AGENTS

Chemotherapy is significantly associated with two fatal second malignancies: acute leukemia and myelodysplastic syndromes. Two types of leukemia have been described. In patients treated with alkylating agents, acute myeloid leukemia is associated with deletions in chromosomes 5 or 7. The lifetime risk is about 1–5%, is increased by radiation therapy, and increases with age. The incidence of these leukemias peaks at 4–6 years, with risk returning close to baseline at 10 years. The other type of acute myeloid leukemia is related to therapy with topoisomerase inhibitors, is associated with chromosome 10q23 translocations, has an incidence <1%, and generally occurs 1.5–3 years after treatment. Both of these acute leukemias are refractory to treatment and have a high mortality rate. The development of myelodysplastic syndromes is increased after chemotherapy, particularly chronic alkylating agent therapy, and these syndromes often are associated with leukemic progression with a dismal prognosis.

RADIATION THERAPY

Patients receiving radiation have an increasing and lifelong risk of second malignancies that is 1–2% per year in the second decade after treatment but increases to >25% after 25 years. These malignancies include cancers of the thyroid and breast, sarcomas, and CNS cancers, which often tend to be aggressive and have a poor prognosis. An example of organ-, age-, and sex-dependent radiation-induced secondary malignancy is breast cancer, in which the risk is small with radiation <age 30 but increases about twentyfold over baseline in women >30 years. A 25-year-old woman treated with mantle radiation for Hodgkin's lymphoma has a 29% actuarial risk of developing breast cancer by age 55 years.

HORMONAL THERAPY

Treatment of breast cancer with tamoxifen for 5 years or longer is associated with a 1–2% risk of endometrial cancer. Surveillance is generally effective at finding these cancers at an early stage. The risk of mortality from tamoxifen-induced endometrial cancer is low compared with the benefit of tamoxifen as adjuvant therapy for breast cancer.

IMMUNOSUPRESSIVE THERAPY

Immunosupressive therapy, as used in allogeneic bone marrow transplantation, particularly with T cell depletion and using antithymocyte globulin or other means, increases the risk of Epstein Barr virus–associated B cell lymphoproliferative disorder. The incidence at 10 years after T cell depletion is 9–12%. Discontinuation of immunosuppressive therapy, if possible, often is associated with complete disease regression.

RECOMMENDATIONS FOR FOLLOW-UP

All former cancer patients should be followed indefinitely. This is done most often by oncologists, but demographic changes suggest that more primary care physicians will need to be trained in the follow-up of treated cancer patients in remission. Cancer patients need to be educated about signs and symptoms of recurrence and potentially adverse effects related to therapy. Localized pain or palpable abnormality in a previously radiated field should prompt radiographic evaluation. Screening tests, when available and validated, should be used on a routine and regular basis, for example, mammography and Pap smear, particularly in patients receiving radiation to specific organs. Annual mammography should start no later than 10 years after breast radiation. Patients receiving radiation fields that encompass thyroid tissue should have regular thyroid exams and TSH testing. Patients treated with alkylating agents or topoisomerase inhibitors should have a complete blood count every 6–12 months, and cytopenias, abnormal cells on peripheral smear, or macrocytosis should be evaluated with bone marrow biopsy and aspirate, along with cytogenetics, flow cytometry, or fluorescence in situ hybridization (FISH) studies as appropriate.

Cancer survival, as the population lives longer and expands, has become an increasingly recognized subject. The Institute of Medicine and the National Research Council of the National Academy of Sciences have published a monograph titled *From Cancer Patient to Cancer Survivor: Lost in Transition*. It proposes a plan to inform clinicians caring for cancer survivors in complete detail about their previous treatments, the complications of those treatments, signs and symptoms of late effects, and recommended screening and follow-up procedures. Table 55-2 describes long-term treatment effects by cancer type.

TABLE 55-2

LONG-TERM TREATMENT EFFECTS BY CANCER TYPE

CANCER TYPE	LATE EFFECTS
Pediatric cancers	Majority have at least one late effect; 30% with moderate/severe problems Cardiovascular: radiation, anthracyclines Lungs: radiation Skeletal abnormalities: radiation Psychological, cognitive, and sexual problems Second neoplasms significant cause of death
Hodgkin's lymphoma	Thyroid dysfunction: radiation Premature coronary artery disease: radiation Gonadal dysfunction: chemotherapy Postsplenectomy sepsis Myelodysplasia Acute myeloid leukemia Non-Hodgkin's lymphomas Breast cancer, lung cancer, and melanoma Fatigue, psychological and sexual problems Peripheral neuropathy
Non-Hodgkin's lymphoma	Myelodysplasia Acute leukemia Bladder cancer Peripheral neuropathy
Acute leukemia	Second malignancies: hematologic, solid tumors Neurophychiatric dysfunction Subnormal growth Thyroid abnormalities Infertility
Bone marrow stem cell transplantation	Infertility Graft vs host disease (allogeneic transplant) Psychosexual dysfunction
Head and neck cancer	Poor dentition, dry mouth, poor nutrition: radiation
Breast cancer	Tamoxifen: endometrial cancer, blood clots Aromatase inhibitors: osteoporosis, arthritis. Cardiomyopathy: anthracycline ± radiation, trastuzaumab Acute leukemia Hormone-deficiency symptoms: hot flashes, vaginal dryness, dyspareunia Psychosocial dysfunction "Chemo brain"
Testicular cancer	Raynaud's phenomenon Renal dysfunction Pulmonary dysfunction Retrograde ejaculation: surgery Sexual dysfunction (15%)
Colon cancer	Major risk is second colon cancer Quality of life high in survivors
Prostate cancer	Impotence Urinary incontinence (0–15%) Chronic prostatitis or cystitis: radiation

OUTLOOK

Clearly, the challenge for the future is to combine chemotherapy, targeted agents, biologic therapies, radiation, and surgery to produce better outcomes with less toxicity, including late effects of therapy. This is easily said and less easily accomplished. As treatment becomes more effective in new patient populations (ovarian, bladder, anal, and laryngeal cancers, for example), one can expect to discover new populations at risk for late effects. These populations will have to be followed carefully so that such effects are recognized and treated. Cancer survivors represent an underutilized resource for prevention studies. Childhood cancer survivors especially have multiple chronic health impairments. The incidence of these late treatment consequences appears to have no plateau with age, throwing in stark relief the necessity of close monitoring and therapies with fewer late consequences of treatment.

APPENDIX

LABORATORY VALUES OF CLINICAL IMPORTANCE

Alexander Kratz ■ Michael A. Pesce ■ Robert C. Basner ■ Andrew J. Einstein

This Appendix contains tables of reference values for laboratory tests, special analytes, and special function tests. A variety of factors can influence reference values. Such variables include the population studied, the duration and means of specimen transport, laboratory methods and instrumentation, and even the type of container used for the collection of the specimen. The reference or "normal" ranges given in this appendix may therefore not be appropriate for all laboratories, and these values should only be used as general guidelines. Whenever possible, reference values provided by the laboratory performing the testing should be utilized in the interpretation of laboratory data. Values supplied in this Appendix reflect typical reference ranges in adults. Pediatric reference ranges may vary significantly from adult values.

In preparing the Appendix, the authors have taken into account the fact that the system of international units (SI, système international d'unités) is used in most countries and in some medical journals. However, clinical laboratories may continue to report values in "traditional" or conventional units. Therefore, both systems are provided in the Appendix. The dual system is also used in the text except for (1) those instances in which the numbers remain the same but only the terminology is changed (mmol/L for meq/L or IU/L for mIU/mL), when only the SI units are given, and (2) most pressure measurements (e.g., blood and cerebrospinal fluid pressures), when the traditional units (mmHg, mmH_2O) are used. In all other instances in the text, the SI unit is followed by the traditional unit in parentheses.

REFERENCE VALUES FOR LABORATORY TESTS

TABLE 1

HEMATOLOGY AND COAGULATION

ANALYTE	SPECIMEN	SI UNITS	CONVENTIONAL UNITS
Activated clotting time	WB	70–180 s	70–180 s
Activated protein C resistance (factor V Leiden)	P	Not applicable	Ratio >2.1
ADAMTS13 activity	P	≥0.67	≥67%
ADAMTS13 inhibitor activity	P	Not applicable	≤0.4 U
ADAMTS13 antibody	P	Not applicable	≤18 U
Alpha$_2$ antiplasmin	P	0.87–1.55	87–155%
Antiphospholipid antibody panel			
PTT-LA (lupus anticoagulant screen)	P	Negative	Negative
Platelet neutralization procedure	P	Negative	Negative
Dilute viper venom screen	P	Negative	Negative
Anticardiolipin antibody	S		
IgG		0–15 arbitrary units	0–15 GPL
IgM		0–15 arbitrary units	0–15 MPL

(continued)

TABLE 1

HEMATOLOGY AND COAGULATION (*CONTINUED*)

ANALYTE	SPECIMEN	SI UNITS	CONVENTIONAL UNITS
Antithrombin III	P		
Antigenic		220–390 mg/L	22–39 mg/dL
Functional		0.7–1.30 U/L	70–130%
Anti-Xa assay (heparin assay)	P		
Unfractionated heparin		0.3–0.7 kIU/L	0.3–0.7 IU/mL
Low-molecular-weight heparin		0.5–1.0 kIU/L	0.5–1.0 IU/mL
Danaparoid (Orgaran)		0.5–0.8 kIU/L	0.5–0.8 IU/mL
Autohemolysis test	WB	0.004–0.045	0.4–4.50%
Autohemolysis test with glucose	WB	0.003–0.007	0.3–0.7%
Bleeding time (adult)		<7.1 min	<7.1 min
Bone marrow: See Table 7			
Clot retraction	WB	0.50–1.00/2 h	50–100%/2 h
Cryofibrinogen	P	Negative	Negative
D-dimer	P	220–740 ng/mL FEU	220–740 ng/mL FEU
Differential blood count	WB		
Relative counts:			
Neutrophils		0.40–0.70	40–70%
Bands		0.0–0.05	0–5%
Lymphocytes		0.20–0.50	20–50%
Monocytes		0.04–0.08	4–8%
Eosinophils		0.0–0.6	0–6%
Basophils		0.0–0.02	0–2%
Absolute counts:			
Neutrophils		1.42–6.34 × 10^9/L	1420–6340/mm^3
Bands		0–0.45 × 10^9/L	0–450/mm^3
Lymphocytes		0.71–4.53 × 10^9/L	710–4530/mm^3
Monocytes		0.14–0.72 × 10^9/L	140–720/mm^3
Eosinophils		0–0.54 × 10^9/L	0–540/mm^3
Basophils		0–0.18 × 10^9/L	0–180/mm^3
Erythrocyte count	WB		
Adult males		4.30–5.60 × 10^{12}/L	4.30–5.60 × 10^6/mm^3
Adult females		4.00–5.20 × 10^{12}/L	4.00–5.20 × 10^6/mm^3
Erythrocyte life span	WB		
Normal survival		120 days	120 days
Chromium labeled, half-life ($t_{1/2}$)		25–35 days	25–35 days
Erythrocyte sedimentation rate	WB		
Females		0–20 mm/h	0–20 mm/h
Males		0–15 mm/h	0–15 mm/h
Euglobulin lysis time	P	7200–14400 s	120–240 min
Factor II, prothrombin	P	0.50–1.50	50-150%
Factor V	P	0.50–1.50	50-150%
Factor VII	P	0.50–1.50	50–150%
Factor VIII	P	0.50–1.50	50–150%
Factor IX	P	0.50–1.50	50–150%
Factor X	P	0.50–1.50	50–150%
Factor XI	P	0.50–1.50	50–150%
Factor XII	P	0.50–1.50	50–150 %
Factor XIII screen	P	Not applicable	Present
Factor inhibitor assay	P	<0.5 Bethesda Units	<0.5 Bethesda Units
Fibrin(ogen) degradation products	P	0–1 mg/L	0–1 µg/mL
Fibrinogen	P	2.33–4.96 g/L	233–496 mg/dL
Glucose-6-phosphate dehydrogenase (erythrocyte)	WB	<2400 s	<40 min
Ham's test (acid serum)	WB	Negative	Negative

(*continued*)

TABLE 1

HEMATOLOGY AND COAGULATION (*CONTINUED*)

ANALYTE	SPECIMEN	SI UNITS	CONVENTIONAL UNITS
Hematocrit	WB		
Adult males		0.388–0.464	38.8–46.4
Adult females		0.354–0.444	35.4–44.4
Hemoglobin			
Plasma	P	6–50 mg/L	0.6–5.0 mg/dL
Whole blood:	WB		
Adult males		133–162 g/L	13.3–16.2 g/dL
Adult females		120–158 g/L	12.0–15.8 g/dL
Hemoglobin electrophoresis	WB		
Hemoglobin A		0.95–0.98	95–98%
Hemoglobin A_2		0.015–0.031	1.5–3.1%
Hemoglobin F		0–0.02	0–2.0%
Hemoglobins other than A, A_2, or F		Absent	Absent
Heparin-induced thrombocytopenia antibody	P	Negative	Negative
Immature platelet fraction (IPF)	WB	0.011–0.061	1.1–6.1%
Joint fluid crystal	JF	Not applicable	No crystals seen
Joint fluid mucin	JF	Not applicable	Only type I mucin present
Leukocytes			
Alkaline phosphatase (LAP)	WB	0.2–1.6 μkat/L	13–100 μ/L
Count (WBC)	WB	$3.54–9.06 \times 10^9$/L	$3.54–9.06 \times 10^3$/mm^3
Mean corpuscular hemoglobin (MCH)	WB	26.7–31.9 pg/cell	26.7–31.9 pg/cell
Mean corpuscular hemoglobin concentration (MCHC)	WB	323–359 g/L	32.3–35.9 g/dL
Mean corpuscular hemoglobin of reticulocytes (CH)	WB	24–36 pg	24–36 pg
Mean corpuscular volume (MCV)	WB	79–93.3 fL	79–93.3 μm^3
Mean platelet volume (MPV)	WB	9.00–12.95 fL	9.00–12.95
Osmotic fragility of erythrocytes	WB		
Direct		0.0035–0.0045	0.35–0.45%
Indirect		0.0030–0.0065	0.30–0.65%
Partial thromboplastin time, activated	P	26.3–39.4 s	26.3–39.4 s
Plasminogen	P		
Antigen		84–140 mg/L	8.4–14.0 mg/dL
Functional		0.70–1.30	70–130%
Plasminogen activator inhibitor 1	P	4–43 μg/L	4–43 ng/mL
Platelet aggregation	PRP	Not applicable	>65% aggregation in response to adenosine diphosphate, epinephrine, collagen, ristocetin, and arachidonic acid
Platelet count	WB	$165–415 \times 10^9$/L	$165–415 \times 10^3$/mm^3
Platelet, mean volume	WB	6.4–11 fL	6.4–11.0 μm^3
Prekallikrein assay	P	0.50–1.5	50–150%
Prekallikrein screen	P		No deficiency detected
Protein C	P		
Total antigen		0.70–1.40	70–140%
Functional		0.70–1.30	70–130%
Protein S	P		
Total antigen		0.70–1.40	70–140%
Functional		0.65–1.40	65–140%
Free antigen		0.70–1.40	70–140%
Prothrombin gene mutation G20210A	WB	Not applicable	Not present
Prothrombin time	P	12.7–15.4 s	12.7–15.4 s

(*continued*)

TABLE 1

HEMATOLOGY AND COAGULATION (*CONTINUED*)

ANALYTE	SPECIMEN	SI UNITS	CONVENTIONAL UNITS
Protoporphyrin, free erythrocyte	WB	0.28–0.64 μmol/L of red blood cells	16–36 μg/dL of red blood cells
Red cell distribution width	WB	<0.145	<14.5%
Reptilase time	P	16–23.6 s	16–23.6 s
Reticulocyte count	WB		
Adult males		0.008–0.023 red cells	0.8–2.3% red cells
Adult females		0.008–0.020 red cells	0.8–2.0% red cells
Reticulocyte hemoglobin content	WB	>26 pg/cell	>26 pg/cell
Ristocetin cofactor (functional von Willebrand factor)	P		
Blood group O		0.75 mean of normal	75% mean of normal
Blood group A		1.05 mean of normal	105% mean of normal
Blood group B		1.15 mean of normal	115% mean of normal
Blood group AB		1.25 mean of normal	125% mean of normal
Serotonin release assay	S	<0.2 release	<20% release
Sickle cell test	WB	Negative	Negative
Sucrose hemolysis	WB	<0.1	<10% hemolysis
Thrombin time	P	15.3–18.5 s	15.3–18.5 s
Total eosinophils	WB	150–300 × 10^6/L	150–300/mm^3
Transferrin receptor	S, P	9.6–29.6 nmol/L	9.6–29.6 nmol/L
Viscosity			
Plasma	P	1.7–2.1	1.7–2.1
Serum	S	1.4–1.8	1.4–1.8
von Willebrand factor (vWF) antigen (factor VIII:R antigen)			
Blood group O		0.75 mean of normal	75% mean of normal
Blood group A		1.05 mean of normal	105% mean of normal
Blood group B		1.15 mean of normal	115% mean of normal
Blood group AB		1.25 mean of normal	125% mean of normal
von Willebrand factor multimers	P	Normal distribution	Normal distribution
White blood cells: see "Leukocytes"			

Abbreviations: JF, joint fluid; P, plasma; PRP, platelet-rich plasma; S, serum; WB, whole blood.

TABLE 2

CLINICAL CHEMISTRY AND IMMUNOLOGY

ANALYTE	SPECIMEN	SI UNITS	CONVENTIONAL UNITS
Acetoacetate	P	49–294 μmol/L	0.5–3.0 mg/dL
Adrenocorticotropin (ACTH)	P	1.3–16.7 pmol/L	6.0–76.0 pg/mL
Alanine aminotransferase (ALT, SGPT)	S	0.12–0.70 μkat/L	7–41 U/L
Albumin	S	40–50 g/L	4.0–5.0 mg/dL
Aldolase	S	26–138 nkat/L	1.5–8.1 U/L
Aldosterone (adult)			
Supine, normal sodium diet	S, P	<443 pmol/L	<16 ng/dL
Upright, normal	S, P	111–858 pmol/L	4–31 ng/dL
Alpha fetoprotein (adult)	S	0–8.5 μg/L	0–8.5 ng/mL
$Alpha_1$ antitrypsin	S	1.0–2.0 g/L	100–200 mg/dL
Ammonia, as NH_3	P	11–35 μmol/L	19–60 μg/dL
Amylase (method dependent)	S	0.34–1.6 μkat/L	20–96 U/L

(*continued*)

TABLE 2

CLINICAL CHEMISTRY AND IMMUNOLOGY (*CONTINUED*)

ANALYTE	SPECIMEN	SI UNITS	CONVENTIONAL UNITS
Androstendione (adult)	S		
Males		0.81–3.1 nmol/L	23–89 ng/dL
Females			
Premenopausal		0.91–7.5 nmol/L	26–214 ng/dL
Postmenopausal		0.46–2.9 nmol/L	13–82 ng/dL
Angiotensin-converting enzyme (ACE)	S	0.15–1.1 μkat/L	9–67 U/L
Anion gap	S	7–16 mmol/L	7–16 mmol/L
Apolipoprotein A-1	S		
Male		0.94–1.78 g/L	94–178 mg/dL
Female		1.01–1.99 g/L	101–199 mg/dL
Apolipoprotein B	S		
Male		0.55–1.40 g/L	55–140 mg/dL
Female		0.55–1.25 g/L	55–125 mg/dL
Arterial blood gases	WB		
$[HCO_3^-]$		22–30 mmol/L	22–30 meq/L
P_{CO_2}		4.3–6.0 kPa	32–45 mmHg
pH		7.35–7.45	7.35–7.45
P_{O_2}		9.6–13.8 kPa	72–104 mmHg
Aspartate aminotransferase (AST, SGOT)	S	0.20–0.65 μkat/L	12–38 U/L
Autoantibodies	S		
Anti-centromere antibody IgG		≤29 AU/mL	≤29 AU/mL
Anti-double-strand (native) DNA		<25 IU/L	<25 IU/L
Anti-glomerular basement membrane antibodies			
Qualitative IgG, IgA		Negative	Negative
Quantitative IgG antibody		≤19 AU/mL	≤19 AU/mL
Anti-histone antibodies		<1.0 U	<1.0 U
Anti-Jo-1 antibody		≤29 AU/mL	≤29 AU/mL
Anti-mitochondrial antibody		Not applicable	<20 Units
Anti-neutrophil cytoplasmic autoantibodies		Not applicable	<1:20
Serine proteinase 3 antibodies		≤19 AU/mL	≤19 AU/mL
Myeloperoxidase antibodies		≤19 AU/mL	≤19 AU/mL
Antinuclear antibody		Not applicable	Negative at 1:40
Anti-parietal cell antibody		Not applicable	None detected
Anti-RNP antibody		Not applicable	<1.0 U
Anti-Scl 70 antibody		Not applicable	<1.0 U
Anti-Smith antibody		Not applicable	<1.0 U
Anti–smooth muscle antibody		Not applicable	<1.0 U
Anti-SSA antibody		Not applicable	<1.0 U
Anti-SSB antibody		Not applicable	Negative
Anti-thyroglobulin antibody		<40 kIU/L	<40 IU/mL
Anti-thyroid peroxidase antibody		<35 kIU/L	<35 IU/mL
B-type natriuretic peptide (BNP)	P	Age and gender specific: <100 ng/L	Age and gender specific: <100 pg/mL
Bence Jones protein, serum qualitative	S	Not applicable	None detected
Bence Jones protein, serum quantitative	S		
Free kappa		3.3–19.4 mg/L	0.33–1.94 mg/dL
Free lambda		5.7–26.3 mg/L	0.57–2.63 mg/dL
K/L ratio		0.26–1.65	0.26–1.65
Beta-2-microglobulin	S	1.1–2.4 mg/L	1.1–2.4 mg/L
Bilirubin	S		
Total		5.1–22 μmol/L	0.3–1.3 mg/dL
Direct		1.7–6.8 μmol/L	0.1–0.4 mg/dL
Indirect		3.4–15.2 μmol/L	0.2–0.9 mg/dL

(continued)

TABLE 2

CLINICAL CHEMISTRY AND IMMUNOLOGY (*CONTINUED*)

ANALYTE	SPECIMEN	SI UNITS	CONVENTIONAL UNITS
C peptide	S	0.27–1.19 nmol/L	0.8–3.5 ng/mL
C1-esterase-inhibitor protein	S	210–390 mg/L	21–39 mg/dL
CA 125	S	<35 kU/L	<35 U/mL
CA 19-9	S	<37 kU/L	<37 U/mL
CA 15-3	S	<33 kU/L	<33 U/mL
CA 27-29	S	0–40 kU/L	0–40 U/mL
Calcitonin	S		
Male		0–7.5 ng/L	0–7.5 pg/mL
Female		0–5.1 ng/L	0–5.1 pg/mL
Calcium	S	2.2–2.6 mmol/L	8.7–10.2 mg/dL
Calcium, ionized	WB	1.12–1.32 mmol/L	4.5–5.3 mg/dL
Carbon dioxide content (TCO_2)	P (sea level)	22–30 mmol/L	22–30 meq/L
Carboxyhemoglobin (carbon monoxide content)	WB		
Nonsmokers		0.0–0.015	0–1.5%
Smokers		0.04–0.09	4–9%
Loss of consciousness and death		>0.50	>50%
Carcinoembryonic antigen (CEA)	S		
Nonsmokers		0.0–3.0 μg/L	0.0–3.0 ng/mL
Smokers		0.0–5.0 μg/L	0.0–5.0 ng/mL
Ceruloplasmin	S	250–630 mg/L	25–63 mg/dL
Chloride	S	102–109 mmol/L	102–109 meq/L
Cholesterol: see Table 5			
Cholinesterase	S	5–12 kU/L	5–12 U/mL
Chromogranin A	S	0–50 μg/L	0–50 ng/mL
Complement	S		
C3		0.83–1.77 g/L	83–177 mg/dL
C4		0.16–0.47 g/L	16–47 mg/dL
Complement total		60–144 CAE units	60–144 CAE units
Cortisol			
Fasting, 8 A.M.–12 noon	S	138–690 nmol/L	5–25 μg/dL
12 noon–8 P.M.		138–414 nmol/L	5–15 μg/dL
8 P.M.–8 A.M.		0–276 nmol/L	0–10 μg/dL
C-reactive protein	S	<10 mg/L	<10 mg/L
C-reactive protein, high sensitivity	S	Cardiac risk Low: <1.0 mg/L Average: 1.0–3.0 mg/L High: >3.0 mg/L	Cardiac risk Low: <1.0 mg/L Average: 1.0–3.0 mg/L High: >3.0 mg/L
Creatine kinase (total)	S		
Females		0.66–4.0 μkat/L	39–238 U/L
Males		0.87–5.0 μkat/L	51–294 U/L
Creatine kinase-MB	S		
Mass		0.0–5.5 μg/L	0.0–5.5 ng/mL
Fraction of total activity (by electrophoresis)		0–0.04	0–4.0%
Creatinine	S		
Female		44–80 μmol/L	0.5–0.9 mg/dL
Male		53–106 μmol/L	0.6–1.2 mg/dL
Cryoglobulins	S	Not applicable	None detected
Cystatin C	S	0.5–1.0 mg/L	0.5–1.0 mg/L

(*continued*)

TABLE 2

CLINICAL CHEMISTRY AND IMMUNOLOGY (*CONTINUED*)

ANALYTE	SPECIMEN	SI UNITS	CONVENTIONAL UNITS
Dehydroepiandrosterone (DHEA) (adult)			
Male	S	6.2–43.4 nmol/L	180–1250 ng/dL
Female		4.5–34.0 nmol/L	130–980 ng/dL
Dehydroepiandrosterone (DHEA) sulfate	S		
Male (adult)		100–6190 µg/L	10–619 µg/dL
Female (adult, premenopausal)		120–5350 µg/L	12–535 µg/dL
Female (adult, postmenopausal)		300–2600 µg/L	30–260 µg/dL
11-Deoxycortisol (adult) (compound S)	S	0.34–4.56 nmol/L	12–158 ng/dL
Dihydrotestosterone			
Male	S, P	1.03–2.92 nmol/L	30–85 ng/dL
Female		0.14–0.76 nmol/L	4–22 ng/dL
Dopamine	P	0–130 pmol/L	0–20 pg/mL
Epinephrine	P		
Supine (30 min)		<273 pmol/L	<50 pg/mL
Sitting		<328 pmol/L	<60 pg/mL
Standing (30 min)		<491 pmol/L	<90 pg/mL
Erythropoietin	S	4–27 U/L	4–27 U/L
Estradiol	S, P		
Female			
Menstruating:			
Follicular phase		74–532 pmol/L	<20–145 pg/mL
Midcycle peak		411–1626 pmol/L	112–443 pg/mL
Luteal phase		74–885 pmol/L	<20–241 pg/mL
Postmenopausal		217 pmol/L	<59 pg/mL
Male		74 pmol/L	<20 pg/mL
Estrone	S, P		
Female			
Menstruating:			
Follicular phase		<555 pmol/L	<150 pg/mL
Luteal phase		<740 pmol/L	<200 pg/mL
Postmenopausal		11–118 pmol/L	3–32 pg/mL
Male		33–133 pmol/L	9–36 pg/mL
Fatty acids, free (nonesterified)	P	0.1–0.6 mmol/L	2.8–16.8 mg/dL
Ferritin	S		
Female		10–150 µg/L	10–150 ng/mL
Male		29–248 µg/L	29–248 ng/mL
Follicle-stimulating hormone (FSH)	S, P		
Female			
Menstruating			
Follicular phase		3.0–20.0 IU/L	3.0–20.0 mIU/mL
Ovulatory phase		9.0–26.0 IU/L	9.0–26.0 mIU/mL
Luteal phase		1.0–12.0 IU/L	1.0–12.0 mIU/mL
Postmenopausal		18.0–153.0 IU/L	18.0–153.0 mIU/mL
Male		1.0–12.0 IU/L	1.0–12.0 mIU/mL
Fructosamine	S	<285 umol/L	<285 umol/L
Gamma glutamyltransferase	S	0.15–0.99 µkat/L	9–58 U/L
Gastrin	S	<100 ng/L	<100 pg/mL
Glucagon	P	40–130 ng/L	40–130 pg/mL

(*continued*)

TABLE 2

CLINICAL CHEMISTRY AND IMMUNOLOGY (*CONTINUED*)

ANALYTE	SPECIMEN	SI UNITS	CONVENTIONAL UNITS
Glucose	WB	3.6–5.3 mmol/L	65–95 mg/dL
Glucose (fasting)	P		
Normal		4.2–5.6 mmol/L	75–100 mg/dL
Increased risk for diabetes		5.6–6.9 mmol/L	100–125 mg/dL
Diabetes mellitus		Fasting >7.0 mmol/L A 2-hour level of >11.1 mmol/L during an oral glucose tolerance test A random glucose level of ≥11.1 mmol/L in patients with symptoms of hyperglycemia	Fasting >126 mg/dL A 2-hour level of ≥200 mg/dL during an oral glucose tolerance test A random glucose level of ≥200 mg/dL in patients with symptoms of hyperglycemia
Growth hormone	S	0–5 μg/L	0–5 ng/mL
Hemoglobin A_{1c}	WB	0.04–0.06 HgB fraction	4.0–5.6%
Pre-diabetes		0.057–0.064 HgB fraction	5.7–6.4%
Diabetes mellitus		A hemoglobin A_{1c} level of ≥0.065 Hgb fraction as suggested by the American Diabetes Association	A hemoglobin A_{1c} level of ≥6.5% as suggested by the American Diabetes Association
Hemoglobin A_{1c} with estimated average glucose (eAg)	WB	eAg (mmoL/L) = 1.59 × HbA_{1c} – 2.59	eAg (mg/dL) = 28.7 × HbA_{1c} – 46.7
High-density lipoprotein (HDL) (see Table 5)			
Homocysteine	P	4.4–10.8 μmol/L	4.4–10.8 μmol/L
Human chorionic gonadotropin (HCG)	S		
Nonpregnant female		<5 IU/L	<5 mIU/mL
1–2 weeks postconception		9–130 IU/L	9–130 mIU/mL
2–3 weeks postconception		75–2600 IU/L	75–2600 mIU/mL
3–4 weeks postconception		850–20,800 IU/L	850–20,800 mIU/mL
4–5 weeks postconception		4000–100,200 IU/L	4000–100,200 mIU/mL
5–10 weeks postconception		11,500–289,000 IU/L	11,500–289,000 mIU/mL
10–14 weeks post conception		18,300–137,000 IU/L	18,300–137,000 mIU/mL
Second trimester		1400–53,000 IU/L	1400–53,000 mIU/mL
Third trimester		940–60,000 IU/L	940–60,000 mIU/mL
β-Hydroxybutyrate	P	60–170 μmol/L	0.6–1.8 mg/dL
17-Hydroxyprogesterone (adult)	S		
Male		<4.17 nmol/L	<139 ng/dL
Female			
Follicular phase		0.45–2.1 nmol/L	15–70 ng/dL
Luteal phase		1.05–8.7 nmol/L	35–290 ng/dL
Immunofixation	S	Not applicable	No bands detected
Immunoglobulin, quantitation (adult)			
IgA	S	0.70–3.50 g/L	70–350 mg/dL
IgD	S	0–140 mg/L	0–14 mg/dL
IgE	S	1–87 kIU/L	1–87 IU/mL
IgG	S	7.0–17.0 g/L	700–1700 mg/dL
IgG_1	S	2.7–17.4 g/L	270–1740 mg/dL
IgG_2	S	0.3–6.3 g/L	30–630 mg/dL
IgG_3	S	0.13–3.2 g/L	13–320 mg/dL
IgG_4	S	0.11–6.2 g/L	11–620 mg/dL
IgM	S	0.50–3.0 g/L	50–300 mg/dL
Insulin	S, P	14.35–143.5 pmol/L	2–20 μU/mL
Iron	S	7–25 μmol/L	41–141 μg/dL

(*continued*)

TABLE 2

CLINICAL CHEMISTRY AND IMMUNOLOGY (*CONTINUED*)

ANALYTE	SPECIMEN	SI UNITS	CONVENTIONAL UNITS
Iron-binding capacity	S	45–73 μmol/L	251–406 μg/dL
Iron-binding capacity saturation	S	0.16–0.35	16–35%
Ischemia modified albumin	S	<85 KU/L	<85 U/mL
Joint fluid crystal	JF	Not applicable	No crystals seen
Joint fluid mucin	JF	Not applicable	Only type I mucin present
Ketone (acetone)	S	Negative	Negative
Lactate	P, arterial P, venous	0.5–1.6 mmol/L 0.5–2.2 mmol/L	4.5–14.4 mg/dL 4.5–19.8 mg/dL
Lactate dehydrogenase	S	2.0–3.8 μkat/L	115–221 U/L
Lipase	S	0.51–0.73 μkat/L	3–43 U/L
Lipids: see Table 5			
Lipoprotein (a)	S	0–300 mg/L	0–30 mg/dL
Low-density lipoprotein (LDL) (see Table 5)			
Luteinizing hormone (LH)	S, P		
Female			
Menstruating			
Follicular phase		2.0–15.0 U/L	2.0–15.0 mIU/mL
Ovulatory phase		22.0–105.0 U/L	22.0–105.0 mIU/mL
Luteal phase		0.6–19.0 U/L	0.6–19.0 mIU/mL
Postmenopausal		16.0–64.0 U/L	16.0–64.0 mIU/mL
Male		2.0–12.0 U/L	2.0–12.0 mIU/mL
Magnesium	S	0.62–0.95 mmol/L	1.5–2.3 mg/dL
Metanephrine	P	<0.5 nmol/L	<100 pg/mL
Methemoglobin	WB	0.0–0.01	0–1%
Myoglobin	S		
Male		20–71 μg/L	20–71 μg/L
Female		25–58 μg/L	25–58 μg/L
Norepinephrine	P		
Supine (30 min)		650–2423 pmol/L	110–410 pg/mL
Sitting		709–4019 pmol/L	120–680 pg/mL
Standing (30 min)		739–4137 pmol/L	125–700 pg/mL
N-telopeptide (cross-linked), NTx	S		
Female, premenopausal		6.2–19.0 nmol BCE	6.2–19.0 nmol BCE
Male		5.4–24.2 nmol BCE	5.4–24.2 nmol BCE
NT-Pro BNP	S, P	<125 ng/L up to 75 years <450 ng/L >75 years	<125 pg/mL up to 75 years <450 pg/mL >75 years
5′ Nucleotidase	S	0.00–0.19 μkat/L	0–11 U/L
Osmolality	P	275–295 mOsmol/kg serum water	275–295 mOsmol/kg serum water
Osteocalcin	S	11–50 μg/L	11–50 ng/mL
Oxygen content	WB		
Arterial (sea level)		17–21	17–21 vol%
Venous (sea level)		10–16	10–16 vol%
Oxygen saturation (sea level)	WB	Fraction:	Percent:
Arterial		0.94–1.0	94–100%
Venous, arm		0.60–0.85	60–85%
Parathyroid hormone (intact)	S	8–51 ng/L	8–51 pg/mL

(*continued*)

TABLE 2

CLINICAL CHEMISTRY AND IMMUNOLOGY (*CONTINUED*)

ANALYTE	SPECIMEN	SI UNITS	CONVENTIONAL UNITS
Phosphatase, alkaline	S	0.56–1.63 μkat/L	33–96 U/L
Phosphorus, inorganic	S	0.81–1.4 mmol/L	2.5–4.3 mg/dL
Potassium	S	3.5–5.0 mmol/L	3.5–5.0 meq/L
Prealbumin	S	170–340 mg/L	17–34 mg/dL
Procalcitonin	S	<0.1 μg/L	<0.1 ng/mL
Progesterone	S, P		
Female: Follicular		<3.18 nmol/L	<1.0 ng/mL
Midluteal		9.54–63.6 nmol/L	3–20 ng/mL
Male		<3.18 nmol/L	<1.0 ng/mL
Prolactin	S		
Male		53–360 mg/L	2.5–17 ng/mL
Female		40–530 mg/L	1.9–25 ng/mL
Prostate-specific antigen (PSA)	S	0.0–4.0 μg/L	0.0–4.0 ng/mL
Prostate-specific antigen, free	S	With total PSA between 4 and 10 μg/L and when the free PSA is: >0.25 decreased risk of prostate cancer <0.10 increased risk of prostate cancer	With total PSA between 4 and 10 ng/mL and when the free PSA is: >25% decreased risk of prostate cancer <10% increased risk of prostate cancer
Protein fractions:	S		
Albumin		35–55 g/L	3.5–5.5 g/dL (50–60%)
Globulin		20–35 g/L	2.0–3.5 g/dL (40–50%)
$Alpha_1$		2–4 g/L	0.2–0.4 g/dL (4.2–7.2%)
$Alpha_2$		5–9 g/L	0.5–0.9 g/dL (6.8–12%)
Beta		6–11 g/L	0.6–1.1 g/dL (9.3–15%)
Gamma		7–17 g/L	0.7–1.7 g/dL (13–23%)
Protein, total	S	67–86 g/L	6.7–8.6 g/dL
Pyruvate	P	40–130 μmol/L	0.35–1.14 mg/dL
Rheumatoid factor	S	<15 kIU/L	<15 IU/mL
Serotonin	WB	0.28–1.14 umol/L	50–200 ng/mL
Serum protein electrophoresis	S	Not applicable	Normal pattern
Sex hormone–binding globulin (adult)	S		
Male		11–80 nmol/L	11–80 nmol/L
Female		30–135 nmol/L	30–135 nmol/L
Sodium	S	136–146 mmol/L	136–146 meq/L
Somatomedin-C (IGF-1) (adult)	S		
16 years		226–903 μg/L	226–903 ng/mL
17 years		193–731 μg/L	193–731 ng/mL
18 years		163–584 μg/L	163–584 ng/mL
19 years		141–483 μg/L	141–483 ng/mL
20 years		127–424 μg/L	127–424 ng/mL
21–25 years		116–358 μg/L	116–358 ng/mL
26–30 years		117–329 μg/L	117–329 ng/mL
31–35 years		115–307 μg/L	115–307 ng/mL
36–40 years		119–204 μg/L	119–204 ng/mL
41–45 years		101–267 μg/L	101–267 ng/mL
46–50 years		94–252 μg/L	94–252 ng/mL
51–55 years		87–238 μg/L	87–238 ng/mL
56–60 years		81–225 μg/L	81–225 ng/mL
61–65 years		75–212 μg/L	75–212 ng/mL

(*continued*)

TABLE 2

CLINICAL CHEMISTRY AND IMMUNOLOGY (*CONTINUED*)

ANALYTE	SPECIMEN	SI UNITS	CONVENTIONAL UNITS
66–70 years		69–200 μg/L	69–200 ng/mL
71–75 years		64–188 μg/L	64–188 ng/mL
76–80 years		59–177 μg/L	59–177 ng/mL
81–85 years		55–166 μg/L	55–166 ng/mL
Somatostatin	P	<25 ng/L	<25 pg/mL
Testosterone, free			
Female, adult	S	10.4–65.9 pmol/L	3–19 pg/mL
Male, adult		312–1041 pmol/L	90–300 pg/mL
Testosterone, total,	S		
Female		0.21–2.98 nmol/L	6–86 ng/dL
Male		9.36–37.10 nmol/L	270–1070 ng/dL
Thyroglobulin	S	1.3–31.8 μg/L	1.3–31.8 ng/mL
Thyroid-binding globulin	S	13–30 mg/L	1.3–3.0 mg/dL
Thyroid-stimulating hormone	S	0.34–4.25 mIU/L	0.34–4.25 μIU/mL
Thyroxine, free (fT_4)	S	9.0–16 pmol/L	0.7–1.24 ng/dL
Thyroxine, total (T_4)	S	70–151 nmol/L	5.4–11.7 μg/dL
Thyroxine index (free)	S	6.7–10.9	6.7–10.9
Transferrin	S	2.0–4.0 g/L	200–400 mg/dL
Triglycerides (see Table 5)	S	0.34–2.26 mmol/L	30–200 mg/dL
Triiodothyronine, free (fT_3)	S	3.7–6.5 pmol/L	2.4–4.2 pg/mL
Triiodothyronine, total (T_3)	S	1.2–2.1 nmol/L	77–135 ng/dL
Troponin I (method dependent)	S, P		
99th percentile of a healthy population		0–0.04 μg/L	0–0.04 ng/mL
Troponin T	S, P		
99th percentile of a healthy population		0–0.01 μg/L	0–0.01 ng/mL
Urea nitrogen	S	2.5–7.1 mmol/L	7–20 mg/dL
Uric acid	S		
Females		0.15–0.33 mmol/L	2.5–5.6 mg/dL
Males		0.18–0.41 mmol/L	3.1–7.0 mg/dL
Vasoactive intestinal polypeptide	P	0–60 ng/L	0–60 pg/mL
Zinc protoporphyrin	WB	0–400 μg/L	0–40 μg/dL
Zinc protoporphyrin (ZPP)-to-heme ratio	WB	0–69 μmol ZPP/mol heme	0–69 μmol ZPP/mol heme

Abbreviations: BCE, bone collagen equivalent; IGF, insulin-like growth factor; P, plasma; S, serum; WB, whole blood.

TABLE 3

TOXICOLOGY AND THERAPEUTIC DRUG MONITORING

	THERAPEUTIC RANGE		TOXIC LEVEL	
DRUG	**SI UNITS**	**CONVENTIONAL UNITS**	**SI UNITS**	**CONVENTIONAL UNITS**
Acetaminophen	66–199 µmol/L	10–30 µg/mL	>1320 µmol/L	>200 µg/mL
Amikacin				
Peak	34–51 µmol/L	20–30 µg/mL	>60 µmol/L	>35 µg/mL
Trough	0–17 µmol/L	0–10 µg/mL	>17 µmol/L	>10 µg/mL
Amitriptyline–nortriptyline (total drug)	430–900 nmol/L	120–250 ng/mL	>1800 nmol/L	>500 ng/mL
Amphetamine	150–220 nmol/L	20–30 ng/mL	>1500 nmol/L	>200 ng/mL
Bromide	9.4–18.7 mmol/L	75–150 mg/dL	>18.8 mmol/L	>150 mg/dL
Mild toxicity			6.4–18.8 mmol/L	51–150 mg/dL
Severe toxicity			>18.8 mmol/L	>150 mg/dL
Lethal			>37.5 mmol/L	>300 mg/dL
Caffeine	25.8–103 µmol/L	5–20 µg/mL	>206 µmol/L	>40 µg/mL
Carbamazepine	17–42 µmol/L	4–10 µg/mL	>85 µmol/L	>20 µg/mL
Chloramphenicol				
Peak	31–62 µmol/L	10–20 µg/mL	>77 µmol/L	>25 µg/mL
Trough	15–31 µmol/L	5–10 µg/mL	>46 µmol/L	>15 µg/mL
Chlordiazepoxide	1.7–10 µmol/L	0.5–3.0 µg/mL	>17µmol/L	>5.0 µg/mL
Clonazepam	32–240 nmol/L	10–75 ng/mL	>320 nmol/L	>100 ng/mL
Clozapine	0.6–2.1 µmol/L	200–700 ng/mL	>3.7 µmol/L	>1200 ng/mL
Cocaine			>3.3 µmol/L	>1.0 µg/mL
Codeine	43–110 nmol/mL	13–33 ng/mL	>3700 nmol/mL	>1100 ng/mL (lethal)
Cyclosporine				
Renal transplant				
0–6 months	208–312 nmol/L	250–375 ng/mL	>312 nmol/L	>375 ng/mL
6–12 months after transplant	166–250 nmol/L	200–300 ng/mL	>250 nmol/L	>300 ng/mL
>12 months	83–125 nmol/L	100–150 ng/mL	>125 nmol/L	>150 ng/mL
Cardiac transplant				
0–6 months	208–291 nmol/L	250–350 ng/mL	>291 nmol/L	>350 ng/mL
6–12 months after transplant	125–208 nmol/L	150–250 ng/mL	>208 nmol/L	>250 ng/mL
>12 months	83–125 nmol/L	100–150 ng/mL	>125 nmol/L	150 ng/mL
Lung transplant				
0–6 months	250–374 nmol/L	300–450 ng/mL	>374 nmol/L	>450 ng/mL
Liver transplant				
Initiation	208–291 nmol/L	250–350 ng/mL	>291 nmol/L	>350 ng/mL
Maintenance	83–166 nmol/L	100–200 ng/mL	>166 nmol/L	>200 ng/mL
Desipramine	375–1130 nmol/L	100–300 ng/mL	>1880 nmol/L	>500 ng/mL
Diazepam (and metabolite)				
Diazepam	0.7–3.5 µmol/L	0.2–1.0 µg/mL	>7.0 µmol/L	>2.0 µg/mL
Nordiazepam	0.4–6.6 µmol/L	0.1–1.8 µg/mL	>9.2 µmol/L	>2.5 µg/mL
Digoxin	0.64–2.6 nmol/L	0.5–2.0 ng/mL	>5.0 nmol/L	>3.9 ng/mL
Disopyramide	5.3–14.7 µmol/L	2–5 µg/mL	>20.6 µmol/L	>7 µg/mL
Doxepin and nordoxepin				
Doxepin	0.36–0.98 µmol/L	101–274 ng/mL	>1.8 µmol/L	>503 ng/mL
Nordoxepin	0.38–1.04 µmol/L	106–291 ng/mL	>1.9 µmol/L	>531 ng/mL
Ethanol				
Behavioral changes			>4.3 mmol/L	>20 mg/dL
Legal limit			≥17 mmol/L	≥80 mg/dL
Critical with acute exposure			>54 mmol/L	>250 mg/dL
Ethylene glycol				
Toxic			>2 mmol/L	>12 mg/dL
Lethal			>20 mmol/L	>120 mg/dL

(*continued*)

TABLE 3

TOXICOLOGY AND THERAPEUTIC DRUG MONITORING (*CONTINUED*)

	THERAPEUTIC RANGE		TOXIC LEVEL	
DRUG	**SI UNITS**	**CONVENTIONAL UNITS**	**SI UNITS**	**CONVENTIONAL UNITS**
Ethosuximide	280–700 μmol/L	40–100 μg/mL	>700 μmol/L	>100 μg/mL
Everolimus	3.13–8.35 nmol/L	3–8 ng/mL	>12.5 nmol/L	>12 ng/mL
Flecainide	0.5–2.4 μmol/L	0.2–1.0 μg/mL	>3.6 μmol/L	>1.5 μg/mL
Gentamicin				
Peak	10–21 μmol/mL	5–10 μg/mL	>25 μmol/mL	>12 μg/mL
Trough	0–4.2 μmol/mL	0–2 μg/mL	>4.2 μmol/mL	>2 μg/mL
Heroin (diacetyl morphine)			>700 μmol/L	>200 ng/mL (as morphine)
Ibuprofen	49–243 μmol/L	10–50 μg/mL	>970 μmol/L	>200 μg/mL
Imipramine (and metabolite)				
Desimipramine	375–1130 nmol/L	100–300 ng/mL	>1880 nmol/L	>500 ng/mL
Total imipramine + desimipramine	563–1130 nmol/L	150–300 ng/mL	>1880 nmol/L	>500 ng/mL
Lamotrigine	11.7–54.7 μmol/L	3–14 μg/mL	>58.7 μmol/L	>15 μg/mL
Lidocaine	5.1–21.3 μmol/L	1.2–5.0 μg/mL	>38.4 μmol/L	>9.0 μg/mL
Lithium	0.5–1.3 mmol/L	0.5–1.3 meq/L	>2 mmol/L	>2 meq/L
Methadone	1.0–3.2 μmol/L	0.3–1.0 μg/mL	>6.5 μmol/L	>2 μg/mL
Methamphetamine	0.07–0.34 μmol/L	0.01–0.05 μg/mL	>3.35 μmol/L	>0.5 μg/mL
Methanol			>6 mmol/L	>20 mg/dL
Methotrexate				
Low-dose	0.01–0.1 μmol/L	0.01–0.1 μmol/L	>0.1 mmol/L	>0.1 mmol/L
High-dose (24 h)	<5.0 μmol/L	<5.0 μmol/L	>5.0 μmol/L	>5.0 μmol/L
High-dose (48 h)	<0.50 μmol/L	<0.50 μmol/L	>0.5 μmol/L	>0.5 μmol/L
High-dose (72 h)	<0.10 μmol/L	<0.10 μmol/L	>0.1 μmol/L	>0.1 μmol/L
Morphine	232–286 μmol/L	65–80 ng/mL	>720 μmol/L	>200 ng/mL
Mycophenolic acid	3.1–10.9 μmol/L	1.0–3.5 ng/mL	>37 μmol/L	>12 ng/mL
Nitroprusside (as thiocyanate)	103–499 μmol/L	6–29 μg/mL	860 μmol/L	>50 μg/mL
Nortriptyline	190–569 nmol/L	50–150 ng/mL	>1900 nmol/L	>500 ng/mL
Phenobarbital	65–172 μmol/L	15–40 μg/mL	>258 μmol/L	>60 μg/mL
Phenytoin	40–79 μmol/L	10–20 μg/mL	>158 μmol/L	>40 μg/mL
Phenytoin, free	4.0–7.9 μg/mL	1–2 μg/mL	>13.9 μg/mL	>3.5 μg/mL
% Free	0.08–0.14	8–14%		
Primidone and metabolite				
Primidone	23–55 μmol/L	5–12 μg/mL	>69 μmol/L	>15 μg/mL
Phenobarbital	65–172 μmol/L	15–40 μg/mL	>215 μmol/L	>50 μg/mL
Procainamide				
Procainamide	17–42 μmol/L	4–10 μg/mL	>43 μmol/L	>10 μg/mL
NAPA (*N*-acetylprocainamide)	22–72 μmol/L	6–20μg/mL	>126 μmol/L	>35 μg/mL
Quinidine	6.2–15.4 μmol/L	2.0–5.0 μg/mL	>19 μmol/L	>6 μg/mL
Salicylates	145–2100 μmol/L	2–29 mg/dL	>2900 μmol/L	>40 mg/dL
Sirolimus (trough level)				
Kidney transplant	4.4–15.4 nmol/L	4–14 ng/mL	>16 nmol/L	>15 ng/mL
Tacrolimus (FK506) (trough)				
Kidney and liver				
Initiation	12–19 nmol/L	10–15 ng/mL	>25 nmol/L	>20 ng/mL
Maintenance	6–12 nmol/L	5–10 ng/mL	>25 nmol/L	>20 ng/mL
Heart				
Initiation	19–25 nmol/L	15–20 ng/mL		
Maintenance	6–12 nmol/L	5–10 ng/mL		

(*continued*)

TABLE 3

TOXICOLOGY AND THERAPEUTIC DRUG MONITORING (*CONTINUED*)

	THERAPEUTIC RANGE		TOXIC LEVEL	
DRUG	**SI UNITS**	**CONVENTIONAL UNITS**	**SI UNITS**	**CONVENTIONAL UNITS**
Theophylline	56–111 μg/mL	10–20 μg/mL	>168 μg/mL	>30 μg/mL
Thiocyanate				
After nitroprusside infusion	103–499 μmol/L	6–29 μg/mL	860 μmol/L	>50 μg/mL
Nonsmoker	17–69 μmol/L	1–4 μg/mL		
Smoker	52–206 μmol/L	3–12 μg/mL		
Tobramycin				
Peak	11–22 μg/L	5–10 μg/mL	>26 μg/L	>12 μg/mL
Trough	0–4.3 μg/L	0–2 μg/mL	>4.3 μg/L	>2 μg/mL
Valproic acid	346–693 μmol/L	50–100 μg/mL	>693 μmol/L	>100 μg/mL
Vancomycin				
Peak	14–28 μmol/L	20–40 μg/mL	>55 μmol/L	>80 μg/mL
Trough	3.5–10.4 μmol/L	5–15 μg/mL	>14 μmol/L	>20 μg/mL

TABLE 4

VITAMINS AND SELECTED TRACE MINERALS

		REFERENCE RANGE	
SPECIMEN	**ANALYTE**	**SI UNITS**	**CONVENTIONAL UNITS**
Aluminum	S	<0.2 μmol/L	<5.41 μg/L
Arsenic	WB	0.03–0.31 μmol/L	2–23 μg/L
Cadmium	WB	<44.5 nmol/L	<5.0 μg/L
Coenzyme Q10 (ubiquinone)	P	433–1532 μg/L	433–1532 μg/L
β-Carotene	S	0.07–1.43 μmol/L	4–77 μg/dL
Copper	S	11–22 μmol/L	70–140 μg/dL
Folic acid	RC	340–1020 nmol/L cells	150–450 ng/mL cells
Folic acid	S	12.2–40.8 nmol/L	5.4–18.0 ng/mL
Lead (adult)	S	<0.5 μmol/L	<10 μg/dL
Mercury	WB	3.0–294 nmol/L	0.6–59 μg/L
Selenium	S	0.8–2.0 umol/L	63–160 μg/L
Vitamin A	S	0.7–3.5 μmol/L	20–100 μg/dL
Vitamin B_1 (thiamine)	S	0–75 nmol/L	0–2 μg/dL
Vitamin B_2 (riboflavin)	S	106–638 nmol/L	4–24 μg/dL
Vitamin B_6	P	20–121 nmol/L	5–30 ng/mL
Vitamin B_{12}	S	206–735 pmol/L	279–996 pg/mL
Vitamin C (ascorbic acid)	S	23–57 μmol/L	0.4–1.0 mg/dL
Vitamin D_3,1,25-dihydroxy, total	S, P	36–180 pmol/L	15–75 pg/mL
Vitamin D_3, 25-hydroxy, total	P	75–250 nmol/L	30–100 ng/mL
Vitamin E	S	12–42 μmol/L	5–18 μg/mL
Vitamin K	S	0.29–2.64 nmol/L	0.13–1.19 ng/mL
Zinc	S	11.5–18.4 μmol/L	75–120 μg/dL

Abbreviations: P, plasma; RC, red cells; S, serum; WB, whole blood.

TABLE 5

CLASSIFICATION OF LDL, TOTAL, AND HDL CHOLESTEROL

LDL Cholesterol	
<70 mg/dL	Therapeutic option for very high risk patients
<100 mg/dL	Optimal
100–129 mg/dL	Near optimal/above optimal
130–159 mg/dL	Borderline high
160–189 mg/dL	High
≥190 mg/dL	Very high
Total Cholesterol	
<200 mg/dL	Desirable
200–239 mg/dL	Borderline high
≥240 mg/dL	High
HDL Cholesterol	
<40 mg/dL	Low
≥60 mg/dL	High

Abbreviations: LDL, low-density lipoprotein; HDL, high-density lipoprotein.

Source: Executive summary of the third report of the National Cholesterol Education Program (NCEP) expert panel on detection, evaluation, and treatment of high blood cholesterol in adults (adult treatment panel III). JAMA 2001; 285:2486–97. Implications of Recent Clinical Trials for the National Cholesterol Education Program Adult Treatment Panel III Guidelines. SM Grundy et al for the Coordinating Committee of the National Cholesterol Education Program: Circulation 110:227, 2004.

REFERENCE VALUES FOR SPECIFIC ANALYTES

TABLE 6

CEREBROSPINAL FLUID[a]

	REFERENCE RANGE	
CONSTITUENT	**SI UNITS**	**CONVENTIONAL UNITS**
Osmolarity	292–297 mmol/kg water	292–297 mOsm/L
Electrolytes		
Sodium	137–145 mmol/L	137–145 mEq/L
Potassium	2.7–3.9 mmol/L	2.7–3.9 mEq/L
Calcium	1.0–1.5 mmol/L	2.1–3.0 mEq/L
Magnesium	1.0–1.2 mmol/L	2.0–2.5 mEq/L
Chloride	116–122 mmol/L	116–122 mEq/L
CO_2 content	20–24 mmol/L	20–24 mEq/L
P_{CO_2}	6–7 kPa	45–49 mm Hg
pH	7.31–7.34	
Glucose	2.22–3.89 mmol/L	40–70 mg/dL
Lactate	1–2 mmol/L	10–20 mg/dL
Total protein:		
Lumbar	0.15–0.5 g/L	15–50 mg/dL
Cisternal	0.15–0.25 g/L	15–25 mg/dL
Ventricular	0.06–0.15 g/L	6–15 mg/dL
Albumin	0.066–0.442 g/L	6.6–44.2 mg/dL
IgG	0.009–0.057 g/L	0.9–5.7 mg/dL
IgG index[b]	0.29–0.59	
Oligoclonal bands (OGBs)	<2 bands not present in matched serum sample	
Ammonia	15–47 μmol/L	25–80 μg/dL
Creatinine	44–168 μmol/L	0.5–1.9 mg/dL
Myelin basic protein	<4 μg/L	
CSF pressure		50–180 mm H_2O
CSF volume (adult)	~150 mL	
Red blood cells	0	0
Leukocytes		
Total	0–5 mononuclear cells per μL	
Differential		
Lymphocytes	60–70%	
Monocytes	30–50%	
Neutrophils	None	

[a]Since cerebrospinal fluid (CSF) concentrations are equilibrium values, measurements of the same parameters in blood plasma obtained at the same time are recommended. However, there is a time lag in attainment of equilibrium, and CSF levels of plasma constituents that can fluctuate rapidly (such as plasma glucose) may not achieve stable values until after a significant lag phase.

[b]IgG index = CSF IgG (mg/dL) × serum albumin (g/dL)/serum IgG (g/dL) × CSF albumin (mg/dL).

TABLE 7A

DIFFERENTIAL NUCLEATED CELL COUNTS OF BONE MARROW ASPIRATES[a] 2 AND 6

	OBSERVED RANGE (%)	95% RANGE (%)	MEAN (%)
Blast cells	0–3.2	0–3.0	1.4
Promyelocytes	3.6–13.2	3.2–12.4	7.8
Neutrophil myelocytes	4–21.4	3.7–10.0	7.6
Eosinophil myelocytes	0–5.0	0–2.8	1.3
Metamyelocytes	1–7.0	2.3–5.9	4.1
Neutrophils			
Males	21.0–45.6	21.9–42.3	32.1
Females	29.6–46.6	28.8–45.9	37.4
Eosinophils	0.4–4.2	0.3–4.2	2.2
Eosinophils plus eosinophil myelocytes	0.9–7.4	0.7–6.3	3.5
Basophils	0–0.8	0–0.4	0.1
Erythroblasts			
Male	18.0–39.4	16.2–40.1	28.1
Females	14.0–31.8	13.0–32.0	22.5
Lymphocytes	4.6–22.6	6.0–20.0	13.1
Plasma cells	0–1.4	0–1.2	0.6
Monocytes	0–3.2	0–2.6	1.3
Macrophages	0–1.8	0–1.3	0.4
M:E ratio			
Males	1.1–4.0	1.1–4.1	2.1
Females	1.6–5.4	1.6–5.2	2.8

[a]Based on bone marrow aspirate from 50 healthy volunteers (30 men, 20 women).

Abbreviation: M:E, myeloid to erythroid ratio.

Source: BJ Bain: Br J Haematol 94:206, 1996.

TABLE 7B

BONE MARROW CELLULARITY

AGE	OBSERVED RANGE	95% RANGE	MEAN
Under 10 years	59.0–95.1%	72.9–84.7%	78.8%
10–19 years	41.5–86.6%	59.2–69.4%	64.3%
20–29 years	32.0–83.7%	54.1–61.9%	58.0%
30–39 years	30.3–81.3%	41.1–54.1%	47.6%
40–49 years	16.3–75.1%	43.5–52.9%	48.2%
50–59 years	19.7–73.6%	41.2–51.4%	46.3%
60–69 years	16.3–65.7%	40.8–50.6%	45.7%
70–79 years	11.3–47.1%	22.6–35.2%	28.9%

Source: From RJ Hartsock et al: Am J Clin Pathol 1965; 43:326, 1965.

TABLE 8

STOOL ANALYSIS

	REFERENCE RANGE	
	SI UNITS	CONVENTIONAL UNITS
Alpha-1-antitrypsin	≤540 mg/L	≤54 mg/dL
Amount	0.1–0.2 kg/d	100–200 g/24 h
Coproporphyrin	611–1832 nmol/d	400–1200 μg/24 h
Fat		
Adult		<7 g/d
Adult on fat-free diet		<4 g/d
Fatty acids	0–21 mmol/d	0–6 g/24 h
Leukocytes	None	None
Nitrogen	<178 mmol/d	<2.5 g/24 h
pH	7.0–7.5	
Potassium	14–102 mmol/L	14–102 mmol/L
Occult blood	Negative	Negative
Osmolality	280–325 mosmol/kg	280–325 mosmol/kg
Sodium	7–72 mmol/L	7–72 mmol/L
Trypsin		20–95 U/g
Urobilinogen	85–510 μmol/d	50–300 mg/24 h
Uroporphyrins	12–48 nmol/d	10–40 μg/24 h
Water	<0.75	<75%

Source: Modified from: FT Fishbach, MB Dunning III: *A Manual of Laboratory and Diagnostic Tests*, 7th ed. Philadelphia, Lippincott Williams & Wilkins, 2004.

TABLE 9

URINE ANALYSIS AND RENAL FUNCTION TESTS

	REFERENCE RANGE	
	SI UNITS	**CONVENTIONAL UNITS**
Acidity, titratable	20–40 mmol/d	20–40 meq/d
Aldosterone	Normal diet: 6–25 μg/d Low-salt diet: 17–44 μg/d High-salt diet: 0–6 μg/d	Normal diet: 6–25 μg/d Low-salt diet: 17–44 μg/d High-salt diet: 0–6 μg/d
Aluminum	0.19–1.11 μmol/L	5–30 μg/L
Ammonia	30–50 mmol/d	30–50 meq/d
Amylase		4–400 U/L
Amylase/creatinine clearance ratio ($[Cl_{am}/Cl_{cr}] \times 100$)	1–5	1–5
Arsenic	0.07–0.67 μmol/d	5–50 μg/d
Bence Jones protein, urine, qualitative	Not applicable	None detected
Bence Jones protein, urine, quantitative		
Free Kappa	1.4–24.2 mg/L	0.14–2.42 mg/dL
Free Lambda	0.2–6.7 mg/L	0.02–0.67 mg/dL
K/L ratio	2.04–10.37	2.04–10.37
Calcium (10 mEq/d or 200 mg/d dietary calcium)	<7.5 mmol/d	<300 mg/d
Chloride	140–250 mmol/d	140–250 mmol/d
Citrate	320–1240 mg/d	320–1240 mg/d
Copper	<0.95 μmol/d	<60 μg/d
Coproporphyrins (types I and III)	0–20 μmol/mol creatinine	0–20 μmol/mol creatinine
Cortisol, free	55–193 nmol/d	20–70 μg/d
Creatine, as creatinine		
Female	<760 μmol/d	<100 mg/d
Male	<380 μmol/d	<50 mg/d
Creatinine	8.8–14 mmol/d	1.0–1.6 g/d
Dopamine	392–2876 nmol/d	60–440 μg/d
Eosinophils	<100 eosinophils/mL	<100 eosinophils/mL
Epinephrine	0–109 nmol/d	0–20 μg/d
Glomerular filtration rate	>60 mL/min/1.73 m^2 For African Americans, multiply the result by 1.21	>60 mL/min/1.73 m^2 For African Americans, multiply the result by 1.21
Glucose (glucose oxidase method)	0.3–1.7 mmol/d	50–300 mg/d
5-Hydroindoleacetic acid (5-HIAA)	0–78.8 μmol/d	0–15 mg/d
Hydroxyproline	53–328 μmol/d	53–328 μmol/d
Iodine, spot urine		
WHO classification of iodine deficiency:		
Not iodine deficient	>100 μg/L	>100 μg/L
Mild iodine deficiency	50–100 μg/L	50–100 μg/L
Moderate iodine deficiency	20–49 μg/L	20–49 μg/L
Severe iodine deficiency	<20 μg/L	<20 μg/L
Ketone (acetone)	Negative	Negative
17 Ketosteroids	3–12 mg/d	3–12 mg/d
Metanephrines		
Metanephrine	30–350 μg/d	30–350 μg/d
Normetanephrine	50–650 μg/d	50–650 μg/d

(continued)

TABLE 9

URINE ANALYSIS AND RENAL FUNCTION TESTS (*CONTINUED*)

	REFERENCE RANGE	
	SI UNITS	**CONVENTIONAL UNITS**
Microalbumin		
Normal	0.0–0.03 g/d	0–30 mg/d
Microalbuminuria	0.03–0.30 g/d	30–300 mg/d
Clinical albuminuria	>0.3 g/d	>300 mg/d
Microalbumin/creatinine ratio		
Normal	0–3.4 g/mol creatinine	0–30 μg/mg creatinine
Microalbuminuria	3.4–34 g/mol creatinine	30–300 μg/mg creatinine
Clinical albuminuria	>34 g/mol creatinine	>300 μg/mg creatinine
β_2-Microglobulin	0–160 μg/L	0–160 μg/L
Norepinephrine	89–473 nmol/d	15–80 μg/d
N-telopeptide (cross-linked), NTx		
Female, premenopausal	17–94 nmol BCE/mmol creatinine	17–94 nmol BCE/mmol creatinine
Female, postmenopausal	26–124 nmol BCE/mmol creatinine	26–124 nmol BCE/mmol creatinine
Male	21–83 nmol BCE/mmol creatinine	21–83 nmol BCE/mmol creatinine
Osmolality	100–800 mosm/kg	100–800 mosm/kg
Oxalate		
Male	80–500 μmol/d	7–44 mg/d
Female	45–350 μmol/d	4–31 mg/d
pH	5.0–9.0	5.0–9.0
Phosphate (phosphorus) (varies with intake)	12.9–42.0 mmol/d	400–1300 mg/d
Porphobilinogen	None	None
Potassium (varies with intake)	25–100 mmol/d	25–100 meq/d
Protein	<0.15 g/d	<150 mg/d
Protein/creatinine ratio	Male: 15–68 mg/g Female: 10–107 mg/g	Male: 15–68 mg/g Female: 10–107 mg/g
Sediment		
Red blood cells	0–2/high-power field	
White blood cells	0–2/high-power field	
Bacteria	None	
Crystals	None	
Bladder cells	None	
Squamous cells	None	
Tubular cells	None	
Broad casts	None	
Epithelial cell casts	None	
Granular casts	None	
Hyaline casts	0–5/low-power field	
Red blood cell casts	None	
Waxy casts	None	
White cell casts	None	
Sodium (varies with intake)	100–260 mmol/d	100–260 meq/d
Specific gravity:		
After 12-h fluid restriction	>1.025	>1.025
After 12-h deliberate water intake	≤1.003	≤1.003
Tubular reabsorption, phosphorus	0.79–0.94 of filtered load	79–94% of filtered load
Urea nitrogen	214–607 mmol/d	6–17 g/d
Uric acid (normal diet)	1.49–4.76 mmol/d	250–800 mg/d
Vanillylmandelic acid (VMA)	<30 μmol/d	<6 mg/d

Abbreviations: BCE, bone collagen equivalent; WHO, World Health Organization.

TABLE 10

NORMAL PRESSURES IN HEART AND GREAT VESSELS

PRESSURE (mm Hg)	AVERAGE	RANGE
Right Atrium		
Mean	2.8	1–5
a Wave	5.6	2.5–7
c Wave	3.8	1.5–6
x Wave	1.7	0–5
v Wave	4.6	2–7.5
y Wave	2.4	0–6
Right Ventricle		
Peak systolic	25	17–32
End-diastolic	4	1–7
Pulmonary Artery		
Mean	15	9–19
Peak systolic	25	17–32
End-diastolic	9	4–13
Pulmonary Artery Wedge		
Mean	9	4.5–13
Left Atrium		
Mean	7.9	2–12
a Wave	10.4	4–16
v Wave	12.8	6–21
Left Ventricle		
Peak systolic	130	90–140
End-diastolic	8.7	5–12
Brachial Artery		
Mean	85	70–105
Peak systolic	130	90–140
End-diastolic	70	60–90

Source: Reproduced from: MJ Kern *The Cardiac Catheterization Handbook*, 4th ed. Philadelphia, Mosby, 2003.

TABLE 11

CIRCULATORY FUNCTION TESTS

	RESULTS: REFERENCE RANGE	
TEST	**SI UNITS (RANGE)**	**CONVENTIONAL UNITS (RANGE)**
Arteriovenous oxygen difference	30–50 mL/L	30–50 mL/L
Cardiac output (Fick)	2.5–3.6 L/m^2 of body surface area per min	2.5–3.6 L/m^2 of body surface area per min
Contractility indexes		
Max. left ventricular *dp/dt* (*dp/dt*)	220 kPa/s (176–250 kPa/s)	1650 mmHg/s (1320–1880 mmHg/s)
DP when DP = 5.3 kPa	(37.6 ± 12.2)/s	(37.6 ± 12.2)/s
(40 mm Hg)	3.32 ± 0.84 end-diastolic volumes per second	3.32 ± 0.84 end-diastolic volumes per second
Mean normalized systolic ejection rate (angiography)	1.83 ± 0.56 circumferences per second	1.83 ± 0.56 circumferences per second
Mean velocity of circumferential fiber shortening (angiography)		
Ejection fraction: stroke volume/end-diastolic volume (SV/EDV)	0.67 ± 0.08 (0.55–0.78)	0.67 ± 0.08 (0.55–0.78)
End-diastolic volume	70 ± 20.0 mL/m^2 (60–88 mL/m^2)	70 ± 20.0 mL/m^2 (60–88 mL/m^2)
End-systolic volume	25 ± 5.0 mL/m^2 (20–33 mL/m^2)	25 ± 5.0 mL/m^2 (20–33 mL/m^2)
Left ventricular work		
Stroke work index	50 ± 20.0 (g·m)/m^2 (30–110)	50 ± 20.0 (g·m)/m^2 (30–110)
Left ventricular minute work index	1.8–6.6 [(kg·m)/m^2]/min	1.8–6.6 [(kg·m)/m^2]/min
Oxygen consumption index	110–150 mL	110–150 mL
Maximum oxygen uptake	35 mL/min (20–60 mL/min)	35 mL/min (20–60 mL/min)
Pulmonary vascular resistance	2–12 (kPa·s)/L	20–130 (dyn·s)/cm^5
Systemic vascular resistance	77–150 (kPa·s)/L	770–1600 (dyn·s)/cm^5

Abbreviations: DP, developed left ventricular pressure.
Source: E Braunwald et al: *Heart Disease*, 6th ed. Philadelphia, W.B. Saunders Co., 2001.

TABLE 12

NORMAL ECHOCARDIOGRAPHIC REFERENCE LIMITS AND PARTITION VALUES IN ADULTS

	WOMEN REFERENCE RANGE	MILDLY ABNORMAL	MODERATELY ABNORMAL	SEVERELY ABNORMAL	MEN REFERENCE RANGE	MILDLY ABNORMAL	MODERATELY ABNORMAL	SEVERELY ABNORMAL
Left ventricular dimensions								
Septal thickness, cm	0.6–0.9	1.0–1.2	1.3–1.5	≥1.6	0.6–1.0	1.1–1.3	1.4–1.6	≥1.7
Posterior wall thickness, cm	0.6–0.9	1.0–1.2	1.3–1.5	≥1.6	0.6–1.0	1.1–1.3	1.4–1.6	≥1.7
Diastolic diameter, cm	3.9–5.3	5.4–5.7	5.8–6.1	≥6.2	4.2–5.9	6.0–6.3	6.4–6.8	≥6.9
Diastolic diameter/BSA, cm/m^2	2.4–3.2	3.3–3.4	3.5–3.7	≥3.8	2.2–3.1	3.2–3.4	3.5–3.6	≥3.7
Diastolic diameter/height, cm/m	2.5–3.2	3.3–3.4	3.5–3.6	≥3.7	2.4–3.3	3.4–3.5	3.6–3.7	≥3.8
Left ventricular volumes								
Diastolic, mL	56–104	105–117	118–130	≥131	67–155	156–178	179–201	≥202
Diastolic/BSA, mL/m^2	35–75	76–86	87–96	≥97	35–75	76–86	87–96	≥97
Systolic, mL	19–49	50–59	60–69	≥70	22–58	59–70	71–82	≥83
Systolic/BSA, mL/m^2	12–30	31–36	37–42	≥43	12–30	31–36	37–42	≥43
Left ventricular mass, 2D method								
Mass, g	66–150	151–171	172–182	≥183	96–200	201–227	228–254	≥255
Mass/BSA, g/m^2	44–88	89–100	101–112	≥113	50–102	103–116	117–130	≥131
Left ventricular function								
Endocardial fractional shortening (%)	27–45	22–26	17–21	≤16	25–43	20–24	15–19	≤14
Midwall fractional shortening (%)	15–23	13–14	11–12	≤10	14–22	12–13	10–11	≤9
Ejection fraction, 2D method (%)	≥55	45–54	30–44	≤29	≥55	45–54	30–44	≤29
Right heart dimensions (cm)								
Basal RV diameter	2.0–2.8	2.9–3.3	3.4–3.8	≥3.9	2.0–2.8	2.9–3.3	3.4–3.8	≥3.9
Mid-RV diameter	2.7–3.3	3.4–3.7	3.8–4.1	≥4.2	2.7–3.3	3.4–3.7	3.8–4.1	≥4.2
Base-to-apex length	7.1–7.9	8.0–8.5	8.6–9.1	≥9.2	7.1–7.9	8.0–8.5	8.6–9.1	≥9.2
RVOT diameter above aortic valve	2.5–2.9	3.0–3.2	3.3–3.5	≥3.6	2.5–2.9	3.0–3.2	3.3–3.5	≥3.6
RVOT diameter above pulmonic valve	1.7–2.3	2.4–2.7	2.8–3.1	≥3.2	1.7–2.3	2.4–2.7	2.8–3.1	≥3.2
Pulmonary artery diameter below pulmonic valve	1.5–2.1	2.2–2.5	2.6–2.9	≥3.0	1.5–2.1	2.2–2.5	2.6–2.9	≥3.0
Right ventricular size and function in 4-chamber view								
Diastolic area, cm^2	11–28	29–32	33–37	≥38	11–28	29–32	33–37	≥38
Systolic area, cm^2	7.5–16	17–19	20–22	≥23	7.5–16	17–19	20–22	≥23
Fractional area change, %	32–60	25–31	18–24	≤17	32–60	25–31	18–24	≤17
Atrial sizes								
LA diameter, cm	2.7–3.8	3.9–4.2	4.3–4.6	≥4.7	3.0–4.0	4.1–4.6	4.7–5.2	≥5.3
LA diameter/BSA, cm/m^2	1.5–2.3	2.4–2.6	2.7–2.9	≥3.0	1.5–2.3	2.4–2.6	2.7–2.9	≥3.0
RA minor axis, cm	2.9–4.5	4.6–4.9	5.0–5.4	≥5.5	2.9–4.5	4.6–4.9	5.0–5.4	≥5.5
RA minor axis/BSA, cm/m^2	1.7–2.5	2.6–2.8	2.9–3.1	≥3.2	1.7–2.5	2.6–2.8	2.9–3.1	≥3.2

(*continued*)

TABLE 12

NORMAL ECHOCARDIOGRAPHIC REFERENCE LIMITS AND PARTITION VALUES IN ADULTS (*CONTINUED*)

	WOMEN REFERENCE RANGE	MILDLY ABNORMAL	MODERATELY ABNORMAL	SEVERELY ABNORMAL	MEN REFERENCE RANGE	MILDLY ABNORMAL	MODERATELY ABNORMAL	SEVERELY ABNORMAL
LA area, cm^2	<20	20–30	30–40	≥41	<20	20–30	30–40	≥41
LA volume, mL	22–52	53–62	63–72	≥73	18–58	59–68	69–78	≥79
LA volume/BSA, mL/m^2	16–28	29–33	34–39	≥40	16–28	29–33	34–39	≥40
Aortic stenosis, classification of severity								
Aortic jet velocity, m/s		2.6–2.9	3.0–4.0	>4.0		2.6–2.9	3.0–4.0	>4.0
Mean gradient, mm Hg		<20	20–40	>40		<20	20–40	>40
Valve area, cm^2		>1.5	1.0–1.5	<1.0		>1.5	1.0–1.5	<1.0
Indexed valve area, cm^2/m^2		>0.85	0.60–0.85	<0.6		>0.85	0.60–0.85	<0.6
Velocity ratio		>0.50	0.25–0.50	<0.25		>0.50	0.25–0.50	<0.25
Mitral stenosis, classification of severity								
Valve area, cm^2		>1.5	1.0–1.5	<1.0		>1.5	1.0–1.5	<1.0
Mean gradient, mm Hg		<5	5–10	>10		<5	5–10	>10
Pulmonary artery pressure, mm Hg		<30	30–50	>50		<30	30–50	>50
Aortic regurgitation, indices of severity								
Vena contracta width, cm		<0.30	0.30–0.60	≥0.60		<0.30	0.30–0.60	≥0.60
Jet width/LVOT width, %		<25	25–64	≥65		<25	25–64	≥65
Jet CSA/LVOT CSA, %		<5	5–59	≥60		<5	5–59	≥60
Regurgitant volume, mL/beat		<30	30–59	≥60		<30	30–59	≥60
Regurgitant fraction, %		<30	30–49	≥50		<30	30–49	≥50
Effective regurgitant orifice area, cm^2		<0.10	0.10–0.29	≥0.30		<0.10	0.10–0.29	≥0.30
Mitral regurgitation, indices of severity								
Vena contracta width, cm		<0.30	0.30–0.69	≥0.70		<0.30	0.30–0.69	≥0.70
Regurgitant volume, mL/beat		<30	30–59	≥60		<30	30–59	≥60
Regurgitant fraction, %		<30	30–49	≥50		<30	30–49	≥50
Effective regurgitant orifice area, cm^2		<0.20	0.20–0.39	≥0.40		<0.20	0.20–0.39	≥0.40

Abbreviations: BSA, body surface area; CSA, cross-sectional area; LA, left atrium; LVOT, left ventricular outflow tract; RA, right atrium; RV, right ventricle; RVOT, right ventricular outflow tract; 2D, 2-dimensional.

Source: Values adapted from: American Society of Echocardiography, Guidelines and Standards. *http://www.asecho.org/i4a/pages/index.cfm?pageid=3317*. Accessed February 23, 2010.

TABLE 13

SUMMARY OF VALUES USEFUL IN PULMONARY PHYSIOLOGY

	SYMBOL	TYPICAL VALUES: MAN AGED 40, 75 kg, 175 cm TALL	TYPICAL VALUES: WOMAN AGED 40, 60 kg, 160 cm TALL
Pulmonary Mechanics			
Spirometry—volume-time curves			
Forced vital capacity (FVC)	FVC	5.0 L	3.4 L
Forced expiratory volume in 1 s (FEV_1)	FEV_1	4.0 L	2.8 L
FEV_1/FVC	FEV_1%	80%	78%
Maximal midexpiratory flow rate	MMEF (FEF 25–75)	4.1 L/s	3.2 L/s
Maximal expiratory flow rate	MEFR (FEF 200–1200)	9.0 L/s	6.1 L/s
Spirometry—flow-volume curves			
Maximal expiratory flow at 50% of expired vital capacity	V_{max} 50 (FEF 50%)	5.0 L/s	4.0 L/s
Maximal expiratory flow at 75% of expired vital capacity	V_{max} 75 (FEF 75%)	2.1 L/s	2.0 L/s
Resistance to airflow:			
Pulmonary resistance	RL (R_L)	<3.0 (cm H_2O/s)/L	
Airway resistance	Raw	<2.5 (cm H_2O/s)/L	
Specific conductance	SGaw	>0.13 cm H_2O/s	
Pulmonary compliance			
Static recoil pressure at total lung capacity	Pst TLC	25 ± 5 cm H_2O	
Compliance of lungs (static)	CL	0.2 L cm H_2O	
Compliance of lungs and thorax	C(L + T)	0.1 L cm H_2O	
Dynamic compliance of 20 breaths per minute	C dyn 20	0.25 ± 0.05 L/cm H_2O	
Maximal static respiratory pressures:			
Maximal inspiratory pressure	MIP	>110 cm H_2O	>70 cm H_2O
Maximal expiratory pressure	MEP	>200 cm H_2O	>140 cm H_2O
Lung Volumes			
Total lung capacity	TLC	6.9 L	4.9 L
Functional residual capacity	FRC	3.3 L	2.6 L
Residual volume	RV	1.9 L	1.5 L
Inspiratory capacity	IC	3.7 L	2.3 L
Expiratory reserve volume	ERV	1.4 L	1.1 L
Vital capacity	VC	5.0 L	3.4 L
Gas Exchange (Sea Level)			
Arterial O_2 tension	Pa_{O_2}	12.7 ± 0.7 kPa (95 ± 5 mm Hg)	
Arterial CO_2 tension	Pa_{CO_2}	5.3 ± 0.3 kPa (40 ± 2 mm Hg)	
Arterial O_2 saturation	Sa_{O_2}	0.97 ± 0.02 (97 ± 2%)	
Arterial blood pH	pH	7.40 ± 0.02	
Arterial bicarbonate	HCO_3^-	24 + 2 mEq/L	
Base excess	BE	0 ± 2 mEq/L	
Diffusing capacity for carbon monoxide (single breath)	DL_{CO}	37 mL CO/min/mmHg	27 mL CO/min/mmHg
Dead space volume	V_D	2 mL/kg body wt	
Physiologic dead space; dead space-tidal volume ratio	V_D/V_T		
Rest		≤35% V_T	
Exercise		≤20% V_T	
Alveolar–arterial difference for O_2	$P(A-a)_{O_2}$	≤2.7 kPa ≤20 kPa (≤24 mm Hg)	

Source: Based on: AH Morris et al: *Clinical Pulmonary Function Testing. A Manual of Uniform Laboratory Procedures*, 2nd ed. Salt Lake City, Utah, Intermountain Thoracic Society, 1984.

TABLE 14

GASTROINTESTINAL TESTS

TEST	RESULTS	
	SI UNITS	**CONVENTIONAL UNITS**
Absorption tests		
D-Xylose: after overnight fast, 25 g xylose given in oral aqueous solution		
Urine, collected for following 5 h	25% of ingested dose	25% of ingested dose
Serum, 2 h after dose	2.0–3.5 mmol/L	30–52 mg/dL
Vitamin A: a fasting blood specimen is obtained and 200,000 units of vitamin A in oil is given orally	Serum level should rise to twice fasting level in 3–5 h	Serum level should rise to twice fasting level in 3–5 h
Bentiromide test (pancreatic function): 500 mg bentiromide (chymex) orally; *p*-aminobenzoic acid (PABA) measured		
Plasma		>3.6 (±1.1) μg/mL at 90 min
Urine	>50% recovered in 6 h	>50% recovered in 6 h
Gastric juice		
Volume		
24 h	2–3 L	2–3 L
Nocturnal	600–700 mL	600–700 mL
Basal, fasting	30–70 mL/h	30–70 mL/h
Reaction		
pH	1.6–1.8	1.6–1.8
Titratable acidity of fasting juice	4–9 μmol/s	15–35 mEq/h
Acid output		
Basal		
Females (mean ± 1 SD)	0.6 ± 0.5 μmol/s	2.0 ± 1.8 mEq/h
Males (mean ± 1 SD)	0.8 ± 0.6 μmol/s	3.0 ± 2.0 mEq/h
Maximal (after SC histamine acid phosphate, 0.004 mg/kg body weight, and preceded by 50 mg promethazine, or after betazole, 1.7 mg/kg body weight, or pentagastrin, 6 μg/kg body weight)		
Females (mean ± 1 SD)	4.4 ± 1.4 μmol/s	16 ± 5 mEq/h
Males (mean ± 1 SD)	6.4 ± 1.4 μmol/s	23 ± 5 mEq/h
Basal acid output/maximal acid output ratio	≤0.6	≤0.6
Gastrin, serum	0–200 μg/L	0–200 pg/mL
Secretin test (pancreatic exocrine function): 1 unit/kg body weight, IV		
Volume (pancreatic juice) in 80 min	>2.0 mL/kg	>2.0 mL/kg
Bicarbonate concentration	>80 mmol/L	>80 mEq/L
Bicarbonate output in 30 min	>10 mmol	>10 mEq

MISCELLANEOUS

TABLE 15

BODY FLUIDS AND OTHER MASS DATA

	REFERENCE RANGE	
	SI UNITS	CONVENTIONAL UNITS
Ascitic fluid		
Body fluid		
Total volume (lean) of body weight	50% (in obese) to 70%	
Intracellular	30-40% of body weight	
Extracellular	20-30% of body weight	
Blood		
Total volume		
Males	69 mL/kg body weight	
Females	65 mL/kg body weight	
Plasma volume		
Males	39 mL/kg body weight	
Females	40 mL/kg body weight	
Red blood cell volume		
Males	30 mL/kg body weight	1.15–1.21 L/m^2 of body surface area
Females	25 mL/kg body weight	0.95–1.00 L/m^2 of body surface area
Body mass index	18.5–24.9 kg/m^2	18.5–24.9 kg/m^2

TABLE 16

RADIATION-DERIVED UNITS

QUANTITY	MEASURES	OLD UNIT	SI UNIT	SPECIAL NAME FOR SI UNIT (ABBREVIATION)	CONVERSION
Activity	Rate of radioactive decay	curie (Ci)	Disintegrations per second (dps)	becquerel (Bq)	1 Ci = 3.7×10^{10} Bq 1 mCi = 37 MBq 1 Bq = 2.703×10^{-11} Ci
Exposure	Amount of ionizations produced in dry air by x-rays or gamma rays, per unit of mass	roentgen (R)	Coulomb per kilogram (C/kg)	none	1 C/kg = 3876 R 1 R = 2.58×10^{-4} C/kg 1 mR = 258 pC/kg
Air kerma	Sum of initial energies of charged particles liberated by ionizing radiation in air, per unit of mass	rad	Joule per kilogram (J/kg)	gray (Gy)	1 Gy = 100 rad 1 rad = 0.01 Gy 1 mrad = 10 μGy
Absorbed dose	Energy deposited per unit of mass in a medium, e.g., an organ/tissue	rad	Joule per kilogram (J/kg)	gray (Gy)	1 Gy = 100 rad 1 rad = 0.01 Gy 1 mrad = 10 μGy
Equivalent dose	Energy deposited per unit of mass in a medium, e.g., an organ/tissue, weighted to reflect type(s) of radiation	rem	Joule per kilogram (J/kg)	sievert (Sv)	1 Sv = 100 rem 1 rem = 0.01 Sv 1 mrem = 10 μSv
Effective dose	Energy deposited per unit of mass in a reference individual, doubly weighted to reflect type(s) of radiation and organ(s) irradiated	rem	Joule per kilogram (J/kg)	sievert (Sv)	1 Sv = 100 rem 1 rem = 0.01 Sv 1 mrem = 10 μSv

Acknowledgments

The contributions of Drs. Daniel J. Fink, Patrick M. Sluss, James L. Januzzi, and Kent B. Lewandrowski to this chapter in previous editions of Harrison's Principles of Internal Medicine are gratefully acknowledged. We also express our gratitude to Drs. Amudha Palanisamy and Scott Fink for careful review of tables and helpful suggestions.

REVIEW AND SELF-ASSESSMENT[a]

Charles Wiener ■ Cynthia D. Brown ■ Anna R. Hemnes

QUESTIONS

DIRECTIONS: Choose the **one best** response to each question.

1. For each patient, choose the most likely peripheral blood smear:

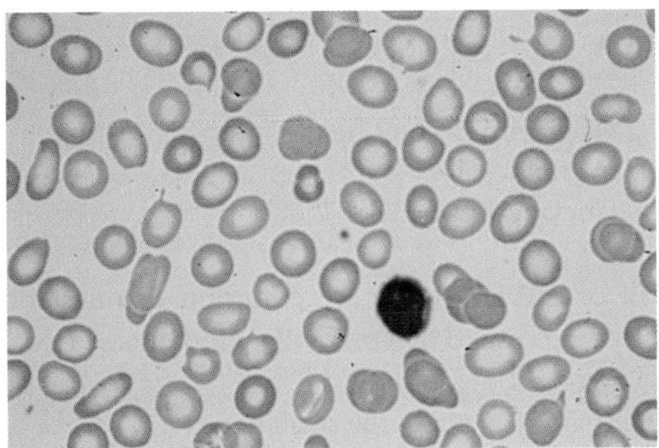

A

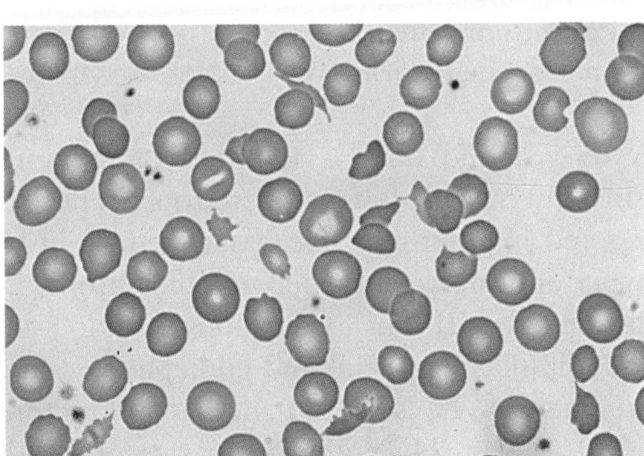

B

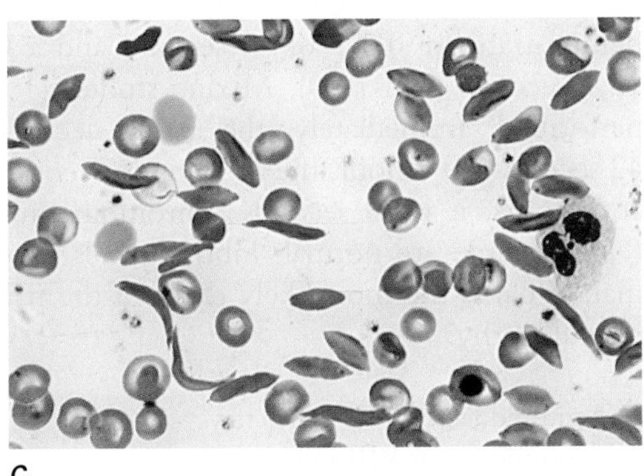

C

1. (*Continued*)

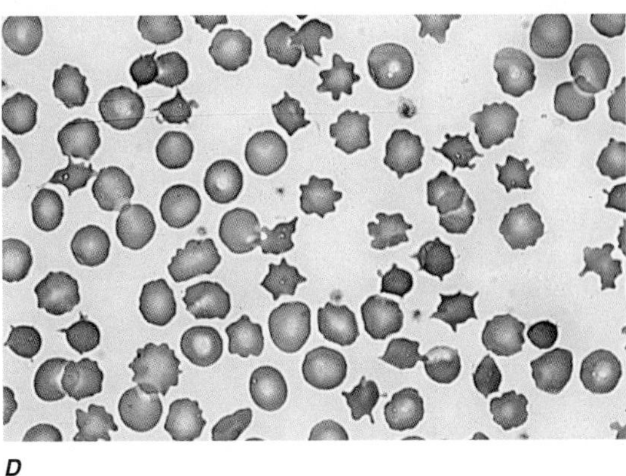

D

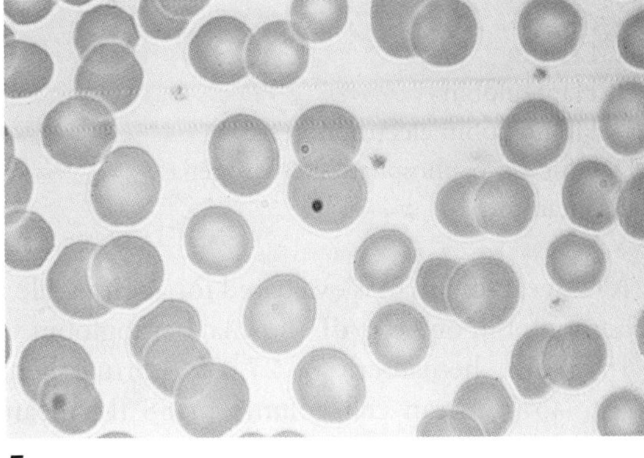

E

1. A 22-year-old man with a hematocrit of 17%. He has sickle cell disease and is admitted with a vaso-occlusive crisis after an upper respiratory illness.
2. A 36-year-old woman with a hematocrit of 32%. She had a splenectomy 5 years ago after a motor vehicle crash.
3. A 55-year-old man with a hematocrit of 28%. He has advanced alcoholic liver disease with cirrhosis and is awaiting liver transplantation.
4. A 64-year-old woman with a hematocrit of 28%. She has heme-positive stool and a 2-cm adenomatous colonic polyp at colonoscopy.
5. A 72-year-old man a hematocrit of 33%. Four years ago, he received a mechanical prosthetic aortic valve because of aortic stenosis caused by a congenital bicuspid valve.

[a]Questions and answers were taken from Wiener C et al (eds): *Harrison's Principles of Internal Medicine Self-Assessment and Board Review*, 18th ed. New York: McGraw-Hill, 2012.

2. A 39-year-old woman is evaluated for anemia. Her laboratory studies reveal a hemoglobin of 7.4 g/dL, hematocrit of 23.9%, mean corpuscular volume of 72 fL, mean cell hemoglobin of 25 pg, and mean cell hemoglobin concentration of 28%. The peripheral smear is shown in Figure 2. Which of the following tests is most likely to be abnormal in this patient?

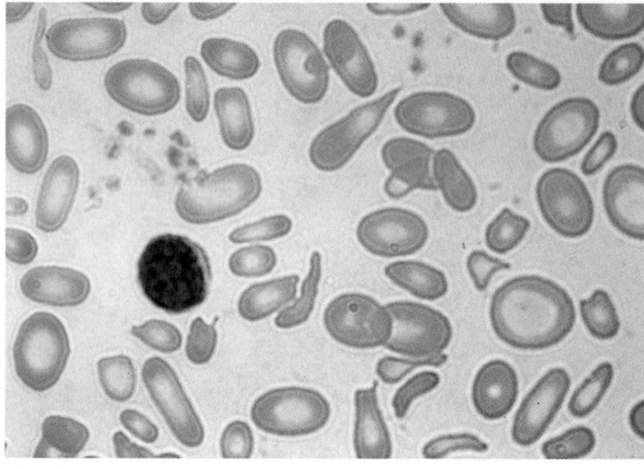

FIGURE 2

A. Ferritin
B. Haptoglobin
C. Hemoglobin electrophoresis
D. Glucose-6-phosphate dehydrogenase
E. Vitamin B_{12}

3. A 62-year-old man is evaluated for anemia. He has a hemoglobin of 9.0 g/dL (normal hemoglobin value, 15 g/dL), hematocrit of 27.0% (normal hematocrit, 45%), mean cell volume of 88 fL, mean cell hemoglobin of 28 pg, and mean cell hemoglobin concentration of 30%. On peripheral blood smear, polychromatophilic macrocytes are seen. The reticulocyte count is 9%. What is the reticulocyte production index?

A. 0.54
B. 1.67
C. 2.7
D. 4.5
E. 5.4

4. You are asked to review the peripheral blood smear from a patient with anemia (Figure 4). Serum lactate dehydrogenase is elevated, and there is hemoglobinuria. This patient is likely to have which physical examination finding?

A. Goiter
B. Heme-positive stools

4. *(Continued)*

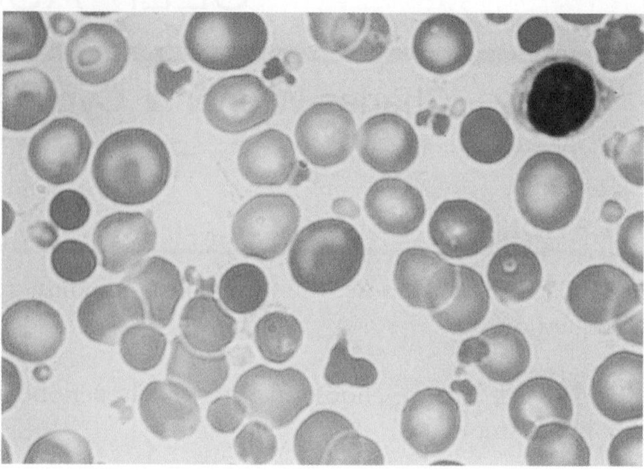

FIGURE 4

C. Mechanical second heart sound
D. Splenomegaly
E. Thickened calvarium

5. All of the following are common manifestations of bleeding caused by von Willebrand disease EXCEPT:

A. Angiodysplasia of the small bowel
B. Epistaxis
C. Menorrhagia
D. Postpartum hemorrhage
E. Spontaneous hemarthrosis

6. A 68-year-old man is admitted to the intensive care unit with spontaneous retroperitoneal bleeding and hypotension. He has a medical history of hypertension, diabetes mellitus, and chronic kidney disease stage III. His medications include lisinopril, amlodipine, sitagliptin, and glimepiride. On initial presentation, he is in pain and has a blood pressure of 70/40 mm Hg with a heart rate of 132 beats/min. His hemoglobin on admission is 5.3 g/dL and hematocrit is 16.0%. His coagulation studies demonstrate an aPTT of 64 seconds and a PT of 12.1 seconds (INR 1.0). Mixing studies (1:1) are performed. Immediately, the aPTT decreases to 42 seconds. At 1 hour, the aPTT is 56 seconds, and at 2 hours, it is 68 seconds. Thrombin time and reptilase time are normal. Fibrinogen is also normal. What is the most likely cause of the patient's coagulopathy?

A. Acquired factor VIII deficiency
B. Acquired factor VIII inhibitor
C. Heparin
D. Lupus anticoagulant
E. Vitamin K deficiency

7. A 54-year-old man is seen in the clinic complaining of painless enlargement of lymph nodes in his neck. He has not otherwise been ill and denies fevers, chills, weight loss, and fatigue. His past medical history is remarkable for pulmonary tuberculosis that was treated 10 years previously under directly observed therapy. He currently takes no medications. He is a heterosexual man in a monogamous relationship for 25 years. He denies illicit drug use. He has smoked 1½ packs of cigarettes daily since 16 years of age. He works as a logger. On physical examination, the patient is thin but not ill-appearing. He is not febrile and has normal vital signs. He has dental caries noted with gingivitis. In the right supraclavicular area, there is a hard and fixed lymph node measuring 2.5 × 2.0 cm in size. Lymph nodes <1 cm in size are noted in the anterior cervical chain. There is no axillary or inguinal lymphadenopathy. His liver and spleen are not enlarged. Which of the following factors in history or physical examination increases the likelihood that the lymph node enlargement is caused by malignancy?

A. Age older than 50 years
B. Location in the supraclavicular area
C. Presence of a lymph node that is hard and fixed
D. Size >2.25 cm^2 (1.5 × 1.5 cm)
E. All of the above

8. A 24-year-old woman presents for a routine checkup and complains only of small masses in her groin. She states that they have been present for at least 3 years. She denies fever, malaise, weight loss, and anorexia. She works as a sailing instructor and competes in triathlons. On physical examination, she is noted to have several palpable 1-cm inguinal lymph nodes that are mobile, nontender, and discrete. There is no other lymphadenopathy or focal findings on examination. What should be the next step in management?

A. Bone marrow biopsy
B. CT scan of the chest, abdomen, and pelvis
C. Excisional biopsy
D. Fine-needle aspiration for culture and cytopathology
E. Pelvic ultrasonography
F. Reassurance

9. All of the following diseases are associated with massive splenomegaly (spleen extends 8 cm below the costal margin or weighs >1000 g) EXCEPT:

A. Autoimmune hemolytic anemia
B. Chronic lymphocytic leukemia

9. (*Continued*)
C. Cirrhosis with portal hypertension
D. Marginal zone lymphoma
E. Myelofibrosis with myeloid metaplasia

10. The presence of Howell-Jolly bodies, Heinz bodies, basophilic stippling, and nucleated red blood cells in a patient with hairy cell leukemia before any treatment intervention implies which of the following?

A. Diffuse splenic infiltration by tumor
B. Disseminated intravascular coagulation (DIC)
C. Hemolytic anemia
D. Pancytopenia
E. Transformation to acute leukemia

11. Which of the following is true regarding infection risk after elective splenectomy?

A. Patients are at no increased risk of viral infection after splenectomy.
B. Patients should be vaccinated 2 weeks after splenectomy.
C. Splenectomy patients over the age of 50 are at greatest risk for postsplenectomy sepsis.
D. *Staphylococcus aureus* is the most commonly implicated organism in postsplenectomy sepsis.
E. The risk of infection after splenectomy increases with time.

12. An 18-year-old man is seen in consultation for a pulmonary abscess caused by infection with *Staphylococcus aureus*. He had been in his usual state of health until 1 week ago when he developed fevers and a cough. He has no ill contacts and presents in the summer. His medical history is significant for episodes of axillary and perianal abscesses requiring incision and drainage. He cannot specifically recall how often this has occurred, but he does know it has been more than five times that he can recall. In one instance, he recalls a lymph node became enlarged to the point that it "popped" and drained spontaneously. He also reports frequent aphthous ulcers and is treated for eczema. On physical examination, his height is 5′3″. He appears ill with a temperature of 39.6°C. Eczematous dermatitis is present in the scalp and periorbital area. There are crackles at the left lung base. Axillary lymphadenopathy is present bilaterally and is tender. The spleen in enlarged. His laboratory studies show a white blood cell count of 12,500/µL (94% neutrophils), hemoglobin of 11.3 g/dL, hematocrit of 34.2%, and platelets of 320,000/µL. Granulomatous inflammation is seen on lymph

12. (*Continued*)
node biopsy. Which of the following tests are most likely found in this patient?

A. Elevated angiotensin-converting enzyme level
B. Eosinophilia
C. Giant primary granules in neutrophils
D. Mutations of the tumor necrosis factor-alpha receptor
E. Positive nitroblue tetrazolium dye test

13. A 72-year-old man with chronic obstructive pulmonary disease and stable coronary disease presents to the emergency department with several days of worsening productive cough, fevers, malaise, and diffuse muscle aches. A chest radiograph demonstrates a new lobar infiltrate. Laboratory measurements reveal a total white blood cell count of 12,100 cells/μL with a neutrophilic predominance of 86% and 8% band forms. He is diagnosed with community-acquired pneumonia, and antibiotic treatment is initiated. Under normal, or "nonstress," conditions, what percentage of the total body neutrophils are present in the circulation?

A. 2%
B. 10%
C. 25%
D. 40%
E. 90%

14. A patient with longstanding HIV infection, alcoholism, and asthma is seen in the emergency department for 1–2 days of severe wheezing. He has not been taking any medicines for months. He is admitted to the hospital and treated with nebulized therapy and systemic glucocorticoids. His CD4 count is 8 and viral load is >750,000. His total white blood cell (WBC) count is 3200 cells/μL with 90% neutrophils. He is accepted into an inpatient substance abuse rehabilitation program and before discharge is started on opportunistic infection prophylaxis, bronchodilators, a prednisone taper over 2 weeks, ranitidine, and highly active antiretroviral therapy. The rehabilitation center pages you 2 weeks later; a routine laboratory check reveals a total WBC count of 900 cells/μL with 5% neutrophils. Which of the following new drugs would most likely explain this patient's neutropenia?

A. Darunavir
B. Efavirenz
C. Ranitidine
D. Prednisone
E. Trimethoprim–sulfamethoxazole

15. All the following are suggestive of iron-deficiency anemia EXCEPT:

A. Koilonychia
B. Pica
C. Decreased serum ferritin
D. Decreased total iron-binding capacity (TIBC)
E. Low reticulocyte response

16. A 24-year-old man with a history of poorly treated chronic ulcerative colitis is found to have anemia with a hemoglobin of 9 g/dL and a reduced mean corpuscular volume. His ferritin is 250 μg/L. Which of the following is the most likely cause of his anemia?

A. Folate deficiency
B. Hemoglobinopathy
C. Inflammation
D. Iron deficiency
E. Sideroblastic anemia

17. All of the following statements regarding the anemia of chronic kidney disease are true EXCEPT:

A. The degree of anemia correlates with the stage of chronic kidney disease.
B. Erythropoietin levels are reduced.
C. Ferritin is reduced.
D. It is typically normocytic and normochromic.
E. Reticulocytes are decreased.

18. All of the following statements regarding the utility of hydroxyurea in patients with sickle cell disease are true EXCEPT:

A. It is effective in reducing painful crises.
B. It produces a chimeric state with partial production of hemoglobin A by the bone marrow.
C. It should be considered in patients with repeated acute chest syndrome episodes.
D. Its mechanism involves increasing production of fetal hemoglobin.
E. The major adverse effect is a reduction in white blood cell count.

19. Which of the following is the most cost-effective test to evaluate a patient for suspected cobalamin (vitamin B_{12}) deficiency?

A. Red blood cell folate
B. Serum cobalamin
C. Serum homocysteine
D. Serum methylmalonate
E. Serum pepsinogen

20. A patient being evaluated for anemia has the peripheral blood smear shown in **Figure 20**. Which of the following is the most likely cause of the anemia?

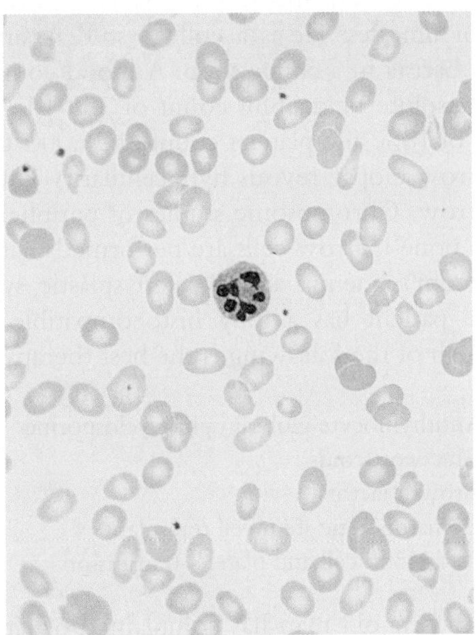

FIGURE 20

A. Acute lymphocytic leukemia
B. Autoantibodies to ADAMTS-13
C. Cobalamin deficiency
D. Epstein-Barr virus infection
E. Iron deficiency

21. Patients from which of the following regions need not be screened for glucose-6-phosphate dehydrogenase (G6PD) deficiency when starting a drug that carries a risk for G6PD-mediated hemolysis?

A. Brazil
B. Russia
C. Southeast Asia
D. Southern Europe
E. Sub-Saharan Africa
F. None of the above

22. A 36-year-old African American woman with systemic lupus erythematosus presents with the acute onset of lethargy and jaundice. On initial evaluation, she is tachycardic and hypotensive, appears pale, is dyspneic, and is somewhat difficult to arouse. Physical examination reveals splenomegaly. Her initial hemoglobin is 6 g/dL, white blood cell count is 6300/μL, and platelets are 294,000/μL. Her total bilirubin is 4 g/dL, reticulocyte count is 18%, and haptoglobin is not detectable. Renal function is normal, as is urinalysis. What would you expect on her peripheral blood smear?

22. (*Continued*)

A. Macrocytosis and polymorphonuclear leukocytes with hypersegmented nuclei
B. Microspherocytes
C. Schistocytes
D. Sickle cells
E. Target cells

23. A 22-year-old pregnant woman of northern European descent presents 3 months into her first pregnancy with extreme fatigue, pallor, and icterus. She reports being previously healthy. On evaluation, her hemoglobin is 8 g/dL with a normal mean corpuscular volume and an elevated mean corpuscular hemoglobin concentration, reticulocyte count of 9%, and indirect bilirubin of 4.9 mg/dL; serum haptoglobin is not detectable. Her peripheral smear is shown in **Figure 23**. Her physical examination is notable for splenomegaly and a normal 3-month uterus. What is the most likely diagnosis?

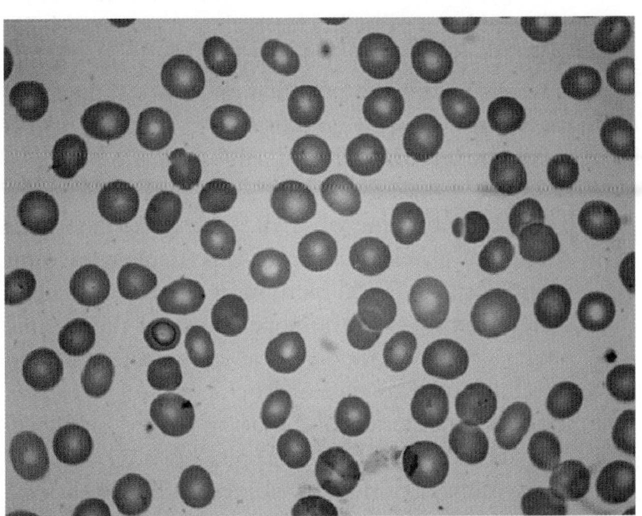

FIGURE 23

A. Colonic polyp
B. G6PD deficiency
C. Hereditary spherocytosis
D. Parvovirus B19 infection
E. Thrombotic thrombocytopenic purpura

24. The triad of portal vein thrombosis, hemolysis, and pancytopenia suggests which of the following diagnoses?

A. Acute promyelocytic leukemia
B. Hemolytic uremic syndrome (HUS)
C. Leptospirosis
D. Paroxysmal nocturnal hemoglobinuria (PNH)
E. Thrombotic thrombocytopenic purpura (TTP)

25. All of the following laboratory values are consistent with an intravascular hemolytic anemia EXCEPT:

A. Increased haptoglobin
B. Increased lactate dehydrogenase (LDH)
C. Increased reticulocyte count
D. Increased unconjugated bilirubin
E. Increased urine hemosiderin

26. Which of the following hemolytic anemias can be classified as extracorpuscular?

A. Elliptocytosis
B. Paroxysmal nocturnal hemoglobinuria
C. Pyruvate kinase deficiency
D. Sickle cell anemia
E. Thrombotic thrombocytopenic purpura

27. A 34-year-old woman with a medical history of sickle cell anemia presents with a 5-day history of fatigue, lethargy, and shortness of breath. She denies chest pain and bone pain. She has had no recent travel. Of note, the patient's 4-year-old daughter had a "cold" 2 weeks before the presentation. On examination, the woman has pale conjunctiva, is anicteric, and is mildly tachycardic. Abdominal examination is unremarkable. Laboratory studies show a hemoglobin of 3 g/dL; her baseline is 8 g/dL. The white blood cell count and platelets are normal. Reticulocyte count is undetectable. Total bilirubin is 1.4 mg/dL. Lactic dehydrogenase is at the upper limits of the normal range. Peripheral blood smear shows a few sickled cells but a total absence of reticulocytes. The patient is given a transfusion of 2 units of packed red blood cells and admitted to the hospital. A bone marrow biopsy shows a normal myeloid series but an absence of erythroid precursors. Cytogenetics are normal. What is the most appropriate next management step?

A. Make arrangements for exchange transfusion.
B. Tissue type her siblings for a possible bone marrow transplant.
C. Check parvovirus titers.
D. Start prednisone and cyclosporine.
E. Start broad-spectrum antibiotics.

28. Aplastic anemia has been associated with all of the following EXCEPT:

A. Carbamazepine therapy
B. Methimazole therapy
C. Nonsteroidal anti-inflammatory drugs
D. Parvovirus B19 infection
E. Seronegative hepatitis

29. A 23-year-old man presents with diffuse bruising. He otherwise feels well. He takes no medications, does not use dietary supplements and does not use illicit drugs. His medical history is negative for any prior illnesses. He is a college student and works as a barista in a coffee shop. A blood count reveals an absolute neutrophil count of 780/μL, hematocrit of 18%, and platelet count of 21,000/μL. Bone marrow biopsy reveals hypocellularity with a fatty marrow. Chromosome studies of peripheral blood and bone marrow cells are performed that exclude Fanconi's anemia and myelodysplastic syndrome. The patient has a fully histocompatible brother. Which of the following is the best therapy?

A. Antithymocyte globulin plus cyclosporine
B. Glucocorticoids
C. Growth factors
D. Hematopoietic stem cell transplant
E. Red blood cell and platelet transfusion

30. A 73-year-old man has complained of fatigue and worsening dyspnea on exertion for the past 2 to 3 months. His medical history is only notable for hypertension and hypercholesterolemia. He is an active golfer who notes that lately he has difficulty walking 18 holes. His handicap has increased by 5 strokes over this time period. Physical examination reveals normal vital signs and is unremarkable except for pallor. His laboratory examination is remarkable for a hematocrit of 25% with a platelet count of 185,000/μL and low normal white cell count. There are no circulating blasts. These abnormalities were not present 1 year ago. Bone marrow reveals a hypercellular marrow with fewer than 5% blasts and the 5q-cytogenetic abnormality. All of the following statements regarding this patient's condition are true EXCEPT:

A. He has myelofibrosis.
B. He is most likely to die as a result of leukemic transformation.
C. His median survival is >12 months.
D. Lenalidomide is effective in reversing the anemia.
E. Only stem cell transplantation offers a cure.

31. All of the following are considered myeloproliferative disorders in the WHO classification system EXCEPT:

A. Chronic myeloid leukemia (bcr-abl positive)
B. Essential thrombocytosis
C. Mastocytosis
D. Polycythemia vera
E. Primary effusion lymphoma

32. Which of the following statements regarding polycythemia vera is correct?

A. An elevated plasma erythropoietin level excludes the diagnosis.
B. Transformation to acute leukemia is common.
C. Thrombocytosis correlates strongly with thrombotic risk.
D. Aspirin should be prescribed to all of these patients to reduce thrombotic risk.
E. Phlebotomy is used only after hydroxyurea and interferon have been tried.

33. A 68-year-old man seeks evaluation for fatigue, weight loss, and early satiety that have been present for about 4 months. On physical examination, his spleen is noted to be markedly enlarged. It is firm to touch and crosses the midline. The lower edge of the spleen reaches to the pelvis. His hemoglobin is 11.1 g/dL and hematocrit is 33.7%. The leukocyte count is 6200/μL and platelet count is 220,000/μL. The white cell count differential is 75% polymorphonuclear leukocytes, 8% myelocytes, 4% metamyelocytes, 8% lymphocytes, 3% monocytes, and 2% eosinophils. The peripheral blood smear shows teardrop cells, nucleated red blood cells, and immature granulocytes. Rheumatoid factor is positive. A bone marrow biopsy is attempted, but no cells are able to be aspirated. No evidence of leukemia or lymphoma is found. What is the most likely cause of the splenomegaly?

A. Chronic primary myelofibrosis
B. Chronic myeloid leukemia
C. Rheumatoid arthritis
D. Systemic lupus erythematosus
E. Tuberculosis

34. A 50-year-old woman presents to your clinic for evaluation of an elevated platelet count. The latest complete blood count is white blood cells (WBC), 7000/μL; hematocrit, 34%; and platelets, 600,000/μL. All the following are common causes of thrombocytosis EXCEPT:

A. Iron-deficiency anemia
B. Essential thrombocytosis
C. Chronic myeloid leukemia
D. Myelodysplasia
E. Pernicious anemia

35. A 38-year-old woman is referred for evaluation of an elevated hemoglobin and hematocrit that was discovered during an evaluation of recurrent headaches. Until about 8 months previously, she was in good health, but she developed increasingly persistent headaches with intermittent vertigo and tinnitus. She was originally prescribed sumatriptan for presumed migraine headaches but did not experience relief of her symptoms. A CT scan of the brain showed no evidence of mass lesion. During evaluation of her headaches, she was found to have a hemoglobin of 17.3 g/dL and a hematocrit of 52%. Her only other symptom is diffuse itching after hot showers. She is a nonsmoker. She has no history pulmonary or cardiac disease. On physical examination, she appears well. Her body mass index is 22.3 kg/m^2. Vital signs are blood pressure of 148/84 mm Hg, heart rate of 86 beats/min, respiratory rate of 12 breaths/min, and SaO2 of 99% on room air. She is afebrile. The physical examination, including full neurologic examination, is normal. There are no heart murmurs. There is no splenomegaly. Peripheral pulses are normal. Laboratory studies confirm elevated hemoglobin and hematocrit. She also has a platelet count of 650,000/μL. Leukocyte count is 12,600/μL with a normal differential. Which of the following tests should be performed next in the evaluation of this patient?

A. Bone marrow biopsy
B. Erythropoietin level
C. Genetic testing for *JAK2 V617F* mutation
D. Leukocyte alkaline phosphatase
E. Red blood cell mass and plasma volume determination

36. A 45-year-old man is evaluated by his primary care physician for complaints of early satiety and weight loss. On physical examination, his spleen is palpable 10 cm below the left costal margin and is mildly tender to palpation. His laboratory studies show a leukocyte count of 125,000/μL with a differential of 80% neutrophils, 9% bands, 3% myelocytes, 3% metamyelocytes, 1% blasts, 1% lymphocytes, 1% eosinophils, and 1% basophils. Hemoglobin is 8.4 g/dL, hematocrit is 26.8%, and platelet count is 668,000/μL. A bone marrow biopsy demonstrates increased cellularity with an increased myeloid to erythroid ratio. Which of the following cytogenetic abnormalities is most likely to be found in this patient?

A. Deletion of a portion of the long arm of chromosome 5, del(5q)
B. Inversion of chromosome 16, inv(16)
C. Reciprocal translocation between chromosomes 9 and 22 (Philadelphia chromosome)
D. Translocations of the long arms of chromosomes 15 and 17
E. Trisomy 12

37. All of the following statements regarding the epidemiology of and risk factors for acute myeloid leukemias are true EXCEPT:

A. Anticancer drugs such as alkylating agents and topoisomerase II inhibitors are the leading cause of drug-associated myeloid leukemias.
B. Individuals exposed to high-dose radiation are at risk for acute myeloid leukemia, but individuals treated with therapeutic radiation are not unless they are also treated with alkylating agents.
C. Men have a higher incidence of acute myeloid leukemia than women.
D. The incidence of acute myeloid leukemia is greatest in individuals younger than 20 years of age.
E. Trisomy 21 (Down syndrome) is associated with an increased risk of acute myeloid leukemia.

38. A 56-year-old woman is diagnosed with chronic myeloid leukemia, Philadelphia chromosome positive. Her presenting leukocyte count was 127,000/μL, and her differential shows <2% circulating blasts. Her hematocrit is 21.1% at diagnosis. She is asymptomatic except for fatigue. She has no siblings. What is the best initial therapy for this patient?

A. Allogeneic bone marrow transplant
B. Autologous stem cell transplant
C. Imatinib mesylate
D. Interferon-α
E. Leukapheresis

39. A 48-year-old woman is admitted to the hospital with anemia and thrombocytopenia after complaining of profound fatigue. Her initial hemoglobin is 8.5 g/dL, hematocrit is 25.7%, and platelet count is 42,000/μL. Her leukocyte count is 9540/μL, but 8% blast forms are noted on peripheral smear. A chromosomal analysis shows a reciprocal translocation of the long arms of chromosomes 15 and 17, t(15;17), and a diagnosis of acute promyelocytic leukemia is made. The induction regimen of this patient should include which of the following drugs?

A. Arsenic
B. Cyclophosphamide, daunorubicin, vinblastine, and prednisone
C. Rituximab
D. Tretinoin
E. Whole-body irradiation

40. The patient in question 39 is started on the appropriate induction regimen. Two weeks after initiation of treatment, the patient develops acute onset of shortness of breath, fever, and chest pain. Her chest radiograph shows bilateral alveolar infiltrates and moderate bilateral pleural effusions. Her leukocyte count is now 22,300/μL, and she has a neutrophil count of 78%, bands of 15%, and lymphocytes 7%. She undergoes bronchoscopy with lavage that shows no bacterial, fungal, or viral organisms. What is the most likely diagnosis in this patient?

A. Arsenic poisoning
B. Bacterial pneumonia
C. Cytomegalovirus pneumonia
D. Radiation pneumonitis
E. Retinoic acid syndrome

41. A 76-year-old man is admitted to the hospital with complaints of fatigue for 4 months and fever for the past week. His temperature has been as high as 38.3°C at home. During this time, he intermittently has had a 5.5-kg weight loss, severe bruising with minimal trauma, and an aching sensation in his bones. He last saw his primary care physician 2 months ago and was diagnosed with anemia of unclear etiology at that time. He has a history of a previous left middle cerebral artery cerebrovascular accident, which has left him with decreased functional status. At baseline, he is able to ambulate in his home with the use of a walker and is dependent on a caregiver for assistance with his activities of daily living. His vital signs are blood pressure of 158/86 mm Hg, heart rate of 98 beats/min, respiratory rate of 18 breaths/min, SaO_2 95%, and temperature of 38°C. He appears cachectic with temporal muscle wasting. He has petechiae on his hard palate. He has no lymph node enlargement. On cardiovascular examination, there is a II/VI systolic ejection murmur present. His lungs are clear. The liver is enlarged and palpable 6 cm below the right costal margin. In addition, the spleen is enlarged, with a palpable spleen tip felt about 4 cm below the left costal margin. There are multiple hematomas and petechiae present in the extremities. Laboratory examination reveals the following: hemoglobin, 5.1 g/dL; hematocrit, 15%; platelets, 12,000/μL; and white blood cell (WBC) count, 168,000/μL with 45% blast forms, 30% neutrophils, 20% lymphocytes, and 5% monocytes. Review of the peripheral blood smear confirms acute myeloid leukemia (M1 subtype, myeloblastic leukemia without maturation) with complex chromosomal abnormalities on cytogenetics. All of the following confer a poor prognosis for this patient EXCEPT:

A. Advanced age
B. Complex chromosomal abnormalities on cytogenetics

41. (*Continued*)
C. Hemoglobin below 7 g/dL
D. Prolonged interval between symptom onset and diagnosis
E. WBC count above 100,000/μL

42. The evaluation in a newly diagnosed case of acute lymphoid leukemia should routinely include all of the following EXCEPT:

A. Bone marrow biopsy
B. Cell-surface phenotyping
C. Cytogenetic testing
D. Lumbar puncture
E. Plasma viscosity

43. All of the following infectious agents have been associated with development of a lymphoid malignancy EXCEPT:

A. *Helicobacter pylori*
B. Hepatitis B
C. Hepatitis C
D. HIV
E. Human herpes virus 8 (HHV8)

44. A 64-year-old man with chronic lymphoid leukemia and chronic hepatitis C presents for his yearly follow-up. His white blood cell count is stable at 83,000/μL, but his hematocrit has dropped from 35–26%, and his platelet count also dropped from 178,000/μL to 69,000/μL. His initial evaluation should include all of the following EXCEPT:

A. AST, ALT, and prothrombin time
B. Bone marrow biopsy
C. Coombs test
D. Peripheral blood smear
E. Physical examination

45. During a routine visit, a 68-year-old woman complains of 3 months of fatigue, abdominal fullness, and bilateral axillary adenopathy. On physical examination, vital signs are normal, and she has bilateral palpable axillary and cervical adenopathy and an enlarged spleen. A complete blood count is notable for a white cell count of 88,000 with 99% lymphocytes. A peripheral smear is shown in Figure 45. Which of the following is the most likely diagnosis?

A. Acute lymphoblastic leukemia
B. Acute myelogenous leukemia
C. Chronic lymphocytic lymphoma
D. Hairy cell leukemia
E. Mononucleosis

45. (*Continued*)

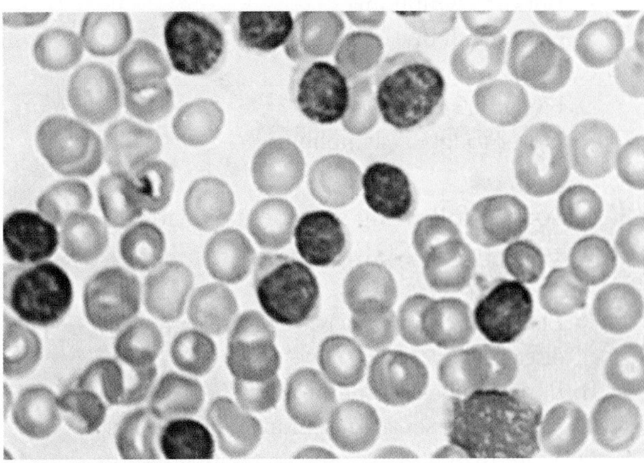

FIGURE 45

46. Which of the following carries the best disease prognosis with appropriate treatment?

A. Burkitt's lymphoma
B. Diffuse large B-cell lymphoma
C. Follicular lymphoma
D. Mantle cell lymphoma
E. Nodular sclerosing Hodgkin's disease

47. A 27-year-old man seeks medical attention for enlarging nodules in his neck. He reports they are nontender and have been growing for >1 month. At first he thought they were caused by a sore throat, but over the past 3 weeks, he has felt well with no fever, chills, throat pain, or other associated symptoms. He notes a slightly diminished appetite but no weight loss. He works as a video game developer, does not smoke or use illicit drugs, and is sexually active with numerous female partners. He has never been tested for HIV. A lymph node biopsy is performed and is shown in Figure 47. Which of the following is the most likely diagnosis?

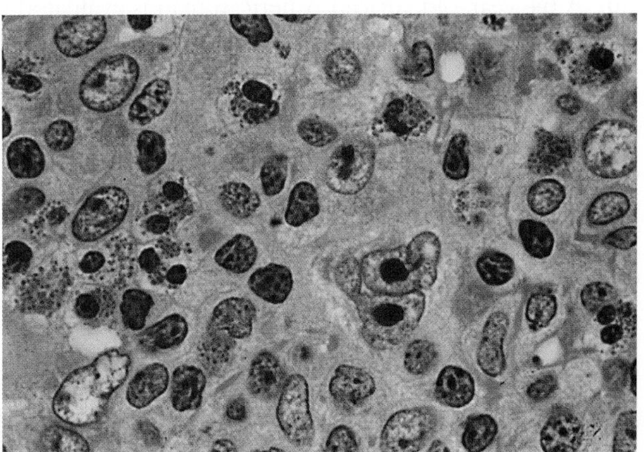

FIGURE 47

47. (*Continued*)
A. Burkitt's lymphoma
B. Cat scratch disease
C. CMV infection
D. Hodgkin's disease
E. Non-Hodgkin's lymphoma

48. All of the following statements regarding mastocytosis are true EXCEPT:

A. Elevated serum tryptase suggests aggressive disease.
B. Eosinophilia is common.
C. It is often associated with myeloid neoplasm.
D. More than 90% of cases are confined to the skin.
E. Urticaria pigmentosa is the most common clinical manifestation.

49. A 58-year-old man is evaluated in the emergency department for sudden onset cough with yellow sputum production and dyspnea. Aside from systemic hypertension, he is otherwise healthy. His only medication is amlodipine. Chest radiograph shows a right upper lobe alveolar infiltrate, and laboratory test results are notable for a blood urea nitrogen of 53 mg/dL, creatinine of 2.8 mg/dL, calcium of 12.3 mg/dL, total protein of 9 g/dL, and albumin of 3.1 g/dL. Sputum culture grows *Streptococcus pneumonia*. Which of the following tests will confirm the underlying condition predisposing him to pneumococcal pneumonia?

A. Bone marrow biopsy
B. Computed tomography of the chest, abdomen, and pelvis with contrast
C. HIV antibody
D. Sweat chloride testing
E. Videoscopic swallow study

50. A 64-year-old African American man is evaluated in the hospital for congestive heart failure, renal failure, and polyneuropathy. Physical examination on admission was notable for these findings and raised waxy papules in the axilla and inguinal region. Admission laboratories showed a blood urea nitrogen of 90 mg/dL and a creatinine of 6.3 mg/dL. Total protein was 9.0 g/dL with an albumin of 3.2 g/dL. Hematocrit was 24%, and white blood cell and platelet counts were normal. Urinalysis was remarkable for 3+ proteinuria but no cellular casts. Further evaluation included an echocardiogram with a thickened left ventricle and preserved systolic function. Which of the following tests is most likely to diagnose the underlying condition?

50. (*Continued*)
A. Bone marrow biopsy
B. Electromyogram (EMG) with nerve conduction studies
C. Fat pad biopsy
D. Right heart catheterization
E. Renal ultrasonography

51. A 75-year-old man is hospitalized for treatment of a deep-vein thrombosis. He had recently been discharged from the hospital about 2 months ago. At that time, he had been treated for community-acquired pneumonia complicated by acute respiratory failure requiring mechanical ventilation. He was hospitalized for 21 days at that time and had discharged from a rehabilitation 2 weeks ago. On the day before admission, he developed painful swelling of his left lower extremity. Lower extremity Doppler ultrasonography confirmed an occlusive thrombus of his deep femoral vein. After an initial bolus, he is started on a continuous infusion of unfractionated heparin at 1600 U/hr because he has end-stage renal disease on hemodialysis. His activated partial thromboplastin time is maintained in the therapeutic range. On day 5, it is noted that his platelets have fallen from 150,000/μL to 88,000/μL. What is the most appropriate action at this time?

A. Continue heparin infusion at the current dose and assess for anti-heparin/platelet factor 4 antibodies.
B. Stop all anticoagulation while awaiting results of anti-heparin/platelet factor 4 antibodies.
C. Stop heparin infusion and initiate argatroban.
D. Stop heparin infusion and initiate enoxaparin.
E. Stop heparin infusion and initiate lepirudin.

52. A 48-year-old woman is evaluated by her primary care physician for a complaint of gingival bleeding and easy bruising. She has noted the problem for about 2 months. Initially, she attributed it to aspirin that she was taking intermittently for headaches, but she stopped all aspirin and nonsteroidal anti-inflammatory drug use 6 weeks ago. Her only medical history is an automobile accident 12 years previously that caused a liver laceration. It required surgical repair, and she did receive several transfusions of red blood cells and platelets at that time. She currently takes no prescribed medications and otherwise feels well. On physical examination, she appears well and healthy. She has no jaundice or scleral icterus. Her cardiac and pulmonary examination results are normal. The abdominal examination shows a liver span of 12 cm to percussion, and the edge is palpable 1.5 cm below the right costal

52. (*Continued*)
margin. The spleen tip is not palpable. There are petechiae present on her extremities and hard palate with a few small ecchymoses on her extremities. A complete blood count shows a hemoglobin of 12.5 g/dL, hematocrit of 37.6%, white blood cell count of 8400/μL with a normal differential, and a platelet count of 7500/μL. What tests are indicated for the workup of this patient's thrombocytopenia?

A. Antiplatelet antibodies
B. Bone marrow biopsy
C. Hepatitis C antibody
D. Human immunodeficiency antibody
E. C and D
F. All of the above

53. A 54-year-old woman presents acutely with alterations in mental status and fever. She was well until 4 days previously when she began to develop complaints of myalgia and fever. Her symptoms progressed rapidly, and today her husband noted her to be lethargic and unresponsive when he awakened. She has recently felt well otherwise. Her only current medication is atenolol 25 mg daily for hypertension. On physical examination, she is responsive only to sternal rub and does not vocalize. Her vital signs are blood pressure of 165/92 mm Hg, heart rate of 114 beats/min, temperature of 38.7°C (101.7°F), respiratory rate of 26 breaths/min, and oxygen saturation of 92% on room air. Her cardiac examination shows a regular tachycardia. Her lungs have bibasilar crackles. The abdominal examination is unremarkable. No hepatosplenomegaly is present. There are petechiae on the lower extremities. Her complete blood count has a hemoglobin of 8.8 g/dL, hematocrit of 26.4%, white blood cell count of 10.2/μL (89% polymorphonuclear cells, 10% lymphocytes, 1% monocytes), and a platelet count of 54,000/μL. A peripheral blood smear is shown in Figure 53. Her basic metabolic panel has a sodium of 137 meq/L, potassium of 5.4 meq/L, chloride of 98 meq/L, bicarbonate of 18 meq/L, BUN of 89 mg/dL, and creatinine of 2.9 mg/dL. Which statement most correctly describes the pathogenesis of the patient's condition?

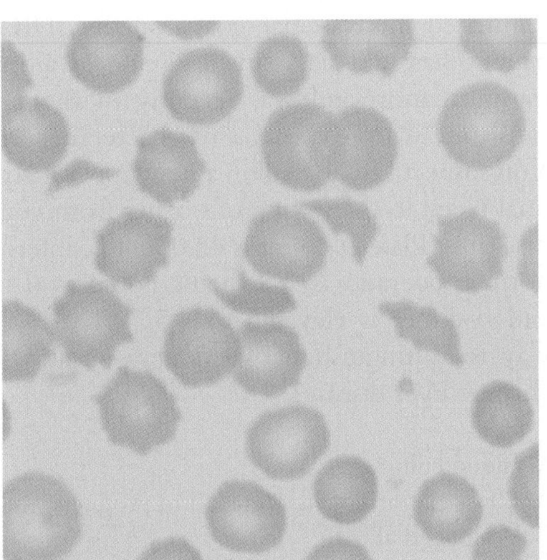

FIGURE 53

A. Development of autoantibodies to a metalloproteinase that cleaves von Willebrand factor
B. Development of autoantibodies to the heparin-platelet factor 4 complex
C. Direct endothelial toxicity initiated by an infectious agent
D. Inherited disorder of platelet granule formation
E. Inherited disorder of von Willebrand factor that precludes binding with factor VIII

54. What is the best initial treatment for the patient in question 53?

A. Acyclovir 10 mg/kg intravenously every 8 hours
B. Ceftriaxone 2 g intravenously daily plus vancomycin 1 g intravenously twice daily
C. Hemodialysis
D. Methylprednisolone 1 g intravenously
E. Plasma exchange

55. Which of the following statements regarding hemophilia A and B is TRUE?

A. Individuals with factor VIII deficiency have a more severe clinical course than those with factor IX deficiency.
B. Levels of factor VIII or IX need to be measured before administration of replacement therapy in patients presenting with acute bleeding to calculate the appropriate dose of factor.
C. Primary prophylaxis against bleeding is never indicated.
D. The goal level of factor VIII or IX is >50% in the setting of large-volume bleeding episodes.
E. The life expectancy of individuals with hemophilia is about 50 years.

56. A 24-year-old man is admitted to the hospital with circulatory collapse in the setting of disseminated meningococcemia. He is currently intubated, sedated, and on mechanical ventilation. He has received over 6 L of intravenous saline in the past 6 hours but remains hypotensive, requiring treatment with norepinephrine and vasopressin at maximum doses. He is making <20 mL of urine each hour. Blood is noted to be oozing from all

56. (*Continued*)
of IV sites. His endotracheal secretions are blood tinged. His laboratory studies show a white blood cell count of 24,300/μL (82% neutrophils, 15% bands, 3% lymphocytes), hemoglobin of 8.7 g/dL, hematocrit of 26.1%, and platelets of 19,000/μL. The international normalized ratio is 3.6, the activated partial thromboplastin time is 75 seconds, and fibrinogen is 42 mg/dL. The lactate dehydrogenase level is 580 U/L, and the haptoglobin is <10 mg/dL. The peripheral smear shows thrombocytopenia and schistocytes. All of the following treatments are indicated in this patient EXCEPT:

A. Ceftriaxone 2 g intravenously twice daily
B. Cryoprecipitate
C. Fresh-frozen plasma
D. Heparin
E. Platelets

57. All the following are vitamin K–dependent coagulation factors EXCEPT:

A. Factor X
B. Factor VII
C. Protein C
D. Protein S
E. Factor VIII

58. A 31-year-old man with hemophilia A is admitted with persistent gross hematuria. He denies recent trauma and any history of genitourinary pathology. The examination is unremarkable. Hematocrit is 28%. All the following are treatments for hemophilia A EXCEPT:

A. Desmopressin (DDAVP)
B. Fresh-frozen plasma
C. Cryoprecipitate
D. Recombinant factor VIII
E. Plasmapheresis

59. All of the following statements regarding the lupus anticoagulant (LA) are true EXCEPT:

A. LAs typically prolong the activated partial thromboplastin time.
B. A 1:1 mixing study will not correct in the presence of LAs.
C. Bleeding episodes in patients with LAs may be severe and life threatening.
D. Female patients may experience recurrent midtrimester abortions.
E. LAs may occur in the absence of other signs of systemic lupus erythematosus.

60. All the following cause prolongation of the activated partial thromboplastin time that does not correct with a 1:1 mixture with pooled plasma EXCEPT:

A. Lupus anticoagulant
B. Factor VIII inhibitor
C. Heparin
D. Factor VII inhibitor
E. Factor IX inhibitor

61. You are evaluating a 45-year-old man with an acute upper gastrointestinal (GI) bleed in the emergency department. He reports increasing abdominal girth over the past 3 months associated with fatigue and anorexia. He has not noticed any lower extremity edema. His medical history is significant for hemophilia A diagnosed as a child with recurrent elbow hemarthroses in the past. He has been receiving infusions of factor VIII for most of his life and received his last injection earlier that day. His blood pressure is 85/45 mm Hg with a heart rate of 115 beats/min. His abdominal examination is tense with a positive fluid wave. Hematocrit is 21%. Renal function and urinalysis results are normal. His activated partial thromboplastin time is minimally prolonged, his international normalized ratio is 2.7, and platelets are normal. Which of the following is most likely to yield a diagnosis for the cause of his GI bleeding?

A. Factor VIII activity level
B. *Helicobacter pylori* antibody test
C. Hepatitis B surface antigen
D. Hepatitis C RNA
E. Mesenteric angiogram

62. You are managing a patient with suspected disseminated intravascular coagulopathy (DIC). The patient has end-stage liver disease awaiting liver transplantation and was recently in the intensive care unit with *Escherichia coli* bacterial peritonitis. You suspect DIC based on a new upper gastrointestinal bleed in the setting of oozing from venipuncture sites. Platelet count is 43,000/μL, international normalized ratio is 2.5, hemoglobin is 6 mg/dL, and D-dimer is elevated to 4.5. What is the best way to distinguish between new-onset DIC and chronic liver disease?

A. Blood culture
B. Elevated fibrinogen degradation products
C. Prolonged aPTT
D. Reduced platelet count
E. Serial laboratory analysis

63. All of the following genetic mutations are associated with an increased risk of deep-vein thrombosis EXCEPT:

A. Factor V Leiden mutation
B. Glycoprotein 1b platelet receptor
C. Heterozygous protein C deficiency
D. Prothrombin 20210G
E. Tissue plasminogen activator

64. A 76-year-old man presents to an urgent care clinic with pain in his left leg for 4 days. He also describes swelling in his left ankle, which has made it difficult for him to ambulate. He is an active smoker and has a medical history remarkable for gastroesophageal reflux disease, deep-vein thrombosis (DVT) 9 months ago that resolved, and well-controlled hypertension. Physical examination is revealing for 2+ edema in his left ankle. A D-dimer is ordered and is elevated. Which of the following makes D-dimer less predictive of DVT in this patient?

A. Age older than 70 years
B. History of active tobacco use
C. Lack of suggestive clinical symptoms
D. Negative Homan's sign on examination
E. Previous DVT in the past year

65. A 22-year-old woman comes to the emergency department complaining of 12 hours of shortness of breath. The symptoms began toward the end of a long car ride home from college. She has no medical history, and her only medication is an oral contraceptive. She smokes occasionally, but the frequency has increased recently because of examinations. On physical examination, she is afebrile with respiratory rate of 22 breaths/min, blood pressure of 120/80 mm Hg, heart rate of 110 beats/min, and oxygen saturation on room air of 92%. The rest of her physical examination findings are normal. A chest radiograph and complete blood count are normal. Her serum pregnancy test result is negative. Which of the following is the indicated management strategy?

A. Check D-dimer and, if normal, discharge with nonsteroidal anti-inflammatory therapy.
B. Check D-dimer and, if normal, obtain lower extremity ultrasound.
C. Check D-dimer and, if abnormal, treat for deep-vein thrombosis/pulmonary embolism.
D. Check D-dimer and, if abnormal, obtain a contrast multislice computed tomography scan of the chest.
E. Obtain a contrast multislice computed tomography scan of the chest.

66. All of the anticoagulant or antiplatelet drugs listed are correctly matched with their mechanisms of action EXCEPT:

A. Abciximab—Glycoprotein IIb/IIIa receptor inhibitor
B. Clopidogrel—Adenosine diphosphate receptor blockade
C. Enoxaparin—Direct thrombin inhibition
D. Rivaroxaban—Factor Xa inhibition
E. Warfarin—Inhibition of production of the vitamin K–dependent clotting factors

67. A 66-year-old woman is prescribed clopidogrel and aspirin after implantation of a bare metal stent in her right coronary artery. Two weeks after the procedure, the woman presents to the emergency department with acute-onset chest pain and electrocardiographic changes consistent with an acute inferior myocardial infarction. Emergent cardiac catheterization confirms in-stent restenosis. The patient insists she has been adherent to her prescribed therapy. Which of the following statements most correctly described the most likely cause of the patient's restenosis despite her current therapy?

A. She likely has aspirin resistance and should be treated with higher doses of aspirin to prevent a recurrence.
B. She likely has clopidogrel resistance caused by a genetic polymorphism of the CYP pathway.
C. She should have been treated with low-molecular-weight heparin to prevent this complication.
D. She should have been treated with warfarin to prevent this complication.
E. Because she has demonstrated resistance to clopidogrel, switching to prasugrel would not be useful to prevent further complications.

68. A 48-year-old woman is diagnosed with a deep-vein thrombosis of her left lower extremity. When considering initial anticoagulant therapy, all of the following are advantages of low-molecular-weight heparins over heparin EXCEPT:

A. Better bioavailability
B. Dose-dependent clearance
C. Longer half-life after subcutaneous injection
D. Lower risk of heparin-induced thrombocytopenia
E. Predictable anticoagulant effect

69. In which of the following patients presenting with acute dyspnea would a positive D-dimer prompt additional testing for a pulmonary embolus?

69. (*Continued*)

A. A 24-year-old woman who is 32 weeks pregnant
B. A 48-year-old man with no medical history who presents with calf pain following prolonged air travel; the alveolar–arterial oxygen gradient is normal
C. A 56-year-old woman undergoing chemotherapy for breast cancer
D. A 62-year-old man who underwent hip replacement surgery 4 weeks previously
E. A 72-year-old man who had an acute myocardial infarction 2 weeks ago

70. A 62-year-old woman is hospitalized following an acute pulmonary embolism. All of the following would typically indicate a massive pulmonary embolism EXCEPT:

A. Elevated serum troponin levels
B. Initial presentation with hemoptysis
C. Initial presentation with syncope
D. Presence of right ventricular enlargement on CT scan of the chest
E. Presence of right ventricular hypokinesis on echocardiogram

71. Which of the following statements regarding diagnostic imaging in pulmonary embolism is TRUE?

A. A high probability ventilation–perfusion scan is one that has at least one segmental perfusion defect in the setting of normal ventilation.
B. If a patient has a high probability ventilation–perfusion scan, there is a 90% likelihood that the patient does indeed have a pulmonary embolism.
C. Magnetic resonance angiography provides excellent resolution for both large proximal and smaller segmental pulmonary emboli.
D. Multidetector-row spiral CT imaging is suboptimal for detecting small peripheral emboli, necessitating the use of invasive pulmonary angiography.
E. None of the routinely used imaging techniques provide adequate evaluation of the right ventricle to assist in risk stratification of the patient.

72. A 53-year-old woman presents to the hospital following an episode of syncope, with ongoing lightheadedness and shortness of breath. She had a history of antiphospholipid syndrome with prior pulmonary embolism and has been nonadherent to her anticoagulation medication recently. She has been prescribed warfarin, 7.5 mg daily, but reports taking it only intermittently. She does not know her most recent INR. On presentation to the emergency department, she appears diaphoretic and tachypneic. Her vital signs are as follows: blood pressure of 86/44 mm Hg, heart rate of 130 beats/min, respiratory rate of 30 breaths/min, and oxygen saturation of 85% on room air. Cardiovascular examination shows a regular tachycardia without murmurs, rubs, or gallops. The lungs are clear to auscultation. On extremity examination, there is swelling of her left thigh with a positive Homan's sign. Chest CT angiography confirms a saddle pulmonary embolus with ongoing clot seen in the pelvic veins on the left. Anticoagulation with unfractionated heparin is administered. After a fluid bolus of 1 L, the patient's blood pressure remains low at 88/50 mm Hg. Echocardiogram demonstrates hypokinesis of the right ventricle. On 100% non-rebreather mask, the oxygen saturation is 92%. What is the next best step in the management of this patient?

A. Continue current management.
B. Continue IV fluids at 500 mL/h for a total of 4 L of fluid resuscitation.
C. Refer for inferior vena cava filter placement and continue current management.
D. Refer for surgical embolectomy.
E. Treat with dopamine and recombinant tissue plasminogen activator, 100 mg IV.

73. A 42-year-old woman presents to the emergency department with acute onset of shortness of breath. She recently had been to visit her parents out of state and rode in a car for about 9 hours each way. Two days ago, she developed mild calf pain and swelling, but she thought that this was not unusual after having been sitting with her legs dependent for the recent trip. On arrival to the emergency department, she is noted to be tachypneic. The vital signs are as follows: blood pressure of 98/60 mm Hg, heart rate of 114 beats/min, respiratory rate of 28 breaths/min, oxygen saturation of 92% on room air, and weight of 89 kg. The lungs are clear bilaterally. There is pain in the right calf with dorsiflexion of the foot, and the right leg is more swollen compared with the left. An arterial blood gas measurement shows a pH of 7.52, PCO_2 25 mm Hg, and PO_2 68 mm Hg. Kidney and liver function are normal. A helical CT scan confirms a pulmonary embolus. All of the following agents can be used alone as initial therapy in this patient EXCEPT:

A. Enoxaparin 1 mg/kg SC twice daily
B. Fondaparinux 7.5 mg SC once daily
C. Tinzaparin 175 U/kg SC once daily
D. Unfractionated heparin IV adjusted to maintain activated partial thromboplastin time (aPTT) two to three times the upper limit of normal
E. Warfarin 7.5 mg PO once daily to maintain INR at 2–3

74. In general, which of the following is the greatest risk factor for the development of cancer?

A. Age
B. Alcohol use
C. Cigarette smoking
D. Female sex
E. Obesity

75. Among women younger than 60 years of age who die from cancer, which of the following is the most common primary organ of origin?

A. Breast
B. Cervix
C. Colon
D. Bone marrow
E. Lung

76. A 68-year-old woman is diagnosed with stage II breast cancer. She has a history of severe chronic obstructive pulmonary disease with an FEV_1 of 32% predicted, coronary artery disease with prior stenting of the left anterior descending artery, peripheral vascular disease, and obesity. She continues to smoke 1 to 2 packs of cigarettes every day. She requires oxygen at 2 L/min continuously and is functionally quite limited. She currently is able to attend to all of her activities of daily living, including showering and dressing. She retired from her work as a waitress 10 years previously because of her lung disease. At home, she does attend to some of the household chores but is not able to use a vacuum. She goes out once or twice weekly to run typical errands and drives. She feels short of breath with most of these activities and often uses a motorized chair when out and about. How would you categorize her performance status and prognosis for treatment taking this into consideration?

A. She has an Eastern Cooperative Oncology Group (ECOG) grade of 1 and has a good prognosis with appropriate therapy.
B. She has an ECOG grade of 2 and has a good prognosis with appropriate therapy.
C. She has an ECOG grade of 3 and has a good prognosis with appropriate therapy.
D. She has an ECOG grade of 3 and has a poor prognosis despite therapy.
E. She has an ECOG grade of 4 and has a poor prognosis that precludes therapy.

77. Which of the following tumor markers is appropriately matched with the cell type cancer and can be followed during treatment as an adjunct to assess disease burden?

77. (*Continued*)
A. CA-125—Colon cancer
B. Calcitonin—Follicular carcinoma of the thyroid
C. CD30—Hairy cell leukemia
D. Human chorionic gonadotropin—Gestational trophoblastic disease
E. Neuron-specific enolase—Non–small cell carcinoma of the lung

78. Which of the following statements regarding current understanding of the genetic changes that must occur for a cell to become cancerous is TRUE?

A. Caretaker genes determine when a cell enters into a replicative phase and must acquire mutations to allow unregulated cell growth.
B. For a cell to become cancerous, it is estimated that a minimum of 20 mutations must occur.
C. For a tumor suppressor gene to become inactivated and allow unregulated cell growth, both copies of the gene must have mutations.
D. Oncogenes act in an autosomal recessive fashion.
E. Within a cancer, there are generally two to five cells of origin.

79. All the following conditions are associated with an increased incidence of cancer EXCEPT:

A. Down syndrome
B. Fanconi's anemia
C. von Hippel–Lindau syndrome
D. Neurofibromatosis
E. Fragile X syndrome

80. Cancer therapy is increasingly personalized with targeted small molecule therapies that are directed against specific signal transduction pathways that are commonly activated in a particular cell type of cancer. Which of the following therapies is correctly matched with its molecular target?

A. Bevacizumab—EGFR
B. Erlotinib—VEGF
C. Imatinib—Bcr-Abl
D. Rituximab—CD45
E. Sunitinib—RAF

81. Which of the following defines the term epigenetics?

A. Changes that alter the pattern of gene expression caused by mutations in the DNA code
B. Changes that alter the pattern of gene expression that persist across at least one cell division but are not caused by changes in the DNA code

81. (*Continued*)

C. Irreversible changes of the chromatin structure that regulates gene transcription and cell proliferation without permanent alteration of the DNA code

82. Which of the following patients with metastatic disease is potentially curable by surgical resection?

A. A 24-year-old man with a history of osteosarcoma of the left femur with a 1-cm metastasis to his right lower lobe referred for right lower lobectomy
B. A 56-year-old woman with a history of colon cancer with three metastases to the left lobe of the liver referred for left hepatic lobectomy
C. A 72-year-old man with metastatic prostate cancer to several vertebrae referred for orchiectomy
D. All of the above
E. None of the above

83. You are studying a new chemotherapeutic agent for use in advanced colorectal carcinoma and have completed a phase II clinical trial. Which of the following factors indicates that the drug is suitable for study in a phase III clinical trial?

A. Complete response rates of 10–15%
B. Increased disease-free survival rates by 1 month
C. Increased overall survival by 1 month
D. Partial response rate of 20–25%
E. Partial response rates of 50% or more

84. Match the following chemotherapeutic agents with their mechanisms of action:

1. Cisplatin	A. Antimetabolite agent
2. Daunorubicin	B. Antimitotic agent
3. 5-Fluorouracil	C. Antitumor antibiotic
4. Gefitinib	D. DNA alkylator
5. Paclitaxel	E. Tyrosine kinase inhibitor

85. A 48-year-old woman with stage III breast cancer is undergoing chemotherapy with a regimen that includes doxorubicin. She presents 8 days after her last treatment to the emergency department with a fever of 104.1°F (40.1°C). She has chills, rigors, and a headache. Her chest radiograph, urinalysis, and tunneled intravenous catheter site show no obvious evidence of infection. Her white blood cell count upon presentation is 500/μL (0% neutrophils, 50% monocytes, 50% lymphocytes). Blood cultures are drawn peripherally and through the catheter. What is the next step in the treatment of this patient?

85. (*Continued*)

A. Broad-spectrum antibiotics with ceftazidime and vancomycin
B. Broad-spectrum antibiotics with ceftazidime, vancomycin, and voriconazole
C. Granulocyte-macrophage colony-stimulating factor after subsequent cycles of chemotherapy only
D. Granulocyte-macrophage colony-stimulating factor now and after subsequent cycles of chemotherapy
E. A and C
F. A and D

86. What is the most common side effect of chemotherapy?

A. Alopecia
B. Diarrhea
C. Febrile neutropenia
D. Mucositis
E. Nausea with or without vomiting

87. A 24-year-old woman is seen in follow-up 12 months after an allogeneic stem cell transplant for acute myeloid leukemia. She is doing well without evidence of recurrent disease but has had manifestations of chronic graft-versus-host disease. She should be administered all of the following vaccines EXCEPT:

A. Diphtheria–tetanus
B. Influenza
C. Measles, mumps, and rubella
D. Poliomyelitis via injection
E. 23-Valent pneumococcal polysaccharide

88. A 66-year-old woman has chronic lymphocytic leukemia with a stable white blood cell count of between 60,000 and 70,000/μL. She is currently hospitalized with pneumococcal pneumonia. This is the patient's third episode of pneumonia within the past 12 months. What finding on laboratory testing would be most likely in this patient?

A. Granulocytopenia
B. Hypogammaglobulinemia
C. Impaired T-cell function with normal T-lymphocyte counts
D. Low CD4 count
E. No specific abnormality is expected.

89. A 63-year-old man is treated with chemotherapy for stage IIIB adenocarcinoma of the lung with paclitaxel and carboplatin. He presents for evaluation of a fever of 38.3°C (100.9°F). He is found

89. (*Continued*)
to have erythema at the exit site of his tunneled catheter, although the tunnel itself is not tender or red. Blood cultures are negative at 48 hours. His neutrophil count is 1,550/μL. What is the best approach to the management of this patient?

A. Removal of catheter alone
B. Treatment with ceftazidime and vancomycin
C. Treatment with topical antibiotics at the catheter site
D. Treatment with vancomycin alone
E. Treatment with vancomycin and removal of catheter

90. All of the following statements regarding the difference between breast cancer in pregnant versus nonpregnant women are true EXCEPT:

A. Estrogen-positive tumors are more common in pregnant women.
B. Her-2 positivity is more common in pregnant women.
C. A higher stage is more common in pregnant women.
D. Positive lymph nodes are more common in pregnant women.
E. Tumor size at diagnosis is larger in pregnant women.

91. You are caring for a 56-year-old woman who was admitted to the hospital with a change in mental status. She underwent a right-sided mastectomy and axillary lymph node dissection 3 years previously for stage IIIB ductal carcinoma. Serum calcium is elevated at 15.3 mg/dL. A chest radiograph demonstrates innumerable pulmonary nodules, and a head CT shows a brain mass in the right frontal lobe with surrounding edema. Despite correcting her calcium and treating cerebral edema, the patient remains confused. You approach the family to discuss the diagnosis of widely metastatic disease and the patient's poor prognosis. Which of the following is NOT a component of the seven elements for communicating bad news (P-SPIKES approach)?

A. Assess the family's perception of her current illness and the status of her underlying cancer diagnosis.
B. Empathize with the family's feelings and provide emotional support.
C. Prepare mentally for the discussion.
D. Provide an appropriate setting for discussion.
E. Schedule a follow-up meeting in 1 day to reassess whether there are additional informational and emotional needs.

92. Which of the following is not a component of a living will?

A. Delineation of specific interventions that would be acceptable to the patient under certain conditions
B. Description of values that should guide discussions regarding terminal care
C. Designation of a health care proxy
D. General statements regarding whether the patient desires receipt of life-sustaining interventions such as mechanical ventilation

93. A 72-year-old woman has stage IV ovarian cancer with diffuse peritoneal studding. She is developing increasing pain in her abdomen and is admitted to the hospital for pain control. She previously was treated with oxycodone 10 mg orally every 6 hours as needed. Upon admission, she is initiated on morphine intravenously via patient-controlled analgesia. During the first 48 hours of her hospitalization, she received an average daily dose of morphine 90 mg and reports adequate pain control unless she is walking. What is the most appropriate opioid regimen for transitioning this patient to oral pain medication?

	SUSTAINED-RELEASE MORPHINE	IMMEDIATE-RELEASE MORPHINE
A.	None	15 mg every 4 hours as needed
B.	45 mg twice daily	5 mg every 4 hours as needed
C.	45 mg twice daily	15 mg every 4 hours as needed
D.	90 mg twice daily	15 mg every 4 hours as needed
E.	90 mg three time daily	15 mg every 4 hours as needed

94. You are asked to consult on 62-year-old man who was recently found to have newly metastatic disease. He was originally diagnosed with cancer of the prostate 5 years previously and presented to the hospital with back pain and weakness. Magnetic resonance imaging (MRI) demonstrated bony metastases to his L2 and L5 vertebrae with spinal cord compression at the L2 level only. On bone scan images, there was evidence of widespread bony metastases. He has been started on radiation and hormonal therapy, and his disease has shown some response. However, he has become quite depressed since the metastatic disease was found.

94. (*Continued*)
His family reports that he is sleeping for 18 or more hours daily and has stopped eating. His weight is down 12 lb over 4 weeks. He expresses profound fatigue, hopelessness, and a feeling of sadness. He claims to have no interest in his usual activities and no longer interacts with his grandchildren. What is the best approach to treating this patient's depression?

A. Do not initiate pharmacologic therapy because the patient is experiencing an appropriate reaction to his newly diagnosed metastatic disease.
B. Initiate therapy with doxepin 75 mg nightly.
C. Initiate therapy with fluoxetine 10 mg daily.
D. Initiate therapy with fluoxetine 10 mg daily and methylphenidate 2.5 mg twice daily in the morning and at noon.
E. Initiate therapy with methylphenidate 2.5 mg twice daily in the morning and at noon.

95. You are treating a 76-year-old woman with Alzheimer's disease admitted to the intensive care unit for aspiration pneumonia. After 7 days of mechanical ventilation, her family requests that care be withdrawn. The patient is palliated with fentanyl intravenously at a rate of 25 μg/hr and midazolam intravenously at 2 mg/hr. You are urgently called to the bedside 15 minutes after the patient is extubated because the patient's daughter is distraught. She states that you are "drowning" her mother and is upset because her mother appears to be struggling to breathe. When you enter the room, you hear a gurgling noise that is coming from accumulated secretions in the oropharynx. You suction the patient for liberal amounts of thin salivary secretions and reassure the daughter that you will make her mother as comfortable as possible. Which of the following interventions may help with the treatment of the patient's oral secretions?

A. Increased infusion rate of fentanyl
B. *N*-acetylcysteine nebulized
C. Pilocarpine drops
D. Placement of a nasal trumpet and oral airway to allow easier access for aggressive suctioning
E. Scopolamine patches

96. A 48-year-old woman presents to her physician with a complaint of an enlarging mole on her right lower extremity. She had noticed the area about 1 year previously and believes it has enlarged. She also notes that it recently has become itchy and occasionally bleeds. On physical examination, the lesion is located on the right mid-thigh. It measures 7.5 × 6 mm with irregular borders and a variegated hue with some areas appearing quite black. A biopsy confirms nodular melanoma. Which of the following is the best predictor of metastatic risk in this patient?

A. Breslow thickness
B. Clark level
C. Female gender
D. Presence of ulceration
E. Site of lesion

97. A 53-year-old man with a history of superficial spreading melanoma is diagnosed with disease metastatic to the lungs and bones. Genetic testing confirms the presence of the *BRAF V600E* mutation. What do you recommend for treatment of this patient?

A. Dacarbazine
B. Hospice care
C. Interleukin-2
D. Ipilimumab
E. Vemurafenib

98. A 65-year-old man presents to his primary care physician complaining of a hoarse voice for 6 months. He smokes 1 pack of cigarettes daily and drinks at least a six pack of beer daily. His physical examination reveals a thin man with a weak voice in no distress. No stridor is heard. The head and neck examination is normal. No cervical lymphadenopathy is present. He is referred to otolaryngology where a laryngeal lesion is discovered. Biopsy reveals squamous cell carcinoma. On imaging, the mass measures 2.8 cm. No suspicious lymphadenopathy is present on PET imaging. What is the best choice of therapy in this patient?

A. Concomitant chemotherapy and radiation therapy
B. Chemotherapy alone
C. Radiation therapy alone
D. Radical neck dissection alone
E. Radical neck dissection followed by concomitant chemotherapy and radiation

99. Which of the following statements is true with regard to the solitary pulmonary nodule?

A. A lobulated and irregular contour is more indicative of malignancy than a smooth one.
B. About 80% of incidentally found pulmonary nodules are benign.

99. (*Continued*)

C. Absence of growth over a period of 6 to 12 months is sufficient to determine if a solitary pulmonary nodule is benign.
D. Ground-glass nodules should be regarded as benign.
E. Multiple nodules indicate malignant disease.

100. A 64-year-old man seeks evaluation for a solitary pulmonary nodule that was found incidentally. He had presented to the emergency department for shortness of breath and chest tightness. A CT pulmonary angiogram did not show any evidence of pulmonary embolism. However, a 9-mm nodule is seen in the periphery of the left lower lobe. No enlarged mediastinal lymph nodes are present. He is a current smoker of 2 packs of cigarettes daily and has done so since the 16 years of age. He generally reports no functional limitation related to respiratory symptoms. His FEV_1 is 88% predicted, FVC is 92% predicted, and diffusion capacity is 80% predicted. He previously had normal chest radiography findings 3 years previously. What is the next best step in the evaluation and treatment of this patient?

A. Perform a bronchoscopy with biopsy for diagnosis.
B. Perform a combined PET and CT to assess for uptake in the nodule and assess for lymph node metastases.
C. Perform a follow-up CT scan in 3 months to assess for interval growth.
D. Refer the patient to radiation oncology for stereotactic radiation of the dominant nodule.
E. Refer the patient to thoracic surgery for video-assisted thoracoscopic biopsy and resection of lung nodule if malignancy is diagnosed.

101. A 62-year-old man presents to the emergency department complaining of a droopy right eye and blurred vision for the past day. The symptoms started abruptly, and he denies any antecedent illness. For the past 4 months, he has been complaining of increasing pain in his right arm and shoulder. His primary care physician has treated him for shoulder bursitis without relief. His medical history is significant for COPD and hypertension. He smokes 1 pack of cigarettes daily. He has chronic daily sputum production and has stable dyspnea on exertion. On physical examination, he has right eye ptosis with unequal pupils. On the right, his pupil is 2 mm and not reactive; on the left, the pupil is 4 mm and reactive. However, his ocular movements appear intact. His lung fields are clear to auscultation. On extremity examination, there is wasting of the intrinsic muscles of the hand. Which of the following would be most likely to explain the patient's constellation of symptoms?

101. (*Continued*)

A. Enlarged mediastinal lymph nodes causing occlusion of the superior vena cava
B. Metastases to the midbrain from small cell lung cancer
C. Paraneoplastic syndrome caused by antibodies to voltage-gated calcium channels
D. Presence of a cervical rib on chest radiography
E. Right apical pleural thickening with a mass-like density measuring 1 cm in thickness

102. A 55-year-old man presents with superior vena cava syndrome and is diagnosed with small cell lung cancer. Which of the following tests are indicated to properly stage this patient?

A. Bone marrow biopsy
B. CT scan of the abdomen
C. CT or MRI of the brain with intravenous contrast
D. Lumbar puncture
E. B and C
F. All of the above

103. As an oncologist, you are considering treatment options for your patients with lung cancer, including small molecule therapy targeting the epidermal growth factor receptor (EGFR). Which of the following patients is most likely to have an EGFR mutation?

A. A 23-year-old man with a hamartoma
B. A 33-year-old woman with a carcinoid tumor
C. A 45-year-old woman who has never smoked with an adenocarcinoma
D. A 56-year-old man with a 100 pack-year history of tobacco with small cell lung carcinoma
E. A 76-year-old man with squamous cell carcinoma and a history of asbestos exposure

104. Given that most individuals with lung cancer present with advanced disease and have a high mortality rate, much research has investigated methods for early detection of lung cancer. Which of the following approaches is most likely to impact disease-related mortality from lung cancer?

A. Carefully design and implement low-dose chest CT screening in individuals with >30 pack years of cigarette smoking.
B. Continue annual screening with chest radiography for individuals with >30 pack years of cigarette smoking
C. Do not recommend any screening because 30 years of research has not demonstrated any effect on mortality from lung cancer.

104. (*Continued*)

D. Offer screening with low-dose CTs to all current or former smokers.
E. Offer screening with combined PET and CT to individuals with >30 pack years of tobacco use.

105. All of the following conditions may be associated with a thymoma EXCEPT:

A. Erythrocytosis
B. Hypogammaglobulinemia
C. Myasthenia gravis
D. Polymyositis
E. Pure red blood cell aplasia

106. A 52-year-old woman has been having worsening cough for the past month. She is a nonsmoker and has no known health problems. The cough is nonproductive and present throughout the day and night. It worsens when lying on her back. She has also noticed some upper chest pain and dyspnea on exertion for the past week. A chest radiograph shows a large mass (>5 cm) confined to the anterior mediastinum. Which of the following diagnoses is most likely?

A. Hodgkin's lymphoma
B. Non-Hodgkin's lymphoma
C. Teratoma
D. Thymoma
E. Thyroid carcinoma

107. Which of the following is the most likely finding in a patient with a "dry" bone marrow aspiration?

A. Chronic myeloid leukemia
B. Hairy cell leukemia
C. Metastatic carcinoma infiltration
D. Myelofibrosis
E. Normal bone marrow

108. All of the following statements are true regarding the criteria to diagnose hypereosinophilic syndrome EXCEPT:

A. Increased bone marrow eosinophils must be demonstrated.
B. It is not necessary to have increased circulating eosinophils.
C. Primary myeloid leukemia must be excluded.
D. Reactive eosinophilia (e.g., parasitic infection, allergy, collagen vascular disease) must be excluded.
E. There must be <20% myeloblasts in blood or bone marrow.

109. A 34-year-old woman is seen by her internist for evaluation of right breast mass. This was noted approximately 1 week ago when she was showering. She has not had any nipple discharge or discomfort. She has no other medical problems. On examination, her right breast has a soft 1 cm × 2 cm mass in the right upper quadrant. There is no axillary lymphadenopathy present. The contralateral breast is normal. The breast is reexamined in 3 weeks, and the same findings are present. The cyst is aspirated, and clear fluid is removed. The mass is no longer palpable. Which of the following statements is true?

A. Breast MRI should be obtained to discern for residual fluid collection.
B. Mammography is required to further evaluate the lesion.
C. She should be evaluated in 1 month for recurrence.
D. She should be referred to a breast surgeon for resection.
E. She should not breastfeed any more children.

110. Which of the following women has the lowest risk of breast cancer?

A. A woman with menarche at 12 years, first child at 24 years, and menopause at 47 years
B. A woman with menarche at 14 years, first child at 17 years, and menopause at 52 years
C. A woman with menarche at 16 years, first child at 17 years, and menopause at 42 years
D. A woman with menarche at 16 years, first child at 32 years, and menopause at 52 years
E. They are all equal

111. Which of the following tumor characteristics confers a poor prognosis in patients with breast cancer?

A. Estrogen receptor positive
B. Good nuclear grade
C. Low proportion of cells in S-phase
D. Overexpression of erbB2 (HER-2/neu)
E. Progesterone receptor positive

112. A 56-year-old man presents to a physician with weight loss and dysphagia. He feels that food gets stuck in his mid-chest such that he no longer is able to eat meats. He reports his diet consists primarily of soft foods and liquids. The symptoms have progressively worsened over 6 months. During this time, he has lost about 50 lb. He occasionally gets pain in his mid-chest that radiates to his back and also occasionally feels that he regurgitates undigested foods. He does not have a history

112. *(Continued)*
of gastroesophageal reflux disease. He does not regularly seek medical care. He is known to have hypertension but takes no medications. He drinks 500 cc or more of whiskey daily and smokes 1.5 packs of cigarettes per day. On physical examination, the patient appears cachectic with temporal wasting. He has a body mass index of 19.4 kg/m^2. His blood pressure is 198/110 mm Hg, heart rate is 110 beats/min, respiratory rate is 18 breaths/min, temperature is 37.4°C (99.2°F), and oxygen saturation is 93% on room air. His pulmonary examination shows decreased breath sounds at the apices with scattered expiratory wheezes. His cardiovascular examination demonstrates an S4 gallop with a hyperdynamic precordium. A regular tachycardia is present. Blood pressures are equal in both arms. Liver span is not enlarged. There are no palpable abdominal masses. What is the most likely cause of the patient's presentation?

A. Adenocarcinoma of the esophagus
B. Ascending aortic aneurysm
C. Esophageal stricture
D. Gastric cancer
E. Squamous cell carcinoma of the esophagus

113. A 64-year-old woman presents with complaints of a change in stool caliber for the past 2 months. The stools now have a diameter of only the size of her fifth digit. Over this same period, she feels she has to exert increasing strain to have a bowel movement and sometimes has associated abdominal cramping. She often has blood on the toilet paper when she wipes. During this time, she has lost about 20 lb. On physical examination, the patient appears cachectic with a body mass index of 22.5 kg/m^2. The abdomen is flat and nontender. The liver span is 12 cm to percussion. On digital rectal examination, a mass lesion is palpated approximately 8 cm into the rectum. A colonoscopy is attempted, which demonstrates a 2.5-cm sessile mass that narrows the colonic lumen. The biopsy confirms adenocarcinoma. The colonoscope is not able to traverse the mass. A CT scan of the abdomen does not show evidence of metastatic disease. Liver function test results are normal. A carcinoembryonic antigen level is 4.2 ng/mL. The patient is referred for surgery and undergoes rectosigmoidectomy with pelvic lymph node dissection. Final pathology demonstrates extension of the primary tumor into the muscularis propria but not the serosa. Of 15 lymph nodes removed, two are positive for tumor. What do you recommend for this patient after surgery?

113. *(Continued)*

A. Chemotherapy with a regimen containing 5-fluorouracil
B. Complete colonoscopy within 3 months
C. Measurement of CEA levels at 3-month intervals
D. Radiation therapy to the pelvis
E. All of the above

114. A healthy 62-year-old woman returns to your clinic after undergoing routine colonoscopy. Findings included two 1.3-cm sessile (flat-based), villous adenomas in her ascending colon that were removed during the procedure. What is the next step in management?

A. Colonoscopy in 3 years
B. Colonoscopy in 10 years
C. CT scan of the abdomen
D. Partial colectomy
E. Reassurance

115. Which of the following should prompt investigation for hereditary nonpolyposis colon cancer screening in a 32-year-old man?

A. Father, paternal aunt, and paternal cousin with colon cancer with ages of diagnosis of 54, 68, and 37 years, respectively
B. Innumerable polyps visualized on routine colonoscopy
C. Mucocutaneous pigmentation
D. New diagnosis of ulcerative colitis
E. None of the above

116. All of the following statements regarding pancreatic cancer are true EXCEPT:

A. Alcohol consumption is not a risk factor for pancreatic cancer.
B. Cigarette smoking is a risk factor for pancreatic cancer.
C. Despite accounting for fewer than 5% of malignancies diagnosed in the United States, pancreatic cancer is the fourth leading cause of cancer death.
D. If detected early, the 5-year survival rate is up to 20%.
E. The 5-year survival rates for pancreatic cancer have improved substantially in the past decade.

117. A 65-year-old man is evaluated in clinic for 1 month of progressive painless jaundice and 10 lb of unintentional weight loss. His physical examination is unremarkable. A dual-phase contrast CT shows a suspicious mass in the head of the pancreas with biliary ductal dilation. Which of the following is the best diagnostic test to evaluate for suspected pancreatic cancer?

117. (*Continued*)
A. CT-guided percutaneous needle biopsy
B. Endoscopic ultrasound-guided needle biopsy
C. ERCP with pancreatic juice sampling for cytopathology
D. FDG-PET imaging
E. Serum CA 19-9

118. A 63-year-old man complains of notable pink-tinged urine for the past month. At first he thought it was caused by eating beets, but has not cleared. His medical history is notable for hypertension and cigarette smoking. He does report some worsening urinary frequency and hesitancy over the past 2 years. Physical examination is unremarkable. Urinalysis is notable for gross hematuria with no white blood cells or casts. Renal function is normal. Which of the following statements regarding this patient is true?

A. Cigarette smoking is not a risk for bladder cancer.
B. Gross hematuria makes prostate cancer more likely than bladder cancer.
C. If invasive bladder cancer with nodal involvement but no distant metastases is found, the 5-year rate survival is 20%.
D. If superficial bladder cancer is found, intravesicular BCG may be used as adjuvant therapy.
E. Radical cystectomy is generally recommended for invasive bladder cancer.

119. A 68-year-old man comes to his physician complaining of 2 months of increasing right flank pain with 1 month of worsening hematuria. He was treated for cystitis at a walk-in clinic 3 weeks ago with no improvement. He also reports poor appetite and 5 lb of weight loss. His physical examination is notable for a palpable mass in the right flank measuring >5 cm. His renal function is normal. All of the following are true about this patient's likely diagnosis EXCEPT:

A. Anemia is more common than erythrocytosis.
B. Cigarette smoking increased his risk.
C. If his disease has metastasized, with best therapy 5-year survival is >50%.
D. If his disease is confined to the kidney, the 5-year survival rate is >80%.
E. The most likely pathology is clear cell carcinoma.

120. In the patient described in question 119, imaging shows a 10-cm solid mass in the right kidney and multiple nodules in the lungs consistent with metastatic disease. Needle biopsy of a lung lesion confirms the diagnosis of renal cell carcinoma. Which of the following is recommended therapy?

120. (*Continued*)
A. Gemcitabine
B. Interferon-gamma
C. Interleukin-2
D. Radical nephrectomy
E. Sunitinib

121. Which of the following has been shown in randomized trials to reduce the future risk of pancreatic cancer diagnosis?

A. Finasteride
B. Selenium
C. Testosterone
D. Vitamin C
E. Vitamin E

122. A 54-year-old man is evaluated in an executive health program. On physical examination, he is noted to have an enlarged prostate with a right lobe nodule. He does not recall his last digital rectal examination and has never had prostate-specific antigen (PSA) tested. Based on this evaluation, which of the following is next recommended?

A. Bone scan to evaluate for metastasis
B. PSA
C. PSA now and in 3 months to measure PSA velocity
D. Repeat digital rectal examination in 3 months
E. Transrectal ultrasound-guided biopsy

123. Which of the following statements describes the relationship between testicular tumors and serum markers?

A. Pure seminomas produce α-fetoprotein (AFP) or beta human chorionic gonadotropin (β-hCG) in >90% of cases.
B. More than 40% of nonseminomatous germ cell tumors produce no cell markers.
C. Both β-hCG and AFP should be measured in following the progress of a tumor.
D. Measurement of tumor markers the day after surgery for localized disease is useful in determining the completeness of the resection.
E. β-hCG is limited in its usefulness as a marker because it is identical to human luteinizing hormone.

124. A 32-year-old man presents complaining of a testicular mass. On examination, you palpate a 1 cm × 2 cm painless mass on the surface of the left testicle. A chest x-ray shows no lesions, and a CT scan of the abdomen and pelvis shows no evidence of retroperitoneal adenopathy. The α-fetoprotein (AFP) level is elevated at 400 ng/mL. Beta human

124. (*Continued*)
chorionic gonadotropin (β-hCG) is normal, as is lactate dehydrogenase (LDH). You send the patient for an orchiectomy. The pathology comes back as seminoma limited to the testis alone. The AFP level declines to normal at an appropriate interval. What is the appropriate management at this point?

A. Radiation to the retroperitoneal lymph nodes
B. Adjuvant chemotherapy
C. Hormonal therapy
D. Retroperitoneal lymph node dissection (RPLND)
E. Positron emission tomography (PET) scan

125. Which of the following statements regarding the relationship between ovarian cancer and *BRCA* gene mutations is true?

A. Most women with *BRCA* mutations have a family history that is strongly positive for breast or ovarian cancer (or both).
B. More than 30% of women with ovarian cancer have a somatic mutation in either *BRCA1* or *BRCA2*.
C. Prophylactic oophorectomy in patients with *BRCA* mutations does not protect against the development of breast cancer.
D. Screening studies with serial ultrasound and serum CA-125 tumor marker studies are effective in detecting early stage disease.
E. Women with known mutations in a single *BRCA1* or *BRCA2* allele have a 75% lifetime risk of developing ovarian cancer.

126. All of the following statements regarding the diagnosis of uterine cancer are true EXCEPT:

A. The 5-year survival rate after surgery in disease confined to the corpus is approximately 90%.
B. Endometrial carcinoma is the most common gynecologic malignancy in the United States.
C. Most women present with amenorrhea.
D. Tamoxifen is associated with an increased risk of endometrial carcinoma.
E. Unopposed estrogen exposure is a risk factor for developing endometrial carcinoma.

127. A 73-year-old man presents to the clinic with 3 months of increasing back pain. He localizes the pain to the lumbar spine and states that the pain is worst at night while he is lying in bed. It is improved during the day with mobilization. Past history is notable only for hypertension and remote cigarette smoking. Physical examination is normal. Laboratory studies are notable for an elevated

127. (*Continued*)
alkaline phosphatase. A lumbar radiogram shows a lytic lesion in the L3 vertebra. Which of the following malignancies is most likely?

A. Gastric carcinoma
B. Non–small cell lung cancer
C. Osteosarcoma
D. Pancreatic carcinoma
E. Thyroid carcinoma

128. A primary tumor of which of these organs is the *least likely* to metastasize to bone?

A. Breast
B. Colon
C. Kidney
D. Lung
E. Prostate

129. A 22-year-old man comes into clinic because of a swollen leg. He does not remember any trauma to the leg, but the pain and swelling began 3 weeks ago in the anterior shin area of his left foot. He is a college student and is active in sports daily. A radiograph of the right leg shows a destructive lesion with a "moth-eaten" appearance extending into the soft tissue and a spiculated periosteal reaction. Codman's triangle (a cuff of periosteal bone formation at the margin of the bone and soft tissue mass) is present. Which of the following are the most likely diagnosis and optimal therapy for this lesion?

A. Chondrosarcoma; chemotherapy alone is curative
B. Chondrosarcoma; radiation with limited surgical resection
C. Osteosarcoma; preoperative chemotherapy followed by limb-sparing surgery
D. Osteosarcoma; radiation therapy
E. Plasma cell tumor; chemotherapy

130. A 42-year-old man presented to the hospital with right upper quadrant pain. He was found to have multiple masses in the liver that were found to be malignant on H&E staining of a biopsy sample. Your initial history, physical examination, and laboratory tests, including prostate-specific antigen, are unrevealing. Lung, abdominal, and pelvic CT scans are unremarkable. He is an otherwise healthy individual with no chronic medical problems. Which immunohistochemical markers should be obtained from the biopsy tissue?

A. α-Fetoprotein
B. Cytokeratin

130. (*Continued*)
C. Leukocyte common antigen
D. Thyroglobulin
E. Thyroid transcription factor 1

131. A 52-year-old woman is evaluated for abdominal swelling with a computed tomogram that shows ascites and likely peritoneal studding of tumor but no other abnormality. Paracentesis shows adenocarcinoma but cannot be further differentiated by the pathologist. A thorough physical examination, including breast and pelvic examination, shows no abnormality. CA-125 levels are elevated. Pelvic ultrasonography and mammography findings are normal. Which of the following statements is true?

A. Compared with other women with known ovarian cancer at a similar stage, this patient can be expected to have a less than average survival.
B. Debulking surgery is indicated.
C. Surgical debulking plus cisplatin and paclitaxel is indicated.
D. Bilateral mastectomy and bilateral oophorectomy will improve survival.
E. Fewer than 1% of patients with this disorder will remain disease free 2 years after treatment.

132. A 29-year-old man is found on routine chest radiography for life insurance to have left hilar adenopathy. CT scanning confirms enlarged left hilar and paraaortic nodes. He is otherwise healthy. Besides biopsy of the lymph nodes, which of the following is indicated?

A. Angiotensin-converting enzyme (ACE) level
B. β-hCG
C. Thyroid-stimulating hormone (TSH)
D. PSA
E. C-reactive protein

133. A 49-year-old man is admitted to the hospital with a seizure. He does not have a history of seizures and he currently takes no medications. He has AIDS and is not under any care at this time. His physical examination is most notable for small, shoddy lymphadenopathy in the cervical region. A head CT shows a ring-enhancing lesion in the right temporal lobe, with edema but no mass effect. A lumbar puncture shows no white or red blood cells, and the Gram stain is negative. His serum *Toxoplasma* IgG is positive. He is treated with pyrimethamine, sulfadiazine, and levetiracetam. After 2 weeks of therapy the central nervous system (CNS) lesion has not changed in size and he has not had any more seizures. All microbiologic cultures and viral studies, including Epstein-Barr virus DNA from the cerebrospinal fluid, are negative. What is the best course of action for this patient at this time?

A. Continue treatment for CNS toxoplasmosis
B. Dexamethasone
C. IV acyclovir
D. Stereotactic brain biopsy
E. Whole-brain radiation therapy

134. A young man with a history of a low-grade astrocytoma comes into your office complaining of weight gain and low energy. He is status post resection of his low-grade astrocytoma and had a course of whole-brain radiation therapy 1 year ago. A laboratory workup reveals a decreased morning cortisol level of 1.9 μg/dL. In addition to depressed adrenocorticotropic hormone function, which of the following hormones is most sensitive to damage from whole-brain radiation therapy?

A. Growth hormone
B. Follicle-stimulating hormone
C. Prolactin
D. Thyroid-stimulating hormone

135. A 37-year-old woman with a history of 6 months of worsening headache is admitted to the hospital after a tonic-clonic seizure that occurred at work. The seizure lasted a short time and terminated spontaneously. On examination, her vital signs are normal, she is somnolent but awake, and there are no focal abnormalities. Her initial CT scan showed no acute hemorrhage but was abnormal. An MRI is obtained and is shown in **Figure 135**. What is the most likely diagnosis in this patient?

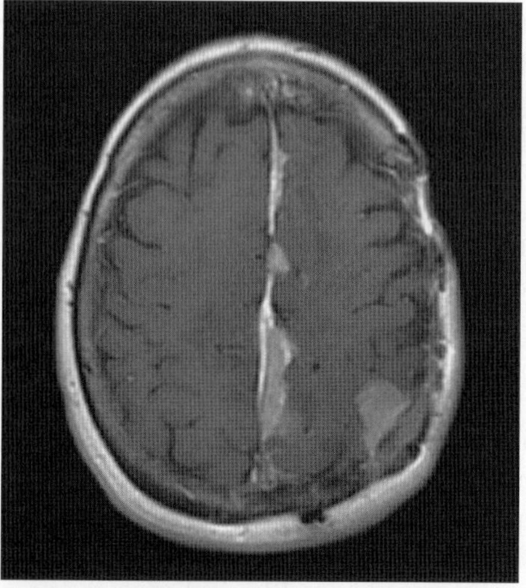

FIGURE 135

135. *(Continued)*
A. Brain abscess
B. Glioblastoma
C. Low-grade astrocytoma
D. Meningioma
E. Oligodendroglioma

136. A healthy 53-year-old man comes to your office for an annual physical examination. He has no complaints and has no significant medical history. He is taking an over-the-counter multivitamin and no other medicines. On physical examination he is noted to have a nontender thyroid nodule. His thyroid-stimulating hormone (TSH) level is checked and is found to be low. What is the next step in his evaluation?

A. Close follow-up and measure TSH in 6 months
B. Fine-needle aspiration
C. Low-dose thyroid replacement
D. Positron emission tomography followed by surgery
E. Radionuclide thyroid scan

137. All of the following statements regarding asymptomatic adrenal masses (incidentalomas) are true EXCEPT:

A. All patients with incidentalomas should be screened for pheochromocytoma.
B. Fine-needle aspiration may distinguish between benign and malignant primary adrenal tumors.
C. In patients with a history of malignancy, the likelihood that the mass is a metastasis is approximately 50%.
D. The majority of adrenal incidentalomas are nonsecretory.
E. The vast majority of adrenal incidentalomas are benign.

138. A 35-year-old man is seen in the emergency department for evaluation of epigastric pain, diarrhea, and reflux. He reports frequent similar episodes and has undergone multiple endoscopies. In each case he was told that he has a duodenal ulcer. He has become quite frustrated because he was told that ulcers are usually due to a bacteria that can be treated, but he does not have *Helicobacter pylori* present on any of his ulcer biopsies. His current medications are high-dose omeprazole and oxycodone/acetaminophen. He is admitted to the hospital for pain control. Which of the following is the most appropriate next step in his diagnostic evaluation?

A. CT scan of the abdomen.
B. Discontinue omeprazole for 1 week and measure plasma gastrin level.
C. Gastric pH measurement.
D. Plasma gastrin level.
E. Screen for parathyroid hyperplasia.

139. A 48-year-old female is undergoing evaluation for flushing and diarrhea. Physical examination is normal except for nodular hepatomegaly. A CT scan of the abdomen demonstrates multiple nodules in both lobes of the liver consistent with metastases in the liver and a 2-cm mass in the ileum. The 24-hour urinary 5-HIAA excretion is markedly elevated. All the following treatments are appropriate EXCEPT:

A. Diphenhydramine
B. Interferon α
C. Octreotide
D. Ondansetron
E. Phenoxybenzamine

140. While undergoing a physical examination during medical student clinical skills, the patient in question 139 develops severe flushing, wheezing, nausea, and lightheadedness. Vital signs are notable for a blood pressure of 70/30 mm Hg and a heart rate of 135 beats/min. Which of the following is the most appropriate therapy?

A. Albuterol
B. Atropine
C. Epinephrine
D. Hydrocortisone
E. Octreotide

141. A 49-year-old male is brought to the hospital by his family because of confusion and dehydration. The family reports that for the last 3 weeks he has had persistent copious, watery diarrhea that has not abated with the use of over-the-counter medications. The diarrhea has been unrelated to food intake and has persisted during fasting. The stool does not appear fatty and is not malodorous. The patient works as an attorney, is a vegetarian, and has not traveled recently. No one in the household has had similar symptoms. Before the onset of diarrhea, he had mild anorexia and a 5-lb weight loss. Since the diarrhea began, he has lost at least 5 kg. The physical examination is notable for blood pressure of 100/70 mm Hg, heart rate of 110 beats/min, and temperature of 36.8°C (98.2°F). Other than poor skin turgor, confusion, and diffuse muscle weakness, the physical examination is unremarkable. Laboratory studies are notable for a normal complete blood count and the following chemistry results:

141. (*Continued*)

Na^+	146 mEq/L
K^+	3.0 mEq/L
Cl^-	96 mEq/L
HCO_3^-	36 mEq/L
BUN	32 mg/dL
Creatinine	1.2 mg/dL

A 24-hour stool collection yields 3 L of tea-colored stool. Stool sodium is 50 meq/L, potassium is 25 mEq/L, and stool osmolality is 170 mosmol/L. Which of the following diagnostic tests is most likely to yield the correct diagnosis?

A. Serum cortisol
B. Serum TSH
C. Serum VIP
D. Urinary 5-HIAA
E. Urinary metanephrine

142. An 18-year-old girl is evaluated at her primary care physician's office for a routine physical. She is presently healthy. Her family history is notable for a father and two aunts with MEN 1, and the patient has undergone genetic testing and carries the *MEN 1 gene*. Which of the following is the first and most common presentation for individuals with this genetic mutation?

A. Peptic ulcer disease
B. Hypercalcemia
C. Hypoglycemia
D. Amenorrhea
E. Uncontrolled systemic hypertension

143. A 35-year-old man is referred to your clinic for evaluation of hypercalcemia noted during a health insurance medical screening. He has noted some fatigue, malaise, and a 4-lb weight loss over the past 2 months. He also has noted constipation and "heartburn." He is occasionally nauseated after large meals and has water brash and a sour taste in his mouth. The patient denies vomiting, dysphagia, or odynophagia. He also notes decreased libido and a depressed mood. Vital signs are unremarkable. Physical examination is notable for a clear oropharynx, no evidence of a thyroid mass, and no lymphadenopathy. Jugular venous pressure is normal. Heart sounds are regular with no murmurs or gallops. The chest is clear. The abdomen is soft with some mild epigastric tenderness. There is

143. (*Continued*)
no rebound or organomegaly. Stool is guaiac positive. Neurologic examination is nonfocal. Laboratory values are notable for a normal complete blood count. Calcium is 11.2 mg/dL, phosphate is 2.1 mg/dL, and magnesium is 1.8 meq/dL. Albumin is 3.7 g/dL, and total protein is 7.0 g/dL. TSH is 3 μIU/mL, prolactin is 250 μg/L, testosterone is 620 ng/dL, and serum insulin-like growth factor 1 (IGF-1) is normal. Serum intact parathyroid hormone level is 135 pg/dL. In light of the patient's abdominal discomfort and heme-positive stool, you perform an abdominal computed tomography (CT) scan that shows a lesion measuring 2 × 2 cm in the head of the pancreas. What is the diagnosis?

A. Multiple endocrine neoplasia (MEN) type 1
B. MEN type 2a
C. MEN type 2b
D. Polyglandular autoimmune syndrome
E. Von Hippel–Lindau (VHL) syndrome

144. A 43-year-old man with episodic, severe hypertension is referred for evaluation of possible secondary causes of hypertension. He reports feeling well generally, except for episodes of anxiety, palpitations, and tachycardia with elevation in his blood pressure during these episodes. Exercise often brings on these events. The patient also has mild depression and is presently taking sertraline, labetalol, amlodipine, and lisinopril to control his blood pressure. Urine 24-hour total metanephrines are ordered and show an elevation of 1.5 times the upper limit of normal. Which of the following is the next most appropriate step?

A. Hold labetalol for 1 week and repeat testing.
B. Hold sertraline for 1 week and repeat testing.
C. Immediately refer for surgical evaluation.
D. Measure 24-hour urine vanillymandelic acid level.
E. Send for MRI of the abdomen.

145. A 45-year-old man is diagnosed with pheochromocytoma after presentation with confusion, marked hypertension to 250/140 mm Hg, tachycardia, headaches, and flushing. His fractionated plasma metanephrines show a normetanephrine level of 560 pg/mL and a metanephrine level of 198 pg/mL (normal values: normetanephrine: 18–111 pg/mL; metanephrine: 12–60 pg/mL). CT scanning of the abdomen with IV contrast demonstrates a 3-cm mass in the right adrenal gland. A brain MRI with gadolinium shows edema of the white matter near the parietooccipital junction consistent with reversible

145. *(Continued)*
posterior leukoencephalopathy. You are asked to consult regarding management. Which of the following statements is true regarding management of pheochromocytoma is this individual?

A. Beta-blockade is absolutely contraindicated for tachycardia even after adequate alpha-blockade has been attained.
B. Immediate surgical removal of the mass is indicated, because the patient presented with hypertensive crisis with encephalopathy.
C. Salt and fluid intake should be restricted to prevent further exacerbation of the patient's hypertension.
D. Treatment with phenoxybenzamine should be started at a high dose (20–30 mg three times daily) to rapidly control blood pressure, and surgery can be undertaken within 24–48 hours.
E. Treatment with IV phentolamine is indicated for treatment of the hypertensive crisis. Phenoxybenzamine should be started at a low dose and titrated to the maximum tolerated dose over 2–3 weeks. Surgery should not be planned until the blood pressure is consistently below 160/100 mm Hg.

146. An 81-year-old man is admitted to the hospital for altered mental status. He was found at home, confused and lethargic, by his son. His medical history is significant for metastatic prostate cancer. The patient's medications include periodic intramuscular goserelin injections. On examination, he is afebrile. Blood pressure is 110/50 mm Hg, and the pulse rate is 110 beats/min. He is lethargic and minimally responsive to sternal rub. He has bitemporal wasting, and his mucous membranes are dry. On neurologic examination, he is obtunded. The patient has an intact gag reflex and withdraws to pain in all four extremities. Rectal tone is normal. Laboratory values are significant for a creatinine of 4.2 mg/dL, a calcium level of 14.4 mEq/L, and an albumin of 2.6 g/dL. All the following are appropriate initial management steps EXCEPT:

A. Normal saline
B. Pamidronate
C. Furosemide when the patient is euvolemic
D. Calcitonin
E. Dexamethasone

147. A 55-year-old man is found to have a serum calcium of 13.0 mg/dL after coming to clinic complaining of fatigue and thirst for the past month. A chest radiograph demonstrates a 4-cm mass in the right lower lobe. Which of the following serum tests is most likely to reveal the cause of his hypercalcemia?

147. *(Continued)*
A. Adrenocorticotropic hormone (ACTH)
B. Antidiuretic hormone (ADH)
C. Insulin-like growth factor
D. Parathyroid hormone (PTH)
E. Parathyroid hormone related protein (PTH-rp)

148. A 55-year-old woman presents with progressive incoordination. Physical examination is remarkable for nystagmus, mild dysarthria, and past pointing on finger-to-nose testing. She also has an unsteady gait. MRI reveals atrophy of both lobes of the cerebellum. Serologic evaluation reveals the presence of anti-Yo antibody. Which of the following is the most likely cause of this clinical syndrome?

A. Non–small cell cancer of the lung
B. Small cell cancer of the lung
C. Breast cancer
D. Non-Hodgkin's lymphoma
E. Colon cancer

149. A 58-year-old woman with known stage IV breast cancer presents to the emergency department with an inability to move her legs. She has had lower back pain for the past 4 days and has found it difficult to lie down. There is no radiating pain. Earlier today, the patient lost the ability to move either of her legs. In addition, she has been incontinent of urine recently. She has been diagnosed previously with metastatic disease to the lung and pleura from her breast cancer but was not known to have spinal or brain metastases. Her physical examination confirms absence of movement in the bilateral lower extremities associated with decreased to absent sensation below the umbilicus. There is increased tone and 3+ deep tendon reflexes in the lower extremities with crossed adduction. Anal sphincter tone is decreased, and the anal wink reflex is absent. What is the most important first step to take in the management of this patient?

A. Administer dexamethasone 10 mg intravenously.
B. Consult neurosurgery for emergent spinal decompression.
C. Consult radiation oncology for emergent spinal radiation.
D. Perform MRI of the brain.
E. Perform MRI of the entire spinal cord.

150. A 64-year-old man presents to the emergency department complaining of shortness of breath and facial swelling. He smokes 1 pack of cigarettes daily and has done so since the age of 16 years. On physical examination, he has dyspnea at an angle of 45 degrees or less. His vital signs are heart rate of 124

150. (*Continued*)
beats/min, blood pressure of 164/98 mm Hg, respiratory rate of 28 breaths/min, temperature of 37.6°C (99.6°F), and oxygen saturation of 89% on room air. Pulsus paradoxus is not present. His neck veins are dilated and do not collapse with inspiration. Collateral venous dilation is noted on the upper chest wall. There is facial edema and 1+ edema of the upper extremities bilaterally. Cyanosis is present. There is dullness to percussion and decreased breath sounds over the lower half of the right lung field. Given this clinical scenario, what would be the most likely finding on CT examination of the chest?

A. A central mass lesion obstructing the right mainstem bronchus
B. A large apical mass invading the chest wall and brachial plexus
C. A large pericardial effusion
D. A massive pleural effusion leading to opacification of the right hemithorax
E. Enlarged mediastinal lymph nodes causing obstruction of the superior vena cava

151. In the scenario in question 152, the initial therapy of this patient includes all of the following EXCEPT:

A. Administration of furosemide as needed to achieve diuresis
B. Elevation of the head of the bed to 45 degrees

151. (*Continued*)
C. Emergent radiation
D. Low-sodium diet
E. Oxygen

152. A 21-year-old man is treated with induction chemotherapy for acute lymphoblastic leukemia. His initial white blood cell count before treatment was 156,000/μL. All of the following are expected complications during his treatment EXCEPT:

A. Acute kidney injury
B. Hypercalcemia
C. Hyperkalemia
D. Hyperphosphatemia
E. Hyperuricemia

153. All of the following would be important for prevention of these complications EXCEPT:

A. Administration of allopurinol 300 mg/m^2 daily
B. Administration of intravenous fluids at a minimum of 3000 mL/m^2 daily
C. Alkalinization of the urine to a pH of >7.0 by administration of sodium bicarbonate
D. Frequent monitoring of serum chemistries every 4 hours
E. Prophylactic hemodialysis before initiating chemotherapy

ANSWERS

1. The answers are 1—C, 2—E, 3—D, 4—A, and 5—B.
(Chap. 6) Patients with homozygous sickle cell disease have red blood cells (RBCs) that are less pliable and more "sticky" than normal RBCs. Vaso-occlusive crisis is often precipitated by infection, fever, excessive exercise, anxiety, abrupt changes in temperature, hypoxia, or hypertonic dyes. Peripheral blood smear will show the typical elongated, crescent-shaped RBCs. There is also a nucleated RBC at the bottom of the figure, which may occur attributable to increased bone marrow production. Howell-Jolly bodies, small nuclear remnants normally removed by the intact spleen, are seen in RBCs in patients after splenectomy and with maturation or dysplastic disorders characterized by excess production. Acanthocytes are contracted dense RBCs with irregular membrane projections that vary in width and length. They are seen in patients with severe liver disease and abetalipoproteinemia and in rare patients with McLeod blood group. Iron deficiency, often caused by chronic stool blood loss in patients with colonic polyps or adenocarcinoma, causes a hypochromic microcytic anemia characterized by small, pale RBCs (a small lymphocyte is present on the smear to assess RBC size). RBCs are never hyperchromic; if more than the normal amount of hemoglobin is made, the cells get larger, not darker. Fragmented RBCs, or schistocytes, are helmet-shaped cells that reflect microangiopathic hemolytic anemia (e.g., thrombotic thrombocytopenic purpura, disseminated intravascular coagulation, hemolytic uremic syndrome, scleroderma crisis) or shear damage from a prosthetic heart valve.

2. The answer is A.
(Chap. 2) This patient with anemia demonstrates a low mean cell volume, low mean cell hemoglobin, and low mean cell hemoglobin concentration. The peripheral smear demonstrates microcytic and hypochromic cells, which would be expected given these laboratory findings. In addition, there is marked variation in size

(anisocytosis) and shape (poikilocytosis). These findings are consistent with severe iron-deficiency anemia, and serum ferritin would be expected to be <10 to 15 μg/L. A low haptoglobin level would be seen in cases of hemolysis, which can be intravascular or extravascular in origin. In intravascular hemolysis, the peripheral smear would be expected to show poikilocytosis with the presence of schistocytes (fragmented red blood cells [RBCs]). In extravascular hemolysis, the peripheral smear would typically shows spherocytes. Hemoglobin electrophoresis is used to determine the presence of abnormal hemoglobin variants. Sickle cell anemia is the most common form and demonstrates sickled RBCs. Thalassemias are also common inherited hemoglobinopathies. The peripheral smear in thalassemia often shows target cells. Glucose-6-phosphate dehydrogenase deficiency leads to oxidant-induced hemolysis with presence of bite cells or blister cells. Vitamin B_{12} deficiency leads to macrocytosis, which is not consistent with this case.

3. The answer is C.

(Chap. 2) The reticulocyte index and reticulocyte production index are useful in the evaluation of anemia to determine the adequacy of bone marrow response to the anemia. A normal reticulocyte count is 1–2%, and in the presence of anemia, this would be expected to rise to more than two to three times the normal value (the reticulocyte index). The reticulocyte index is calculated as Reticulocyte count × (Patient's hemoglobin/Normal hemoglobin). In this case, the reticulocyte index would be 5.4%. A second correction is further necessary in this patient given the presence of polychromatophilic macrocytes on peripheral smear. This finding indicates premature release of reticulocytes from the bone marrow ("shift cells"), and thus these cells have a longer life span. It is recommended to further divide the reticulocyte index by a factor of 2, which is known as the reticulocyte production index. In this case, the value would be 2.7%.

4. The answer is C.

(Chap. 2) This blood smear shows fragmented red blood cells (RBCs) of varying size and shape. In the presence of a foreign body within the circulation (prosthetic heart valve, vascular graft), RBCs can become destroyed. Such intravascular hemolysis will also cause serum lactate dehydrogenase to be elevated and hemoglobinuria. In isolated extravascular hemolysis, there is no hemoglobin or hemosiderin released into the urine. The characteristic peripheral blood smear in splenomegaly is the presence of Howell-Jolly bodies (nuclear remnants within red blood cells). Certain diseases are associated with extramedullary hematopoiesis (e.g., chronic hemolytic anemias), which can be detected by an enlarged spleen, thickened calvarium, myelofibrosis, or hepatomegaly. The peripheral blood smear may show teardrop cells or nucleated RBCs. Hypothyroidism is associated with macrocytosis, which is not demonstrated here. Chronic gastrointestinal blood loss will cause microcytosis, not schistocytes.

5. The answer is E.

(Chap. 3) von Willebrand disease (VWD) is an inherited disorder of platelet adhesion that has several types. The most common type is inherited in an autosomal dominant fashion and is associated with low levels of qualitatively normal von Willebrand factor. As a disorder primary hemostasis associated with the development of a platelet plug, VWD is primarily associated with mucosal bleeding. General bleeding symptoms that are more common in VWD include prolonged bleeding after surgery or dental procedures, menorrhagia, postpartum hemorrhage, and large bruises. However, easy bruising and menorrhagia are common complaints and are not specific for VWD in isolation. Factors that raise concern for VWD in women with menstrual symptoms include iron-deficiency anemia, need for blood transfusion, passage of clots >1 inch in diameter, and need to change a pad or tampon more than hourly. Epistaxis is also a very common occurrence in the general population, but it is the most common complaint of males with VWD. Concerning features of epistaxis that may be more likely to indicate an underlying bleeding diathesis are lack of seasonal variation and bleeding that requires medical attention. Although most gastrointestinal bleeding in individuals with VWD is unrelated to the bleeding diathesis, VWD types 2 and 3 are associated with angiodysplasia of the bowel and gastrointestinal bleeding. Spontaneous hemarthroses or deep muscle hematomas are seen in clotting factor deficiencies and not seen VWD except severe VWD with associated decreased factor VIII levels <5%.

6. The answer is B.

(Chap. 3) The activated partial thromboplastin time (aPTT) measures the integrity of the intrinsic and common coagulation pathways, and as such, is affected by all of the coagulation factors, except factor VII. The aPTT reagent contains phospholipids derived from animal or vegetable sources and includes an activator of the intrinsic coagulation system, such as nonparticulate ellagic acid or kaolin. The phospholipid reagent frequently varies from laboratory to laboratory. Thus, an aPTT measured in one hospital may differ from another. Isolated elevations in the aPTT can be related to factor deficiencies, heparin or direct thrombin inhibitors, lupus anticoagulant, or the presence of a specific factor inhibitor. To differentiate between the presence of factor deficiencies and inhibitors, mixing studies should be performed. Mixing studies are performed by mixing normal plasma and the patient's plasma in a 1:1 ratio. The aPTT and prothrombin time (PT) are incubated at

37°C, and levels are measured immediately and serially thereafter for about 2 hours. If the cause is an isolated factor deficiency, the aPTT should correct to normal values and remain normal throughout the incubation period. In the presence of an acquired inhibitor, the aPTT may or may not correct immediately, but upon incubation, the inhibitor becomes more active, and the aPTT will progressively prolong. In contrast, the aPTT does not correct immediately or with incubation in the presence of lupus anticoagulants. The presence of serious bleeding in the presence of mixing studies suggesting an inhibitor should further rule out lupus anticoagulant as a cause because the lupus anticoagulant typically presents with no symptoms or as a thrombotic disorder. The mixing studies do not, however, eliminate the presence of heparin as a cause of the prolonged aPTT. If heparin were present, the thrombin time, but not the reptilase time, would be prolonged. In this scenario, both values were normal, ruling out the presence of heparin or a direct thrombin inhibitor. Likewise, disseminated intravascular coagulation can be ruled out in the presence of normal fibrinogen levels. In serious vitamin K deficiency, both the PT and aPTT should be prolonged.

7. The answer is E.

(Chap. 4) Lymphadenopathy has many causes, including infections, immunologic diseases, and malignancy among others. In the vast majority of cases, the cause of enlarged lymph nodes is a benign process. In the primary care practice, fewer than 1% of individuals will have malignancy, and in individuals referred for lymphadenopathy, this number rises only to 16%. Some features on history and physical examination lead to an increased likelihood that the cause of lymphadenopathy is infectious. Fevers and chills are more commonly present in benign respiratory illness but can be present in malignancy. Thus, fever is a nonspecific symptom. Likewise, generalized versus focal lymphadenopathy is also not specific. The site of lymph node enlargement can be important and raise the risk of malignancy. The presence of supraclavicular lymphadenopathy is never normal. These lymph nodes drain the thoracic cavity and retroperitoneal space and are most commonly enlarged in malignancy. However, infectious etiologies can also cause supraclavicular lymphadenopathy. The size and texture of the lymph nodes also provide important information. Nodes <1.0 cm × 1.0 cm are almost always benign, but lymph nodes >2.0 cm in maximum diameter or with an area of 2.25 cm^2 (1.5 × 1.5 cm) are more likely to be malignant. Nodes containing metastatic cancer tend to be described as hard, fixed, and nontender. In lymphoma, however, the nodes can be tender because of rapid enlargement of the node with subsequent stretching of the capsule of the lymph nodes. Lymphomatous nodes are also frequently described as firm, rubbery, and mobile.

8. The answer is F.

(Chap. 4) This patient's lymphadenopathy is benign. Inguinal nodes smaller than 2 cm are common in the population at large and need no further workup provided that there is no other evidence of disseminated infection or tumor and that the nodes have qualities that do not suggest tumor (not hard or matted). A practical approach would be to measure the nodes or even photograph them if visible and follow them serially over time. Occasionally, inguinal lymph nodes can be associated with sexually transmitted diseases. However, these are usually ipsilateral and tender, and evaluation includes bimanual examination and appropriate cultures, not necessarily pelvic ultrasonography. A total-body CT scan would be indicated if other pathologic nodes suggestive of lymphoma or granulomatous disease are present in other anatomic locations. Bone marrow biopsy would be indicated only if a diagnosis of lymphoma is made first.

9. The answer is C.

(Chap. 4) Portal hypertension causes splenomegaly via passive congestion of the spleen. It generally causes only mild enlargement of the spleen because expanded varices provide some decompression for elevated portal pressures. Myelofibrosis necessitates extramedullary hematopoiesis in the spleen, liver, and even other sites such as the peritoneum, leading to massive splenomegaly caused by myeloid hyperproduction. Autoimmune hemolytic anemia requires the spleen to dispose of massive amounts of damaged red blood cells, leading to reticuloendothelial hyperplasia and frequently an extremely large spleen. Chronic myeloid leukemia and other leukemias and lymphomas can lead to massive splenomegaly caused by infiltration with an abnormal clone of cells. Marginal zone lymphoma typically presents with splenomegaly. If a patient with cirrhosis or right heart failure has massive splenomegaly, a cause other than passive congestion should be considered.

10. The answer is A.

(Chap. 4) The presence of Howell-Jolly bodies (nuclear remnants), Heinz bodies (denatured hemoglobin), basophilic stippling, and nucleated red blood cells (RBCs) in the peripheral blood implies that the spleen is not properly clearing senescent or damaged RBCs from the circulation. This usually occurs because of surgical splenectomy but is also possible when there is diffuse infiltration of the spleen with malignant cells. Hemolytic anemia can have various peripheral smear findings depending on the etiology of the hemolysis. Spherocytes and bite cells are an example of damaged RBCs that might appear because of autoimmune hemolytic anemia and oxidative damage, respectively. Disseminated intravascular coagulation is characterized by schistocytes and thrombocytopenia on smear with an elevated international normalized ratio

and activated partial thromboplastin time as well. However, in these conditions, damaged RBCs are still cleared effectively by the spleen. Transformation to acute leukemia does not lead to splenic damage.

11. The answer is A.

(Chap. 4) Splenectomy leads to an increased risk of overwhelming postsplenectomy sepsis, an infection that carries an extremely high mortality rate. The most commonly implicated organisms are encapsulated. *Streptococcus pneumoniae*, *Haemophilus influenzae*, and sometime gram-negative enteric organisms are most frequently isolated. There is no known increased risk for any viral infections. Vaccination for *S. pneumoniae*, *H. influenzae*, and *Neisseria meningitidis* is indicated for any patient who may undergo splenectomy. The vaccines should be given at least 2 weeks before surgery. The highest risk of sepsis occurs in patients younger than 20 years of age because the spleen is responsible for first-pass immunity, and younger patients are more likely to have primary exposure to implicated organisms. The risk is highest during the first 3 years after splenectomy and persists at a lower rate until death.

12. The answer is E.

(Chap. 5) Chronic granulomatous disease (CGD) is an inherited disorder of abnormal phagocyte function. Seventy percent of cases are inherited in an X-linked fashion with the other 30% being autosomal recessive. Affected individuals are susceptible to infectious with catalase-positive organisms, especially *Staphylococcus aureus*. Other organisms that can be seen include *Burkholderia cepacia*, *Aspergillus* spp., and *Chromobacterium violaceum*. Most individuals present in childhood, and infections commonly affect the skin, ears, lungs, liver, and bone. Excessive inflammatory reaction can lead to suppuration of lymph nodes, and granulomatous inflammation can be seen on lymph node biopsy and found in the gastrointestinal and genitourinary tracts. Aphthous ulcers and eczematous skin rash can also be seen. The underlying genetic defect in CGD is the inability of neutrophils and monocytes to generate the appropriate oxidative burst in response to infectious organisms. Several mutations can lead to the disease, and these affect one of the five subunits of the NADPH (nicotinamide adenine dinucleotide phosphate) oxidase enzyme. The test of choice to diagnose chronic granulomatous disease is the nitroblue tetrazolium dye test, which demonstrates lack of superoxide and hydrogen peroxide production in the face of an appropriate stimulus.

13. The answer is A.

(Chap. 5) Under normal or nonstress conditions, roughly 90% of the neutrophil pool is in the bone marrow, 2–3% in the circulation, and the remainder in the tissues. The circulating pool includes the freely flowing cells in the bloodstream and the others are marginated in close proximity to the endothelium. Most of the marginated pool is in the lung, which has a vascular endothelium surface area. Margination in the postcapillary venules is mediated by selectins that cause a low-affinity neutrophil–endothelial cell interaction that mediates "rolling" of the neutrophils along the endothelium. A variety of signals, including interleukin 1, tumor necrosis factor α, and other chemokines, can cause leukocytes to proliferate and leave the bone marrow and enter the circulation. Neutrophil integrins mediate the stickiness of neutrophils to endothelium and are important for chemokine-induced cell activation. Infection causes a marked increase in bone marrow production of neutrophils that marginate and enter tissue. Acute glucocorticoids increase neutrophil count by mobilizing cells from the bone marrow and marginated pool.

14. The answer is E.

(Chap. 5) Many drugs can lead to neutropenia, most commonly via retarding neutrophil production in the bone marrow. Of the list in the answer choices, trimethoprim–sulfamethoxazole is the most likely culprit. Other common causes of drug-induced neutropenia include alkylating agents such as cyclophosphamide or busulfan, antimetabolites including methotrexate and 5-flucytosine, penicillin and sulfonamide antibiotics, antithyroid drugs, antipsychotics, and anti-inflammatory agents. Prednisone, when used systemically, often causes an increase in the circulating neutrophil count because it leads to demargination of neutrophils and bone marrow stimulation. Ranitidine, an H_2 blocker, is a well-described cause of thrombocytopenia but has not been implicated in neutropenia. Efavirenz is a nonnucleoside reverse transcriptase inhibitor whose main side effects include a morbilliform rash and central nervous system effects, including strange dreams and confusion. The presence of these symptoms does not require drug cessation. Darunavir is a new protease inhibitor that is well tolerated. Common side effects include a maculopapular rash and lipodystrophy, a class effect for all protease inhibitors.

15. The answer is D.

(Chap. 7) Iron-deficiency anemia is a condition consisting of anemia and clear evidence of iron deficiency. It is one of the most prevalent forms of malnutrition. Globally, 50% of anemia is attributable to iron deficiency and accounts for approximately 841,000 deaths annually worldwide. Africa and parts of Asia bear 71% of the global mortality burden; North America represents only 1.4% of the total morbidity and mortality associated with iron deficiency. Initially, a state of negative iron balance occurs during which iron stores become slowly depleted. Serum ferritin may decrease, and the presence of stainable iron on bone marrow preparation decreases. When

iron stores are depleted, serum iron begins to fall. Total iron-binding capacity (TIBC) starts to increase, reflecting the presence of circulating unbound transferrin. When the transferrin saturation falls to 15–20%, hemoglobin synthesis is impaired. The peripheral blood smear reveals the presence of microcytic and hypochromic red blood cells. Reticulocytes may also become hypochromic. Reticulocyte numbers are reduced relative to the level of anemia, reflecting a hypoproduction anemia secondary to iron deficiency. Clinically, these patients exhibit the usual signs of anemia, which are fatigue, pallor, and reduced exercise capacity. Cheilosis and koilonychia are signs of advanced tissue iron deficiency. Some patients may experience pica, a desire to ingest certain materials, such as ice (pagophagia) and clay (geophagia).

16. The answer is C.

(Chap. 7) (See Table 7-4.) The differential diagnosis of microcytic anemia includes iron deficiency, hemoglobinopathy (e.g., thalassemia), myelodysplastic syndromes (including sideroblastic anemia), and chronic inflammation. Inflammation can be distinguished from iron deficiency because iron deficiency typically includes a very low ferritin level (<50 μg/L) and iron binding saturation, but in inflammation, they are normal or increased. Any chronic inflammatory state may cause a hypoproliferative anemia caused by inadequate marrow utilization of iron related to hyperproduction of a number of cytokines, including tumor necrosis factor, interferon-gamma, and interleukin-1. The anemia of chronic disease may be normocytic/normochromic or microcytic. Serum iron and iron binding are normal to high in thalassemia and sideroblastic anemia. Folate deficiency causes macrocytic anemia.

17. The answer is C.

(Chap. 7) Progressive chronic kidney disease (CKD) is usually associated with a moderate to severe hypoproliferative anemia. The level of the anemia correlates with the stage of CKD. Red blood cells (RBCs) are typically normocytic and normochromic, and reticulocytes are decreased. The anemia is primarily caused by a failure of erythropoietin (EPO) production by the diseased kidney and a reduction in RBC survival. Polycystic kidney disease shows a smaller degree of EPO deficiency for a given level of renal failure. By contrast, patients with diabetes or myeloma have more severe EPO deficiency for a given level of renal failure. Assessment of iron status provides information to distinguish the anemia of CKD from other forms of hypoproliferative anemia and to guide management. Patients with the anemia of CKD usually present with normal serum iron, total iron-binding capacity, and ferritin levels. However, those maintained on chronic hemodialysis may develop iron deficiency from blood loss through the dialysis procedure. EPO therapy is effective in correcting the anemia of CKD. Iron must be replenished in patients with concomitant iron deficiency to ensure an adequate response to EPO therapy.

18. The answer is B.

(Chap. 8, MM Hsieh et al: N Engl J Med *2009;361:2309–2317)* The most significant recent advance in the therapy of sickle cell anemia has been the introduction of hydroxyurea as a mainstay of therapy for patients with severe symptoms. Hydroxyurea increases fetal hemoglobin and may exert beneficial effects on red blood cell (RBC) hydration, vascular wall adherence, and suppression of the granulocyte and reticulocyte counts. Hemoglobin F levels increase in most patients within a few months. Hydroxyurea should be considered in patients experiencing repeated episodes of acute chest syndrome or with more than three crises per year requiring hospitalization. The utility of this agent for reducing the incidence of other complications (priapism, retinopathy) is under evaluation, as are the long-term side effects. Hydroxyurea offers broad benefits to most patients whose disease is severe enough to impair their functional status, and it may improve survival. The main adverse effect is a reduction in white blood cell (WBC) count; dosage should be titrated to maintain a WBC count at 5000 to 8000/μL. WBCs and reticulocytes may play a major role in the pathogenesis of sickle cell crisis, and their suppression may be an important benefit of hydroxyurea therapy. A recent study demonstrated that nonmyeloablative bone marrow transplantation in patients with sickle cell disease could produce a stable chimera that corrected RBC counts and reversed the sickle cell phenotype.

19. The answer is B.

(Chap. 9) Serum cobalamin is measured by an enzyme-linked immunosorbent assay test and is the most cost-effective test to rule out deficiency. Normal serum levels are typically above 200 ng/L. In patients with megaloblastic anemia caused by cobalamin deficiency, the level is usually <100 ng/L. In general, the more severe the deficiency, the lower the serum cobalamin level. In patients with spinal cord damage caused by the deficiency, levels are very low even in the absence of anemia. Borderline low levels may occur in pregnancy in patients with megaloblastic anemia caused by folate deficiency. In patients with cobalamin deficiency sufficient to cause anemia or neuropathy, the serum methylmalonate (MMA) level is increased. Serum MMA and homocysteine levels have been proposed for the early diagnosis of cobalamin deficiency even in the absence of hematologic abnormalities or subnormal levels of serum cobalamin. Serum MMA levels fluctuate, however, in patients with renal failure. Mildly elevated serum MMA or homocysteine levels occur in up to 30% of apparently healthy volunteers and 15% of elderly subjects. These findings bring into question the exact cutoff points for

normal MMA and homocysteine levels. It is also unclear at present whether these mildly increased metabolite levels have clinical consequences. Serum homocysteine is increased in both early cobalamin and folate deficiency but may also be increased in other conditions (e.g., chronic renal disease; alcoholism; smoking; pyridoxine deficiency; hypothyroidism; and therapy with steroids, cyclosporine, and other drugs). The red blood cell folate assay is a test of body folate stores. It is less affected than the serum assay by recent diet and traces of hemolysis. Subnormal levels occur in patients with megaloblastic anemia caused by folate deficiency but also in nearly two-thirds of patients with severe cobalamin deficiency. False-normal results may occur if a folate-deficient patient has received a recent blood transfusion or if a patient has an increased reticulocyte count. Serum pepsinogen may be low in patients with pernicious anemia.

20. The answer is C.

(Chap. 9) The peripheral blood smear shows hypochromasia, macrocytosis, and a hypersegmented (>five lobes) neutrophil. These findings are typical for a megaloblastic anemia as seen in cobalamin or folate deficiency. The mean corpuscular volume is typically >100 fL, and there is significant anisocytosis and poikilocytosis. There may also be leukopenia and thrombocytopenia that correlate with the degree of deficiency. Other less common causes of megaloblastic anemia include therapy with drugs that interfere with folate metabolism (methotrexate) or DNA synthesis (hydroxyurea, AZT, cytosine arabinoside, 6-mercaptopurine) and some cases of acute myeloblastic leukemia or myelodysplasia. Autoantibodies to ADAMTS-13 are associated with thrombotic thrombocytopenic purpura, which causes a microangiopathic hemolytic anemia. Epstein-Barr virus infection is associated with large atypical lymphocytes, not hypersegmented neutrophils. Iron-deficiency anemia causes a microcytic hypochromic anemia.

21. The answer is B.

(Chap. 10) Red blood cells (RBCs) use glutathione produced by the hexose monophosphate shunt to compensate for increased production of reactive oxygen species (oxidant stress), usually induced by drugs or toxins. Defects in glucose-6-phosphate dehydrogenase (G6PD) are the most common congenital hexose monophosphate shunt defect. If the RBC is unable to maintain an adequate level of glutathione during oxidant stress, hemoglobin precipitates in the RBC, producing Heinz bodies. Because the G6PD gene is on the X chromosome, almost all affected patients are males. G6PD deficiency is widely distributed throughout regions that are currently or were once highly malarial endemic. It is common in males of African, African American, Sardinian, and Sephardic descent. In most persons with G6PD deficiency, there is no evidence of symptomatic disease. However, infection, ingestion of fava beans, or exposure to an oxidative agent (drug or toxin) can trigger an acute hemolytic event. Bite cells, Heinz bodies, and bizarre poikilocytes may be evident on smear. The drugs that most commonly precipitate a G6PD crisis include dapsone, sulfamethoxazole, primaquine, and nitrofurantoin. The anemia is often severe with rapid onset after drug ingestion, and renal failure can occur.

22. The answer is B.

(Chap. 10) This patient's lupus and her rapid development of truly life-threatening hemolytic anemia are both very suggestive of autoimmune hemolytic anemia. Diagnosis is made by a positive Coombs test result documenting antibodies to the red cell membrane, but smear will often show microspherocytes, indicative of the damage incurred to the red cells in the spleen. Schistocytes are typical for microangiopathic hemolytic anemias such as hemolytic uremic syndrome or thrombotic thrombocytopenic purpura. The lack of thrombocytopenia makes these diagnoses considerably less plausible. Macrocytosis and polymorphonuclear leukocytes with hypersegmented nuclei are very suggestive of vitamin B_{12} deficiency, which causes more chronic, non–life-threatening anemia. Target cells are seen in liver disease and thalassemias. Sickle cell anemia is associated with aplastic crises, but this patient has no known diagnosis of sickle cell disease and is showing evidence of erythropoietin response based on the presence of elevated reticulocyte count.

23. The answer is C.

(Chap. 10) The peripheral blood smear shows microspherocytes, small densely staining red blood cells (RBCs) that have lost their central pallor characteristic of hereditary spherocytosis. Spherocytosis is almost the only condition with an increased mean corpuscular hemoglobin concentration. Hereditary spherocytosis is a heterogeneous RBC membranopathy that can be either congenital (usually autosomal dominant) or acquired; it is characterized by predominantly extravascular hemolysis in the spleen caused by defects in membrane structural proteins. This spleen-mediated hemolysis leads to the conversion of classic biconcave RBCs on smear to spherocytes. Splenomegaly is common. This disorder can be severe, depending on the site of mutation, but is often overlooked until some stressor such as pregnancy leads to a multifactorial anemia, or an infection such as parvovirus B19 transiently eliminates RBC production altogether. Acute treatment is with transfusion. Glucose-6-phosphate dehydrogenase (G6PD) deficiency is a cause of hemolysis that is usually triggered by the presence of an offending oxidative agent. The peripheral blood smear may show Heinz bodies. Parvovirus infection may cause a pure RBC aplasia. The presence of active reticulocytosis and laboratory findings consistent

with hemolysis are not compatible with that diagnosis. Chronic gastrointestinal blood loss, such as caused by a colonic polyp, would cause a microcytic, hypochromic anemia without evidence of hemolysis (indirect bilirubin, haptoglobin abnormalities).

24. The answer is D.

(Chap. 10) Each of the listed diagnoses has a rather characteristic set of laboratory findings that are virtually diagnostic for the disease once the disease has progressed to a severe stage. The combination of portal vein thrombosis, hemolysis, and pancytopenia is typical for paroxysmal nocturnal hemoglobinuria (PNH). PNH is a rare disorder characterized by hemolytic anemia (particularly at night), venous thrombosis, and deficient hematopoiesis. It is a stem cell–derived intracorpuscular defect. Anemia is usually moderate in severity, and there is often concomitant granulocytopenia and thrombocytopenia. Venous thrombosis occurs much more commonly than in the population at large. The intraabdominal veins are often involved, and patients may present with Budd-Chiari syndrome. Cerebral sinus thrombosis is a common cause of death in patients with PNH. The presence of pancytopenia and hemolysis should raise suspicion for this diagnosis even before the development of a venous thrombosis. In the past, PNH was diagnosed by abnormalities on the Ham or sucrose lysis test; however, currently flow cytometry analysis of glycosylphosphatidylinositol (GPI) linked proteins (e.g., CD55 and CD59) on red blood cells and granulocytes is recommended. Hemolytic uremic syndrome (HUS) and thrombotic thrombocytopenic purpura (TTP) both cause hemolysis and thrombocytopenia, as well as fevers. Cerebrovascular events and mental status change occur more commonly in TTP, and renal failure is more common in HUS. Severe leptospirosis, or Weil's disease, is notable for fevers, hyperbilirubinemia, and renal failure. Conjunctival suffusion is another helpful clue. Acute promyelocytic leukemia is notable for anemia, thrombocytopenia, and either elevated or a decreased white blood cell count, all in the presence of disseminated intravascular coagulation.

25. The answer is A.

(Chap. 10) Haptoglobin is an α-globulin normally present in serum. It binds specifically to the globin portion of hemoglobin, and the complex is cleared by the mononuclear cell phagocytosis. Haptoglobin is reduced in all hemolytic anemias because it binds free hemoglobin. It can also be reduced in cirrhosis and so is not diagnostic of hemolysis outside of the correct clinical context. Assuming normal bone marrow and iron stores, the reticulocyte count will be elevated as well to try to compensate for the increased red blood cell (RBC) destruction of hemolysis. Release of intracellular contents from the RBC (including hemoglobin and lactate dehydrogenase) induces heme metabolism, producing unconjugated bilirubinemia. If the haptoglobin system is overwhelmed, the kidney will filter free hemoglobin and reabsorb it in the proximal tubule for storage of iron by ferritin and hemosiderin. Hemosiderin in the urine is a marker of filtered hemoglobin by the kidneys. In massive hemolysis, free hemoglobin may be excreted in urine.

26. The answer is E.

(Chap. 10) Hemolytic anemias may be classified as intracorpuscular or extracorpuscular. In intracorpuscular disorders, the patient's red blood cells (RBCs) have an abnormally short life span because of an intrinsic RBC factor. In extracorpuscular disorders, the RBC has a short life span because of a nonintrinsic RBC factor. Thrombotic thrombocytopenic purpura (TTP) is an acquired disorder in which red blood cell and platelet destruction occur not because of defects of these cell lines but rather as a result of microangiopathy leading to destructive shear forces on the cells. Other clinical signs and symptoms include fever; mental status change; and, less commonly, renal impairment. Most acquired adult cases of TTP are associated with autoantibodies to ADAMTS-13 (or von Willebrand factor–cleaving protease). All cases of hemolysis in conjunction with thrombocytopenia should be rapidly ruled out for TTP by evaluation of a peripheral smear for schistocytes because plasmapheresis is lifesaving. Other causes of extravascular hemolytic anemia include hypersplenism, autoimmune hemolytic anemia, disseminated intravascular coagulation, and other microangiopathic hemolytic anemias. The other four disorders listed in the question all refer to some defect of the RBC itself that leads to hemolysis. Elliptocytosis is a membranopathy that leads to varying degrees of destruction of the RBC in the reticuloendothelial system. Sickle cell anemia is a congenital hemoglobinopathy classified by recurrent pain crises and numerous long-term sequelae that is caused by a well-defined β-globin mutation. Pyruvate kinase deficiency is a rare disorder of the glycolytic pathway that causes hemolytic anemia. Paroxysmal nocturnal hemoglobinuria (PNH) is a form of acquired hemolysis caused by an intrinsic abnormality of the RBCs. It also often causes thrombosis and cytopenias. Bone marrow failure is a feared association with PNH.

27. The answer is C.

(Chap. 11) Pure red blood cell aplasia (PRCA) is a condition characterized by the absence of reticulocytes and erythroid precursors. A variety of conditions may cause PRCA. It may be idiopathic. It may be associated with certain medications, such as trimethoprim–sulfamethoxazole (TMP-SMX) and phenytoin. It can be associated with a variety of neoplasms, either as a precursor to a hematologic malignancy such as leukemia or myelodysplasia or as part of an autoimmune phenomenon,

as in the case of thymoma. Infections also may cause PRCA. Parvovirus B19 is a single-strand DNA virus that is associated with erythema infectiosum, or fifth disease in children. It is also associated with arthropathy and a flulike illness in adults. It is thought to attack the P antigen on proerythroblasts directly. Patients with a chronic hemolytic anemia, such as sickle cell disease, or with an immunodeficiency are less able to tolerate a transient drop in reticulocytes because their red blood cells do not survive in the peripheral blood for an adequate period. In this patient, her daughter had an illness before the appearance of her symptoms. It is reasonable to check her parvovirus immunoglobulin M (IgM) titers. If the results are positive, a dose of intravenous Ig is indicated. Because her laboratory test results and smear are not suggestive of dramatic sickling, an exchange transfusion is not indicated. Immunosuppression with prednisone, cyclosporine, or both may be indicated if another etiology of the PRCA is identified. However, that would not be the next step. Similarly, a bone marrow transplant might be a consideration in a young patient with myelodysplasia or leukemia, but there is no evidence of that at this time. Antibiotics have no role in light of her normal white blood cell count and the lack of evidence for a bacterial infection.

28. The answer is D.

(Chap. 11) Aplastic anemia is defined as pancytopenia with bone marrow hypocellularity. Aplastic anemia may be acquired, iatrogenic (chemotherapy), or genetic (e.g., Fanconi's anemia). Acquired aplastic anemia may be caused by drugs or chemicals (expected toxicity or idiosyncratic effects), viral infections, immune diseases, paroxysmal nocturnal hemoglobinuria, pregnancy, or idiopathic causes. Aplastic anemia from idiosyncratic drug reactions (including those listed as well others, including as quinacrine, phenytoin, sulfonamides, or cimetidine) are uncommon but may be encountered given the wide usage of some of these agents. In these cases, there is usually not a dose-dependent response; the reaction is idiosyncratic. Seronegative hepatitis is a cause of aplastic anemia, particularly in young men who recovered from an episode of liver inflammation 1 to 2 months earlier. Parvovirus B19 infection most commonly causes pure red blood cell (RBC) aplasia, particularly in patients with chronic hemolytic states and high RBC turnover (e.g., sickle cell anemia).

29. The answer is D.

(Chap. 11) This patient has aplastic anemia. In the absence of drugs or toxins that cause bone marrow suppression, it is most likely that he has an immune-mediated injury. Growth factors are not effective in the setting of hypoplastic bone marrow. Transfusion should be avoided unless emergently needed to prevent the development of alloantibodies. Glucocorticoids have no efficacy in aplastic anemia. Immunosuppression with antithymocyte globulin and cyclosporine is a therapy with proven efficacy for this autoimmune disease with a response rate of up to 70%. Relapses are common, and myelodysplastic syndrome or leukemia may occur in approximately 15% of treated patients. Immunosuppression is the treatment of choice for patients without suitable bone marrow transplant donors. Bone marrow transplantation is the best current therapy for young patients with matched sibling donors. Allogeneic bone marrow transplants from matched siblings result in long-term survival in more than 80% of patients, with better results in children than adults. The effectiveness of androgens has not been verified in controlled trials, but occasional patients will respond or even demonstrate blood count dependence on continued therapy. Sex hormones upregulate telomerase gene activity in vitro, possibly also their mechanism of action in improving marrow function. For patients with moderate disease or those with severe pancytopenia in whom immunosuppression has failed, a 3 to 4-month trial is appropriate.

30. The answer is B.

(Chap. 11) Myelodysplasia, or the MDSs, are a heterogeneous group of hematologic disorders broadly characterized by cytopenias associated with a dysmorphic (or abnormal appearing) and usually cellular bone marrow and by consequent ineffective blood cell production. The mean onset of age is after 70 years. MDS is associated with environmental exposures such as radiation and benzene; other risk factors have been reported inconsistently. Secondary MDS occurs as a late toxicity of cancer treatment, usually with a combination of radiation and the radiomimetic alkylating agents such as busulfan, nitrosourea, or procarbazine (with a latent period of 5–7 years) or the DNA topoisomerase inhibitors (2 years). Both acquired aplastic anemia after immunosuppressive treatment and Fanconi's anemia can evolve into MDS. MDS is a clonal hematopoietic stem cell disorder leading to impaired cell proliferation and differentiation. Cytogenetic abnormalities are found in approximately half of patients, and some of the same specific lesions are also seen in frank leukemia. Anemia dominates the early course. Most symptomatic patients complain of the gradual onset of fatigue and weakness, dyspnea, and pallor, but at least half of patients are asymptomatic, and their MDS is discovered only incidentally on routine blood counts. Previous chemotherapy or radiation exposure is an important historic fact. Fever and weight loss should point to a myeloproliferative rather than myelodysplastic process. About 20% of patients have splenomegaly. Bone marrow is typically hypercellular. Median survival varies from months to years, depending on the number of blasts in marrow and the specific cytogenetic abnormality. Isolated 5q- is associated with a median survival in years. Most patients die as a result of complications of pancytopenia and not because of leukemic

transformation; perhaps one-third succumb to other diseases unrelated to their MDS. Precipitous worsening of pancytopenia, acquisition of new chromosomal abnormalities on serial cytogenetic determination, increase in the number of blasts, and marrow fibrosis are all poor prognostic indicators. The outlook in therapy-related MDS, regardless of type, is extremely poor, and most patients progress within a few months to refractory acute myeloid leukemia. Historically, the therapy of MDS has been unsatisfactory. Only stem cell transplantation offers cure. Survival rates of 50% at 3 years have been reported, but older patients are particularly prone to develop treatment-related mortality and morbidity. Results of transplant using matched unrelated donors are comparable, although most series contain younger and more highly selected cases. However, multiple new drugs have been approved for use in MDS. Several regimens appear to not only improve blood counts but also to delay onset of leukemia and to improve survival.

Lenalidomide, a thalidomide derivative with a more favorable toxicity profile, is particularly effective in reversing anemia in MDS patients with 5q- syndrome; a high proportion of these patients become transfusion independent.

31. The answer is E.

(Chap. 13) The World Health Organization's classification of the chronic myeloproliferative diseases (MPDs) includes eight disorders, some of which are rare or poorly characterized but all of which share an origin in a multipotent hematopoietic progenitor cell, overproduction of one or more of the formed elements of the blood without significant dysplasia, a predilection to extramedullary hematopoiesis or myelofibrosis, and transformation at varying rates to acute leukemia. Within this broad classification, however, significant phenotypic heterogeneity exists. Some diseases such as chronic myeloid leukemia (CML), chronic neutrophilic leukemia (CNL), and chronic eosinophilic leukemia (CEL) express primarily a myeloid phenotype, but in others, such as polycythemia vera (PV), primary myelofibrosis (PMF), and essential thrombocytosis (ET), erythroid or megakaryocytic hyperplasia predominates. The latter three disorders, in contrast to the former three, also appear capable of transforming into each other. Such phenotypic heterogeneity has a genetic basis. CML is the consequence of the balanced translocation between chromosomes 9 and 22 (t[9;22][q34;11]), CNL has been associated with a t(15;19) translocation, and CEL occurs with a deletion or balanced translocations involving the *PDGFR-alpha* gene. By contrast, to a greater or lesser extent, PV, PMF, and ET are characterized by expression of a *JAK2* mutation, V617F, that causes constitutive activation of this tyrosine kinase that is essential for the function of the erythropoietin and thrombopoietin receptors but not the granulocyte colony-stimulating factor receptor. This essential distinction is also reflected in the natural history of CML, CNL, and CEL, which is usually measured in years, and their high rate of transformation into acute leukemia. By contrast, the natural history of PV, PMF, and ET is usually measured in decades, and transformation to acute leukemia is uncommon in the absence of exposure to mutagenic agents. Primary effusion lymphoma is not a myeloproliferative disease. It is one of the diseases (Kaposi's sarcoma, multicentric Castleman's disease) associated with infection with human herpes virus-8, particularly in immunocompromised hosts.

32. The answer is A.

(Chap. 13) Polycythemia vera (PV) is a clonal disorder that involves a multipotent hematopoietic progenitor cell. Clinically, it is characterized by a proliferation of red blood cells (RBCs), granulocytes, and platelets. The precise etiology is unknown. Unlike chronic myeloid leukemia, no consistent cytogenetic abnormality has been associated with the disorder. However, a mutation in the autoinhibitory, pseudokinase domain of the tyrosine kinase JAK2—that replaces valine with phenylalanine (V617F), causing constitutive activation of the kinase—appears to have a central role in the pathogenesis of PV. Erythropoiesis is regulated by the hormone erythropoietin. Hypoxia is the physiologic stimulus that increases the number of cells that produce erythropoietin. Erythropoietin may be elevated in patients with hormone-secreting tumors. Levels are usually "normal" in patients with hypoxic erythrocytosis. In PV, however, because erythrocytosis occurs independently of erythropoietin, levels of the hormone are usually low. Therefore, an elevated level is *not* consistent with the diagnosis. PV is a chronic, indolent disease with a low rate of transformation to acute leukemia, especially in the absence of treatment with radiation or hydroxyurea. Thrombotic complications are the main risk for PV and correlate with the erythrocytosis. Thrombocytosis, although sometimes prominent, does not correlate with the risk of thrombotic complications. Salicylates are useful in treating erythromelalgia but are not indicated in asymptomatic patients. There is no evidence that thrombotic risk is significantly lowered with their use in patients whose hematocrits are appropriately controlled with phlebotomy. Phlebotomy is the mainstay of treatment. Induction of a state of iron deficiency is critical to prevent a reexpansion of the RBC mass. Chemotherapeutics and other agents are useful in cases of symptomatic splenomegaly. Their use is limited by side effects, and there is a risk of leukemogenesis with hydroxyurea.

33. The answer is A.

(Chap. 13) Chronic primary myelofibrosis (PMF) is the least common myeloproliferative disorder and is considered

a diagnosis of exclusion after other causes of myelofibrosis have been ruled out. The typical patient with PMF presents in the sixth decade of life, and the disorder is asymptomatic in many patients. Fevers, fatigue, night sweats, and weight loss may occur in PMF, but these symptoms are rare in other myeloproliferative disorders. However, no signs or symptoms are specific for the diagnosis of PMF. Often marked splenomegaly is present and may extend across the midline and to the pelvic brim. A peripheral blood smear demonstrates the typical findings of myelofibrosis, including teardrop-shaped red blood cells (RBCs), nucleated RBCs, myelocytes, and metamyelocytes that are indicative of extramedullary hematopoiesis. Anemia is usually mild, and platelet and leukocyte counts are often normal. About 50% of patients with PMF have the *JAK2 V617F* mutation. Bone marrow aspirate is frequently unsuccessful because the extent of marrow fibrosis makes aspiration impossible. When a bone marrow biopsy is performed, it demonstrates hypercellular marrow with trilineage hyperplasia and increased number of megakaryocytes with large dysplastic nuclei. Interestingly, individuals with PMF often have associated autoantibodies, including rheumatoid factor, antinuclear antibodies, or positive Coombs test results. To diagnose someone as having PMF, it must be shown that he or she does not have another myeloproliferative disorder or hematologic malignancy that is the cause of myelofibrosis. The most common disorders that present in a similar fashion to PMF are polycythemia vera and chronic myeloid leukemia. Other nonmalignant disorders that can cause myelofibrosis include HIV infection, hyperparathyroidism, renal osteodystrophy, systemic lupus erythematosus, tuberculosis, and bone marrow replacement in other cancers such as prostate and breast cancer. In the patient described here, there is no other identifiable cause of myelofibrosis; thus, chronic PMF can be diagnosed.

34. The answer is E.

(Chap. 13) Thrombocytosis may be "primary" or "secondary." Essential thrombocytosis is a myeloproliferative disorder that involves a multipotent hematopoietic progenitor cell. Unfortunately, no clonal marker can reliably distinguish it from more common nonclonal, reactive forms of thrombocytosis. Only 50% of patients with essential (primary) thrombocytosis have the *JAK2 V617F* mutation. Therefore, the diagnosis is one of exclusion. Common causes of secondary thrombocytosis include infection, inflammatory conditions, malignancy, iron deficiency, hemorrhage, and postsurgical states. Other myeloproliferative disorders, such as chronic myeloid leukemia and myelofibrosis, may result in thrombocytosis. Similarly, myelodysplastic syndromes, particularly the 5q-syndrome, may cause thrombocytosis. Pernicious anemia caused by vitamin B_{12} deficiency does not typically cause thrombocytosis. However, correction of vitamin B_{12} deficiency or folate deficiency may cause a "rebound" thrombocytosis. Similarly, cessation of chronic ethanol use may also cause rebound thrombocytosis.

35. The answer is E.

(Chap. 13) In a patient presenting with an elevated hemoglobin and hematocrit, the initial step in the evaluation is to determine whether erythrocytosis represents a true elevation in red blood cell (RBC) mass or whether spurious erythrocytosis is present because of plasma volume contraction. (See Figure 35.) This step may be not necessary, however, in individuals with hemoglobin >20 g/dL. After absolute erythrocytosis has been determined by measurement of RBC mass and plasma volume, the cause of erythrocytosis must be determined. If there is not an obvious cause of the erythrocytosis, an erythropoietin level should be checked. An elevated erythropoietin level suggests hypoxia or autonomous production of erythropoietin as the cause of erythrocytosis. However, a normal erythropoietin level does not exclude hypoxia as a cause. A low erythropoietin level should be seen in the myeloproliferative disorder polycythemia vera (PV), the most likely cause of erythrocytosis in this patient. PV is often discovered incidentally when elevated hemoglobin is found during testing for other reasons. When symptoms are present, the most common complaints are related to hyperviscosity of the blood and include vertigo, headache, tinnitus, and transient ischemic attacks. Patients may also complain of pruritus after showering. *Erythromelalgia* is the term give to the symptom complex of burning, pain, and erythema in the extremities and is associated with thrombocytosis in PV. Isolated systolic hypertension and splenomegaly may be found. In addition to elevated red RBC mass and low erythropoietin levels, other laboratory findings in PV include thrombocytosis and leukocytosis with abnormal leukocytes present. Uric acid levels and leukocyte alkaline phosphatase may be elevated but are not diagnostic for PV. Approximately 30% of individuals with PV are homozygous for the *JAK2 V617F* mutation, and >90% are heterozygous for this mutation. This mutation located on the short arm of chromosome 9 causes constitutive activation of the Janus kinase (JAK) protein, a tyrosine kinase that renders erythrocytes resistant to apoptosis and allows them to continue production independently from erythropoietin. However, not every patient with PV expresses this mutation, and approximately 50% of patients with chronic myelofibrosis and essential thrombocytosis express this mutation. Thus, it is not recommended as an initial diagnostic test for PV but may be used for confirmatory purposes. Bone marrow biopsy provides no specific information in PV and is not recommended.

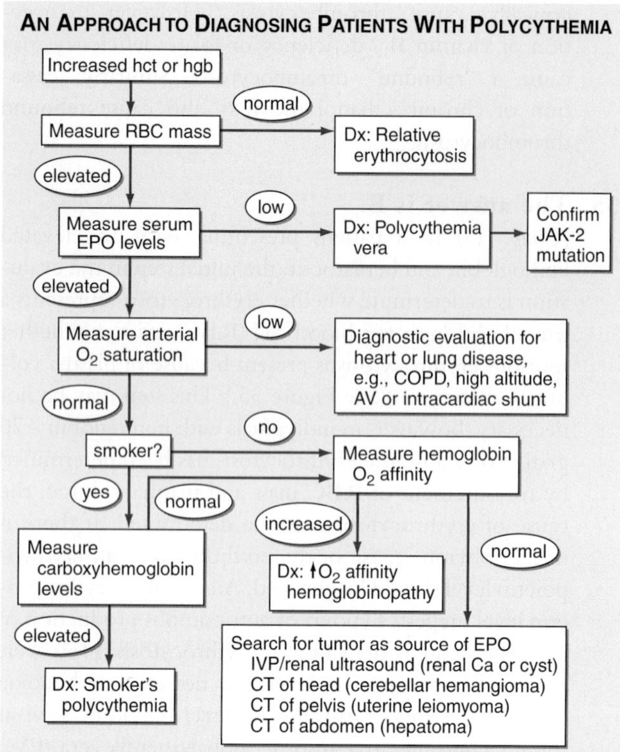

36. The answer is C.

(Chap. 14) This patient presents with typical findings of chronic myeloid leukemia (CML), which has an incidence of 1.5 per 100,000 people yearly. The typical age of onset is in the mid forties, and there is a slight male predominance. Half of individuals are asymptomatic at the time of diagnosis. If symptoms are present, they are typically nonspecific and include fatigue and weight loss. Occasionally, patients have symptoms related to splenic enlargement such as early satiety and left upper quadrant pain. Laboratory findings are suggestive of CML. A high leukocyte count of 100,000/μL is typical, with a predominant granulocytic differential, including neutrophils, myelocytes, metamyelocytes, and band forms. The circulating blast count should be <5%. Anemia and thrombocytosis are also common. The bone marrow demonstrates nonspecific increase in cellularity with an increase in the myeloid-to-erythroid ratio. The diagnosis of CML is established by identifying a clonal expansion of a hematopoietic stem cell possessing a reciprocal translocation between chromosomes 9 and 22. This translocation results in the head-to-tail fusion of the breakpoint cluster region (*BCR*) gene on chromosome 22q11 with the *ABL1* (named after the Abelson murine leukemia virus) gene located on chromosome 9q34. The bcr-abl fusion protein results in constitutive activation of abl tyrosine kinase enzyme that prevents apoptosis and leads to increased survival of the cells containing the mutation. Ultimately, untreated CML develops into an accelerated phase with increasing numbers of mutations and leads to acute blast crisis. The deletion of the long arm of chromosome 5 is present in some individuals with acute myeloid leukemias and is associated with older age at diagnosis. The inversion of chromosome 16 is typically present in acute myelomonocytic leukemia (M4 subtype). The translocation of the long arms of chromosomes 15 and 17 is the mutation associated with acute promyelocytic anemia that results in arrest of cellular differentiation that can be treated with pharmacologic doses of ATRA (all-*trans* retinoic acid). Finally, trisomy 12 is one of several mutations that may result in the development of chronic lymphocytic leukemia.

37. The answer is D.

(Chap. 14) The acute myeloid leukemias (AMLs) are a group of hematologic malignancies derived from hematologic stem cells that have acquired chromosomal mutations that prevent differentiation into mature myeloid cells. The specific chromosomal abnormalities predict in which stage of differentiation the cell is arrested and are associated with the several subtypes of AML that have been identified. In the United States, >16,000 new cases of AML are diagnosed yearly, and the numbers of new cases of AML has increased in the past 10 years. Men are diagnosed with AML more frequently than women (4.6 cases per 100,000 population vs 3.0 cases per 100,000, respectively). In addition, older age is associated with increased incidence of AML, with an incidence of 18.6 cases per 100,000 population in those older than 65 years of age. AML is uncommon in adolescents. Other known risk factors for the development of AML include hereditary genetic abnormalities, radiation and chemical exposures, and drugs. The most common hereditary abnormality linked to AML is trisomy 21 (Down syndrome). Other hereditary syndromes associated with an increase of AML include diseases associated with defective DNA repair such as Fanconi's anemia and ataxia telangiectasia. Survivors of the atomic bomb explosions in Japan were found to have a high incidence of AML as have survivors of other high-dose radiation exposures. However, therapeutic radiation is not associated with an increased risk of AML unless the patient was also treated concomitantly with alkylating agents. Anticancer drugs are the most common causes of drug-associated AML. Of the chemotherapeutic agents, alkylating agents and topoisomerase II inhibitors are the drugs most likely to be associated with AML.

38. The answer is C.

(Chap. 14) The goal of therapy in chronic myeloid leukemia (CML) is to achieve prolonged, durable, non-neoplastic, nonclonal hematopoiesis, which entails the eradication of any residual cells containing the *BCR-ABL1* transcript. Hence, the goal is complete molecular remission and cure. Therapy of CML has changed in recent years because of the presence of a proven curative

treatment (allogeneic transplantation) that has significant toxicity and a targeted treatment (imatinib) with outstanding outcome based on 8-year follow-up data. New tyrosine kinase inhibitors are becoming available, making this a dynamic topic. Many experts currently recommend initiating therapy with a tyrosine kinase inhibitor and reserving allogeneic transplantation for those who develop drug resistance. Imatinib mesylate is a tyrosine kinase inhibitor that acts to decrease the activity of the bcr-abl fusion protein that results from the reciprocal translocation of chromosomes 9 and 22 (Philadelphia chromosome). It acts as a competitive inhibitor of the abl kinase at its ATP binding site and thus leads to inhibition of tyrosine phosphorylation of proteins in *bcr-abl* signal transduction. In newly diagnosed CML, imatinib results in a complete hematologic remission in 95% of patients initially and 76% at 18 months. Low-risk patients have a higher durable remission rate. All imatinib-treated patients who achieved major molecular remission (26%), defined as 3 log or greater reduction in *BCR-ABL1* transcript level at 18 months compared with pretreatment level, were progression free at 5 years. There is a consensus that molecular responses can be used as a treatment goal in CML. Imatinib, taken orally, has limited side effects that include nausea, fluid retention, diarrhea, and skin rash and is usually well tolerated. Interferon-α was previously the first-line chemotherapy if bone marrow transplant was not an option, but it has been replaced by imatinib mesylate. Autologous stem cell transplant is not currently used for treatment of CML because there is no reliable way to select residual normal hematopoietic progenitor cells. Leukopheresis is used for control of leukocyte counts when the patient is experiencing complications such as respiratory failure or cerebral ischemia related to the high white blood cell count.

39. and 40. The answers are D and E, respectively.
(Chap. 14) Treatment of acute promyelocytic leukemia (PML) is an interesting example of how understanding the function of the protein produced by the genetic abnormality can be used to develop a treatment for the disease. The translocation of the long arms of chromosomes 15 and 17, t(15;17), results in the production of a chimeric protein called promyelocytic leukemia (Pml)/retinoic acid receptor α (Rar-α). The Pml-Rar-α fusion protein suppresses gene transcription and arrests differentiation of the cells in an immature state, leading to promyelocytic leukemia. Pharmacologic doses of the ligand of the Rar-α receptor, tretinoin, stimulate the cells to resume differentiation. With use of tretinoin, the leukemic cells differentiate to mature neutrophils and undergo subsequent apoptosis. Tretinoin plus concurrent anthracycline-based chemotherapy appears to be among the most effective treatments for APL, leading to complete remission (CR) rates of 90–95%. The primary side effect of tretinoin is the development of retinoic acid syndrome. The onset of retinoic acid syndrome from ATRA (all-*trans* retinoic acid) is usually within the first 3 weeks of treatment. Typical symptoms are chest pain, fever, and dyspnea. Hypoxia is common, and chest radiography usually shows diffuse alveolar infiltrates with pleural effusions. Pericardial effusions may also occur. The cause of retinoic acid syndrome is possibly related to the adhesion of the differentiated leukemia cells to the pulmonary endothelium or the release of cytokines by these cells to cause vascular leak. The mortality rate for patients with retinoic acid syndrome is 10%. High-dose glucocorticoid therapy is usually effective in the treatment of retinoic acid syndrome. Arsenic trioxide has antileukemic activity and may be used in tretinoin refractory cases. It is also under investigation for combination chemotherapy. Cyclophosphamide, daunorubicin, vinblastine, and prednisone are the constituents of the combination chemotherapy commonly known as CHOP, which is indicated for the treatment of B-cell lymphomas. Rituximab is most commonly used as a treatment of B-cell non-Hodgkin's lymphoma and a variety of autoimmune disorders. Rituximab is a monoclonal antibody directed against the CD20 cell-surface molecule of B lymphocytes. It has no current role in the treatment of acute myeloid leukemias. Whole-body irradiation is used primarily before bone marrow transplant to ensure complete eradication of cancerous leukemic cells in the bone marrow.

41. The answer is C.
(Chap. 14) Patients with acute leukemia frequently present with nonspecific symptoms of fatigue and weight loss. In addition, weight loss and anorexia are also common. About half have had symptoms for >3 months at the time of presentation. Fever is present in only about 10% of patients at presentation, and 5% have evidence of abnormal hemostasis. On physical examination, hepatomegaly, splenomegaly, sternal tenderness, and evidence of infection or hemorrhage are common presenting signs. Laboratory studies are confirmatory with evidence of anemia, thrombocytopenia, and leukocytosis often present. The median presenting leukocyte count at presentation is 15,000/μL. About 20–40% have presenting leukocyte counts <5000/μL, and another 20% have counts >100,000/μL. Review of the peripheral smear confirms leukemia in most cases. If Auer rods are seen, the diagnosis of acute myeloid leukemia (AML) is virtually certain. Thrombocytopenia (platelet count <100,000/μL) is seen in >75% of individuals with AML. After the diagnosis of AML has been confirmed, rapid evaluation and treatment should be undertaken. The general health of the cardiovascular, pulmonary, hepatic, and renal systems should be evaluated because chemotherapy has adverse effects that may cause organ dysfunction in any of these systems. Overall, chromosome findings at diagnosis are currently the most important independent prognostic factor. Patients with t(15;17) have a very good prognosis

(~85% cured), and those with t(8;21) and inv(16) have a good prognosis (~55% cured), but those with no cytogenetic abnormality have a moderately favorable outcome (~40% cured). Patients with a complex karyotype, t(6;9), inv(3), or −7, have a very poor prognosis. Among the prognostic factors that predict poor outcomes in AML, age at diagnosis is one of the most important because individuals of advanced age tolerate induction chemotherapy poorly. In addition, advanced age is more likely to be associated with multiple chromosomal abnormalities that predict poorer response to chemotherapy, although some chromosomal markers predict a better response to chemotherapy. Poor performance status independent of age also decreases survival in AML. Responsiveness to chemotherapy and survival are also worse if the leukocyte count is >100,000/μL or the antecedent course of symptoms is prolonged. Anemia, leukopenia, or thrombocytopenia present for >3 months is a poor prognostic indicator. However, there is no absolute degree of anemia or thrombocytopenia that predicts worse outcomes.

42. The answer is E.

(Chap. 15) Viscosity testing is typically reserved for cases of multiple myeloma in which paraproteins (particularly immunoglobulin M) can lead to vascular sludging and subsequent tissue ischemia. Acute lymphoid leukemia (ALL) can lead to end-organ abnormalities in the kidney and liver; therefore, routine chemistry tests are indicated. A lumbar puncture must be performed in cases of newly diagnosed ALL to rule out spread of disease to the central nervous system. Bone marrow biopsy reveals the degree of marrow infiltration and is often necessary for classification of the tumor. Immunologic cell-surface marker testing often identifies the cell lineage involved and the type of tumor, information that is often impossible to discern from morphologic interpretation alone. Cytogenetic testing provides prognostic information on the disease natural history. In ALL, the prognosis depends on the genetic characteristics of the tumor, the patient's age, the white blood cell count, and the patient's overall clinical status and major organ function.

43. The answer is B.

(Chap. 15) Hepatitis B and C are both common causes of cirrhosis and are strongly associated with the development of hepatocellular carcinoma. Hepatitis C, but not hepatitis B, can also lead to a lymphoplasmacytic lymphoma, often in the spleen, that resolves with cure of hepatitis C. Epstein-Barr virus has been associated with a large number of lymphoid malignancies, including posttransplant lymphoproliferative disease (PTLD), Hodgkin's disease, central nervous system lymphoma, and Burkitt's lymphoma. *Helicobacter pylori* infection is necessary and sufficient for gastric mucosa-associated lymphoid tissue (MALT) lymphoma development, and cure can be achieved with eradication of the organism in some cases. HHV8 is a known cause of body cavity lymphoma, including primary pleural lymphoma. In addition to those listed, human T-lymphotropic virus type 1 is associated with adult T-cell lymphoma or leukemia. Other disorders associated with lymphoma include celiac sprue, autoimmune disease, and biologic therapies for autoimmune disease. Celiac sprue has been associated with gastrointestinal tract lymphoma. Many collagen vascular diseases (e.g., Sjogren's disease) and anti–tumor necrosis factor therapies have been associated with the development of lymphoma.

44. The answer is B.

(Chap. 15) Autoimmune hemolytic anemia and thrombocytopenia are common, and a peripheral blood smear and a Coombs test help evaluate their presence. Hypersplenism is also seen in chronic lymphoid leukemia (CLL) as the spleen sequesters large numbers of circulating blood cells and enlarges. Hence, a careful left upper quadrant examination looking for a palpable splenic tip is the standard of care in this situation. This patient is at risk of hepatic decompensation as well, given his hepatitis C that can also cause anemia and thrombocytopenia. Bone marrow infiltration of tumor cells can lead to cytopenias in CLL. However, this is in effect a diagnosis of exclusion. After these three possibilities have been ruled out, a bone marrow biopsy is a reasonable next step. This initial evaluation before presuming spread of CLL is critical for therapy because each possibility requires different therapy (glucocorticoids or rituximab for hemolysis, hepatology referral for liver failure, and splenectomy for symptomatic hypersplenism).

45. The answer is C.

(Chap. 15) The peripheral smear shows increased numbers of small, well-differentiated, normal-appearing lymphocytes characteristic of chronic lymphocytic leukemia, the most common leukemia or lymphoma in adults. Common presenting complaints typically include fatigue, frequent infections, new lymphadenopathy, and abdominal complaints relating to splenomegaly. Hairy cell leukemia is a rare disease that presents predominantly in older men. The typical presentation involves pancytopenia, although occasional patients will have a leukemic presentation. Splenomegaly is usual. The malignant cells appear to have "hairy" projections on light and electron microscopy. Patients with this disorder are prone to unusual infections, including infection by *Mycobacterium avium intracellulare*, and to vasculitic syndromes. Hairy cell leukemia is responsive to chemotherapy with cladribine with clinical complete remissions in the majority of patients and frequent long-term disease-free survival.

46. The answer is E.

(Chap. 15) Classical Hodgkin's disease carries a better prognosis than all types of non-Hodgkin's lymphoma.

Patients with good prognostic factors can achieve cure with extended field radiation alone, but those with a higher risk disease often achieve cure with high-dose chemotherapy and sometimes radiation. The chance of cure is so high (>90%) that many protocols are now considering long-term sequelae of current therapy such as carcinomas, hypothyroidism, premature coronary disease, and constrictive pericarditis in those receiving radiation therapy. A variety of chemotherapy regimens are effective with long-term disease-free survival in patients with advanced disease achieved in >75% of patients who lack systemic symptoms and in 60–70% of patients with systemic symptoms.

47. The answer is D.

(Chap. 15) The large cell with a bilobed nucleus and prominent nucleoli giving an "owl's eyes" appearance near the center of the field is a Reed-Sternberg cell, confirming the diagnosis of Hodgkin's disease. Hodgkin's disease occurs in 8000 patients in the United States each year, and the disease does not appear to be increasing in frequency. Most patients present with palpable lymphadenopathy that is nontender; in most patients, these lymph nodes are in the neck, supraclavicular area, and axilla. More than half the patients have mediastinal adenopathy at diagnosis, and this is sometimes the initial manifestation. A subdiaphragmatic presentation of Hodgkin's disease is unusual and more common in older men. One-third of patients present with fevers, night sweats, or weight loss, which are B symptoms in the Ann Arbor staging classification. Occasionally, Hodgkin's disease can present as a fever of unknown origin. This is more common in older patients who are found to have mixed cellularity Hodgkin's disease in an abdominal site. Rarely, the fevers persist for days to weeks followed by afebrile intervals and then recurrence of the fever (Pel-Ebstein fever). The differential diagnosis of a lymph node biopsy suspicious for Hodgkin's disease includes inflammatory processes, mononucleosis, non-Hodgkin's lymphoma, phenytoin-induced adenopathy, and nonlymphomatous malignancies.

48. The answer is D.

(Chap. 16) Mastocytosis is a proliferation and accumulation of mast cells in one or more organ systems. Only the skin is involved in approximately 80% of cases with the other 20% being defined as systemic mastocytosis caused by the involvement of another organ system. The most common manifestation of mastocytosis is cutaneous urticaria pigmentosa, a maculopapular pigmented rash involving the papillary dermis. Other cutaneous forms include diffuse cutaneous mastocytosis (almost entirely in children) and mastocytoma. Clinical manifestations of systemic mastocytosis are related to either cellular infiltration of organs or release of histamine, proteases, eicosanoids, or heparin from mast cells. Therefore, signs and symptoms may include constitutional symptoms, skin manifestations (pruritus, dermatographia, rash), mediator-related symptoms (abdominal pain, flushing, syncope, hypertension, diarrhea), and bone-related symptoms (fracture, pain, arthralgia). In a recent series, 40% of patients with systemic mastocytosis had an associated myeloid neoplasm, most commonly myeloproliferative syndrome, chronic myeloid leukemia, or myelodysplastic syndrome. Eosinophilia was present in approximately one-third of patients. Elevated serum tryptase, bone marrow involvement, splenomegaly, skeletal involvement, cytopenia, and malabsorption predict more aggressive disease and a worse prognosis. Many patients with systemic mastocytosis have an activating mutation of c-Kit, a kinase inhibited by imatinib; however, the mutation appears relatively resistant to this agent.

49. The answer is A.

(Chap. 17) The patient presents with pneumococcal pneumonia and evidence of hypercalcemia, renal failure, and a wide protein gap suggestive of an M protein. These findings are classic for multiple myeloma. Although the patient appears to be making large quantities of immunoglobulins, they are in fact generally monoclonal, and patients actually have functional hypogammaglobulinemia related to both decreased production and increased destruction of normal antibodies. This hypogammaglobulinemia predisposes patients to infections, most commonly pneumonia with pneumococcus or *Staphylococcus aureus* or gram-negative pyelonephritis. Bone marrow biopsy would confirm the presence of clonal plasma cells and define the quantity, which will help define treatment options. A serum protein electrophoresis would also be indicated to prove the presence of the M protein suspected by the wide protein gap. Although HIV may be associated with kidney injury, both acute and chronic, hypercalcemia would be an unusual feature. There is no clinical history of aspiration, and the location of infiltrate, upper lobe, is unusual for aspiration. Sweat chloride testing is not indicated because there is no suspicion for cystic fibrosis. Because solid organ malignancy is not suspected, computed tomography of the body is unlikely to be helpful.

50. The answer is A.

(Chap. 18) This patient presents with a multisystem illness involving the heart, kidneys, and peripheral nervous system. The physical examination is suggestive of amyloidosis with classic waxy papules in the folds of his body. The laboratory test results are remarkable for renal failure of unclear etiology with significant proteinuria but no cellular casts. A possible etiology of the renal failure is suggested by the elevated gamma globulin fraction and low hematocrit, bringing to mind a monoclonal gammopathy perhaps leading to renal failure through amyloid AL deposition. This could also account for the

enlarged heart seen on the echocardiography and the peripheral neuropathy. The fat pad biopsy is generally reported to be 60–80% sensitive for amyloid; however, it would not allow a diagnosis of this patient's likely myeloma. A right heart catheterization probably would prove that the patient has restrictive cardiomyopathy secondary to amyloid deposition; however, it too would not diagnose the underlying plasma cell dyscrasia. Renal ultrasonography, although warranted to rule out obstructive uropathy, would not be diagnostic. Similarly, the electromyographic and nerve conduction studies would not be diagnostic. The bone marrow biopsy is about 50–60% sensitive for amyloid, but it would allow evaluation of the percent of plasma cells in the bone marrow and allow the diagnosis of multiple myeloma to be made. Multiple myeloma is associated with amyloid AL in approximately 20% of cases. Light chains most commonly deposit systemically in the heart, kidneys, liver, and nervous system, causing organ dysfunction. In these organs, biopsy would show the classic eosinophilic material that, when exposed to Congo red stain, has a characteristic apple-green birefringence.

51. The answer is C.

(Chap. 19) Heparin-induced thrombocytopenia (HIT) is a clinical diagnosis that must not be missed because life-threatening thrombosis can occur if not treated appropriately. The cause of HIT is the formation of antibodies to the complex of heparin and platelet factor 4 (PF4). This complex is able to activate platelets, monocytes, and endothelial cells. Many patients exposed to heparin will develop antibodies to the heparin–PF4 complex, but only a few of these will progress to develop thrombocytopenia or thrombocytopenia with thrombosis (HITT). The typical patient will develop evidence of HIT 5 to 14 days after exposure to heparin, although it can occur within 5 days in individuals exposed to heparin within about the previous 100 days as would be expected in this patient given his recent hospitalization. The nadir platelet count is typically >20,000/μL. When HIT is suspected, one should not delay treatment for laboratory testing because no currently available test has adequate sensitivity or specificity for the diagnosis. The antiheparin/PF4 antibody test result is positive in many individuals who have been exposed to heparin regardless of whether HIT is present. The platelet activation assay is more specific but less sensitive for HIT. As soon as HIT is suspected, heparin should be discontinued and replaced with an alternative form of anticoagulation to protect against development of new thromboses. Low-molecular-weight heparins (LMWHs) such as enoxaparin are not appropriate treatment options in individuals with HIT. Although heparin is 10 times more likely to cause HIT, LMWHs also cause the illness and should not be used. The primary agents used for HIT in the United States are the direct thrombin inhibitors argatroban and lepirudin. Argatroban is the preferred agent for this patient because of his renal failure. The drug is not excreted by the kidneys, and no dosage adjustment is required. In contrast, lepirudin is markedly increased in renal failure, and a significant dosage adjustment is required. Danaparoid has previously been used frequently for HIT and HITT, but this medication is no longer available in the United States. Other anticoagulants that are used for treatment of HITT include bivalirudin and fondaparinux, but these also are not currently approved for use in the United States.

52. The answer is E.

(Chap. 19) This patient presents with symptoms of thrombocytopenia, including bleeding gums and easy bruising. The only finding on physical examination may be petechiae at points of increased venous pressure, especially in the feet and ankles. The laboratory findings confirm thrombocytopenia but show no abnormalities in other cell lines. When evaluating isolated thrombocytopenia, one must initially consider whether an underlying infection or medication is causing the platelet count to fall. There is a long list of medications that are implicated in thrombocytopenia, including aspirin, acetaminophen, penicillins, H_2 blockers, heparin, and many others. This patient discontinued all medications over 6 weeks previously, and the platelet count would be expected to recover if a medication reaction were the cause. She gives no signs of any acute infection. Thus, the most likely diagnosis is immune thrombocytopenia purpura (ITP). This disorder is also known as idiopathic thrombocytopenia purpura and refers to an immune-mediated destruction of platelets and possible inhibition of platelet release from megakaryocytes. ITP can truly be idiopathic, or it can be secondary to an underlying disorder, including systemic lupus erythematosus (SLE), HIV, or chronic hepatitis C virus (HCV) infection. The platelet count can be quite low (<5000/μL) in patients with ITP and usually presents with mucocutaneous bleeding. Laboratory testing for ITP should include a peripheral smear that typically demonstrates large platelets with otherwise normal morphology. Initial testing should evaluate for secondary causes of ITP, including HIV antibodies, HCV antibodies, serologic testing for SLE, serum protein electrophoresis, and immunoglobulins. If anemia is also present, a direct Coombs test is indicated to assess whether there is a combined autoimmune hemolytic anemia with ITP (Evans syndrome). Antiplatelet antibody testing is not recommended because these tests have low sensitivity and specificity for ITP. In addition, bone marrow biopsy is typically not performed unless there are other abnormalities that are not explained by ITP or the patient has failed to respond to usual therapy.

53 and 54. The answers are A and E, respectively.

(Chap. 19) This patient presents with the classic pentad of thrombotic thrombocytopenic purpura (TTP), which

is fever, neurologic symptoms, acute renal failure, thrombocytopenia, and microscopic angiopathic hemolytic anemia (MAHA). Although this is the classic presentation, it is not necessary to have all five characteristics for an individual to be diagnosed with TTP. In recent years, the pathogenesis of inherited and idiopathic TTP has been discovered to be attributable to a deficiency of or antibodies directed against the ADAMTS-13 protein. The ADAMTS-13 protein is a metalloproteinase that cleaves von Willebrand factor (VWF). In the absence of ADAMTS-13, ultra-large VWF multimers circulate in the blood and can cause pathogenic platelet adhesion and activation, resulting in microvascular ischemia and microangiopathic hemolytic anemia. However, it appears as if there is a necessary inciting event because not all individuals with an inherited deficiency of ADAMTS-13 develop TTP. Some drugs have been implicated as causative agents in TTP. Ticlopidine and possibly clopidogrel cause TTP by inducing antibody formation. Other drugs, including mitomycin C, cyclosporine, and quinine, can cause TTP by causing direct endothelial toxicity.

A diagnosis of TTP can be made based on clinical factors. It should be differentiated from disseminated intravascular coagulation, which causes MAHA but has a predominant coagulopathy. Hemolytic uremic syndrome also causes MAHA and appears very similar to TTP in clinical presentation, although neurologic symptoms are less prominent. Often a preceding diarrheal illness alerts one to hemolytic syndrome as the cause of MAHA. It is important to make a prompt and correct diagnosis because the mortality rate for patients with TTP without treatment is 85–100%, decreasing to 10–30% with treatment. The primary treatment for TTP remains plasma exchange. Plasma exchange should be continued until the platelet count returns to the normal range and there is no further evidence of hemolysis for at least 2 days. Glucocorticoids can be used as adjunctive treatment in TTP but are not effective as the sole therapy. Recent research suggests that rituximab may be useful in primary treatment of TTP. However, relapse is common with rituximab.

55. The answer is D.

(Chap. 20) The hemophilias are X-linked inherited disorders that cause deficiency of factor VIII (hemophilia A) or factor 9 (hemophilia B). The hemophilias affect about 1 in 10,000 males worldwide with hemophilia A responsible for 80% of cases. Clinically, there is no difference between hemophilia A and B. The disease presentation largely depends on the residual activity of factor VIII or factor IX. Severe disease is typically seen when factor activity is <1%, and moderate disease appears when the levels range between 1% and 5%. The clinical manifestation of moderate and severe disease is commonly bleeding into the joints, soft tissues, and muscles that occurs after minimal trauma or even spontaneously. When factor activity is >25%, bleeding would occur only after major trauma or surgery, and the diagnosis may not be made unless a prolonged activated partial thromboplastin time is seen on routine laboratory examination. To make a definitive diagnosis, one would need to measure specific levels of factor VIII and IX. Without treatment, life expectancy is limited, but given the changes in therapy since the 1980s, the life span is about 65 years. Early treatment of hemophilia required the use of pooled plasma that was used to make factor concentrates. Given the large number of donors required to generate the factor concentrates and the frequent need for transfusion in some individuals, bloodborne pathogens such as HIV and hepatitis C are among the leading cause of death in patients with hemophilia. In the 1990s, recombinant factor VIII and IX were developed. Primary prophylaxis is given to individuals with baseline factor activity levels of <1% to prevent spontaneous bleeding, especially hemarthroses. Although this strategy is highly recommended, only about 50% of eligible patients receive prophylactic therapy because of the high costs and need for regular intravenous infusions. When an individual is suspected of having a bleed, the treatment should begin as soon as possible and not delayed until factor activity levels return. Factor concentrates should be given to raise the activity level to 50% for large hematomas or deep muscle bleeds, and an individual may require treatment for a period of 7 days or more. For milder bleeds, including uncomplicated hemarthrosis, the goal factor activity level is 30–50% with maintenance of levels between 15% and 25% for 2 to 3 days after the initial transfusions. In addition to treatment with factor concentrates, care should be taken to avoid medications that inhibit platelet function. DDAVP, a desmopressin analogue, can be given as adjunctive therapy for acute bleeding episodes in hemophilia A because this may cause a transient rise in factor VIII levels and von Willebrand factor because of release from endothelial cells. This medication is typically only useful in mild to moderate disease. Antifibrinolytic drugs such as tranexamic acid or ε-amino caproic acid are helpful in promoting hemostasis for mucosal bleeding.

56. The answer is D.

(Chap. 20) Disseminated intravascular coagulation (DIC) is a consumptive coagulopathy that is characterized by diffuse intravascular fibrin formation that overcomes the body's natural anticoagulant mechanisms. DIC is most commonly associated with sepsis, trauma, or malignancy or in obstetric complications. The pathogenesis of DIC is not completely elucidated, but it involves intravascular exposure to phospholipids from damaged tissue, hemolysis, and endothelial damage. This leads to stimulation of procoagulant pathways with uncontrolled thrombin generation and microvascular ischemia. A secondary hyperfibrinolysis subsequently occurs. The primary clinical

manifestations of DIC are bleeding at venipuncture sites, petechiae, and ecchymoses. Severe gastrointestinal and pulmonary hemorrhage can occur. The clinical diagnosis of DIC is based on laboratory findings in the appropriate clinical setting, such as severe sepsis. Although there is no single test for DIC, the common constellation of findings is thrombocytopenia (<100,000/μL), elevated prothrombin time and activated partial thromboplastin time, evidence of microangiopathic hemolytic anemia, and elevated fibrin degradation productions and D-dimer. The fibrinogen level may be <100 mg/dL but often does not decrease acutely unless the DIC is very severe. The primary treatment of DIC is to treat the underlying cause, which in this case would be antibiotic therapy directed against *Neisseria meningitidis*. For patients such as this one who are experiencing bleeding related to the DIC, attempts to correct the coagulopathy should be undertaken. Platelet transfusions and fresh-frozen plasma (FFP) should be given. In addition, cryoprecipitate is indicated as the fibrinogen level is <100 mg/dL. In general, 10 U of cryoprecipitate are required for every 2 to 3 units of FFP. In acute DIC, heparin is not been demonstrated to be helpful and may increase bleeding. Low-dose heparin therapy (5–10 U/kg) is used for chronic low-grade DIC such as that seen in acute promyelocytic leukemia or removal of a dead fetus.

57. The answer is E.

(Chap. 20) Vitamin K is a fat-soluble vitamin that plays an essential role in hemostasis. It is absorbed in the small intestine and stored in the liver. It serves as a cofactor in the enzymatic carboxylation of glutamic acid residues on prothrombin-complex proteins. The three major causes of vitamin K deficiency are poor dietary intake, intestinal malabsorption, and liver disease. The prothrombin complex proteins (factors II, VII, IX, and X and protein C and protein S) all decrease with vitamin K deficiency. Factor VII and protein C have the shortest half-lives of these factors and therefore decrease first. Therefore, vitamin K deficiency manifests with prolongation of the prothrombin time first. With severe deficiency, the activated partial thromboplastin time will be prolonged as well. Factor VIII is not influenced by vitamin K.

58. The answer is E.

(Chap. 20) Hemophilia A results from a deficiency of factor VIII. Replacement of factor VIII is the centerpiece of treatment. Cessation of aspirin or nonsteroidal anti-inflammatory drugs is highly recommended. Fresh-frozen plasma (FFP) contains pooled plasma from human sources. Cryoprecipitate refers to FFP that is cooled, resulting in the precipitation of material at the bottom of the plasma. This product contains about half the factor VIII activity of FFP in a tenth of the volume. Both agents are therefore reasonable treatment options. DDAVP (desmopressin) causes the release of a number of factors and von Willebrand factor from the liver and endothelial cells. This may be useful for patients with mild hemophilia. Recombinant or purified factor VIII (i.e., Humate P) is indicated in patients with more severe bleeding. Therapy may be required for weeks, with levels of factor VIII kept at 50%, for postsurgical or severe bleeding. Plasmapheresis has no role in the treatment of patients with hemophilia A.

59. The answer is C.

(Chap. 20) Lupus anticoagulants (Las) cause prolongation of coagulation tests by binding to phospholipids. Although most often encountered in patients with systemic lupus erythematosus, they may also develop in normal individuals. The diagnosis is first suggested by prolongation of coagulation tests. Failure to correct with incubation with normal plasma confirms the presence of a circulating inhibitor. Contrary to the name, patients with LA activity have normal hemostasis and are not predisposed to bleeding. Instead, they are at risk for venous and arterial thromboembolisms. Patients with a history of recurrent unplanned abortions or thrombosis should undergo lifelong anticoagulation. The presence of LAs or anticardiolipin antibodies without a history of thrombosis may be observed because many of these patients will not go on to develop a thrombotic event.

60. The answer is D.

(Chap. 20) The activated partial thromboplastin time (aPTT) involves the factors of the intrinsic pathway of coagulation. Prolongation of the aPTT reflects either a deficiency of one of these factors (factor VIII, IX, XI, XII, and so on) or inhibition of the activity of one of the factors or components of the aPTT assay (i.e., phospholipids). This may be further characterized by the "mixing study" in which the patient's plasma is mixed with pooled plasma. Correction of the aPTT reflects a deficiency of factors that are replaced by the pooled sample. Failure to correct the aPTT reflects the presence of a factor inhibitor or phospholipid inhibitor. Common causes of a failure to correct include the presence of heparin in the sample, factor inhibitors (factor VIII inhibitor being the most common), and the presence of antiphospholipid antibodies. Factor VII is involved in the extrinsic pathway of coagulation. Inhibitors to factor VII would result in prolongation of the prothrombin time.

61. The answer is D.

(Chap. 20) This patient presents with a significant upper gastrointestinal (GI) bleed with a prolonged prothrombin time (PT). Hemophilia should not cause a prolonged PT. This and the presence of ascites raise the possibility of liver disease and cirrhosis. The contamination of blood products in the 1970s and 1980s resulted in widespread transmission of HIV and hepatitis C virus (HCV) within the hemophilia population receiving factor infusions.

It is estimated in 2006, that >80% of hemophilia patients older than 20 years old are infected with HCV. Viral inactivation steps were introduced in the 1980s, and recombinant factor VIII and IX were first produced in the 1990s. HCV is the major cause of morbidity and the second leading cause of death in patients exposed to older factor concentrates. Patients develop cirrhosis and complications that include ascites and variceal bleeding. End-stage liver disease requiring a liver transplant is curative for the cirrhosis and the hemophilia (the liver produces factor VIII). Hepatitis B was not transmitted in significant numbers to patients with hemophilia. Diverticular disease or peptic ulcer disease would not explain the prolonged PT. Patients with inadequately repleted factor VIII levels are more likely to develop hemarthroses than GI bleeds, and the slightly prolonged activated partial thromboplastin time makes this unlikely.

62. The answer is E.
(Chap. 20) The differentiation between disseminated intravascular coagulation (DIC) and severe liver disease is challenging. Both entities may manifest with similar laboratory findings, which are elevated fibrinogen degradation products, prolonged activated partial thromboplastin time and prothrombin time, anemia, and thrombocytopenia. When suspecting DIC, these tests should be repeated over a period of 6 to 8 hours because abnormalities may change dramatically in patients with severe DIC. In contrast, these test results should not fluctuate as much in patients with severe liver disease. Bacterial sepsis with positive blood cultures is a common cause of DIC but is not diagnostic.

63. The answer is B.
(Chap. 21) Venous thrombosis occurs through activation of the coagulation cascade primarily through the exposure to tissue factor, and the genetic factors that contribute to a predisposition to venous thrombosis typically are polymorphisms affecting procoagulant or fibrinolytic pathways. In contrast, arterial thrombosis occurs in the setting a platelet activation, and the genetic predisposition for arterial thrombosis includes mutations that affect platelet receptors or redox enzymes. The most common inherited risk factors for venous thrombosis are the factor V Leiden mutation and prothrombin 20210 mutation. Other mutations predisposing an individual to venous thrombosis include inherited deficiency of protein C or S and mutations of fibrinogen, tissue plasminogen activator, thrombomodulin, or plasminogen activator inhibitor. The glycoprotein 1b platelet receptor mutation would increase the risk of arterial, but not venous, thrombosis.

64. The answer is A.
(Chap. 21) D-Dimer is a degradation product of cross-linked fibrin and is elevated in conditions of ongoing thrombosis. Low concentrations of D-dimer are considered to indicate the absence of thrombosis. Patients older than the age of 70 years frequently have elevated D-dimers in the absence of thrombosis, making this test less predictive of acute disease. Clinical symptoms are often not present in patients with deep-vein thrombosis (DVT) and do not affect interpretation of a D-dimer. Tobacco use, although frequently considered a risk factor for DVT, and previous DVT should not affect the predictive value of D-dimer. Homan's sign, calf pain elicited by dorsiflexion of the foot, is not predictive of DVT and is unrelated to D-dimer.

65. The answer is E.
(Chaps. 21 and 22) The clinical probability of pulmonary embolism (pulmonary embolism) can be delineated into low to high likelihood using the clinical decision rule shown in Table 22-1. In those with a score of 3 or less, pulmonary embolism is low or moderately likely, and a D-dimer test should be performed. A normal D-dimer result combined with a low to moderate clinical probability of pulmonary embolism identifies patients who do not need further testing or anticoagulation therapy. Those with either a likely clinical probability (score >3) or an abnormal D-dimer (with unlikely clinical probability) require an imaging test to rule out pulmonary embolism. Currently, the most attractive imaging method to detect pulmonary embolism is the multislice computed tomography (CT). It is accurate and, if the result is normal, safely rules out pulmonary embolism. This patient has a clinical probability score of 4.5 because of her resting tachycardia and the lack of an alternative diagnosis at least as likely as pulmonary embolism. Therefore, there is no indication for measuring D-dimer, and she should proceed directly to multislice CT of the chest. If this cannot be performed expeditiously, she should receive one dose of low-molecular-weight heparin while awaiting the test.

66. The answer is C.
(Chap. 23) In recent years, a variety of new anticoagulant and antiplatelet drugs have been developed for clinical use. Platelets play an important role in arterial thrombosis, particularly in coronary artery and cerebrovascular disease. Aspirin is the most widely used antiplatelet drug worldwide. Aspirin exerts its effects through inhibition of cyclooxygenase-1. Other commonly used oral antiplatelet agents are clopidogrel and dipyridamole. Clopidogrel is in a class of agents called thienopyridines along with ticlopidine. Thienopyridines act to block a specific adenosine diphosphate receptor ($P2Y_{12}$) and inhibit platelet aggregation. Dipyridamole inhibits phosphodiesterase to decrease the breakdown of cyclic adenosine monophosphate (cAMP) to decrease platelet aggregation. Intravenous antiplatelet agents have also become increasingly important in the treatment of acute coronary syndromes. All of the intravenous agents act to inhibit platelet aggregation by blocking the glycoprotein (Gp) IIb/IIIa receptor. The

three agents in clinical use as Gp IIb/IIIa inhibitors are abciximab, eptifibatide, and tirofiban.

Anticoagulant agents are primarily used for the prevention and treatment of venous thrombosis. Many anticoagulants are available and act by a variety of mechanisms. Heparin has been used for many years but requires frequent monitoring to be used safely. More recently, low-molecular-weight heparins (LMWHs) have been introduced. These agents are given subcutaneously and generally preferred in many instances over heparin given a more predictable anticoagulant effect. Both heparin and the LMWHs are indirect thrombin inhibitors that act primarily through activation of antithrombin. When activated, antithrombin inhibits clotting enzymes, especially thrombin and factor Xa. Fondaparinux is a newer anticoagulant that inhibits only factor Xa, although it is a synthetic analogue of the pentasaccharide sequence in heparin that binds antithrombin. However, it is too short to bridge antithrombin to thrombin. The direct thrombin inhibitors bind directly to thrombin (rather than antithrombin) to exert their activity. The direct thrombin inhibitors include lepirudin, argatroban, and bivalirudin. The most commonly used oral anticoagulant is warfarin, which inhibits the production of vitamin K–dependent clotting factors. Given the need for frequent monitoring and extensive drug interactions, developing other oral anticoagulants that are safe and effective has been desired for many years. No oral drug has yet been introduced into the market. However, several are in the final stages of development. These include two factor Xa inhibitors (rivaroxaban and apixaban) and one factor IIa inhibitor (dabigatran etexilate).

67. The answer is B.

(Chap. 23) After implantation of a bare metal coronary artery stent, aspirin and clopidogrel are recommended for at least 4 weeks to decrease the risk of in-stent restenosis. This patient, however, developed the complication despite adherence to her therapy. This generally suggests resistance to clopidogrel with a decreased ability of clopidogrel to inhibit platelet aggregation. There is a known genetic component to clopidogrel resistance related to specific genetic polymorphisms of the CYP isoenzymes. Up to 25% of whites, 30% of African Americans, and 50% of Asians may carry an allele that renders them resistant to clopidogrel. These polymorphisms are less important in the activation of prasugrel. Thus, in individuals who have evidence of clopidogrel resistance, switching to prasugrel should be considered.

Aspirin resistance is a more controversial subject. It is defined simply in clinical terms as failure of aspirin to prevent ischemic vascular events. Biochemically, aspirin resistance can be defined by failure of usual doses of the drug to produce inhibitory effects on platelet function. However, resistance to aspirin is not reversed by higher doses of aspirin or adding another antiplatelet agent. Because the primary mechanism of arterial thrombosis is platelet aggregation, the anticoagulant agents warfarin and low-molecular-weight heparin are not indicated.

68. The answer is B.

(Chap. 23) Low-molecular-weight heparins (LMWHs) have largely replaced heparin for most indications if a patient does not have any contraindications to therapy. LMWHs have better bioavailability and longer half-lives after subcutaneous injection. Thus, they can be given at routine intervals for both prophylaxis and treatment. In addition, dosing of LMWHs is simplified because these drugs have a dose-independent clearance, and predictable anticoagulant effects means that monitoring of anticoagulant effect is not required in most patients. Finally, LMWHs have a lower risk of heparin-induced thrombocytopenia, which is important in both short- and long-term administration.

69. The answer is B.

(Chap. 22) The D-dimer measured by enzyme-linked immunosorbent assay (ELISA) is elevated in the setting of breakdown of fibrin by plasmin, and the presence of a positive D-dimer can prompt the need for additional imaging for deep-vein thrombosis and/or pulmonary embolus in specific clinical situations in which the patient would be considered to have an elevation in D-dimer. However, one must be cautious about placing value on an elevated D-dimer in other situations when there can be an alternative explanation for the elevated level. Of the scenarios listed in the question, the only patient who would be expected to have a negative D-dimer result would be the patient with calf pain and recent air travel. The presence of a normal alveolar–arterial oxygen gradient cannot reliably differentiate between those with and without pulmonary embolism. In all the other scenarios, elevations in D-dimer could be related to other medical conditions and provide no diagnostic information to inform the clinician regarding the need for further evaluation. Some common clinical situations in which the D-dimer is elevated include sepsis, myocardial infarction, cancer, pneumonia, the postoperative state, and the second and third trimesters of pregnancy.

70. The answer is B.

(Chap. 22) Clinically, individuals with massive pulmonary embolus present with hypotension, syncope, or cyanosis. The hypotension and syncope occur due to acute right ventricular overload, and elevated troponin or amino terminal (NT)-pro-brain natriuretic peptide can result from this right ventricular strain. Both elevated troponin and NT-pro-brain natriuretic peptide predict worse outcomes in pulmonary embolism. Further prognostic signs of massive pulmonary embolism include the presence of right ventricular enlargement on computed tomography of the chest or right ventricular hypokinesis on echocardiography. The presence of hemoptysis, pleuritic chest pain, or

cough in association with pulmonary embolism most commonly indicates a small peripheral lesion.

71. The answer is B.

(Chap. 22) For many years, ventilation–perfusion imaging (V-Q) was the standard for the diagnosis of pulmonary embolism (pulmonary embolism). Determination of abnormal V-Q imaging can be difficult. To call a V-Q scan a high-probability scan, one needs to see two or more segmental perfusion defects in the setting of normal ventilation. In patients with underlying lung disease, however, ventilation is frequently abnormal, and most patients with pulmonary embolism do not actually have high-probability V-Q scans. When there is a high-probability V-Q scan, the likelihood of pulmonary embolism is 90% or greater. Alternatively, patients with normal perfusion imaging have a very low likelihood of pulmonary embolism. Most patients fall into either the low or intermediate probability of having a pulmonary embolism by V-Q imaging. In this setting, 40% of patients with a high clinical suspicion of pulmonary embolism are determined by pulmonary angiography to indeed have a pulmonary embolism despite having a low-probability V-Q scan. At the present time, V-Q scanning is largely supplanted by multidetector-row spiral computed tomography (CT) angiography of the chest. Compared with conventional CT scanning with intravenous contrast, the multidetector spiral CT can provide evaluation of the pulmonary arteries to the sixth-order branches, a level of resolution that is as good as or exceeds that of conventional invasive pulmonary angiography. In addition, the CT allows evaluation of the right and left ventricles as well as the lung parenchyma to provide additional information regarding prognosis in acute pulmonary embolism or alternative diagnosis in the patient with dyspnea. Magnetic resonance angiography is a rarely used alternative to the above modalities in patients with contrast dye allergy. This technique provides the ability to detect large proximal PEs but lacks reliability for segmental and subsegmental pulmonary embolism.

72. The answer is E.

(Chap. 22) This patient is presenting with massive pulmonary embolus (pulmonary embolism) with ongoing hypotension, right ventricular dysfunction, and profound hypoxemia requiring 100% oxygen. In this setting, continuing with anticoagulation alone is inadequate, and the patient should receive circulatory support with fibrinolysis if there are no contraindications to therapy. The major contraindications to fibrinolysis include hypertension >180/110 mm Hg, known intracranial disease or prior hemorrhagic stroke, recent surgery, or trauma. The recommended fibrinolytic regimen is recombinant tissue plasminogen activator (rTPA), 100 mg IV over 2 hours. Heparin should be continued with the fibrinolytic to prevent a rebound hypercoagulable state with dissolution of the clot. There is a 10% risk of major bleeding with fibrinolytic therapy, with a 1–3% risk of intracranial hemorrhage. The only indication approved by the U.S. Food and Drug Administration for fibrinolysis in pulmonary embolism is for massive pulmonary embolism presenting with life-threatening hypotension, right ventricular dysfunction, and refractory hypoxemia. In submassive pulmonary embolism presenting with preserved blood pressure and evidence of right ventricular dysfunction on echocardiogram, the decision to pursue fibrinolysis is made on a case-by-case basis. In addition to fibrinolysis, the patient should also receive circulatory support with vasopressors. Dopamine and dobutamine are the vasopressors of choice for the treatment of shock in pulmonary embolism. Caution should be taken with ongoing high-volume fluid administration, as a poorly functioning right ventricle may be poorly tolerant of additional fluids. Ongoing fluids may worsen right ventricular ischemia and further dilate the right ventricle, displacing the interventricular septum to the left to worsen cardiac output and hypotension. If the patient had contraindications to fibrinolysis and was unable to be stabilized with vasopressor support, referral for surgical embolectomy should be considered. Referral for inferior vena cava filter placement is not indicated at this time. The patient should be stabilized hemodynamically as a first priority. The indications for inferior vena cava filter placement are active bleeding, precluding anticoagulation, and recurrent deep-vein thrombosis on adequate anticoagulation.

73. The answer is E.

(Chap. 22) Warfarin should not be used alone as initial therapy for the treatment of venous thromboembolic disease (VTE) for two reasons. First, warfarin does not achieve full anticoagulation for at least 5 days, as its mechanism of action is to decrease the production of vitamin K–dependent coagulation factors in the liver. Second, a paradoxical reaction that promotes coagulation may also occur upon initiation of warfarin as it also decreases the production of the vitamin K–dependent anticoagulants protein C and protein S, which have shorter half-lives than the procoagulant factors. For many years, unfractionated heparin delivered intravenously was the treatment of choice for VTE. However, it requires frequent monitoring of activated partial thromboplastin time (aPTT) levels and hospitalization until therapeutic international normalized ratio (INR) is achieved with warfarin. There are now several safe and effective alternatives to unfractionated heparin that can be delivered SC. Low-molecular-weight heparins (enoxaparin, tinzaparin) are fragments of unfractionated heparin with a lower molecular weight. These compounds have a greater bioavailability, longer half-life, and more predictable onset of action. Their use in renal insufficiency should be considered with caution because low-molecular-weight heparins are renally cleared. Fondaparinux is a direct factor Xa inhibitor that, like low-molecular-weight heparins, requires no

monitoring of anticoagulant effects and has been demonstrated to be safe and effective in treating both deep-vein thrombosis and pulmonary embolism.

74. The answer is A.

(Chap. 26) Although cigarette smoking is the greatest modifiable risk factor for the development of cancer, the most significant risk factor for cancer in general is age. Two-thirds of all cancers are diagnosed in individuals older than 65 years, and the risk of developing cancer between the ages of 60 and 79 years is one in three in men and one in five in women. In contrast, the risk of cancer between birth and age 49 years is one in 70 for boys and men and one in 48 for girls and women. Overall, men have a slightly greater risk of developing cancer than women (44% vs 38% lifetime risk).

75. The answer is A.

(Chap. 26) The cause of cancer death differs across the life span. In women who are younger than 20 years of age, the largest cause of cancer death is leukemia. Between the ages of 20 and 59 years, breast cancer becomes the leading cause of cancer death. However, lung cancer is the leading cause of cancer death after the age of 60 years and is overall the number one cause of cancer death in women.

76. The answer is B.

(Chap. 26) Although tumor burden is certainly a major factor in determining cancer outcomes, it is also important to consider the functional status of the patient when considering the therapeutic plan. The physiologic stresses of undergoing surgical interventions, radiation therapy, and chemotherapy can exhaust the limited reserves of a patient with multiple medical problems. It is clearly difficult to adequately measure the physiologic reserves of a patient, and most oncologists use performance status measures as a surrogate. Two of the most commonly used measures of performance status are the Eastern Cooperative Oncology Group (ECOG) and Karnofsky performance status. The ECOG scale provides a grade between 0 (fully active) and 5 (dead). Most patients are considered to have adequate reserve for undergoing treatment if the performance status is 0 to 2, with a grade 2 indicating someone who is ambulatory and capable of all self-care but unable carry out work activities. These individuals are up and about >50% of waking hours. A grade 3 performance score indicates someone who is capable of only limited self-care and is confined to a bed or chair >50% of waking hours. The Karnofsky score ranges from 0 (dead) to 100 (normal) and is graded at 10-point intervals. A Karnofsky score of <70 also indicates someone with poor performance status.

77. The answer is D.

(Chap. 26) Tumor markers are proteins produced by tumor cells that can be measured in the serum or urine. These markers are neither sensitive nor specific enough to be useful for diagnosis or screening of cancer. However, in an individual with a known malignancy, rising or falling levels may be helpful for determining disease activity and response to therapy. Common tumor markers with associated diseases are shown in Table 26-6. Of the tumor pairs listed, only human chorionic gonadotropin is correctly paired with its association with gestational trophoblastic disease.

78. The answer is C.

(Chap. 24) Cancer occurs when a single cell acquires a series of genetic mutations that allow the cell to proliferate without regulation. The clonal nature of cancer is a key feature that allows a malignancy to be differentiated from hyperplasia, in which polyclonality is seen. Significant research has occurred over the past decades that allows us to understand the genetic causes of cancer in greater detail, and new research is providing a growing knowledge of cancer of any number of cell types with the hopes that future therapies can be personalized to the mutations that are present in the individual cancer. Based on laboratory research, it is thought that five to 10 mutations are needed for a cell to transform into a malignant cancer, although often many more mutations can be seen. The major genes involved in cancer are oncogenes and tumor-suppressor genes. Both of these types of genes contribute to the malignant phenotype by leading to unregulated cell division or the ability to avoid programmed cell death. Oncogenes require only a single mutation to become activated and act in an autosomal dominant fashion. In contrast, tumor-suppressor genes require both copies of the allele to become inactivated to lose their protective effects against unregulated cell growth. Caretaker genes are a subset of tumor-suppressor genes and have no direct effect on cell growth. These genes function to help the cell protect the integrity of its genome by repairing DNA defects that occur.

79. The answer is E.

(Chap. 24) A small proportion of cancers occur in patients with a genetic predisposition. Roughly 100 syndromes of familial cancer have been reported. Recognition allows for genetic counseling and increased cancer surveillance. Down syndrome, or trisomy 21, is characterized clinically by a variety of features, including moderate to severe learning disability, facial and musculoskeletal deformities, duodenal atresia, congenital heart defects, and an increased risk of acute leukemia. Fanconi's anemia is a condition that is associated with defects in DNA repair. There is a higher incidence of cancer, with leukemia and myelodysplasia being the most common cancers. von Hippel–Lindau syndrome is associated with hemangioblastomas, renal cysts, pancreatic cysts and carcinomas, and renal cell cancer. Neurofibromatosis (NF) types I and II are both associated with increased tumor formation. NF II is more associated with schwannoma.

Both carry a risk of malignant peripheral nerve sheath tumors. Fragile X is a condition associated with chromosomal instability of the X chromosome. These patients have mental retardation; typical morphologic features, including macro-orchidism and prognathia; behavioral problems; and occasionally seizures. Increased cancer incidence has not been described.

80. The answer is C.

(Chap. 25) Cancer treatment is undergoing a revolution with an increasing number of therapies that are directed specifically against signal transduction pathways. These pathways are often activated in cancer cells and contribute to the malignant phenotype of the cell. One commonly affected signal transduction pathway is that of tyrosine kinase. Typically, tyrosine kinase is only active for a very short period. However, in malignant cells, the tyrosine kinase pathway can be constitutively activated through mutation, gene amplification, or gene translocation. Small molecule therapy that can inhibit a tyrosine kinase pathway can lead to decreased proliferation of malignant cells, decreased survival, and impeded angiogenesis. Examples of targeted small molecule therapies and their molecular targets can be found in Table 25-2. These include drugs as well as monoclonal antibodies. Among the first small molecule therapies to be used in malignancy was imatinib, which has dramatically changed therapy in chronic myeloid leukemia. This drug targets the activated tyrosine kinase pathway activated by the Bcr-Abl mutation that is present in this disease.

Bevacizumab is a monoclonal antibody targeted against pathways in vascular endothelial growth factor (VEGF) and is used in lung and colon cancer. It had previously been used for breast cancer, but the U.S. Food and Drug Administration has recommended against its use in breast cancer as of November 2011 (*www.fda.gov*, accessed December 1, 2011). Erlotinib and gefitinib are active against tumors carrying mutations of the epidermal growth factor receptor, especially in lung cancer. Rituximab has been used for many years and is an anti-CD20. Its most common use is in B-cell lymphomas and leukemias, but it is undergoing trials for use in autoimmune disease as well. Sunitinib and sorafenib both have activity against a large number of kinases. Whereas sunitinib targets c-Kit, VEGFR-2, PDGFR-β, and Fit-3, sorafenib targets RAF, VEGFR-2, PDGFR-α/β, Fit-3, and c-Kit.

81. The answer is B.

(Chap. 25) Epigenetics is a term that refers to changes in the chromatin structure of the cell that lead to alterations in gene expression without underlying changes in the DNA code. As such, these changes are potentially reversible and may be targets for cancer therapy. An example of an important epigenetic change is hypermethylation of promoter regions (so-called CpG islands) in tumor-suppressor genes that lead to the inactivation of one allele of the gene.

82. The answer is A.

(Chap. 28) Generally, when metastatic disease is observed, surgical interventions do not change the outcome of a particular cancer. However, in a few instances, one should consider surgery as potentially curative. One example is metastatic osteosarcoma to the lung, which can be cured by resection of the lung lesion. There are other instances in which surgery may be effective in patients with metastatic disease. In non–small cell lung cancer, individual with a solitary brain metastasis at the time of diagnosis may also be treated with resection of the brain and lung lesions in a staged fashion. In colon cancer with liver metastases, hepatic lobectomy may produce long-term disease-free survival in as many as 25% of individuals if fewer than five lesions are observed in a single hepatic lobe. Another role for surgical resection in metastatic disease is to remove the source of hormone production that can stimulate cancer growth. This is occasionally recommended in prostate cancer, although antiandrogen therapy is most commonly used.

83. The answer is D.

(Chap. 28) Clinical trials in cancer drug discovery follows a stepwise process before the drug is determined to be safe and effective for treatment of a specific cancer. Before proceeding to trials in human, cancer drugs must demonstrate antitumor activity with a specific dose and interval in animal trials. After this, drugs enter phase I trials to establish safe dosage range and side effects in humans. Clinical antitumor effect is observed, but phase II trials enroll a larger group of people to more rigorously quantify antitumor effects in humans. Further side effect data is collected as well. The dose given in phase II trials is the maximal tolerated dose determined in phase I trials. Although phase I trials often given escalating doses of an agent, phase II trials use a fixed dose, and the drug is given to only a very select and homogeneous group of patients. An agent is determined to be "active" and may proceed to a phase III trial if there is a partial regression rate of at least 20–25% with reversible non–life-threatening side effects. Phase III trials enroll the largest numbers of patients and often compare the drug with standard therapies for the particular cancer. Phase IV trials occur after release of the drug and are called postmarketing studies. These trials provide important information about risks, benefits, and optimal use in the general population of patients with a particular cancer, which can often be quite different than those patients enrolled in a clinical trial.

84. The answers are 1—D, 2—C, 3—A, 4—E, and 5—B.

(Chap. 28) Cancer chemotherapy typically requires actively dividing cells to exert their actions to kill the cancer cells. The mechanism of action of the majority of

chemotherapeutic agents can be broadly categorized as those affecting DNA, those affecting microtubules, and molecularly targeted agents. Within each of these broad categories, several common families of drugs operating have distinct mechanisms of action. DNA alkylating agents are cell cycle phase nonspecific agents that covalently modify DNA bases and lead to cross-linkage of DNA strands. These cells become unable to complete normal cell division. Examples of common DNA alkylating agents are cyclophosphamide, chlorambucil, dacarbazine, and the platinum agents (carboplatin, cisplatin, and oxaliplatin). Antitumor antibiotics are naturally occurring substances typically produced by bacteria that bind to DNA directly and cause free radical damage that leads to DNA breakage. Included in this group are topoisomerase poisons that are derived from plants that prevent DNA unwinding and replication. Examples of agents in this category are bleomycin, etoposide, topotecan, irinotecan, doxorubicin, daunorubicin, and mitoxantrone. Other drugs that are common anticancer agents affect DNA indirectly, especially through interference in the synthesis of purines or pyrimidines. This category of agents is known as antimetabolites and includes methotrexate, azathioprine, 5-fluorouracil, cytosine arabinoside, gemcitabine, fludarabine, asparaginase, and pemetrexed, among others.

Chemotherapeutics agents that target the microtubules interfere with cell division by inhibiting the mitotic spindle. These antimitotic agents include vincristine, vinblastine, vinorelbine, paclitaxel, and docetaxel, among others.

Molecularly targeted agents are relatively new agents for the treatment of malignancy. When compared with traditional cancer chemotherapy, these agents are directed against specific proteins within cells that are important in cell signal processing. There are many different types of molecularly targeted agents with the largest class being tyrosine kinase inhibitors. Commonly used tyrosine kinase inhibitors include imatinib, gefitinib, erlotinib, sorafenib, and sunitinib. All-*trans* retinoic acid is another example of a molecularly targeted agent that attaches to the promyelocytic leukemia–retinoic acid receptor fusion protein to stimulate differentiation of the promyelocytes to mature granulocytes. Other categories of targeted agents include histone deacetylase inhibitors and mTOR (mammalian target of rapamycin) inhibitors.

85. The answer is E.

(Chap. 28) Myelosuppression predictably occurs after administration of a variety of chemotherapeutic agents. Antimetabolites and anthracyclines (including doxorubicin) typically cause neutropenia between 6 and 14 days after administration of the agent. Febrile neutropenia is diagnosed based on a single temperature >38.5°C or three temperatures >38.0°C. Treatment of febrile neutropenia conventionally includes initiation of treatment with broad-spectrum antibiotics. If there is no obvious site of infection, then coverage for *Pseudomonas aeruginosa* is recommended. Active antibiotics include third- or fourth-generation cephalosporins (including ceftazidime), antipseudomonal penicillins, carbapenems, and aminoglycosides. Vancomycin should be considered in this patient because of her tunneled intravenous catheter despite the apparent lack of cutaneous infection and would be continued until culture demonstrated the absence of a resistant organism. There is no need for an antifungal agent because this patient has not had prolonged neutropenia, and this is the first fever recorded. Moreover, given the chemotherapy given, the expected duration of neutropenia is expected to be relatively brief. In many instances such as this, oral antibiotics such as ciprofloxacin can be given.

There is no role for granulocyte transfusions in the treatment. However, the use of colony-stimulating factors often is considered. These agents have historically been overused, and the American Society of Clinical Oncology has developed practice guidelines to assist in determining which patients should receive colony-stimulating factors. Briefly, there is no evidence for benefit in either febrile or afebrile neutropenic patients, and they should not routinely be used in acute myeloid leukemia or myelodysplastic syndromes. The only therapeutic use is in individuals who have undergone bone marrow or stem cell transplantation to speed myeloid recovery. The primary use of colony-stimulating factors is in the setting of prevention. Because this patient has now experienced an episode of febrile neutropenia, she should be given colony-stimulating factors beginning 24 to 72 hours after chemotherapy administration, and the medication should continue until the neutrophil count is 10,000/μL or greater. Colony-stimulating factors may be given after the first cycle of chemotherapy if the likelihood of febrile neutropenia is >20%, if the patient has preexisting neutropenia or active infection, if the patient is older than 65 years of age and is being treated for lymphoma, or if the patient has a poor performance status or has had extensive prior chemotherapy.

86. The answer is E.

(Chap. 28) Nausea with or without vomiting is the most common side effect of chemotherapy. It can be anticipatory in nature, acute, or occur >24 hours after administration. Patients at increased risk of nausea include younger patients, women, and those with a history of motion or morning sickness. The chemotherapeutic agents used also alter the risk of nausea and vomiting. Highly emetogenic drugs include high-dose cyclophosphamide and cisplatin. Low-risk drugs include fluorouracil, taxanes, and etoposide. In patients receiving high-risk regimens, prophylactic treatment with a combination of medications acting at different sites is recommended. Typically, the regimen would include

a serotonin antagonist such as dolasetron, a neurokine receptor antagonist such are aprepitant, and potent corticosteroids such as dexamethasone.

87. The answer is C.

(Chap. 29) Patients who have undergone allogeneic stem cell transplant remain at risk for infectious complications for an extended period despite engraftment and apparent return of normal hematopoietic capacity. Individuals with graft-versus-host disease (GVHD) often require immunosuppressive treatment that further increases their infectious risk. Prevention of infection is the goal in these individuals, and the clinician should ensure appropriate vaccinations for all patients who have undergone intensive chemotherapy, have been treated for Hodgkin's disease, or have undergone hematopoietic stem cell transplant. No vaccines except influenza should be given before 12 months after transplant. Then the only vaccines that should be given are inactivated vaccines. Therefore, oral vaccine for poliomyelitis and the varicella zoster vaccine are contraindicated. The measles, mump, and rubella vaccine is also a live virus vaccine but can be safely given after 24 months if the patient does not have GVHD. Other recommended vaccines include diphtheria–tetanus, inactivated poliomyelitis (by injection), *Haemophilus influenzae* type B, hepatitis B, and 23-valent pneumococcal polysaccharide vaccine. Meningococcal vaccination is recommended in splenectomized patients and in those living in endemic areas, including college dormitories.

88. The answer is B.

(Chap. 29) Specific malignancies are associated with underlying immune dysfunction and infection with specific organisms. Chronic lymphocytic leukemia and multiple myeloma may have an associated hypogammaglobulinemia. Individuals with these disorders are at risk of infections with *Streptococcus pneumoniae, Haemophilus influenzae,* and *Neisseria meningitidis.* Although immunoglobulin therapy is effective, it is more cost effective to give prophylactic antibiotics in these patients. Acute myeloid or lymphocytic leukemias often have an associated neutropenia and may present with overwhelming infection from extracellular bacteria and fungi, especially if the duration of neutropenia is prolonged. Patients with lymphomatous disorders often have abnormal T cell function despite normal numbers of T cells. Moreover, most patients also receive treatment with high doses of glucocorticoids that further impair T cell function. These individuals have an increased risk of infection with intracellular pathogens and may contract pneumonia with *Pneumocystis jiroveci.*

89. The answer is D.

(Chap. 29) Clinicians are often faced with treatment decisions regarding catheter-related infections in patients who are immunocompromised from cancer and chemotherapy. Because many patients require several weeks of chemotherapy, tunneled catheters are often placed, and determining the need for catheter removal is an important consideration. When blood culture results are positive or there is evidence of infection along the track of the tunnel, catheter removal is recommended. When the erythema is limited to the exit site only, then it is not necessary to remove the catheter unless the erythema fails to respond to treatment. The recommended treatment for an exit site infection should be directed against coagulase-negative staphylococci. In the options presented, vancomycin alone is the best option for treatment. There is no need to add therapy for gram-negative organisms because the patient does not have neutropenia and has negative culture results.

90. The answer is A.

(Chap. 31) Breast cancer in pregnant women is defined as cancer diagnosed during pregnancy or up to 1 year after delivery. Only about 5% of all breast cancers occur in women younger than 40 years of age, and of those, approximately 25% are pregnancy-associated cancer. Needle biopsy of breast masses in pregnant women is often nondiagnostic, and false-positive test results may occur. Breast cancers diagnosed during pregnancy have a worse outcome than other breast cancers. The cancers tend to be diagnosed at a later stage (often the signs are thought to be related to pregnancy) and tend to have a more aggressive behavior. Approximately 30% of breast cancers found in pregnancy are estrogen receptor positive in contrast to 60–70% being estrogen receptor positive overall. Larger tumor size, positive axillary nodes, Her-2 positivity, and higher stage are all more common in pregnant women.

91. The answer is E.

(Chap. 32) Communication of bad news is an inherent component of the physician–patient relationship, and these conversations often occur in a hospital setting where the treating provider is not the primary care provider for the patient. Many physicians struggle with providing clear and effective communication to patients who are seriously ill and their family members. In the scenario presented in this case, it is necessary to have a discussion about the patient's poor prognosis and determine the goals of care without the input of the patient because her mental status remains altered. Failure to provide clear communication in the appropriate environment can lead to tension in the relationship between the physician and patient and may lead to overly aggressive treatment. The P-SPIKES approach (Table 32-2) has been advocated as a simple framework to assist physicians in effectively communicating bad news to patients. The components of this communication tool are:

- Preparation—Review what information needs to be communicated and plan how emotional support will be provided.
- Setting of interaction—This step is often the most neglected. Ensure a quiet and private environment and attempt to minimize any interruptions.
- Patient (or family) perceptions and preparation—Assess what the patient and family know about the current condition. Use open-ended questions.
- Invitation and information needs—Ask the patient or family what they would like to know and also what limits they want regarding bad information
- Knowledge of the condition—Provide the patient and family with the bad news and assess understanding.
- Empathy and exploration—Empathize with the patient and family's feelings and offer emotional support. Allow plenty of time for questions and exploration of their feelings.
- Summary and planning—Outline the next steps for the patient and family. Recommend a timeline to achieve the goals of care.

Setting a follow-up meeting is not a primary component of the P-SPIKES framework but may be necessary when a family or patient is not emotionally ready to discuss the next steps in the care plan.

92. The answer is C.
(Chap. 32) Advance care planning documentation is an increasing component of medical practice. As of 2006, 48 states and the District of Columbia had enacted legislation regarding advance care planning. The two broad types of advance care planning documentation are living wills and designation of a health care proxy (option C). Although these two documents are often combined into a single document, designation of a health care proxy is not one of the primary components of a living will. The living will (or instructional directive) delineates the patient's preferences (option A) regarding treatment under different scenarios (e.g., whether condition is perceived as terminal). These documents can be very specific to a condition such as cancer but may also be very broad in the case of elderly individuals who do not currently have a terminal condition but want to outline their wishes for care in the event of an unexpected health crisis. Examples of what this might include general statements regarding the receipt of life-sustaining therapies (option D) and the values that should guide the decisions regarding terminal care (option B).

93. The answer is C.
(Chap. 32) A primary goal of palliative care medicine is to control pain in patients who are terminally ill. Surveys have found that 36–90% of individuals with advanced cancer have substantial pain, and an individualized treatment plan is necessary for each patient. For individuals with continuous pain, opioid analgesics should be administered on a scheduled basis around the clock at an interval based on the half-life of the medication chosen. Extended-release preparations are frequently used because of their longer half-lives. However, it is inappropriate to start immediately with an extended-release preparation. In this scenario, the patient was treated with a continuous intravenous infusion via patient-controlled analgesia for 48 hours to determine her baseline opioid needs. The average daily dose of morphine required was 90 mg. This total dose should be administered in divided doses two or three times daily (either 45 mg twice daily or 30 mg three times daily). In addition, an immediate-release preparation should be available for administration for breakthrough pain. The recommended dose of the immediate-release preparation is 20% of the baseline dose. In this case, the dose would be 18 mg and could be given as either 15 or 20 mg four times daily as needed.

94. The answer is D.
(Chap. 32) Depression is difficult to diagnose in individuals with terminal illness and is often an overlooked symptom by physicians because many individual believe it a normal component of terminal illness. Furthermore, symptoms commonly associated with depression such as insomnia and anorexia are also frequently seen in serious illness or occur as a side effect of treatment. Although about 75% of terminally ill patients express some depressive symptoms, only 25% or fewer have major depression. When assessing depression in terminally ill individuals, one should focus on symptoms pertaining to the dysphoric mood, including helplessness, hopelessness, and anhedonia. It is inappropriate to do nothing in when one believes major depression is occurring (option A). The approach to treatment should include nonpharmacologic and pharmacologic therapies. The pharmacologic approach to depression should be the same in terminally ill individuals as in non–terminally ill individuals. If an individual has a prognosis of several months or longer, selective serotonin reuptake inhibitors (fluoxetine, paroxetine) or serotonin–noradrenaline reuptake inhibitors (venlafaxine) are the preferred treatment because of their efficacy and side effect profile. However, these medications take several weeks to become effective. Thus, starting fluoxetine alone (option C) is not preferred. In patients with major depression and fatigue or opioid-induced somnolence, combining a traditional antidepressant with a psychostimulant is appropriate (option D). Psychostimulants are also indicated in individuals with a poor prognosis who are not expected to live long enough to experience the benefits of treatment with a traditional antidepressant. A variety of psychostimulant medications are available, including methylphenidate, modafinil, dextroamphetamine, and pemoline. Because this patient has a prognosis of several

months or longer, methylphenidate alone is not recommended (option E). Because of their side effect profile, tricyclic antidepressants (option A) are not used in the treatment of depression in terminally ill patients unless they are used as adjunctive treatment for chronic pain.

95. The answer is E.

(Chap. 32) Withdrawal of care is a common occurrence in intensive care units. More than 90% of Americans die without performance of cardiopulmonary resuscitation. When a family decides to withdraw care, the treating care team of doctors, nurses, and respiratory therapists must work together to ensure that the dying process will be comfortable for both the patient and the family. Commonly, patients receive a combination of anxiolytics and opioid analgesics. These medications also provide relief of dyspnea in the dying patient. However, they have little effect on oropharyngeal secretions (option A). The accumulation of secretions in the oropharynx can produce agitation, labored breathing, and noisy breathing that has been labeled the "death rattle." This can be quite distressing to the family. Treatments for excessive oropharyngeal secretions are primarily anticholinergic medications, including scopolamine delivered transdermally (option E) or intravenously, atropine, and glycopyrrolate. Although placement of a nasal trumpet or oral airway (option D) may allow better access for suctioning of secretions, these can be uncomfortable or even painful interventions that are typically discouraged in a palliative care situation. *N*-acetylcysteine (option B) can be used as a mucolytic agent to thin lower respiratory secretions. Pilocarpine (option C) is a cholinergic stimulant and increases salivary production.

96. The answer is A.

(Chap. 33) The staging criteria for melanoma include the thickness of the lesion, the presence of ulceration, and the presence and number of involved lymph nodes. Of these, the single best predictor of metastatic risk is the Breslow thickness, particularly >4 mm, although the other factors also provide additional predictive value. Other factors that predict survival in melanoma are younger age, gender with female sex predicting a better survival, and anatomic site with favorable sites being the forearm and leg. The Clark level defined melanoma based on the layer of skin to which a melanoma had invaded, but this has been found to be not predictive of metastatic risk.

97. The answer is E.

(Chap. 33, PB Chapman et al: N Engl J Med *2011;364: 2507–2516)* Treatment of metastatic melanoma has largely shown very little improvements on mortality in this disease. The median survival time after diagnosis of metastatic disease is typically 6 to 15 months. Until August 2011, the only Food and Drug Administration (FDA)–approved chemotherapy for the treatment of metastatic disease was dacarbazine, although response rates are about 20% or less. Interleukin-2 (IL-2) therapy has also been attempted alone or in combination with interferon-α. This therapy has led to long-term disease-free survival in about 5% of treated patients but is associated with significant toxicity that limits its usefulness. IL-2 should only be administered to patients with good performance status and at centers experienced in the treatment of IL-2 toxicity. Most recently in August 2011, the FDA approved the drug vemurafenib (PLX4032) for the treatment of metastatic melanoma. This drug targets *BRAF*, which is a common mutation in melanoma that results in constitutive activation of the mitogen-activated protein (MAP) kinase pathway. Vemurafenib has specifically demonstrated to have the best activity against the BRAF V600E mutation, the most common kinase mutation in metastatic melanoma. Data published in 2011 demonstrated that individuals with this specific mutation have response rates of 48% to the drug compared with only 5% for dacarbazine. Furthermore, the 6-month survival was rate 84% in the vemurafenib group compared with only 64% in the dacarbazine group. Ipilimumab is another promising new therapy for the treatment of metastatic melanoma. This treatment is a monoclonal antibody that blocks cytotoxic T-cell antigen 4 (CTLA-4), and a recent clinical trial demonstrated improved overall survival rates in patients treated with ipilimumab plus dacarbazine compared with dacarbazine alone (C Robert et al: *N Engl J Med* 2011,364. 2517–25).

98. The answer is C.

(Chap. 34) Head and neck cancers account for about 3% of all malignancies in the United States and comprise a varied site of tumors, including those of the nasopharynx, oropharynx, hypopharynx, and larynx. Squamous cell history is the predominant cell type at all sites, but there are different risk factors by site. Nasopharyngeal cancers are rare in the United States but are endemic in the Mediterranean and Far East, where they are associated with Epstein-Barr virus infection. Oropharyngeal cancers are associated with tobacco use, especially smokeless tobacco, and increasing numbers of oropharyngeal cancers are found to be associated with human papilloma virus (HPV). The association with HPV virus infection, particularly serotypes 16 and 18, characterizes these oropharyngeal cancers as a form of sexually transmitted disease and is associated with oral sexual practices and an increased number of sexual partners. However, the predominant risk factors for head and neck cancers, particularly those of the hypopharynx and larynx, are alcohol and tobacco use. Cancers of the larynx often present with the subacute onset of hoarseness that does not resolve over time, but symptoms of head and neck cancer can be rather nonspecific. In more advanced cases, pain, stridor, dysphagia, odynophagia, and cranial neuropathies can occur. Diagnosis of head and neck cancer should include computed tomography of the head

and neck and endoscopic examination under anesthesia to perform biopsies. Positron emission tomography scans may be used as adjunctive therapy. The staging of head and neck cancers follows a TNM (tumor, node, metastasis) staging guideline. This patient would be staged as T2N0M0 based on a tumor size without evidence of lymph node involvement or distant metastatic disease. With this designation, the patient's overall stage would be stage II and classified as localized disease. The intent of therapy at this stage of disease is cure of cancer, and the overall 5-year survival is 60–90%. The choice of therapy for laryngeal cancer is radiation therapy to preserve the voice. Surgical therapy could be chosen by the patient as well but is less desirable. In locally or regionally advanced disease, patients can still be approached with curative intent, but this requires multimodality therapy with surgery followed by concomitant chemotherapy and radiation treatment.

99. The answer is A.

(Chap. 35) Solitary pulmonary nodules are frequent causes of referral to a pulmonologist, but most solitary pulmonary nodules are benign. In fact, >90% of incidentally identified nodules are of benign origin. Features that are more likely to be present in a malignant lesion are size larger than 3 cm, eccentric calcification, rapid doubling time, and lobulated and irregular contour. Ground-glass appearance on computed tomography can be either malignant or benign. Among malignant lesions, it is seen more commonly in bronchoalveolar cell carcinoma. When multiple pulmonary nodules are identified, it most commonly represents prior granulomatous disease from healed infections. If multiple nodules are malignant in origin, it usually indicates disease metastatic to the lung but can be simultaneous lung primary lesions or lesions metastatic from a primary lung cancer. Many incidentally identified nodules are too small to be diagnosed by biopsy and are nonspecific in nature. In this situation, it is prudent to follow the lesions for 2 years, especially in a patient who is high risk for lung cancer to allow for a proper doubling time to occur. If the lesion remains stable for 2 years, it is most likely benign, although some slow-growing tumors such bronchoalveolar cell carcinoma can have a slower growth rate.

100. The answer is E.

(Chap. 35) The evaluation and treatment of solitary pulmonary nodules is important to understand. This patient has a long smoking history with a new nodule that was not apparent by chest radiography 3 years previously. This should be assumed to be a malignant nodule, and definitive diagnosis and treatment should be attempted. The option for diagnostic and staging procedures include positron emission tomography (PET) and computed tomography (CT), bronchoscopic biopsy, percutaneous needle biopsy, and surgical biopsy with concomitant resection if positive. PET and CT would be low yield in this patient given the small size of the primary lesion (<1 cm) and the lack of enlarged mediastinal lymph nodes. Likewise, bronchoscopy would not provide a good yield because the lesion is very peripheral in origin, and a negative biopsy result for malignancy would not be definitive. Appropriate approaches would be to either perform a percutaneous needle biopsy with CT guidance or perform a surgical biopsy with definitive resection if positive. Because this patient has preserved lung function, surgical biopsy and resection is a good treatment option. A repeat CT scan assessing for interval growth would only be appropriate if the patient declined further workup at this time. Referral for treatment with radiation therapy is not appropriate in the absence of tissue diagnosis of malignancy, and surgical resection is the preferred primary treatment because the patient has no contraindications to surgical intervention.

101. The answer is E.

(Chap. 35) Pancoast syndrome results from apical extension of a lung mass into the brachial plexus with frequent involvement of the eighth cervical and first and second thoracic nerves. As the tumor continues to grow, it will also involve the sympathetic ganglia of the thoracic chain. The clinical manifestations of a Pancoast tumor include shoulder and arm pain and Horner's syndrome (ipsilateral ptosis, miosis, and anhidrosis). Often, the shoulder and arm pain presents several months before diagnosis. The most common cause of Pancoast syndrome is an apical lung tumor, usually non–small cell lung cancer. Other causes include mesothelioma and infection, among others. Although midbrain lesions can cause Horner's syndrome, other cranial nerve abnormalities would be expected.

Enlarged mediastinal lymph nodes and masses in the middle mediastinum can occlude the superior vena cava (SVC), leading to SVC syndrome. Individuals with SVC syndrome typically present with dyspnea and have evidence of facial and upper extremity swelling. Eaton Lambert myasthenic syndrome is caused by antibodies to voltage-gated calcium channels and is characterized by generalized weakness of muscles that increases with repetitive nerve stimulation. Cervical ribs can cause thoracic outlet syndrome by compression of nerves or vasculature as they exit the chest. This typically presents with ischemic symptoms to the affected limb, but intrinsic wasting of the muscles of the hand can be seen because of neurologic compromise.

102. The answer is E.

(Chap. 35) At the time of diagnosis, 70% of small cell lung cancers have metastasized. In contrast to non–small cell lung cancer, small cell lung cancer is staged as limited or extensive disease based on the spread of disease in the body rather than size of the tumor burden or extent of lymph node involvement. Common sites of metastases in small cell lung cancer are thoracic lymph nodes, brain, adrenal glands, and liver. All patients diagnosed with small cell lung cancer should undergo chest and

abdominal computed tomography (CT) scans as well as CT or magnetic resonance imaging (MRI) imaging of the brain. If bone pain is present, radionuclide bone scans should be performed. Bone marrow biopsies are not typically indicated as isolated bone marrow metastases are rare. If there are signs of spinal cord compression or leptomeningeal involvement, imaging of the spine by MRI or CT and lumbar puncture are indicated, respectively.

103. The answer is C.

(Chap. 35) Mutations of the epidermal growth factor receptor (EGF-R) have recently been recognized as important mutations that affect the response of non–small cell lung cancers to treatment with EGF-R tyrosine kinase inhibitors. Initial studies of erlotinib in all patients with advanced non–small cell lung cancer failed to show a treatment benefit; however, when only patients with EGF-R mutations were considered, treatment with anti-EGF-R therapy improved progression-free and overall survival. Patients who are more likely to have EGF-R mutations are women, nonsmokers, Asians, and those with adenocarcinoma histopathology.

104. The answer is B.

(Chap. 35, National Lung Screening Trial Research Team, DR Aberle et al: N Engl J Med *2011;365: 395–409)* Screening for lung cancer in high-risk individuals has been investigated for many years. Screening trials require large numbers of participants that can be followed for long periods of time and are expensive to conduct. Until 2011, no screening trial had been able to demonstrate any decrease in lung cancer mortality. Previous screening modalities have been primarily chest radiographs with or without sputum cytology. In June 2011, the main results of the National Lung Cancer Screening Trial (NLST) were published in the *New England Journal of Medicine.* The trial enrolled >50,000 individuals with a >30 pack-year history of cigarette smoking and randomized the individuals to yearly chest radiographs or low-dose computed tomography (CT) scans for a period of 3 years. Outcomes in the individuals continued to be followed for a total of almost 8 years, when the trial was stopped early. Individuals receiving low-dose CT scans demonstrated a 20% mortality reduction from lung cancer compared with those receiving chest radiographs alone, and more individuals receiving CT scans were diagnosed at early stages of disease. A caveat in broadly applying these results in clinical practice is that >90% of positive scans proved to be false positives. At this point, more research on the cost effectiveness of CT scans and the appropriate population to which to offer scans needs to be done before widespread screening is recommended.

105. The answer is A.

(Chap. 36) About 40% of patients with thymoma have another systemic autoimmune illness related to the thymoma. About 30% of patients with thymoma have myasthenia gravis, 5–8% have pure red blood cell (RBC) aplasia, and about 5% have hypogammaglobulinemia. Thymectomy results in the resolution of pure RBC aplasia in about 30% of patients but rarely benefits patients with hypogammaglobulinemia. Among patients with myasthenia gravis, about 10–15% have a thymoma. Thymectomy produces at least some symptomatic improvement in about 65% of patients with myasthenia gravis. In one large series, thymoma patients with myasthenia gravis had a better long-term survival from thymoma resection than did those without myasthenia gravis. Thymoma more rarely may be associated with polymyositis, systemic lupus erythematosus, thyroiditis, Sjögren's syndrome, ulcerative colitis, pernicious anemia, Addison's disease, scleroderma, and panhypopituitarism. In one series, 70% of patients with thymoma were found to have another systemic illness. Erythrocytosis caused by ectopic production of erythropoietin is often seen in conjunction with renal cell and hepatocellular carcinomas.

106. The answer is D.

(Chap. 36) Thymoma is the most common cause of an anterior mediastinal mass in adults, accounting for about 40% of all mediastinal masses. The other major causes of anterior mediastinal masses are lymphomas, germ cell tumors, and substernal thyroid tumors. Carcinoid tumors, lipomas, and thymic cysts also may produce radiographic masses. After combination chemotherapy for another malignancy, teenagers and young adults may develop a rebound thymic hyperplasia in the first few months after treatment. Granulomatous inflammatory diseases (tuberculosis, sarcoidosis) can produce thymic enlargement. Thymomas are most common in the fifth and sixth decades of life, are uncommon in children, and are distributed evenly between men and women. About 40–50% of patients are asymptomatic; masses are detected incidentally on routine chest radiographs. When symptomatic, patients may have cough, chest pain, dyspnea, fever, wheezing, fatigue, weight loss, night sweats, or anorexia. Occasionally, thymomas may obstruct the superior vena cava. After a mediastinal mass has been detected, a surgical procedure is required for definitive diagnosis. An initial mediastinoscopy or limited thoracotomy can be undertaken to get sufficient tissue to make an accurate diagnosis. Fine-needle aspiration is poor at distinguishing between lymphomas and thymomas but is more reliable in diagnosing germ cell tumors and metastatic carcinoma. Thymomas and lymphomas require sufficient tissue to examine the tumor architecture to ensure an accurate diagnosis and obtain prognostic information. Thymomas are epithelial tumors, and all of them have malignant potential. It is not worthwhile to try to divide them into benign and malignant forms. Staging systems are based on degree of invasiveness and correlate with prognosis. About 65% of thymomas are encapsulated and noninvasive, and about

35% are invasive. Tumors that are encapsulated and noninvasive (stage 1) have a 96% 5-year survival rate after complete resection surgery.

107. The answer is E.

(Chap. 36) A "dry tap" is defined as the inability to aspirate bone marrow and is reported in approximately 5% of attempts. It is rare in the case of normal bone marrow. The differential diagnosis includes metastatic carcinoma infiltration (17%); chronic myeloid leukemia (15%); myelofibrosis (14%); hairy cell leukemia (10%); acute leukemia (10%); and lymphomas, including Hodgkin's disease (9%).

108. The answer is B.

(Chap. 36) The diagnostic criteria for chronic eosinophilic leukemia and the hypereosinophilic syndrome first requires the presence of persistent eosinophilia >1500/μL in blood, increased marrow eosinophils, and <20% myeloblasts in blood or marrow. Additional disorders that must be excluded include all causes of reactive eosinophilia, primary neoplasms associated with eosinophilia (e.g., T-cell lymphoma, Hodgkin's disease, acute lymphoid leukemia, mastocytosis, chronic myeloid leukemia, acute myeloid leukemia [AML], myelodysplasia, and myeloproliferative syndromes), and T-cell reaction with increased interleukin-5 or cytokine production. If these entities have been excluded and the myeloid cells show a clonal chromosome abnormality and blast cells (>2%) are present in peripheral blood or are increased in marrow (but <20%), then the diagnosis is chronic eosinophilic leukemia. Patients with hypereosinophilic syndrome and chronic eosinophilic leukemia may be asymptomatic (discovered on routine testing) or present with systemic findings such as fever, shortness of breath, new neurologic findings, or rheumatologic findings. The heart, lungs, and central nervous system are most often affected by eosinophil-mediated tissue damage.

109. The answer is C.

(Chap. 37) The patient has a breast cyst. This has a benign feel on examination, and aspiration of the mass showed nonbloody fluid with resolution of the mass. If there were residual mass or bloody fluid, mammography and biopsy would be the next step. In patients such as this with nonbloody fluid in whom aspiration clears the mass, reexamination in 1 month is indicated. If the mass recurs, then aspiration should be repeated. If fluid recurs, mammography and biopsy would be indicated at that point. There is no indication at this point to refer for advanced imaging or surgical evaluation. Breastfeeding is not affected by the presence of a breast cyst.

110. The answer is C.

(Chap. 37) Breast cancer risk is related to many factors, but age of menarche, age of first full-term pregnancy, and age at menopause together account for 70–80% of all breast cancer risk. The lowest risk patients have the shortest duration of total menses (i.e., later menarche and earlier menopause), as well as an early first full-term pregnancy. Specifically, the lowest risks are menarche at age 16 years old or older, first pregnancy by the age of 18 years, and menopause that begins 10 years before the median age of menopause of 52 years. Thus, patient C meets these criteria.

111. The answer is D.

(Chap. 37) Pathologic staging remains the most important determinant of overall prognosis. Other prognostic factors have an impact on survival and the choice of therapy. Tumors that lack estrogen or progesterone receptors are more likely to recur. The presence of estrogen receptors, particularly in postmenopausal women, is also an important factor in determining adjuvant chemotherapy. Tumors with a high growth rate are associated with early relapse. Measurement of the proportion of cells in S-phase is a measure of the growth rate. Tumors with more than the median number of cells in S-phase have a higher risk of relapse and an improved response rate to chemotherapy. Histologically, tumors with a poor nuclear grade have a higher risk of recurrence than do tumors with a good nuclear grade. At the molecular level, tumors that overexpress erbB2 (HER-2/neu) or that have a mutated p53 gene portend a poorer prognosis for patients. The overexpression of erbB2 is also useful in designing optimal treatment regimens, and a human monoclonal antibody to erbB2 (Herceptin) has been developed.

112. The answer is E.

(Chap. 38) Esophageal cancer is an uncommon gastrointestinal malignancy with a high mortality rate because most patients do not present until advanced disease is present. The typical presenting symptoms of esophageal cancer are dysphagia with significant weight loss. Dysphagia is typically fairly rapidly progressive over a period of weeks to months. Dysphagia initially in only to solid foods but progresses to include semisolids and liquids. For dysphagia to occur, an estimated 60% of the esophageal lumen must be occluded. Weight loss occurs because of decreased oral intake in addition to the cachexia that is common with cancer. Associated symptoms may include pain with swallowing that can radiate to the back, regurgitation or vomiting of undigested food, and aspiration pneumonia. The two major cell types of esophageal cancer in the United States are adenocarcinoma and squamous cell carcinoma, which have different risk factors. Individuals with squamous cell carcinomas typically have a history of both tobacco and alcohol abuse, but those with adenocarcinoma more often have a history of long-standing gastroesophageal reflux disease and Barrett's esophagitis. Among those

with a history of alcohol and tobacco abuse, there is an increased risk with increased intake and interestingly is more associated with whiskey drinking compared with wine or beer. Other risk factors for squamous cell carcinoma of the esophagus include ingestion of nitrites, smoked opiates, fungal toxins in pickled vegetables, and physical insults that include long-standing ingestion of very hot tea or lye.

113. The answer is E.

(Chap. 38) Colorectal cancer is the second most common cause of cancer death in the United States, and the mortality rate related to the disease has been decreasing in recent years. When colorectal cancer is identified, patients should be referred for surgical intervention because proper staging and prognosis cannot be determined without pathologic specimens if there is no gross evidence of metastatic disease. The preoperative workup to assess for metastatic or synchronous disease includes a complete colonoscopy if possible, chest radiography, liver function testing, carcinoembryonic antigen (CEA) testing, and computed tomography of the abdomen. Staging of colorectal cancer follows a TNM (tumor, node, metastasis) staging system. However, the T staging is not based on absolute size of the tumor rather it is based upon the extension of the tumor through the colonic wall. T1 tumors can extend into the submucosa but not beyond, T2 tumors extend into the muscularis propria, and T3 tumors involve the serosa and beyond. Nodal metastases are graded as N1 (one to three lymph nodes positive) and N2 (≥four lymph nodes positive). This patient's stage of cancer would be T2N1M0 and would be staged as a stage III cancer. Despite the relatively advanced stage, the overall 5-year survival rate would be 50–70% because of improvements in overall care of the patient with colorectal cancer. Because the patient had an occluding lesion that prevents preoperative colonoscopy, the patient needs to have a complete colonoscopy performed within the first several months after surgery and every 3 years thereafter. Serial measurements of CEA every 3 months have also been advocated by some specialists. Annual computed tomography may be performed for the first 3 years after resection, although the utility of the practice is debated. Radiation therapy to the pelvis is recommended for all patients with rectal cancer because it reduces the local recurrence rate, especially in stage II and III tumors. When postoperative radiation therapy is combined with chemotherapeutic regimens containing 5-fluorouracil, the local recurrence rate is further reduced and overall survival is increased as well.

114. The answer is A.

(Chap. 38) Most colorectal cancers arise from adenomatous polyps. Only adenomas are premalignant, and only a minority of these lesions becomes malignant. Most polyps are asymptomatic, causing occult bleeding in fewer than 5% of patients. Sessile (flat-based) polyps are more likely to become malignant than pedunculated (stalked) polyps. Histologically, villous adenomas are more likely to become malignant than tubular adenomas. The risk of containing invasive carcinoma in the polyp increases with size with <2% in polyps <1.5 cm, 2%–10% in polyps 1.5 to 2.5 cm, and 10% in polyps >2. 5 cm. This patient had two polyps that were high risk based on histology (villous) and appearance (sessile) but only moderate risk by size (<1.5 cm). Polyps, particularly those larger than 2.5 cm in size, sometimes contain cancer cells but usually progress to cancer quite slowly over an approximate 5-year period. Patients with adenomatous polyps should have a follow-up colonoscopy or radiographic study in 3 years. If no polyps are found on initial study, the test (endoscopic or radiographic) should be repeated in 10 years. Computed tomography is only warranted for staging if there is a diagnosis of colon cancer, not for the presence of polyps alone.

115. The answer is A.

(Chap. 38) A strong family history of colon cancer should prompt consideration for hereditary nonpolyposis colon cancer (HNPCC), or Lynch syndrome, particularly if diffuse polyposis is not noted on colonoscopy. HNPCC is characterized by (1) three or more relatives with histologically proven colorectal cancer, one of whom is a first-degree relative and of the other two, at least one with the diagnosis before age 50 years, and (2) colorectal cancer in at least two generations. The disease is an autosomal dominant trait and is associated with other tumors, including in the endometrium and ovary. The proximal colon is most frequently involved, and cancer occurs with a median age of 50 years, 15 years earlier than in sporadic colon cancer. Patients with HNPCC are recommended to receive biennial colonoscopy and pelvic ultrasonography beginning at age 25 years. Innumerable polyps suggest the presence of one of the autosomal dominant polyposis syndromes, many of which carry a high malignant potential. These include familial adenomatous polyposis, Gardner's syndrome (associated with osteomas, fibromas, epidermoid cysts), or Turcot's syndrome (associated with brain cancer). Peutz-Jeghers syndrome is associated with mucocutaneous pigmentation and hamartomas. Tumors may develop in the ovary, breast, pancreas, and endometrium; however, malignant colon cancers are not common. Ulcerative colitis is strongly associated with development of colon cancer, but it is unusual for colon cancer to be the presenting finding in ulcerative colitis. Patients are generally symptomatic from their inflammatory bowel disease long before cancer risk develops.

116. The answer is E.

(Chap. 40) Pancreatic cancer is the fourth leading cause of cancer death in the United States despite representing

only 3% of all newly diagnosed malignancies. Infiltrating ductal adenocarcinomas account for the vast majority of cases and arise most frequently in the head of pancreas. At the time of diagnosis, 85–90% of patients have inoperable or metastatic disease, which is reflected in the 5-year survival rate of only 5% for all stages combined. An improved 5-year survival of up to 20% may be achieved when the tumor is detected at an early stage and when complete surgical resection is accomplished. Over the past 30 years, 5-year survival rates have not improved substantially. Cigarette smoking may be the cause of up to 20–25% of all pancreatic cancers and is the most common environmental risk factor for this disease. Other risk factors are not well established because of inconsistent results from epidemiologic studies, but they include chronic pancreatitis and diabetes. Alcohol does not appear to be a risk factor unless excess consumption gives rise to chronic pancreatitis.

117. The answer is B.

(Chap. 40) Dual-phase, contrast-enhanced spiral computed tomography (CT) is the imaging modality of choice to visualize suspected pancreatic masses. In addition to imaging the pancreas, it also provides accurate visualization of surrounding viscera, vessels, and lymph nodes. In most cases, this study can determine surgical resectability. There is no advantage of magnetic resonance imaging (MRI) over CT in predicting tumor resectability, but selected cases may benefit from MRI to characterize the nature of small indeterminate liver lesions and to evaluate the cause of biliary dilation when no obvious mass is seen on CT. Preoperative confirmation of malignancy is not always necessary in patients with radiologic appearances consistent with operable pancreatic cancer. Endoscopic ultrasound-guided needle biopsy is the most effective technique to evaluate the mass for malignancy. It has an accuracy of approximately 90% and has a smaller risk of intraperitoneal dissemination compared with CT-guided percutaneous biopsy. Endoscopic retrograde cholangiopancreatography (ERCP) is a useful method for obtaining ductal brushings, but the diagnostic value of pancreatic juice sampling is only 25–30%. CA 19-9 is elevated in approximately 70–80% of patients with pancreatic carcinoma, but ERCP is not recommended as a routine diagnostic or screening test because its sensitivity and specificity are inadequate for accurate diagnosis. Preoperative CA 19-9 levels correlate with tumor stage and prognosis. It is also an indicator of asymptomatic recurrence in patients with completely resected tumors. Fluorodeoxyglucose positron emission tomography (FDG-PET) should be considered before surgery for detecting distant metastases.

118. The answer is D.

(Chap. 41) Bladder cancer is the fourth most common cancer in men and the thirteenth most common cancer in women. Cigarette smoking has a strong association with bladder cancer, particularly in men. The increased risk persists for at least 10 years after quitting. Bladder cancer is a small cause of cancer deaths because most detected cases are superficial with an excellent prognosis. Most cases of bladder cancer come to medical attention by the presence of gross hematuria emanating from exophytic lesions. Microscopic hematuria is more likely caused by prostate cancer than bladder cancer. Cystoscopy under anesthesia is indicated to evaluate for bladder cancer. In cases of superficial disease, bacille Calmette-Guérin is an effective adjuvant to decrease recurrence or treat unresectable superficial disease. In the United States, cystectomy is generally recommended for invasive disease. Even invasive cancer with nodal involvement has a >40% 10-year survival after surgery and adjuvant therapy.

119 and 120. The answers are C and E, respectively.

(Chap. 41) The incidence of renal cell carcinoma continues to rise and is now nearly 58,000 cases annually in the United States, resulting in 13,000 deaths. The male-to-female ratio is 2 to 1. Incidence peaks between the ages of 50 and 70 years, although this malignancy may be diagnosed at any age. Many environmental factors have been investigated as possible contributing causes; the strongest association is with cigarette smoking. Risk is also increased for patients who have acquired cystic disease of the kidney associated with end-stage renal disease and for those with tuberous sclerosis. Most renal cell carcinomas are clear cell tumors (60%) with papillary and chromophobic tumors less common. Clear cell tumors account for >80% of patients who develop metastases. The classic triad of hematuria, flank pain, and a palpable mass is only present in 10–20% of patients initially. Most cases currently are found as incidental findings on computed tomography or ultrasonography done for different reasons. The increasing number of incidentally discovered low-stage tumors has contributed to an improved 5-year survival rate. The paraneoplastic phenomenon of erythrocytosis caused by increased production of erythropoietin is only found in 3% of cases; anemia caused by advanced disease is far more common. Stage 1 and 2 tumors are confined to the kidney and have a >80% survival after radical nephrectomy. Stage 4 tumors with distant metastases have a 50-year survival of 10%. Renal cell carcinoma is notably resistant to traditional chemotherapeutic agents. Cytokine therapy with interleukin-2 or interferon-gamma produces regression in 10–20% of patients with metastatic disease. Recently, the advent of antiangiogenic medications has changed the treatment of advance renal cell carcinoma. Sunitinib was demonstrated to be superior to interferon-gamma, and it (or sorafenib) is now first-line therapy for patients with advanced metastatic disease.

121. The answer is A.

(Chap. 42) The results from several large double-blind, randomized chemoprevention trials have established 5 alpha-reductase inhibitors as the predominant therapy to reduce the future risk of a prostate cancer diagnosis. Randomized placebo-controlled trials have shown that finasteride and dutasteride reduce the period prevalence of prostate cancer. Trials of selenium, vitamin C, and vitamin E have shown no benefit versus placebo.

122. The answer is E.

(Chap. 42) As shown in Figure 42-2, transrectal ultrasound-guided biopsy is recommended for men with either an abnormal digital rectal examination (DRE) or abnormal serum prostate-specific antigen (PSA) results. Twenty-five percent of men with a PSA above 4 ng/mL and abnormal DRE results have cancer, as do 17% of men with a PSA of 2.5 to 4 ng/mL and normal DRE results.

123. The answer is C.

(Chap. 43) Ninety percent of persons with nonseminomatous germ cell tumors produce either α-fetoprotein (AFP) or beta human chorionic gonadotropin (β-hCG); in contrast, persons with pure seminomas usually produce neither. These tumor markers are present for some time after surgery; if the presurgical levels are high, 30 days or more may be required before meaningful postsurgical levels can be obtained. The half-lives of AFP and β-hCG are 6 days and 1 day, respectively. After treatment, unequal reduction of β-hCG and AFP may occur, suggesting that the two markers are synthesized by heterogeneous clones of cells within the tumor; thus, both markers should be followed. β-hCG is similar to luteinizing hormone except for its distinctive beta subunit.

124. The answer is D.

(Chap. 43) Testicular cancer occurs most commonly in the second and third decades of life. The treatment depends on the underlying pathology and the stage of the disease. Germ cell tumors are divided into seminomatous and nonseminomatous subtypes. Although the pathology of this patient's tumor was seminoma, the presence of α-fetoprotein (AFP) is suggestive of occult nonseminomatous components. If there are any nonseminomatous components, the treatment follows that of a nonseminomatous germ cell tumor. This patient therefore has a clinical stage I nonseminomatous germ cell tumor. Because his AFP returned to normal after orchiectomy, there is no obvious occult disease. However, between 20% and 50% of these patients will have disease in the retroperitoneal lymph nodes. Numerous trials have indicated no overall survival difference in this cohort between observation and retroperitoneal lymph node dissection (RPLND). Because of the potential side effects of RPLND, the choice of surveillance or RPLND is based on the pathology of the primary tumor. If the primary tumor shows no evidence for lymphatic or vascular invasion and is limited to the testis, then either option is reasonable. If lymphatic or vascular invasion is present or the tumor extends into the tunica, spermatic cord, or scrotum, then surveillance should not be offered. Either approach should cure >95% of patients. Radiation therapy is the appropriate choice for stage I and stage II seminoma. It has no role in nonseminomatous lesions. Adjuvant chemotherapy is not indicated in early-stage testicular cancer. Hormonal therapy is effective for prostate cancer and receptor-positive breast cancer but has no role in testicular cancer. Positron emission tomography may be used to locate viable seminoma in residua which mandates surgical excision or biopsy.

125. The answer is A.

(Chap. 44) Approximately 10% of women with ovarian cancer have a somatic mutation in one of two DNA repair genes, *BRCA1* (chromosome 17q12-21) or *BRCA2* (chromosome 13q12-13). Individuals inheriting a single copy of a mutant allele have a very high incidence of breast and ovarian cancer. Most of these women have a family history that is notable for multiple cases of breast or ovarian cancer (or both), although inheritance through male members of the family can camouflage this genotype through several generations. The most common malignancy in these women is breast carcinoma, although women harboring germ-line *BRCA1* mutations have a marked increased risk of developing ovarian malignancies in their forties and fifties with a 30–50% lifetime risk of developing ovarian cancer. Women harboring a mutation in *BRCA2* have a lower penetrance of ovarian cancer with perhaps a 20–40% chance of developing this malignancy, with onset typically in their fifties or sixties. Women with a *BRCA2* mutation also are at slightly increased risk of pancreatic cancer. Screening studies in this select population suggest that current screening techniques, including serial evaluation of the CA-125 tumor marker and ultrasound, are insufficient at detecting early-stage and curable disease, so women with these germ-line mutations are advised to undergo prophylactic removal of their ovaries and fallopian tubes typically after completing childbearing and ideally before ages 35 to 40 years. Early prophylactic oophorectomy also protects these women from subsequent breast cancer with a reduction of breast cancer risk of approximately 50%.

126. The answer is C.

(Chap. 44) Endometrial carcinoma is the most common gynecologic malignancy in the United States. Most are adenocarcinomas. Development of these tumors is a multistep process with estrogen playing an important early role in driving endometrial gland proliferation. Relative overexposure to this class of hormones is a risk factor for the subsequent development of endometrial tumors.

In contrast, progestins drive glandular maturation and are protective. Hence, women with high endogenous or pharmacologic exposure to estrogens, especially if unopposed by progesterone, are at high risk for endometrial cancer. Obese women, women treated with unopposed estrogens, and women with estrogen-producing tumors (e.g., granulosa cell tumors of the ovary) are at higher risk for endometrial cancer. In addition, treatment with tamoxifen, which has anti-estrogenic effects in breast tissue but estrogenic effects in uterine epithelium, is associated with an increased risk of endometrial cancer. The majority of women with tumors of the uterine corpus present with postmenopausal vaginal bleeding caused by shedding of the malignant endometrial lining. Premenopausal women often present with atypical bleeding between typical menstrual cycles. These signs typically bring a woman to the attention of a health care professional, and hence the majority of women present with early-stage disease in which the tumor is confined to the uterine corpus. For patients with disease confined to the uterus, hysterectomy with removal of the fallopian tubes and ovaries results in approximately 90% 5-year survival.

127. The answer is B.

(Chap. 45) Bone pain resulting from metastatic lesions may be difficult to distinguish from degenerative disease, osteoporosis, or disk disease in elderly individuals. Generally, these patients present with insidious worsening localized pain without fevers or signs of infection. In contrast to pain related to disk disease, the pain of metastatic disease is worse when the patient is lying down or at night. Neurologic symptoms related to metastatic disease constitute an emergency. Lung, breast, and prostate cancers account for approximately 80% of bone metastases. Thyroid carcinoma, renal cell carcinoma, lymphoma, and bladder carcinoma may also metastasize to bone. Metastatic lesions may be lytic or blastic. Most cancers cause a combination of both, although prostate cancer is predominantly blastic. Either lesion may cause hypercalcemia, although lytic lesions more commonly do this. Lytic lesions are best detected with plain radiography. Blastic lesions are prominent on radionuclide bone scans. Treatment and prognosis depend on the underlying malignancy. Bisphosphonates may reduce hypercalcemia, relieve pain, and limit bone resorption.

128. The answer is B.

(Chap. 45) Metastatic tumors of bone are more common than primary bone tumors. Prostate, breast, and lung primaries account for 80% of all bone metastases. Tumors from the kidney, bladder, and thyroid and lymphomas and sarcomas also commonly metastasize to bone. Metastases usually spread hematogenously. In decreasing order, the most common sites of bone metastases include the vertebrae, proximal femur, pelvis, ribs, sternum, proximal humerus, and skull. Pain is the most common symptom. Hypercalcemia may occur with bone destruction. Lesions may be osteolytic, osteoblastic, or both. Osteoblastic lesions are associated with a higher level of alkaline phosphatase. Colon cancer typically metastasizes initially via lymphatic spread, making the liver and lungs common sites of secondary disease.

129. The answer is C.

(Chap. 45) The most common malignant tumors of bone are plasma cell tumors related to multiple myeloma. The bone lesions are lytic lesions caused by increased osteoclast activity without osteoblastic new bone formation. Of the nonhematopoietic tumors, the most common are osteosarcoma, chondrosarcoma, Ewing's sarcoma, and malignant fibrous histiocytoma. Osteosarcomas account for 45% of bone sarcomas and produce osteoid (unmineralized bone) or bone. They typically occur in children, adolescents, and adults up to the third decade of life. The "sunburst" appearance of the lesion and Codman's triangle in this young man are indicative of an osteosarcoma. Whereas osteosarcomas have a predilection for long bones, chondrosarcomas are more often found in flat bones, especially the shoulder and pelvic girdles. Osteosarcomas are radioresistant. Long-term survival with combined chemotherapy and surgery is 60–80%. Chondrosarcomas account for 20–25% of bone sarcomas and are most common in adults in the fourth to sixth decades of life. They typically present indolently with pain and swelling. They are often difficult to distinguish from benign bone lesions. Most chondrosarcomas are chemoresistant, and the mainstay of therapy is resection of the primary as well as metastatic sites.

130. The answer is B.

(Chap. 47) Patients with cancer from an unknown primary site present a common diagnostic dilemma. Initial evaluation should include history, physical examination, appropriate imaging, and blood studies based on gender (e.g., prostate-specific antigen in men, mammography in women). Immunohistochemical staining of biopsy samples using antibodies to specific cell components may help elucidate the site of the primary tumor. Although many immunohistochemical stains are available, a logical approach is represented in Figure 47-1. Additional tests may be helpful based on the appearance under light microscopy or the results of the cytokeratin stains. In cases of cancer of unknown primary, cytokeratin staining is usually the first branch point from which the tumor lineage is determined. Cytokeratin is positive in carcinoma because all epithelial tumors contain this protein. Subsets of cytokeratin, such as CK7 and CK20, may be useful to determine the likely etiology of the primary tumor. Leukocyte common antigen, thyroglobulin, and thyroid transcription factor 1 are characteristic of lymphoma, thyroid cancer, and lung or thyroid cancer,

respectively. α-Fetoprotein staining is typically positive in germ cell, stomach, and liver carcinoma.

131. The answer is C.

(Chap. 47) The patient presents with symptoms suggestive of ovarian cancer. Although her peritoneal fluid is positive for adenocarcinoma, further speciation cannot be done. Surprisingly, the physical examination and imaging do not show a primary source. Although the differential diagnosis of this patient's disorder includes gastric cancer or another gastrointestinal malignancy and breast cancer, peritoneal carcinomatosis is most commonly caused by ovarian cancer in women even when the ovaries are normal at surgery. Elevated CA-125 levels or the presence of psammoma bodies is further suggestive of an ovarian origin, and such patients should receive surgical debulking and carboplatin or cisplatin plus paclitaxel. Patients with this presentation have a similar stage-specific survival compared with other patients with known ovarian cancer. Ten percent of patients with this disorder, also known as primary peritoneal papillary serous carcinoma, will remain disease free 2 years after treatment.

132. The answer is B.

(Chap. 47) The patient is a young man with asymmetric hilar adenopathy. The differential diagnosis would include lymphoma; testicular cancer; and, less likely, tuberculosis or histoplasmosis. Because of his young age, testicular examination and ultrasonography would be indicated, as would measurement of α-fetoprotein (AFP) or beta human chorionic gonadotropin (β-hCG), which are generally markedly elevated. In men with carcinoma of unknown primary source, AFP and β-hCG should be checked because the presence of testicular cancer portends an improved prognosis compared with possible primary sources. Biopsy would show lymphoma. The ACE level may be elevated but is not diagnostic of sarcoidosis. Sarcoidosis should not be considered likely in the presence of asymmetric hilar adenopathy. Thyroid disorders are not likely to present with unilateral hilar adenopathy. Finally, prostate-specific antigen is not indicated in this age category, and C-reactive protein would not differentiate any of the disorders mentioned above. Biopsy is clearly the most important diagnostic procedure.

133. The answer is D.

(Chap. 46) Distinguishing central nervous system (CNS) toxoplasmosis from primary CNS lymphoma in a patient with HIV infection is often difficult. The standard approach in a neurologically stable patient is to treat the patient for toxoplasmosis for 2–3 weeks then repeat neuroimaging. If the imaging shows clear improvement, continue antibiotics. If there is no response to therapy after 2 weeks, therapy does not need to be continued and a stereotactic brain biopsy is indicated. In this immunocompromised patient who has not responded to treatment for CNS toxoplasmosis, a positive CNS EBV DNA would be diagnostic of CNS lymphoma. Whole-brain radiation therapy is part of the treatment for CNS lymphoma, which is not yet diagnosed in this patient, and should not be instituted empirically. Treatments directed at viral infections of the CNS or CNS lymphomas are not indicated at this time since a diagnosis is still yet to be made. In the absence of a change in neurologic status or evidence of mass effect on CT, there is no indication for dexamethasone. Of note, the incidence of primary CNS lymphoma appears to be increasing in immunocompetent individuals for unclear reasons.

134. The answer is A.

(Chap. 46) Endocrine dysfunction resulting in hypopituitarism frequently follows exposure of the hypothalamus or pituitary gland to therapeutic radiation. Growth hormone is the most sensitive to the damaging effects of whole-brain radiation therapy, and thyroid-stimulating hormone is the least sensitive. Adrenocorticotropic hormone, prolactin, and gonadotropins have an intermediate sensitivity. Other complications of radiation therapy to the brain include acute radiation injury manifest by headache, sleepiness, and worsening of preexisting neurologic defects. Early delayed radiation injury occurs within the first 4 months after therapy. It is associated with increased white matter signal on magnetic resonance imaging and is steroid responsive. Late delayed radiation injury occurs >4 months after therapy, typically 8–24 months. There may be dementia, gait apraxia, focal necrosis (after focal irradiation), or the development of secondary malignancies.

135. The answer is D.

(Chap. 46) The postgadolinium magnetic resonance imaging (MRI) shows multiple meningiomas along the falx and left parietal cortex. Meningiomas derive from the cells that give rise to the arachnoid granulations. They are now the most common primary brain tumor, accounting for approximately 32% of the total, and occur more commonly in women than men. They are usually benign (World Heatlh Organization classification grade 1) and attached to the dura. They rarely invade the brain. Meningiomas are diagnosed with increasing frequency as more people undergo neuroimaging studies for various indications. Their incidence increases with age, and they are more common in patients with a history of cranial irradiation. They are most commonly located over the cerebral convexities, especially adjacent to the sagittal sinus, but can also occur in the skull base and along the dorsum of the spinal cord. Many meningiomas are found incidentally following neuroimaging for unrelated reasons. They can also present with headaches, seizures, or focal neurologic deficits. On imaging studies

they have a characteristic appearance usually consisting of a partially calcified, densely enhancing extra-axial tumor arising from the dura. The main differential diagnosis of meningioma is a dural metastasis. Total surgical resection of a meningioma is curative. Low-grade astrocytoma and high-grade astrocytoma (glioblastoma) often infiltrate into adjacent brain and rarely have the clear margins seen in Figure 135. Oligodendroma comprise approximately 15% of all gliomas and show calcification in roughly 30% of cases. They have a more benign course and are more responsive than other gliomas to cytotoxic therapy. For low-grade oligodendromas, the median survival is 7–8 years. Brain abscess will have distinctive ring-enhancing features with a capsule, will often have mass effect, and will have evidence of inflammation on MRI scanning.

136. The answer is E.

(Chap. 48) Thyroid nodules are found in 5% of patients. Nodules are more common with age, in women, and in iodine-deficient areas. Given their prevalence, the cost of screening, and the generally benign course of most nodules, the choice and order of screening tests have been very contentious. A small percentage of incidentally discovered nodules will represent thyroid cancer, however. A TSH should be the first test to check after detection of a thyroid nodule. A majority of patients will have normal thyroid function tests. In the case of a normal TSH, fine-needle aspiration or ultrasound-guided biopsy can be pursued. If the TSH is low, a radionuclide scan should be performed to determine if the nodule is the source of thyroid hyperfunction (a "hot" nodule). In this case, this is the best course of action. "Hot" nodules can be treated medically, resected, or ablated with radioactive iodine. "Cold" nodules should be further evaluated with a fine-needle aspiration. Four percent of nodules undergoing biopsy are malignant, 10% are suspicious for malignancy, and 86% are indeterminate or benign.

137. The answer is B.

(Chap. 51) Incidental adrenal masses are often discovered during radiographic testing for another condition and are found in approximately 6% of adult subjects at autopsy. Fifty percent of patients with a history of malignancy and a newly discovered adrenal mass will actually have an adrenal metastasis. Fine-needle aspiration of a suspected metastatic malignancy will often be diagnostic. In the absence of a suspected nonadrenal malignancy, most adrenal incidentalomas are benign. Primary adrenal malignancies are uncommon (<0.01%), and fine-needle aspiration is not useful to distinguish between benign and malignant primary adrenal tumors. Although 90% of these masses are nonsecretory, patients with an incidentaloma should be screened for pheochromocytoma and hypercortisolism with plasma free metanephrines and an overnight dexamethasone suppression test, respectively. When radiographic features suggest a benign neoplasm (<3 cm), scanning should be repeated in 3–6 months. When masses are > 6 cm, surgical removal (if more likely to be primary adrenal malignancy) or fine-needle aspiration (if more likely to be metastatic malignancy) is preferred.

138. The answer is B.

(Chap. 49) The patient presents with recurrent peptic ulcers without evidence of *Helicobacter pylori* infection. The diagnosis of Zollinger-Ellison syndrome (ZES) should be obtained. Additional features that suggest nonclassic idiopathic ulcer disease include the presence of diarrhea, which is commonly present in ZES, but not idiopathic ulcers. The diagnosis is commonly made through measurement of plasma gastrin levels, which should be markedly elevated, but common use of proton pump inhibitors (PPIs) that potently suppress gastric acid secretion confound this measurement. Because PPI use suppresses gastric acid production, gastrin rises. Thus PPI use should be discontinued for 1 week prior to measurement of gastrin in plasma. Often this requires collaboration with gastroenterologists to ensure safety and potentially offer alternative pharmacology during this time. Once hypergastrinemia is confirmed, the presence of low gastric pH must be confirmed, as the most common cause of elevated gastrin is achlorhydria due to pernicious anemia. Imaging of the abdomen is indicated after demonstration of hypergastrinemia. Finally, although ZES may be associated with multiple endocrine neoplasia type 1, which often has parathyroid hyperplasia or adenoma, this is less likely than isolated ZES.

139 and 140. The answers are E and E, respectively.

(Chap. 49) In patients with a nonmetastatic carcinoid, surgery is the only potentially curative therapy. The extent of surgical resection depends on the size of the primary tumor because the risk of metastasis is related to the size of the tumor. Symptomatic treatment is aimed at decreasing the amount and effect of circulating substances. Drugs that inhibit the serotonin 5-HT_1 and 5-HT_2 receptors (methysergide, cyproheptadine, ketanserin) may control diarrhea but not flushing. 5-HT_3 receptor antagonists (ondansetron, tropisetron, alosetron) control nausea and diarrhea in up to 100% of these patients and may alleviate flushing. A combination of histamine H_1 and H_2 receptor antagonists may control flushing, particularly in patients with foregut carcinoid tumors. Somatostatin analogues (octreotide, lanreotide) are the most effective and widely used agents to control the symptoms of carcinoid syndrome, decreasing urinary 5-HIAA excretion and symptoms in 70–80% of patients. Interferon α, alone or combined with hepatic artery embolization, controls flushing and diarrhea in 40–85% of these patients. Phenoxybenzamine is an α_1-adrenergic receptor blocker that is used in the treatment of pheochromocytoma.

Carcinoid crisis is a life-threatening complication of carcinoid syndrome. It is most common in patients with intense symptoms from foregut tumors or markedly high levels of urinary 5-HIAA. The crisis may be provoked by surgery, stress, anesthesia, chemotherapy, or physical trauma to the tumor (biopsy or, in this case, physical compression of liver lesions). These patients develop severe typical symptoms plus systemic symptoms such as hypotension and hypertension with tachycardia. Synthetic analogues of somatostatin (octreotide, lanreotide) are the treatment of choice for carcinoid crisis. They are also effective in preventing crises when administered before a known inciting event. Octreotide 150–250 μg subcutaneously every 6–8 hours should be started 24–48 h before a procedure that is likely to precipitate a carcinoid crisis.

141. The answer is C.

(Chap. 49) This patient presents with the classic findings of a VIPoma, including large-volume watery diarrhea, hypokalemia, dehydration, and hypochlorhydria (WDHA, or Verner-Morrison syndrome). Abdominal pain is unusual. The presence of a secretory diarrhea is confirmed by a stool osmolal gap (2[stool Na + stool K] – [stool osmolality]) below 35 and persistence during fasting. In osmotic or laxative-induced diarrhea, the stool osmolal gap is over 100. In adults, over 80% of VIPomas are solitary pancreatic masses that usually are larger than 3 cm at diagnosis. Metastases to the liver are common and preclude curative surgical resection. The differential diagnosis includes gastrinoma, laxative abuse, carcinoid syndrome, and systemic mastocytosis. Diagnosis requires the demonstration of large-volume secretory diarrhea (>700 mL/d) and elevated serum VIP. Computed tomography of the abdomen will often demonstrate the pancreatic mass and liver metastases.

142. The answer is B.

(Chap. 50) Multiple endocrine neoplasia (MEN) syndrome is defined as a disorder with neoplasms affecting two or more hormonal tissues in several members of the family. The most common of these is MEN 1, which is caused by the gene coding the nuclear protein called Menin. MEN 1 is associated with tumors or hyperplasia of the parathyroid, pancreas, pituitary, adrenal cortex, and foregut, and/or subcutaneous or visceral lipomas. The most common and earliest manifestation is hyperparathyroidism with symptomatic hypercalcemia. This most commonly occurs in the late teenage years and 93–100% of mutation carriers develop this complication. Gastrinomas, insulinomas, and prolactinomas are less common and tend to occur in patients in their 20s, 30s, and 40s. Pheochromocytoma may occur in MEN 1, but is more commonly found in MEN 2A or von Hippel–Lindau syndrome.

143. The answer is A.

(Chap. 50) This patient's clinical scenario is most consistent with multiple endocrine neoplasia (MEN) 1, or the "3 Ps": parathyroid, pituitary, and pancreas. MEN 1 is an autosomal dominant genetic syndrome characterized by neoplasia of the parathyroid, pituitary, and pancreatic islet cells. Hyperparathyroidism is the most common manifestation of MEN 1. The neoplastic changes affect multiple parathyroid glands, making surgical care difficult. Pancreatic islet cell neoplasia is the second most common manifestation of MEN 1. Increased pancreatic islet cell hormones include pancreatic polypeptide, gastrin, insulin, vasoactive intestinal peptide, glucagons, and somatostatin. Pancreatic tumors may be multicentric, and up to 30% are malignant, with the liver being the first site of metastases. The symptoms depend on the type of hormone secreted. The Zollinger-Ellison syndrome causes elevations of gastrin, resulting in an ulcer diathesis. Conservative therapy is often unsuccessful. Insulinoma results in documented hypoglycemia with elevated insulin and C-peptide levels. Glucagonoma results in hyperglycemia, skin rash, anorexia, glossitis, and diarrhea. Elevations in vasoactive intestinal peptide result in profuse watery diarrhea. Pituitary tumors occur in up to half of patients with MEN 1. Prolactinomas are the most common. The multicentricity of the tumors makes resection difficult. Growth hormone–secreting tumors are the next most common, with adrenocorticotropic hormone– and corticotropin-releasing hormone–secreting tumors being more rare. Carcinoid tumors may also occur in the thymus, lung, stomach, and duodenum.

144. The answer is A.

(Chap. 51) When the diagnosis of pheochromocytoma is entertained, the first step is measurement of catecholamines and/or metanephrines. This can be achieved by urinary tests for vanillylmandelic acid, catecholamines, fractionated metanephrines, or total metanephrines. Total metanephrines have a high sensitivity and therefore are frequently used. A value of three times the upper limit of normal is highly suggestive of pheochromocytoma. Borderline elevations, as this patient had, are likely to be false positives. The next most appropriate step is to remove potentially confounding dietary or drug exposures, if possible, and repeat the test. Likely culprit drugs include levodopa, sympathomimetics, diuretics, tricyclic antidepressants, and alpha and beta blockers (labetalol in this case). Sertraline is a selective serotonin reuptake inhibitor antidepressant, not a tricyclic. Alternatively, a clonidine suppression test may be ordered.

145. The answer is E.

(Chap. 51) Complete removal of the pheochromocytoma is the only therapy that leads to a long-term cure, although 90% of tumors are benign. However, preoperative control of hypertension is necessary to prevent surgical complications and lower mortality. This patient is presenting with encephalopathy in a hypertensive crisis. The hypertension should be managed initially with IV medications to lower the mean arterial pressure by approximately 20% over the initial 24-hour period.

Medications that can be used for hypertensive crisis in pheochromocytoma include nitroprusside, nicardipine, and phentolamine. Once the acute hypertensive crisis has resolved, transition to oral α-adrenergic blockers is indicated. Phenoxybenzamine is the most commonly used drug and is started at low doses (5–10 mg three times daily) and titrated to the maximum tolerated dose (usually 20–30 mg daily). Once alpha blockers have been initiated, beta blockade can safely be utilized and is particularly indicated for ongoing tachycardia. Liberal salt and fluid intake helps expand plasma volume and treat orthostatic hypotension. Once blood pressure is maintained below 160/100 mm Hg with moderate orthostasis, it is safe to proceed to surgery. If blood pressure remains elevated despite treatment with alpha blockade, addition of calcium channel blockers, angiotensin receptor blockers, or angiotensin-converting enzyme inhibitors should be considered. Diuretics should be avoided, as they will exacerbate orthostasis.

146. The answer is E.

(Chap. 52) Hypercalcemia is a common oncologic complication of metastatic cancer. Symptoms include confusion, lethargy, change in mental status, fatigue, polyuria, and constipation. Regardless of the underlying disease, the treatment is similar. These patients are often dehydrated because hypercalcemia may cause nephrogenic diabetes insipidus and are often unable to take fluids orally. Therefore, the primary management entails reestablishment of euvolemia. Often hypercalcemia resolves with hydration alone. Patients should be monitored for hypophosphatemia. Bisphosphonates are now the mainstay of therapy because they stabilize osteoclast resorption of calcium from the bone. However, their effects may take 1 to 2 days to manifest. Care must be taken in cases of renal insufficiency because rapid administration of pamidronate may exacerbate renal failure. When euvolemia is achieved, furosemide may be given to increase calciuresis. Nasal or subcutaneous calcitonin further aids the shift of calcium out of the intravascular space. Since the advent of bisphosphonates, calcitonin is only used in severe cases of hypercalcemia because of its rapid effect. Glucocorticoids may be useful in patients with lymphoid malignancies because the mechanism of hypercalcemia in these conditions is often related to excess hydroxylation of vitamin D. However, in this patient with prostate cancer, dexamethasone will have little effect on the calcium level and may exacerbate the altered mental status.

147. The answer is E.

(Chap. 52) A variety of hormones are produced ectopically by tumors that may cause symptomatic disease. Eutopic production of parathyroid hormone (PTH) by the parathyroid gland is the most common cause of hypercalcemia. Hypercalcemia may rarely be produced by ectopic hyperparathyroid production but is most often caused by parathyroid hormone related protein (PTH-rp) production by squamous cell (head and neck, lung, skin), breast, genitourinary, and gastrointestinal tumors. This protein can be measured as a serum assay. Antidiuretic hormone, causing hyponatremia, is commonly produced by lung (squamous, small cell), gastrointestinal, genitourinary, and ovary tumors. Adrenocorticotropic hormone, causing Cushing's syndrome, is commonly produced by tumors in the lung (small cell, bronchial carcinoid, adenocarcinoma, squamous), thymus, pancreatic islet, and medullary thyroid carcinoma. Insulin-like growth factor secreted by mesenchymal tumors, sarcomas, and adrenal, hepatic, gastrointestinal, kidney, or prostate tumors may cause symptomatic hypoglycemia.

148. The answer is C.

(Chap. 53) One of the better characterized paraneoplastic neurologic syndromes is cerebellar ataxia caused by Purkinje cell drop-out in the cerebellum; it is manifested by dysarthria, limb and gait ataxia, and nystagmus. Radiologic imaging reveals cerebellar atrophy. Many antibodies have been associated with this syndrome, including anti-Yo, anti-Tr, and antibodies to the glutamate receptor. Although lung cancer, particularly small cell cancer, accounts for a large number of patients with neoplasm-associated cerebellar ataxia, those with the syndrome who display anti-Yo antibodies in the serum typically have breast or ovarian cancer. Cerebellar ataxia may also be seen in Hodgkin's lymphoma in association with anti-Tr antibodies.

149. The answer is A.

(Chap. 54) This patient presents with symptoms of spinal cord compression in the setting of known stage IV breast cancer. This represents an oncologic emergency because only 10% of patients presenting with paraplegia regain the ability to walk. Most commonly, patients develop symptoms of localized back pain and tenderness days to months before developing paraplegia. The pain is worsened by movement, cough, or sneezing. In contrast to radicular pain, the pain related to spinal cord metastases is worse with lying down. Patients presenting with back pain alone should have a careful examination to attempt to localize the lesion before development of more severe neurologic symptoms. In this patient with paraplegia, there is an definitive level at which sensation is diminished. This level is typically one to two vertebrae below the site of compression. Other findings include spasticity, weakness, and increased deep tendon reflexes. In those with autonomic dysfunction, bowel and bladder incontinence occur with decreased anal tone, absence of the anal wink and bulbocavernosus reflexes, and bladder distention. The most important initial step is the administration of high-dose intravenous corticosteroids to minimize associated swelling around the lesion and prevent paraplegia while allowing further

evaluation and treatment. Magnetic resonance imaging (MRI) should be performed of the entire spinal cord to evaluate for other metastatic disease that may require therapy. Although a brain MRI may be indicated in the future to evaluate for brain metastases, it is not required in the initial evaluation because the bilateral nature of the patient's symptoms and sensory level clearly indicate the spinal cord as the site of the injury. After an MRI has been performed, a definitive treatment plan can be made. Most commonly, radiation therapy is used with or without surgical decompression.

150 and 151. The answers are E and C, respectively. *(Chap. 54)* This clinical scenario describes an individual with superior vena cava (SVC) syndrome, which is an oncologic emergency. Eighty-five percent of cases of SVC syndrome are caused by either small cell or squamous cell cancer of the lung. Other causes of SVC syndrome include lymphoma, aortic aneurysm, thyromegaly, fibrosing mediastinitis, thrombosis, histoplasmosis, and Behçet's syndrome. The typical clinical presentation is dyspnea, cough, and facial and neck swelling. Symptoms are worsened by lying flat or bending forward. As the swelling progresses, it can lead to glossal and laryngeal edema with symptoms of hoarseness and dysphagia. Other symptoms can include headaches, nasal congestion, pain, dizziness, and syncope. In rare cases, seizures can occur from cerebral edema, although this is more commonly associated with brain metastases. On physical examination, dilated neck veins with collateralization on the anterior chest wall are frequently seen. There is also facial and upper extremity edema associated with cyanosis. The diagnosis of SVC syndrome is a clinical diagnosis. A pleural effusion is seen in about 25% of cases, more commonly on the right. A chest computed tomography scan would demonstrate decreased or absent contrast in the central veins with prominent collateral circulation and would help elucidate the cause. Most commonly this would be mediastinal adenopathy or a large central tumor obstructing venous flow. The immediate treatment of SVC syndrome includes oxygen, elevation of the head of the bed, and administration of diuretics in combination with a low-sodium diet. Conservative treatment alone often provides adequate relief of symptoms and allows determination of the underlying cause of the obstruction. In this case, this would include histologic confirmation of cell type of the tumor to provide more definitive therapy. Radiation therapy is the most common treatment modality and can be used in an emergent situation if conservative treatment fails to provide relief to the patient.

152 and 153. The answers are B and E, respectively. *(Chap. 54)* Tumor lysis syndrome occurs most commonly in individuals undergoing chemotherapy for rapidly proliferating malignancies, including acute leukemias and Burkitt's lymphoma. In rare instances, it can be seen in chronic lymphoma or solid tumors. As the chemotherapeutic agents act on these cells, there is massive tumor lysis that results in release of intracellular ions and nucleic acids. This leads to a characteristic metabolic syndrome of hyperuricemia, hyperphosphatemia, hyperkalemia, and hypocalcemia. Acute kidney injury is frequent and can lead to renal failure, requiring hemodialysis if uric acid crystallizes within the renal tubules. Lactic acidosis and dehydration increase the risk of acute kidney injury. Hyperphosphatemia occurs because of the release of intracellular phosphate ions and causes a reciprocal reduction in serum calcium. This hypocalcemia can be profound, leading to neuromuscular irritability and tetany. Hyperkalemia can become rapidly life threatening and cause ventricular arrhythmia.

Knowing the characteristics of tumor lysis syndrome, one can attempt to prevent the known complications from occurring. It is important to monitor serum electrolytes very frequently during treatment. Laboratory studies should be obtained no less than three times daily, but more frequent monitoring is often needed. Allopurinol should be administered prophylactically at high doses. If allopurinol fails to control uric acid to <8 mg/dL, rasburicase, a recombinant urate oxidase, can be added at a dose of 0.2 mg/kg. Throughout this period, the patient should be well hydrated with alkalinization of the urine to a pH of >7.0. This is accomplished by administration of intravenous normal or ½ normal saline at a dose of 3000 mL/m^2 daily with sodium bicarbonate. Prophylactic hemodialysis is not performed unless there is underlying renal failure before starting chemotherapy.

INDEX

Bold number indicates the start of the main discussion of the topic; numbers with "f "and "t"refer to figure and table pages.